Infectious Disease
in Emergency Medicine

Infectious Disease in Emergency Medicine

Edited by

Judith C. Brillman, M.D., F.A.C.E.P.
Assistant Professor of Emergency Medicine,
University of New Mexico School of Medicine;
Clinical Director,
Department of Emergency Medicine,
University of New Mexico Hospital, Albuquerque

Ronald W. Quenzer, M.D.
Associate Professor of Medicine, University of New Mexico
School of Medicine; Chief, Division of General Medicine, and
Medical Director, Primary Care Initiative, University of New
Mexico Hospital, Albuquerque

Little, Brown and Company
Boston/Toronto/London

Library of Congress Cataloging-in-Publication Data

Infectious disease in emergency medicine / edited by Judith C.
    Brillman, Ronald W. Quenzer.
        p.   cm.
    Includes bibliographical references and index.
    ISBN 0-316-10838-3
    1. Communicable diseases.   2. Emergency medicine.   I. Brillman.
Judith C.   II. Quenzer, Ronald W.
    [DNLM: 1. Communicable Diseases.   2. Emergencies.   WC 100 I432]
RC112.I458   1992
616—dc20
DNLM/DLC
for Library of Congress   92-17541
                                                                         CIP

Printed in the United States of America

MV-NY

To Jack and Ruth, who took me away from this book
—J. C. B.

To Ginny, Barth, Branson, and Nick for their inspiration
and patience
—R. W. Q.

Contents

Preface

The emergency physician is constantly confronted by patients with the acute onset of undiagnosed symptoms that are likely caused by an infectious disease. The successful practitioner of emergency medicine has mastered the art of knowing when to look up things. This practitioner, when presented with a problem relating to infectious disease, is at a disadvantage, as infectious disease texts are classically organized by organism and organ system. However, the etiologic organism is rarely known while the patient is in the emergency department.

The mission of *Infectious Disease in Emergency Medicine* is to address common, practical, clinical infectious disease issues that arise in the emergency department. It is a reference appropriate for practicing emergency physicians, residents and students in emergency medicine, other physicians practicing in ambulatory care settings, and the infectious disease consultant in the emergency department.

The book is organized into three parts. Part I, Principles of Infectious Disease, discusses decision making in the emergency department, including workup, immediate treatment, and disposition decision making. The significance of abnormal vital signs and laboratory data is considered. Principles of anti-infective therapy and infection control and prophylaxis are explored.

In Part II we attempt to model the clinical diagnostic problems with which the emergency practitioner is confronted. Specific symptoms are discussed in individual chapters, with regard to the historical, physical examination, and laboratory data that are most appropriate to gather for that symptom. A complete differential diagnosis for each symptom is generally provided within the tables, which offer quick reference. Other chapters address infection in specific hosts, emphasizing infectious disease processes and disposition decisions that are unique to the host. The patient with unusual exposures, or living circumstances, is also addressed. This part should allow the practitioner to create an appropriate differential diagnosis based on presenting symptoms, host characteristics, and circumstances.

Part III contains a definitive discussion of the etiology, diagnosis, and treatment of specific infectious diseases by organ system. Disposition decision making and treatment are emphasized. Tables guide the reader to understand likely organisms and appropriate antibiotics for specific populations at risk.

J.C.B.
R.W.Q.

Acknowledgments

Infectious Disease in Emergency Medicine is the product of the contributions of many individuals. We would like to thank our assistants who edited, checked, corrected, and typed draft after draft. These include Jan Frank, Kathie Geiser, Linda Bailey, Nancy Bannister, Shelli Doyle, Paula Hinote, Monique Chavez, Jeff Lauer, Julie Kesti, and Tanya Moraga. Sarah Langwell and Barth Quenzer through their medical illustrations enhanced the understanding of the text. We appreciate the advice, contributions, and patience of our colleagues. This project could not have been done without the support of our respective chairmen, Paul B. Roth and Robert G. Strickland. It has been a pleasure to work with Susan Pioli, our editor at Little, Brown and Company.

Contributing Authors

Michael Jay Bresler, M.D., F.A.C.E.P.
Associate Clinical Professor of Surgery, Stanford University School of Medicine; Attending Physician, Department of Emergency Services, Stanford University Medical Center, Stanford, California

Judith C. Brillman, M.D., F.A.C.E.P.
Assistant Professor of Emergency Medicine, University of New Mexico School of Medicine; Clinical Director, Department of Emergency Medicine, University of New Mexico Hospital, Albuquerque

Charles K. Brown, M.D., F.A.C.E.P.
Assistant Professor of Emergency Medicine and Assistant Residency Director, East Carolina University School of Medicine; Attending Physician, Department of Emergency Medicine, Pitt County Memorial Hospital, Greenville

Myron S. Cohen, M.D.
Professor of Medicine, University of North Carolina at Chapel Hill School of Medicine; Chief, Division of Infectious Disease, University of North Carolina Hospitals, Chapel Hill

Larry E. Davis, M.D., F.A.C.P.
Professor of Neurology and Microbiology, University of New Mexico School of Medicine; Chief, Neurology Service, New Mexico Regional Federal Medical Center, Albuquerque

Robin L. Davis, Pharm.D.
Associate Professor, University of New Mexico School of Pharmacy, Albuquerque

Thomas A. Deutsch, M.D., F.A.C.S.
Associate Professor of Ophthalmology, Rush Medical College of Rush University; Associate Attending Physician, Department of Ophthalmology, Rush-Presbyterian-St. Luke's Medical Center, Chicago

David Doezema, M.D., F.A.C.E.P.
Associate Professor of Emergency Medicine, University of New Mexico School of Medicine; Clinical Director, Department of Emergency Medicine, University of New Mexico Hospital, Albuquerque

Cathy L. Drake, M.D., F.A.C.E.P.
Assistant Professor of Emergency Medicine, University of New Mexico School of Medicine; Staff Physician, Emergency Department, Lovelace Medical Center, Albuquerque

Donald E. Fry, M.D., F.A.C.S.
Professor of Surgery, University of New Mexico School of Medicine; Chairman, Department of Surgery, University of New Mexico Hospital, Albuquerque

Jack Fuhrer, M.D.
Assistant Professor of Medicine, Division of Infectious Diseases, State University of New York at Stony Brook, Health Sciences Center School of Medicine; Clinical Director, AIDS Center, The University Hospital at Stony Brook

Raquel L. Gibly, M.D.
Resident Physician, University of New Mexico School of Medicine; Attending Physician, Department of Emergency Medicine, University of New Mexico Hospital, Albuquerque

Larry J. Goodman, M.D.
Associate Professor of Medicine, Section of Infectious Disease, Rush Medical College of Rush University; Associate Attending Physician, Department of Internal Medicine, Section of Infectious Disease, Rush-Presbyterian-St. Luke's Medical Center, Chicago

L. Clark Hansbarger, M.D., F.A.A.P.
Associate Professor of Pediatrics and Program Director, Residency Training, University of New Mexico School of Medicine; Director of General Pediatrics, University of New Mexico Hospital, Albuquerque

Mark Hauswald, M.D., F.A.C.E.P.
Associate Professor of Emergency Medicine,
University of New Mexico School of Medicine,
Albuquerque

Robert D. Herr, M.D., F.A.C.E.P., F.A.C.P.
Assistant Professor (Clinical) of Surgery, Division of
Emergency Medicine and Adjunct Assistant Professor
(Clinical) of Medicine, University of Utah School of
Medicine; Attending Physician, University Hospital,
Salt Lake City

Fred S. Herzon, M.D., F.A.C.S.
Professor and Chief, Division of Otolaryngology, Head
and Neck Surgery, University of New Mexico School
of Medicine; Attending Surgeon and Chief, Ear,
Nose, and Throat Division, University of New
Mexico Hospital, Albuquerque

Lourdes Irizarry, M.D.
Assistant Professor of Medicine, University of New
Mexico School of Medicine; Attending Physician,
Section of Infectious Diseases, New Mexico Regional
Federal Medical Center, Albuquerque

David R. Johnson, M.D.
Assistant Professor of Emergency Medicine, University
of New Mexico School of Medicine; Attending
Physician, Department of Emergency Medicine,
University of New Mexico Hospital, Albuquerque

Steven M. Joyce, M.D., F.A.C.E.P.
Associate Professor of Surgery, University of Utah
School of Medicine; Attending Physician, Emergency
Department, University Hospital, Salt Lake City

Harold A. Kessler, M.D.
Associate Professor of Medicine and Immunology/
Microbiology, Rush Medical College of Rush
University; Senior Attending Physician, Department
of Internal Medicine, Rush-Presbyterian-St. Luke's
Medical Center, Chicago

Eric M. Koscove, M.D., F.A.C.E.P.
Clinical Faculty, Department of Emergency Medicine,
Harbor-UCLA Medical Center, Torrance, California

Frederick T. Koster, M.D.
Professor of Medicine, University of New Mexico
School of Medicine; Attending Physician,
Department of Medicine, University of New Mexico
Hospital, Albuquerque

**Douglas Lindsey, M.D., Dr.P.H., F.A.C.S.,
F.A.C.E.P.**
Professor of Surgery Emeritus, University of Arizona
College of Medicine; Attending Physician, Emergency
Department, University Medical Center, Tucson

Chien Liu, M.D.
Professor Emeritus of Medicine and Pediatrics,
University of Kansas School of Medicine, Kansas City

Christopher M. Lowther, M.D.
Assistant Professor of Medicine, University of Kansas
School of Medicine, Kansas City

Peter P. McKellar, M.D.
Clinical Associate Professor of Internal Medicine,
University of Arizona College of Medicine, Tucson;
Director, Division of Infectious Diseases and Associate
Director, Medical Residency Program, Good
Samaritan Regional Medical Center, Phoenix

Darwin L. Palmer, M.D., F.A.C.P.
Professor of Medicine, University of New Mexico
School of Medicine; Chief, Division of Infectious
Diseases, University of New Mexico Hospital and
New Mexico Regional Federal Medical Center,
Albuquerque

John C. Pottage, Jr., M.D., F.A.C.P.
Associate Professor of Medicine, Rush Medical
College of Rush University; Associate Attending
Physician, Department of Internal Medicine, Rush-
Presbyterian-St. Luke's Medical Center, Chicago

Ronald W. Quenzer, M.D.
Associate Professor of Medicine, University of New
Mexico School of Medicine; Chief, Division of
General Medicine, and Medical Director, Primary
Care Initiative, University of New Mexico Hospital,
Albuquerque

William P. Reed, M.D.
Professor of Medicine, University of New Mexico
School of Medicine; Associate Chief of Staff for
Research, New Mexico Regional Federal Medical
Center, Albuquerque

Robert L. Rhyne, M.D.
Associate Professor of Family and Community
Medicine, University of New Mexico School of
Medicine; Attending Physician, Department of Family
Medicine, University of New Mexico Hospital,
Albuquerque

Richard J. Roche, M.D.
Assistant Professor of Medicine, University of New Mexico School of Medicine; Attending Physician, Gerontology Division, University of New Mexico Hospital, Albuquerque

John Segreti, M.D.
Assistant Professor of Medicine, Rush Medical College of Rush University; Associate Attending Physician, Department of Internal Medicine, Section of Infectious Disease, Rush-Presbyterian-St. Luke's Medical Center, Chicago

Jonathan S. Serody, M.D.
Postdoctoral Fellow in Infectious Diseases and Hematology, University of North Carolina at Chapel Hill School of Medicine, Chapel Hill

Suzanne M. Shepherd, M.D., F.A.C.E.P.
Associate Professor of Emergency Medicine, East Carolina University School of Medicine; Attending Physician, Department of Emergency Medicine, Pitt County Memorial Hospital, Greenville

Gary L. Simpson, M.D., Ph.D., M.P.H., F.A.C.P.
Clinical Associate Professor of Medicine, University of New Mexico School of Medicine, Albuquerque; Medical Director, Bureau of Infectious Diseases, Department of Health, Santa Fe, New Mexico

David P. Sklar, M.D., F.A.C.E.P.
Associate Professor and Vice Chairman of Emergency Medicine, University of New Mexico School of Medicine; Attending Physician, Department of Emergency Medicine, University of New Mexico Hospital, Albuquerque

Russell D. Snyder, M.D.
Professor of Pediatrics and Neurology, University of New Mexico School of Medicine; Director, Division of Pediatric Neurology, University of New Mexico Hospital, Albuquerque

J. Stephan Stapczynski, M.D., F.A.C.E.P.
Associate Professor and Chair of Emergency Medicine, University of Kentucky College of Medicine; Attending Physician and Medical Director, Department of Emergency Medicine, University of Kentucky Medical Center, Lexington

George L. Sternbach, M.D., F.A.C.E.P.
Clinical Associate Professor of Surgery, Stanford University School of Medicine, Stanford; Emergency Physician, Seton Medical Center, Daly City, California

Charles Stewart, M.D., F.A.C.E.P.
Associate Regional Medical Director, EMSA Limited Partnership, Western Region, Denver

David A. Talan, M.D., F.A.C.E.P.
Associate Professor of Medicine, University of California, Los Angeles, UCLA School of Medicine, Los Angeles; Associate Director, Department of Emergency Medicine, Olive View Medical Center, Sylmar, California

Dan Tandberg, M.D., F.A.C.E.P.
Professor of Emergency Medicine, University of New Mexico School of Medicine; Attending Physician, Department of Emergency Medicine, University of New Mexico Hospital, Albuquerque

Knox H. Todd, M.D.
Research Fellow, Division of Emergency Medicine, University of California, Los Angeles, UCLA School of Medicine, Los Angeles; Attending Physician, UCLA Emergency Medicine Center, Los Angeles

Peter Viccellio, M.D., F.A.C.E.P.
Assistant Professor of Emergency Medicine, State University of New York at Stony Brook, Health Sciences Center School of Medicine; Vice Chairman, Department of Emergency Medicine, The University Hospital at Stony Brook

Melvin P. Weinstein, M.D.
Professor of Medicine and Pathology, University of Medicine and Dentistry of New Jersey, Robert Wood Johnson Medical School; Director, Microbiology Laboratory, Robert Wood Johnson University Hospital, New Brunswick

Josephine M. Williams, M.D.
Adjunct Assistant Professor of Medicine, University of New Mexico School of Medicine; Director, STD Clinic, Bernalillo County Health Office, Albuquerque

I

Principles of
Infectious Disease

1

Critical Decisions in Emergency Medicine Treatment of Infectious Disease

PETER VICCELLIO
JACK FUHRER

The infectious diseases encompass a prodigious number of entities with highly variable presentations. The diagnosis of infection is entertained in a substantial portion of patient visits to an emergency department. Most patients, having relatively benign infections, will enjoy recovery regardless of proper diagnosis or type of treatment. From this larger set of patients, the emergency physician must determine which patients require more specific diagnosis or specific therapy. The physician's task for such patients is directed at answering the following questions:

1. Are a patient's symptoms caused by infection?
2. If so, what class or type of infection is causing the symptoms?
3. Can a specific diagnosis be made?
4. What system or systems in the body are being affected?
5. Are other coexisting illnesses present?
6. Is this patient a compromised host?
7. What treatment has the patient already received, and what has been the response to therapy?
8. Would the patient benefit from specific therapy?
9. Is inpatient therapy warranted?
10. How rapidly should therapy be initiated?

11. Should consultation be obtained?
12. Are other individuals at risk from exposure?
13. What follow-up care needs to be done?
14. Is this a reportable disease?

In addition to the physician's thorough grounding in infectious diseases, the answers to these questions are derived from, if the patient's clinical status allows it, a complete history, a physical examination, and an appropriate laboratory evaluation. In those patients presenting with overwhelming infection, the treating physician should be familiar with the typical causative agents given the patient's clinical presentation, age, and other relevant factors. In those cases, the initial evaluating physician is responsible for rapid institution of appropriate therapy.

The History

Proper diagnosis demands a thorough elicitation from the patient of the nature of the current complaint, associated complaints, preexisting medical and surgical problems, medications, an exposure and travel history, an immunization history, and a history of allergies. In addition, a sexual history and a history of alcohol, tobacco, and other drug use may be essential. A carefully obtained history can provide clues that may lead to the diagnosis of a relatively exotic infectious disease that would not otherwise be given consideration.

Specific Symptoms

The nature of the patient's current symptoms must be thoroughly explored. What exactly caused the patient to seek medical attention at this time? What is the duration and the rate of development of these symptoms? Are other complaints associated with these symptoms? Are there factors that exacerbate or mitigate these symptoms? Has any treatment been attempted? If so, what has been the response to that treatment? Have these symptoms been present in the past? If so, how have they been evaluated and treated?

General Symptoms

General symptoms that suggest infection include fever, sweats, weakness, malaise, anorexia, change in mental status, and worsening of a preexisting medical condition. If the infection is localized, symptoms at that site will usually dominate the clinical picture. However, complaints or physical findings remote from that area may provide crucial diagnostic information.

Past Medical History

The patient's medical history is critical in determining unusual susceptibility to infection, such as a history of diabetes, AIDS, alcoholism, IV drug abuse, past splenectomy, chronic institutionalization, or cancer, particularly in those recently treated with chemotherapeutic agents. Artificial valves, joints, and other foreign bodies provide a locus for infection that the host cannot eliminate. A history of medications is crucial. Particular attention should be given to whether the patient has been taking antibiotics prior to presentation, which may alter the presenting symptoms as well as prevent positive cultures. Medications such as steroids, chemotherapeutic agents, and other immunosuppressive drugs can alter the patient's ability to resist infection and suppress symptoms. Drug-induced fever can confuse the

clinical picture. Finally, several agents at toxic levels, particularly salicylate and anticholinergic agents, produce a syndrome that may mimic overwhelming infection. Exposure through occupation, hobby, or environment can provide clues to the presence of more unusual infecting agents. Travel history is crucial; the physician should determine typical infectious agents endemic to the region through which the patient has traveled.

Review of Systems

A review of systems may reveal a cause of the infection. Examples include a history of murmur, a recent dental extraction (endocarditis), pharyngitis (rheumatic fever), urethritis (disseminated gonococcemia), gastroenteritis (postinfectious enthesiopathies), recent antibiotic therapy (Clostridium difficile), post gastrectomy (salmonella), and recent instrumentation.

Social History

Finally a proper social history can provide clues to the physician regarding the likelihood of successful outpatient therapy. The physician is obligated to determine whether the patient can afford the medications being prescribed, whether appropriate follow-up is available to the patient, and whether the patient will reliably take the medication prescribed.

The Physical Examination

The first step in the physical exam should be to identify those patients in need of emergency therapy. Those patients with unstable vital signs, rapidly deteriorating mental status, or symptoms and physical findings suggestive of bacterial meningitis, septic shock, or acute bacterial endocarditis should be immediately cultured and have parenteral antibiotic therapy initiated, ideally within the first 10–15 minutes of presentation. Those not falling into this group can undergo a more detailed history and physical examination. When evaluating a patient, the physician should remember that symptoms can be vague and nonspecific and that the patient may appear quite stable in the face of grave infection.

Vital Signs

TEMPERATURE MEASUREMENT AND FEVER

Oral temperatures are notoriously inaccurate, particularly in those patients with a respiratory rate of 20 or greater and those who have recently ingested food or drink [1]. Tympanic membrane temperatures are highly accurate if properly obtained, although questions exist as to their accuracy when taken on small infants or in ear canals occluded by cerumen [2, 3]. Rectal temperatures, considered the "gold standard," may be falsely low if the thermometer is inserted directly into stool in the rectum. Immediate temperature measurement of freshly voided urine has been described as a useful technique in patients suspected of factitious fever [4] (see Chap. 2).

Although fever (temperature > 37°C) is a cardinal sign of infection, several precautionary comments should be made. In those serious infections usually associated with a significant fever, absence of fever may reflect an inability of the host to mount a febrile response. Fever typically is not present throughout a 24-hour period, even in serious infection, and the patient may present to the emergency department while afebrile. Patients who have taken antipyretics may be afebrile at the time of evaluation, or they may have a blunted fever curve. The history of fever provided by the patient may be inaccurate, particularly in those patients who have not actually measured their temperature. However, it is difficult for the treating physician to ignore such a history in any particular patient. The pattern of the fever may provide a clue to more unusual infections such as malaria, but in general it does not distinguish one infection from another or distinguish infectious causes from noninfectious ones. The extremes of age can alter response to infection. Baseline temperature in the elderly may be more than a degree lower compared with that of younger patients [5].

HEART RATE

Tachycardia (heart rate > 100 beats per minute) can result from fever, anxiety, pain, hypoxia, cardiac involvement, or significant dehydration and, as such, requires careful evaluation. Bradycardia in the face of an elevated temperature is relatively unusual and might suggest infection from typhoid

fever, infection with an intracellular organism, or myocardial involvement from any of a number of infectious agents (Table 1-1).

RESPIRATORY RATE

Respiratory rate can be elevated (> 18 respirations per minute) from anxiety, infection of the respiratory tract, hypoxia, sepsis, or metabolic acidosis. Hypoxemia can be a manifestation of infection-induced adult respiratory distress syndrome (ARDS). Tachypnea can also be an early manifestation of the sepsis syndrome. Like tachycardia, it deserves careful assessment.

HYPOTENSION

Frank hypotension (blood pressure < 90/60 mm Hg) can reflect severe hypovolemia, septic shock, or a noninfectious cause. Hypovolemia should be corrected quickly. If the clinician truly cannot determine the nature and the type of shock, Swan-Ganz catheterization will be necessary to direct treatment. The patient who does not respond rapidly to appropriate fluid therapy should be considered to have life-threatening infection and should be cultured emergently and administered intravenous antibiotics. Short of frank supine hypotension, the patient may exhibit more moderate signs of decreased circulating blood volume. Although many texts provide formal guidelines for interpretation of postural signs, surprisingly little literature validates those guidelines. A recent study [6] involving the removal of two units of whole blood (1000 ml) from healthy volunteers found that symptoms of lightheadedness or a reflex tachycardia greater than 30 BPM were far more accurate than any type or degree of change in the blood pressure in identifying those who had this amount of blood removed. This has not been validated for intravascular depletion from other causes. Along similar lines, a formal study of capillary refill did not vali-

Table 1-1. Infections exhibiting relative bradycardia

Dengue fever	Psittacosis
Legionnaires' disease	Typhoid fever
Leptospirosis	Epidemic typhus
Malaria	Yellow fever
Mycoplasma syndromes	

date the usefulness of this sign in assessing the adequacy of perfusion [7].

The General Physical Examination

SKIN

The skin should be carefully searched for the presence of cellulitis, lymphangitis, abscess, rash, petechiae or purpura, nodules, Janeway's lesions, Osler's nodes, and splinter hemorrhages. A number of infections can be diagnosed by the appearance of the skin findings alone. The presence of a petechial rash should alert the physician to the possibility of meningococcemia or Rocky Mountain spotted fever. (Dermatologic manifestations of infectious diseases are covered extensively in Chap. 9.) Jaundice is evidence of hepatobiliary disease (such as cholangitis) or hemolysis (such as in clostridial sepsis).

LYMPH NODES

Diffuse involvement is typical of viral syndromes but is also consistent with a number of other infections. Posterior cervical adenopathy in a patient with pharyngitis is suggestive of mononucleosis or toxoplasmosis. A solitary enlarged node is characteristic of cat scratch disease and scrofula, or it may result from drainage of a local infection to that node or group of nodes (see Chap. 10).

EYES

The differential diagnosis of "red eye" is covered in Chap. 35. Conjunctival ulcerations may be seen in oculoglandular tularemia, lymphogranuloma venereum, and tuberculosis. Corneal ulcers must be distinguished from more benign corneal abrasions. Penetration of the globe may not be evident from routine inspection but may cause severe endophthalmitis. The presence of a hypopyon signals iridocyclitis, endophthalmitis, and corneal disease. Periorbital cellulitis may drain through the ophthalmic veins into the cavernous sinus, causing septic cavernous sinus thrombosis. Retrobulbar infections can be associated with proptosis of the globe, edema of the lids, and pain on movement of extraocular muscles. Limited range of motion or frank ophthalmoplegia in any direction suggests a serious retro-orbital or CNS infection or meningeal irritation. The sclerae are the best sites for determi-

nation of the presence of jaundice, which can usually be appreciated with bilirubin above 2 mg/dl; jaundice is better appreciated in natural light than in fluorescent light. A fundoscopic exam can reveal infection within the globe, and a retinal exam can reveal Roth's spots, septic emboli, or a primary infection in the retina or choroid, such as toxoplasmosis.

EARS

Inspection of the ear canal can reveal otitis externa, characterized by an inflamed ear canal, exudate, and pain with traction of the tragus. An invasive otitis externa caused by pseudomonas (malignant otitis externa) is seen particularly in diabetics. Otitis media, far more common in children than in adults, causes bulging and redness of the tympanic membrane; landmarks are obscured, the light reflex is often lost, and air conduction is significantly impaired. (See Chap. 34.)

NOSE AND SINUSES

The nose and sinuses should be evaluated as potential sources of infection. Absence of percussive tenderness over the maxillary or frontal sinuses in an alert patient makes significant infection in these areas unlikely. Conversely positive percussive tenderness is suggestive, but not diagnostic, for sinusitis and does not distinguish viral from bacterial sinusitis. Infection of the ethmoid and sphenoid sinuses cannot be directly determined by physical exam. Mild pain elicited from extraocular movement is typical of sinusitis in the periorbital region, which can also be seen in retro-orbital infections and meningeal irritation. (See Chap. 34.)

OROPHARYNX

Careful inspection of the entire oropharynx can reveal signs of local or systemic infection and contribute to making a specific diagnosis. Enanthems suggest viral illness such as herpangina, herpes simplex, and measles. (See Chaps. 21 and 36.) Teeth must be inspected to identify dental abscess and evidence sought for spread to the floor of the mouth or buccal area. The pharynx and retropharynx may demonstrate exudate or abscess. Throat pain in the absence of oropharyngeal abnormality on gross inspection must raise suspicion of involvement of the epiglottis, larynx, trachea, or esophagus. (See Chap. 22.)

LUNGS

Examination of the lungs should be directed at assessing underlying cardiopulmonary disease, as well as evidence of consolidation and effusion (see Chap. 23). It is important to note that perihilar infections often reveal a normal pulmonary exam. Mycoplasma and other atypical pneumonias, for instance, may have dramatic radiographic findings but minimal findings on physical exam. Auscultation of breath sounds does not constitute an adequate exam, and many findings will be missed in a careless exam. The examiner should evaluate for dullness on percussion, tactile fremitus, vocal fremitus, egophony, whispered pectoriloquy, and presence of bronchial breath sounds and listen for the presence of a friction rub.

Auscultatory percussion (performed by lightly percussing the patient's sternum with the index finger while listening with the stethoscope in comparable areas on both sides of the chest; a difference in transmission of sound is considered to be a positive finding) in one study was found to be the single most accurate method for distinguishing a normal from an abnormal examination and required minimal cooperation from the patient [8]. Overall, given the significant number of false negative physical findings in patients with pneumonia, a normal physical exam should not obviate the need for a chest x-ray (nor should a normal chest x-ray eliminate the diagnosis of pneumonia) [9–11].

In the patient with signs of infection, pleural effusions should be considered to be infected until proved otherwise. In the patient with congestive heart failure, benign right-sided or bilateral effusion are typical and should clear or at least decrease with appropriate therapy; isolated left-sided effusions should always be considered pathologic. The patient who presents with high-grade sepsis, severe chest pain, and a left-sided pleural effusion should be assumed to have a ruptured or perforated esophagus until proved otherwise.

HEART

The presence of a significant murmur should heighten the clinician's suspicion of endocarditis. In subacute endocarditis, most commonly the murmur is preexisting. Acute endocarditis typically causes murmurs of insufficiency; thus, the examiner should carefully evaluate neck veins for Cannon waves of tricuspid insufficiency (which may otherwise be silent) and should auscultate the heart with the patient upright and at maximal exhalation (for pulmonary and aortic regurgitation) and in the left lateral decubitus position (for mitral insufficiency). In acute endocarditis the murmur may worsen over a period of several hours. In pericarditis a friction rub may be heard and may vary in intensity with respirations. (See Chap. 24.)

ABDOMEN

Massive hepatomegaly may be noted with acute right-sided endocarditis, due to tricuspid insufficiency. The liver typically exhibits punch tenderness in hepatitis (see Chap. 26). Acute cholecystitis characteristically has a positive Murphy's sign. In Fitz-Hugh-Curtis syndrome a friction rub over the liver can be elicited with respirations. Splenomegaly may be noted in a number of viral illnesses, particularly mononucleosis, and also in subacute endocarditis. Any of a number of causes of acute abdomen can be associated with fever and are discussed in Chap. 27. Costovertebral (CVA) tenderness should be sought, although this is neither necessary nor sufficient to make the diagnosis of pyelonephritis (see Chap. 28).

Gastroenteritis can be associated with mild to moderate diffuse tenderness, but findings of ileus or rebound are not characteristic of this diagnosis. It is particularly hazardous to make such a diagnosis in elderly patients. Any findings of rigidity or rebound tenderness should be assumed to be peritonitis and can be from any of a variety of causes. In patients with preexisting ascites, an increase in girth may be the only sign of spontaneous bacterial peritonitis, the patient otherwise lacking in pain, fever, or elevated white count. Rectal examination may reveal a tender prostate, blood or mucus in the stool, perirectal abscess, or proctitis from a variety of causes.

GENITALIA

Orchitis, epididymitis, urethritis, and other sexually transmitted diseases are commonly found and can give rise to systemic symptoms (see Chaps. 28–30). In a woman any cervical, vaginal, or urethral discharge should be noted and appropriately cultured. Cervical motion tenderness is the hallmark of pelvic inflammatory disease, but it is not diagnostic for this entity. Conversely, absence of tenderness does not exclude significant occult infection.

Spine and Extremities

Pain, swelling, erythema, warmth, and limited range of motion in a peripheral joint are highly suggestive of infection. The pattern of joint involvement (monarticular vs. polyarticular, symmetric vs. asymmetric, with or without skin rash, migratory vs. fixed) is crucial to the differential diagnosis. (See Chap. 33.) Infection of the hip joint characteristically is associated with limited range of motion and pain with movement; the pain radiates to the anterior and medial portion of the thigh to the knee or may be located purely in the knee. It should be noted that the knee itself is normally cooler to the touch than the thigh, and loss of this coolness may signify inflammation and infection of the joint.

The distinction of septic from aseptic bursitis is a difficult one. In the past it has been distinguished only by aspiration, Gram's stain, and culture of the bursal fluid. A recent study suggests that a distinction can be made between the two in the case of olecranon bursitis by measuring the skin temperature differential between the affected elbow and the unaffected elbow; a difference of greater than 2°C is highly suggestive of infection [12]. (See Chap. 33.)

Localized muscle tenderness is characteristic of fasciitis and myositis, which, in spite of their overwhelming nature, can be quite difficult to diagnose without a high index of suspicion; such patients typically are quite toxic (see Chap. 32).

Localized bony tenderness can signify the presence of infection. Awaiting positive x-ray findings guarantees disastrous consequences. Osteomyelitis of the vertebral column, similar to osteomyelitis in other areas, is characterized by localized pain in the area of infection. This diagnosis should always be considered in a patient who presents with unexplained back pain, particularly if it is well localized. Thoracic vertebral involvement is characteristic of tuberculosis, whereas lumbar involvement is characteristic of the more usual organisms, particularly

Escherichia coli and *Staphylococcus aureus.* Early diagnosis of bone and joint infection serves as the only protection against irreversible destruction. (See Chap. 33.)

Nervous System

An altered mental status should heighten the suspicion of a CNS infection, although many infections outside the nervous system can be associated with a decreased mental status, particularly in the very old and the very young. Absence of nuchal rigidity does not eliminate the possibility of meningitis. Meningeal irritation characteristically worsens with flexion of the head onto the chest and is relieved by extension. Mild meningeal irritation can be distinguished from osteoarthritis of the cervical spine in the following manner: In osteoarthritis the neck typically flexes to a fixed point and then stops; in meningitis the neck tends to flex to a certain point and "catch" but then flexes a bit farther. Also the pain in meningeal irritation tends to radiate down the neck and into the back. Upper-lobe pneumonias, particularly in children, can cause reflex irritation of the underlying musculature and thus mimic the findings of meningeal irritation. The patient's response to lateral rotation or abduction of the head is not helpful in distinguishing benign conditions from serious ones. Focal supratentorial neurological manifestations are suggestive of a mass lesion; the presence of focal cranial nerve abnormalities is characteristic of basilar meningitis and cavernous sinus thrombosis. In the absence of meningeal symptoms, cranial neuropathies, particularly of the facial nerve, should raise the suspicion of Lyme disease. (See Chaps. 7, 8, and 31.)

Laboratory Analysis

The debate regarding appropriate workup of minor outpatient infections is beyond the scope of this chapter. However, any time a diagnosis of serious infection is entertained, at the very least a complete blood count (CBC) with differential, a chest x-ray, urinalysis, and blood cultures should be obtained. Properly collected specimens from the site of suspected infection should be cultured and gram stained, if possible before initiation of antibiotics (see Chap. 3). In suspected cases of meningitis where the physician chooses to delay lumbar puncture until a CT scan is obtained, blood cultures should be obtained and antibiotic therapy initiated immediately. Most cultures of spinal fluid obtained after initiation of antibiotics will still be positive if obtained within 2–3 hours [13]. More extensive or sophisticated evaluation is determined by the suspected site and the nature of the infection.

WBC Count

The WBC count and differential cannot be reliably used to support the presence or absence of serious infection. There appears to be an increasing chance of significant bacterial infection associated with a high WBC count, a shift to the left, prominent bandemia, and elevated erythrocyte sedimentation rate (ESR), and this appears to be true across all age groups [14–17]. However, these are neither sensitive or specific enough for certain diagnosis. (See Chap. 3.)

Acute Phase Reactants

The ESR is somewhat useful if it is exceptionally high (> 100); in those circumstances, the ESR suggests a limited infectious differential, including TB, subacute endocarditis, chronic abscess, and other infections of a chronic nature, as well as collagen vascular diseases and neoplasms (see Chap. 3). Measurement of the C-reactive protein has enjoyed a resurgence of interest in recent years, but it provides no specific answers.

Arterial Blood Gas

Either an arterial blood gas (ABG) or pulse oximetry can be used to assess the patient's level of oxygenation. It is important to note that clinical assessment of hypoxia is grossly inaccurate [18]. An ABG will also assess the patient's acid-base status.

Coagulation Studies

If the patient is considered to have sepsis, viral hemorrhagic fever, or thrombocytopenia, then prothrombin time, platelet count, and fibrin split products should be measured.

Other more extensive workup should proceed as

indicated by the diagnoses being considered, and the patient's clinical status. Appropriate serological and immunological tests should be obtained as indicated.

Diagnosis and Management Decisions

Diagnostic Considerations

A careful history, comprehensive physical examination, and appropriate laboratory testing should limit the differential and establish the likelihood of serious infection. The most critical decisions then become whether the patient should be admitted to the hospital and whether the patient should be started on antimicrobial therapy. In many instances, the appearance of the patient is the crucial factor that determines the need for admission and more aggressive therapy. The decision to treat the patient outside the hospital assumes that the host is mightier than the infection, that there will be little or no benefit from hospitalization, and that therapy will safely eradicate or control the disease of concern.

In the well-appearing patient, the clinician must keep in mind those entities that require inpatient treatment in spite of the patient's appearance (Table 1-2). Examples include endopthalmitis, subacute or acute bacterial endocarditis, spontaneous bacterial peritonitis, intra-abdominal abscess, and fever in the asplenic patient, the neutropenic or immunosuppressed patient, the IV drug abuser, the alcoholic, and the elderly patient. The physician must consider noninfectious causes of fever, such as drug fever, immunologic disease, pulmonary embolus, or subarachnoid hemorrhage, before concluding that infection of some type is the cause of the patient's symptoms.

In many patients, particularly those with minor infections, a definitive diagnosis is not possible but, fortunately, also not necessary. The ubiquitous upper respiratory infection, sore throat, and gastroenteritis generally are straightforward diagnoses as clinical syndromes and respond either to treatment or to the passage of time. The physician's goal, other than providing relief and specific therapy where necessary, is to ensure that serious illness is

Table 1-2. Infectious syndromes generally
requiring admission

Nervous System Infections
Meningitis
Encephalitis
Cerebral abscess
Transverse myelitis
Guillain-Barré

Head and Neck Infections
Endopthalmitis
Epiglottitis
Malignant otitis externa
Cervical fascial plane infection

Lower Respiratory Tract Infections
Necrotizing pneumonia
ARDS
Pneumonia in the immunocompromised patient
Empyema

Cardiovascular and Mediastinal Infections
Endocarditis
Pericarditis/myocarditis (except viral w/hemodynamic
    stability)
Mediastinitis
Supporative thrombophlebitis
Rheumatic fever

Abdominal Infections
Peritonitis (except in chronic ambulatory peritoneal
    dialysis)
Intra-abdominal abscess
Cholangitis
Appendicitis

Genitourinary Tract Infections
Complicated pyelonephritis
Complicated prostatitis
Renal abscess
Complicated pelvic inflammatory disease

Skin and Soft-Tissue Infections
Lymphangitis
Cellulitis in the immunocompromised patient
Necrotizing cellulitis
Fetid foot
Erysipelas
Infected burns
Necrotizing fasciitis/gangrene

Musculoskeletal Infections
Acute osteomyelitis
Septic arthritis

Tenosynovitis of the hand
Myositis
Paraspinal/paravertebral infections

Infections of the Lymphatic System
Buboes
Fever in the asplenic patient

General Infections
Undiagnosed fever in the immunocompromised
    patient
Bacteremia
Septic emboli
Prosthetic device infections
Toxic shock syndrome
Opportunistic infections
Fever in the IV drug user

not buried beneath apparently benign symptoms. One must not forget that diagnoses of viral infection are often well-educated guesses and essentially diagnoses of exclusion in the emergency department environment.

Immediate Therapy

Many patients with infectious disease, whether confirmed or suspected, require immediate treatment. Obviously any patient who is grossly toxic or who exhibits hemodynamic instability or hypoxia deserves a rapid workup and the institution of appropriate therapy, including antibiotics. Often the need for emergent treatment necessarily precedes the establishment of a specific diagnosis such as urosepsis or meningococcemia. Also certain diseases, confirmed or suspected, dictate an emergent workup and the rapid initiation of therapy, such as meningitis, sepsis, endopthalmitis, and acute carditis (Table 1-3).

Admission Criteria

GENERAL CONSIDERATIONS
The decision to admit or discharge a given patient is sometimes a complex one, often based more on local practice than scientific rigor. As a general statement of principle, patients with infection should be admitted if they are at risk for significant morbidity or mortality. This risk is determined by

Table 1-3. Infectious diseases requiring immediate therapy

Acute endocarditis	Necrotizing fasciitis
Endopthalmitis	Meningitis
Epiglottitis	Sepsis

factors that are specific to the presumptive disease process, to the individual host, and to the interaction of the host and the disease.

DISEASE-SPECIFIC FACTORS

Specific diseases and syndromes that generally require admission for treatment are listed in Table 1-2.

Presumptive Site of Infection. The presumptive site of infection is one of the more important criteria for determining admission to the hospital. The site of infection may be evidence of deep tissue infection in areas where antibiotics penetrate poorly or where infection commonly leads to great morbidity or mortality.

Patients with infectious diseases such as viral syndromes, streptococcal pharyngitis, otitis media, sinusitis, some pneumonias, infectious diarrhea, urinary tract infections, and sexually transmitted diseases (STDs) often can be treated with oral antibiotics and managed as outpatients. For many infections, such as pneumonia, pyelonephritis, and pelvic inflammatory disease, the need for admission is often determined by the status and the underlying susceptibility of the host more than the disease per se. It is possible that long-term morbidity may be decreased in a subset of these infections by parenteral therapy. Other infections clearly require admission to the hospital.

CNS INFECTIONS. A patient who has meningitis, a brain abscess, a subdural abscess, or encephalitis should be admitted to the hospital for initial evaluation and treatment. In the patient with suspected acute meningitis, a thorough neurologic and fundoscopic evaluation should be performed to rule out increased intracranial pressure secondary to mass effect, followed by a lumbar puncture. It is appropriate to initiate antibiotic therapy in the emergency department based on cerebrospinal fluid analysis,

age, host risk factors, and epidemiologic history. (See Chap. 31.)

HEAD AND NECK INFECTIONS. Because of fascial planes of the head and neck, some infections in this region spread more rapidly and have the ability to cause airway compromise. For instance, acute epiglottitis is a rapidly progressive cellulitis of the epiglottis and can cause abrupt, complete airway obstruction. To breathe, the patient will prefer to lean forward while drooling oral secretions [19–21]. Recognition of this entity is critical, as are decisions regarding airway management and appropriate antibiotics [22, 23]. The decision to intubate should take into account the age of the patient and the likelihood of an acute obstruction. Children under 4 years of age in the same household should be given *Hemophilus influenzae* prophylaxis (rifampin) and followed closely [24]. (See Chap. 36.)

PNEUMONIA. Community-acquired pneumonia secondary to *Streptococcus pneumoniae*, *Mycoplasma pneumoniae*, and *H. influenzae* can often be adequately treated with oral antibiotics in the home setting. The patient who presents with respiratory compromise as evidenced by a significant degree of hypoxemia or who has a parapneumonic pleural effusion would best be served by admission to the hospital. Patients with underlying lung disease, for example, chronic obstructive pulmonary disease (COPD), asthma, and cystic fibrosis, are more likely to have respiratory insufficiency resulting from pneumonia and generally should be hospitalized for this diagnosis. Patients with AIDS are at risk for *Pneumocystis carinii* pneumonia (PCP) as well as other opportunistic pathogens (e.g., cytomegalovirus and *Mycobacterium tuberculosis*) and common bacterial pathogens [25]. Patients with mild PCP (A-a oxygen gradient on room air of < 30 mm Hg) can often be cared for in the home setting; however, patients with moderate to severe PCP can have rapid deterioration and may benefit from adjunctive corticosteroids [26] and admission to the hospital. Other immunosuppressed patients, for example, cancer patients and asplenic patients, are best treated in the hospital setting when presenting with pneumonia. All patients with suspected empyema require admission. (See Chap. 23.)

CARDIAC INFECTIONS. A patient with a presumptive diagnosis of endocarditis should initially be treated in the hospital. Included in this group is any patient with a fever and an artificial valve or fever and a history of recent IV drug use [27]. Complications of endocarditis are serious and include embolic episodes, mycotic aneurysms, CNS manifestations, mural and valve ring abscesses, and arrhythmias. The patient with subacute bacterial endocarditis (e.g., secondary to viridans *streptococci*) may not appear toxic, whereas the patient with acute endocarditis (e.g., secondary to *S. aureus*) may look very ill. Patients with a history of illicit drug use are at increased risk for right-sided endocarditis and embolic phenomena to the lungs. Most commonly *S. aureus* is the offending organism [28]. Patients with acute myopericarditis similarly would benefit from hospitalization. Such patients are at increased risk for arrhythmias as well as cardiac dysfunction and should be monitored for such. (See Chap. 24.)

INTRA-ABDOMINAL INFECTIONS. In assessing the patient with abdominal pain and fever, the physician needs to ask several questions. Does the patient have an intra-abdominal catastrophe, for example, a perforated viscus? Is the patient dehydrated or likely to become dehydrated in the next 24 hours if discharged from the hospital? Is there evidence of ascites and concern for bacterial peritonitis (e.g., in an alcoholic with abdominal pain)? Is the working diagnosis acute cholecystitis, appendicitis, or tubo-ovarian abscess? Is the patient toxic in appearance? If the answer to any of these questions is yes, the patient would best be served by admission to the hospital. (See Chap. 27.)

BONE, JOINT, AND MUSCLE INFECTIONS. Any patient suspected of having an acute bacterial infection of bone, joint, or muscle requires admission, definitive diagnosis, and treatment. Chronic osteomyelitis can often be evaluated and treated in the outpatient setting. (See Chap. 33.)

Natural Course of Suspected Diagnosis. Effective emergency physicians need to understand the natural course of a suspected disease to make an appropriate disposition. This holds true whether the patient is a trauma patient, a patient with a cardiac problem, or a patient with an infectious disease. A patient's appearance at the moment of arrival at the emergency department does not necessarily predict the patient's outcome.

The patient with pyelonephritis and urinary obstruction may appear well at the moment but is at risk for urosepsis if not aggressively treated. Conversely the patient with viral gastroenteritis or streptococcal pharyngitis may look toxic but will recover quickly if appropriate therapy is initiated prior to discharge from the emergency department.

Although the emergency physician will rarely be certain about the etiologic agent, clinical clues may point to infection by a particularly virulent organism. Concern about the presence of a virulent organism mandates admission and emergent antibiotic therapy. *S. aureus* may be suspected in the patient with pneumonia accompanied by pleural effusion and abscess on a chest x-ray. A Gram's stain of the sputum may confirm this suspicion. Purpuric cutaneous lesions should lead to concern about meningococcemia. Jaundice in the patient with a septic abortion suggests clostridial sepsis with hemolysis. A bluish periorbital cellulitis in a young child points to *H. influenzae* infection.

HOST-SPECIFIC FACTORS

The importance of host factors is reflected in a broad literature of medicine that documents the presence of serious infection in patients who appear to have trivial illness. Thus, fever alone indicates the need for admission for IV drug abusers, neutropenic patients, and patients at particularly high risk for endocarditis, regardless of clinical symptoms or certainty on the part of the physician of minor illness. The physician who chooses to discharge a febrile diabetic, alcoholic, or elderly patient does so at significant risk to the patient.

Age of Patient. The age of the patient is important from several perspectives. Both the very young and the very old are at greater risk for infection. Children who have lost maternal antibodies and have not produced their own antibodies can develop infections with encapsulated bacteria, for example, *H. influenzae* and *Neisseria meningitidis* [29, 30]. In young infants (< 3 months old), clinical evaluation is a poor predictor of serious illness; fever in this age group necessitates either admission or close, reliable, and frequent follow-up [31]. (See Chap. 14.) The immune defect in the elderly is felt to be secondary to a functional decline in cell-mediated immunity as well as to reduction of organ-specific physiologic function [32]. Symptoms of infection may be less dramatic and poorly localized. Diagnosis of a benign viral syndrome in an elderly patient should be made with the greatest caution. (See Chap. 15.)

The age of the patient should guide the physician as to the organisms more commonly associated with the suspected site of infection. For instance, a neonate presenting with meningitis needs to be treated with antibiotics that will cover *Listeria monocytogenes* [33], Group B streptococcus [34, 35], *E. coli* [36], and enterococcus [37], whereas in older children *H. influenzae* are the most common bacterial cause of meningitis between the neonatal period and age 6 years [38]. In adults meningitis is most commonly caused by *S. pneumoniae* [39]. Although the decision to admit these patients is obvious, the choice of antibiotics will be guided by their age, spinal fluid Gram's stain, or positive bacterial antigens present in the cerebrospinal fluid.

The choice and the dosage of antibiotics are based on the age and the weight of the patient. Tetracyclines and quinolones should be avoided if possible in children. Tetracyclines can result in discoloration of teeth, and quinolones may affect the articular growth plate.

Underlying Disease. It is critical to obtain an adequate history to determine if the patient has any underlying diseases that would predispose to certain types of infection. It is also important for the emergency physician to be familiar with the types of infection seen in a compromised host. For instance, the asplenic or functionally asplenic patient is at risk for bacterial infection secondary to encapsulated organisms like *S. pneumoniae*, *H. influenzae*, and *N. meningitidis*. Infections due to *S. pneumoniae* can result in an overwhelming pneumococcal sepsis syndrome. Splenectomized patients and alcoholics bitten by a dog can develop shock and disseminated intravascular coagulation secondary to the DF-2 bacillus (*Capnocytophaga* species), a slowly growing gram-negative organism [40, 41]. In addition, babesiosis in an asplenic individual is often more serious, with increased morbidity. Patients who are neutropenic are at increased risk from gram-negative bacillary infections as well as fungal infections. Because of their significantly high morbidity and

mortality, febrile neutropenic patients should be treated with parenteral broad-spectrum antibiotics in the hospital setting. Patients with lymphoma and patients on steroids may be at increased risk for intracellular organisms, for example, *L. monocytogenes*, *Cryptococcus neoformans*, and *M. tuberculosis*. Patients with HIV infection are at increased risk for opportunistic pathogens, such as *P. carinii*, *M. tuberculosis*, *Mycobacteria avium intracellulare*, cytomegalovirus, and *Toxoplasmosis gondii*, as well as bacterial infections secondary to pneumococcus and *H. influenzae* (see Chap. 17). Other underlying conditions that impair host defenses include diabetes mellitus, alcoholism, and IV drug abuse (see Chaps. 16 and 18).

Compliance. The physician must determine that the patient can acquire the necessary medications, can and will use them appropriately, understands the diagnosis and expected course, and knows which symptoms dictate immediate follow-up. The patient must also be given explicit instructions concerning appropriate outpatient follow-up, and follow-up should be provided for those patients not already linked to appropriate resources. Remembering that "the doctor proposes and the patient disposes," the physician must adequately discuss therapy and provide clear, written instructions. A simple and clearly directed therapeutic regimen will greatly enhance patient compliance. (See Chap. 20.)

INTERACTION OF DISEASE AND HOST

Acuity and Duration of Symptoms. The patient who appears acutely ill when infected is likely to benefit most from admission to the hospital and treatment with parenteral antibiotics. As mentioned earlier, the patient with hemodynamic instability must be treated immediately and admitted. In less ill patients, determining the acuity of illness may be subjective and is often based on history and physical examination. The more rapid the onset of symptomatology, the more aggressively the patient must be treated because, for whatever reason, the patient is unable to contain the infection. The patient who presents with a cellulitis that is rapidly progressing often appears toxic. Group A streptococci and *S. aureus* are responsible for the overwhelming majority of cases of cellulitis [42]. If a history of a cat or dog bite is obtained, then infection with *Pasteurella mutocida* should be considered. Patients compromised by acute pneumonia may be cyanotic or tachypneic or simply tell the physician they are dyspneic. One the other hand, patients with chronic symptomatology, for example, those with pulmonary tuberculosis, usually appear chronically ill but nonetheless may merit admission to the hospital.

The duration and acuity of illness should be confirmed with friends or family when possible. Acute mental dysfunction and hemodynamic instability can be suggestive of sepsis in the febrile patient or even in the afebrile patient with a localized site of infection. In addition, hypothermia may be seen in septic patients as well.

Oral versus Parenteral Antibiotic Therapy. The emergency physician more often will prescribe oral antimicrobial agents than parenteral agents. The appropriateness of oral therapy versus parenteral therapy is based on the previously mentioned factors such as site of infection, natural course of infection, and host factors. Parenteral therapy must be used if a patient is unable to take medication orally, such as in the patient with repetitive vomiting. In prescribing oral antimicrobial agents, the emergency physician should be comfortable with the diagnosis, having defined the most likely bacterial pathogens causing the infection in the patient and knowing the antimicrobial agent's spectrum of activity and tissue penetration. Similarly if antimicrobial therapy needs to be immediately initiated by the emergency department physician, the choice of antibiotic(s) should also be based on these factors. (See Chap. 4.)

In critically ill patients, timely administration of appropriate antibiotics is the single most important intervention and should be implemented at the earliest moment feasible. Care should be taken that appropriate cultures are obtained, when possible, to confirm the diagnosis and to guide therapy. At minimum, two sets of blood cultures should be drawn, even in the most critical patient. For suspected bacterial meningitis, sepsis, or acute endocarditis, the first dose of intravenous antibiotic should be administered within the first half hour. Definitive intervention cannot await admission to

an inpatient area. Such interventions, including antibiotic administration, should occur in the emergency department. The majority of patients not in these categories can undergo a more methodical workup, but in most cases they should have appropriate therapy initiated within 6 hours of presentation.

Disease Reporting

There are a number of infectious diseases whose diagnoses (or suspected diagnoses) require reporting. The basic responsibility for reporting these diseases lies with the individual licensed clinicians. In addition to the public health benefits of disease reporting (including the detection of common-source outbreaks, the control and prevention of the spread of communicable infections, and appropriate allocation of public health resources), the timely notification of health offices offers the emergency department physician a range of resources that can immediately benefit individual patients. These resources include assistance in handling and processing diagnostic specimens and in the clinical management and surveillance of individuals exposed to the index case and at risk for a potentially communicable disease.

Considerable interstate variation exists regarding specific infections to be reported, the mechanisms of reporting, and the range of resources available. Each emergency department should have a mechanism that ensures the reporting of appropriate entities. Such a mechanism should be coordinated with the clinical laboratory in which the diagnosis of many of these infectious diseases will be confirmed. The most common manner in which diseases are reported involves telephoning a toll-free health department number or filling out a card. Physicians can contact their state health department to find out the reportable diseases and reporting mechanisms in their particular state. Table 1-4 lists the address and telephone number for the health department in each state and territory. Specific notifiable diseases tracked by the Centers for Disease Control (CDC) and published weekly in the *Morbidity and Mortality Weekly Report* (MMWR) are listed in Table 1-5. The CDC also maintains a physician hotline, 404-332-4555.

Table 1-4. State and territorial health departments

Alabama
Department of Public Health
State Office Building
Montgomery, AL 36130-1701
205-261-5052

Alaska
Department of Health & Social
  Services
Alaska Office Building
Pouch H 06
Juneau, AK 99811
907-465-3090

Arizona
Department of Health Services
1740 W Adams Street
Phoenix, AZ 85007
602-255-1024

Arkansas
Department of Health
4815 W Markham Street
Little Rock, AR 72205-3867
501-661-2000

California
Department of Health Services
714 P Street Room 1253
Sacramento, CA 95814
916-445-1248

Colorado
Department of Health
4210 E 11th Avenue
Denver, CO 80220
303-320-8333

Connecticut
State Department of Health
  Services
150 Washington Street
Hartford, CT 06106
203-566-2279

Delaware
Department of Health & Social
  Services
Division of Public Health
Jesse Cooper Building
Capitol Square
Dover, DE 19901
302-736-4701

District of Columbia
Department of Human Services
Commission of Public Health
1875 Connecticut Avenue, NW
Room 825
Washington, DC 20009
202-673-7700

Florida
Department of Health &
  Rehabilitative Services
Building 1, Room 115
1323 Winewood Boulevard
Tallahassee, FL 32301
904-487-2705

Georgia
Department of Human Resources
Division of Public Health
878 Peachtree Street, NE
Atlanta, GA 30309
404-894-7505

Hawaii
Department of Health
PO Box 3378
Honolulu, HI 96801
808-548-6505

Idaho
Department of Health & Welfare
Division of Health
State House
Boise, ID 83720-9990
208-334-5930

Illinois
Department of Public Health
535 W Jefferson Street
Springfield, IL 62761
217-782-4977

Indiana
State Board of Health
1330 W Michigan Street
PO Box 1964
Indianapolis, IN 46206-1964
317-633-8400

Iowa
Department of Health
Robert Lucas State Office Building
Des Moines, IA 50319-0075
515-281-5605

Kansas
State Department of Health &
  Environment
Forbes Field, Building 321
Topeka, KA 66620-0001
913-862-9360

Kentucky
Cabinet for Human Resources
Department of Health Services
275 E Main Street
Frankfort, KY 40621
502-564-3970

Louisiana
Department of Health & Human
  Resources
Office of Health Services &
  Environmental Quality
325 Loyola Avenue
PO Box 60630
New Orleans, LA 70160
504-568-5052

Maine
Department of Human Services
Bureau of Health
State House, Station 11
157 Capital Street
Augusta, ME 04333
207-289-3201

Maryland
State Department of Health &
  Mental Hygiene
201 W Preston Street
Baltimore, MD 21201
301-225-6500

Massachusetts
Department of Public Health
150 Tremont Street
Boston, MA 02111
617-727-2700

Michigan
Department of Public Health
3500 N Logan Street
PO Box 30035
Lansing, MI 48909
517-335-8024

Minnesota
Department of Health
717 Delaware Street, SE
Minneapolis, MN 55440
612-623-5100

Mississippi
State Department of Health
Felix J Underwood Building
2423 N State Street
PO Box 1700
Jackson, MS 39215-1700
601-960-7634

Missouri
Department of Health
1738 E Elm
PO Box 570
Jefferson City, MO 65102-0570
314-751-6400

Table 1-4. (*continued*)

Montana
State Department of Health &
  Environmental Sciences
Cogswell Building
Helena, MT 59620
406-444-2544

Nebraska
State Department of Health
301 Centennial Mall South
PO Box 95007
Lincoln, NE 68509-5007
402-471-2133

Nevada
State Department of Human
  Resources
Division of Health
505 E King Street, Room 201
Capitol Complex
Carson City, NV 89710
702-885-4740

New Hampshire
State Department of Health &
  Welfare
Division of Public Health Services
Health & Welfare Building
Hazen Drive
Concord, NH 03301
603-271-4477

New Jersey
State Department of Health
C N 360
John Fitch Plaza
Trenton, NJ 08625
609-292-7837

New Mexico
Health & Environment
  Department
1190 St. Francis Drive
PO Box 968
Santa Fe, NM 87504-0968
505-827-2615

New York
State Department of Health
Empire State Plaza
Tower Building, 14th Floor
Albany, NY 12237
518-474-2011

Department of Health
125 Worth Street
New York, NY 10013
212-566-7132

North Carolina
Department of Human Resources
Division of Health Services
225 N McDowell Street
PO Box 2091
Raleigh, NC 27602-2091
919-733-3446

North Dakota
State Department of Health
State Capitol Building
Bismarck, ND 58505
701-224-2372

Ohio
Department of Health
246 N High Street
PO Box 118
Columbus, OH 43266-0118
614-466-2253

Oklahoma
State Department of Health
1000 NE 10th
PO Box 53551
Oklahoma City, OK 73152
405-271-4200

Oregon
Department of Human Resources
State Health Division
1400 SW 5th Avenue
Portland, OR 97201
503-229-5032

Pennsylvania
State Department of Health
PO Box 90
Harrisburg, PA 17108
717-787-6436

Rhode Island
Department of Health
75 Davis Street, Room 401
Providence, RI 02908
401-277-2231

South Carolina
Department of Health &
  Environmental Control
J Marion Sims Building
2600 Bull Street
Columbia, SC 29201
803-734-4880

South Dakota
State Department of Health
Joe Foss Building
523 E Capitol Avenue
Pierre, SD 57501
605-773-3361

Tennessee
Department of Health &
  Environment
Cordell Hull Building, Room 344
Sixth Avenue North
Nashville, TN 37219
614-741-3111

Texas
Department of Health
1100 W 49th Street
Austin, TX 78756
512-458-7375

Utah
Department of Health
PO Box 16700
Salt Lake City, UT 84116-0700
801-538-6111

Vermont
Department of Health
60 Main Street
PO Box 70
Burlington, VT 05402
802-863-7200

Virginia
State Department of Health
The James Madison Building
109 Governor Street
Richmond, VA 23219
804-786-3561

Washington
Department of Social & Health
  Services
Division of Health
Mail Stop ET-21
Olympia, WA 98504
206-753-5871

West Virginia
State Department of Health
1800 Washington Street,
  Room 206
Charleston, WV 25305
304-348-2971

Wisconsin
Department of Health & Social
  Services
Division of Health
One W Wilson Street
PO Box 309
Madison, WI 53701-0309
608-266-1511

Table 1-4. (*continued*)

Wyoming
Department of Health & Social
  Services
Division of Health and Medical
  Services
Hathaway Building
Cheyenne, WY 82002
307-777-7121

Puerto Rico
Department of Health
GPO Box 70184
San Juan, PR 00936
809-766-2240

Virgin Islands of the United States
Department of Health
PO Box 7309
St. Thomas, USVI 00801
809-774-6097

American Samoa
Government of American Samoa
Department of Health
LBJ Tropical Medicine Center
Pago Pago, American Samoa
  96799
Overseas 011-684-633-4590

Guam
Department of Public Health &
  Social Services
Government of Guam
PO Box 2816
Agana, Guam 96910
Overseas 011-671-734-2931-39
011-671-734-2951-59

*Commonwealth of the Northern
  Mariana Islands*
Department of Health Services
Office of the Governor
Saipan, Mariana Islands 96950
Overseas 011-670-6234-8951,
  8952, 8953, 8954
TELEX 783744

Table 1-5. Notifiable diseases tabulated
weekly by the CDC

AIDS
Aseptic meningitis
Encephalitis (primary, post-infectious)
Gonorrhea (civilian)
Hepatitis (viral, by type: A, B, NA-NB, unspecified)
Legionnaires' disease
Leprosy
Malaria
Measles (Rubeola: indigenous, imported)
Meningococcal infections
Mumps
Pertussis
Rubella
Syphilis
Toxic shock syndrome
Tuberculosis
Tularemia
Typhoid fever
Typhus fever (tick-borne, RMSF)
Rabies (animal)

References

1. Terndrup TE, Allegra JR, Kealy JA. A Comparison of oral, rectal and tympanic membrane-derived temperature changes after ingestion of liquids and smoking. *Am J Emerg Med* 7:150–54, 1989.
2. Kenney RD et al. Evaluation of an infrared tympanic membrane thermometer in pediatric patients. *Pediatrics* 85:854–57, 1990.
3. Shinozaki T, Deane R, Perkins FM. Infrared tympanic thermometer: evaluation of a new clinical thermometer. *Crit Care Med* 16:148–50, 1988.
4. Murray HW et al. Urinary temperature: a clue to early diagnosis of factitious fever. *N Engl J Med* 296:23–24, 1977.
5. Castle SC et al. Fever response in elderly nursing home residents: are the older truly colder? *J Am Geriatr Soc* 39:853–57, 1991.
6. Knopp R, Claypool R, Leonardi D. Use of the tilt test in measuring acute blood loss. *Ann Emerg Med* 9:72–75, 1980.
7. Schriger DL, Baraff L. Defining normal capillary refill; variation with age, sex and temperature. *Ann Emerg Med* 17:932–35, 1988.
8. Guarino JR. Auscultatory percussion of the chest. *Lancet* 1332–34, 1980.
9. Kennedy J et al. Should a lateral chest radiograph be routine in suspected pneumonia? *Aust Pediatr J* 22(4):299, 1986.
10. Patterson RJ et al. Chest radiographs in the evaluation of the febrile patient. *Am J Roent* 155(4):833, 1990.
11. Leventhal JM. Clinical predictors of pneumonia as a guide to ordering chest roentgenograms. *Clin Pediatr* 21:730, 1982.
12. Smith DL et al. Septic and nonseptic olecranon bursitis: utility of the surface temperature probe in the early differentiation of septic and nonseptic cases. *Arch Intern Med* 149:1581, 1989.
13. Talan DA et al. Role of empiric parenteral antibiotics prior to lumbar puncture in suspected bacte-

rial meningitis: state of the art. *Rev Infect Dis* 10(2):365, 1988.

14. Tinetti ME et al. Use of the erythrocyte sedimentation rate in chronically ill, elderly patients with a decline in health status. *Am J Med* 80:844, 1986.

15. Mellors JW et al. A simple index to identify occult bacterial infection in adults with acute unexplained fever. *Arch Intern Med* 147(4):666, 1987.

16. Leibovici L, Cohen O, Wysenbeek AJ. Occult bacterial infection in adults with unexplained fever: validation of a diagnostic index. *Arch Intern Med* 150:1270, 1990.

17. Wasserman J et al. Utility of fever, white blood cells and differential count in predicting bacterial infections in the elderly. *J Am Geriatr Soc* 37:537–43, 1989.

18. Mihm FG, Halperin BD. Noninvasive detection of profound arterial desaturation using a pulse oximetry device. *Anesthesiology* 62:85–87, 1985.

19. Sendi K, Crysdale WS. Acute epiglottitis: decade of change—a 10 year experience with 242 children. *J Otolaryngol* 196–202, 1987.

20. McGuire TJ, Pointer JE. Evaluation of a pulse oximeter in the prehospital setting. *Ann Emerg Med* 17:1058–62, 1988.

21. Jones J et al. Continuous emergency department monitoring of arterial saturation in adult patients with respiratory distress. *Ann Emerg Med* 17:463–68, 1988.

22. Battaglia JD, Lockhart CH. Management of acute epiglottitis by nasotracheal intubation. *Am J Dis Child* 129:334–36, 1975.

23. McCracken GH Jr. Commentary. *J Pediatr* 94:987, 1979.

24. Klein JO (ed.). *Report of the Committee on Infectious Diseases*. Evanston, IL.: American Academy of Pediatrics, 1982. P. 105.

25. Murray JF et al. Pulmonary complications of the acquired immunodeficiency syndrome: report of a National Heart, Lung and Blood Institute workshop. *N Engl J Med* 310:1682–88, 1984.

26. Bozzette SA, et al. A controlled trial of early adjunctive treatment with corticosteroids for pneumocystis carinii pneumonia in the acquired immunodeficiency syndrome. *N Engl J Med* 323:1451–57, 1990.

27. Samet JH et al. Hospitalization decision in febrile intravenous drug users. *Am J Med* 89:53–57, 1990.

28. Watanakunakorn C. Changing epidemiology and newer aspects of infective endocarditis. *Adv Intern Med* 22:21, 1977.

29. Tramont, EC. General or nonspecific host defense mechanisms. In GL Mandell, RG Douglas, JE Bennett (eds.), *Principles and Practice of Infectious Diseases*. New York: Churchill Livingstone 1990. Pp. 33–41.

30. Goldschneide I, Gotschlich ED, Artenstein MS. Human immunity to the meningococcus. *J Exp Med* 129:1307, 1969.

31. Baker MD, Avner JR, Bell LM. Failure of infant observation scales in detecting serious illness in febrile, 4- to 8-week old infants. *Pediatrics* 85:1040–43, 1990.

32. Saltzman RL, Peterson PK. Immunodeficiency of the elderly. *Rev Infect Dis* 9(6):1127–39, 1987.

33. Iwarson S, Ludin-Janson G, Svensson R. Listeria meningitis in the noncompromised host. *Infection* 5:204, 1977.

34. Baker CJ et al. Suppurative meningitis due to streptococci of Lancefield group B: a study of 33 infants. *J Pediatr* 82:724–29, 1973.

35. Chin KD, Fitzhardinge PM. Sequelae of early-onset group B streptococcal neonatal meningitis. *J Pediatr* 106:819–22, 1985.

36. Haggerty RJ, Ziai M. Acute bacterial meningitis. *Adv Pediatr* 13:129, 1964.

37. Klein JO, Marcy SM. Bacterial sepsis and meningitis. In JS Remington, JD Klein (eds.), *Infectious Diseases of the Fetus and Newborn Infant*. Philadelphia: Saunders, 1983. Pp. 679–734.

38. Swartz MN, Dodge PR. Bacterial meningitis: a review of selected aspects. *N Engl J Med*: 272(2):725–31, 1965.

39. Bolan G, Barza M. Acute bacterial meningitis in children and adults. A perspective. *Med Clin North Am* 69:231, 1985.

40. Hinrichs JH, Dunkelberg WE. DF-2 septicemia after splenectomy: epidemiology and immunologic response. *South Med J* 73:1638–40, 1980.

41. Chaudhuris AK, Hartley RB, Maddocks AC. Waterhouse-Friederichsen syndrome caused by a DF-2 bacterium in a splenectomized host. *J Clin Pathol* 34:172–73, 1981.

42. Swartz MN. Cellulitis and superficial infections. In GL Mandell, RG Douglas, JE Bennett (eds.), *Principles and Practice of Infectious Diseases*. New York: Churchill Livingstone, 1990. Pp. 796–807.

2

Temperature Measurement and the Clinical Significance of Fever

DAVID P. SKLAR
DAN TANDBERG

As one of the four vital signs, usually measured before the emergency physician begins an evaluation, a patient's body temperature often influences the subsequent course of evaluation, the final diagnosis, and decisions regarding admission to the hospital. Understanding the mechanisms of body temperature elevation, the methods of measuring temperature, patterns of fever, and the prognostic value of elevated temperature can help the emergency physician caring for a febrile patient. The normal basal body temperature is considered to be 37°C when determined orally but may vary from 36°–37.8°C. Rectal temperature is 0.6°C higher. Table 2-1 shows temperature conversions from centigrade to Fahrenheit.

Mechanisms of Body Temperature Elevation

Homeostatic Mechanisms

The human body regulates the core temperature at approximately 37°C through activity occurring in the hypothalamus. Thermosensitive neurons discharge at a rate that varies with the temperature of the blood in surrounding vessels [1]. If the blood reaching the hypothalamus is cooler than the set point of this part of the brain, several mechanisms that conserve or produce heat occur, including vasoconstriction, piloerection, increased muscle tone, and shivering. During fever the hypothalamic set point first rises, then the thermoregulatory neurons of the hypothalamus initiate warming after being stimulated by blood that is cooler than the set point. The core temperature rises to the new set point and a new equilibrium is reached.

Circadian Variability

The hypothalamic set point exhibits daily variability; it reaches its lowest level in the early morning hours and its highest elevation in the late afternoon [2] in response to circadian variations of growth hormone, cortisol, and sleep (Fig. 2-1). During fever there is persistence of this variability, which can be as much as 2°C [3]. Therefore, fever can best be defined as a core temperature elevation outside the range of normal daily variation. It should be clear that, depending on the time of day that the temperature is measured, specific elevations may be more or less easily distinguished from background variability of temperature. Thus, a patient with an oral temperature of 37.5°C measured at 6:00 AM may have clinically important fever, whereas a patient with a temperature of 38°C measured at 6:00 PM may not.

19

Table 2-1. Body temperature conversions from centigrade to Fahrenheit

°C	°F
35.6	96.1
35.8	96.4
36.0	96.8
36.2	97.1
36.4	97.5
36.6	97.8
36.8	98.2
37.0	98.6
37.2	98.9
37.4	99.3
37.6	99.6
37.8	100.0
38.0	100.4
38.2	100.7
38.4	101.1
38.6	101.4
38.8	101.8
39.0	102.2
39.2	102.5
39.4	102.9
39.6	103.2
39.8	103.6
40.0	104.0
40.2	104.3
40.4	104.7
40.6	105.1
40.8	105.4
41.0	105.8
41.2	106.1
41.4	106.5
41.6	106.8
41.8	107.2

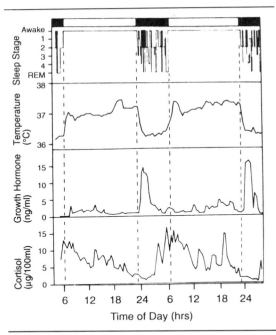

Fig. 2-1. Circadian variations in temperature, sleep, growth hormone, and cortisol. (Source: Moore-Ede MC, Czeisler CA, Richardson GS. *N Engl J Med* 309:468–70, 1983. Used with permission)

Temperature elevations not due to increases in the hypothalamic set point can occur when the body's homeostatic mechanisms are overwhelmed. This condition can occur in hot environments in which body heat–losing mechanisms such as sweating fail, when internal heat production cannot be controlled (as in status epilepticus), or when drugs such as atropine impair the usual physiologic responses to increased temperature. Body temperature elevations also can occur after CNS alterations due to traumatic, infectious, neoplastic, immu-

nologic, or toxic conditions and usually represent failure of the thermoregulatory system. It is important that temperature elevations caused by the overwhelming of hemostatic mechanisms rather than the alteration of the hypothalamic set point be distinguished, since rapid cooling of the patient in such cases can be lifesaving.

Pathophysiology of Temperature Elevation in Infections

The importance of fever to the emergency physician is due primarily to its association with human infectious diseases. Whether fever has a beneficial effect in infected humans is not known. In reptiles, however, prevention of a febrile response has been shown to lower survival after bacterial injection [4].

PYROGENS
There are several mechanisms by which infections cause fever in humans; one is by endotoxin derived from the cell walls of gram-negative bacteria. Endo-

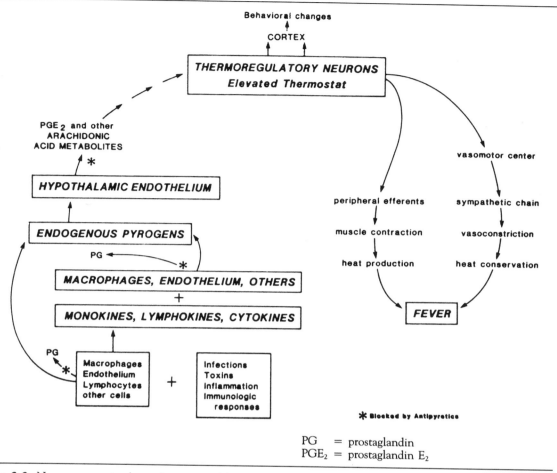

Fig. 2-2. New concepts in the pathogenesis of fever. (Source: Dinarello CA, Cannon JG, Wolff SM. New concepts in the pathogenesis of fever. *Rev Infect Dis* 10:168–89, 1988. Used with permission)

toxin has a direct effect on the hypothalamus, resulting in a rapid biphasic elevation of temperature [5]. Another mechanism is mediated by a substance derived primarily from macrophages that can be stimulated by bacteria, toxins, or endogenously produced molecules such as antigen-antibody complexes, complement components, and some lymphocytic products. This endogenous pyrogen has been identified as interleukin-1 and appears to act by stimulating prostaglandin E_2 synthesis in the hypothalamus (Figure 2-2) [6]. Interleukin-1 is released into the circulation after the onset of an infectious or inflammatory disease and reaches the hypothalamic regulatory center through the hypothalamic arterioles. Arachidonic acid is liberated and metabolized to prostaglandin E_1, and the hypothalamic set point is raised. This initiates an increase of heat production or conservation. Other molecules released by macrophages also cause fever by direct action on the hypothalamus or by stimulating interleukin-1 release. Tumor necrosis factor, which has a cytotoxic effect on some tumor cells and is associated with weight loss, also induces a febrile response [7]. Finally, interferons also appear to induce fever through mechanisms similar to interleukin-1 [8].

IMMUNOLOGIC EFFECT

Although fever has not been associated convincingly with increased survival in humans, interleukin-1, which stimulates fever, also appears to increase activation of lymphocytes as temperature is raised from 37° to 39°C [9]. Elevated temperature also increases the induction of cytotoxic T cells and helper T cells. The immunologic products of B cells are also increased at higher body temperatures [1].

ANTIPYRETICS

Whether antipyretics, such as aspirin, acetaminophen, or nonsteroidal anti-inflammatory drugs (NSAIDs) that act by blocking prostaglandin synthesis and thus blocking changes in the hypothalamic set point, have an important clinical effect on a person's ability to respond to infection is not clear. Aspirin use lengthens the time of rhinovirus shedding in humans [10]. Prostaglandin inhibitors increase survival in endotoxin-induced shock in sheep [11], but similar results in humans have not been demonstrated. The body temperature response to antipyretics does not seem to differ between patients with bacterial and nonbacterial infections in a clinically useful way [12, 13]. Thus, antipyretics cannot be justified as a diagnostic test. Antipyretic types and dosages are listed in Table 2-2. Aspirin, acetaminophen, and nonsteroid anti-inflammatory drugs (NSAIDs) are equally effective as antipyretic agents.

Physical methods of antipyresis should be used in conjunction with antipyretics, because with the altered hypothalamic set point, the body is already responding to a cooler environment. Some studies have suggested that these methods do not hasten defervescence but may promote discomfort [14]. The body can be sponged with tepid water and cooled as the water evaporates. This method is used most often in children. Cold water is not used, as it can lead to vasoconstriction or increased heat production through shivering. Isopropyl alcohol is also avoided because it can be absorbed through a child's skin and lead to toxicity. Cooling blankets should be removed when the temperature is below 38.3°C to avoid undershooting the normal temperature. A variety of methods are used to treat patients with heat stroke, including placing ice over large blood vessels (neck and groin areas), using fans, lavage with cool water, and ice water baths. Corticosteroids also reduce fever, but their use is contraindicated in symptomatic relief of fever because of their potential detrimental effect on host defenses.

Other reasons for using antipyretics include prevention of febrile seizures, the comfort of the patient, and reduction of the cardiovascular stress of a febrile response. Prevention of febrile seizures by the

Table 2-2. Antipyretic agents

| Agent | Dosage | |
	Adults	Children
Aspirin[a]	325–650 mg po/pr q4–6h	10–20 mg/kg q6h (not to exceed 3.6 g/d)
Acetaminophen	325–650 mg po/pr q4–6h	10–15 mg/kg q4–6h
NSAIDs		
Ibuprofen[b]	200–400 mg po q6h	5mg/kg for T < 102.5°C, 10 mg/kg for T > 102.5°C (not to exceed 40 mg/kg/d)

Physical Methods of Antipyresis
Sponging body with tepid water
Cooling blanket
Ice water over vascular areas

[a] Avoid the use of aspirin in viral-type illnesses because of the risk of Reye's syndrome. Also avoid in patients with allergy, hemostatic or platelet abnormalities, or gastrointestinal tract ulcers and in patients receiving anticoagulation therapy. May lead to abrupt hypothermia and hypotension in patients with lymphoproliferative disorders.
[b] Avoid the use of ibuprofen in patients with allergy, syndrome of nasal polyps, angioedema and bronchospastic reaction to aspirin or other NSAIDs, gastrointestinal tract ulcers, hemostatic abnormalities, or renal dysfunction and in patients receiving anticoagulation therapy.

use of antipyretics has not been proved, and a recent review suggests that vasopressin (which acts as an endogenous antipyretic) may be a precipitating factor in febrile seizures. Blocking vasopressin might be more important than lowering temperature [14]. As for comfort and cardiovascular stress, only at extreme levels of febrile response are major effects noticeable, and even in these situations it is unclear how much spontaneous defervescence might have occurred without antipyretic therapy. A recent review concludes, "There is no evidence that fever is detrimental or that antipyretic therapy offers any significant benefit . . . fever usually does more good than harm [14]."

Blunting of Febrile Response

Although anything that causes tissue destruction and macrophage activity can stimulate the release of interleukin-1 and other endogenous pyrogenic substances, it is the potential presence of microbial agents that is of greatest concern to the emergency physician managing a febrile patient. Because infectious agents can rapidly overwhelm the body's defenses but can be quickly killed with antibiotics, the recognition of fever and the rapid evaluation and management of the febrile patient who may have an infectious cause for fever are imperative. Symptomatic antipyretic therapy limits the usefulness of temperature measurement as an early indication of serious infection.

Temperature Measurement and Recognition

Thermometer Types

Because fever is such an important early sign of microbial disease, rapid, accurate methods for temperature measurement are exceptionally important in the emergency department. The ideal technique of temperature measurement should precisely reflect the core temperature, be easily and quickly performed, and be associated with little or no risk or discomfort to the patient [15]. Historically the core temperature has been estimated by measuring the esophageal [16], rectal [17], oral [18], pulmonary artery, skin [19], urinary bladder [20], or tympanic membrane [21] temperature. Simultaneous mea-

surements at multiple sites during heating or cooling of the body allow for comparison of the various sites and an estimation of response time as core temperature changes [22]. Several varieties of thermometers are used in emergency medicine, with the liquid-in-glass type in use the longest [23]. A newer method to measure body temperature employs a transducer or a probe connected through an analog or digital converter to a microprocessor. Light-emitting diodes or a liquid crystal display provide a digital readout of the temperature. Commonly used transducers include resistance coils, thermocouples, thermistors, and infrared detectors.

GLASS THERMOMETERS

Glass thermometers contain a fluid such as alcohol, pentane, or mercury, which expands with increasing temperature. Mercury is most often used in clinical emergency medicine since it combines the advantages of a low freezing and a high boiling point, uniform expansion characteristics, rapid heat conduction, good visibility, and high cohesiveness in glass. Mercury-in-glass thermometers have a narrow constriction between the reservoir and the scale to help prevent the mercury from leaking back into the reservoir, which is why they must be shaken down firmly prior to use. The glass of the front of the thermometer is configured into a lens to increase ease of reading. The response time is at least 90 seconds, but equilibrium may require from 3 to as long as 9 minutes to be achieved [18, 24, 25]. Typical mercury thermometers have a narrow calibrated range of 34°–41°C and can mislead the clinician if severe hypothermia or hyperthermia is present. Errors of 0.5°C occur in the normal range, and larger errors may occur at the extremes of measurement [26]. Mercury thermometers in compliance with criteria developed by the National Bureau of Standards read within 0.1°C in the range of 37–39 and within 0.2°C at 41 [27].

THERMISTOR PROBES

Older clinical temperature probes typically used resistance coils or the thermocouple [28]. Thermistors are semiconductor devices that, for the most part, have replaced resistance coils and thermocouples in emergency care. Thermistors are made from oxides of heavy transition metals such as iron, zinc, manganese, and cobalt. The metal is compressed, heated, and fused into a bead; leads are then sintered to the semiconductive material and a protective coating is applied. The resistance across the device decreases with temperature elevation. The response to temperature change is rapid, often less than 1 second, but the presence of a protective plastic or metal probe cover can increase this time considerably. Thermistors are not linear devices; their resistance varies exponentially with the inverse absolute temperature [29], but this nonlinearity can be corrected with electronic circuitry. It is also difficult to manufacture thermistor probes with identical characteristics; each must be calibrated individually. Commercially available digital electronic thermometers use these devices, as do modern rectal probes and pulmonary artery catheters.

LIQUID CRYSTAL THERMOMETERS

Liquid crystal thermometers are plastic strips that contain cholesteric compounds that alter their molecular structure and change color in response to varying temperature [19]. Commercially available devices record in the range of 34°–40°C, usually in six or eight equal divisions. However, their imprecision causes some investigators to question their clinical usefulness [30].

INFRARED DETECTORS

Infrared detectors that measure energy emitted by the eardrum without actually touching the eardrum recently have been introduced into emergency medicine. These devices consist of an otoscope-like ear speculum, a handle containing a microprocessor, and a digital display. The detector itself is a disk of thin plastic film coated with black material with nearly complete infrared absorption characteristics. About 50 tiny bismuth-antimony thermocouples are attached at the perimeter and connected in series. Equilibrium is reached in 1–2 seconds, and accuracy is to within 0.1°C.

Body Location of Temperature Measurement

ORAL VERSUS RECTAL AND TYMPANIC

The oral temperature measurement is convenient and is preferred by most patients and staff. It can, however, be misleading if the patient is breathing rapidly [31], has smoked recently, or has ingested hot or cold liquids [32]. The oral temperature generally is no more than 0.6°C lower than the rectal or infrared tympanic membrane temperature, but much greater differences have been found in patients who are tachypneic. Tachypnea has been found to lower measured oral temperature by an average of 0.5°C for every increase of 10 respirations per minute [31]. The rectal temperature reflects core temperature more accurately than the oral determination, but its measurement requires privacy and added staff effort and may not be as practical for routine ambulatory patients. Infrared tympanic membrane temperature measurement is fast, convenient, and well accepted by staff and patients [33] and offers the theoretical advantage of a shared blood supply with the brain [34]. Several studies have found strong correlation of tympanic membrane temperature measurement with core temperature estimated by rectal or pulmonary artery temperature [21, 32, 35–37]. Green et al. [21] studied oral, rectal, and tympanic temperatures in 411 patients. Tympanic and rectal temperatures correlated closely with no significant difference. Tympanic and oral temperatures varied significantly, as did rectal and oral temperatures. One study [38] in adults disputes the accuracy of the tympanic membrane temperature. Those authors, however, combined oral and rectal temperatures as the control group; the difficulties with such a grouping are well described by Terndrup [39] and Benincasa [37], who reiterate the difference in temperature measured at the oral and the rectal sites and the potential confounding by the ingestion of hot or cold liquid and tachypnea.

A study in children by Rhoads and Grandner [40] suggests that higher temperatures were missed by the tympanic probe. In that study of 113 children between 1 month and 10 years of age either oral or rectal temperatures were compared with tympanic membrane temperatures. Rectal temperatures averaged 0.76°C higher than tympanic, and oral temperatures averaged 0.53°C higher than tympanic. Another study by Muma et al. demonstrated similar discrepancies between tympanic membrane temperatures and rectal temperatures in children less than 3 years old [41]. Such discrepancies are worrisome, since higher levels of fever might be missed if tympanic probes are used. The authors suggest that the large size of the probe might make proper positioning difficult in children, leading to faulty readings.

Another pediatric study [36], that included 964 children, demonstrated no difference in tympanic membrane measurements between ears in spite of the presence of acute suppurative otitis media or nonsuppurative otitis media. The difference between tympanic and rectal temperatures was 0.05°C in 623 children (95% confidence interval of 0.01–0.09); in 341 children who had oral temperatures compared, the difference was 0.08°C (95% confidence interval 0.03–0.13). Thus, the measurement of tympanic membrane temperatures in children should be used with caution until more validation of their accuracy in the outpatient setting is available. In addition, the effects of improper aiming of the device, eardrum perforation and impacted cerumen, have not been carefully investigated using the commonly employed devices in an outpatient setting.

CORE TEMPERATURE

Esophageal, pulmonary artery, and urinary bladder temperatures are not used often in emergency care because of their invasiveness. Temperature measurement of freshly voided urine, however, can be useful in cases of suspected factitious fever [42].

SKIN TEMPERATURE

Skin temperature is often estimated during the course of physical examination as the physician touches the patient's forehead, chest, or abdomen. The perception of warmth greater than that of the examiner's fingers is a useful bedside indicator of fever. It is best to estimate a patient's temperature with the dorsum of the fingers since the skin there is much thinner than on the palmar surface. Skin temperature can also be estimated with liquid crystal thermometry. Such measurement, however, is about 2.2°C less than core temperature, and appropriate correction must be made for clinical use [19].

Continuous measurement of skin temperature is helpful in identifying patients who become febrile while in the emergency department. A liquid crystal device placed on the forehead will demonstrate a color change as the temperature changes [43]. Additional temperature measurements should be made

if the patient's skin feels warm, if other clinical findings suggest a strong likelihood of a fever or an infectious process, or if antipyretic drugs were ingested before presentation.

Preferred Methods of Measurement

Considering all the possible advantages and disadvantages of the various body temperature measurement methods, we suggest the following: For routine screening of adults, we prefer infrared tympanic membrane temperature measurement, because of its speed and convenience. The ear canal, however, must be visualized and the absence of obstructing debris confirmed before this measurement is interpreted. Oral temperature measurement with a digital electronic thermometer is a convenient alternative in patients who are cooperative, who are not tachypneic, and who have not recently smoked or ingested hot or cold liquids. Oral measurement with a mercury-in-glass thermometer is our third choice for ED screening because of its slow response time.

We must reemphasize that while infrared tympanic membrane temperature measurement appears to accurately reflect core body temperature, this technique has not been investigated to the same extent as oral and rectal determinations. Future research may uncover additional situations in which it does not accurately reflect core temperature.

For children under the age of 3 years, we believe that rectal temperatures should continue to be the standard measurement of potentially febrile patients until the accuracy of the tympanic measurement is proven in ambulatory children.

For precise temperature determinations in patients with fever, we prefer rectal measurements taken with a mercury-in-glass thermometer.

Fever Magnitude as a Diagnostic Sign

Once the temperature has been accurately measured and is found to be elevated, the emergency physician must evaluate the significance of this finding. How does the magnitude of temperature elevation correlate with the presence of serious infection, septicemia, or prognosis? In children the extent of fever has been found to be associated with increasing risk of bacteremia [44] and meningitis [45]. However, even in cases of extreme (> 41°C) hyperpyrexia the incidence of bacteremia is only 20% [45]. Patients with noninfectious causes of fever, such as malignancy, connective tissue disease, or cirrhosis, are unlikely to mount a febrile response above 38.6°C. Infections such as viral hepatitis, tuberculosis, Legionnaire's disease, and the zoonoses are unlikely to result in a temperature above 38.6°C.

Adults

In adults an association between the extent of a fever and an infection is more controversial [46, 47]. The correlation of fever and advanced age with incidence of serious bacterial infection has been made in outpatient populations [48]. In IV drug abusers, those with endocarditis seem to have a slightly higher temperature than those with other conditions, but the difference is too small to be clinically useful [49].

Previous studies have been weakened by the indiscriminate use of oral and rectal temperature measurements, thus making interpretation of their conclusions difficult. Even if an association between elevated temperature and septicemia in adults exists, the large fraction of patients with septicemia at lower temperature levels suggests a significant overlap between bacteremic and nonbacteremic groups. This suggests that fever is neither a sensitive nor a specific marker for bacteremia and that at high temperature levels specificity increases at the cost of sensitivity.

Children

The data presented by McGowen et al. [44] illustrates the difficulty of using temperature elevation to assist in decisions concerning possible sepsis in children. In their study, out of 708 children they found 31 patients (4.4%) with true positive blood cultures. Also, 43 patients (6.1%) had contaminated blood cultures and were analyzed in the negative culture group. Septicemia rates ranged from 0.94% below 38.9°C to 8.7% between 39.4°C and 39.9°C. Even above 40°C the bacteremia rate was only 8.0%. Thus, although bacteremia rates increased as fever increased, they were still relatively

low, and fever by itself was not a very helpful predictor of sepsis.

McCarthy and Dolan [45] demonstrated a 13% bacteremia rate for children with temperatures between 40.5°C and 41.0°C and a 20% rate of bacteremia when temperatures were greater than 41.1°C. Their study, however, did not report the rate of false positive blood cultures (contaminants), nor did it explain the selection criteria for blood cultures since all children with very great temperature elevations did not have cultures drawn. Thus, a true estimate of bacteremia rates at selected temperatures was not possible from their data.

What should be clear from these studies is that even at very high temperatures only a small percentage of patients will have positive blood cultures. Using McGowan's data, even at a temperature of greater than 40°C the specificity of temperature as an indicator for bacteremia is 82%, while the sensitivity is only 31%. If a threshold temperature of 39.4°C is used, sensitivity for bacteremia increases to 76% but specificity drops to 60%. These data in children suggest that very high temperature elevations correlate directly with bacteremia, but the lower levels of fever that are more common also are compatible with sepsis—even children without fever occasionally are bacteremic. Although less conclusive than the data in children, a recent study of 1225 hospitalized adult patients demonstrated that a temperature greater than or equal to 38.3°C is a strong predictor of bacteremia [50]. However, a temperature greater than 38.3°C only increases the probability of bacteremia from a baseline of 7% to a probability of 10%. Bacteremia also occurs in adults with slight or no temperature elevation. Physicians who detect risk factors for bacteremia in febrile or only slightly febrile adults should recognize the low but real potential for bacteremia in this population [51].

Extreme Hyperpyrexia

Extreme hyperpyrexia (temperature > 41°C) should alert the physician to the possibility of the loss of the CNS autoregulatory mechanism through either CNS injury or infection. Alternatively environmental heat exposure, internal heat production from continuous muscular activity, and drugs such as antipsychotics or stimulants can cause extreme temperature elevations and require a high index of suspicion if they are to be detected quickly and treated. Once these conditions are eliminated from consideration, the physician can then attempt to sort out infectious causes of very high fever and strongly consider blood stream infection.

Fever as a Prognostic or Diagnostic Sign

Mortality

The effect of temperature on mortality is complex. Since the presence of fever increases the risk of sepsis and the presence of sepsis increases the risk of death, it would seem clear that increased temperature would increase the risk of death. However, in populations of patients who are established as septic, elevated temperature may actually increase survival, possibly by providing a better environment for leukocyte activity. Conversely a correlation between fever elevation and mortality has been made in elderly adults [48]. In patients with sepsis and altered mental status, a temperature lower than normal is associated with increased mortality [52]. The question of fever and mortality is important since it may affect the decision of whether to use antipyretic therapy. At this time, however, the effect of elevated temperature on mortality requires further elucidation before definitive recommendations can be made.

Diagnosis

In general pyogenic infections of major organ systems, such as the lungs, kidneys, or hepatobiliary system, are accompanied by fevers. Intravascular infections such as from endocarditis, catheter-related infections, or mycotic aneurysm, are accompanied by sustained fevers. Localized, contained, or focal infections, such as cystitis, osteomyelitis, cutaneous abscess, sinusitis, and otitis media in adults, often are not associated with fevers. In children, because infections are poorly contained, these same infections are more likely to be accompanied by fever.

In the emergency department the conditions most commonly associated with high temperature include pneumonia, pyelonephritis, streptococcal pharyngitis, and viral upper respiratory illness [48]. In children the disease spectrum is somewhat different and varies with age. Otitis media, streptococcal pharyngitis, and viral syndromes occur most commonly in association with elevated temperature, although the probability of meningitis and septicemia appears to increase as fever rises over 40°C [45, 53]. In both children and adults, however, the relatively low prevalence of life-threatening infection in the population of febrile patients and the occurrence of some life-threatening infections in nonfebrile patients make fever alone not very helpful in sorting the potentially very ill from those not so sick.

Diagnosis and treatment of the patient with a fever and localized source are relatively straightforward, compared to the febrile patient without an obvious source. Risk factors for sepsis, such as age [47], IV drug abuse [49, 50], an abnormal heart valve [51], diabetes mellitus [47], altered mental status [52], temperature greater than or equal to 38.3°C [50], underlying fatal disease [50], major comorbidity, and acute abdomen, can be helpful in suggesting the need for blood cultures and the probability of sepsis. The patient in whom a source for fever cannot be identified, who is ill appearing, or who has a risk factor for sepsis may require admission for observation and further diagnostic maneuvers.

Noninfectious causes of fever can occur in emergency department patients, but they frequently are unrecognized because of the brevity of the encounters and the lack of follow-up. Drugs, neoplasms, and immunologic disorders occasionally are found, along with a variety of miscellaneous disorders. Representative causes are shown in Table 2-3.

Patterns of Fever

Certain diseases, such as malaria and typhoid fever, have long been associated with specific temporal patterns of fever. In the emergency department, however, multiple temperature measurements are not routinely made at regular intervals, and patients are not evaluated for long enough periods of time for recognizable patterns to become evident. The frequent use of antipyretics makes the interpretation of specific fever patterns even more difficult. Finally, modern investigation has been unsuccess-

Table 2-3. Noninfectious causes of fever

Drugs	Thyroid supplements	Miscellaneous
Allopurinol	Vancomycin	Acute gout
Amphetamines		Acute porphyria
Amphotericin B	Neoplasms	Alcoholic hepatitis
Anticholinergic agents	Acute lymphocytic leukemia	Atropine poisoning
Antihistamines	Disseminated carcinomatosis	CNS hemorrhage
Asparaginase	Eosinophilic granuloma	Cholecystitis
Azathioprine	Ewing's sarcoma	Crush injury
Barbiturates	Hepatoma	Dehydration (children)
Bleomycin	Hodgkin's disease	Delirium tremens
Cephalosporins	Hypernephroma	Factitious fever
Cimetidine	Liver adenoma	Heat stroke
Cocaine	Lung carcinoma	Hemolytic anemia
Cyclic antidepressants	Lymphoma	Inflammatory bowel disease
Dinitrophenol	Myelomonocytic leukemia	Malignant hyperthermia
Ethanol withdrawal	Pancreatic cancer	Myelofibrosis
Hydralazine		Myocardial infarction
Iodides	Immunologic	Pancreatitis
Isoniazid	Blood transfusion reaction	Periodic disease
LSD	Cranial arteritis	Pheochromocytoma
Methyldopa	(giant cell, temporal)	Pulmonary embolization
Nitrofurantoin	Erythema multiforme	Rupture of the spleen
Para-aminosalicylic acid	Erythema nodosum	Sarcoidosis
Penicillins	Giant cell arteritis	Thyroiditis
Phencyclidine	Granulomatous hepatitis	Thyrotoxicosis
Phenytoin	Hypersensitivity states	Weber-Christian disease
Procainamide	Polyarteritis nodosa	
Propylthiouracil	Rheumatic fever	
Quinidine	Rheumatoid arthritis	
Rifampicin	Still's disease	
Salicylates	Systemic lupus erythematosus	
Streptokinase	Systemic vasculitis	
Streptomycin	Wegener's granulomatosis	
Sulfonamides		
Sympathomimetics		

ful in demonstrating any usefulness of fever patterns, even in hospitalized patients [54].

Afebrile Infectious Syndromes

It is clear that some patients may be suffering from major infectious problems yet fail to mount a febrile response. In a review of 600 patients with gram-negative bacteremia, 13% had temperatures less than 36.4°C and 5% were afebrile [55]. In a study of 216 patients with unperforated diverticular disease, the mean temperature was 37.7°C [56]. A study of 187 patients with pneumococcal bacteremia dem-

onstrated that 3% had temperatures less than 97°F, and 17% had temperatures between 97°F and 100°F on admission [57]. In a community hospital 9% of bacteremic patients were afebrile [58].

Failure to mount a febrile response has been particularly well documented in the elderly. In two studies afebrile bacteremia was demonstrated in 29% and 13% of bacteremic patients 65 years or older versus 11% and 4% of patients less than 65 years old [57, 58]. In a study of 221 patients evaluated for bacterial infection, 48% of elderly patients with bacterial infection were afebrile [47].

Other populations may fail to mount a febrile

Table 2-4. Agents and conditions
that blunt febrile response

Agents
Aspirin
Acetaminophen
NSAIDs
Corticosteroids
Immunosuppressive agents used in transplant
   recipients and cancer patients

Conditions
Granulocytopenia
Extremes of age
Debilitation
Liver failure
Renal failure

response, including patients who are immunosuppressed or debilitated (e.g., with hepatic or renal failure). Agents and conditions that can mask or blunt a febrile response are listed in Table 2-4. Further confounding this issue is the reality that fever may be intermittent, such as in malaria or bacterial endocarditis. Of course fever is only one indication of infection. Other signs include elevated WBC count, elevated erythrocyte sedimentation rate, tachycardia, tachypnea, or constitutional symptoms such as headache, malaise, arthralgias, and myalgias. It behooves the physician to exhaust the possibility of infection in patients with suggestive conditions, symptoms, or signs, despite the absence of fever. Examples of other indicators of infection include tachypnea in the potentially septic patient, change in mental status in the elderly, and abdominal pain in the patient with ascites.

References

1. Dinarello CA, Cannon JG, Wolff SM. New concepts on the pathogenesis of fever. *Rev Infect Dis* 10:168–89, 1988.
2. Reinberg A. Circadian changes in the temperature of human beings. *Bibliotheca Radiologica* 6:128–39, 1975.
3. Dinarello CA, Wolff SM. Pathogenesis of fever in man. *N Engl J Med* 298:607–12, 1978.
4. Kluger MJ, Ringler DH, Anver MR. Fever and survival. *Science* 188:166–68, 1975.
5. Atkins E. Fever: the old and the new. *J Infect Dis* 149:339–48, 1984.
6. Dinarello CA. Interleukin-1 and the pathogenesis of the acute-phase response. *N Engl J Med* 311:1415–18, 1984.
7. Beutler B, Cerami A. Cachectin and tumor necrosis factor as two sides of the same biological coin. *Nature* 320:584–88, 1986.
8. Horning SJ et al. Clinical and immunologic effects of recombinant leukocyte A interferon in eight patients with advanced cancer. *JAMA* 247:1718–22, 1982.
9. Duff GW, Duran SK. The pyrogenic and mitogenic actions of interleukin-1 are related. *Nature* 304:449–51, 1983.
10. Stanley ED et al. Increased virus shedding with aspirin treatment of rhinovirus infection. *JAMA* 231:1248–51, 1975.
11. Jacobs ER et al. Ibuprofen improves survival in sheep endotoxin shock. *J Crit Care* 3:142, 1986.
12. Torrey SB et al. Temperature response to antipyretic therapy in children. *Am J Emerg Med* 3:190–92, 1985.
13. Baker MD, Fosarelli PD, Carpenter RO. Childhood fever, correlation of diagnosis with temperature response to acetaminophen. *Pediatrics* 80:315–18, 1987.
14. Styrt B, Sugarman B. Antipyresis and fever. *Arch Intern Med* 150:1589–97, 1990.
15. Togawa T. Body temperature measurement. *Clin Phys Physiol Meas* 6:83–108, 1985.
16. Whitby JD, Dunkin LJ. Temperature differences in the oesophagus. *Br J Anaesth* 40:991–95, 1968.
17. DuBois FF. The many different temperatures of the human body and its parts. *West J Surg* 59:470–90, 1951.
18. Nichols GA et al. Oral, axillary and rectal temperature determinations and relationships. *Nurs Res* 15(4):307–10, 1966.
19. Burgess GE et al. Continuous monitoring of skin temperature using a liquid crystal thermometer during anesthesia. *South Med J* 71:516–18, 1978.
20. Lilly JK, Borland JP, Zekan S. Urinary bladder temperature monitoring: a new index of body core temperature. *Crit Care Med* 8:742–44, 1980.
21. Green MM, Danzl DF, Praszkier H. Infrared tympanic thermography in the emergency department. *J Emerg Med* 7:437–40, 1989.
22. Otto RJ, Metzler MH. Rewarming from experimental hypothermia: comparison of heated aerosol inhalation, peritoneal lavage and pleural lavage. *Crit Care Med* 16:869–75, 1988.
23. Benzinger TH. Temperature: Part 1. Arts and concepts. In TH Benzinger (ed.), *Benchmark Papers in*

Human Physiology. Vol. 9. Stroudsberg, PA.: Dowden, Hutchinson & Ross, 1977.

24. Nichols GA. Taking adult temperatures: rectal measurements. *Am J Nurs* 72(6):1092–93, 1972.

25. Nichols GA, Kucha DH. Taking adult temperatures: oral measurements. *Am J Nurs* 72(6):1092–93, 1972.

26. Knapp HA. Accuracy of glass clinical thermometers compared to electronic thermometers. *Am J Surg* 112:139–41, 1966.

27. US Department of Commerce. National Bureau of Standards: *Clinical Thermometers (Maximum-Self-Registering, Mercury-in-Glass)*. Voluntary Product Standards PS 39–70. Washington, DC: Government Printing Office: May 1971.

28. Holdcroft A. Methods of measuring body temperature. In A Holdcroft (ed.), *Body Temperature Control In Anaesthesia, Surgery and Intensive Care*. London: Bailliere Tindall, 1981.

29. Eggers DF Jr et al. Statistical thermodynamics. In *Physical Chemistry*. New York: Wiley, 1964.

30. Ellis GL, Williamson B, White J. Liquid crystal thermometer strips [letter]. *J Emerg Med* 1989; 7:675–76.

31. Tandberg D, Sklar D. Effect of tachypnea on the estimation of body temperature by an oral thermometer. *N Engl J Med* 308:945–46, 1983.

32. Terndrup TE, Alegra JR, Kealy JA. A comparison of oral, rectal and tympanic membrane-derived temperature changes after ingestion of liquids and smoking. *Am J Emerg Med* 7(2):150–54, 1989.

33. Barber N, Kilmon CA. Reactions to tympanic temperature measurement in an ambulatory setting. *Pediatr Nurs* 15:477–81, 1989.

34. Benzinger TH. Heat regulation: homeostasis of central temperature in men. *Physiol Rev* 49:671–759, 1969.

35. Shinozaki T, Deane R, Perkins FM. Infrared tympanic thermometer: evaluation of a new clinical thermometer. *Crit Care Med* 16:148–50, 1988.

36. Kenney RD et al. Evaluation of an infrared tympanic membrane thermometer in pediatric patients. *Pediatrics* 85:854–58, 1990.

37. Benincasa RM. FirstTemp paper problems [letter]. *Ann Emerg Med* 19:734–35, 1990.

38. Ros SP. Evaluation of a tympanic membrane thermometer in an outpatient clinical setting. *Ann Emerg Med* 18:1004–06, 1989.

39. Terndrup TE. Tympanic membrane thermometers [letter]. *Ann Emerg Med* 19:341–42, 1990.

40. Rhoads FA, Grandner J. Assessment of an aural infrared sensor for body temperature measurement in children. *Clin Pediatr* (Phila) 29:112–15, 1990.

41. Muma BK et al. Comparison of rectal, axillary, and tympanic membrane temperatures in infants and young children. *Ann Emerg Med* 20:41–44, 1991.

42. Fox RH et al. Body temperature in the elderly: a natural study of physiological, social and environmental conditions. *Br Med J* 1:200, 1973.

43. Dart RC et al. Liquid crystal thermometry for continuous temperature measurement in emergency department patients. *Ann Emerg Med* 14:1188–90, 1985.

44. McGowan JE et al. Bacteremia in febrile children seen in a walk-in pediatric clinic. *N Engl J Med* 288:1309–12, 1973.

45. McCarthy P, Dolan T. Hyperpyrexia in children. *Am J Dis Child* 130:849–51, 1976.

46. Wasserman M et al. Utility of fever, white blood cells and differential count in predicting bacterial infections in the elderly. *J Am Geriatr Soc* 37:537–43, 1989.

47. Mellors JW et al. A simple index to identify occult bacterial infection in adults with acute unexplained fever. *Arch Intern Med* 147:666–71, 1987.

48. Keating HJ et al. Effect of aging on the clinical significance of fever in ambulatory adult patients. *J Am Geriatr Soc* 32:282–87, 1984.

49. Marantz PR et al. Inability to predict diagnosis in febrile intravenous drug abusers. *Ann Intern Med* 1987; 106:823–28.

50. Bates DW, Cook EF, Goldman L, et al. Predicting bactermia in hospitalized patients. *Ann Intern Med* 113:495–550, 1990.

51. Sklar DP, Rusnik R. The value of outpatient blood cultures in the emergency department. *Am J Emerg Med* 5:95–100, 1987.

52. Spray CL et al. Impact of encephalopathy or mortality in the sepsis syndrome. *Crit Care Med* 18:801–06, 1990.

53. Wright PF et al. Pattern of illness in the highly febrile young child: epidemiologic, clinical and laboratory correlates. *Pediatrics* 67:694–700, 1981.

54. Musher DM et al. Fever patterns: their lack of clinical significance. *Arch Intern Med* 139:1225–28, 1979.

55. Kreger BE et al. Gram negative bacteremia-III. Reassessment of etiology, epidemiology and ecology in 612 patients. *Am J Emerg Med* 68:332–43, 1980.

56. Wahlby L, Knutsen OH. Leukocyte counts, ESR and fever in the diagnosis of diverticulitis. *Acta Chir Scand* 148:623–24, 1982.

57. Finkelstein MS et al. Pneumococcal bacteremia in adults: age-dependent differences in presentation and outcome. *J Am Geriatr Soc* 31:19–27, 1983.

58. Gleckman R, Hibert D. Afebrile bacteremia: a phenomenon in geriatric patients. *JAMA* 248:1478–81, 1982.

3

Laboratory Tests in the Diagnosis of Infectious Disease in the Emergency Department

MELVIN P. WEINSTEIN
RONALD W. QUENZER

The clinical laboratory has long provided the standard underpinnings for the diagnosis of many infectious diseases. Microbiology laboratories, in particularly, are relied on to determine the etiology; consequently in most hospitals they handle large numbers of specimens, often with multiple tests requested on each specimen. With the advent of diagnosis-related groups (DRGs) each test uses more of an institution's increasingly limited resources and thus makes appropriate use of the laboratory of greater importance. In this chapter we review important principles of and provide directives to etiologic diagnosis that should enhance appropriate use of the laboratory for infectious diseases problems seen in the emergency department.

Nonmicrobiologic Tests

Hematologic indices, urinalysis, measurement of certain blood chemistries, and tests for acute phase reactants are all used to assist in the diagnosis of infectious diseases. In the emergency department these tests can take on added value because the results are available sooner than those of microbiologic cultures that require growth of organisms for diagnosis.

The WBC Count

A WBC count is commonly ordered in the emergency department, but its use is problematic because it is neither a specific nor a sensitive test. The range for "normal" WBC counts (within 95% confidence limits) varies in the literature from 3487–4300/μl for the lower limit to 9206–10,900/μl for the upper limit [1]. The ranges of normal values for the components of the WBC count also vary. If 100 cells are counted, chance variation can cause the percentage of cells attributed to a particular cell line to vary by as much as 15% [1]. Observer variability as to what constitutes a mature neutrophil or monocyte contributes to difficulties in interpretation of this test. Also the impact of computerized cell line recognition has not yet been well defined. Several physiologic variations independent of infection can alter the WBC count. For example, WBC counts rise in the afternoon, and blacks tend to have lower WBC counts than whites [1]. The changes in the WBC count and its components by age are listed in Table 3-1. A rise in leukocyte count appears to be a nonspecific response to illness or other conditions of physiologic stress. Noninfectious causes of an elevated WBC count are listed in Table 3-2. Numerous studies have demonstrated that the range of overlap of the

Table 3-1. Normal leukocyte counts

Age	Total leukocytes		Neutrophils[a]			Lymphocytes			Monocytes		Eosinophils	
	Mean	Range	Mean	Range	%	Mean	Range	%	Mean	%	Mean	%
Birth	—[b]	—	4.0	2.0–6.0	—	4.2	2.0–7.3	—	0.6	—	0.1	—
12 hours	—	—	11.0	7.8–14.5	—	4.2	2.0–7.3	—	0.6	—	0.1	—
24 hours	—	—	9.0	7.0–12.0	—	4.2	2.0–7.3	—	0.6	—	0.1	—
1–4 weeks	—	—	3.6	1.8–5.4	—	5.6	2.9–9.1	—	0.7	—	0.2	—
6 months	11.9	6.0–17.5	3.8	1.0–8.5	32	7.3	4.0–13.5	61	0.6	5	0.3	3
1 year	11.4	6.0–17.5	3.5	1.5–8.5	31	7.0	4.0–10.5	61	0.6	5	0.3	3
2 years	10.6	6.0–17.0	3.5	1.5–8.5	33	6.3	3.0–9.5	59	0.5	5	0.3	3
4 years	9.1	5.5–15.5	3.8	1.5–8.5	42	4.5	2.0–8.0	50	0.5	5	0.3	3
6 years	8.5	5.0–14.5	4.3	1.5–8.0	51	3.5	1.5–7.0	42	0.4	5	0.2	3
8 years	8.3	4.5–13.5	4.4	1.5–8.0	53	3.3	1.5–6.8	39	0.4	4	0.2	2
10 years	8.1	4.5–13.5	4.4	1.8–8.0	54	3.1	1.5–6.5	38	0.4	4	0.2	2
16 years	7.8	4.5–13.0	4.4	1.8–8.0	57	2.8	1.2–5.2	35	0.4	5	0.2	3
21 years	7.4	4.5–11.0	4.4	1.8–7.7	59	2.5	1.0–4.8	34	0.3	4	0.2	3

[a]Neutrophils include band cells at all ages and a small number of metamyelocytes and myelocytes in the first few days of life.
[b]Numbers of leukocytes are in thousands per μl; ranges are estimates of 95% confidence limits; and percentages refer to differential counts.
Data on infants under the age of 1 month are derived from Monroe et al., *J Pediatr* 95:89, 1979, *and* Weinberg et al., *J Pediatr* 106:462, 1985. Other values are from Albritton EC (ed.), *Standard Value in Blood.* Philadelphia: Saunders, 1952.
Adapted from R. Dallnean, White blood cells, developmental changes in number. In AM Rudolph (ed.), *Pediatrics* (18th ed.). Norwalk, CT: Appleton and Lange East, 1987. Pp. 1060–61.

Table 3-2. Noninfectious causes of leukocytosis

Emotional or physical stress	Pregnancy
Inflammation	Recent surgery (36 hours)
Malignancy	Exercise
Blood loss	Sickle cell disease
Myeloproliferative disorder	Sickle cell crisis
Drugs, e.g., epinephrine, lithium, steroids	Diabetic ketoacidosis
	Trauma
Presentation to the ED	Cigarette smoking
Seizures	

WBC count is too great to allow discrimination between pathophysiologic processes on the basis of the WBC count. Wenz and colleagues studied 486 patients with infections, inflammatory processes, trauma, and malignant diseases in whom a WBC count was drawn [2]. They failed to demonstrate a statistically significant difference among the WBC count, the percent of granulocytes, and the percent of band forms between any of the patient groups.

Callaham studied 860 emergency department patients in whom WBC counts had been obtained; 128 of those counts were greater than 11,000/μl. Patients with elevated WBC counts were grouped by diagnosis: bacterial, viral, uncertain etiology, or noninfectious. There was no significant difference in WBC counts between groups [3]. Much energy has been devoted to determining if the WBC count can predict bacteremia, especially in children. A WBC count greater than 15,000/μl has been found to increase the likelihood that a febrile child is bacteremic. In children with a temperature higher than 40°C and a WBC count greater than 15,000/μl, McCarthy found that 50% were bacteremic [4]. However, one-half of bacteremic children have WBC counts less than 15,000/μl [5]. Studies of WBC counts in adults have similar results. Depending on age, 26%–40% of bacteremic patients reported by Finkelstein et al. had WBC counts less than 10,000/μl [6]. In 121 adults presenting with unexplained fever, occult bacterial infection was found in 56% of those with a WBC count greater than 15,000/μl and in 32% of those with lower WBC counts [7]. These authors agree with Shapiro et al. that "the leukocyte count may provide useful confirmatory information when an infection is suspected, but when the diagnosis is clear from other data, documentation of leukocytosis is less likely to affect management" [1]. Furthermore, the WBC count is not of sufficient sensitivity to exclude significant bacterial disease when it is within normal ranges, nor is it specific enough to indicate that infection is present when it is elevated. However, marked neutrophilic leukocytosis (> 25,000/μl) from any cause, an indicator of the severity of an illness, has been associated with poor outcome with an overall mortality rate of almost 30% and can be used as a prognostic marker in the emergency department [8].

Strand et al. reported that the presence of cytoplasmic vacuolization of neutrophils (sensitivity = 90.5%) was significantly ($P > .001$) more sensitive for bloodstream infection than an elevated granulocyte count (sensitivity = 66.7%) or a band count alone (sensitivity = 72.0%) [9]. Cytoplasmic vacuolization was also found in 15.9% of a group of healthy persons in this study, so it cannot be relied on singularly to diagnose infected patients. Some patients with serious infections, particularly those who are elderly, alcoholic, or otherwise significantly debilitated (e.g., patients with end-stage malignancies), may fail to mount a leukocytosis and may, in fact, have leukopenia because fewer white blood cells are available for mobilization. Often such individuals will have a shift to the left in the absence of leukocytosis. Whether this abnormality will be detected in an era when differential counts in many laboratories are done by instruments rather than technologists is problematic.

Other hematologic abnormalities are useful for the diagnosis of infection. Lymphocytopenia has been noted in nearly 50% of a group of septic patients [9]. Atypical lymphocytosis is present in many viral infections, particularly those due to Epstein-Barr virus and cytomegalovirus, and also may be seen in patients with pertussis and listeriosis. Anemia itself characteristically is present in patients with infections of longer duration at the time of presentation; examples include subacute bacterial endocarditis, tuberculosis, and HIV infection. Finally, direct examination of the blood smear, especially the buffy coat, rarely provides the etiologic diagnosis of infection because it requires the presence of more than 1,000,000 microorganisms per milliliter for visualization in a peripheral smear and at least 40,000 microorganisms per milliliter to visualize in a buffy coat [10]. Such a high grade of bacteremia or fungemia is unusual. The finding of organisms on the peripheral smear should be validated by a Gram's stain and the physician notified immediately, since the mortality is over 50% [11–13]. Buffy coat examination may be worthwhile in patients who have had splenectomies and those with overwhelming sepsis, including neonates.

Urinalysis

Direct examination of the urine continues to be valuable for the early diagnosis of bacterial infections of the genitourinary tract. Pyuria and WBC casts suggest the presence of urinary infection; casts suggest upper-tract disease (e.g., pyelonephritis). Infection with urea-splitting bacteria, such as *Proteus mirabilis*, typically is associated with an alkaline pH in the urine. A normal urinalysis in a patient with signs and symptoms of pyelonephritis may be an indication of ureteral obstruction, the normal bladder urine representing urine flow from the uninfected contralateral kidney. The triad of pyuria, hematuria, and sterile urine should suggest the possibility of genitourinary tuberculosis. The presence of 1 to 2 leukocytes per high-power field (40 × objective) or bacteria seen under oil immersion (100 × objective) in unspun urine examined microscopically has a 95% correlation with the presence of 100,000, as in 10^5, colony-forming units (CFU) or more bacteria per ml [14]. Thus, microscopy is a good screen for high colony count urinary tract infection.

Blood Chemistry

Blood chemistry results can be useful for the early diagnosis and management of infection in the emergency department. An abnormal blood glucose may indicate the presence of previously unsuspected diabetes mellitus, a disease associated with increased risk of certain infections (e.g., cellulitis, chronic foot infections, and osteomyelitis) or specific microorganisms (e.g., group B streptococci, yeasts, and phycomycetes). Knowledge of the blood glucose level also is necessary for proper interpretation of the glucose concentration in the cerebrospinal fluid. Abnormal liver function tests may suggest hepatitis due to the hepatitis viruses or other infectious agents that are associated with hepatic inflammation (see Chap. 26). Extrahepatic infections such as sepsis, bacterial pneumonia involving the lower lobes, and legionellosis may also present with elevated liver enzymes as a nonspecific finding. The presence of diminished renal or liver function can influence the selection and the dosage of antimicrobial therapy in some patients.

Acute Phase Reactants

Acute phase reactants, particularly the erythrocyte sedimentation rate (ESR) and the C-reactive protein (CRP), have been used for the diagnosis of infectious diseases as well as other inflammatory disorders. These as well as other serum proteins are elevated in response to nonspecific inflammation. The CRP increases in response to any inflammatory process within hours and gradually decreases over days; the ESR increases more slowly over several days and then returns to baseline as the inflammation resolves. In the emergency department both tests have limited utility because of their lack of specificity for etiologic diagnosis [15]. An erythrocyte sedimentation rate (ESR) that exceeds 100 mm/hr is usually associated with infection (33%), malignancy (17%), renal disease (17%), or connective tissue disease (14%) [16, 17]. The measurement of CRP in the cerebrospinal fluid (CSF) has been used by some to diagnose bacterial meningitis, high levels suggesting bacterial infection. The practical usefulness of the test in this situation is controversial, and no firm recommendation can be made.

Microbiologic Tests

For the most part the laboratory diagnosis of infectious diseases remains the responsibility of the clinical microbiology laboratory. The traditional diagnostic studies, including microscopic examinations and cultures, have been supplemented more recently by the availability of tests for microbial antigens and nucleic acid probes for more rapid diag-

nosis. Nevertheless, microscopy and cultures remain the key studies for diagnosis. In the emergency department the physician's knowledge of the value and the limitations of these tests assumes great importance, because early diagnosis and appropriate initial management of patients with serious infections often make the difference between life and death or at least between shorter and uncomplicated versus longer and more complicated illnesses.

Specimen Collection and Processing

COLLECTION AND EVALUATION OF SPECIMENS
The laboratory diagnosis of infectious diseases begins with the collection of an appropriate sample for laboratory testing. That the culture is only as good as the sample obtained deserves repeating. Whenever possible the specimens for culture should be obtained prior to antimicrobial therapy. Antibiotics retard or prevent the growth of organisms, thus delaying or inhibiting the etiologic diagnosis. When specimens are obtained for culture, care must be taken to avoid contamination of the sample with normal colonizing flora of the skin, mucous membranes, wound surfaces, or extraneous foreign matter. Failure to do so lends to misinterpretation or difficulty in interpretation of the culture results. A Gram's stain of a specimen that shows the presence of polymorphonuclear leukocytes and the absence of squamous cells suggests a good-quality sample. If a predominant organism can be detected on the Gram's stain of a good sample, the emergency medicine physician can make a better selection of empiric therapy. Swabs, most frequently used to collect specimens, are particularly suitable for specimens from the pharynx and external genitalia. Swabs tipped with rayon, calcium alginate, or polyester are less toxic to most organisms and are preferred to cotton swabs (cotton tips are acceptable for pharyngeal specimens). Swabs must immediately be placed in media to prevent drying during transportation. Most microorganisms are very susceptible to desiccation.

Second only to the importance of obtaining an adequate specimen is the necessity to label properly all material submitted to the laboratory. The patient's name, identifying hospital number, physician's name, date and time of collection, source of the specimen, test(s) desired, and clinical diagnosis are all imperative information for the laboratory personnel. Requests for special tests or unusual pathogens should be communicated directly by phone or in person to the laboratory personnel as well as on the requisition. Specimens from individuals suspected of having highly contagious diseases (e.g., plague, diphtheria, and yellow fever) must be labeled as such as well as communicated directly to the laboratory supervisor.

Transport of Specimens

Prolonged transport delays are commonplace in medical facilities and may lead to false-negative or false-positive results. This is particularly true of specimens submitted for culture. Long delays permit some microorganisms to multiply rapidly, resulting in aberrant results. For example, a urine sample contaminated with a few bacteria will support their multiplication at room temperature so that within 2 hours these colonizing bacteria will number more than $10^4–10^5$ as if etiologically significant. This leads to inappropriate antibiotic therapy. On the other hand long delays may allow certain fastidious microorganisms to die, hardy microorganisms to overgrow, or specimens to desiccate.

It is good practice for the emergency department to have a policy and a procedure to ensure that all culture samples arrive at the microbiology laboratory within 1 hour of collection. If delay is anticipated, the sample generally should be stored refrigerated (2–8°C) until transportation. Cultures for gonorrhea, *Trichomonas vaginalis*, and anaerobes, however, may not survive refrigerator temperatures and must be transported directly at room temperature. Blood cultures should be incubated at 35°C. Some laboratories reject specimens with prolonged transport times as well as specimens collected improperly or incompletely labeled.

Identification of Organisms

Microscopy

Microscopy, Gram's stains, and other microscopic preparations are capable of providing the clinician with information almost immediately about the nature of the infectious process. Moreover, such examinations aid in evaluating the quality of the

specimen. Determination of specimen quality is important, since poor-quality specimens may provide both misleading smear and culture results. Preparation of the smear itself requires care; an improperly prepared or stained smear that misleads the clinician will lead to improper diagnosis and therapy for the patient. A good smear should be thick enough to show representative quantitation of organisms in a specimen and thin enough to see individual cells. Some body fluids (e.g., joint, pleural) can be very viscous due to high protein content, and dilution may be necessary for the smears to be interpreted. Smears of purulent material (e.g., pus from an abscess or a urethral exudate) should be made by gently rolling the swab once or twice across the slide so that the characteristic arrangement of the cells is not destroyed. During examination of the microscopic characteristics of specimens, several areas of the slide are evaluated. This procedure ensures that judgments are made on the basis of representative areas of the specimen. One of the most frequent uses of microscopy is in the examination of smears of expectorated sputum from patients with suspected pneumonia. Specimens that contain more than 10 squamous epithelial cells per low-power field (10 × objective) likely are contaminated with oropharyngeal flora and saliva; these specimens will not predict reliably the etiologic agent of the patient's infection. Indeed many laboratories will reject such specimens for culture based on the known poor quality of the specimen. If a better specimen cannot be obtained, therapeutic management without benefit of sputum culture may be necessary.

Gram's Stain. The most common stain used is a Gram's stain, which classifies microorganisms by their morphology and by their reaction to the stain (i.e., gram positive vs. gram negative). After a representative portion of the specimen is placed on the slide and allowed to air-dry, the specimen is fixed by gentle heating over a flame. If the slide is heated for too long, cellular material may be destroyed, making the slide more difficult to interpret. An alternative fixation technique used in some laboratories consists of flooding the air-dried smear with methanol for 2 minutes, then draining the slide and allowing it to air-dry again. This latter technique more consistently preserves the cellular morphology of the smear. Once fixed the slide is then, in sequence, flooded with crystal violet for 15 seconds, rinsed with tap water, drained of excess water, flooded with Gram's iodine for 15 seconds, rinsed with tap water and drained, decolorized with acetone until no more purple dye washes off the slide (a few seconds), rinsed with tap water again and drained, flooded with safranin for 15 seconds, rinsed with tap water, and blotted dry. To determine whether the stained specimen has been adequately decolorized, thereby ensuring adequate visualization and interpretation of gram-negative bacteria, nuclei of polymorphonuclear neutrophils should be examined. In an adequately decolorized stain the nuclei stain pink or red; the nuclei stain purple if the decolorization step was not adequate. Underdecolorized stains can be decolorized further by repeating the staining procedure, starting with the decolorization step.

Methylene Blue Stain. When considerable background material is present, Gram's-stain smears can be difficult to interpret. The methylene blue stain facilitates examination for bacteria and leukocytes, which stain dark blue, in contrast to mucus and other cellular material, which stain light blue. The stain is easy to perform; after methanol or heat fixation of the smear, the slide is flooded with methylene blue for 30–60 seconds, rinsed, drained, and blotted dry. The stain also can be used to examine diarrheal stool for the presence of fecal leukocytes, the presence of which suggests invasive bacterial infection or colitis (due to inflammatory bowel disease, *Clostridium difficile*, ischemia, etc.) as opposed to viral gastroenteritis or parasitic infection, in which the presence of fecal leukocytes would be unusual (see Chap. 25). Other uses of the methylene blue stain are for showing characteristic morphology of *Haemophilus* organisms, *Neisseria* organisms, the characteristic metachromatic granules of *Corynebacterium diphtheriae*, and gram-negative bacteria, which can be hard to demonstrate in Gram's stains.

Acridine Orange Stain. The acridine orange (AO) stain has particular value in the examination of body fluids in which there may be relatively few organisms. Because a fluorescence microscope must be used, AO stains usually must be performed in the

laboratory by a technologist experienced with the technique. Nonetheless, clinicians should be aware of the stain and request that it be performed if, for example, a Gram's stain shows the presence of leukocytes but no bacteria, and infection is suspected. Since bacteria usually can be detected at 400 × magnification (using the 40 × high dry lens of the microscope), greater areas of the smear can be scanned in a short time span. Microorganisms detected by the AO stain cannot be assessed with regard to the characteristics of a Gram's stain unless, having determined that organisms are present, reexamination of the Gram's stain results in detection of microorganisms.

Acid-Fast Stains. In general acid-fast stains (Ziehl-Neelson, Kinyoun) are not useful for the diagnosis of mycobacterial disease in the emergency department. Most laboratories process specimens for acid-fast microscopy and culture in a batch mode once or twice a week after concentrating and decontaminating the specimens, a laborious process. Because acid-fast stains have such poor sensitivity and are time-consuming for the microbiology laboratory, requests for them should be limited to patients in whom there is high clinical suspicion of tuberculosis. More important for the emergency physician is the knowledge that the diagnostic yield from unconcentrated specimens, the so-called direct acid-fast smear, is so low that the results are virtually always negative, even when the clinical probability of mycobacterial disease is high. Thus, most laboratories are reluctant to comply with requests for STAT acid-fast smears.

KOH Wet Preparation. A potassium hydroxide (KOH) preparation (using 10% KOH) is used primarily to detect fungal elements in skin scrapings, hair, or nails. The KOH dissolves keratinized cells, leaving a clear background in which hyphae can be seen more easily. A drop of KOH is placed on a large slide with a fragment of the tissue to be examined, the latter teased or separated enough to allow a thin preparation over which a cover slip can be placed. The preparation is gently heated by passing it through a flame two or three times, then examined using the 10 × (low power) objective and reduced illumination. Artifacts such as cotton or elastic fibers, feathers, and bubbles (air, oil, or grease) can interfere with interpretation.

India Ink Preparation. An India ink preparation is used to detect capsules of *Cryptococcus neoformans* in cerebrospinal and other body fluids, including urine. The sensitivity of this test for cryptococcal meningitis in non-HIV patients is 25%–50%, whereas it is 70%–80% in HIV-infected individuals because of their higher concentration of organisms [18]. A drop of sediment from a centrifuged specimen is mixed with a small drop of India ink on a clean slide and overlaid with a cover slip. The slide then is scanned under low power using reduced illumination. The mucoid capsules of cryptococci appear as clear halos that surround the yeast cells and in turn are surrounded by the black mass of India ink particles. The most helpful diagnostic finding is the presence of budding yeast forms; buds can be detached from the mother cell but enclosed in the same capsule. White blood cells may give the appearance of a capsule and be difficult to differentiate from yeast cells if budding is not seen. However, leukocytes usually disintegrate after 10 or more minutes, and the preparation can be reexamined after this short delay. The cryptococcal antigen test is much more sensitive and should replace the India ink preparation in laboratories.

Dark-Field Exams. The diagnosis of primary syphilis and some cases of secondary syphilis (e.g., mucous patches, condyloma lata) can be made using the dark-field microscopy exam (see Fig. 30-10; also Chap. 30). Most clinicians and increasing numbers of technologists have little or no experience with dark-field microscopy. For that reason dark-field exams should be done only by individuals with experience. If a technologist with experience is available, that person should perform the test in the laboratory. Some city and state health departments provide on-call service for these examinations.

Malaria Smears. The diagnosis of malaria almost always rests on the visualization of parasites in the peripheral blood; in many cases the diagnosis is made by routine review of the peripheral smear during evaluation of a febrile patient. However, as more laboratories switch to automated leukocyte differential exams, this diagnostic bonus may be lost. Most laboratories have a standard procedure for obtaining and staining specimens when malaria smears are requested. Thus, when malaria is suspected, the laboratory should be consulted. In general a drop of capillary blood from a finger puncture smeared directly on several slides is preferred over blood drawn by venipuncture and sent to the laboratory for smears. If venipuncture is the method by which blood is obtained, an anticoagulant-containing tube should be used.

CULTURES

Bacterial Cultures. Although cultures are not useful for making immediate diagnoses or therapeutic decisions in the emergency department, clinicians must know the value and the limitations of cultures for the diagnoses of infectious diseases. Moreover, early and accurate diagnosis rests on prompt and appropriate culturing when the patient is first seen; thus, the role played by emergency department professionals is crucial. It is key that the specimen obtained is representative of the disease process. Normal colonizing flora and contamination must be avoided when the specimen is obtained. Otherwise, culture results will be difficult if not impossible to interpret. Specimens obtained prior to administration of antibiotics are more likely to reflect the true microbiology of the infection. Since there may be relatively few microorganisms present per gram of tissue or per milliliter of body fluid, larger quantities of material are preferred over smaller quantities.

Prompt transport of specimens to the laboratory increases the chance that fastidious pathogens such as pneumococci, meningococci, and gonococci, if present, will be detected and not overgrown by hardier commensal flora. Cultures most often are obtained for the detection of bacterial pathogens. The so-called routine cultures for aerobic and facultative bacteria can be obtained by using swabs (e.g., throat cultures) or by direct placement of specimens in sterile containers (e.g., urine, sputum, and stool). Material for anaerobic culture is best obtained by using needle and syringe (e.g., abscess contents, normally sterile body fluid); swabs are discouraged because organisms are more likely to be exposed to oxygen and drying. In general, anaerobic cultures of sputum, urine, the vagina and endometrium, and decubitus wounds should not be done because the presence of commensal anaerobic bacteria is predictable, and interpretation of culture results—pathogens versus colonizers—is not possible. Gram stains, however, may provide important information to direct initial empiric therapy.

Fungal Cultures. Fungal cultures are obtained in the same manner as routine bacterial cultures, except cotton swabs are not acceptable. Indeed, assuming specimen quantity is adequate, the same specimen can be used for both bacterial and fungal isolation in the laboratory. It is important to note, however, that specimens from patients with fungal infections may contain not only the etiologic agent but also contaminating bacteria that may overgrow the slower-growing fungus. Therefore, prompt transport of specimens to and prompt processing by the laboratory increase diagnostic yield.

Mycobacterial Cultures. Mycobacterial cultures in the emergency department most often are obtained from patients with suspected pulmonary tuberculosis or subacute meningitis syndrome or from HIV-infected individuals with suspected disseminated mycobacterial infection. For the diagnosis of pulmonary tuberculosis, 5–10 ml of expectorated sputum should be collected and sent in a screw-capped container to the laboratory. For the diagnosis of tuberculous meningitis, 5–10 ml of cerebrospinal fluid should be provided for the laboratory personnel to centrifuge to concentrate the sample. Modest delays in transport are acceptable as long as the specimen is refrigerated, since most laboratories batch mycobacterial cultures rather than processing them in sequence as they arrive. In HIV-infected patients the most frequent culture sources are blood. The procedure for mycobacterial blood culture depends on the system used in individual hospitals, and emergency department personnel should consult the lab for direction when such cultures are needed.

Viral and Chlamydial Cultures. Viral and chlamydial cultures are the "gold standard" for etiologic diagnosis of infections due to these microorganisms. Not all hospitals, however, have the laboratory facilities or the technical staff to perform cell culture techniques for these agents. Specimens can be sent to reference laboratories, or other diagnostic modalities (e.g., enzyme immunoassays and nucleic acid probes) can be used. (These techniques are discussed later in this chapter.) Where culture is available, laboratories usually provide transport media in which swabs are placed. It is important to remember that these microbes most often are present intracellularly; thus, cellular material must be obtained by more vigorous swabbing than ordinarily is done for bacterial culture.

SPECIMEN COLLECTION AND CULTURES FROM SELECTED ANATOMIC SITES

Blood Cultures. Detection of bacteremia or fungemia has great clinical and prognostic importance. A blood culture essentially is a venipuncture obtained in a sterile fashion, the blood specimen being inoculated to one or more (usually two) broth-containing bottles or transport tubes, which are then sent to the laboratory for processing. Sterile technique in obtaining the blood specimen reduces the chance that skin flora will contaminate the specimen and provide confusing test results. Most institutions use iodophors to scrub the venipuncture site before blood is obtained; these compounds exert their antiseptic effect 1–2 minutes after contact. A good rule of thumb is to let the iodophor dry completely before proceeding with the venipuncture. Because the chance of contamination is greatly increased (making positive culture results more difficult to interpret), obtaining blood for culture from indwelling catheters (e.g., Hickman catheters in cancer patients) is discouraged. Venipuncture from a peripheral site always is preferable. Separate needles are used for each venipuncture. A single needle and syringe can be used both to obtain the blood and to inoculate the culture bottles; contamination is no greater than with the two-needle technique recommended formerly.

Some patients with signs and symptoms of sepsis already may have received antibiotics prior to arriving in the emergency department. Reagents and blood culture broths are available that contain resins that bind antibiotics present in the blood, thereby (in theory) increasing the probability of detecting bacteremia [19]. Studies of the efficacy of resin bottles or media are inconclusive, and the cost of the reagents is high. It should be remembered that blood inoculated for culture usually is diluted five- to tenfold, and the concentration of any antimicrobial present in the blood is reduced by the same proportion. The final judgment as to the utility of these systems is not yet available. In adults the number of blood cultures needed to detect bloodstream infection depends in part on the volume of blood obtained for each culture. In general 30 ml of blood will detect 99% of bacteremias [20, 21, 22, 23]. Thus, if 10 ml of blood is obtained per culture, three separate culture sets (i.e., venipunctures) should be obtained; if 15 ml of blood or more is obtained per culture, only two culture sets are recommended. In small children 1–5 ml of blood should be obtained per culture set. Paired rather than single blood cultures make results more easily interpreted. Timing of blood cultures depends in large measure on the acuity of the patient. Acutely septic patients should have two or three blood culture sets obtained in rapid sequence, after which empiric antimicrobial therapy can be started promptly (see Chap. 6). In contrast, less ill patients can have their blood cultures done in sequence over several hours or days.

CSF Cultures. Bacterial meningitis is a medical emergency. Lumbar puncture is done using sterile technique, and CSF is rushed to the laboratory for examination and culture. In many cases the diagnosis of bacterial meningitis can be made based on the sediment after centrifugation of small volumes of CSF (e.g., 1 ml for a Gram's stain and culture). However, few organisms are present in many patients, and larger volumes (2–4 ml) are preferred. Moreover, when the differential diagnosis is broad, fungal, mycobacterial, and viral cultures also may be requested, in which case 5–10 ml of CSF is needed. In infants and young children smaller volumes are acceptable.

Throat Cultures. In patients with pharyngitis the most important differential diagnosis is between viral etiologies and the group A streptococcus (see Chap. 21). Indeed, most laboratories screen throat cultures only for group A streptococci. When a diagnosis of gonococcal pharyngitis, pertussis, or diphtheria is considered, the laboratory should be consulted. Gonococcal culture media are routinely available, whereas cultures for *Bordetella pertussis* and *C. diphtheriae* require special media that may not be immediately available. Throat cultures are

obtained by swabbing vigorously in the areas of exudate or inflammation and placing the swab in a liquid medium for transport to the laboratory. Newer direct tests for group A streptococcal antigen are done in some institutions, but they are less sensitive than cultures for detection of group A streptococci. A positive antigen test usually confirms the diagnosis of "strep throat," but a negative antigen test requires a backup culture before group A streptococcal infection can be ruled out.

Ear, Nose, and Sinus Cultures. Cultures from the nose and the ear canal rarely provide any useful information about the etiology of upper respiratory, inner ear, and sinus infections. Sinus cultures obtained surgically by direct sinus puncture and aspiration avoid the normal nasopharyngeal flora and represent the etiologic agent. Nasopharyngeal cultures are not useful for determining the etiology of otitis media. When bacteriologic diagnosis is crucial, tympanocentesis with culture of the middle ear fluid is mandated. A scraping of the external ear canal can provide the etiologic agent in diabetics with persistent otitis externa at risk for serious otitis externa. *Staphylococcus aureus* and *Pseudomonas aeruginosa* are the frequent pathogens.

Sputum Cultures. Most sputum specimens, whether obtained by expectoration or by suctioning (in the obtunded host), are contaminated to some degree with oropharyngeal flora. Thus, screening the sputum specimen for contamination using the Gram's stain smear is crucial for assessing the quality of the specimen [24, 25]. Specimens with more than 25 leukocytes and fewer than 10 squamous epithelial cells per low-power field (10 × objective) more accurately reflect the etiologic agent(s). The quality of expectorated specimens can be enhanced if the patient first rinses the mouth with water and then coughs deeply and provides only that material in the specimen container. The specimen should be transported to the laboratory promptly, since dominant but fastidious pathogens such as the pneumococcus may be overgrown by oropharyngeal commensals when delays in transport are long. When the etiologic diagnosis is critical and a good specimen cannot be obtained by noninvasive methods, transtracheal aspiration, which avoids the oropharyngeal flora, can be performed in the emergency department. Other specimens obtained by flexible bronchoscopy with shielded catheter to diminish oropharyngeal contamination, transthoracic lung aspiration, and open-lung biopsies are associated with more risk and expense and are postadmission procedures usually reserved for difficult pneumonias. In addition to evaluating sputum for quality of the specimen, the Gram's stain smear is useful in guiding initial therapy. False-negative interpretations do occur, particularly in pneumococcal pneumonia [26]. However, the etiologic pathogens in pneumonia identified by blood cultures or by transthoracic needle aspirate are almost always present in the sputum, either as the sole isolate or as the predominant organism in mixed flora [27].

Urine Cultures. Many patients who present to the emergency department with symptoms and signs of urinary tract infection will have a culture obtained. The most common and least invasive specimen for diagnosis is the midstream clean catch urine, which is obtained after appropriate cleansing of the external genitalia and urethral orifice and ideally at least 2 hours after the previous voiding [28]. Other acceptable specimens include those obtained from single catheterization, direct aspiration from an existing indwelling catheter (e.g., in a patient arriving from a nursing home), or suprapubic bladder aspiration. Not acceptable are specimens obtained without appropriate cleansing prior to urination or those taken from a catheter drainage bag.

Since the criteria for significant bacteriuria are based on quantitation, cultures must be promptly submitted to and processed by the laboratory; alternatively specimens can be refrigerated (4°C) or processed in preservative kits [29]. Bacterial counts should remain stable for up to 24 hours at 4°C. Delay in culturing urine left standing at room temperature for more than 2 hours after collection has been shown to significantly increase urinary colony counts [30]. The enteric bacteria that cause most urinary infections multiply rapidly at room temperature, and processing delays can permit bacterial growth and confuse the diagnosis. Interpretation of colony counts depends on the patient's clinical features and the manner in which the specimen was obtained. Any bacteria found in urine from a suprapubic aspirate are significant, whereas 10^5 or more colony-forming units (CFUs) per milliliter in a

midstream urine specimen from an asymptomatic patient are reliably associated with infection [31]. In women with acute dysuria, the presence of 10^2 or fewer CFUs per milliliter of urine correlates with infection [32]. Most laboratories routinely identify and perform antimicrobial susceptibility tests on microorganisms present in numbers greater than 10^4 per milliliter unless mixed flora is present. If polymicrobial bacteriuria is anticipated (e.g., chronic indwelling catheter, neurogenic bladder), a special request to identify more than one microorganism should be made at the time the urine is submitted. This is appropriate only if the sample was obtained by suprapubic aspirate or in-and-out straight catheter procedure.

Stool Cultures. The best specimens for stool culture are fresh, unformed stools. Rectal swabs are inferior for the diagnosis of clinical disease and should not be used; the bacterial inoculum in such specimens may be insufficient for detection of the pathogen. The exception to utilizing rectal swabs is in the diagnosis of proctitis caused by *Neisseria gonorrhea*, chlamydia, or the herpes simplex virus. In practice the swab tip is passed one to two inches beyond the anal sphincter and then rotated to sample the anal crypts. Most laboratories do not culture stool routinely for *Vibrio* species or *Yersinia* species; thus, if cholera or yersinia dysentery is suspected, the laboratory personnel should be notified so that appropriate media will be used. In patients who have received antimicrobials within the prior 6–8 weeks, the possibility of C. *difficile* diarrhea should be considered, and toxin assay for this pathogen obtained.

Skin, Soft-Tissue, Decubitus, and Superficial Wound Cultures. Many infections are accompanied by skin lesions; also many patients with minor injuries present only after they have developed skin and soft tissue infection. Thus, cultures of the skin and the soft tissues commonly are obtained in the emergency department. For the laboratory to process these specimens appropriately, good communication is needed. For example, selective media for *Vibrio* species can be used if the laboratory personnel are made aware that the culture comes from a lesion that may have been contaminated by seawater or brackish water, where marine vibrios are common. Similarly technologists will look for

Eikenella corrodens in cultures from human bite wounds and *Pasteurella multocida* in cultures from animal bite wounds. Tissue itself or pus aspirated in a syringe always is preferred. To avoid desiccation, tissue samples should be placed in a sterile container, such as a urine cup, containing a few milliliters of sterile nonbacteriostatic saline. Some lesions (e.g., puncture wounds associated with bites) may be small and require use of a swab. In those cases the surrounding skin should be cleansed thoroughly to reduce the presence of surface commensals that will contaminate the culture specimen.

When vesicles or bullae are present, as may be the case in some systemic bacterial infections, they should be aspirated in an attempt to provide the etiologic diagnosis. Aspiration of the subcutaneous tissue with needle and syringe (sometimes after injection of 0.5 ml of nonbacteriostatic saline) occasionally will be useful in cases of cellulitis. Swab cultures of draining sinuses or fistulae have poor predictive value for deep infection owing to virtually universal contamination with colonizing surface flora. Likewise, surface cultures of decubitus and neuropathic ulcers are virtually useless, again owing to the omnipresence of fecal and other flora. Deep-tissue cultures from surgical debridement or punch biopsies are satisfactory [33]. In septic patients with open bedsores or draining lesions, the etiology for infection is best determined by blood cultures (if positive) or by needle aspiration through normal skin to get to the infected tissues, punch biopsies, or surgical debridement.

Genital Cultures. Of all the sexually transmitted diseases, only gonorrhea is diagnosed primarily by culture. Appropriate sites for culture in women include not only the urethra and cervix but also the anus and the throat. In heterosexual men only the urethra need be cultured; cultures of the anus and the throat should be added in homosexual men. Gonorrhea cultures should be obtained using swabs made of materials that are not toxic to the fastidious gonococci, such as cotton or rayon. Specimens should be inoculated promptly to transport media that will support the organisms, or they should be swabbed directly to agar (chocolate and Thayer-Martin or other modified chocolate agar) with prompt incubation in a 5%–10% carbon dioxide atmosphere. Although the diagnosis of gonococcal urethritis in males can be made by a Gram's stain

smear, culture is required for detection of penicillin-resistant strains.

The gold standard for detection of *Chlamydia trachomatis* is cell culture, but many laboratories do not have cell culture capabilities. Other means of diagnosis include immunoassay techniques and direct detection using fluorescein-conjugated monoclonal antibodies and fluorescence microscopy. These techniques approach the sensitivity of culture in populations with a high prevalence of chlamydial infection but are of substantially less value in low-prevalence populations [34]. When specimens are obtained for the detection of chlamydiae, it should be remembered that this microbe is an intracellular pathogen. Thus, a technique vigorous enough to yield epithelial cells on the swab must be used. In practice, swabs for gonorrhea culture and stain can be obtained first, thus clearing secretions for ease of recovery of epithelial cells.

In the authors' view, the diagnosis of genital herpes simplex infection most often is made clinically, and culture seldom should be necessary. When laboratory corroboration is necessary, the base of an ulcer is swabbed and the swab placed in a viral transport medium for cell culture. In institutions without cell culture facilities, the specimen can be sent to a reference laboratory, or nonculture-based methods can be used. Women with pelvic inflammatory disease sometimes have cultures obtained from the endocervix. These cultures frequently are contaminated by the normal anaerobic and enteric flora of the female genital tract, and cultures yielding these organisms are uninterpretable. Endocervical cultures yielding gonococci, *S. aureus* (in suspected toxic shock syndrome), *Listeria monocytogenes*, or group A or B streptococci in women with puerperal or postoperative infections may be of value. When specimens are obtained from the endocervix, the speculum should be inserted without the use of lubricants, which contain antibacterial agents and may interfere with culture results. Warm water should be used instead of a lubricant.

Cultures of Other Body Fluids. Fluid may accumulate in virtually any body organ or cavity in response to infection, and aspiration of such potentially infected collections in the emergency department may provide the critical information needed to treat the patient appropriately. Thus, thoracentesis, paracentesis, arthrocentesis, and even pericardiocentesis are performed in the emergency department. In each instance, the fluid obtained should be placed in a sterile container and transported to the laboratory for stains and culture. It also is acceptable to leave the fluid in the syringe, cap the syringe, and send it to the laboratory. As has been emphasized previously, volume is important. Samples from closed, normally sterile sites are appropriate for aerobic and anaerobic setup. Gram's stain and cultures for aerobic and anaerobic bacteria are usually routine, but they should be noted on the requisition. Additional stains and cultures for mycobacteria, fungi, parasites, and viruses are directed by the clinical circumstances. It is always a good idea to ask the laboratory to save an aliquot for possible later stains or serologic assays.

Nonculture-Based Tests

Laboratory medicine has entered an era in which new technologies are being utilized for clinical diagnosis. Potentially these new methods can provide results earlier than traditional cultures. Moreover, they provide an alternative diagnostic tool when culture is not technically feasible (e.g., virus, chlamydia, and mycoplasma cultures). These new, rapid diagnostic tests have special utility in the emergency department setting. It is important to note that the predictive value of any rapid diagnostic method is related to the prevalence in the target population. If the prevalence of the infection is low, then a very sensitive and specific test is required for predictive values to be useful. Most of the assays utilizing nonculture-based diagnostic methods that are currently marketed represent first-generation efforts. We can expect more and better tests in the reasonably near future.

Bacterial Meningitis. Because of the emergent nature of bacterial meningitis, early diagnosis and correct therapy are essential. Since Gram's stains are positive in only 80%–85% of cases, alternative methods for rapid etiologic diagnosis have been sought. For the most part assays for the presence of bacterial antigens have been the focus, first using countercurrent immunoelectrophoresis (CIE) and now latex agglutination (LA) or coagglutination (CoA). Several kits are marketed that are designed to detect the antigens of *Haemophilus influenzae*

type B, *Neisseria meningitidis*, *Streptococcus pneumoniae*, and the group B streptococcus. Overall these kits have comparable sensitivity to the Gram's stain. The tests utilizing LA for the pneumococcus and meningococcus are considerably less sensitive and specific than the Gram's stain [35, 36]. Detection of pneumococcal antigen by enzyme immunoassay (EIA) has improved sensitivity and specificity; with increasing availability it may be the preferred test in this circumstance [37]. A DNA probe for identification of *S. pneumoniae* is available and may soon be very useful in detecting meningitis [38]. Similarly detection of *N. meningitidis* antigen in CSF by EIA is probably more sensitive than a Gram's stain, with a positive predictive value of at least 81% and a negative predictive value of 96% [37]. Bacterial antigen assays work best when CSF is tested and less well when serum or urine is tested, the latter having a substantial increase in nonspecific agglutination reactions [39]. Given the test limitations some laboratories do not offer these assays. When they are used, their greatest value may be in patients in whom there is strong clinical evidence of meningitis but a negative Gram's stain or in patients in whom partially treated meningitis is suspected. Nonetheless, clinical judgment is more important than the results of these tests.

Another laboratory test that has been advocated by some for the diagnosis of bacterial meningitis is the limulus lysate assay [40–42]. This test detects the presence of endotoxin and, therefore, gram-negative bacteria, including *H. influenzae* and *N. meningitidis*. The assay is extremely sensitive, perhaps too much so since false positive tests can be a problem. Also problematic is the technical difficulty of running the assay and the nonspecific nature of positive test results. Positive limulus tests can be due to the presence of endotoxin from any gram-negative microorganism.

Cryptococcal Meningitis. In contrast to the limited value of bacterial antigen testing in meningitis, detection of cryptococcal antigen by LA in the CSF is both highly sensitive and specific. This assay has a sensitivity of 95%–100%, which exceeds the India ink test and therefore is preferred [43, 44]. False-positive results are unusual but occur with the slide LA in neurosyphilis, infection from other fungi (e.g., *Trichosporon beigleii*), or patients with IgM rheumatoid factor [45–47]. The usefulness of this test is enhanced in that cultures may be negative or slow to grow, and the titer is useful in determining response to therapy. High CSF titers correlate with high concentration of organisms in the CSF; both tend to increase with disease progression and decrease with recovery from therapy [48–50]. Detection of cryptococcal antigen in CSF or serum is a reliable test for the diagnosis of cryptococcosis.

Streptococcal Pharyngitis. In recent years there has been a proliferation of commercial test kits that detect the presence of group A streptococcal antigen in throat swabs. Using either LA methods or an enzyme immunoassay technique, these tests are capable of diagnosing strep throat in as short a period as 15–20 minutes (assuming personnel are available to perform the test immediately). Potentially these assays have particular value for patients who present to the emergency department with complaints of sore throat. Virtually all the kits have good specificity (> 90%); that is, a positive test truly represents the presence of group A streptococci [51, 52]. The main limitation of the tests is their less-than-optimal sensitivity, ranging from as low as 40% in some studies to as high as 99% in others [53–56]. It is the authors' view that none of these assays should be used alone for diagnosis. If one of these tests is used, a two-swab technique is recommended: the first swab is used for antigen detection; if the antigen test is negative, the second swab is used for culture. If the antigen test is positive, a presumptive diagnosis of group A streptococcal pharyngitis can be made.

Sexually Transmitted Diseases. The major focus of nonculture-based diagnosis for sexually transmitted diseases has been for the detection of *C. trachomatis* and herpes simplex virus. Researchers, however, are investigating assay systems that are capable of detecting the presence of multiple sexually transmitted pathogens using a single specimen. Nongonococcal urethritis in men and genital tract infection in women due to *C. trachomatis* now can be detected using commercially available fluorescein-conjugated monoclonal antibody kits, EIA methods, and nucleic acid probes. The sensitivity of these methods compared with culture varies considerably. For example, the tests approach the sensitivity of culture (i.e., 90% sensitivity) in symptomatic women from populations

with a high prevalence of chlamydial infection [57]. Predictive value is considerably lower (i.e., 65%–70%) in populations with a low prevalence of chlamydial infection and in asymptomatic women screened during pregnancy [58]. The differing sensitivities may relate in part to the number of organisms present in the specimen, larger numbers of organisms being present in symptomatic patients and, therefore, having a greater likelihood of detection by these methods. Overall the sensitivities and specificities for chlamydia antigen detection assays are, respectively, as follows: direct fluorescent antibody (DFA) technique 56%–100% and 82%–100%, EIA 44%–100% and 93%–98%, and DNA probe 60%–88% and 95%–99% [58–62]. Awareness of the assay used in individual hospitals permits a more accurate interpretation of the results.

The diagnosis of genital herpes infection is by viral culture technique, but it also can be made using fluorescein-labeled monoclonal or polyclonal antibody kits. Published reports have suggested sensitivity of 70%–90% compared to culture [63]. Considerations in deciding about the usefulness of these tests are similar to those for chlamydia. At this time, the availability of herpes immunoassay for clinicians is limited. The authors emphasize, however, that diagnoses of the great majority of genital herpes infections can be made without the need for laboratory confirmation.

At the time of this writing there are nonculture-based kits available for the diagnosis of gonorrhea. One test utilizes EIA technology and approximates the sensitivity of culture for the diagnosis of gonococcal urethritis in males. When compared to urethral culture in males, the sensitivity is 94%–97% and the specificity is 96%–98% [64, 65]. It is less sensitive (78%–79%) and specific (87%–98%) than culture in asymptomatic women, and it should not be used to diagnose gonococcal pharyngitis or proctitis because of inadequate sensitivity [64, 65]. The EIA may remain positive after treatment, so it cannot be used as a test of cure. A DNA probe is 93% sensitive and 99% specific compared to culture, but it is not commercially available [66].

Screening Tests for Bacteriuria. Because urine cultures represent the most frequent tests sent to the microbiology laboratory and because the great majority of specimens, perhaps 80%–90%, are negative by the usual quantitative culture methods, techniques for detecting "significant" bacteriuria have been marketed. These techniques include several variations of the leukocyte esterase and nitrate test strips, bioluminescence systems, and a calorimetric test device. Each of these screening techniques has been shown to correlate reasonably well with the presence of 100,000 or more bacteria per milliliter of urine [67]. The sensitivity of the leukocyte esterase–nitrate test most commonly used in outpatient settings is about 85% for detecting 10^5 or more CFUs. However, sensitivity for detection of low-colony-count urinary infection ($< 10^3$ CFU/ml) is limited. Physicians working in institutions with laboratories that use these screening techniques should be aware of the limitations. The predictive values for positive tests are much lower (25%–50%) than the predictive values for negative tests. The data for the screening tests show sensitivities as well as predictive values for negative results of less than 90% [68].

Detection of C. Difficile Diarrhea. Laboratory confirmation of diarrhea due to C. *difficile*, the causal organism of pseudomembranous enterocolitis, and 20%–30% of antibiotic-associated diarrhea is suboptimal [69]. The culture requires selective media that are not used routinely in most laboratories and storage and transport of stool specimens at 4°C [70]. Moreover, although sensitive, the culture lacks sufficient specificity for diagnosis. Assays for the toxins produced by C. *difficile* are used most often for diagnosis. Probably the best assay is that which detects toxin B (cytotoxin) largely and toxin A (enterotoxin); however, tissue culture techniques are required, but they are not available in many laboratories [71]. Also marketed is a rapid LA method that detects an organism-associated protein; the value of this test has been controversial, and its clinical value remains uncertain. Some have suggested that it be used as a screening test and that a second positive test by another method be required before diagnosis can be considered confirmed. Indeed, there is currently no one laboratory test for C. *difficile* considered sufficiently sensitive and specific for diagnosis. An EIA kit that measures the combination of toxin A and toxin B in the stool is 95% sensitive compared to tissue culture assay

and is becoming available commercially [72]. Other promising tests include DNA probes for toxin A, detection of C. *difficile* antigens in feces, and immunoblot detection of C. *difficile*–reactive antibodies in serum [73–75].

Detection of Legionella Pneumophila. L. *pneumophila* can be detected in respiratory specimens by DFA technique. Sputum as well as bronchoscopic, transtracheal, and open lung biopsy samples are all acceptable. However, the sensitivity is only about 70% but with a 97% specificity [76]. Therefore, a negative DFA in no way excludes the diagnosis of Legionnaires' disease. At the time of this writing a nucleic acid probe (sensitivity = 70%; specificity = 99%) is under investigation [77, 78]. Utilizing EIA and radioimmunoassay (RIA) techniques, L. *pneumophila*–soluble antigen can be detected in the urine of patients with acute infection (< 7 days from onset) and may provide additional diagnostic information. The sensitivities and specificities for EIA are 70% and 99% and for RIA 93% and 100%, respectively [79–81].

Diagnosis of Mycoplasma Pneumoniae. The gold standard for diagnosis of M. *pneumoniae* infections has been via serology because isolation of the organism and interpretation of that isolation are difficult. More rapid tests employ antigen detection by immunoblotting sputum or throat swabs for polypeptide, but they are not routinely available. Probes to detect M. *pneumoniae* DNA are now available [82] and have been reported to have good sensitivity and specificity but need to be better confirmed by careful clinical field trials [83].

References

1. Shapiro MF, Greenfield S. The complete blood count and leukocyte differential count: an approach to their rational application. *Ann Int Med* 106:65–74, 1987.
2. Wenz B et al. The clinical utility of leukocyte differential in emergency medicine. *Am J Clin Pathol* 86:298–303, 1986.
3. Callaham M. Inaccuracy and expense of the leukocyte count in making urgent clinical decisions. *Ann Emerg Med* 15:774–81, 1986.
4. McCarthy PL, Jekel JF, Dolan TF. Temperature greater than or equal to 40 C in children less than 24

months of age: a prospective study. *Pediatrics* 59:663–68, 1977.

5. McGowan JE Jr et al. Bacteremia in febrile children seen in a "walk-in" pediatric clinic. *N Engl J Med* 288:1309–12, 1973.

6. Finkelstein MS et al. Pneumococcal bacteremia in adults: age dependent differences in presentation and in outcome. *J Am Geriatr Soc* 31:19–27, 1983.

7. Mellors JW et al. A simple index to identify occult bacterial infection in adults with acute unexplained fever. *Arch Intern Med* 147:666–72, 1987.

8. Chang R, Wong G. Prognostic significance of marked leukocytosis in hospitalized patients. *J Gen Int Med* 6:199–203, 1991.

9. Strand CL, Goldstein D, Castella A. Value of cytoplasmic vacuolization of neutrophils in the diagnosis of bloodstream infection. *Lab Med* 22:263–66, 1991.

10. Reik H, Rubin SJ. Evaluation of the buffy coat smear for rapid detection of bacteremia. *JAMA* 245:357–59, 1981.

11. Smith H. Leukocytes containing bacteria in plain blood films from patients with septicemia. *Aust Am Med* 15:210–19, 1966.

12. Brooks GF, Pribble AH, Beaty HN. Early diagnosis of bacteremia by buffy coat examinations. *Arch Intern Med* 132:673–75, 1973.

13. Barenfanger JE, Dick BW, Rabinovich S. Significance of visualization of bacteria in blood smears. *Lab Med* 21:579–81, 1990.

14. Robins DG et al. Urine microscopy as an aid to detection of bacteriuria. *Lancet* 1:476–78, 1975.

15. Sox HC, Liang MH. The erythrocyte sedimentation rate: guidelines for rational use. *Ann Intern Med* 104:515, 1986.

16. Fincher R-ME, Page MI. Clinical significance of extreme elevation of the erythrocyte sedimentation rate. *Arch Intern Med* 146:1581, 1986.

17. Bedell SE, Bush BJ. Erythrocyte sedimentation rate. *Am J Med* 78:1001, 1985.

18. Kovacs JA et al. Cryptococcosis in the acquired immunodeficiency syndrome. *Ann Intern Med* 103:533, 1985.

19. Washington JA, Ilstrup DM. Blood cultures: issues and controversies. *Rev Infect Dis* 8:792–802, 1986.

20. Tenney JH et al. Controlled evaluation of the volume of blood cultured in detection of bacteremia and fungemia. *J Clin Microbiol* 15:558–61, 1982.

21. Washington JA. Blood cultures: principles and techniques. *Mayo Clin Proc* 50:91–98, 1975.

22. Weinstein MP et al. The clinical significance of positive blood cultures: a comprehensive analysis of 500 episodes of bacteremia and fungemia in adults. I. Laboratory and epidemiologic observations. *Rev Infect Dis* 5:35–53, 1983.

23. Ilstrup DM, Washington JA. The importance of volume of blood cultured in the detection of bacteremia and fungemia. *Diagn Microbiol Infect Dis* 1:107–10, 1983.

24. Murray PR, Washington JA. Microscopic and bacteriologic analysis of expectorated sputum. *Mayo Clin Proc* 50:339–44, 1975.

25. Van Scoy RE. Bacterial sputum cultures. *Mayo Clin Proc* 52:39–41, 1977.

26. Barrett-Connor E. The nonvalue of sputum culture in the diagnosis of pneumococcal pneumonia. *Am Rev Respir Dis* 103:845–48, 1971.

27. Davidson M, Tempest B, Palmer DL. Bacteriologic diagnosis of acute pneumonia. *JAMA* 235:158–63, 1976.

28. Roberts AP, Robinson RE, Beard RW. Some factors affecting bacterial colony counts in urinary infection. *Br Med J* 1:400–03, 1967.

29. Weinstein MP. Clinical evaluation of a urine transport kit with lyophilized preservative for culture, urinalysis, and sediment microscopy. *Diagn Microbiol Infect Dis* 3:501–08, 1985.

30. Hindman R, Tronic B, Bartlett R. Effect of delay on culture of urine. *J Clin Microbiol* 4:102–03, 1976.

31. Kass EH. Asymptomatic infections of the urinary tract. *Trans Assoc Am Physicians* 69:56–64, 1956.

32. Stamm WE et al. Diagnosis of coliform infection in acutely dysuric women. *N Engl J Med* 307:463–68, 1982.

33. Robson MC, Heggers JP. Surgical infection. I. Single bacterial species or polymicrobic in origin? *Surgery* 65:608–10, 1969.

34. Lipkin ES et al. Comparison of monoclonal antibody staining and culture in diagnosing cervical chlamydial infection. *J Clin Microbiol* 23:114–17, 1986.

35. Morissey AM, Jacobs MR, Boxerbaum B. Value of bacterial antigen latex agglutination tests of body fluids in a teaching institution. In *Abstracts of the 1986 ICAAC.* Washington, DC: American Society for Microbiology, 1986. No. 71, p. 109.

36. Cuevas LE, Hart CA, Mughogho G. Latex particle agglutination tests as an adjunct to the diagnosis of bacterial meningitis: a study from Malawi. *Ann Trop Med Parasitol* 83:375–79, 1989.

37. Salih MAM et al. Rapid diagnosis of bacterial meningitis by an enzyme immunoassay of cerebrospinal fluid. *Epidemiol Infect* 103:301–10, 1989.

38. Pozzi G, Oggioni MR, Tomasz A. DNA probe for identification of Streptococcus pneumoniae. *J Clin Microbiol* 27:370–72, 1989.

39. Woodhead MA et al. A comparison of countercurrent immunoelectrophoresis and latex agglutination for the detection of pneumococcal antigen in a com-

munity based pneumonia study. *Serodiagn Immunother Infect Dis* 4:159–65, 1990.

40. Brandtzaeg P et al. Plasma endotoxin as a predictor of multiple organ failure and death in systemic meningococcal disease. *J Infect Dis* 159:195–204, 1989.

41. Arditi M, Ables L, Yogev R. Cerebrospinal fluid endotoxin levels in children with H. influenzae meningitis before and after administration of intravenous ceftriaxone. *J Infect Dis* 160:1005–11, 1989.

42. Bayston KF, Cohen J. Bacterial endotoxin and current concepts in the diagnosis and treatment of endotoxemia. *J Med Microbiol* 31:73–83, 1990.

43. Muchmore HG, Felton FG, Scott EN. Rapid presumptive identification of Cryptococcus neoformans. *J Clin Microbiol* 8:166–70, 1978.

44. Coovadia YM, Solwa Z. Sensitivity and specificity of a latex agglutination test for detection of cryptococcal antigen in meningitis. *S Afr Med J* 71:510–12, 1987.

45. Campbell CK et al. Cryptococcal latex antigen test positive in patient with Trichosporon beigelii infection [letter]. *Lancet* 2:43–44, 1985.

46. Eng RHK, Person A. Serum cryptococcal antigen determination in the presence of rheumatoid factor. *J Clin Microbiol* 14:700–02, 1981.

47. Stockman L, Roberts GD. Specificity of the latex test for cryptococcal antigen: a rapid, simple method for eliminating interference factors. *J Clin Microbiol* 17:945–47, 1983.

48. Goodman JS, Kaufman L, Koenig MG. Diagnosis of cryptococcal meningitis. *N Engl J Med* 285:434–46, 1971.

49. Perfect JR, Durack DT, Gallis HA. Cryptococcemia. *Medicine* 62:98–109, 1983.

50. Gordon MA, Vedder DK. Serologic tests in diagnosis and prognosis of cryptococcosis. *JAMA* 197:961–67, 1966.

51. Kellogg JA, Manzella JP. Detection of group A streptococci in the laboratory or physician's office. Culture vs. antibody methods. *JAMA* 255:2638–42, 1986.

52. Miller JM et al. Evaluation of the directigen group A strep test kit. *J Clin Microbiol* 20:846–48, 1984.

53. Wegner DL, Witte DL, Schrantz RD. Insensitivity of rapid antigen detection methods and single blood agar plate culture for diagnosing streptococcal pharyngitis. *JAMA* 267:695–97, 1992.

54. Slifkin M, Gil GM. Evaluation of the Culturette Brand Ten-Minute Strep ID technique. *J Clin Microbiol* 20:12–14, 1984.

55. Manasse RJ. Evaluation of the Pacific Biotech Cards Strep A test for detecting group A streptococci from throat cultures. *J Clin Microbiol* 27:1657–58, 1989.

56. Gerber MA et al. Antigen detection test for strep-

tococcal pharyngitis: evaluation of sensitivity with respect to true infections. *J Pediatr* 108:654–57, 1986.

57. Barnes R. Laboratory diagnosis of human chlamydial infections. *Clin Microbiol Rev* 2:119–36, 1989.

58. Gann PH et al. Accuracy of Chlamydia trachomatis antigen detection methods in a low-prevalence population in a primary care setting. *J Clin Microbiol* 28:1580–85, 1990.

59. Peterson EM et al. Molecular techniques for the detection of Chlamydia trachomatis. *J Clin Microbiol* 27:2359–63, 1989.

60. LeBar W et al. Comparison of DNA probe, monoclonal antibody enzyme immunoassay, and cell culture for the detection of Chlamydia trachomatis. *J Clin Microbiol* 27:826–28, 1989.

61. Wiesmeier E et al. Enzyme-linked immunosorbent assays in the detection of Chlamydia trachomatis: how valid are they? *Diagn Microbiol Infect Dis* 9:213–23, 1988.

62. Kellogg JA, Seiple JW, Levisky JS. Efficacy of duplicate genital specimens and repeated testing for confirming positive results for chlamydiazyme detection of Chlamydia trachomatis antigen. *J Clin Microbiol* 27:1218–21, 1989.

63. Sunstrum J. Herpes simplex infections: a review. *J Clin Immunoassay* 12:175–78, 1989.

64. Stamm WE et al. Antigen detection for the diagnosis of gonorrhea. *J Clin Microbiol* 19:399–403, 1984.

65. Papasian CJ, Bartholomew WR, Amsterdam D. Validity of an enzyme immunoassay for detection of Neisseria gonorrhoeae antigens. *J Clin Microbiol* 19:347–50, 1984.

66. Granato PA, Franz MR. Evaluation of a prototype DNA probe test for the noncultural diagnosis of gonorrhea. *J Clin Microbiol* 27:632–35, 1989.

67. Pezzlo M. Detection of urinary tract infections by rapid methods. *Clin Microbiol Rev* 1:268, 1988.

68. Brooks GF, York MK. Cost-effective clinical microbiology and newer tests of importance to the practitioner. In JS Remington, MN Swartz (eds.), *Current Clinical Topics in Infectious Diseases*. New York: McGraw-Hill, 1986.

69. Bowman RA, Riley TV. Routine culturing for Clostridium difficile? *Pathology* 16:240–42, 1984.

70. Bowman RA, Riley TV. Isolation of Clostridium difficile from stored specimens and comparative susceptibility of various tissue cell lines to cytotoxin. *FEMS Microbiology Letters* 34:31–35, 1986.

71. Bowman RA, Riley TV. Laboratory diagnosis of Clostridium difficile-associated diarrhoea. *Eur J Clin Microbiol Infect Dis* 7:476–84, 1988.

72. Laughon BE et al. Enzyme immunoassays for detec-

tion of Clostridium difficile toxins A and B in faecal specimens. *J Infect Dis* 149:781–88, 1984.

73. Pantosti A et al. Immunoblot analysis of serum immunoglobulin G response to surface proteins of Clostridium difficile in patients with antibiotic-associated diarrhea. *J Clin Microbiol* 27:2594–97, 1989.

74. Yolken RH et al. Enzyme immunoassay for the detection of Clostridium difficile antigen. *J Infect Dis* 144:378, 1981.

75. Tabaqchali S. Epidemiologic markers of Clostridium difficile. *Rev Infect Dis* 12 (suppl 2):S192–99, 1990.

76. Edelstein PH et al. Clinical utility of a monoclonal direct fluorescent reagent specific for Legionella pneumophila: comparative study with other reagents. *J Clin Microbiol* 22:419–21, 1985.

77. Pfaller MA. Laboratory diagnosis of infections due to Legionella species: practical application of DNA probes in the clinical microbiology laboratory. *Lab Med* 19:301–04, 1988.

78. Pasculle AW et al. Laboratory and clinical evalua-

tion of a commercial DNA probe for the detection of Legionella spp. *J Clin Microbiol* 27:2350–58, 1989.

79. Tang PW, Toma S, Rajkumar WD. Detection of urinary antigens of Legionella pneumophila serogroup 12 by broad-spectrum enzyme-linked immunosorbent assay. *J Clin Microbiol* 27:783–84, 1989.

80. Sathapatayavongs B et al. Rapid diagnosis of Legionnaire's disease by urinary antigen detection. *Am J Med* 72:576–82, 1982.

81. Tang PW, Toma S. Broad-spectrum enzyme-linked immunosorbent assay for detection of Legionella soluble antigens. *J Clin Microbiol* 24:556–58, 1986.

82. Bernet C et al. Detection of Mycoplasma pneumoniae by using the polymerase chain reaction. *J Clin Microbiol* 27:2492–96, 1989.

83. Marjaana Kleemola SR, Karjalainen JE, Raty RKH. Rapid diagnosis of Mycoplasma pneumoniae infection: clinical evaluation of a commercial probe test. *J Infect Dis* 162:70–75, 1990.

4

Anti-Infective Therapy in the Emergency Department

ROBIN L. DAVIS

Selection of an Antimicrobial Agent

Selection of an appropriate antimicrobial agent for the patient in the emergency department involves many considerations. The availability of new classes of antimicrobial agents, drugs that are well absorbed after oral administration (thus achieving serum concentrations that are effective for the treatment of a variety of disease states), and the changing pattern of pathogenic microbes and their antimicrobial susceptibility make the choice of an antimicrobial agent ever changing. Antimicrobial therapy should be tailored to the individual patient to achieve the most effective, least toxic, and most cost-effective therapy. The emergency department physician must take into consideration the site of infection, the clinical status of the patient, and the presumptive pathogen. Whenever possible the physician should use Gram's stains or other rapid methods for the identification of bacteria to help guide initial therapy. In most cases identification of the pathogen causing the infection will not be available for 24–48 hours. To avoid treatment delay and illness progression, empirical therapy of the most likely affecting organisms based on a variety of host and epidemiologic factors should be initiated.

The widespread indiscriminate use of antibiotics has led to increasing bacterial resistance. In selecting antibiotics, physicians should take into consid-

eration local resistance patterns in the community. For most uncomplicated community acquired infections, the use of a single agent is generally effective. For immunocompetent patients with uncomplicated infections, a bacteriostatic agent often is adequate to treat infection because of the contribution of the host defenses to the eradication of the organism. For immunocompromised patients or for life-threatening infections, a bactericidal agent is more appropriate. Antimicrobial agents are listed by their bactericidal or bacteriostatic activity in Table 4-1. It should be noted that drugs that generally achieve bactericidal activity may be bacteriostatic against some organisms, for example, vancomycin against enterococci.

Antibiotic combinations can be used to prevent the emergence of resistant organisms (such as in the treatment of tuberculosis), to broaden coverage against polymicrobial infections (such as peritoneal or pelvic infections), for presumptive initial therapy in neutropenic or other patients with multiple possible pathogens, or to achieve synergistic activity. Although synergism is frequently observed in vitro, only a few combinations achieve synergism clinically. Furthermore, synergistic combinations are drug and organism specific, and synergy will not necessarily be achieved with two drugs against all organisms. Clinical examples of synergistic drug combinations resulting in improved outcome are

Table 4-1. Effects of antimicrobial agents
on susceptible bacteria

Bactericidal Drugs
Aminoglycosides
Carbapenems
Cephalosporins
Glycopeptides (vancomycin, teicoplanin)
Metronidazole
Penicillin
Quinolones

Bacteriostatic Drugs
Chloramphenicol
Clindamycin
Macrolides (erythromycin, azithromycin)
Sulfonamides
Tetracyclines

the combination of an aminoglycoside with penicillin for the treatment of *Streptococcus viridans* or enterococcal endocarditis, a penicillinase-resistant penicillin against *Staphylococcus aureus* infections, and an antipseudomonal penicillin such as ticarcillin against *Pseudomonas aeruginosa*. A synergistic fixed combination of trimethoprim and sulfamethoxazole is available for the treatment of urinary tract infections. Amphotericin B and flucytosine are synergistic therapy for the treatment of cryptococcal meningitis [1]. Reasons to avoid using combinations of antibiotics include possible antimicrobial antagonism, additive toxicity, increased cost, increased drug preparation and administration time in hospitalized patients, and possibly poor compliance with the more complicated regimen in outpatients.

Pharmacologic properties of a drug are an important consideration to ensure that adequate concentrations of bacteriologically active drugs are achieved at the site of infection. A list of excellent pharmacology references is provided in Table 4-2. Also, many hospitals have clinical pharmacists or drug information centers.

Presumptive Therapy

The physician prescribing antimicrobial therapy in the emergency department rarely has the benefit of culture and sensitivity data as a guide in antibiotic selection. The prescribed regimen must be based on the most likely pathogens that could infect that anatomical site in that patient, which will vary with patient age, clinical status, and the severity of infection. More virulent, antibiotic-resistant, or opportunistic organisms cause infection in immunocompromised, elderly, or institutionalized patients. Pathogens for common infections are listed in Table 4-3. Initial or presumptive therapy should be broad enough to cover the most likely pathogens in a patient and narrowed after the infecting organism and its antibiotic susceptibility pattern have been identified.

Pharmacokinetics

The discipline of pharmacokinetics is the study of the absorption, distribution, metabolism, and excretion of a drug and the relationship of these processes to the time course of the drug in the body. Because of the complexities of the human body, these factors may differ among individuals and thus lead to vastly different antimicrobial concentrations and the resultant effects at the site of infection [2].

ABSORPTION

The rate and the extent of absorption of a drug often determine its utility for the treatment of serious infections. The *bioavailability* of an agent is the fraction absorbed after oral or parenteral administration compared to the same drug given intravenously. For some antibiotics, such as penicillin and dicloxacillin, poor or erratic absorption after oral administration limits their use in most situations to the treatment of mild to moderate infections caused by extremely susceptible organisms such that concentration of drug at the site of infection exceeds the minimum inhibitory concentration (MIC) for that organism by several fold [3, 4]. Other agents, such as metronidazole and trimethoprim-sulfamethoxazole, are well absorbed after oral administration [5, 6]. When taken less than one hour before or less than two hours after a meal, the absorption of some agents, such as dicloxacillin [4] and ampicillin [7], may be dramatically decreased while it may be enhanced for other drugs, such as griseofulvin [8] and cefuroxime axetil [9]. Food may slow the rate but not the extent of absorption for

Table 4-2. Useful pharmacology references

Reference	Comments
Drug Facts and Comparisons, Facts and Comparisons, Inc.	Groups drugs by therapeutic class, lists mechanism of action, indications, contraindications, warnings, adverse reactions, dosage and administration, and patient information. Unique advantages include monthly updates, tables comparing drugs within classes, relative cost index, and monographs on drugs prior to FDA approval.
American Hospital Formulary Service, American Society of Hospital Pharmacists	Published annually. Similar to *Drug Facts and Comparisons* but provides more detailed information on pharmacology, clinical use, and dosages used by their advisors. Computerized version lists references.
Martindale's: *The Extra Pharmacopoeia*, Pharmaceutical Press	Good resource for foreign compounds, unapproved uses, and unusual adverse reactions. Includes references.
The Use of Antibiotics, J. B. Lippincott, Inc.	Published approximately every 10 years; provides detailed, well-referenced information on all aspects of a drug.
Handbook of Clinical Drug Data, Drug Intelligence Publications, Inc.	Useful pocket-sized text. Provides practical information on all drug classes. Unique advantages include tables on drug-induced diseases, drugs in pregnancy and lactation, and drug interactions as well as drug monographs.
Guide to Antimicrobial Therapy, Antimicrobial Therapy, Inc.	Published annually; inexpensive, practical pocket resource.
Medical Letter Handbook of Antimicrobial Therapy, The Medical Letter, Inc.	Published every 2 years; inexpensive pocket-sized reference containing useful reviews from the Medical Letter.
Drug Interaction Facts, Facts and Comparisons, Inc., and *Drug Interactions*, Applied Therapeutics, Inc.	Updated quarterly; both provide referenced comprehensive lists of drug interactions, including the onset and clinical significance. Both also available on disk for personal computers.

other drugs, such as cephalexin [10] and ciprofloxacin [11]. Ketoconazole requires an acid environment for absorption, and its effectiveness may be diminished in patients with achlorhydria or receiving drugs that decrease or neutralize gastric acid secretion [12]. Table 4-4 lists some of commonly used antibiotics and when they should be taken in regard to meals. Absorption may increase linearly over the dosage range, as is the case with ketoconazole [13]. The extent of absorption may also be dose dependent. The bioavailability of acyclovir decreases with increasingly larger doses [14].

DISTRIBUTION

Once a drug reaches the blood stream, either by intravenous injection or by absorption from the gastrointestinal tract or tissue from a parenteral injection, to be effective in the treatment of an infection it must diffuse, or distribute, from the blood stream to the site of infection and achieve concentrations high enough at that site to have an antimicrobial effect. High serum concentrations do not necessarily ensure adequate antibiotic concentrations at the infected tissue site.

The distribution of a drug in the body is described by the term *volume of distribution*. This is not an actual volume but rather a proportionality constant that relates the amount of drug in the body to its concentration in the serum. The volume of distribution is therefore often referred to as an "apparent" volume, since it does not represent a true physiologic space [2]. Drugs that bind avidly to plasma proteins, such as ceftriaxone [15], are held in the central circulation and exhibit small volumes of distribution. Polar agents, like aminoglycosides, distribute to extracellular fluid [16]. Patients with disease states that have increased extracellular fluid, such as ascites or congestive heart failure, require larger doses given at less frequent intervals to achieve the same peak serum concentrations and

Table 4-3. Usual pathogens that cause common infections

Site and type of infection	Suspected organisms
Respiratory	
Pharyngitis	Group A streptococci
Bronchitis, otitis, sinusitis	H. influenzae, S. pneumoniae
Pneumonia	
Community-acquired	
Normal host	S. pneumoniae
Aspiration	Normal oropharyngeal flora
Pediatrics	S. pneumoniae, H. influenzae
COPD	S. pneumoniae, H. influenzae
Alcoholic	S. pneumoniae, K. pneumoniae
Hospital-acquired	
Aspiration	Mouth anaerobes, gram-negative aerobic bacilli, S. aureus
Neutropenic	Fungi, gram-negative aerobic bacilli, S. aureus
AIDS	Fungi, pneumocystis, legionellae, nocardiae, H. influenzae, pneumococci
Urinary Tract	
Community-acquired	E. coli, other gram-negative bacilli
Hospital-acquired	Resistant gram-negative bacilli
Skin/Soft Tissue	
Cellulitis	Group A streptococci
IV catheter site	S. aureus, S. epidermidis
Surgical wound	S. aureus, gram-negative bacilli
Diabetic ulcer	S. aureus, gram-negative bacilli, anaerobes
Furuncle	S. aureus
Intra-abdominal	B. fragilis, E. coli, enterococci
Gastroenteritis	Salmonella, Shigella, Campylobacter, amoebae, giardia, viruses
Endocarditis	
Subacute	S. viridans
Acute	S. aureus
IV drug abuser	S. aureus, gram-negative aerobic bacilli
Osteomyelitis/Septic Arthritis	S. aureus, streptococci, gram-negative aerobic bacilli
Meningitis	
<2 months	E. coli, group B streptococci, listeriae
2 months to 12 years	H. influenzae, S. pneumoniae, N. meningiditis
Adults	S. pneumoniae, N. meningiditis
Elderly, immuno-compromised	S. pneumoniae, listeriae, gram-negative bacilli

Adapted from BJ Guglielmo. Principles of antimicrobial therapy. In *Applied Therapeutics: The Clinical Use of Drugs* (4th ed.). Applied Therapeutics, Inc., 1988, P. 723; and DP Alexander. Central nervous system infections. In ET Herfindal, DR Gourley, LL Hart (eds.), *Clinical Pharmacy and Therapeutics* (4th ed.). Baltimore: Williams & Wilkins, 1988, pp. 780–91.

the same trough serum concentrations as other patients. Many drugs do not readily penetrate into the cerebrospinal fluid (CSF) and are either ineffective (e.g., clindamycin, first-generation cephalosporins, and erythromycin) or require very high doses (e.g., penicillin) for the treatment of meningitis.

Lipophilic agents, such as acyclovir and chloramphenicol, as well as the less lipophilic third-generation cephalosporins, readily cross cell membranes and achieve relatively high concentrations in most tissues, including the CNS [17]. The CSF penetration of commonly used antimicrobial agents

Table 4-4. Guidelines on food intake and absorption of orally administered antimicrobial agents

Drugs That Can Be Taken Without Regard to Meals	
Acyclovir	Doxycycline
Amoxicillin	Erythromycin estolate
Cefaclor	Fluconazole
Cefixime	Metronidazole
Cephradine, cephalexin	Minocycline
Ciprofloxacin	Ofloxacin
Clindamycin	Penicillin V

Drugs That Should Be Taken on an Empty Stomach[a]
Ampicillin
Dicloxacillin, oxacillin
Erythromycin base and stearate
Ketoconazole
Norfloxacin
Sulfonamides
Tetracycline

Drugs for Which Absorption Is Enhanced by Food
Cefuroxime axetil
Griseofulvin[b]

[a] At least one hour before or two hours after meals.
[b] Absorption is enhanced by ingestion with a high-fat meal.

is listed in Table 4-5. Other sites, such as the prostate, may be difficult to penetrate because of the pH of the local environment and therefore may not be treated effectively with many drugs that the laboratory reports as microbiologically sensitive. The new fluoroquinolones [18] and trimethoprim-sulfamethoxazole [6] are useful agents for acute and chronic prostatic infections because of their excellent penetration.

METABOLISM AND EXCRETION

Anti-infectives are categorized by the primary route of elimination, as shown in Table 4-6. The majority of antimicrobial agents are eliminated by the kidneys, so dosages need to be adjusted in patients with renal dysfunction. Dosage recommendations for those patients are often available in the manufacturers' product literature, in nomograms, and in a variety of secondary references [19, 20]. For drugs that undergo hepatic metabolism, fewer guidelines for dosage recommendations exist. The elimination of drugs such as erythromycin, ketoconazole, and rifampin is prolonged in patients with hepatic failure and may require dosage adjustments in those patients.

Host Factors

EPIDEMIOLOGY

A number of patient-specific factors may limit the response to an antibiotic. The clinical setting in which the organism was acquired may influence the resistance patterns of the infecting organism. Infections that occur while patients are in nursing homes or hospitalized are likely to be caused by organisms more resistant to antibiotics than those acquired in the community. Infections in immunocompromised hosts may be due to opportunistic organisms that do not normally cause infection in immunocompetent hosts. For example, *Pneumocystis carinii* rarely causes disease in normal hosts, but it is a common respiratory pathogen in patients with AIDS [21]. Patients who have received recent courses of antimicrobial therapy may develop infections with organisms resistant to that drug. For example, a patient with recurrent urinary tract infections treated with ampicillin may subsequently develop an infection caused by an ampicillin-resistant organism. Cultures obtained after antibiotic therapy has begun can yield misleading negative results. A history of adverse reactions with classes of drugs can also limit the usefulness of certain agents. Drugs that frequently cause an adverse reaction, such as erythromycin, should be avoided if possible in patients who report a prior history of intolerance to that drug.

SITE OF INFECTION

The site of infection is of paramount importance in the choice of an antibiotic, the route of administration, the need for combination therapy with more than one agent, the dosage, and the duration of therapy. Infections for which it is difficult to achieve therapeutic concentrations of antibiotics, such as meningitis or the vegetation of bacterial endocarditis, usually require high-dosage, parenteral antibiotic therapy.

Therapeutic serum concentrations of antibiotics may not ensure microbiologically active concentrations at the site of infection. For example, aminoglycosides have reduced antibacterial activity at purulent sites of infection and require high concentrations of drug to treat pneumonia compared to other sites [22, 23]. Conversely the concentrations of aminoglycosides achieved in the urine greatly exceed serum concentrations. Lower dosages can be used to treat uncomplicated lower urinary tract in-

Table 4-5. CSF concentration of antimicrobial agents

Agent	CSF/serum concentration with inflamed meningitis (%)	Agent	CSF/serum concentration with inflamed meningitis (%)
Penicillins		*Antimycobacterial Agents*	
Ampicillin	8–13	Cycloserine	100
Methicillin	3–12	Ethambutol	25–30
Mezlocillin	14	Isoniazid	100
Nafcillin	9–20	Para-amino salicylic acid	poor
Penicillin G	3	Pyrazinamide	100
Piperacillin	16	Rifampin	10–30
Ticarcillin	10	Streptomycin	10–40
Cephalosporins		*Miscellaneous Antibacterials*	
Cefamandole	1–20	Aminoglycosides	10–30
Cefazolin	1–4	Clindamycin	minimal
Cefoperazone	2–3	Chloramphenicol	45–99
Cefotaxime	10–25	Ciprofloxacin	15–40
Cefotetan	1–4	Erythromycin	6–10
Ceftazidime	22	Tetracycline/doxycycline	10–25
Ceftriaxone	7–11	Vancomycin	7–21
Cefuroxime	11–56	*Antifungal Agents*	
Cephalothin	1–6	Amphotericin B	2–3
Beta-lactamase Inhibitors		Fluconazole	50–90
Clavulanate	8	Flucytosine	70
Sulbactam	2–20	Itraconazole	not detected
Sulfonamides		Ketoconazole	poor
Sulfadiazine	50–80	*Antiviral Agents*	
Sulfamethoxazole	25–30	Acyclovir	50
Trimethoprim	30–50	Amantadine	50–60
		Ganciclovir	24–67
		Zidovudine	50–100

Adapted from S Norris, CH Mandell. Tables of antimicrobial agent pharmacology. In GL Mandell, RG Douglas Jr, JE Bennett (eds.), *Principles and Practice of Infectious Diseases* (3rd ed.). New York: Churchill-Livingstone, 1990.

fections in patients with normal renal function [15]. Patients with uncomplicated cystitis can be adequately treated in as few as 3 days, while patients with pyelonephritis require 14 days of therapy [24]. Bacterial endocarditis is generally treated with high-dosage parenteral combination therapy [25].

AGE

The organisms that cause disease, the dosage of antimicrobials used to treat infection, and drug toxicities are influenced by the age of the patient. For example, neonatal meningitis is most com-

monly caused by group B streptococci, *Escherichia coli*, and *Listeria monocytogenes*. *Haemophilus influenzae* type B, *Neisseria meningitidis*, and *Streptococcus pneumoniae* are the major pathogens that cause meningitis in children aged 2 months to 5 years. In older children and adults meningococcus and pneumococcus are the major pathogens. In adults over age 60 years pneumococcus, *L. monocytogenes*, and gram-negative bacilli once again become important pathogens [26].

Children should not receive treatment with certain drugs, because of age-related toxicity. Tetra-

Table 4-6. Major routes of elimination for antimicrobial agents

Renal	Hepatic	Renal and hepatic
Antibacterial Agents		
Aminoglycosides	Clindamycin	Azlocillin
Cephalosporins[a]	Chloramphenicol	Cefotaxime[b]
Ethambutol	Cefaperazone (biliary)	Ciprofloxacin
Penicillins[a]	Erythromycin	Dicloxacillin
Sulfasoxazole	Metronidazole	Doxycycline
Tetracycline	Rifampin	Mezlocillin
Trimethoprim	Isoniazid[c]	Nafcillin
Vancomycin		Piperacillin
		Sulfamethoxazole[d]
Antifungal Agents		
Fluconazole	Ketoconazole	
Flucytosine		
Antiviral Agents		
Acyclovir	Zidovudine	
Amantadine		
Ganciclovir		

[a] See exceptions in other categories.
[b] Active des-acetyl metabolite accumulates in end-stage renal disease.
[c] Renal route (30%) in slow acetylators.
[d] Renal route in slow acetylators.

cyclines bind avidly to developing bone and tooth structures and can cause a brownish discoloration of the teeth or enamel hypoplasia if administered to children or to pregnant women [27]. Quinolones are reported to cause arthropathy, gait abnormalities, and articular cartilage lesions in weight-bearing joints in young animals and have not been approved by the FDA for the use in children [28]. Age-dependent pharmacokinetic differences affect the dosages of drugs needed to achieve similar serum concentrations in different groups. Neonates and premature infants have a larger proportion of their body weight as water compared to adults. The resulting increased volume of distribution for water-soluble drugs requires larger dosages of drugs given less frequently to neonates compared to older children and adults. Decreased hepatic metabolism necessitates lower dosages of hepatically eliminated drugs to avoid toxicity (e.g., "gray syndrome" associated with the use of chloramphenicol). Undeveloped renal function requires a reduction in dosages of drugs eliminated by the kidney, such as

aminoglycosides, penicillin, and cephalosporins [1, 29].

Elderly patients may require lower dosages of drugs than older children and adults because they may have longer drug half-lives due to reduced hepatic and renal function. Elderly patients may also suffer a higher frequency of adverse effects from therapeutic serum concentrations than younger patients. Although gastric hydrochloric acid secretion diminishes with increasing age, the absorption of antibiotics (except ketoconazole, which requires acidity for absorption) is unchanged compared to younger patients. A reduction in the percentage of body weight as water and an increase in the percentage of fat alter the volume of distribution of many drugs. Drugs like aminoglycosides that distribute to extracellular fluid may be given in lower dosages to achieve the same serum concentrations as in younger patients. Lipophilic drugs distribute to fat tissue, yielding longer half-lives. Lower dosages and longer intervals between doses may be needed for drugs eliminated by the kidneys, such

as penicillins, cephalosporins, and the fluoroquinolones [29].

RENAL AND HEPATIC FUNCTION

Antimicrobial agents are listed by their primary
route of elimination in Table 4-6. Dosages of most
antimicrobial agents should be individualized for
each patient, based on hepatic or renal function.
Most antimicrobial agents are largely eliminated by
the kidneys. It is therefore desirable to estimate the
glomerular filtration rate for patients in whom impaired renal function is suspected by calculating an
estimated creatinine clearance before prescribing
the dosage of a drug. Since creatinine is a by-
product of normal muscle metabolism and is eliminated by the kidneys, its serum concentration depends on its rate of production (i.e., muscle mass)
and its elimination (renal function). It should be
noted that a normal serum creatinine, especially in
the upper end of the normal range, may be a reflection of decreased renal function in the patient with
decreased muscle mass or a cachectic or elderly
patient. Therefore, it is desirable to calculate a
creatinine clearance, formulas for which are readily
available [30]. Drug dosages in patients with decreased renal function can be found in the manufacturers' product literature or any variety of secondary
references [19, 20]. Examples of drugs that require
no modification in impaired renal function are
erythromycin, clindamycin, orally administered
chloramphenicol, cefoperazone, and metronidazole. In general most penicillins, cephalosporins,
quinolones, vancomycin, and fluconazole require
some modification in dosage, especially in patients
with severe renal impairment.

Drugs that undergo hepatic metabolism should
be given in reduced dosages in patients with hepatic
dysfunction. Examples of these drugs are chloramphenicol and ketoconazole. Unfortunately no
clear guidelines for dosage reduction in these patients exist but must be made based on an evaluation of the patient's clinical status and clinical response. Drugs that undergo hepatic metabolism
should be used cautiously in patients with severe
liver dysfunction, and patients should be closely
evaluated for signs and symptoms of toxicity [1, 29].

PREGNANCY

Physiologic changes during pregnancy may necessitate changes in drug regimens. Absorption of drugs
administered orally may be slowed or decreased.

The volume of distribution for most drugs is increased. Decreased plasma protein binding during
pregnancy may also increase the volume of distribution for some drugs. Increases in renal blood flow
result in enhanced clearance of drugs eliminated by
the kidneys, altering dosage requirements. Combined, these factors can result in the need to administer larger doses in pregnant women. The hepatic
metabolism of antimicrobials in pregnancy, however, does not appear to be affected for most drugs
[29]. Virtually all antibiotics cross the placenta,
exposing the fetus to potential adverse drug effects.
Pregnancy status should always be considered in
women of childbearing age. Few large-scale studies
evaluating the safety of antimicrobials during pregnancy have been done. Drugs must therefore be
used judiciously in the pregnant patient.

Risk factors have been defined by the Food and
Drug Administration (FDA) [31] based on the
strength of the data supporting the relative risk or
safety of a drug during pregnancy and lactation.
These categories range from controlled studies in
humans demonstrating no fetal risk in the first
trimester with the possibility of fetal harm remote
(category A) to animal or human studies demonstrating fetal abnormalities where the risk outweighs any potential benefit from the use of the
drug (category X). Unfortunately few drugs have
been assigned risk factors by their manufacturers.
However, the available data have been reviewed,
and risk factors for many drugs have been assigned
by the authors of a recent publication [32]. Other
sources provide frequently updated lists of antimicrobials that can be used safely in pregnancy
[19]. It appears that most penicillins, cephalosporins, and erythromycin are safe to use in pregnancy. Metronidazole and ticarcillin are teratogenic in animals and should be avoided. The
potential for teratogenicity of many other antimicrobials is unclear [1, 29]. Based on the best
currently available data, antimicrobials that appear
safe and those that should be avoided in pregnancy
are listed in Table 4-7.

LACTATION

Most antimicrobial agents administered in therapeutic doses to lactating women appear in measurable concentrations in their breast milk. Normally
the concentrations of drugs that appear in the
breast milk are low, but they may still cause adverse

Table 4-7. Safety of antimicrobial agents in pregnancy

Contraindicated	Use with caution[a]		Probably safe
Amantadine	Acyclovir	Iodoquinol	Aztreonan
Griseofulvin	Aminoglycosides	Ketoconazole	Cephalosporins
Lindane	Amphotericin B	Mebendazole	Chloroquine (low doses)
Quinolones	Antituberculars	Mefloquine	Erythromycin (except estolate)
Ribavirin	Clindamycin	Metronidazole	Methenamine
Tetracyclines	Crotamiton	Pentamidine	Nystatin
	Dapsone[b]	Quinacrine	Pencillins
	Fluconazole	Trimethoprim	Permethrin
	Flucytosine	Vancomycin	Praziquantel
	Furazolidone[c]	Zidoviol	Sulfonamides[c]
	Ganciclovir		

[a] Use only if there is a strong indication and no alternative agent; many of these agents are animal teratogens.
[b] Especially at term.
[c] Contraindicated at term.
Adapted from The Medical Letter, Inc., *The Medical Letter Handbook of Antimicrobial Therapy.* New York: The Medical Letter Inc., 1990.

Table 4-8. Safety of drugs in lactation

Effect	Drug	
Effects unknown but may be of concern	Chlorampenicol, metronidazole	
Hemolysis reported in G6PD-deficient infants	Nalidixic acid, nitrofurantoin	
Caution in G6PD-deficient, jaundiced, premature, ill, or stressed infants	Sulfonamide	
Usually compatible with breast-feeding with no reported adverse effects on infants	Acyclovir	Ethambutol
	Amoxicillin	Hydroxychloroquine
	Aztreonam	Isoniazid
	Cefadroxil	Pyrimethamine
	Cefazolin	Quinine
	Cefotaxime	Rifampin
	Cefoxitin	Streptomycin
	Ceftazidime	Sulbactam
	Ceftriaxone	Tetracycline
	Chloroquine	Ticarcillin
	Clindamycin	Trimethoprim/sulfamethoxazole
	Cycloserine	
	Dapsone	
	Erythromycin	

Adapted from American Academy of Pediatrics Committee on Drugs. Transfer of drugs and other chemicals into human milk. *Pediatr* 84:924–36, 1989.

effects in the nursing infant. The percentage of a drug excreted into breast milk depends on its ionization, molecular weight, and lipophilicity. Drugs that are lipophilic and neutral or basic in blood accumulate in acidic breast milk. Nalidixic acid has been reported to cause hemolysis in infants deficient in glucose-6-phosphate dehydrogenase (G6PD). Sul-

fonamides may displace bilirubin in hypoalbuminemic infants, causing kernicterus [1, 29]. Even small amounts in breast milk may be dangerous to those infants. Extensive evaluations· of the safety of drugs in lactation have recently been published [32, 33] (see Chap. 29). The effects of certain drugs on lactation are listed in Table 4-8.

Cost

Because of the growing number of antimicrobial agents that have become available, the clinician often has several drugs to choose from that could be equally effective in the treatment of an infection. The cost of the antibiotic then, either to the patient or to the institution, should be an important consideration in the selection of a drug. The costs for several antibiotics that are equally effective in treating an uncomplicated urinary tract infection are listed in Table 4-9. As illustrated in the table, the costs of treatments differ widely.

Other factors may also contribute to the total cost of a course of therapy. Hospitalized patients receiving intravenous antibiotic therapy will also have associated costs of drug preparation and administration. Laboratory monitoring for adverse effects, such as renal function in patients on aminoglycoside therapy, also leads to increased costs. Oral therapy, even with an expensive agent, is almost always less expensive than parenteral therapy. Generic drugs are less costly than brand-name agents. References are available that provide the average wholesale cost to the pharmacy or the relative cost of a product (see Table 4-2). Patient charges may vary based on the additional dispensing charges added by the pharmacy. Average wholesale costs for oral and parenteral anti-infectives are listed in Tables 4-10 and 4-11.

Toxicity

Antimicrobial agents can cause drug-specific direct toxic effects or adverse effects that could be caused by any antimicrobial agent. Many drugs can cause a hypersensitivity reaction, with symptoms ranging from fever to mild rash to anaphylaxis. A careful drug history should be taken to avoid the administration of a drug class to which the patient previously has suffered a hypersensitivity reaction. Although the absolute occurrence rate of hypersensitivity reactions with various classes of antibiotics is not clear, they are more common with penicillins and sulfonamides but occur rarely with aminoglycosides [1, 29]. Vancomycin can cause a nonallergic rash that can be avoided by slowing the rate of infusion [34]. It was previously estimated that 5%–10% of penicillin-allergic patients are also allergic to cephalosporins. More recently this figure has been lowered to less than 2% [35]. In a series of 62 patients with positive penicillin skin tests given cephalosporins on the day of skin testing, only 1 patient developed a reaction (mild urticaria and bronchospasm) [35].

Many infectious disease specialists hold that cephalosporins can be given to a penicillin-allergic patient if the patient has a history of only a minor allergic reaction, for example, minor urticaria, without any major anaphylactic reaction with bronchospasm or hypotension. Although the incidence of cross-reactivity may be low, because of the life-threatening nature of anaphylaxis and the lack of proven tests that predict cephalosporin hypersensitivity, the most prudent course would be never to give a cephalosporin to a patient with a history of type I hypersensitivity reactions to penicillin (or with a positive reaction to any penicillin reagent on skin testing), unless alternative drugs are unacceptable or less desirable. This issue remains unsettled, and each situation must be analyzed individually. Cephalosporin use in these patients is guided by the severity of the previous allergic reaction, the availability of acceptable alternative agents, and clinical judgment. It should be noted that most fatal allergic reactions to B-lactam antibiotics occur in individuals who have never had a previous allergic reaction [36]. In clinical practice the majority of patients with a history of "allergy to penicillin" receive cephalosporins without any adverse reaction. While some specialists advocate documenting a history of penicillin allergy with skin testing, this procedure is not appropriate in an emergency department [37]. It should also be noted that the commercially available penicillin skin-testing

Table 4-9. Pharmacy costs for similar 10-day courses of antibiotic therapy

Drug	Dosage	Cost* ($)
Amoxicillin	250 mg po q8h	2.43
Cephradine	250 mg po q6h	11.37
Trimethoprim/ sulfamethoxazole	1 DS q12h	1.35
Ciprofloxacin	250 mg po q12h	21.36

* Cost to pharmacy; patient charges will be higher.
Source: Medi-Span, Inc., *Medi-Span Prescription Pricing Guide.* Indianapolis: Medi-Span, Inc., April 1991.

Table 4-10. Dosages and costs of oral anti-infectives

Drug	Adult dosage	Cost for 10 days of therapy ($)[*]
Penicillins		
Amoxicillin (generic)	250–500 mg q6h	5–10
Amoxicillin-clavulanic acid (Augmentin)	250–500 mg q8h	39–79
Ampicillin (generic)	500–1000 mg q6h	7–13
Carbenicillin	382–764 mg q6h	53–106
Cloxacillin (generic)	500–1000 mg q6h	24–48
Dicloxacillin (generic)	250–500 mg q6h	14–29
Penicillin V (generic)	250–500 mg q6h	3–5
Cephalosporins		
Cefaclor	250–500 mg q8h	45–89
Cefadroxil (generic)	250–500 mg q6h	36–73
Cefixime	400 mg q12–24h	44–88
Cefuroxime axetil	250–500 mg q12h	24–47
Cephalexin (generic)	250–1000 mg q6h	16–54
Cephradine (generic)	250–1000 mg q6h	19–57
Erythromycins		
Base (generic)	250–500 mg q6h	5–10
Enteric-coated base (generic)	250–500 mg q6h	9–19
Ethylsuccinate (generic)	250–500 mg q6h	9–17
Fluoroquinolones		
Ciprofloxacin	250–750 mg q12h	40–91
Norfloxacin	400 mg q12h	39
Sulfonamides and Trimethoprim		
Sulfamethoxazole/trimethoprim (generic)	800/160 mg q12h	8
Sulfasoxazole (generic)	500 mg q6h	2
Trimethoprim (generic)	100 mg q12h	4
Tetracyclines		
Doxycycline (generic)	50–100 mg q12h	3–5
Tetracycline (generic)	250–500 mg q6h	2–5
Miscellaneous Antibacterials		
Clindamycin (generic)	150–450 mg q6h	35–106
Metronidazole (generic)	250–500 mg q6h	6–11
Nitrofurantoin (generic macrocrystals)	50–100 mg q6h	15–29
Vancomycin	125–500 mg q6h	189–370
Antifungal Agents		
Clotrimazole	10 mg 5 times daily	25
Fluconazole	200–400 mg q24h	90–180
Griseofulvin-ultrafine	330–660 mg q24h	23–46
Ketoconazole	200–400 mg q24h	18–37
Nystatin (generic)	500,000u qid	19
Antiviral Agents		
Acyclovir	200–800 mg 5 times daily	34–134
Amantadine	100 mg q12–24h	3–6
Zidovudine	100 mg 3–5 times daily	42–72

[*] Costs are average wholesale prices rounded to the nearest dollar. Generic costs are averages.
Drug Topics Red Book, 1990.

Table 4-11. Dosages and costs of parenteral anti-infectives for moderate and severe infections

| Drug | Dosage | | Cost/day ($)[b] |
	Moderate infection	Severe infection	
Penicillins			
Ampicillin (generic)	0.5–1 g q6h	2 g q4–6h	4–24
Ampicillin/sulbactam	1.5 g q6h	3 g q6h	22–44
Carbenicillin	200 mg/kg/d	400–500 mg/kg/d	27–66
Mezlocillin	3–4 g q6–8h	3–4 g q4–6h	35–86
Nafcillin (generic)	0.5-1 g q6h	2 g q4h	9–52
Penicillin G (generic)	2 mU q6h	2–4 mU q4h	1–15
Piperacillin	3–4 g q6–8h	3–4 g q4–6h	39–78
Ticarcillin	1 g q6h	3 g q4–6h	11–49
Ticarcillin-clavulanate	—	3.1 g q4–6h	44
Aztreonam	1–2 g q8–12h	2 g q6–8h	41–105
Cephalosporins			
Cefazolin (generic)	0.5–1 g q8h	2 g q8h	9–35
Cefotaxime	1–2 g q8–12h	2 g q6h	28–75
Ceftazidime	1 g q8h	2 g q8h	41–83
Ceftriaxone	1–2 g q2–4h	1–2 g q12–24h	28–112
Cefuroxine	750 mg q8h	1.5 g q8h	20–40
Aminoglycosides			
Amikacin	5 mg/kg q8h	5 mg/kg q8h	86
Tobramycin (generic)	1 mg/kg q8h	1.5 mg/kg q8h	22–33
Gentamicin (generic)	1 mg/kg q8h	1.5 mg/kg q8h	4–6
Tetracyclines			
Doxycycline	100 mg q24h	100 mg q12h	20–41
Tetracycline	250–500 mg q12h	500 mg q6h	10–40
Miscellaneous Antibacterials			
Chloramphenicol (generic)	50 mg/kg/d	50–100 mg/kg/d	17–35
Clindamycin (generic)	300–600 mg q6–8h	900 mg q8h	16–32
Erythromycin (generic)	500 mg q6h	1 g q6h	12–24
Metronidazole (generic)	7.5 mg/kg/d q6h	7.5 mg/kg/d q6h	33
Vancomycin (generic)	500 mg q6h or 1 g q12h	500 mg q6h or 1 g q12h	80

[a] Meningitis dosages may be higher for some drugs.
[b] Costs are average wholesale prices, rounded to the nearest dollar, and do not include preparation and administration charges. Prices for generic drugs are averaged.
Source: Drug Topics Red Book, 1991.

product does not test for the antigenic determinant that causes type I hypersensitivity reactions [36]. Periodic review of this issue with local infectious disease subspecialists may be reasonable. As a general rule, in cases of sepsis where this allergic issue arises and the clinician wants to avoid a B-lactam antibiotic (penicillins or cephalosporins) for gram-positive coverage, vancomycin is the antibiotic most frequently recommended as a substitute [38]. Chloramphenicol has also been used in situations where a pneumococcal or meningococcal infection is present in a penicillin-allergic patient [39]. Alternatively patients can be treated with the monobactam antibiotic aztreonam, which is only weakly cross-reactive with penicillin antibiotics and can be safely administered to most penicillin-allergic patients [40, 41]. This agent lacks activity against aerobic gram-positive and anaerobic bacteria. If therapy with penicillins is absolutely necessary, rapid oral or parenteral desensitization methods are available [36].

Any broad-spectrum antibiotic can cause gastrointestinal upset and diarrhea either by direct effect or by alterations in the gastrointestinal microflora. This is normally a benign condition that resolves after discontinuation of the antibiotic and usually does not require a change in therapy. Antibiotic-associated colitis (AAC) and pseudomembranous colitis are the most serious gastrointestinal disorders implicated in antibiotic use. Thought to be due to S. aureus in the 1950s, it is now known to be caused by a cytopathic toxin produced by resistant strains of Clostridium difficile that are allowed to overgrow when antibiotic-sensitive flora are suppressed [42]. The antibiotic-specific relative risk of developing AAC has never been evaluated in controlled clinical trials, but most reported cases in the past decade have been caused by clindamycin, lincomycin, ampicillin, and cephalosporins. Clindamycin has been estimated to cause AAC in 1 in 10 to 1 in 10,000 patients in various reports [42]. The patient typically presents with profuse watery or mucoid green, foul-smelling diarrhea and abdominal pain. Patients may also experience high fevers and bloody diarrhea. These symptoms occur most commonly after several days of antibiotic therapy, but patients may present with symptoms after antibiotic therapy has been discontinued and should be thoroughly questioned for prior antibiotic use over the past several weeks. Untreated disease may resolve when the antimicrobial therapy is discontinued, or it may cause life-threatening colitis. Prompt discontinuation of antimicrobial therapy, if possible, is indicated. Vancomycin and metronidazole have been used successfully to treat infections, but both are associated with relapses after discontinuation of therapy [42].

Changes in resident microflora after treatment with broad-spectrum antibacterials commonly lead to infections due to Candida albicans. Inhibition of the normal vulvovaginal bacterial flora can lead to vaginal candidiasis. Overgrowth by C. albicans can also cause oral thrush or systemic infections.

Interactions of Anti-Infectives with Commonly Used Drugs

Antimicrobials can induce or inhibit the metabolism of other commonly used drugs, causing a reduction in their pharmacologic effect or an increase in their potential toxicity. Examples of important interactions are listed in Table 4-12 [17, 43, 44].

Route of Administration

For most mild to moderate infections, patients can be treated with orally administered antibiotics. This is the preferred route of administration in the outpatient setting. Exceptions to this method would be drugs that are not absorbed when given orally, such as vancomycin, aminoglycosides, and amphotericin B. Serious infections require treatment with parenteral antibiotics. Most drugs can be given by either the intravenous or the intramuscular route of administration. Adequate serum concentrations can be achieved after intramuscular injection in most cases if injected into a well-perfused muscle. Intramuscular injections should not be given to patients in shock. Because of the possibility of tissue necrosis, some drugs, such as vancomycin, amphotericin B, and pentamidine, should not be given by the intramuscular route.

Many clinicians may feel it useful to initiate therapy with a parenteral dose of a drug in the emergency department and follow with oral outpatient treatment. This will not improve outcome in a noncompliant patient, but will result only in a partially treated infection. Similarly no studies indicate that giving a single dose of one class of drugs (e.g., ampicillin and gentamicin) followed by oral therapy with another class (e.g., a sulfonamide) will improve outcome. This approach could result in an infection that is only partially treated by the parenteral agent and make follow-up assessment by the primary care physician difficult to evaluate. It does not speed the onset of the effect of the oral drug, which still requires five elimination half-lives to reach steady-state concentration [2]. In general 24–48 hours of therapy are required before significant improvement is obtained. Therefore, giving one or two doses of an intravenous drug and then

Table 4-12. Interactions of anti-infectives with selected commonly used drugs

Drug	Mechanism	Effect
Cephalosporins with . . .		
Alcohol	Inhibition of intermediary metabolism of alcohol by MTT side chain of cefamandole, cefoperazone, and moxalactam	Disulfiram-like reaction
Anticoagulants	Antiprothrombinemic effect of MTT side chain	Increases degree of anticoagulation and risk of bleeding
Chloramphenicol with . . .		
Hypoglycemics (sulfonylureas)	Decreased sulfonylurea metabolism	Increased hypoglycemic effect
Phenytoin	Decreased phenytoin metabolism	Possible phenytoin toxicity
Theophylline	Decreased theophylline metabolism	Possible theophylline toxicity
Warfarin	Decreased warfarin metabolism	Increased degree of anticoagulation and risk of bleeding
Erythromycin with . . .		
Carbamazepine	Decreased carbamazepine metabolism	Possible carbamazepine toxicity
Cyclosporine	Decreased cyclosporine metabolism	Possible cyclosporine toxicity
Fluconazole with . . .		
Hypoglycemics (sulfonylureas)	Decreased sulfonylurea metabolism	Increased hypoglycemic effect
Phenytoin	Decreased phenytoin metabolism	Possible phenytoin toxicity
Rifampin	Increased fluconazole metabolism	Possible decreased antifungal activity
Warfarin	Decreased warfarin metabolism	Increased anticoagulant effect
Fluoroquinolones with . . .		
Antacids	Decreased quinolone absorption	Decreased antibacterial activity
Theophylline	Decreased theophylline metabolism	Possible theophylline toxicity
Warfarin	Decreased warfarin metabolism	Increased anticoagulant effect
Griseofulvin with . . .		
Oral contraceptives	Increased hormone metabolism	Decreased contraceptive effect
Warfarin	Increased warfarin metabolism	Decreased anticoagulant effect
Ketoconazole with . . .		
Antacids	Decreased ketoconazole absorption	Decreased antifungal effect
Cyclosporine	Decreased cyclosporine metabolism	Increased concentration of cyclosporine in blood
Warfarin	Decreased warfarin metabolism	Increased anticoagulant effect and possible bleeding
H_2 antagonists	Decreased ketoconazole absorption	Possible decreased antifungal effect
Isoniazid	Decreased blood concentrations	Decreased ketoconazole effect
Phenytoin	Altered phenytoin metabolism	Altered effects of one or both drugs
Rifampin	Decreased blood concentrations	Decreased rifampin and ketoconazole effects
Metronidazole with . . .		
Alcohol	Possible inhibition of intermediary metabolism of alcohol	Mild disulfiram-like symptoms
Warfarin	Decreased warfarin metabolism	Increased anticoagulant effect
Nalidixic acid with . . .		
Warfarin	Displacement from binding sites	Increased anticoagulant effect

Table 4-12. (continued)

Drug	Mechanism	Effect
Rifampin with . . .		
Warfarin	Increased warfarin metabolism	Decreased anticoagulant effect
Barbiturates	Increased barbiturate metabolism	Decreased barbiturate effect
Chloramphenicol	Increased chloramphenicol metabolism	Decreased chloramphenicol effect
Contraceptives, oral	Increased hormone metabolism	Decreased contraceptive effect
Digitalis	Increased digitalis metabolism	Decreased digitoxin and digoxin effect
Hypoglycemics (sulfonylurea)	Increased sulfonylurea metabolism	Decreased hypoglycemic effect
Phenytoin	Increased phenytoin metabolism	Decreased phenytoin effect
Quinidine	Increased quinidine metabolism	Decreased quinidine effect
Theophylline	Increased theophylline metabolism	Decreased theophylline effect
Verapamil	Increased verapamil metabolism	Decreased verapamil effect
Tetracyclines with . . .		
Antacids, oral	Decreased tetracycline absorption	Decreased antibacterial effect
Digoxin	Decreased gut metabolism and increased absorption	Increased digoxin effect
Iron, oral	Decreased absorption	Decreased tetracycline effect, but not with doxycycline

Adapted from: S Norris, CH Nightingale, GL Mandell. Tables of antimicrobial agent pharmacology. In GL Mandell, RG Douglas Jr, JE Bennett (eds.), *Principles and Practice of Infectious Diseases* (3rd ed.). New York: Churchill-Livingstone: 1990. Pp. 456–60; and RL Davis. Drug interactions with fluoroquinolone antibiotics. *Drug Interact Newsletter* 8:27–31, 1988; and JD Lazar, KD Wilner. Drug interactions with fluconazole. *Rev Infect Dis* 12(suppl 3):S327–33, 1990.

waiting for improvement of infection to determine the need of intravenous drug therapy or hospitalization also is not rational. A rational approach would be to give intravenous therapy during rehydration or until the patient is stabilized and able to take medications by the oral route, while observing for clinical deterioration or while gathering additional information.

Intravenous doses may result in higher peak serum concentrations simply because larger doses are given or because of the rapid rate of infusion (usually 15–30 minutes) compared to the time required for oral absorption (usually 1/2–2 hours). Giving the same dose of a well-absorbed oral drug results in the same amount of total drug delivered. Gastrointestinal intolerance or incomplete absorption may limit the amount of a drug that is administered orally. Peak concentrations achieved after an intramuscular injection may not be reached much sooner than after an oral dose. It should be noted that the American Heart Association recommends the administration of oral amoxicillin or clindamycin 1 hour before dental, urological, or gastrointestinal procedures or an intravenous drug 30 minutes prior to the procedure [45], a difference of only 30 minutes. Giving adequate oral therapy suffices for most patients, unless hospitalization for intravenous treatment of a serious infection is indicated.

Drugs of Choice for Common Infections

Drugs of choice for common infectious organisms are listed in Table 4-13. See Table 4-11 for antimicrobial dosages by severity of infection.

How to Choose Among Antibiotics

For most infections, there are several agents from which to choose. Since successful treatment of the infection is the reason for therapy, the most efficacious agent should be considered as first choice, provided that its toxicities or contraindications do not prohibit its use in that patient. If several agents are equally effective, then the drug that is least

Table 4-13. Antimicrobial agents of choice for common infections

Organism	Drug of choice	Alternatives
Gram-Positive Cocci		
S. aureus		
Non–penicillinase-producing	Penicillin	Cephalosporin, vancomycin, clindamycin
Penicillinase-producing	Penicillinase resistant penicillin	Cephalosporin, vancomycin, ampicillin-sulbactam
Methicillin-resistant	Vancomycin ± gentamicin ± rifampin	TMP-SMX, ciprofloxacin
Streptococci		
Group A	Penicillin	Erythromycin, cephalosporin
Group B	Penicillin or ampicillin	Erythromycin, cephalosporin
Group D	Penicillin or ampicillin ± gentamicin	Vancomycin, ciprofloxacin ± gentamicin
Viridans group	Penicillin ± gentamicin	Cephalosporin, vancomycin
Pneumococcus	Penicillin	Cephalosporin, erythromycin
Gram-Negative Cocci		
Moraxella (Branhamella) catarrhalis	Amoxicillin-clavulanate	TMP-SMX, erythromycin, second-generation cephalosporin
N. gonorrhea	Ceftriaxone	Spectinomycin, ciprofloxacin, penicillin
N. meningitidis	Penicillin	Cefotaxime, ceftriaxone, chloramphenicol
Gram-Positive Bacilli		
C. difficile	Vancomycin	Metronidazole
L. monocytogenes	Ampicillin ± gentamicin	TMP-SMX
Gram-Negative Bacilli		
Bacteroides		
Oropharyngeal	Penicillin G	Clindamycin, metronidazole, cefoxitin, cefotetan
Gastrointestinal	Metronidazole	Clindamycin, cefoxitin, piperacillin, imipenem
Campylobacter jejuni	Ciprofloxacin, erythromycin	Tetracycline, gentamicin
Enterobacter	Third-generation cephalosporin	Aminoglycoside, antipseudomonal penicillin, ciprofloxacin
E. coli	Cephalosporin	Ampicillin, aminoglycoside, anti-pseudomonal penicillin, ampicillin-sulbactam, ciprofloxacin
K. pneumoniae	Third-generation cephalosporin	Aminoglycoside, ciprofloxacin
Proteus mirabilis	Ampicillin	Cephalosporin, ciprofloxacin
Serratia	Third-generation cephalosporin	Aminoglycoside, antipseudomonal penicillin, ciprofloxacin
Shigella	TMP-SMX	Ciprofloxacin, ampicillin
Other Gram-Negative Bacilli		
H. influenzae		
Life-threatening infection	Cefotaxime, ceftriaxone	Ampicillin plus chloramphenicol
Other infections	Ampicillin or amoxicillin	TMP-SMX, cefaclor, cefuroxime, amoxicillin-clavulanate

Table 4-13. (*continued*)

Organism	Drug of choice	Alternatives
Legionella pneumophilia	Erythromycin ± rifampin	Tetracycline
Pasturella multocida	Penicillin	Tetracycline, cephalosporin, amoxicillin-clavulanate
Pseudomonas aeruginosa	Antipseudomonal penicillin ± aminoglycoside	Ciprofloxacin, imipenem, ceftazidime
Mycoplasma		
M. *pneumoniae*	Erythromycin, tetracycline	
Fungi		
Aspergillus fumigatus	Amphotericin B	
Blastomyces		
Immunocompromised	Amphotericin B	
Immunocompetent	Ketoconazole	
Candida		
Orophageal	Fluconazole or ketoconazole	Low-dose amphotericin B
Deep	Amphotericin B ± flucytosine	
Chromoblastomycoses	Flucytosine	
Coccidiodes immitis		
Immunocompromised	Amphotericin B	
Immunocompetent	Ketoconazole	
Cryptococcus neoformans	Amphotericin B ± flucytosine	Fluconazole
Histoplasma capsulatum		
Immunocompromised	Amphotericin B	
Immunocompetent	Ketoconazole	
Mucor	Amphotericin B	
Sporothrix schenckii		
Cutaneous	Iodides, heat	
Deep	Amphotericin B	

Adapted from: The choice of antimicrobial drugs. *Med Lett Drugs Ther* 32:41–48, 1990; and Drugs for treatment of fungal infections. *Med Lett Drugs Ther* 32:58–60, 1990.

toxic and less costly should be used. One caveat to this would be that the prescriber should take into consideration the likelihood that the patient will be able to comply with the prescribed regimen. For example, a patient may find it difficult to take ampicillin four times daily separated 1 to 2 hours from meals, but may find taking amoxicillin three times daily without regard to food more convenient. Drugs that can be given once or twice daily may increase compliance and are easier to administer to school-age children or children in day care centers. Drug interactions that require dosage modification or additional patient monitoring should be avoided if possible.

Antibacterial Agents

Penicillins

CHEMISTRY

The basic structure shared by all penicillins consists of three components: a five-membered thiazolidine ring connected to a beta-lactam ring to which a side chain is attached. The beta-lactam is required for antibacterial effect; modifications in the side chain determine the bacterial spectrum, the beta-lactamase stability, and the pharmacokinetic properties of the penicillin. Naturally occurring penicillin G (benzylpenicillin) has been modified in the laboratory to yield a variety of penicillins with different pharmacokinetic and antibacterial properties. The penicillins currently available in the United States are listed in Table 4-14 [48].

MECHANISM OF ACTION

Like all beta-lactam antibiotics, penicillins have bactericidal activity against susceptible organisms. Penicillins inhibit the final step in penicillin cell wall synthesis by binding to bacterial penicillin-binding proteins (PBPs) [49, 50].

SPECTRUM OF ACTIVITY

The naturally occurring penicillins, penicillin G and penicillin V, have similar antimicrobial spectra, although penicillin G is 5–10 times more potent than penicillin V. Penicillin has activity against a variety of clinically important gram-positive aerobic cocci, including *S. pneumoniae*, groups A, B, C, and G streptococci, *S. viridans*, and non–penicillinase-producing *S. aureus*. It is active against some strains of group D *Streptococcus faecalis*, although it is usually used in combination with an aminoglycoside for this. Penicillin is effective against a variety of anaerobic bacteria, including anaerobic cocci such as peptostreptococci, *Clostridium perfringens*, and bacteroides (oropharyngeal strains only, although some may be resistant). Penicillin has excellent activity against the gram-negative aerobes *N. meningitidis* and *Pasteurella multocida*. *Treponema pallidum* and non–penicillinase-

Table 4-14. Classification of the penicillins

Type and generic names	Representative brand names	Routes of administration
Natural		
Penicillin G	Pfizerpen	IM, IV, PO
Benzathine penicillin G	Bicillin, Permapen	IM
Procaine penicillin G	Wycillin, Duracillin	IM
Penicillin V	V-Cillin, Pen-Vee K	PO
Penicillinase-resistant		
Methicillin	Staphcillin	IM, IV
Oxacillin	Prostaphlin	IM, IV, PO
Nafcillin	Unipen	IM, IV, PO
Cloxacillin	Tegopen	PO
Dicloxacillin	Dynapen, Dycill	PO
Extended spectrum		
Ampicillin	Polycillin, Omnipen	IM, IV, PO
Amoxicillin	Amoxil, Larotid	PO
Bacampicillin	Spectrobid	PO
Cyclacillin	Cyclapen-W	PO
Antipseudomonal penicillins		
Carbenicillin	Geopen, Geocillin	IM, IV, PO
Ticarcillin	Ticar	IM, IV
Mezlocillin	Mezlin	IM, IV
Azlocillin	Azlin	IM, IV
Piperacillin	Pipracil	IM, IV
Amidinopenicillin		
Amidinocillin	Coactin	IM, IV
Combinations with B-lactamase inhibitors		
Amoxicillin plus potassium clavulanate	Augmentin	PO
Ampicillin plus sulbactam	Unasyn	IM, IV
Ticarcillin plus potassium clavulanate	Timentin	IM, IV

producing strains of Neisseria gonorrhoeae are also susceptible [48, 51].

The naturally occurring penicillins are readily hydrolyzed by bacterial beta-lactamases to inactive compounds. Modifications of the side chain of the penicillin molecule have resulted in agents that are resistant to hydrolysis by beta-lactamases. As a general rule the use of penicillin is preferred for organisms that test susceptible to both penicillin and penicillinase-resistant agents because of superior in vitro activity. Penicillinase-resistant penicillins have in vitro activity against most aerobic streptococci but poor activity against anaerobic species such as peptostreptococcus and other oropharyngeal anaerobic organisms. They are not active against bacteroides and have poor activity against N. gonorrhoeae. They have excellent activity against penicillinase-producing strains of S. aureus and Staphylococcus epidermidis that are resistant to penicillin but do not have activity against methicillin-resistant strains [48, 51].

The aminopenicillins (ampicillin and amoxicillin) have an extended spectrum of activity against some gram-negative aerobic bacteria compared to penicillin G. Ampicillin and amoxicillin have similar activity against most isolates. They are active in vitro against penicillin-susceptible (non-beta-lactamase-producing) staphylococci and streptococci. Unlike penicillinase-resistant penicillins, they retain their activity against S. faecalis and have enhanced activity against L. monocytogenes compared to penicillin G. The gram-negative spectrum of activity of the aminopenicillins is expanded to include E. coli, Proteus mirabilis, and non–penicillinase-producing strains of H. influenzae. Ampicillin and amoxicillin are also active against salmonellae and shigellae, with amoxicillin being twofold more active against the former and twofold less active against the latter [48, 51]. The antipseudomonal penicillins can be separated into two categories based on their in vitro activity. The carboxypenicillins (carbenicillin, ticarcillin) have similar activity, except that ticarcillin is to two to four times more active in vitro against P. aeruginosa than carbenicillin. The piperazine and ureidopenicillins (azlocillin, mezlocillin, piperacillin) have greater potency against some organisms in vitro. Gram-negative aerobic organisms may have resistance to azlocillin but remain susceptible to mezlocillin and piperacillin. All have activity against P. aeruginosa and other nosocomial Enterobacteriaceae that are resistant to ampicillin. They are not active against penicillinase-producing staphylococci, but piperazine and ureidopenicillins are active against S. faecalis. They have activity in vitro against anaerobic gram-negative bacilli, including Bacteroides fragilis [48, 51].

In an effort to minimize bacterial resistance, beta-lactam antibiotics have been combined with the beta-lactam inhibitors clavulanic acid (amoxicillin and ticarcillin) and sulbactam (ampicillin). The inhibitor irreversibly forms a covalent bond with bacterial beta-lactamase, protecting the antibiotic from hydrolysis. The combination of clavulanic acid with ticarcillin extends the spectrum to include beta-lactamase–producing strains of staphylococci, E. coli, H. influenzae, Klebsiella organisms, Proteus, N. gonorrhoeae, Moraxella catarrhalis, and bacteroides. Antibiotic-resistant nosocomial organisms that produce Richmond-Sykes class I beta-lactamases, such as Pseudomonas, Serratia, Citrobacter, and Enterobacter organisms, that are ticarcillin resistant are not susceptible to the combination, nor are methicillin-resistant staphylococci [48].

Combining clavulanic acid with amoxicillin or sulbactam with ampicillin extends the aminopenicillin spectrum to include beta-lactamase–producing strains of S. aureus, H. influenzae, M. catarrhalis, bacteriodes, N. gonorrhoea, Klebsiella organisms, E. coli, and Proteus. The activity against organisms already susceptible to the antibiotic alone is not enhanced by the combination [48].

PHARMACOKINETICS

Penicillin G is acid labile and is poorly absorbed (20%) after oral administration. Penicillin V is acid stable and is better absorbed (60%). Of the beta-lactamase–resistant penicillins, cloxacillin and dicloxacillin have the best oral absorption. Amoxicillin is better absorbed (80%–90%) than ampicillin (30%–70%). Carbenicillin is poorly absorbed after oral administration and achieves concentrations high enough to treat only urinary tract infections. The other antipseudomonal penicillins are not absorbed after oral administration. Food decreases the absorption of the beta-lactamase–stable penicillins and ampicillin, but not penicillin V or amoxicillin [48, 51].

Most of the penicillins are recovered as parent compound in the urine. The penicillinase-resistant penicillins oxacillin and nafcillin and the piperazine and ureidopenicillins undergo some hepatic metabolism as well as renal elimination and do not accumulate in patients with renal dysfunction. Elimination half-lives in patients with normal renal function for penicillins range from 0.5 to 1.2 hours [48, 51]. Penicillin G can be combined with insoluble compounds such as procaine or benzathine for intramuscular administration. These repository forms result in slower absorption and prolonged serum concentrations, such that procaine penicillin G can be administered twice daily and serum concentrations of penicillin are detectable for 3 weeks or more after benzathine penicillin injection [48, 51].

CLINICAL USE
Because of its in vitro and in vivo efficacy, penicillin G remains the agent of choice for the treatment of infections caused by group A streptococci and S. pneumoniae. It is the drug of choice for all stages of syphilis. Procaine penicillin G has been used as single-dose treatment of gonorrhea, although its use has been largely supplanted by ceftriaxone because of the emergence of resistant penicillinase-producing strains. Benzathine penicillin G can be used as single-dose therapy for the treatment of primary syphilis. The drug may persist in the serum for as long as 4 weeks after intramuscular injection. It should not be used for the treatment of gonorrhea because of the low serum concentrations associated with its use. Penicillin V is not a substitute for parenteral therapy, but it is useful for the treatment of mild infections of the mouth, pharynx, respiratory tract, and soft tissue [48, 51].

Penicillinase-resistant penicillins are useful for the treatment of infections due to penicillinase-producing staphylococci. They are not indicated for empiric therapy of infections that may be due to methicillin-resistant staphylococci such as those associated with prosthetic devices or intravenous line infections [46, 48, 51]. The extended-spectrum aminopenicillins are useful for the treatment of community acquired infections in children older than 6 years of age in which beta-lactamase– or amoxicillin-resistant H. influenzae is not suspected, including urinary tract infections, respiratory tract infections, chronic bronchitis, otitis media, and sinusitis, and in combination with probenecid for the treatment of gonorrhea caused by non-penicillinase–producing strains. Because of its superior oral absorption, which is unaffected by food, amoxicillin is the preferred agent for oral administration [46, 48, 51]. Both are indicated for the prevention of endocarditis before dental, gastrointestinal, and urologic procedures (45).

Use of antipseudomonal penicillins is reserved for the treatment of severe infections due to P. aeruginosa and other antibiotic-resistant gram-negative bacteria, usually in combination with an aminoglycoside [48, 51].

The addition of a beta-lactamase inhibitor to amoxicillin and ampicillin makes them useful agents for the treatment of infections where S. aureus, beta-lactamase–producing strains of H. influenzae, and other gram-negative bacilli are present. They are used for the treatment of otitis media; sinusitis; infections of the respiratory tract, skin, soft tissue, and urinary tract; and bite wounds. A combination of ticarcillin plus clavulanate is indicated in clinical situations in which S. aureus, aerobic gram-negative bacilli, and anaerobic organisms are suspected [48, 51, 52].

ADVERSE EFFECTS
Penicillins are well tolerated and cause few serious adverse reactions. The major side effect associated with penicillin use is hypersensitivity, which may manifest as drug-induced fever, rash, angioneurotic edema, or serum sickness. Patients with mononucleosis develop a macular or maculopapular erythematous rash if given ampicillin. Orally administered agents may cause gastrointestinal upset and diarrhea, although this is rarely severe enough to necessitate discontinuing drug therapy. Amoxicillin, because of its superior oral absorption, causes significantly less diarrhea than ampicillin. When penicillin is given in high doses to patients with renal failure, neuromuscular irritability, including seizures, has been reported [48, 51, 52].

When given in large doses, the sodium content of carbenicillin (4.7 meq/g) and ticarcillin (5.2 meq/g) can result in sodium accumulation and fluid overload with possible hypokalemia. An average daily 30-g dose of carbenicillin or 18 g of ticarcillin supplies 141 and 94 meq of sodium, respectively. The ureidopenicillins, piperacillin, mezlocillin, and azlocillin each supply approximately 2 meq/g sodium, delivering significantly less sodium in an average 18 g daily dose. This could be an important consideration in patients with cardiac disease or renal dysfunction. Carbenicillin and ticarcillin, because of the carboxylic acid group on their side chain, have been associated with decreased platelet aggregation, which occurs less frequently with the piperazine and ureidopenicillins [53, 54].

Any penicillin can cause interstitial nephritis, although it has been reported to be more common with methicillin and may not occur with nafcillin [55, 56]. Nafcillin causes a higher incidence of thrombophlebitis when given intravenously. Rarely, penicillins can cause anemia, neutropenia, granulocytopenia, and elevations in hepatic enzymes.

Although most common with ampicillin, any broad-spectrum antibiotic, whether given by the oral or intravenous route, can cause pseudomembranous colitis or AAC [48, 51, 52].

Cephalosporins

The cephalosporins have been grouped into three generations. This classification is based on the activity against gram-negative aerobic bacilli and the resistance to beta-lactamases. The available cephalosprins are shown in Table 4-15.

CHEMISTRY

The cephalosporins are beta-lactam antibiotics like the penicillins. The cephalosporin molecule consists of a six-membered dihydrothiazine ring attached to a beta-lactam ring. Modifications of position 7 of the

Table 4-15. Classification of the cephalosporins

Type and generic names	Representative brand names	Routes of administration
First Generation		
Cefadroxil	Duricef, Clitracef	PO
Cefazolin	Ancef, Kefzol	IM, IV
Cephalexin	Keflex	PO
Cephalothin	Keflin, Selfin	IM, IV
Cephapirin	Cefadyl	IM, IV
Cephradine	Velosef	IM, IV, PO
Second Generation		
Cefaclor	Ceclor	PO
Cefamandole	Mandol	IM, IV
Cefmetazole	Zefazone	IV
Cefotetan	Cefotan	IM, IV
Cefonicid	Monocid	IM, IV
Ceforanide	Precef	IM, IV
Cefoxitin	Mefoxin	IM, IV
Cefuroxime	Zinacef, Kefurox	IM, IV
Cefuroxime axetil	Ceftin	PO
Third Generation		
Cefixime	Suprax	PO
Cefoperazone	Cefobid	IM, IV
Cefotaxime	Claforan	IM, IV
Ceftazidime	Fortaz, Tazidime	IM, IV
Ceftizoxime	Cefizox	IM, IV
Ceftriaxone	Rocephen	IM, IV
Moxalactam	Moxam	IM, IV

7-aminocephalosporanic acid enhances the antibacterial activity, especially against gram-negative bacilli. Modifications at carbon 3 of the dihydrothiazine ring change the pharmacokinetic properties of the drug and have also been associated with adverse reactions. Cephamycins result from the addition of methoxy group at the 7 position of the beta-lactam ring. The oxams (moxalactam) are created by the substitution of an oxygen for the sulfur atom in the dihydrothiazine [49].

MECHANISM OF ACTION
Cephalosporins, oxams (moxalactam), and cephamycins (cefoxitin) are bactericidal against susceptible bacteria by inhibiting bacterial cell wall synthesis through their effects on PBPs in a way similar to penicillins [49, 50].

SPECTRUM OF ACTIVITY
All cephalosporins have a broad spectrum of activity against both gram-positive and gram-negative organisms. The first-generation cephalosporins have the best activity against aerobic gram-positive cocci, while second and third generations of cephalosporins have increasingly superior activity against gram-negative isolates. None of the cephalosporins is active against enterococci (S. faecalis), methicillin-resistant S. aureus, S. epidermidis, penicillin-resistant S. pneumoniae, or L. monocytogenes [57, 58].

The antimicrobial spectrum of first-generation cephalosporins can be considered interchangeable among agents. First-generation drugs are the most active against staphylococci and streptococci. They have good activity against most community acquired strains of E. coli, P. mirabilis, and Klebsiella pneumoniae. They are not effective against Pseudomonas organisms or other antibiotic-resistant or nosocomially acquired strains. They have moderate activity against oropharyngeal anaerobes in vitro but have inferior activity to penicillin G and have not been studied for the treatment of aspiration pneumonia. They are ineffective against beta-lactamase or ampicillin-resistant strains of H. influenzae [57].

Although there are eight second-generation cephalosporins currently available in the United States, cefamandole and cefoxitin are the two prototypes for the generation, to which the other six can be compared. Cefuroxime, cefaclor, cefonicid, and ceforanide are contrasted with cefamandole and cefmetazole and cefotetan to cefoxitin. The cefamandole prototypes have slightly less activity against staphylococci and streptococci than the first-generation agents, although they are still useful for the treatment of infections caused by those bacteria. They have good clinical activity against Enterobacter organisms and beta-lactamase–producing strains of H. influenzae. Compared to first-generation drugs, cefaclor has enhanced activity against H. influenzae [57, 58].

Cefoxitin is less active than the cefamandole group against staphylococci and streptococci. Cefoxitin has excellent activity against first-generation resistant gram-negative organisms, including E. coli, Klebsiella organisms, indole-positive and negative Proteus and Serratia species, but it is less active than cefamandole against Enterobacter species and some strains of H. influenzae. Cefoxitin is effective against anaerobic organisms, including B. fragilis, and therefore is useful for the treatment of mixed aerobic and anaerobic infections. Cefotetan has good activity against B. fragilis but is less active than cefoxitin against other bacteroides [57, 58].

Third-generation cephalosporins are inferior to first-generation agents against streptococci and staphylococci, but they are more resistant to beta-lactamases produced by gram-negative organisms, particularly those that occur in institutional or nosocomial settings. They can be separated into two groups, based on their antipseudomonal activity. Those agents possessing activity against P. aeruginosa include cefoperazone and ceftazidime. Those that do not possess antipseudomonal activity include moxalactam, cefotaxime, ceftizoxime, ceftriaxone, and cefixime. They have antibacterial activity against a variety of aerobic gram-negative bacteria that are resistant to first- and second-generation agents and generally are bactericidal at lower concentrations. All have good activity against N. gonorrhoeae, of which ceftriaxone is the most active. Moxalactam has less activity against aerobic gram-positive cocci but is as active as cefoxitin against B. fragilis. Ceftazidime has the poorest activity of all cephalosporins against aerobic gram-positive organisms but is active against P. aeruginosa. Cefoperazone is less effective than other third-generation cephalosporins against aerobic gram-negative bacilli other than *Pseudomonas* organisms [57, 58].

PHARMACOKINETICS

Many of the cephalosporins are not absorbed and are not available except for administration by the parenteral route. The first-generation oral cephalosporins are well absorbed. Coadministration with food delays but does not affect the total amount of drug absorbed for all oral agents except cefuroxime axetil. Its bioavailability increases from 30% when taken on an empty stomach to 50% when taken with food [9]. The oral absorption of cefixime ranges from 40%–50% [59].

Cephalosporins are widely distributed throughout the body. First-generation agents penetrate poorly into the central nervous system and cannot be used for the treatment of meningitis or other CNS infections. Satisfactory penetration into the CSF has been achieved with cefuroxime, cefotaxime, ceftizoxime, ceftriaxone, moxalactam, and ceftazidime [57].

Most cephalosporins are excreted unchanged by the kidneys and require dosage adjustment in patients with renal dysfunction. Exceptions include ceftriaxone and cefoperazone, which undergo primarily biliary excretion [60, 61]. Cefotaxime is metabolized to desacetylcefotaxime, which accumulates in patients with renal dysfunction [62]. Some agents have prolonged elimination half-lives and can be given in one or two daily doses (ceftriaxone, cefixime, ceforanide, and cefonicid) [57, 58].

CLINICAL USE

Because of their broad spectrum of activity, first-generation cephalosporins are useful agents for empiric therapy of community acquired infections of the respiratory and urinary tracts, skin, and soft tissue. Their use as single agents in hospital acquired infections or immunocompromised hosts is not recommended because of their limited activity against gram-negative organisms. They are useful alternatives for the treatment of staphylococcal and nonenterococcal streptococcal infections in penicillin-allergic patients, although up to 7% will have cross-hypersensitivity with cephalosporins. Patients who have suffered an anaphylactic reaction or angioneurotic edema to penicillins probably should not be prescribed cephalosporins, especially if not given under close supervision [36]. First-generation cephalosporins are the drugs of choice for prophylaxis of cardiovascular, orthopedic, biliary, pelvic, and intra-abdominal surgery. Cefazolin is the preferred agent because it has the longest half-life of the first-generation cephalosporins [57, 58]. The second-generation cephalosporins cefuroxime and cefamandole are effective for the treatment of community acquired infections in which beta-lactamase–producing *H. influenzae* is suspected. Both drugs have been used for the treatment of respiratory tract infections, sinusitis, otitis media, and other infections. Cefuroxime is the preferred agent because of its longer duration of activity and ability to penetrate the CSF [57, 58]. Its use in the treatment of meningitis has been supplanted by third-generation cephalosporins because of faster sterilization of the spinal fluid and milder hearing loss [63, 64].

Third-generation cephalosporins can be used to treat some gram-positive infections, especially cefotaxime or ceftriaxone for meningitis when *S. pneumoniae*, *H. influenzae*, or other gram-negative bacilli are suspected pathogens. However, for the treatment of most gram-positive infections, superior agents such as the penicillins or the first-generation cephalosporins are preferred. The third-generation cephalosporins are the most active against *Enterobacteriaceae*, including nosocomially acquired organisms or those that are resistant to multiple antibiotics. Cefoperazone and moxalactam are the poorest against these strains. Ceftazidime and cefoperazone are especially useful for the treatment of infections where *P. aeruginosa* is suspected, such as in patients with neutropenic sepsis, patients receiving immunosuppressive drugs such as corticosteroids, and other compromised hosts. Because it has less activity than ceftazidime against non-pseudomonal gram-negative bacilli, cefoperazone may not be as effective for this indication [57, 58].

Because of its 8-hour half-life, ceftriaxone can be given in one or two daily doses. It can be administered once daily to treat skin and soft tissue infections in the outpatient setting. Because of its activity against penicillinase-producing strains of *N. gonorrhoeae*, it is the recommended treatment for gonorrhea occurring in all anatomical sites [65].

ADVERSE EFFECTS

Like the penicillins, cephalosporins are well tolerated. The major adverse reaction is hypersensitivity. There is little to no cross-reactivity with aztreonam [36]. Other adverse effects are similar to the penicillins. Cephalosporins containing a methylthiotetrazole (MTT) group (moxalactam, cefamandole, cefotetan, and cefoperazone) can cause hypoprothrombinemia. Bleeding is especially a problem with moxalactam, probably because of the additive effect of its carboxylic acid group causing abnormalities in platelet aggregation. Risk factors for the development of coagulopathies include use of moxalactam [66], critical illness, and malnutrition [67]. The hypoprothrombinemia can be corrected by the use of parenteral vitamin K, which should be administered prophylactically in seriously ill patients receiving any broad-spectrum antibiotic, especially those containing MTT side chains [66, 67]. Disulfiram-like reactions can occur with the cephalosporins containing the MTT side chain if alcohol is ingested, which may be contained in oral medications such as cough suppressants or as a solubilizing agent for other oral or intravenous medications [57, 58]. Other reactions include gastrointestinal disturbances such as diarrhea and AAC. Rarely have cephalosporins been associated with thrombocytopenia, neutropenia, and hepatic or renal dysfunction. Superinfections occur commonly, especially in patients receiving third-generation agents, especially with *P. aeruginosa*, *Candida* organisms, and enterococci [57, 58].

Tetracyclines

CHEMISTRY

The basic structure of the tetracycline molecule consists of a hydronaphthacene nucleus of four fused rings. The generic names of the tetracycline analogues are determined by substitutions on the basic tetracycline molecule at the fifth, sixth, or seventh position [68].

MECHANISM OF ACTION

Tetracyclines inhibit protein synthesis by binding to the 30S ribosomal subunit, blocking the binding of tRNA to the accepter site on the mRNA ribosome complex. They accumulate in bacterial but not mammalian cells by an inactive process, thus they are more toxic to microbes than to human cells [68].

SPECTRUM OF ACTIVITY

Tetracyclines have a broad spectrum of activity. Tetracycline is the least active compound, with minimum inhibitory concentrations two to four times higher than minocycline, the most potent. The activity of doxycycline is close to that of minocycline. Tetracyclines have activity against *H. influenzae* and pneumococci, although some strains are resistant. Up to 40% of *Streptococcus pyogenes* may be resistant to tetracycline. Community acquired *E. coli* are often susceptible to concentrations achieved in the urine. *Brucella* species, *Vibrio cholerae*, and other vibrios are susceptible. *Campylobacter* species and shigella may be resistant. They have activity against penicillin-susceptible gonococci and meningococci. The tetracyclines are also active against anaerobic organisms, including actinomyces and *B. fragilis*, with doxycycline more active than tetracycline. Other susceptible organisms include *Mycoplasma pneumoniae*, *Borrelia burgdorferi*, rickettsiae, and chlamydiae [39, 68].

PHARMACOKINETICS

After oral administration tetracycline, doxycycline, and minocycline are absorbed 77%, 93%, and 95%, respectively. Administration of tetracycline with food reduces its bioavailability by 50% [69]. The absorption of doxycycline and minocycline is not impaired by food [69, 70]. Antacids, iron, and dairy products form divalent and trivalent chelates with all tetracyclines and impair their absorption [39].

Tetracyclines are widely distributed in the body, including the lungs, liver, kidney, brain, and sputum. The more lipophilic minocycline and doxycycline achieve higher concentrations. Concentrations in the CSF for all the drugs are low. Tetracyclines cross the placenta and enter breast milk [39, 68].

CLINICAL USE

Tetracyclines are considered the agents of choice for the treatment of urethritis caused by *Chlamydiae* and *Ureaplasma* organisms. They are an alternative to erythromycin for the treatment of *M. pneumoniae* and *Legionella pneumophilia* infections. They are effective for the treatment of cholera, brucellosis, leptospirosis, the early stages of Lyme disease, and rickettsial diseases such as Rocky Mountain spotted fever, typhus, Q fever, lymphogranuloma venereum, and granuloma inguinale [39, 46, 68]. Tetracyclines can also be used for the treatment of urinary tract infections acquired in the community and chronic pulmonary infections in patients with chronic obstructive lung disease and are an alternative to penicillins for the treatment of gonorrhea and syphilis in patients who are penicillin allergic. Doxycycline can be used for the prevention of traveler's diarrhea [39, 68]. Doxycycline can be administered with food, has a convenient twice-daily dosing schedule, and is available as generic products that are no more expensive than tetracycline.

CONTRAINDICATIONS
Tetracycline accumulates in patients with renal failure and has been implicated in causing further renal damage. Doxycycline accumulates to only a small extent and is the preferred agent in patients with renal disease. Tetracyclines are contraindicated in patients under 12 years of age and pregnant and lactating women because of their effects on developing bones and teeth [39, 68, 71].

ADVERSE EFFECTS
Tetracyclines are irritating compounds that commonly cause gastrointestinal upset. Doxycycline and minocycline can be taken with food (but not dairy products or antacids) to minimize gastrointestinal symptoms [39, 68]. They have been reported to cause esophageal ulcerations. This is especially problematic if medications are taken just before bedtime. Patients should be advised to take their oral drug with an adequate amount of fluid and not to take just before retiring [72]. Intravenous administration of tetracycline frequently causes pain and thrombophlebitis. Intramuscular administration of tetracyclines is painful. The intramuscular formulation contains procaine and should not be administered intravenously.

Because of their broad spectrum of activity, tetracyclines commonly cause *Candida* superinfections of the throat and vulvovaginitis [39, 68]. Tetracyclines, except for doxycycline, can worsen azotemia in patients with renal dysfunction by inhibiting protein synthesis and amino acid metabolism. Demeclocycline can cause diabetes insipidus and is used for the treatment of syndrome of inappropriate antidiuretic hormone (SIADH). Older formulations of tetracycline produced a reversible renal tubular acidosis (Fanconi's syndrome), but newer formulations have been modified to avoid this effect [39, 68]. Tetracyclines can cause photosensitivity reactions. Demeclocycline is the most phototoxic, followed by doxycycline. Minocycline can cause a reversible vertigo that is three times more common in women than men [73]. Hypersensitivity reactions, including rash, urticaria, anaphylaxis, and fixed drug eruptions, occur infrequently [68].

Erythromycin

CHEMISTRY
Erythromycin is a macrolide antibiotic consisting of a 14-membered macrocyclic lactone ring. Macrolides are poorly water soluble, are inactivated by gastric acid, and are poorly absorbed after oral administration. Erythromycin is available as the base and the estolate, ethylsuccinate, and stearate salts for oral administration and water-soluble glucoptate and lactobionate salts for intravenous use [74].

MECHANISM OF ACTION
Erythromycin inhibits bacterial protein synthesis by binding to the 50S ribosomal subunit and inhibiting RNA-dependent protein synthesis. Erythromycin can also inhibit ribosomal binding of chloramphenicol and other macrolide antibiotics [74].

SPECTRUM OF ACTIVITY
Erythromycin can be bacteriostatic or bactericidal, depending on the concentration of the drug. Erythromycin has activity against gram-positive cocci, including group A streptococci, *S. pneumoniae*, *S. viridans*, and community acquired staphylococci. Hospital acquired staphylococci may be resistant. Susceptible gram-positive bacilli include *L. monocytogenes* and *Corynebacterium diphtheriae*. The gram-negative spectrum of erythromycin is limited to *N. meningitidis*, *N. gonorrhoeae*, and *Bordetella pertussis* and marginal activity against *H. influenzae*. Some anaerobic bacilli are susceptible, but *B. fragilis* is resistant. Other susceptible organisms include *T. pallidum*, *L. pneumophilia*, *M. pneumoniae*, *Chlamydia pneumoniae* (TWAR),

Chlamydia trachomatis, Ureaplasma organisms, and rickettsiae [74].

PHARMACOKINETICS

The absorption of oral erythromycin varies widely and depends on the salt form in the dosage form administered. Erythromycin base is hydrolyzed by gastric acid and poorly absorbed, and absorption is decreased by food. Acid-resistant enteric-coated preparations protect from gastric hydrolysis. The estolate salt and some enteric-coated base preparations (E-Mycin and Ery-Tab) can be taken with food and may be better tolerated after oral administration. These two enteric-coated base preparations are recommended in adults unable to tolerate other base formulations. Other salt forms are absorbed better than the base but are not used in adults because of possible cholestatic jaundice. Erythromycin is widely distributed in the body, although it poorly penetrates into the CSF. Erythromycin achieves good intracellular concentrations in alveolar macrophages and polymorphonuclear leukocytes [74, 75].

Erythromycin undergoes some metabolism in the liver, but it is excreted largely as unchanged drug in the feces and bile. Five to 15% is recovered as unchanged drug in the urine, although urine concentrations are variable. The elimination half-life of erythromycin is 1.4 hours, prolonged to 5 hours in anuria [74, 75].

CLINICAL USE

Erythromycin is the drug of choice for the treatment of *M. pneumoniae* infections, *L. pneumophilia*, diphtheria, pertussis, and chlamydial conjunctivitis, pneumonia, or chlamydia infection in pregnancy. Oral erythromycin and ciprofloxacin are both drugs of choice for gastroenteritis due to *Campylobacter jejuni* [46]. Erythromycin can be used for the treatment of mild staphylococcal or streptococcal infections or as an alternative to penicillin in allergic patients. It is not recommended for treatment of infections of the oral cavity or deep fascial spaces because of the emergence of resistant oral anaerobes and streptococci [76]. Erythromycin can be used for the treatment of gonorrhea or nongonococcal urethritis in pregnant patients or patients unable to tolerate penicillin G or tetracycline. It is an alternative to amoxicillin in allergic

patients for the prophylaxis of rheumatic fever and endocarditis [45, 74].

ADVERSE EFFECTS

Erythromycin commonly causes gastrointestinal irritation even after intravenous administration, possibly by increasing gastrointestinal contractility by mimicking the effect of motilin [77, 78]. Thrombophlebitis can occur with intravenous administration. Intramuscular injection is very painful. Intravenous administration is indicated for serious infections requiring large doses that would not be tolerated orally or in patients unable to take or tolerate oral doses. Allergic reactions include fever, skin rash, and eosinophilia. Rare cholestatic jaundice occurs with the estolate and ethylsuccinate salts, usually in adults after 10–14 days of therapy but may occur after the first dose in patients who have previously been treated with the drug [74, 75]. Transient deafness has rarely been reported, some with concurrent CNS changes after high doses or in patients with hepatic or renal dysfunction [79]. As with any antibiotic, gastrointestinal and vaginal *Candida* superinfections and AAC caused by overgrowth of *C. difficile* can occur [74].

Erythromycin has been reported to cause prolongation of the QT interval and torsades de pointes due to direct electrophysiologic effects [80, 81]. The use of erythromycin, especially parenteral forms, should probably be avoided in patients with a long QT syndrome. Some authors recommend monitoring the ECG periodically in patients at risk for a long QT interval, such as patients being treated with type 1A antiarrhythmic agents, amiodarone, hypokalemia, or hypomagnesia [81].

Erythromycin can decrease the hepatic metabolism of drugs metabolized by hepatic microsomal cytochrome P450 enzymes, including warfarin, carbamazepine, phenytoin, and theophylline, and decrease the gastrointestinal metabolism of digoxin, leading to increased absorption [17].

Glycopeptides

CHEMISTRY

Vancomycin is the only glycopeptide antibiotic currently approved by the FDA. When first introduced, vancomycin contained up to 30% impurities. Currently available formulations are purer and have fewer adverse effects. Teicoplanin (formerly teichomycin A) and daptinomycin are related compounds that are currently under investigation in the United States. Glycopeptides are large molecules. The molecular weights of vancomycin and teicoplanin are approximately 1450 and 1560–1891 d, respectively. Teicoplanin is more lipophilic than vancomycin [38].

MECHANISM OF ACTION

The glycopeptide antibiotics inhibit bacterial cell wall synthesis at a different step than the beta-lactam antibiotics. Vancomycin can also inhibit RNA synthesis and alter cell wall permeability [38].

SPECTRUM OF ACTIVITY

Vancomycin has excellent activity against aerobic gram-positive cocci, including S. aureus and methicillin-susceptible and methicillin-resistant coagulase-negative staphylococci (CNS), S. pyogenes, S. pneumoniae, S. viridans, and enterococcal and nonenterococcal strains of group D streptococci. Recently resistant strains of a CNS, Staphylococcus haemolyticus, and enterococci have been identified. Gram-positive bacilli, including group JK corynebacteria, C. difficile, and L. monocytogenes, are susceptible. Organisms that are usually susceptible include anaerobic or microaerophilic streptococci; clostridia, including C. perfringens; Bacillus anthracis; and diphtheroids. Vancomycin is bacteriocidal against most organisms but may be bacteriostatic at clinically achievable concentrations against enterococci and S. viridans [38].

PHARMACOKINETICS

Vancomycin and teicoplanin are poorly absorbed after oral administration. Vancomycin is well distributed to most body tissues except CSF, although bacteriocidal concentrations have been detected in patients with meningitis. Vancomycin is eliminated by the kidneys, with an elimination half-life ranging from 6 hours in normal adults to 5–10 days in anuric patients. Elimination may also be prolonged in patients with hepatic dysfunction [38]. Because of its long half-life, patients with renal failure may be administered vancomycin as infrequently as once weekly. Several nomograms are available for vancomycin dosage modification in patients with varying stages of renal dysfunction [82–84]. Teicoplanin undergoes both renal and hepatic elimination. It has a prolonged elimination half-life of 40–70 hours, allowing once-a-day dosing [38].

CLINICAL USE

Vancomycin is the drug of choice for the treatment of infections due to methicillin-resistant staphylococci, penicillin-resistant group JK corynebacteria, and enterococcal endocarditis in penicillin-allergic patients and is used orally for the treatment of enterocolitis due to C. difficile and S. aureus. Methicillin-resistant staphylococci should be suspected in nosocomial infections or infections associated with indwelling intravenous catheters, prosthetic devices, recent surgery, or sinusitis following intubation [38, 46]. It is a parenteral alternative to oral therapy for prophylaxis of endocarditis in penicillin-allergic patients with valvular heart disease [45].

ADVERSE EFFECTS

Vancomycin is extremely painful when given intramuscularly and can cause thrombophlebitis when given intravenously. The "red neck syndrome" is a nonallergic reaction consisting of pruritus, an erythematous or maculopapular rash on the face, neck, and upper torso with possible hypotension. This adverse effect occurs during or shortly after intravenous infusion and is due to histamine release. In severe cases it can cause cardiovascular collapse. The incidence of this effect is unknown, but it can be treated by slowing the rate of intravenous infusion or by pretreatment with antihistamines [85, 86]. True allergic reactions are uncommon. Administration of standard doses in patients with renal dysfunction have resulted in ototoxicity [79]. Mild reversible nephrotoxicity has been reported. Retrospective reports that vancomycin can increase aminoglycoside-induced nephrotoxicity [38] have been disputed by prospective studies [87].

Teicoplanin causes only mild pain after intramuscular injection and has not caused thrombophlebitis. Rapid infusions are not associated with adverse effects. Ototoxicity has been reported [38].

Sulfonamides and Trimethoprim

CHEMISTRY

Sulfonamides are derivatives of sulfanilamide, which is structurally similar to para-aminobenzoic acid (PABA). Trimethoprim is a 2-4-diamino-5 (3'4'5'-trimethoxybenzyl) pyrimidine.

MECHANISM OF ACTION

Sulfonamides and trimethoprim block sequential steps in folic acid synthesis. Sulfonamides are bacteriostatic. The combination of sulfonamides and trimethoprim acts synergistically against susceptible organisms [88].

SPECTRUM OF ACTIVITY

Sulfonamides are broad-spectrum antibiotics. They are active against streptococci, staphylococci, including many methicillin-resistant strains, and L. monocytogenes. They have excellent activity against gram-negative organisms, including E. coli, K. pneumoniae, P. mirabilis, H. influenzae, M. catarrhalis, and other Enterobacteriaceae. Most strains of N. meningitidis are resistant. Other susceptible organisms include actinomyces, chlamydiae, plasmodia, Toxoplasma species, Nocardia asteroides, and P. carinii [88, 89].

Trimethoprim has a similar spectrum. Combined with sulfamethoxazole, it is active against S. aureus, S. pyogenes, S. pneumoniae, E. coli, P. mirabilis, Shigellae, Salmonellae, Pseudomonas cepacia, Pseudomonas pseudomallei, Yersinia enterocolitica, N. gonorrhoeae, and M. catarrhalis. P. aeruginosa are resistant. The optimal in vitro trimethoprim-sulfamethoxazole ratio is 1:20, which is not always achieved in vivo at all sites of infection [88, 89].

PHARMACOKINETICS

The clinically useful sulfonamides are absorbed almost completely after oral administration. Topical sulfonamides may also be absorbed and achieve detectable serum concentrations. Sulfonamides are widely distributed throughout the body, including the CSF. They readily cross the placenta and enter breast milk. Sulfonamides undergo acetylation and glucuronidation in the liver and are recovered in the urine as parent compound and metabolized drug. The more lipophilic agents have longer elimination half-lives. The short-acting drugs, such as sulfisoxazole, have elimination half-lives of 6 hours; the medium-acting drugs, such as sulfamethoxazole and sulfadiazine, are less soluble and have elimination half-lives of approximately 10–20 hours. Sulfadoxime is a long-acting sulfonamide with an elimination half-life of approximately 100–230 hours [88].

Trimethoprim is well absorbed after oral administration, is widely distributed in most body fluids, including CSF, and is excreted in the urine primarily as unchanged drug. It has an elimination half-life of approximately 10 hours [88].

CLINICAL USE

Sulfonamides are widely used for the treatment of urinary tract infections and can be combined with bladder analgesics for that purpose (e.g., phenazopyridine). They are the drugs of choice for the treatment of infections due to N. asteroides and are used to treat toxoplasmosis and Plasmodium falciparum malaria, lymphogranuloma venereum, and chancroid. They are alternatives to tetracycline or erythromycin for the treatment of infections due to C. trachomatis [46, 88]. The combination of trimethoprim and sulfamethoxazole is useful for the treatment and prophylaxis of upper and lower acute and chronic urinary tract infections caused by susceptible Enterobacteriaceae. It achieves therapeutic concentrations in the prostate and can be used to treat acute and chronic prostatitis [88]. It is the drug of choice for the treatment of gastrointestinal infections due to shigella and Y. enterocolitica [46]. It is used for the treatment of acute otitis media, sinusitis, and bronchitis, including ampicillin-resistant strains of H. influenzae. High dosages are used to treat P. carinii pneumonia in patients with AIDS and other immunocompromised hosts. Oral administration has also been used after cancer chemotherapy to prevent neutropenic sepsis and in AIDS patients to prevent P. carinii infections [88].

CONTRAINDICATIONS

Sulfonamides are contraindicated during the last month of pregnancy and in the neonatal period because they displace bilirubin from its protein-binding sites and can cause kernicterus in the developing fetus or neonate. The teratogenicity of trimethoprim is not established at this point; however, its use in pregnancy is not recommended.

ADVERSE EFFECTS

Trimethoprim and sulfonamides can cause nausea, vomiting, diarrhea, anorexia, and headache. Older, less water-soluble sulfonamide compounds (sulfadiazine, sulfathiazole) were associated with crystalluria; this is less frequent with the newer, more soluble agents (sulfasoxazole and sulfamethoxazole). Trimethoprim-sulfamethoxazole, especially with high doses or prolonged use, can result in thrombocytopenia, leukopenia, and granulocytopenia. Granulocytopenia may improve or resolve with dosage reduction but rarely responds to treatment with folinic acid in patients without folate deficiencies [88, 90]. Folinic acid has not been found to be superior to folic acid in the prevention of cytopenias [91].

Hypersensitivity reactions are not uncommon. Skin rashes, including erythema nodosum and multiforme and Stevens-Johnson syndrome, may occur. Vasculitis and anaphylaxis have also been reported. Renal and hepatic dysfunction occur rarely. Patients with AIDS may experience a higher frequency of adverse skin, blood, hepatic, and renal toxicity, occurring in 30%–70% of patients [92, 93]. Genetic differences may be responsible for the predisposition to hypersensitivity reactions. Acetylator status has been associated with an increased risk of hypersensitivity [94]. Hemolytic anemia may be associated with G6PD deficiency, although hemolysis did not occur in a recent study of G6PD-deficient patients receiving trimethoprim-sulfamethoxazole [95].

Sulfonamides are highly protein bound and may displace other highly protein-bound agents from their albumin-binding sites, transiently increasing their effects. Examples include warfarin, methotrexate, oral hypoglycemic agents, and phenytoin. Sulfonamides may be displaced from their binding sites by other highly protein-bound agents, such as indomethacin, nonsteroidal anti-inflammatory drugs, and probenecid [88].

PABA derivatives, such as procaine and other local anesthetics, may decrease the activity of sulfonamides. Combination with methenamine compounds may lead to insoluble urinary precipitates [88].

Quinolones

CHEMISTRY

The prototype for this group is nalidixic acid. Newer drugs are derived from modifications of the 4-quinolone ring. The fluoroquinolones (all quinolones except nalidixic acid and cinoxacin) have enhanced antimicrobial in vitro activity and pharmacokinetic properties and include norfloxacin, ciprofloxacin, ofloxacin, and lomefloxacin (available in the United States) and investigational agents, including enoxacin, pefloxacin, temafloxacin, lomefloxacin, fleroxacin, and tosulfoxacin [96].

Mechanism of Action

Quinolone antibiotics are DNA gyrase inhibitors (topoisomerase II), the enzyme responsible for introducing negative supercoils into bacterial DNA [96].

SPECTRUM OF ACTIVITY

Nalidixic acid and cinoxacin have activity against most Enterobacteriaceae, including E. coli, Proteus, and Klebsiella and Enterobacter organisms. Some strains of Shigella, Salmonella, and brucella may be sensitive. Pseudomonas and Serratia organisms, streptococci, and staphylococci are resistant. These drugs achieve concentrations adequate to treat only urinary tract infections. Resistance may be acquired during treatment [96].

The fluoroquinolones have an extended spectrum and increased potency compared to the nonfluorinated compounds (nalidixic acid and cinoxacin). Ciprofloxacin is the most potent of the group. Norfloxacin achieves concentrations high enough to treat only infections of the genitourinary and gastrointestinal tracts. All fluoroquinolones have activity against a wide spectrum of aerobic gram-negative and gram-positive bacteria, including most Enterobacteriaceae, Haemophilus species, M. catarrhalis, N. gonorrhoeae, and N. meningitidis. P. aeruginosa is susceptible, but other Pseudomonas species are not. Agents that cause gastroenteritis, including Shigella, Salmonella, and Yersinia, Campylobacter, and Vibrio organisms are very susceptible. Other facultative gram-negative bacilli, including Brucella and Legionella, are susceptible, especially to ciprofloxacin [97, 98].

Fluoroquinolones are less active against gram-positive species. They have good activity against staphylococci, including methicillin-resistant strains, but resistance or decreased susceptibility commonly occurs during treatment. They are less active against streptococci, C. trachomatis, and Ureaplasma urealyticum. Ciprofloxacin and ofloxacin are the most active fluoroquinolones against mycobacteria [97, 98].

PHARMACOKINETICS

All quinolones are well absorbed after oral administration. Bioavailability ranges from 40% (norfloxacin) to 60% (ciprofloxacin) and exceeds 90% for the other compounds. All achieve high concentrations in the urine. Fluoroquinolones have volumes of distribution that exceed total body water (greater than 100 L), illustrating their excellent penetration into most tissues. Concentrations in the lung, prostate, macrophages, and polymorphonuclear leukocytes exceed those achieved in the serum. The CSF penetration is excellent for ofloxacin (90% of serum) and lower for the other drugs [97].

All quinolones are eliminated by both hepatic and renal routes of elimination. Some agents are metabolized to active compounds, and all undergo glomerular filtration and tubular secretion. Elimination half-lives range from 2–4 hours (cinoxacin, ciprofloxacin, norfloxacin) to 5 hours (ofloxacin, enoxacin) to 8 or more hours (other investigational quinolones and nalidixic acid) [96–98].

CLINICAL USE

Because of the rapid emergence of resistance, nalidixic acid and cinoxacin have limited usefulness for the treatment of urinary tract infections caused by susceptible organisms. The fluoroquinolones are effective for the treatment of severe and complicated urinary tract infections, including those caused by P. aeruginosa and other antibiotic-resistant bacteria, although the development of resistance is common. They are the drugs of choice for prostatitis in patients with sulfonamide allergies or sulfonamide-resistant organisms [97, 98].

Fluoroquinolones are effective for the treatment of uncomplicated gonococcal infections, including those caused by penicillinase-producing strains. They are less effective than doxycycline for the treatment of C. trachomatis [97]. They are highly

effective drugs of choice for a variety of gastrointestinal infections, including the prevention and treatment of traveler's diarrhea, Campylobacter organisms, Shigella, Salmonella typhi and other species, and Y. enterocolitica [46, 97]. They have been used in the treatment of respiratory tract infections, including pulmonary exacerbations associated with P. aeruginosa in patients with cystic fibrosis. Because of their poor activity against streptococci, they are not drugs of first choice for the treatment of community acquired infections of the respiratory tract, skin, and soft tissue [97].

Fluoroquinolones have been effective therapy in patients with other gram-negative aerobic infections. As with other classes of drugs, treatment of infections in the lower extremities of diabetic patients has been associated with a low cure rate and the development of resistant organisms. Fluoroquinolones have also been used for the treatment of acute and chronic osteomyelitis in adult patients. Ciprofloxacin and norfloxacin have been used for the prevention of neutropenic sepsis in patients receiving cancer chemotherapy. Only a few patients with meningitis have been treated with quinolones to date [97].

CONTRAINDICATIONS

Because of the damage they cause to the cartilage of weight-bearing joints in animals, quinolones have not been approved by the FDA for use in children. Use in children and pregnant women is not recommended [97].

ADVERSE EFFECTS

The quinolones are well-tolerated agents. The most common adverse effects are gastrointestinal, occurring in 3%–6% of patients. AAC with C. difficile rarely has been reported. CNS toxicity has occurred in 1%–4% of patients, including headache, dizziness, agitation, and sleep disturbances. Seizures have occurred, most commonly in patients with underlying brain disease in combination with the use of other epileptogenic drugs, like theophylline, or when used in combination with nonsteroidal anti-inflammatory drugs (NSAIDs) but also in patients without any known predisposing factors. As with all drugs, hypersensitivity reactions can occur. Photosensitivity reactions have been reported. Mild elevations in liver function tests, mild leukopenia, eosinophilia, hematuria, interstitial nephritis, and acute renal failure occur rarely [97–99]. Quinolones have been reported to interact with a number of other drugs. Nalidixic acid can displace warfarin from its protein-binding sites, causing an increased hypoprothrombinemic effect. Magnesium, aluminum, and possibly calcium antacids and ferrous sulfate dramatically reduce the absorption of orally administered agents. Sucralfate, but not cimetidine or ranitidine, also reduces absorption [17, 43, 97].

Several fluoroquinolones can decrease the metabolism of drugs eliminated by hepatic microsomal oxidative enzymes. Enoxacin is the most potent inhibitor, followed by ciprofloxacin and pefloxacin. Norfloxacin has been shown to have a minimal effect and ofloxacin little or no enzyme-inhibiting effect. Drugs eliminated by this pathway may reach toxic concentrations and toxicity unless appropriate dosage adjustments are made. In vitro studies indicate that quinolones in combination with NSAIDs displace gamma aminobutyric acid (GABA) from its binding sites in the brain, theoretically increasing the risk of seizures. This potentially serious interaction should be monitored for patients being coadministered these two classes of drugs [17, 43, 97].

Clindamycin

CHEMISTRY
Clindamycin is a lincomycin derivative with increased antibacterial potency and oral absorption [74].

MECHANISM OF ACTION
Clindamycin inhibits bacterial protein synthesis by binding to the 50S ribosomal subunit of bacterial RNA. Clindamycin may compete with erythromycin and chloramphenicol for the same binding sites; therefore, coadministration of these agents may result in an antagonistic effect [39].

SPECTRUM OF ACTIVITY
Because clindamycin is more potent and better absorbed than its congener lincomycin, the use of lincomycin is not recommended. Clindamycin has moderate activity against staphylococci and streptococci, although enterococci are usually resistant. Aerobic gram-negative cocci, such as N. meningitidis, and gram-negative bacilli are resistant. Clindamycin is extremely active against most clinically important anaerobic organisms, especially B. fragilis and non-fragilis strains, including Bacteroides vulgatus, Bacteroides thetaiotaomicron, Bacteroides ovatus, and Bacteroides distasonis, although some strains may have up to a 15% rate of resistance. Up to 10% of clostridial species other than C. perfringens and 10% of peptococci may be resistant. Occasional strains of other streptococci and up to 20% of hospital acquired S. aureus may also be resistant to clindamycin [39].

Other anaerobes are generally susceptible. Actinomyces is rarely resistant, and N. asteroides is sensitive. All aerobic gram-negative bacilli are resistant. Strains of Toxoplasma gondii are susceptible [39, 100].

PHARMACOKINETICS
Clindamycin is nearly completely absorbed after oral administration. Food delays but does not decrease absorption. The oral palmitate suspension and phosphate injection are rapidly hydrolyzed by plasma esterases to the inactive ester and clindamycin base. Clindamycin is widely distributed throughout the body but does not penetrate into the CSF. Clindamycin undergoes hepatic and renal clearance. The elimination half-life of clindamycin is 2.4 hours and is somewhat prolonged in renal failure (to 6 hours) and in patients with severe hepatic disease. Significant dosage modification should be made for patients with severe hepatic disease. Significant dosage modification should be made for patients with concomitant renal and hepatic failure [39, 100].

CLINICAL USE
Because of the possibility of serious, potentially fatal pseudomembranous colitis and the drug's limited spectrum of activity, clindamycin is usually reserved as an alternative agent for staphylococcal, streptococcal, and anaerobic infections. Because of its poor penetration into the CNS, it is not indicated for the treatment of bacterial meningitis, although it is useful for the treatment of CNS toxoplasmosis. It is indicated for the treatment of anaerobic infections caused by B. fragilis or other susceptible anaerobic bacteria, especially intra-abdominal or gynecologic pelvic infections when used

in combination with a drug like an aminoglycoside that covers aerobic gram-negative bacilli. It is not superior to penicillin for the treatment of respiratory tract infections, but it has been found to be more effective than penicillin in patients with putrid lung abscess [100, 101]. It is an alternative to penicillin in allergic patients for the treatment of infections of the oral cavity or deep fascial spaces [76], anaerobic respiratory infections, C. *perfringens* infections, and mild to moderate staphylococcal infections and an alternative to amoxicillin for the prophylaxis against endocarditis [46]. It is superior to metronidazole for the treatment of infections where microaerophilic organisms are suspected, such as infections of the mouth or respiratory tract, since metronidazole is active only against obligate anaerobes. It has been used topically for the treatment of acne vulgaris. It has also been used for the treatment of falciparum malaria [39].

ADVERSE EFFECTS

Gastrointestinal irritation, including nausea, vomiting, cramps, and diarrhea, occurs frequently. Pseudomembranous colitis due to overgrowth of toxin-secreting C. *difficile* has been reported in 0.01%–10% of patients being treated with clindamycin. If colitis due to C. *difficile* is suspected, therapy with clindamycin should be promptly discontinued. Oral vancomycin (125 mg) or metronidazole (500 mg) every 6 hours are the treatments of first and second choice, respectively. Relapses commonly occur [39, 46].

Other rare adverse effects include reversible elevations in liver enzymes, neutropenia, thrombocytopenia, and agranulocytosis. Clindamycin rarely causes irritation after intramuscular or intravenous injection [39].

Metronidazole

CHEMISTRY

Metronidazole is a lipophilic nitroimidazole derivative.

MECHANISM OF ACTION

Metronidazole is reduced by susceptible bacterial nitroreductases to reactive compounds that disrupt DNA and nucleic acid synthesis [102].

SPECTRUM OF ACTIVITY

Metronidazole is active against gram-negative obligate anaerobic bacilli, such as B. *fragilis*, and fusobacteria. Anaerobic gram-positive and gram-negative cocci, clostridia, and *Gardnerella vaginalis* are susceptible, as are parasites, including *Trichomonas vaginalis*, *Giardia lamblia* and *Entamoeba histolytica*. Aerobic and microaerophilic cocci are resistant [102, 103].

PHARMACOKINETICS

Metronidazole is almost completely absorbed after oral administration. Its volume of distribution is equal to total body water. It is widely distributed, with therapeutic concentrations achieved in most tissues, including abscesses, bile, bone, and CSF. It undergoes hepatic metabolism by hydroxylation, acetylation, and glucuronidation, although oxidation is the major metabolic pathway. Its elimination half-life is 8 hours in patients with normal and abnormal renal function. Patients with liver dysfunction should receive a reduced dosage [102, 103].

CLINICAL USE

Metronidazole is indicated for the treatment of parasitic infections such as trichomoniasis, amebiasis, and giardiasis. It is useful for the treatment of infections caused by Bacteroides and other anaerobic organisms, including intra-abdominal and pelvic abscesses, osteomyelitis, bacteremia, endocarditis, and brain abscess. Unlike many antibiotics, it retains its activity in environments with a low pH and low oxygen tension and penetrates into abscesses. It is the drug of choice for the treatment of gastrointestinal strains of bacteroides and vaginitis due to G. *vaginalis*. It is an alternative to vancomycin for the treatment of C. *difficile*–induced AAC [102, 103]. Because it is not active against aerobic or microaeophilic bacteria, it cannot be used alone for treatment of oral or other respiratory tract infections.

CONTRAINDICATIONS

Although there are few to no human data to substantiate the risk of malignancy and teratogenicity observed in animals, metronidazole is contraindicated in pregnant and lactating women. Although a long-term study in patients with vaginal trichomoniasis receiving 7–10 days of relatively low doses of metronidazole showed no increase in malignancy, a possibility of cancer in three patients with Crohn's disease receiving long-term metronidazole was suspected [104, 105]. More data are needed to define the teratogenic effect of metronidazole on the human fetus. The drug probably should be avoided in pregnancy, especially the first trimester [106, 107].

ADVERSE EFFECTS

The most common adverse effects associated with oral metronidazole therapy are nausea and vomiting, especially with high doses. These side effects can be minimized by taking the drug with food. Other adverse effects are generally mild and include metallic taste and a mild disulfiram-like reaction when taken with alcohol. Metronidazole can cause reversible neutropenia and peripheral neuropathy. Therapy should be discontinued if symptoms of paresthesia appear [102, 103].

Metronidazole can inhibit the hepatic microsomal enzyme cytochrome P-450, resulting in a decrease in metabolism and an increase in the effect of drugs eliminated by that pathway, such as the anticoagulant warfarin. Because metronidazole itself undergoes oxidative metabolism, its clearance can be increased or decreased by enzyme inducers or inhibitors, such as barbiturates or cimetidine, respectively, resulting in decreased antimicrobial effect or possible metronidazole toxicity [17].

Antifungal Agents

Polyenes

CHEMISTRY

The polyene antifungal agents amphotericin B, nystatin, and natamycin are soluble in water. The antifungal effects of amphotericin are maximal between pH 6.0 and 7.5. The agent is less effective at lower pH [108].

MECHANISM OF ACTION

The polyene antifungal agents have their antifungal effect by binding to the sterol moiety ergosterol of the fungal cell wall, resulting in an increase in the permeability of the cell membrane, leaking of the cytoplasmic components, and cell death [108].

SPECTRUM OF ACTIVITY

Amphotericin B has antifungal activity against most fungi that cause clinically important infections, including *Histoplasma capsulatum*, *Blastomyces dermatitidis*, *Coccidioides immitis*, *Cryptococcus neoformans*, *C. albicans* and other *Candida* species, *Sporothrix schenckii*, *Rhizopus oryzae*, *Mucor heimalis*, and *Aspergillus fumigatus*. Nystatin and natamycin also have a broad antifungal spectrum of activity in vitro [109].

PHARMACOKINETICS

Absorption of the polyene antifungal agents from the gastrointestinal tract is negligible after usual oral doses. After intravenous administration, amphotericin B is detectable in most body fluids and tissues, with highest concentrations found in the liver, lungs, kidneys, and spleen. It undergoes primarily extrarenal routes of elimination. Its elimination is triexponential, with a half-life of 24 hours during the second phase of elimination and a terminal elimination half-life of 15 days [110, 111]. Ophthalmic administration of natamycin results in therapeutic concentrations in the corneal stroma but not in the intraocular fluid [112, 113].

CLINICAL USE

Because it is toxic in concentrations required for the treatment of systemic infections, use of nystatin is limited to the topical treatment of infections of the skin, mucous membranes, and intestinal tract caused by *Candida* organisms. Natamycin ophthalmic suspension is used to treat fungal blepharitis, conjunctivitis, and keratitis [109, 112, 113].

Amphotericin B is the primary therapeutic agent used intravenously to treat a variety of serious systemic fungal infections, including meningitis, bone and joint infections, pneumonia, endocarditis, esophagitis, urinary tract infections, and peritonitis. Amphotericin B also has an important role in the empiric treatment of neutropenic patients who remain febrile despite treatment with broad-spectrum antibacterial agents. It is also used topically to treat a variety of dermatomycoses and as a bladder irrigation for fungal cystitis [109].

ADVERSE EFFECTS

Topical agents usually cause few adverse effects. Amphotericin B can cause an acute reaction during infusion, consisting of chills, fever, rigors, headache, hypotension, tachypnea, and less commonly ventricular fibrillation. A reduction in glomerular filtration (usually reversible) and renal tubular acidosis with associated magnesium and potassium wasting (prolonged or irreversible) occur frequently. Rare effects include leukopenia, thrombocytopenia, and hepatitis [108, 109].

Azoles

CHEMISTRY
The imidazoles ketoconazole, miconazole, econazole, clotrimazole, and the triazole itraconazole are poorly soluble in water. Fluconazole is a triazole that has excellent water solubility [109].

MECHANISM OF ACTION
Imidazole and triazole antifungal agents inhibit the synthesis of ergosterol, the major sterol of the fungal cell wall, by inhibition of lanosterol demethylase, the enzyme responsible for the methylation of the precursor lanosterol to ergosterol. This results in a reduction in cell wall integrity, leading to the leakage of cytoplasmic contents and cell death [108].

SPECTRUM OF ACTIVITY
Azoles have a broad antimycotic spectrum and have activity in vitro against most pathogenic fungi. The minimum concentrations required to kill susceptible fungi vary widely among studies, probably due to the lack of standardization of the various methods used to perform the tests. Therefore, the results of in vitro testing should be viewed cautiously. Ketoconazole has activity in vitro against dermatophytes, B. dermatitidis, C. immitis, H. capsulatum, and C. neoformans. Strains of Candida and Aspergillus species may be resistant. The antifungal spectrum of miconazole includes C. immitis, C. albicans, C. neoformans, and most dermatophytes. Aspergillus organisms may be less susceptible [114]. Fluconazole and itraconazole also are active in vitro against most fungal pathogens. Although itraconazole is fungicidal in vitro at lower concentrations, the excellent penetration of fluconazole into most tissues makes it appear to be equally effective [115]. The imidazoles have a broad antifungal spectrum in vitro and are active against most human pathogens, including dermatophytes and Candida species [109].

PHARMACOKINETICS
Unlike the polyenes, ketoconazole, fluconazole, and itraconazole are well absorbed after oral administration. The other azoles are not absorbed orally [108, 109]. Ketoconazole absorption depends on gastric acidity. Patients taking drugs such as antacids or H_2 antagonists or with disease states that reduce gastric acidity have reduced ketoconazole bioavailability [12].

Ketoconazole distributes well into skin, joint spaces, and tendons. It diffuses into aqueous and vitreous humor. Concentrations in uninfected bone are undetectable. Penetration into the CSF is poor, although it has been detected in some reports. Ketoconazole is metabolized by oxidative enzymes in the liver to inactive metabolites, and 13% of an administered dose excreted in the urine is unchanged drug. The elimination half-life is 3 hours [116].

The absorption of itraconazole is enhanced by administering it with a meal. Itraconazole concentrates in extravascular spaces; measured tissue concentrations are higher than those obtained simultaneously in the serum. Like ketoconazole, the drug is extensively bound to plasma protein (99%) and achieves poor concentrations in the CSF and urine. Elimination is triphasic, with a terminal half-life of 24–36 hours [116, 117].

Fluconazole is only minimally protein bound and does not undergo significant hepatic metabolism. The elimination half-life is 22 hours in subjects with normal renal function, prolonged in those with renal dysfunction [116]. The major pharmacokinetic feature that distinguishes fluconazole from other azoles is its excellent penetration into the CSF, with concentrations to 60%–80% of simultaneous serum concentrations in patients with inflamed or uninflamed meninges [116, 118].

CLINICAL USE
Ketoconazole can be used as an alternative to amphotericin B for the treatment of histoplasmosis, coccidiomycosis, and blastomycosis in immunocompetent hosts. It can be used to treat candida esophagitis. In preliminary studies itraconazole appears to be a promising drug for the treatment of blastomycosis, coccidiomycosis, histoplasmosis, and sporotrichosis. Fluconazole has been shown to be effective for the treatment of oropharyngeal or

esophageal candidiasis and for prevention of relapse of cryptococcal meningitis in AIDS patients [47].

Because of its toxicity and the availability of other safer agents, intravenous miconazole is used rarely. The use of it and the other imidazoles (clotrimazole, miconazole, econazole, terconazole, and butoconazole) is limited to treatment of vulvovaginitis caused by *Candida* and cutaneous infections due to susceptible organisms. All are equally effective. Miconazole and clotrimazole have recently received nonprescription status from the FDA for vulvovaginal and cutaneous administration. Oral clotrimazole troches are available by prescription only and are used for the treatment and prevention of oral candidiasis [108, 109].

ADVERSE EFFECTS

The most common adverse effects associated with ketoconazole use are dosage-dependent gastrointestinal upset and hypersensitivity reactions. High dosages can cause gynecomastia, impotence, decreased libido, and menstrual irregularities. Ketoconazole causes a dosage-dependent suppression of the ACTH response with possible clinical hypoadrenalism. It rarely causes hepatitis and more commonly can cause asymptomatic elevations of transaminases [109, 115].

In preliminary studies itraconazole and fluconazole have been well tolerated in humans. The most common adverse reactions with both drugs have been nausea and other gastrointestinal symptoms. Elevations in liver function tests have been reported in less than 5% of patients. Decreases in cortisol and testosterone have not been observed with either drug [16].

Intravenous miconazole frequently causes nausea, vomiting, anemia, and hyponatremia. Anaphylaxis and CNS reactions, including tremors, euphoria, confusion, hallucinations, and seizures, have been reported. Cardiorespiratory arrest has been reported with rapid infusions [108].

Miconazole, ketoconazole, and fluconazole can inhibit the metabolism of drugs metabolized by hepatic cytochrome P-450, such as phenytoin or warfarin [17, 44]. The effect of itraconazole on hepatic enzyme activity requires further study.

Topical agents are usually well tolerated. Local effects of burning, irritation, erythema, urticaria, pruritus, and rare cases of contact allergy have been reported [108].

Antiviral Agents

Acyclovir

CHEMISTRY

Acyclovir is a purine nucleoside analog in which a linear side chain has been substituted for the cyclic sugar of the guanosine molecule [119].

MECHANISM OF ACTION

Acyclovir is administered as a prodrug that must be phosphorylated by viral thymidine kinase to its active triphosphate form. It inhibits viral DNA polymerase, acts as a chain terminator, and inhibits DNA synthesis [119].

SPECTRUM OF ACTIVITY

Acyclovir has antiviral activity against viruses in the herpevirus family, including herpes simplex virus (HSV) types 1 and 2, varicella zoster virus (VZV), and Epstein-Barr virus. Cytomegalovirus (CMV) is inhibited by much higher concentrations of acyclovir than other herpes viruses [119, 120].

PHARMACOKINETICS

Acyclovir is available in oral and intravenous forms. The bioavailability of the oral agent ranges from 15%–30%, decreasing with increasingly larger doses. Its volume of distribution corresponds to total body water. It is widely distributed to most body fluids, achieving 33%–50% of serum concentrations in the CSF and aqueous humor. The elimination half-life is 2–3 hours in patients with normal renal function. Acyclovir is cleared from the body by glomerular filtration and tubular secretion. Its half-life is prolonged in patients with renal dysfunction [119, 120].

CLINICAL USE

Topical acyclovir ointment has limited efficacy compared to the oral and intravenous forms. Acyclovir is useful for the treatment and prevention of genital HSV infections but offers only modest benefit for the treatment of orolabial lesions. Short-term prophylaxis may reduce the incidence of sun-induced orolabial recurrences. Systemic therapy has been used for the treatment of herpes simplex encephalitis and the treatment and prevention of mucocutaneous infections in immunocompromised patients. It is useful for the treatment of disseminated infections in immunocompromised patients and in the treatment of herpes zoster infections in older adults if begun within 1–2 days of rash onset. It is effective in the prevention of dissemination in immunocompromised patients.

In patients with mononucleosis, acyclovir therapy decreases viral shedding but has not consistently been shown to have any influence on the clinical symptoms or the disease severity. It has no effect on the chronic fatigue syndrome, but it is effective for the treatment of Epstein-Barr virus–induced oral hairy leukoplakia. In controlled trials for the treatment of HSV encephalitis, varicella, and herpes zoster, acyclovir has been found to be either superior to or comparable in efficacy and with significantly less toxicity than the antiviral vidarabine [120].

ADVERSE EFFECTS
Topical acyclovir may cause transient burning on application to genital lesions, especially in primary episodes and in females. Oral acyclovir is generally well tolerated, with infrequent reports of gastrointestinal upset and headache. Acyclovir is relatively insoluble in water at body temperature. Rapid infusions or administration of large intravenous doses in patients not adequately hydrated can result in crystalluria and an increase in serum blood urea nitrogen (BUN) and creatinine that is reversible upon rehydration [120].

Extravasation of intravenous drug may result in inflammation and phlebitis at the injection site. Other uncommon adverse effects include rash, hematuria, hypotension, headache, and nausea. Neurotoxicity has been reported in approximately 1% of patients receiving intravenous therapy, manifested as mental status changes, tremors, seizures, or coma [120].

Ganciclovir

CHEMISTRY
Ganciclovir is a guanine analogue that is structurally similar to acyclovir. It differs only by the addition of a hydroxymethyl group [119].

MECHANISM OF ACTION
Similar to acyclovir, ganciclovir is phosphorylated by viral kinases to its active triphosphate form. The triphosphorylated compound is present in infected cells in a ten-fold-higher concentration than in uninfected cells. Ganciclovir triphosphate inhibits DNA polymerase and is a viral DNA chain terminator. Unlike acyclovir, ganciclovir is incorporated into both host cells and viral DNA [120].

SPECTRUM OF ACTIVITY
Like acyclovir, ganciclovir has antiviral activity against herpes viruses, including HSV 1 and HSV 2, and at higher concentrations against Epstein-Barr virus. It is uniquely active at clinically achievable concentrations against cytomegalovirus [120].

PHARMACOKINETICS
Ganciclovir is not absorbed after oral administration and is available only as an intravenous preparation. The drug is well distributed to body tissues, including CSF, brain tissue, aqueous humor, and subretinal fluid. Ganciclovir is eliminated primarily as unchanged drug by the kidneys, thus dosage adjustment in patients with renal dysfunction is required. Its elimination half-life is 3–4 hours in patients with normal renal function, increasing to 29 hours in severe renal insufficiency [119, 120].

CONTRAINDICATIONS
Ganciclovir is teratogenic and mutagenic and affects the reproductive cells in male and female animals. It is contraindicated in pregnant women and nursing mothers. Because of its effects on the bone marrow, its use is contraindicated in people taking concomitant zidovudine or other myelosuppressive agents [120].

CLINICAL USE
Ganciclovir use has been limited to patients with life- or sight-threatening cytomegalovirus infections. It has been used primarily in AIDS patients with CMV chorioretinitis. Ganciclovir has also been used with some success in uncontrolled studies in pneumonia and other infections caused by CMV in renal, heart, and bone marrow transplantation patients [120–122]. It has also been used to treat CMV gastrointestinal infections in patients with AIDS [123].

ADVERSE EFFECTS
The most common adverse effects caused by ganciclovir are neutropenia, occurring in 40% of patients, and thrombocytopenia, occurring in 20% of

patients. Neurotoxicity ranging from headache to mental status changes, convulsions, and glaucoma has been described in a significant number of patients. Myelosuppression and CNS toxicity necessitate treatment interruption or early discontinuation of therapy. Other reported adverse effects include anemia, rash, fever, elevation in liver function tests, azotemia, gastrointestinal disturbances, and eosinophilia [120].

Zidovudine

CHEMISTRY
Zidovudine (3'-azido-3'-deoxythymidine), formerly called azidothymidine (AZT), is a thymidine analogue in which a hydroxyl moiety is replaced by an azido group [119].

MECHANISM OF ACTION
Zidovudine is the only antiretroviral agent currently approved in the United States for widespread clinical use, although many other drugs are under various stages of investigation. Like acyclovir and ganciclovir, zidovudine is a prodrug that is phosphorylated by viral thymidine kinases to its triphosphate form, which inhibits viral RNA-dependent DNA polymerase or reverse transcriptase. The antiviral activity of zidovudine for infected cells is dependent on its greater affinity for HIV reverse transcriptase than for mammalian DNA [119].

SPECTRUM OF ACTIVITY
Zidovudine inhibits the replication of HIV 1 and other mammalian retroviruses. Higher concentrations are required in vitro to inhibit replication in chronically infected cells compared to exogenously infected cells. Zidovudine is active against human lymphotrophic virus type 1 (HTLV 1), which has been implicated in T-cell leukemias, but it is less active against HIV 2. Although not used for these indications, Epstein-Barr virus is inhibited at higher concentrations. Many Enterobacteriaceae and G. lamblia are also inhibited in vitro [119].

PHARMACOKINETICS
After oral administration approximately 65% of a dose is absorbed. Zidovudine is well distributed in body tissues and fluids. CSF concentrations approach those in the serum. Semen concentrations

exceed serum concentrations by 1.3- to 20-fold, suggesting concentration or accumulation in the prostate [119, 120].

The major route of elimination is hepatic metabolism to the inactive 5'-glucuronide metabolite (GAZT). Both zidovudine and its metabolite undergo renal tubular secretion and glomerular filtration. In patients with severe renal impairment, zidovudine concentrations are moderately increased, but the GAZT metabolite accumulates markedly. Hemodialysis has little effect on removal of the parent compound but significantly removes the inactive metabolite. Therefore, no dosage adjustments need to be made in patients with renal dysfunction or receiving hemodialysis [124]. In contrast the formation of GAZT is markedly reduced in patients with liver cirrhosis in an amount directly proportional to the severity of the cirrhosis. Patients with severe liver dysfunction may require blood-level monitoring or dosage adjustment [125].

CLINICAL USE
Zidovudine has been shown to prolong survival in patients with AIDS, delay a progression to AIDS in patients with the AIDS-related complex (ARC), and delay the progression to AIDS or ARC in HIV-seropositive asymptomatic patients with fewer than 500 CD4 lymphocytes [120, 126, 127, 128]. Although the optimal dosage is not known, it has been administered by continuous infusion safely to children [129] and in reduced doses in both patients with AIDS and patients with ARC [126, 128]. The lowest effective dosage and the time to initiate treatment are not precisely known at the present time [130, 131]. The use of zidovudine to prevent seroconversion in health care workers after occupational exposure to HIV is currently under study. No controlled trials are currently available to evaluate the efficacy for this indication [132].

ADVERSE EFFECTS
The major adverse effects associated with zidovudine use are granulocytopenia and anemia, which occur in up to 45% of patients receiving high-dosage zidovudine therapy. The incidence of hematologic toxicity varies adversely with the patients' pretreatment CD4 lymphocyte count and hematocrit. Other toxicities include severe headache, nausea, insomnia, and myalgia. Neurotox-

icity with seizures has been reported. Many of these symptoms may respond to dosage reduction. In trials in which much lower dosages were used, the incidence and severity of toxicities were less [120, 126, 128].

Little is known about the effects of administration of zidovudine during pregnancy, especially during the first trimester. Zidovudine has been given to a small number of pregnant women with no apparent adverse fetal effects. It does cross the placenta. Because of the paucity of data and the short-term follow-up of children of mothers who received zidovudine during pregnancy, its use in pregnancy should be reserved only for cases where there is clear benefit [133].

Amantadine

CHEMISTRY
Amantadine is not structurally related to other antimicrobial agents. It is a tricyclic amine. Rimantadine is an amantadine analogue under investigation. It has a similar antiviral spectrum but a lower incidence of toxicity.

MECHANISM OF ACTION
The exact mechanism by which amantadine has its antiviral activity is unknown, but it may block the uncoating of the viral genome in lysosomes [120].

SPECTRUM OF ACTIVITY
The antiviral spectrum of amantadine is limited to the inhibition of replication of influenza A. It has no effect on influenza B or other viruses [119].

PHARMACOKINETICS
Amantadine is well absorbed after oral administration. It is widely distributed to body fluids and tissues, including CSF, saliva, nasal secretions, and lung tissue. It is excreted unchanged in the urine by glomerular filtration and possibly tubular secretion. The elimination half-life is variable (mean of 16 hours) but is prolonged in elderly adults and patients with renal dysfunction, requiring dosage adjustment to minimize toxicity [120].

CLINICAL USE
Amantadine is useful for the prevention and treatment of patients with viral infections caused by influenza A. Prophylaxis with amantadine is an alternative to influenza vaccination in patients in whom the vaccine is contraindicated or would be ineffective or during the period after vaccination before an immune response has been provoked. Amantadine treatment should be initiated in unimmunized health care workers and household members with regular contact as soon as influenza has been identified in the community or the home. Controlled studies indicate that treatment is effective in infected patients if therapy is begun within 48 hours of symptom onset, although these studies were done in college students or military recruits and not in elderly or high-risk adults [120].

CONTRAINDICATIONS
Amantadine is teratogenic in animals, and its safety during pregnancy or lactation has not been established.

ADVERSE EFFECTS
The most common adverse effects associated with amantadine use are gastrointestinal upset and CNS agitation, including nervousness, lightheadedness, difficulty concentrating, insomnia, loss of appetite, and nausea. These side effects are concentration dependent and can be minimized by proper dosage reduction adjusted for renal function. The CNS toxicity may be increased by concomitant administration of antihistamines or anticholinergic drugs. Long-term ingestion has caused livedo reticularis, peripheral edema, orthostatic hypotension, and isolated cases of congestive heart failure, vision loss, and urinary retention. Amantadine may increase the frequency of seizures in patients with preexisting seizure disorders [120].

Rimantadine has not yet been approved for use in the United States. Advantages over amantadine include a lower incidence of CNS adverse effects and a nonrenal route of elimination [119].

Antiparasitic Agents

A thorough review of antiparasitic agents is beyond the scope of this chapter. Antiparasitic drugs, indications for their use, and adverse effects are listed in Table 4-16 [134].

Table 4-16. Antiparasitic agents

Generic and brand names	Uses	Adverse effects
Chloroquine (Aralen)	Amebiasis, malaria	*Occasional:* pruritus, vomiting, headache, confusion, depigmentation of hair, skin eruptions, corneal opacity, weight loss, partial alopecia, extraocular muscle palsies, exacerbation of psoriasis, eczema, and other exfoliative dermatoses, myalgias, photophobia *Rare:* irreversible retinal injury (especially when total dosage exceeds 100 grams), discoloration of nails and mucous membranes, nerve-type deafness, peripheral neuropathy and myopathy, heart block, blood dyscrasias, hematemesis
Crotamiton (Eurax)	Scabies	*Occasional:* skin rash, conjunctivitis
Emetine	Amebiasis	*Frequent:* cardiac arrhythmias, precordial pain, muscle weakness, cellulitis at site of injection *Occasional:* diarrhea, vomiting, peripheral neuropathy, heart failure
Furazolidone (Furoxone)	Giardiasis	*Frequent:* nausea, vomiting *Occasional:* allergic reactions, including pulmonary infiltration, hypotension, urticaria, fever, vesicular rash, hypoglycemia, headache *Rare:* hemolytic anemia in G6PD deficiency and neonates, disulfiram-like reaction with alcohol, MAO-inhibitor interactions, polyneuritis
Iodoquinol (Yodoxin)	Amebiasis	*Occasional:* rash, acne, slight enlargement of the thyroid gland, nausea, diarrhea, cramps, anal pruritus *Rare:* optic atrophy, loss of vision, peripheral neuropathy after prolonged use in high dosage (for months), iodine sensitivity
Lindane (Kwell)	Lice, scabies	*Occasional:* eczematous skin rash, conjunctivitis *Rare:* convulsions, aplastic anemia
Malathion (Ovide)	Lice	*Occasional:* local irritation
Mebendazole (Vermox)	Angiostrongyliasis, ascariasis capillariasis, pinworm (enterobiasis), filariasis, hookworm, trichinosis	*Occasional:* diarrhea, abdominal pain *Rare:* leukopenia, agranulocytosis, hypospermia
Mefloquine (Lariam)	Malaria	*Frequent:* vertigo, lightheadedness, nausea, other gastrointestinal disturbances, nightmares, visual disturbances, headache *Occasional:* confusion, psychosis *Rare:* convulsions, coma
Metronidazole (Flagyl)	Amebiasis, giardiasis	*Frequent:* nausea, headache, dry mouth, metallic taste *Occasional:* vomiting, diarrhea, insomnia, weakness, stomatitis, vertigo, paresthesia, rash, dark urine, urethral burning, disulfiram-like reaction with alcohol *Rare:* seizures, encephalopathy, pseudomembranous colitis, ataxia, leukopenia, peripheral neuropathy, pancreatitis
Niclosamide (Niclocide)	Tapeworm	*Occasional:* nausea, abdominal pain
Paromomycin (Humatin)	Amebiasis	*Frequent:* gastrointestinal disturbance *Rare:* eighth-nerve damage (mainly auditory), renal damage

Table 4-16. (*continued*)

Generic and brand names	Uses	Adverse effects
Pentamidine isoethionate (Pentam 300)	Pneumocystis	*Frequent:* hypotension, hypoglycemia often followed by diabetes mellitus, vomiting, blood dyscrasias, renal damage, pain at injection site, gastrointestinal disturbances *Occasional:* may aggravate diabetes, shock, hypocalcemia, liver damage, cardiotoxicity, delirium, rash *Rare:* Herxheimer-type reaction, anaphylaxis, acute pancreatitis, hyperkalemia
Permethrin (Nix)	Lice, scabies	*Occasional:* burning, stinging, numbness, increased pruritus, pain, edema, erythema, rash
Praziquantel (Biltricide)	Chinese liver fluke, intestinal fluke, lung fluke, schistosomiases, tapeworm	*Frequent:* malaise, headache, dizziness *Occasional:* sedation, abdominal discomfort, fever, sweating, nausea, eosinophilia, fatigue *Rare:* pruritus, rash
Primaquine phosphate	Malaria	*Frequent:* hemolytic anemia in G6PD deficiency *Occasional:* neutropenia, gastrointestinal disturbances, methemoglobinemia in G6PD deficiency *Rare:* CNS symptoms, hypertension, arrhythmias
Pryantel pamoate (Antiminth)	Ascariasis, pinworm (enterobiasis), hookworm, moniliforms	*Occasional:* gastrointestinal disturbances, headache, dizziness, rash, fever
Pyrethrins and piperonyl butoxide (Rid)	Lice	*Occasional:* allergic reactions
Pyrimethamine (Daraprim)	Toxoplasmosis	*Occasional:* blood dyscrasias, folic acid deficiency *Rare:* rash, vomiting, convulsions, shock, possibly pulmonary eosinophilia
Pyrimethamine-sulfadoxine (Fansidar)	Malaria	*Frequent:* allergic reactions (rash, photosensitivity, drug fever) *Occasional:* blood dyscrasias, folic acid deficiency, kernicterus in newborns, renal or hepatic damage, Stevens-Johnson syndrome, hemolyticaremea, other blood dyscrasias, rascultitis *Rare:* rash, vomiting, convulsions, shock, possibly pulmonary eosinophilia, pseudomembranous colitis
Quinacrine (Atabrine)	Giardiasis	*Frequent:* dizziness, headache, vomiting, diarrhea *Occasional:* yellow staining of skin, toxic psychosis, insomnia, bizarre dreams, blood dyscrasias, urticaria, blue and black nail pigmentation, psoriasis-like rash *Rare:* acute hepatic necrosis, convulsions, severe exfoliative dermatitis, ocular effects similar to those caused by chloroquine
Quinine sulfate	Malaria	*Frequent:* cinchonism (tinnitus, headache, nausea, abdominal pain, visual disturbance) *Occasional:* hemolytic anemia, other blood dyscrasias, photosensitivity reactions, hypoglycemia, arrhythmias, hypotension, drug fever *Rare:* blindness, sudden death if injected too rapidly
Thiabendazole (Mintezol)	Stronglydiasis, capillariasis	*Frequent:* nausea, vomiting, vertigo *Occasional:* leukopenia, crystalluria, rash, hallucinations, olfactory disturbance, erythema multiforme, Stevens-Johnson syndrome *Rare:* shock, tinnitus, intrahepatic cholestasis, convulsions, angioneurotic edema

Adapted from: Drugs for parasitic infections. *Med Lett Drug Ther* 32:23–32, 1990.

New Macrolide Antibiotics

Background

Interest in macrolide antibiotics has increased in recent years because of their lack of cross-allergenicity with beta-lactam and other classes of antibiotics and the increased recognition of pathogens such as *Legionella*, *Chlamydia*, and *Campylobacter* species. Limitations of erythromycin include its poor bioavailability with certain formulations, its susceptibility to acid hydrolysis in the stomach, significant incidence of gastrointestinal side effects even with intravenous use, and its limited spectrum of activity. Erythromycin's most common use is in the treatment of respiratory tract infections, but its lack of activity against *H. influenzae* seriously limits its usefulness [135, 136]. Two promising macrolide antibiotics in development include the 14-membered macrolide clarithromycin and the 15-membered azithromycin, the first azalide antibiotic.

Spectrum of Activity

Azithromycin and clarithromycin are both active against erythromycin-susceptible staphylococci. Staphylococci that are resistant to erythromycin are also resistant to these compounds. The minimum inhibitory concentrations of azithromycin required against staphylococci are two to four times lower than that of erythromycin; the post-antibiotic effect of clarithromycin against these organisms is three times longer than that observed with erythromycin. Both drugs are active against streptococci, including *S. pyogenes* and *S. pneumoniae*. Azithromycin has variable activity against *L. monocytogenes* and has activity against *C. diphtheriae* similar to erythromycin [135, 136].

Both azithromycin and clarithromycin have excellent activity against most gram-negative bacteria that cause respiratory and other infections, including *H. influenzae*, *M. catarrhalis*, and *B. pertussis*, with clarithromycin having similar activity to erythromycin and azithromycin two- to eight-fold times more active. Azithromycin is very active against organisms found in bite wounds, such as *P. multocida* and *Eikenella corrodens* [135, 136]. Azithromycin has variable activity against *Salmonella*, *Shigella*, and *E. coli*. Other gram-negative organisms such as *Proteus* and *Klebsiella*, *Enterobacter*, *Serratia*, and *Pseudomonas* species are resistant to both drugs.

Because of their excellent intracellular penetration, both drugs are extremely active against intracellular pathogens such as chlamydiae, *Legionella* species, and *M. pneumoniae*. Clarithromycin has activity against anaerobic organisms similar to erythromycin. Azithromycin is more active, inhibiting many anaerobic species at lower concentrations than erythromycin, including *Propionobacterium acnes*, peptococci, peptostreptococci, *C. perfringens*, *C. difficile*, other *clostridia*, *B. fragilis*, and other bacteroides, although some strains of *B. thetaiotaomicron* may be less susceptible. Azithromycin has superior activity to erythromycin against *Borrelia burgdorferi*. Both are active against *Neisseria* species and *Mycobacterium avium-intracellulare*. Neither is active against *Mycobacterium tuberculosis* [135, 136].

Pharmacokinetics

Important pharmacokinetic advantages of these drugs compared to erythromycin include good bioavailability and excellent tissue penetration. Both drugs are stable against gastric acid and do not undergo hydrolysis in the stomach after oral administration. The bioavailability of azithromycin and clarithromycin after oral administration is 37% and 55%, respectively, compared to 25% for erythromycin.

Clarithromycin is metabolized to an active 14-hydroxy derivative. The elimination half-lives of the parent and the metabolite are prolonged in patients with renal dysfunction. Clarithromycin concentrations in tonsillar and lung tissue exceed simultaneous serum concentrations by two- to five-fold. Concentrations inside macrophages and neutrophils exceed extracellular concentrations by nine-fold [136].

After oral administration, azithromycin undergoes polyphasic elimination, characterized by rapid intracellular uptake followed by elimination primarily by biliary excretion, with a terminal elimination half-life of approximately 60 hours. High concentrations exceeding that in the serum by several fold are achieved within phagocytes and transported to the site of infection by chemotactic mechanisms, as well as in pulmonary, urogenital, and lymphatic tissues. Therapeutic azithromycin concentrations are sustained at tissue sites for up to 4–7 days after discontinuing therapy [135, 137].

Clinical Use

Initial studies indicate the effectiveness of these drugs for a variety of clinical uses. Azithromycin has been shown to be effective for the treatment of streptococcal pharyngitis, acute sinusitis, lower respiratory tract infections, skin and skin structure infections, and single-dose treatment of genital chlamydial infections. Clarithromycin has been demonstrated to be an effective agent in the treatment of skin, skin structure, sinus, and lower respiratory tract infections [135, 136]. Preliminary data presented in abstract form indicate that clarithromycin may be a useful adjunct in the treatment of *Mycobacterium avium-intracellulare* infections.

Adverse Effects

Azithromycin and clarithromycin have been well tolerated in published studies. The most common adverse effects reported include diarrhea and other mild gastrointestinal symptoms occurring significantly less (two- to four-fold or more) than seen with erythromycin and other comparative agents. In contrast to erythromycin, neither drug appears to decrease the metabolism of theophylline or other drugs metabolized by the cytochrome P-450 oxidative enzyme system [136, 138].

References

1. Moellering RC. Principles of antiinfective therapy. In GI Mandell, RG Douglas Jr, JE Bennett (eds.), *Principles and Practice of Infectious Diseases* (3rd ed.). New York: Churchill-Livingstone, 1990. Pp. 206–18.
2. Bauer LA. Primer on clinical pharmacokinetics. *Am J Hosp Pharm* 40:1637–41, 1983.
3. McCarthy CG, Finland M. Absorption and excretion of four penicillins: penicillin G, penicillin V, phenethicillin and phenylmercaptomethyl penicillin. *N Engl J Med* 263:315, 1960.
4. Nauta EH, Mattie H. Dicloxacillin and cloxacillin: pharmacokinetics in healthy and hemodialysis subjects. *Clin Pharmacol Ther* 20:98–108, 1976.
5. Bergant T, Bjerke PE, Fausa O. Pharmacokinetics of metronidazole in patients with enteric disease compared to normal volunteers. *Chemotherapy* 27:233–38, 1981.
6. Reeves DS, Wilkinson PJ. The pharmacokinetics of trimethoprim in trimethoprim-sulfonamide combinations, including penetration into body tissues. *Infection* 7:S330–41, 1979.
7. Welling PG, Tse FL. The influence of food on the absorption of antimicrobial agents. *J Antimicrob Chemother* 9:7–27, 1982.
8. Ginsburg CM et al. Effective feeding on bioavailability of griseofulvin in children. *J Pediatr* 102:309–11, 1983.
9. Williams PE, Harding SM. The absolute bioavailability of oral cefuroxime axetil in male and female volunteers after fasting and after food. *J Antimicrob Chemother* 13:191–96, 1984.
10. Tetzlaff TR, McCracken GH Jr, Thomas LL. Bioavailability of cephalexin in children: relationship to drug formulations in males. *J Pediatr* 92:292–94, 1978.
11. Frost RW et al. Ciprofloxacin pharmacokinetics after a standard or high-fat/high-calcium breakfast. *J Clin Pharmacol* 29:953–55, 1989.
12. Van Der Meer et al. The influence of gastric acidity on the bioavailability of ketoconazole. *J Antimicrob Chemother* 6:552–54, 1980.
13. Kucers A, Mc K. Bennett N. Ketoconazole. In *The Use of Antibiotics* (4th ed.). Philadelphia: Lippincott, 1987. Pp. 1506–27.
14. Van Dyke R et al. Pharmacokinetics of increased dose oral acyclovir [abstract]. In Program and abstracts of the 22nd Interscience Conference of Antimicrobial Agents and Chemotherapy. American Society of Microbiology, 1982. P. 139.
15. Stoeckel K et al. Effects of concentration dependent plasma protein finding on ceftriaxone kinetics. *Clin Pharmacol Ther* 29:650–57, 1981.
16. Pechere JC, Dugal R. Clinical pharmacokinetics of aminoglycoside antibiotics. *Clin Pharmacokinet* 4:170–99, 1979.
17. Norris S, Nightingale CH, Mandell GL. Tables of antimicrobial agent pharmacology. In GL Mandell, RG Douglas Jr, JE Bennett (eds.), *Principles and Practice of Infectious Diseases* (3rd ed.). New York: Churchill-Livingstone, 1990. Pp. 456–60.
18. Naber KG. Use of quinolones in urinary tract infections and prostatitis. *Rev Infect Dis* 11(suppl):S1321–37, 1989.
19. The Medical Letter, Inc. *The Medical Letter Handbook of Antimicrobial Therapy.* New York: The Medical Letter Inc., 1990.

20. Bennet WM et al. *Drug Prescribing in Renal Failure: Dosing Guidelines for Adults.* Philadelphia: American College of Physicians, 1987.

21. Davey RT Jr, Masur H. Recent advances in the diagnosis, treatment, and prevention of *Pneumocystis carinii* pneumonia. *Antimicrob Agents Chemother* 34:499–504, 1990.

22. Noone P et al. Experience in monitoring gentamicin therapy during treatment of serious gram-negative sepsis. *Br Med J* 1:477–81, 1974.

23. Moore RD, Smith CR, Lietman PS. Association of aminoglycoside plasma levels with therapeutic outcome in gram-negative pneumonia. *Am J Med* 77:657–62, 1984.

24. Gleckman RA. Treatment duration for urinary tract infections in adults. *Antimicrob Agents Chemother* 31:1–5, 1987.

25. Wilson WR, Geraci JE. Treatment of streptococcal infective endocarditis. *Am J Med* 78(6B):128–37, 1985.

26. Alexander DP. Central nervous system infections. In ET Herfindal, DR Gourley, LL Hart (eds.), *Clinical Pharmacy and Therapeutics* (4th ed.). Baltimore: Williams & Wilkins, 1988. Pp. 780–91.

27. Witkop CJ, Wolf RO. Hypoplasia and intrinsic staining of enamel following tetracycline therapy. *JAMA.* 185:385, 1963.

28. Stahlmann R, Lode H. Safety overview: toxicity, adverse effects and drug interactions. In VT Andriole (ed.), *Quinolones.* London: Academic, 1988. Pp. 201–33.

29. Hoetrich PD. Antimicrobics and anthelmintics for systemic therapy. In PD Hoetrich, MC Jordan (eds.), *Infectious Diseases* (4th ed.). Grand Rapids: Lippincott, 1989. Pp. 206–51.

30. Cockcroft DW, Gault MH. Prediction of creatinine clearance from serum creatinine. *Nephron* 16:31–41, 1976.

31. *Federal Register.* 44:3743–67, 1980.

32. Briggs GG, Freeman RK, Yaffe SJ (eds.). *Drugs in Pregnancy and Lactation* (3rd ed.). Baltimore: Williams & Wilkins, 1990.

33. American Academy of Pediatrics Committee on Drugs. Transfer of drugs and other chemicals into human milk. *Pediatr* 84:924–36, 1989.

34. Newfield P, Roizen MF. Hazards of rapid administration of vancomycin. *Ann Intern Med* 91:581, 1979.

35. Saxon A et al. Immediate hypersensitivity reactions to beta-lactam antibiotics. *Ann Intern Med* 107:204–15, 1987.

36. Weiss ME, Adkinson NF. Beta-lactam allergy. In GL Mandell, RG Douglas Jr, JE Bennett (eds.), *Principles and Practice of Infectious Diseases* (3rd ed.). New York: Churchill-Livingstone, 1990. Pp. 264–69.

37. Donowitz GR, Mandell GL. Cephalosporins. In GL Mandell, RG Douglas Jr, JE Bennett (eds.), *Principles and Practice of Infectious Diseases* (3rd ed.). New York: Churchill-Livingstone, 1990. Pp. 249–59.

38. Fekety R. Vancomycin and teicoplanin. In GL Mandell, RG Douglas Jr, JE Bennett (eds.), *Principles and Practice of Infectious Diseases* (3rd ed.). New York: Churchill-Livingstone, 1990. Pp. 317–23.

39. Wilson WR, Cockerill FR. Tetracyclines, chloramphenicol, erythromycin, and clindamycin. *Mayo Clin Proc* 62:906–15, 1987.

40. Adkinson NF Jr, Mueller B, Swabb EA. Clinical tolerance of the monobactam aztreonam in penicillin allergic subjects [abstract WS 26-4]. Presented at the 14th International Congress of Chemotherapy, Kyoto, Japan, June 23–28, 1985.

41. Saxon A et al. Lack of cross-reactivity between aztreonam, a monobactam antibiotic, and penicillin in penicillin-allergic subjects. *J Infect Dis* 149:16–22, 1984.

42. Fekety R. Antibiotic-associated colitis. In GL Mandell, RG Douglas Jr, JE Bennett (eds.), *Principles and Practice of Infectious Diseases* (3rd. ed.). New York: Churchill-Livingstone, 1990. Pp. 863–70.

43. Davis RL. Drug interactions with fluoroquinolone antibiotics. *Drug Interact Newsletter* 8:27–31, 1988.

44. Lazar JD, Wilner KD. Drug interactions with fluconazole. *Rev Infect Dis* 12(suppl 3):S327–33, 1990.

45. Dajani AS et al. Prevention of bacterial endocarditis. Recommendation by the American Heart Association. *JAMA* 264:2919–21, 1990.

46. The choice of antimicrobial drugs. *Med Lett Drugs Ther* 32:41–48, 1990.

47. Drugs for treatment of fungal infections. *Med Lett Drugs Ther* 32:58–60, 1990.

48. Wright AJ, Wilkowske, CJ. The penicillins. *Mayo Clin Proc* 62:806–20, 1987.

49. Mandell GL, Sande MA. Penicillins, cephalosporins, and other beta-lactam antibiotics. In AG Gilman, TW Rall, AS Nies, P Taylor (eds.), *Pharmacological Basis of Therapeutics* (8th ed.). New York: Pergamon, 1990. Pp. 1065–97.

50. Tomaz ZA. From penicillin-binding proteins to the lysis and death of bacteria: a 1979 view. *Rev Infect Dis* 1:434–67, 1979.

51. Neu HC. Penicillins. In GL Mandell, RG Douglas

Jr, JE Bennett (eds.), *Principles and Practice of Infections Diseases* (3rd. ed.). New York: Churchill-Livingstone, 1990. Pp. 230–46.

52. Bush LM, Calmon J, Johnson CC. Newer penicillins and beta-lactamase inhibitors. *Infect Dis Clin North Am* 38:571–94, 1989.

53. Brown CH 3d et al. The hemostatic defect produced by carbenicillin. *N Engl J Med* 291:265–70, 1974.

54. Fass RJ et al. Platelet-mediated bleeding caused by broad-spectrum penicillins. *J Infect Dis* 6:1242–48, 1987.

55. Barriere Sl, Conte JE Jr. Absence of nafcillin-associated nephritis. A prospective analysis of 210 patients. *West J Med* 133:472–77, 1980.

56. Ditlove J et al. Methicillin nephritis. *Medicine* (Baltimore) 56:483–91, 1977.

57. Thompson RL. Cephalosporin, carbapenem, and monobactam antibiotics. *Mayo Clin Proc* 62:821–34, 1987.

58. Donowitz GR, Mandell GL. Beta-lactam antibiotics. *N Engl J Med* 318:419–26, 1988.

59. Cefixime—a new oral cephalosporin. *Med Lett Drugs Ther* 31:72–74, 1989.

60. Greenfield RA, Gerber AU, Craig WA. Pharmacokinetics of cefoperazone in patients with normal and impaired hepatic and renal function. *Rev Infect Dis* 5(suppl):S127–36, 1983.

61. Stoeckel K, Koup JR. Pharmacokinetics of cefotriaxone in patients with renal and liver insufficiency and correlations with a physiologic nonlinear protein binding model. *Am J Med* 77(4C):26–32, 1984.

62. Ings RM et al. The pharmacokinetics of cefotaxime and its metabolism in subjects with normal and impaired renal function. *Rev Infect Dis* 4(suppl):S379–91, 1982.

63. Schaad UB et al. A comparison of ceftriaxone and cefuroxime for the treatment of bacterial meningitis in children. *N Engl J Med* 322:141–47, 1990.

64. Lebel MH, Hoyt MJ, McCracken GH Jr. Comparative efficacy of ceftriaxone and cefuroxime for treatment of bacterial meningitis. *J Pediatr* 114:1049–54, 1989.

65. 1989 sexually transmitted diseases treatment guidelines. *MMWR* 38(Suppl 8):1–43, 1989.

66. Nichols RL et al. Coagulopathy associated with extended-spectrum cephalosporins in patients with serious infections. *Antimicrob Agents Chemother* 31:281–85, 1987.

67. Grasela TH et al. Prospective surveillance of antibiotic-associated coagulopathy in 970 patients. *Pharmacotherapy* 9:158–64, 1989.

68. Standiford HC. Tetracyclines and chloramphenicol. In GL Mandell, RG Douglas Jr, JE Bennett (eds.), *Principles and Practice of Infectious Diseases* (3rd ed.). New York: Churchill-Livingstone, 1990. Pp. 284–95.

69. Welling PG et al. Bioavailability of tetracycline and doxycycline in fasted and nonfasted subjects. *Antimicrob Agents Chemother* 11:462–69, 1977.

70. Smith C, Woods CG, Woods MJ. Absorption of minocycline [letter]. *J Antimicrob Chemother* 13:93, 1984.

71. Whelton A. Tetracyclines in renal insufficiency: resolution of a therapeutic dilemma. *Bull NY Acad Med* 54:223–36, 1978.

72. Winckler K. Tetracycline ulcers of the oesophagus: endoscopy, histology and reoentgenology in two cases, and review of the literature. *Endoscopy* 13:225–28, 1981.

73. Fanning WL, Gump DW, Sofferman RA. Side effects of minocycline: a double blind study. *Antimicrob Agents Chemother* 11:712–17, 1977.

74. Steigbigel NH. Erythromycin, lincomycin, and clindamycin. In GL Mandell, RG Douglas Jr, JE Bennett (eds.). *Principles and Practice of Infectious Diseases* (3rd ed.). New York: Churchill-Livingstone, 1990. Pp. 308–17.

75. Erythromycin and salts. In JE Knoben, PO Anderson (eds.), *Handbook of Clinical Drug Data* (6th ed.). Hamilton, IL: Drug Intelligence Publications Inc, 1988. Pp. 342–45.

76. Chow AS. Infections of the oral cavity, neck and head. In GL Mandell, RG Douglas Jr, JE Bennett (eds.), *Principles and Practice of Infectious Diseases* (3rd ed.). New York: Churchill-Livingstone, 1990. Pp. 516–25.

77. Klika LJ, Goodman JM. Gastrointestinal tract symptoms from intravenously administered erythromycin [letter]. *JAMA* 248:1309, 1982.

78. Itoh Z et al. Erythromycin mimics exogenous motilin in gastrointestinal contractile activity in the dog. *Am J Physiol* 247:G688–94, 1984.

79. Brummett RE, Fox KE. Vancomycin- and erythromycin-induced hearing loss in humans. *Antimicrob Agents Chemother* 33:791–96, 1989.

80. Lindsay J Jr, Smith MA, Light JA. Torsades de pointes associated with antimicrobial therapy for pneumonia. *Chest* 98:222–23, 1990.

81. Nattel S et al. Erythromycin-induced long QT syndrome: concordance with quinidine and cellular electrophysiologic mechanism. *Am J Med* 89:235–38, 1990.

82. Matzke GR et al. Pharmacokinetics of vancomycin in patients with various degrees of renal function. *Antimicrob Agents Chemother* 15:433–37, 1984.

83. Moellering RC, Krogstad DJ, Greenblatt DJ. Vancomycin therapy in patients with impaired renal function: a nomogram for dosage. *Ann Intern Med* 94:343–46, 1981.

84. Rodvold KA et al. Vancomycin pharmacokinetics in patients with varying degrees of renal function. *Antimicrob Agents Chemother* 32:848–52, 1988.

85. Healy DP et al. Vancomycin-induced histamine release and "red man syndrome": comparison of 1- and 2-hour infusions. *Antimicrob Agents Chemother* 34:550–54, 1990.

86. Sahai J et al. Influence of antihistamine pretreatment on vancomycin-induced red man syndrome. *J Infect Dis* 160:876–81, 1989.

87. Nahata MC. Lack of nephrotoxicity in pediatric patients receiving concurrent vancomycin and aminoglycosides. *Chemotherapy* 330:302–04, 1987.

88. Zinner SH, Mayer KH. Sulfonamides and trimethoprim. In GL Mandell, RG Douglas Jr, JE Bennett (eds.), *Principles and Practice of Infectious Diseases* (3rd ed.). New York: Churchill-Livingstone, 1990. Pp. 325–34.

89. Mandell GL, Sande MA. Sulfonamides, trimethoprim-sulfamethoxazole, quinolones, and agents for urinary tract infections. In AG Gilman, TW Rall, AS Nies, P Taylor (eds.), *Pharmacological Basis of Therapeutics* (4th ed.). New York: Pergamon Press, 1990. Pp. 1047–65.

90. Massur A. Therapy for AIDS. In GL Mandell, RG Douglas Jr, JE Bennett (eds.), *Principles and Practice of Infectious Diseases* (3rd ed.). New York: Churchill-Livingstone, 1990. P. 1105.

91. Bygbjerg IC, Lund JT, Hording M. Effect of folic and folinic acid on cytopenia occurring during co-trimoxazole treatment of *Pneumocystis carinii* pneumonia. *Scand J Infect Dis* 20:685–86, 1988.

92. Small CB et al. The treatment of *Pneumocystis carinii* pneumonia in the acquired immuno-deficiency syndrome. *Arch Intern Med* 145:837–40, 1985.

93. Jaffe HS et al. Complications of co-trimoxazole in the treatment of AIDS associated *Pneumocystis carinii* pneumonia in homosexual men. *Lancet* 2:1109–11, 1983.

94. Shear NH et al. Differences in metabolism of sulfonamides predisposing to idiosyncratic toxicity. *Ann Intern Med* 105:179–84, 1986.

95. Markowitz N, Saravolatz LD. Use of trimethoprim-sulfamethoxazole in a glucose-6-phosphate-dehydrogenenase deficient population. *Rev Infect Dis* 9(suppl):S218–25, 1987.

96. Andriole VT. Quinolones. In GL Mandell, RG Douglas Jr, JE Bennett (eds.), *The Principles and Practice of Infectious Diseases* (3rd ed.). New York: Churchill-Livingstone, 1990. Pp. 334–45.

97. Hooper DC, Wolfson JS. Fluoroquinolone antimicrobial agents. *N Engl J Med* 324:384–94, 1991.

98. Walker RC, Wright AJ. The quinolones. *Mayo Clin Proc* 62:1007–12, 1987.

99. Anastasio GD, Menscer D, Little JM Jr. Norfloxacin and seizures [letter]. *Ann Intern Med* 109:169–70, 1988.

100. Sande MA, Mandell GL. Tetracyclines, chloramphenicol, erythromycin and miscellaneous antibacterial agents. In AG Gilman, TW Rall, AS Nies, P Taylor (eds.), *The Pharmacological Basis of Therapeutics* (8th ed.). New York: Pergamon Press, 1990. Pp. 1134–37.

101. Levison ME et al. Clindamycin compared with penicillin for the treatment of anaerobic lung abscess. *Ann Intern Med* 98:466–71, 1983.

102. Finegold SM, Mathisen GE. Metronidazole. In GL Mandell, RG Douglas Jr, JE Bennett (eds.), *Principles and Practice of Infectious Diseases* (3rd. ed.). New York: Churchill-Livingstone, 1990. Pp. 303–08.

103. Webster LT Jr. Drugs used in the chemotherapy of protozoal infections: amebiasis, giardiasis, and trichononiasis. In AG Gilman, TW Rall, AS Nies, P Taylor (eds.), *The Pharmacological Basis of Therapeutics* (8th ed.). New York: Pergamon Press, 1990. Pp. 998–1007.

104. Beard CM et al. Cancer after exposure to metronidazole. *Mayo Clin Proc* 63:147–53, 1988.

105. Krause JR, Ayuyang HQ, Ellis LD. Occurrence of three cases of carconomia in individuals with Crohn's disease treated with metronidazole. *Am J Gastroenterol* 80:978–82, 1985.

106. Garry VF, Nelson RL. Host mediated transformation: metronidazole. *Mutat Res* 190:289–95, 1987.

107. Robbie MO, Sweet RL. Metronidazole use in obstetrics and gynecology: a review. *Am J Obstet Gynecol* 145:865–81, 1983.

108. Bennett JE. Antifungal agents. In AG Goodman, TW Roll, AS Nies, P. Taylor (eds.), *The Pharmacological Basis of Therapeutics* (8th ed.). New York: Pergamon Press, 1990. Pp. 1165–81.

109. Bennett JE. Antifungal agents. In GL Mandell, RG Douglas Jr, JE Bennett (eds.), *Principles and Practice of Infectious Diseases* (3rd ed.). New York: Churchill-Livingstone 1990. Pp. 361–70.

110. Starke JR et al. Pharmacokinetics of amphotericin B in humans. *Antimicrob Agents Chemother* 13:271–76, 1978.

111. Kucers A, Mc K. Bennett N. Amphotericin B. In *The Use of Antibiotics* (4th ed.). Philadelphia: Lippincott, 1987. Pp. 1441–77.

112. Alcon Laboratories. Natamycin product information. Ft. Worth: Alcon Laboratories, 1989.

113. Kucers A, Mc K. Bennett N. Natamycin. In *The Use of Antibiotics* (4th ed.). Philadelphia: Lippincott, 1987. Pp. 1491–1503.

114. Hume AL, Kerkering TM. Ketoconazole. *Drug Intell Clin Pharm* 17:169, 1983.

115. Bailey EM, Krakovsky DJ, Ryback MJ. The triazole antifungal agents: a review of itraconazole and fluconazole. *Pharmacotherapy* 10:146–53, 1990.

116. Saag MS, Dismukes WE. Azole antifungal agents: emphasis on new triazoles. *Antimicrob Agents Chemother* 32:1–8, 1988.

117. Van Cauteren H et al. Itranconazole pharmacologic studies in animals and humans. *Rev Infect Dis* 9(suppl): S43–46, 1987.

118. Arndt CA et al. Fluconazole penetration into cerebrospinal fluid: implications for treating fungal infections of the central nervous system. *J Infect Dis* 157:178–80, 1988.

119. Douglas RG Jr. Antiviral agents. In AG Gilman, TW Rall, AS Nies, P Taylor (eds.), *The Pharmacological Basis of Therapeutics* (8th ed.). New York: Pergamon Press, 1990. Pp. 1182–1201.

120. Hayden FG, Douglas RG Jr. Antiviral agents. In GL Mandell, RG Douglas Jr, JE Bennett (eds.). *Principles and Practice of Infectious Diseases* (3rd ed.). New York: Churchill-Livingstone, 1990. Pp. 370–93.

121. Winston DJ et al. Ganciclovir therapy for cytomegalovirus infections in recipients of bone marrow transplants and other immunosuppressed patients. *Rev Infect Dis* 10(suppl 3):S547–53, 1988.

122. Snydman DR. Ganciclovir therapy for cytomegalovirus disease associated with renal transplants. *Rev Infect Dis* 10(suppl 3):S554–62, 1988.

123. Dieterich DT et al. Ganciclovir treatment of gastrointestinal infections caused by cytomegalovirus in patients with AIDS. *Rev Infect Dis* 10(suppl 3):S532–37, 1988.

124. Singlas E et al. Zidovudine disposition in patients with severe renal impairment: influence of hemodialysis. *Clin Pharmacol Ther* 46:190–97, 1989.

125. Taburet AM et al. Pharmacokinetics of zidovudine in patients with liver cirrhosis. *Clin Pharmacol Ther* 47:731–39, 1990.

126. Fischl MA et al. A randomized controlled trial of a reduced daily dose of zidovudine in patients with the acquired immunodeficiency syndrome. *N Engl J Med* 323:1009–14, 1990.

127. Volberding PA et al. Zidovudine in asymptomatic human immunodeficiency virus infection: a controlled trial in persons with fewer than 500 CD4-positive cells per cubic millimeter. *N Engl J Med* 322:941–49, 1990.

128. Collier AC et al. A pilot study of low-dose zidovudine in human immunodeficiency virus infection. *N Engl J Med* 323:1115–1121, 1990.

129. Pizzo PA et al. Effect of continuous intravenous infusion of zidovudine (AZT) in children with symptomatic HIV infection. *N Engl J Med* 319:889–96, 1988.

130. Ruedy J, Schecter M, Montaner JSG. Zidovudine for early human immunodeficiency virus (HIV) infection: who, when, and how? [comment]. *Ann Intern Med* 112:721–23, 1990.

131. Friedland GH. Early treatment for HIV: the time has come [editorial]. *N Engl J Med* 322:1000–02, 1990.

132. Public health service statement on management of occupational exposure to human immunodeficiency virus including considerations regarding zidovudine post exposure use. Atlanta, GA: Department of Health and Human Services, Centers for Disease Control. *MMWR* 39:1–14, 1990.

133. Watts DH et al. Pharmacokinetic disposition of zidovudine during pregnancy. *J Infect Dis* 163:226–32, 1991.

134. Drugs for parasitic infections. *Med Lett Drug Ther* 32:23–32, 1990.

135. Moellering RC. Introduction: revolutionary changes in the macrolide and azalide antibiotics. *Am J Med* 91(3A):1S–4S, 1991.

136. Neu HC. The development of macrolides: clarithromycin in prospective. *J Antimicrob Chemother* 27 (suppl A):1–9, 1991.

137. Schentag JJ, Ballow CH. Tissue-directed pharmacokinetics. *Am J Med* 91 (3A):5S–11S, 1991.

138. Hopkins S. Clinical toleration and safety of azithromycin. *Am J Med* 91(3A):40S–45S, 1991.

5

Infection Control and Prophylaxis in the Emergency Department

Darwin L. Palmer

Many patients come to emergency departments with actual or incipient bacterial, viral, and rickettsial infections. While trauma accounts for about one-half of all patient visits to emergency departments, infections are the next most common cause [1]. Since infections may not be recognized, may not have been previously diagnosed, or may be present in an early or atypical form, they can be a contagion risk to both health care workers and other patients. A large proportion of serious infections can be avoided or prevented by simple prophylactic maneuvers or vaccines. For the health care worker, illnesses of major consequence that are preventable include hepatitis, HIV/AIDS, measles, rubella, influenza, polio, diphtheria, meningococcal disease, and tuberculosis. While transmission from patients to health care workers is well documented, infections such as rubella, influenza, and hepatitis can be transmitted from health care worker to patient or patient to patient, sometimes with significant morbidity, high cost, and potential legal consequences. In spite of extensive efforts to immunize health care workers, acceptance of vaccines has been poor; additionally universal precautions to interrupt transmission have not yet been widely implemented.

In addition to prophylaxis for health providers, many emergency patients have injuries or illnesses

that can provide portals of entry for infections. Contaminated open wounds are at preventable risk for tetanus, rabies, and bacterial wound infections. Simple maneuvers such as vaccination, antibiotics, isolation, washing, gloves, and masks are extremely important in interrupting potential infection acquisition by patients in the emergency department.

On the other hand, most patients with infections who arrive in the emergency department present minimal or no risks to the health care worker [2]. Such illnesses as the usual community acquired pneumonia, pharyngitis, urinary tract infections, and most wound and soft tissue infections are not ordinarily contagious. While these conditions do not present infectious risks when they are accurately diagnosed, such diagnosis may not be possible in the brief emergency department encounter. The emphasis of this chapter is on the precautions that preclude infection transmission due to either faulty judgment or an incorrect educated guess.

Finally many patients use an emergency department for much or all of their of health care, including acute and chronic infections. While sound advice and counseling are critical, referral to other sources is advisable for certain illnesses and procedures. These referrals would include the public health service for the long-term care of tuberculosis and the follow-up of sexually transmitted diseases, special infectious disease clinics for travel-associated infections, and private physicians for general preventive vaccinations. Emergency facilities may serve as a source for administration of prophylactic medications (vaccines or antibiotics) for community epidemics such as influenza, measles, typhoid fever, and meningococcal disease. Health care, public safety, and other workers may present for postexposure care for needle sticks, human bites, and other potential exposures to body fluids. Emergency personnel should have ready access to appropriate reference sources such as phone consultation with the Centers for Disease Control (CDC) (404-639-3311; ask for person on call) or the American College of Physicians *Guide for Adult Immunization* [3].

Patient Prophylaxis

Patients with injuries and trauma commonly need wound infection prophylaxis and specific vaccines as preventive measures. In addition, because of the close proximity between patients in waiting rooms and care facilities, the risks of cross-contamination between patients need preventive maneuvers. The latter risks may arise either from emergency department patients with systemic illnesses or from possible bacterial cross-contamination from an infected wound to a clean wound. Physicians and nurses also can be the inadvertent carriers and transmitters of acute systemic or local infections. Transmission by health care workers can generally be prevented by appropriate restriction of work exposure, universal precautions, and the use of vaccines.

Prophylactic Measures for Injuries and Wounds

Traumatic wounds may be contaminated at the time of occurrence with bacterial or fungal pathogens, and often preventive treatment must be given. A careful history of the injury is important to determine how recently the injury was sustained and whether contamination may have occurred through earth, plant, or fecal material, by superficial abrasion or deep puncture, or by bite wound injury (either human or animal). Previous treatment (washing, antiseptics), antibiotic use, and

prior vaccine status must be determined. A wound needs careful examination to detect soilage, presence of pus or foreign bodies, and presence of gas in the tissue. Depending on the type of wound (e.g., blunt vs. penetrating), the anatomic location, and the source of injury, x-rays may be warranted not only to look for traumatic damage to bony structures but also for the presence of foreign bodies and/or gas in the soft tissue. Local wound management and antibiotic therapy are thoroughly discussed in Chap. 13. This chapter focuses on tetanus and rabies prophylaxis for wounds.

TETANUS

Fewer than 100 cases of tetanus have been reported per year in the United States in the past two decades [4]. Most patients who develop tetanus are adults who did not receive adequate wound care or tetanus prophylaxis when medical attention was initially sought. Overall mortality is 30%, but tetanus is completely preventable by vaccination. Tetanus cases most often arise from deep puncture wounds in adults over age 60 with no (or inadequate) prior immunization. An individual with any type of wound should be evaluated for tetanus prophylaxis. Removal of foreign bodies and debridement of devitalized tissue are vital to improve the partial pressure of oxygen in the affected tissues as well as to decrease bacterial contamination. Drainage and irrigation should be performed if necessary. Tetanus immunization, to be complete, must include a primary series of two doses (0.5 ml each) of tetanus vaccine given 4 weeks apart followed by a third dose given 6 to 12 months later. A booster dose of vaccine should be given thereafter every 10 years. Tetanus vaccine in adults preferably should be the absorbed toxoid combined with diphtheria toxoid to give dual protection. Unfortunately many patients are not aware of their tetanus (or diphtheria) immune status, including either the receipt of primary immunization or the interval since the last booster dose of toxoid. If the status is unknown, the recommendation for the use of tetanus toxoid and tetanus immune globulin for wound prophylaxis is to presume no immunity.

Two vaccines are used in various circumstances to induce either (*a*) active, delayed onset immunity (tetanus toxoid) or (*b*) immediate, passive immunity (tetanus immune globulin-TIG). Table 5-1 is a

Table 5-1. Summary guide to tetanus prophylaxis in routine wound management

History of adsorbed tetanus toxoid (doses)	Clean minor wounds		All other wounds[a]	
	Td[b,c]	TIG	Td[c]	TIG
Unknown or <3	Yes	No	Yes	Yes
Three or more[d]	No[e]	No	No[f]	No

[a] Such as, but not limited to, wounds contaminated with dirt, feces, soil, saliva; puncture wounds; avulsions; and wounds resulting from missiles, crushing, burns, and frostbite.
[b] Td = combined tetanus and diphtheria toxoids adsorbed; TIG = tetanus immune globulin.
[c] For persons 7 years of age and older, combined tetanus and diphtheria toxoid adsorbed is preferred to tetanus toxoid alone.
[d] If only three doses of fluid toxoid have been received, a fourth dose of toxoid, preferably an adsorbed toxoid, should be given.
[e] Yes, if more than 10 years since the last dose.
[f] Yes, if more than 5 years since the last dose. More frequent boosters are not needed and can accentuate side effects.
Source: Centers for Disease Control. Diphtheria, tetanus and pertussis: guidelines for vaccine prophylaxis and other preventive measures. *MMWR* 34:405–14, 419–26, 1985.

summary guide to the use of these vaccines. Tetanus toxoid is a purified, formaldehyde-inactivated ("toxoid"), aluminum hydroxide adsorbed preparation. The fluid or adsorbed preparation is available as a single agent or with diphtheria toxoid. The combined vaccine with a reduced concentration of diphtheria toxoid for adults (Td) is recommended for routine use beyond childhood since it provides needed protection for diphtheria in adults at essentially no increase in local or systemic toxicity. The toxoid is given as 0.5 ml intramuscularly. Tetanus immune globulin (TIG) is derived from plasma of hyperimmunized adults by cold ethanol fractionation and does not pose a risk for either hepatitis or HIV transmission. Given intramuscularly at a dose of 250 IU, it provides immediate immunity lasting 28 days, during which time active immunity induced by tetanus toxoid administration has sufficient time to develop. Adverse effects of tetanus toxoid are generally confined to mild or moderate pain at the injection site (reported in 5%–85% of recipients) and may be influenced by the number and recency of prior booster doses; adverse reactions to TIG are rare. With either preparation, the value of the vaccine in appropriate circumstances far outweighs the risk of adverse reactions.

If the wound is clean and the chance of tetanus spores having contaminated the wound is small, Td alone is recommended if the patient has received fewer than three doses of adsorbed toxoid in the past or if it has been more than 10 years since the previous toxoid dose. Most such individuals will have some protective antitoxin levels prior to exposure and those with three or more prior doses of toxoid will respond to an additional dose within 7 days. There is good experimental evidence that protection will begin for tetanus before a measurable level of antitoxin can be detected. If the patient has received complete primary immunization (at least three doses of tetanus toxoid more than five years previously) and has a wound with high risk of contamination, the patient should be given a single dose of toxoid.

Individuals with dirty wounds who indicate that they have received fewer than three toxoid doses should be given TIG as well. TIG does not interfere with the immune response to tetanus toxoid when administered simultaneously but at a separate site. This ensures both passive immunity, starting at the time of TIG injection, and active immunization in the immediate future. In an individual with significant immunosuppression (e.g., HIV infection or cancer chemotherapy) and with a wound that is not clean and minor, the concurrent use of TIG is warranted in all instances since the immune response to tetanus toxoid may be suboptimal.

The dose of TIG is somewhat controversial since circulating levels may be low and there is some concern about the levels necessary to confer protection; however, doses of 250 IU seem to be reasonable in wound prophylaxis. It must be remembered that TIG cannot be given intravenously and does not need to be infused around the wound, but it should be given intramuscularly and at a site separate from tetanus toxoid. It should be further noted that, while antibiotic prophylaxis may be necessary for contaminated wounds to combat bacterial infection, the use of antibiotics does not prevent the development of tetanus.

RABIES

An animal bite wound should prompt consideration for rabies prophylaxis. A careful history as to the species of biting animal, the anatomic location of the bite wound, the severity (deep vs. nonpenetrating) of the bite wound, the locale of the occurrence (urban vs. rural), whether the animal was provoked, and the knowledge of the frequency of rabies in the animals of the vicinity are all vitally important. Although all age groups are susceptible, most human rabies reported to the World Health Organization (WHO) occurs in males younger than 15 years, and 40% of cases occur in children 5–14, undoubtedly due to greater animal exposure. In the United States rabies has been detected most frequently in skunks, raccoons, bats, farm animals (cows, horses), cats, foxes, and dogs. In most of the United States wild animals are more likely sources of rabies exposure than are domestic cats and dogs, since the latter generally are vaccinated. In those states bordering on Mexico (where rabies prophylaxis among dogs and cats is inadequate) dog bites are a high risk. Insectivorous bats in the northern United States are widely infected with rabies but rarely bite humans unless handled directly. Rodents such as squirrels or rats are rarely rabid, although they are susceptible to the virus. A potential rabies exposure has occurred if an animal bite wound has broken the skin or if animal saliva has contaminated the mucous membranes. Rabies prophylaxis is more urgent following bites on proximal portions of extremities or on the head and face. If the exposure was from an urban domestic dog or cat, knowledge of the frequency of local, inner-city rabies may exclude any risk. Rabies vaccine can be deferred if the biting dog or cat can be impounded and observed for signs of rabies. If a patient has been bitten by a wild or domestic skunk or raccoon, the immediate use of rabies vaccine is critical because of their high rate of infection. An unprovoked bite (i.e., an attack by an animal while it was being quietly observed) may be an indication the animal has rabies.

Local treatment of bites and scratches by vigorously cleansing the wound with soap and water followed by irrigation with 70% alcohol or 1% quaternary ammonium compound will reduce the viral inoculum size. Active immunity to rabies is induced by human diploid cell vaccine (HDCV), which has been available since 1980 and which is both more potent and with fewer adverse effects than the older duck embryo preparation. In 1988 a newer adsorbed rabies vaccine, RVA, grown in diploid-cell, fetal rhesus monkey lung cells was licensed for use in the United States and may replace the current HDCV. Available now only in Michigan, dosage scheduling of RVA is the same as for HDCV. Rabies immune globulin (RIG), prepared by fractionation of plasma from hyperimmunized humans, is used to provide immediate, passive immunity. If a significant, high-risk bite wound injury has occurred, RIG at a dose of 20 IU/kg intramuscularly in the deltoid should always be given in combination with HDCV, the latter for five doses (1 ml IM or SC on days 0, 3, 7, 14, and 28). If a patient has been previously vaccinated for preexposure prophylaxis or for a prior bite wound injury, two booster doses of HDCV on days 0 and 3 are sufficient for protection for bite exposure. Injection of HDCV should not be given into the buttocks, since the immune response following an adipose tissue injection is questionable. RIG and HDCV should not be given in the same syringe or into the same anatomical site. Because of the expense of 1.0-ml intramuscular HDCV injections (about $225 in the United States), some patients request use of the lower-dose, 0.1-ml intradermal injections to reduce the cost. While this amount may result in appropriate levels for preexposure prophylaxis (two intradermal doses of 0.1 ml), it is not recommended for bite wound treatment. Table 5-2 summarizes postexposure prophylaxis for rabies.

Because RIG may reduce the antibody response to the vaccine, no more than the recommended dose of RIG should be given. Adverse reactions are significantly less frequent than they were with the previous Semple rabies vaccine. However, approximately 25%–50% of patients who receive the total dose of vaccine will develop mild local reactions at the injection site and up to 20% will have mild headache, nausea, abdominal pain, myalgias and dizziness. Some patients complain of an immune

Table 5-2. Postexposure prophylaxis for rabies

Animal	Condition of animal at time of attack	Treatment of exposed person[*]
Dog, cat	Healthy and available for 10 days of observation.	None unless animal develops rabies.
	Rabid or suspected rabid.	Rabies vaccine and RIG.
	Unknown (escaped).	Consult public health officials; if treatment is indicated, give rabies vaccine and RIG.
Skunk, bat, fox, coyote, raccoon, bobcat, and other carnivores	Regard as rabid unless proven negative by laboratory test.	Rabies vaccine and RIG.
Livestock, rodents, rabbits, hares	Consider individually.	Consult public health officials. Bites of squirrels, hamsters, guinea pigs, gerbils, chipmunks, rats, mice, other rodents, rabbits, and hares almost never require antirabies prophylaxis.

[*] Rabies vaccines include human diploid cell vaccine (HDCV) and rabies vaccine, adsorbed (RVA). RIG indicates rabies-immune globulin. For persons who previously have received preexposure rabies prophylaxis, cleansing the wound and two doses of rabies vaccine (0.1 ml intramuscularly (IM) or subcutaneously (SC), *not* intradermally (ID), on days 0 and 3 are sufficient. For persons who previously have not received preexposure prophylaxis, five doses of rabies vaccine (1.0 ml IM or SC, *not* ID, on days 0, 3, 7, 14, and 28) and one dose of RIG (20 IU/kg IM on day 0) are necessary. See text for details.
Modified from MMWR. 1984; 33:393–402, 407–08.

complex-like syndrome with urticaria, fever, malaise, and arthralgias. These symptoms appear 2–21 days after booster vaccination and are less common with the newer RVA. Local pain and low-grade fever may occur with RIG, but more serious reactions (such as anaphylaxis) are rare except in patients lacking IgA. Immunosuppressive therapy such as corticosteroids should be avoided during preexposure prophylaxis or postexposure treatment, since it may diminish the antibody response to the vaccine. If steroids cannot be avoided, additional doses of HDCV may be given. There is no evidence that administration of rabies vaccination (either HDCV or RIG) during pregnancy causes fetal damage, since neither contains live virus. If the risk of rabies exposure is significant, pregnancy should not be considered a contraindication to postexposure prophylaxis.

Routine Preventive Vaccinations for Adults

Many patients in the United States now receive some or all of their medical care through emergency departments. These patients often need routine preventive vaccinations, which heretofore have been presumably administered under the direction of private physicians. Such routine immunizations include pneumococcal, influenza, mumps, measles, and rubella vaccines. Routine vaccinations for well babies are not covered in this chapter; Table 5-3 provides the recommended immunization schedule. Smallpox vaccination is no longer indicated for any individual since the natural disease has been eradicated worldwide. Tetanus and diphtheria are covered in separate sections in this chapter, as are rabies and hepatitis B.

Of special note are live vaccines, which are generally contraindicated in pregnant or immunocompromised patients. These vaccines are listed in Table 5-4. A pregnancy test and a good history can exclude such individuals from vaccine exposure.

INFLUENZA

Influenza is a disease caused by three major subtypes of virus, A, B, and C. Types A and B cause epidemic and endemic disease throughout the Western world and may result not only in severe clinical disease but major morbidity and mortality in patients with underlying disease and who are not

Table 5-3. Recommended immunization schedule for normal infants and children

Recommended age[a]	Vaccine[b,c]	Comments
2 months	Diphtheria and tetanus toxoids and pertussis vaccine (DTP-1), poliovirus vaccine live oral (OPV-1)	Can be given earlier in areas of high endemicity.
4 months	DTP-2, OPV-2	To avoid viral interference there should be a 6-week to 2-month interval between OPV doses.
6 months	DTP-3	An additional dose of OPV can be useful at this time in areas where there is a high risk for poliovirus exposure.
15 months[d]	Measles, mumps, and rubella virus vaccine, live (MMR-1); DTP-4, OPV-3	Completion of primary series of DTP and OPV.
18 months	Haemophilus influenzae type B polysaccharide conjugate vaccine	
4–6 years	DTP-5, OPV-4, measles or MMR-2	Preferably at or before school entry.
14–16 years	Td-tetanus and diphtheria toxoids adsorbed for adult use	Repeat every 10 years throughout life.

[a] These recommended ages should not be construed as absolute; for example, 2 months can be 6 to 10 weeks.
[b] DTP = diphtheria and tetanus toxoids and pertussis vaccine, OPV = oral poliovirus vaccine, MMR = measles, mumps, and rubella virus vaccine, Td = tetanus and diphtheria toxoid.
[c] For all products used, consult manufacturer's package enclosure for instructions on storage, handling, dosage, and administration. Immunobiologics prepared by different manufacturers may vary, and those of the same manufacturer may change from time to time.
[d] Provided at least 6 months have elapsed since DTP-3, or, if fewer than three DTPs have been received, at least 6 weeks since last dose of DTP or OPV. MMR vaccine should not be delayed to allow simultaneous administration with DTP and OPV. Administering MMR at 15 months and DTP-4 and OPV-3 at 18 months is an acceptable alternative.
Source: Centers for Disease Control. General recommendations on immunization. *MMWR.* 38:205–14, 219–27, 1989.

Table 5-4. Live vaccines contraindicated in pregnant women and immunocompromised patients

Viral	Bacterial
Measles	Bacille Calmette-Guerin
Mumps	
Rubella	
OPV*	
Yellow fever*	

* Indicated in special circumstances (see American College of Physicians, *Guide for Adult Immunization*, 2nd ed. ACP Task Force on Adult Immunization and Infectious Diseases Society of America. Philadelphia: American College of Physicians, 1990).

immune. Influenza viruses tend to have both gradual antigenic changes with time (antigenic drift), as well as major changes approximately every decade in antigenic composition (antigenic shift). These changes can result in lack of protection by either natural immunity from prior disease or by immunity conferred by prior vaccine use. Vaccines

are therefore reviewed on an annual basis and altered when necessary.

Influenza itself is an acute, febrile respiratory illness associated with severe constitutional symptoms, especially retro-orbital headache, fatigue, and severe myalgia. In the Western hemisphere the disease is most common in the fall and winter months; attack rates can be very high, on occasion approaching 20%–30% of a population. Influenza can be severe enough to cause significant mortality, particularly among elderly individuals and patients with underlying medical conditions. Eighty to 90% of the influenza-associated excess mortality occurs among the elderly and those with underlying diseases [5]. Commonly only 20% of these identifiable high-risk individuals are given an annual influenza immunization.

The influenza vaccine is made from egg-grown virus that is highly purified and completely inactivated. As a consequence the current vaccine causes few side effects and cannot cause infection. The vaccine contains two type A strains and one type B strain representing the most recent influenza viruses circulating in the world and likely to cause disease in the United States. It is available in both whole- and split-virus preparations. In adults the antigenicity and frequency of adverse reactions generally are similar with either preparation. Among children the split-virus preparation causes fewer side effects. The protective efficacy of influenza vaccine is correlated with the development of antibodies and results in a 70%–80% reduction in clinical illness. In older patients, such as those in nursing homes, efficacy in protecting against pneumonia, hospitalization, and death remains high, but the vaccine is only 30%–40% effective in preventing clinical illness.

Influenza vaccination has highest priority for all persons who are at risk of severe outcome due to influenza. This includes elderly individuals (more than 65 years of age), patients with cardiorespiratory illness, and patients with immunologic impairment. In addition patients who have a chronic metabolic disorder, such as diabetes, renal disease, or hemoglobinopathies, and patients who need regular medical care should receive immunization. Health care workers and others in critical community jobs, such as police and firemen, also should be immunized to preclude interruption of services during an epidemic. Health care workers can readily transmit the disease to high-risk patients under their care. A single dose (0.5 ml) should be administered intramuscularly on a yearly basis.

Vaccine is generally given in the early fall months to precede the influenza season and will provide effective protection for 6–9 months. Since the immunity wanes after that interval, patients at risk should be vaccinated annually with the latest preparation available. Influenza vaccine can be given simultaneously with pneumococcal vaccine, although they should be injected at separate sites. Reactions to the vaccine are usually minimal and include soreness at the injection site lasting 1 to 2 days, occasional fever, myalgia, and malaise. Severe hypersensitivity reactions are rare. The latter are more likely to occur in individuals who have an underlying allergy to eggs. The occasional respiratory illnesses that occur following vaccination undoubtedly represent coincident infection with viral respiratory agents occurring during the fall and winter season when the influenza vaccine is given. In 1976 the swine influenza vaccine was associated with development of Guillain-Barré syndrome. Careful surveillance of vaccine-associated reactions since that time have shown no relation to serious neurologic disease. Although most physicians prefer to defer use of medications during pregnancy, the vaccine is considered safe for the fetus, and pregnant women with underlying high-risk medical conditions should be vaccinated. Amantadine is an effective prophylactic medication in type A influenza; it can be especially useful as an adjunct to vaccination when a vaccine program is initiated after the onset of a community influenza outbreak.

PNEUMOCOCCAL VACCINE

Pneumococcal infections remain the single most common bacterial cause of lower respiratory tract disease and severe life-threatening pneumonia. Clinical disease ranges from mild acute bacterial bronchitis to severe bacteremic pneumococcal pneumonia [6]. The estimated incidence of pneumonia is 70–250 cases per 100,000 persons per year, with a case fatality rate of approximately 5% in treated patients. Both the incidence and the fatality increase with age over 65 and the presence of chronic cardiac and pulmonary disease, hepatic or renal failure, alcoholism, multiple myeloma, and Hodgkin's disease.

The mortality rate for pneumococcal infections has not improved in recent years, possibly due to the inability to decrease the early fatalities after diagnosis, even with effective antibiotic therapy. Bacteremic pneumonia, occurring in 5%–20% of all pneumococcal pneumonias, still carries an overall case-fatality rate of 15%–25%. A pneumococcal vaccine in use since 1983 contains antigens from the 23 pneumococcal types responsible for 85%–90% of all bacteremic pneumococcal infections. It replaces a vaccine composed of 14 capsular polysaccharide antigens that was licensed in 1977 and widely used until 1983. Pneumococcal vaccine induces type-specific antibodies of the same IgG class induced by infection and acts to increase phagocytosis and the killing of pneumococci by polymorphonuclear cellular mechanisms.

Vaccine effectiveness is highest in young adults, in whom a twofold or greater rise in antibody titer occurs to each antigen in approximately 80% of all recipients. Antibody levels decline progressively over the ensuing 7 to 10 years. Patients who need vaccination because of underlying disease or age should be revaccinated at 10 years. Various studies indicate protective efficacy of pneumococcal vaccine in immunocompromised and elderly patients, patients with alcoholism, patients with chronic cardiopulmonary or renal disease, patients with diabetes, and elderly nursing home residents [7]. The response to pneumococcal vaccine may be suboptimal in the very old, those patients with chronic metabolic disease, and patients with leukemia, lymphoma, multiple myeloma, or HIV infection. Unfortunately no readily available measure of antibody response is clinically available. Patients who need the vaccine because of severe underlying disease may have a suboptimal response to it and possibly deserve revaccination at earlier intervals (5–9 years).

Pneumococcal vaccine should be given as a single intramuscular dose (0.5 ml) in the deltoid. It can be given at the same time as influenza vaccine but at a separate anatomic site. Adverse reactions such as local pain and redness at the injection site are common. They occur in as many as 50% of patients given the earlier 14-valent vaccine but are rarely severe. Severe allergic or systemic reactions, such as a fever or a rash, occur in less than 1% of recipients. The current 23-valent vaccine has fewer problems of severe local reactions than reported with the earlier 14-valent vaccine. No neurologic disorders such as Guillain-Barré syndrome have been reported, and the vaccine is not contraindicated during pregnancy.

MEASLES, MUMPS, AND RUBELLA
Measles, mumps, and rubella vaccines are available as both the univalent single-disease vaccines and as the polyvalent triple (MMR) vaccine. The latter is recommended for most clinical indications for adults since the adverse reaction rate does not increase with polyvalent vaccine over single vaccines and protection is often needed for two or more diseases [8]. All MMR vaccines are live attenuated virus that induce lifelong protection in a large proportion (approximately 95%) of recipients. A single dose of the reconstituted vaccine (0.5 ml) given subcutaneously should provide long lasting, probably lifelong, immunity.

Measles. Measles (rubeola) can be a severe disease, particularly in adults. Encephalitis or death following measles is reported in approximately 1 per 1000 cases. Measles during pregnancy increases the risk of spontaneous abortion, premature labor, and low–birth-weight infants. Approximately 12% of all cases in recent years have occurred in adults age 20 years and older. Indigenous transmission of measles still occurs in the young U.S. adult population; acquisition while traveling abroad and living in close proximity, as in colleges, increase the risk of transmission. Measles vaccine is indicated for all adults born after 1957 who lack documentation of immunization with the live measles vaccine or who do not have laboratory evidence (serology) of immunity [9]. Persons who have received the killed measles vaccine (generally available between 1963 and 1967) should receive a dose of live measles vaccine. In addition susceptible adults who are exposed to measles should be vaccinated, especially if it can be done within the first 72 hours of exposure. Alternatively immune globulin (0.25 ml/kg up to 11.5 ml) can be given to prevent or modify infection if given within the first 6 days of exposure. Vaccination should not be given during severe febrile illness or pregnancy since this is a live virus, although proof of fetal infection and damage is not evident. It should not be given to persons who are immunocompromised as a result of immunodeficiency disease (HIV, leukemia, lymphoma, or generalized malignancy) because of concerns for dissemination.

Mumps. Mumps is generally a self-limited disease, but it can be associated with complications, especially in adults. Such complications include orchitis, occurring in up to 20% of postpubertal males with the disease. More rarely meningitis and nerve deafness complicate infection. Mumps has been decreasing since the introduction of live mumps vaccine, and outbreaks currently occur mostly among adolescents and young adults in high schools, colleges, and occupational settings [10]. A single dose of live attenuated mumps vaccine results in protective immunity and should be given to all adults believed to be susceptible. Persons born in or before 1957 can be considered to be naturally immune; those born after that date are susceptible unless they have had physician-diagnosed mumps, have a record of adequate prior vaccination, or have laboratory evidence of immunity. Special efforts should be made to ensure that high school and college students, as well as hospital workers, are vaccinated. Adverse reactions to mumps vaccine are rare and include rash, pruritus, and CNS dysfunction. Because it is a live virus preparation, mumps vaccine should not be given to pregnant women, although data indicating disease in such individuals are largely lacking.

Rubella. Rubella (German measles) was a frequent childhood illness that has largely been eliminated due to widespread immunization of children throughout most of the United States. The failure to vaccinate all adolescents and young adults has resulted in some continued outbreaks in universities, colleges, and places of employment, including hospitals. Approximately 10%–15% of young adults remain susceptible to rubella [11]. Rubella infections in early pregnancy can result in spontaneous abortions, stillbirth, and fetal infection with the congenital rubella syndrome (see Chap. 29). Vaccination of young women of childbearing age is recommended, unless there is proof of immunity with a documented rubella vaccination or a positive serologic test, or the vaccine is contraindicated. In addition, all health care workers (men and women) who might contract rubella and subsequently expose pregnant patients should be given vaccine [9]. Because of the theoretical risk to the fetus of this live viral vaccine, women of childbearing age should not receive rubella vaccine if they are pregnant. However, the risk of this vaccine appears to be very low. In those pregnant women who have been given vaccine inadvertently, there has been no evidence of malformation in the infants. Adverse reactions to rubella vaccine are seen in up to 40% of adults vaccinated, most commonly joint pain of the hands, transient peripheral neuritis, and, more rarely, frank arthritis.

Infectious Risks from Other Patients

Patients in waiting and treatment areas may be in close contact with individuals having highly contagious and potentially dangerous infectious problems, including such diseases as meningococcal meningitis, diphtheria, or even plague. Fortunately

these severe diseases are infrequent, and the risks are rare for transmission in the waiting area. On the other hand, transmission of milder diseases, such as measles, varicella (chicken pox), and influenza, are very real problems in the emergency department.

Contagion between infected patients in a waiting area can be diminished by adequate space between patients, good ventilation, and rapid turnover of patients to prevent prolonged contact. An alert nurse or other health care worker who is able to triage patients so that those with rash illnesses, high fevers, or persistent and severe coughs are separated may be of help. An appropriate log of patients in any area of the emergency department must be maintained so that if high-risk cross-contamination has occurred, patients placed at risk of serious illness can be contacted later for prophylaxis or treatment.

Prophylactic antibiotics are warranted for close family members and other individuals who have intensive direct contact with patients having meningococcal disease (respiratory infection or meningitis), plague (either bubonic or pneumonic), or diphtheria. When meningococcal prophylaxis is thought necessary, treatment should be started immediately, before results of microbiological testing are obtained. Rifampin is the drug of choice for prophylaxis, because of frequent resistance to sulfonamides and adverse reactions to minocycline. The dose is 600 mg q12h for 2 days for adults and 10 mg/kg q12h for children. Plague contacts, if extensive, close, or unprotected, should be given prophylaxis with oral tetracycline at a dose of 500 mg qid for 5 days in adults. Diphtheria contacts, if not immune, should receive either oral erythromycin 125-500–mg qid for 10 days or benzathine penicillin G (600,000–1,200,000 IU) given intramuscularly.

Fortunately many of the infectious illnesses harbored by patients seeking care at an emergency department are not highly contagious. This is true of common respiratory illnesses such as pneumococcal pneumonia, acute bronchitis caused by *Haemophilus influenzae*, and ordinary cold virus infections. Cross-contamination between patients with most respiratory infections needs prolonged, physical contact. Enteric infections, wound infections, and sexually transmitted diseases also are not readily transmissible in a waiting room area from patient to patient; however, they can be transmitted via health care worker.

Infections from Health Care Workers to Patients

Health care workers are frequent transmitters of infections to patients. Sizable outbreaks as well as individual infections have been traced to health care workers in the emergency department. Streptococcal and staphylococcal infection from asymptomatic carriage in the nasopharynx or perineum can be conveyed to patients via hand contamination and poor washing and gloving techniques. Physicians and nurses who are known to have such carriage, for example, individuals with chronic skin conditions, should have skin lesions cultured and should not have patient contact if a culture is positive for *Staphylococcus aureus* or *Streptococcus pyogenes*. Chronic nasal carriers without active infection pose a lesser risk but must exercise extreme care in hand washing and the use of gloves. Infection surveillance sections should periodically review procedures carried out on patients and infection rates in the emergency section to ensure conformity with universal precautions.

Other infections that on occasion have been documented as being passed from health care worker to patient include herpetic whitlow, varicella zoster, hepatitis B, and influenza. Herpetic whitlow, that is, paronychial infection, is caused by herpes simplex virus type 1. Whitlow can be both chronic and highly contagious. An infected health care worker should either refrain from work related to patient contact or be sure to wear gloves.

A health care worker with varicella zoster (shingles) can transmit this infection to patients during the early course of the disease, before complete crusting and early healing have occurred. The virus is highly contagious. Health care workers with shingles should not be in patient contact during the early phase. There is no evidence that the use of topical agents (acyclovir) prevents transmission or increases healing.

Hepatitis B has been shown to be transmitted by health care workers to patients in the clinical care setting. Outbreaks have been documented to arise from infected emergency department nurses, dental personnel, and surgeons who have been chronic carriers of hepatitis B surface antigen, often un-

known to themselves. The transmission of this highly contagious agent occurs via nicks or cuts on the hands with transfer to the open wounds and mucosal surfaces of a patient. If a chronic hepatitis carrier state is present, the health care worker should exercise extreme caution in the direct care of patients. A single incident of infection with HIV from a health care worker (a dentist) to multiple patients via similar mechanisms recently has been documented.

Health Care Worker–Related Risks

In the emergency department, with its intrinsic large patient volume and short contact, patient infectiousness may go undetected. Health care workers may be at high risk for acquisition of a variety of illnesses from patients. These illnesses can be categorized as those that are vaccine preventable, those that may be preventable by barrier precautions, and those where antibiotics may be appropriate because contact with a contagious bacterial infection has occurred.

Vaccine-Preventable Infections

Emergency personnel are particularly prone to contracting certain vaccine-preventable infectious agents due to their high contact with blood and other body secretions. The risk may be geographically variable and higher in large city hospitals on the East and West coasts.

HEPATITIS B AND C
The most important of these diseases are hepatitis B and hepatitis C. Measures used for protection from hepatitis viruses are discussed in detail in Chap. 26 as well as here. Both forms of hepatitis are transmitted via blood and body secretions and are highly contagious. It is estimated that approximately 20,000–30,000 cases per year of hepatitis B are acquired by health care workers and are the cause of 200–300 deaths per year.

Hepatitis B is almost entirely preventable by use of vaccine. The new recombinant vaccines (Recombivax HB and Engerix-B) are as effective as the previously available plasma-derived vaccine (Heptavax-B) and do not carry risk of transmission of HIV/AIDS or other viral illness [3]. The vaccine confers long-lasting immunity to approximately 95%–98% of those given the standard initial, 1-month, and 6-month primary regimen. All health care workers who have potential contact with blood or body secretions should receive vaccine; this is particularly applicable to emergency personnel, who have among the highest rates of seroprevalence (15%–30%) of any hospital employees

(Table 5-5) [12]. The recombinant vaccine must be given at a dose of 1.0 ml IM in the deltoid (10 μg of the Recombivax HB and 20 μg of Engerix-B) (Table 5-6). Both vaccines have a modest rate of adverse reactions, with local injection site pain in 15%–20% and rare fever, rash, or myalgia in less than 3%.

It is not clear how long protective immunity

Table 5-5. Prevalence of hepatitis B serologic markers in various population groups

Population group	Prevalence of serologic markers of HBV infection	
	HBsAG (%)	Any marker (%)
Immigrants/refugees from areas of high HBV endemicity	13	70–85
Alaskan natives/Pacific Islanders	5–15	40–70
Clients in institutions for the developmentally disabled	10–20	35–80
Users of illicit parenteral drugs	7	60–80
Sexually active homosexual men	6	35–80
Household contacts of HBV carriers	3–6	30–60
Patients of hemodialysis units	3–10	20–80
Health care workers with frequent blood contact	1–2	15–30
Prisoners (male)	1–8	10–80
Staff of institutions for the developmentally disabled	1	10–25
Heterosexuals with multiple partners	0.5	5–20
Health care workers with no or infrequent blood contact	0.3	3–10
General population (NHANES II)*		
Blacks	0.9	14
Whites	0.2	3

*Second National Health and Nutrition Examination Survey.
Source: Centers for Disease Control. Protection against viral hepatitis. MMWR 39 (S-2):1–26, 1990.

Table 5-6. Recommended doses and schedules of currently licensed HB vaccines

Group	Vaccine doses					
	Heptavax-B[a,b] (μg)	(ml)	Recombivax HB[a] (μg)	(ml)	Engerix-B[a,c] (μg)	(ml)
Infants of HBV-carrier mothers	10	0.5	5	0.5	10	0.5
Other infants and children <11 years	10	0.5	2.5	0.25	10	0.5
Children and adolescents 11–19 years	20	1.0	5	0.5	20	1.0
Adults >19 years	20	1.0	10	1.0	20	1.0
Dialysis patients and other immunocompromised persons	40	2.0[d]	40	1.0[e]	40	2.0[d,f]

[a] Usual schedule: three doses at 0, 1, 6 months.
[b] Available only for hemodialysis and other immunocompromised patients and for persons with known allergy to yeast.
[c] Alternative schedule: four doses at 0, 1, 2, 12 months.
[d] Two 1.0-ml doses given at different sites.
[e] Special formulation for dialysis patients.
[f] Four-dose schedule recommended at 0, 1, 2, 6 months.
Source: Centers for Disease Control. Protection against viral hepatitis. MMWR 39 (S-2):1–26, 1990.

persists, but a booster should probably be repeated 10 years after the primary series in individuals who are at risk and should result in a prompt anamnestic response. In health care workers who have been employed in high-risk occupations (e.g., surgery or nursing in the emergency section) for many years, the chances are excellent for prior hepatitis and permanent immunity; hepatitis serology should be checked to preclude the need for vaccination. In workers who have sustained a contaminated, sharp (needle or scalpel) injury and who have had no prior vaccination, use of hepatitis B immune globulins (HBIG), at a dose of 0.06 ml/kg IM, coupled with initial hepatitis vaccine, is indicated to give immediate passive immune protection (Table 5-7) [13]. This regimen is also appropriate for workers who are bitten or have mucous membrane exposure to body fluids from a population in which hepatitis is prevalent. Examples might include an aide bitten by an institutionalized mentally retarded patient or a corrections officer spat at by a prisoner. New employees who have had minimum or no prior contact with blood need not be tested for hepatitis antibody since their chances of having prior hepatitis and current antibody are small. Cost

effectiveness would dictate not testing such employees or routinely following up serologic checking after vaccine administration. However, if an individual is to remain in a field with a very high risk of blood exposure for many years, it is probably wise to check the immune response to hepatitis vaccine at one month following the final (6-month) dose, since a small percentage (approximately 5%) may not develop immunity. About one-half of the initial nonresponders to hepatitis vaccine will respond to one additional dose of vaccine. Use of additional doses thereafter may not increase the response, and such individuals will remain at risk of acquiring hepatitis.

HCV

Parenterally transmitted non-A, non-B (e.g., HCV) hepatitis is usually a transfusion-associated disease. Health care workers who have frequent contact with the blood and body fluids of high-risk patients, for example, transfusion recipients, parenteral drug users, and dialysis patients, are at risk through accidental percutaneous exposure. The value of postexposure prophylaxis with immune globulins (IG) is uncertain at this time, but it may

Table 5-7. Recommendations for hepatitis B prophylaxis following percutaneous or permucosal exposure

Exposed person	Treatment when source is:		
	HBsAg positive	HBsAg negative	Not tested or unknown
Unvaccinated	HBIG × 1[a] and initiate HB vaccine[b]	Initiate HB vaccine[b]	Initiate HB vaccine[b]
Previously vaccinated	Test exposed for anti-HBs	No treatment	No treatment
Known responder	1. If adequate,[c] no treatment 2. If inadequate, HB vaccine booster dose		
Known non-responder	HBIG × 2 or HBIG × 1 plus 1 dose HB vaccine	No treatment	If known high-risk source, *may treat as if source were HBsAg positive*
Response unknown	Test exposed for anti-HBs 1. If inadequate,[c] HBIG × 1 plus HB vaccine booster dose 2. If adequate, no treatment	No treatment	Test exposed for anti-HBs 1. If inadequate,[c] HB vaccine booster dose 2. If adequate, no treatment

[a] HBIG dose 0.06 ml/kg IM.
[b] HB vaccine dose; see Table 5-6.
[c] Adequate anti-HBs is ≥ 10 SRU by RIA or positive by EIA.
Source: Centers for Disease Control. Protection against viral hepatitis. *MMWR* 39 (S-2):1–26, 1990.

be reasonable to administer IG (0.06 ml/kg) as soon as possible after the incident [13].

INFLUENZA

Influenza is a major risk for emergency department personnel because of the high rate of patient contact during an influenza epidemic. All hospital and other health care personnel are routinely advised to receive vaccine to minimize absenteeism among critical care individuals, to provide the best personal protection for employees, and to prevent backspread to the patients under their care. Current killed polyvalent vaccines are about 70%–80% effective in preventing infection and have about a 5% rate of adverse reaction. They provide protection for about 6–9 months and should be administered in the September–November period before the flu season.

DIPHTHERIA

Diphtheria is of small risk in the emergency department. However, because the tetanus/diphtheria vaccine is suggested for all adults, all emergency department personnel should be vaccinated at 10-year intervals with Td vaccine. The adult-preparation Td (with a lower dose of diphtheria toxoid) should be used, to decrease adverse reactions. The vaccine is highly effective, has a small rate of adverse reactions, and should provide approximately 10 years of protective immunity in the adult who has had an earlier primary series.

In the instance of the individual who has not been immunized recently and who is exposed to a patient with diphtheria, use of benzathine penicillin (600,000–1,200,000 units as a single dose or oral erythromycin 125–500 mg qid for 7 days) as prophylaxis should be considered. The duration of antibiotic prophylaxis for diphtheria is 3–5 days.

POLIO

Polio vaccine reimmunization is probably not warranted for any U.S. adults unless they are traveling to areas of polio endemicity or are in contact with large numbers of people arriving from overseas. Health care workers who deal with international travelers, refugees, or immigrants probably should be reimmunized at 10-year intervals. For adults who have not been previously immunized, the new enhanced potency inactivated poliomyelitis vaccine is the preferred primary vaccine in a four-dose regimen [14]. For adults who have had a previous primary series with the oral live virus, a single dose of the oral trivalent vaccine will provide adequate booster responses.

MEASLES AND RUBELLA

Measles and rubella immunity should be required for all health care workers, especially those employed in the emergency section. The chance that a health care worker will be in contact with either measles or rubella is high, and employee immune status should be ensured, either by documentation of prior immunization or by immune status demonstrated by serologic titer. Transmission from patients to health care workers and vice versa is a real possibility; measles is more severe in adults (encephalitis), and rubella can cause development of the rubella syndrome in the fetus of an infected pregnant woman. Vaccine is available as a single agent (measles or rubella), a dual vaccine (MR), and the trivalent product (MMR); MMR vaccine is recommended for most adults. A single dose should provide excellent immune response in adults with a prior primary series. Because MMR is a live attenuated virus preparation, there is a theoretical risk to the developing fetus; thus, it should not be given to pregnant women. The adverse reaction rate to the triple-vaccine preparation is essentially the same as that to the individual vaccines themselves. The reaction rates are small, with slight fever and pain at the injection site seen in 5%–15% of recipients. Transient rashes have developed in 5% of those vaccinated, and reaction rates are higher (40%–50%) in those who have previously received killed measles vaccine. Individuals who were born in or before 1956 do not need vaccination with measles, because contact with the natural disease has probably occurred.

Universal Precautions

A number of illnesses that patients carry and that can be transmitted to health care workers can be adequately guarded against by the use of standard precautions such as hand washing and gloves, gowns, and masks [14]. The AIDS virus (HIV) is not highly contagious, but use of universal precautions will prevent transmission from blood to the health care worker. It is estimated that in some East Coast hospitals as many as 20% of the patients coming into an emergency section with trauma may be HIV infected. Since the infection may not be manifest (or even known to the patient), the need for universal precautions in handling all patients is evident. Hand washing, caution in using needles and sharps, and the use of gloves, gowns, and masks are necessary. Emergency department treatment rooms should be equipped with gloves, masks, protective caps, gowns, and eye goggles. A disposable puncture-resistant container for needles and sharps should be in each room and used for all needles, which should not be recapped.

A more mundane disease of high-transmission rate is tuberculosis. Patients with chronic cough, weight loss, and fever should be presumed to have tuberculosis, and suitable precautions should be taken to prevent transmission to others. A chest x-ray can rapidly confirm a presumptive diagnosis in the emergency department setting. A patient for whom this diagnosis is a possibility should be kept in a single room during examination and should wear a mask, as should the health care provider. It has been demonstrated epidemiologically that patients with active tuberculosis disease who are not suspected of having the disease have the greatest chance of transmitting the infection to others.

Patients with syphilis, genital herpes, or gonorrhea have low risk of transmitting infections to others unless gross contamination of open wounds or blood transmission occurs. The transmission of these diseases can be readily interrupted by the application of universal precautions, especially hand washing and the use of gloves. Health practitioners often fail to glove when touching rashes. Gloving can avoid infection from highly contagious causes of rash, such as secondary syphilis.

Exposure to Needlesticks, Blood, and Body Fluids

All emergency departments should have a policy of and a procedure for reporting incidents and medical management of any employee or patient who is exposed to blood or other body fluids via needlestick or other percutaneous exposure, mucous membrane exposure (e.g., splash to eye or mouth), or a cutaneous exposure involving large amounts of blood or prolonged contacts with blood. The procedure at the University of New Mexico Medical Center requires that health care workers who sustain such an exposure must report it to their supervisor. After a hospital incident report form is completed, the exposed person is referred to the employee health clinic, the emergency department, or an infectious disease specialist for further evaluation and management. The donor (the person to whose blood or body fluids the health care worker or other patient was exposed) is then questioned and his or her record evaluated for possible risk factors for blood borne diseases, hepatitis B surface antigen (HBsAg) status, hepatitis C (HCV) status, and HIV status. High-risk groups are identified in Table 5-8.

If the donor's hepatitis and HIV status are unknown, HBsAg, HCV antibody, and HIV antibody tests should be requested. For high-risk donors or known HBsAg-positive donors serologic testing of the donor or the exposed employee should be set up within 24 hours of exposure. If the health care worker has received vaccine but has not had HBsAb titer done within the last 12 months, a sample should be sent for testing. If the worker has not received vaccine, the HB vaccine series should be initiated. If the donor is HBsAg positive and the worker has not received hepatitis B vaccine, HBIG should be administered at 0.06 ml/kg or 5.0 ml for adults as a single injection in addition to the HB vaccine series being initiated.

If the donor is known to be or is suspected of being HIV positive several additional issues have to be addressed urgently to make the decision whether

Table 5-8. Persons at high risk for HIV and HBV

Persons of Asian, Pacific Island, or Alaskan Eskimo descent, whether immigrant or U.S. born

Persons born in Haiti or sub-Saharan Africa

Persons with a history of any of the following:
  Acute or chronic liver disease
  Rejection as a blood donor
  Blood transfusions on repeated occasions between 1978 and 1985
  Household contact with an HBV carrier
  Multiple episodes of venereal diseases
  Percutaneous use of illicit drugs
  In males, sexual contact with another male since 1978

Hemophiliacs

Prostitutes

Sexual partners of high-risk persons

Children born to high-risk parents

to prescribe zidovudine. The risk from a simple needlestick is 1 in 1000 or less of converting to HIV-seropositive status [15–18]. Persons who experience a deep parenteral injury from donors with AIDS who are not on antiretroviral therapy certainly may present higher-risk odds, and this should be taken into consideration in the management of the patient-employee. Zidovudine prophylaxis, although controversial, is widely practiced. The drug's questionable efficacy, recognized adverse reactions, its unknown long-term safety, as well as its high cost justify considerable discussion before prophylaxis implementation. If zidovudine is prescribed, no more than 6 hours should be allowed to pass before the first dose. Currently the practice is to give the patient-employee zidovudine 200 mg q4h for 72 hours, then 200 mg q4h for five doses each day (omitting the 4 AM dose) for 25 days. If a 200-mg dose cannot be tolerated, it can be changed to 100 mg. A CBC with differential should be ordered at 2 and 4 weeks.

When the donor is HIV positive, the worker must be counseled regarding the risk of infection and what precautions to observe. It is best to request that the patient's primary physician or an infectious disease specialist assume responsibility for such counseling. Clinical and serologic evaluation (HIV antibody test) should be performed, and the employee should be advised to report and seek medical evaluation for any acute febrile illness that occurs within the ensuing 12 weeks. Seronegative employees should be retested at 6, 12, 26, and 52 weeks postexposure.

If the donor or the source of blood or body fluid is unknown, the employee should have the HBV series initiated if he or she is not HBsAb seropositive and should be offered HIV testing.

A procedural flow sheet that addresses all of these circumstances is difficult to design, but it is useful to clinicians who infrequently address the problem. The University of New Mexico Medical Center utilizes the algorithm in Fig. 5-1.

Fig. 5-1. Needlestick or mucous membrane exposure—flow sheet

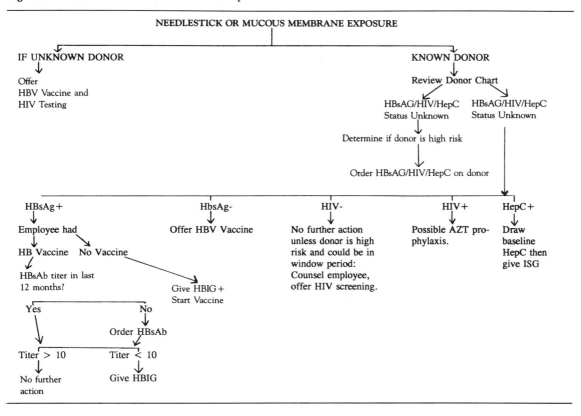

Other Transmissible Infections

A variety of bacterial diseases encountered in acute care patients can be transmitted to health care workers. Meningococcal meningitis is infective probably via fomites to those in close contact with these patients, including health care workers. Health care workers exposed to a patient diagnosed with meningococcal disease should be treated with prophylactic antibiotics (rifampin or sulfonamides). Penicillin is not an appropriate antibiotic for preventive therapy, because it does not penetrate the nasal pharyngeal secretions. In the event that a geographic region has an outbreak or an unusually high rate of neningococcal disease, use of meningococcal vaccine may be considered for all workers who potentially are in contact with infected patients.

Plague is a potential, albeit infrequent, risk during the spring and summer in limited areas of the United States in the Southwest and the far western states, notably New Mexico, Arizona, Colorado, Utah, and California. In a patient presenting with a bubo (painful swelling in a lymph node), fever, and pulmonary symptoms, the consideration must be given to secondary plague pneumonia arising by hematogenous spread from the bubo. This condition presents a highly contagious problem to contacts and must be treated with prophylactic antibiotics (tetracycline 500 mg qid for 5 days). Health care workers should wear a mask, as should the patient, during examination and care.

References

1. Moffett HL. Common infections in ambulatory patients. Ann Intern Med 89:743, 1978.
2. Jackson MR, Lynch P. Ambulatory care settings. In JV Bennett, PH Brachman (eds.). Hospital Infections (2nd ed.). Boston: Little, Brown, 1986.
3. American College of Physicians. Guide for Adult Immunizations. (2nd ed.). Philadelphia: American College of Physicians, 1990.
4. Wassilak SGF, Orenstein WA. Tetanus. In SA Plotkin and EA Mortimer Jr (eds.). Vaccines. Philadelphia: Saunders, 1988.
5. Glezen WP, Couch RB, Six HR. The influenza herald wave. Am J Epidemiol 116:589–98, 1982.
6. Centers for Disease Control. Update: pneumococcal polysaccharide vaccine usage—United States. MMWR 33:273–76, 281, 1984.
7. Davis AL et al. Pneumococcal infection and immunologic response to pneumococcal vaccine in chronic obstructive pulmonary disease. Chest 92:204–12, 1987.
8. Centers for Disease Control. Recommendations of the Immunization Practices Advisory Committee. Measles prevention. MMWR 36:409–18, 423, 425, 1982.
9. Greaves WL et al. Prevention of rubella transmission in medical facilities. JAMA 248:861–64, 1982.
10. Wharton M et al. Mumps transmission in hospitals. Arch Intern Med 150:47–49, 1990.
11. Bart KJ et al. Universal immunization to interrupt rubella. Rev Infect Dis 7S:177–84, 1985.
12. Dienstag JL, Ryan DM. Occupational exposure to hepatitis B virus in hospital personnel: infection or immunization? Am J Epidemiol 26:115–30, 1983.
13. Centers for Disease Control. Protection against viral hepatitis: recommendations of the Immunization Practices Advisory Committee (IPAC). MMWR 39:1–26, 1990.
14. Centers for Disease Control. Poliomyelitis prevention: enhanced-potency inactivated poliomyelitis vaccine—supplementary statement. MMWR 36: 795–98, 1987.
15. Gerberding JL et al. Risk of transmitting the human immunodeficiency virus, cytomegalovirus, and hepatitis B virus to health care workers exposed to patients with AIDS and AIDS-related conditions. J Infect Dis 156:1–8, 1987.
16. Kuhls TL, Viker S, Parris NB, et al. Occupational risk of HIV, HBV and HSV-2 infections in health care personnel caring for AIDS patients. Am J Public Health 77:1306–09, 1987.
17. McEvoy M et al. Prospective study of clinical, laboratory, and ancillary staff with accidental exposures to blood or body fluids from patients infected with HIV. Br Med J 294:1596–97, 1987.
18. Henderson DK et al. Risk for occupational transmission of human immunodeficiency virus type 1 (HIV-1) associated with clinical exposures: a prospective evaluation. Ann Intern Med 113:740–46, 1990.

II

Clinical Syndromes
and Differential Diagnosis

6

Sepsis, Septic Syndrome, and Septic Shock

ERIC M. KOSCOVE

Despite many advances in therapy, septic shock remains an entity with extremely high mortality. It is estimated that 20%–50% of all patients with septic shock die [1]. With the exception of AIDS, the factors that are predisposing to septic shock are found predominantly in middle-aged and elderly patients. An increasing proportion of the U.S. population is elderly. In 1950 10.5% of the population was age 62 or older. In 1988 it was 15%, and it is estimated that by the year 2030 25% of the population will be 62 or older. This "graying of America" is resulting in an increased proportion of patients presenting with sepsis and septic shock. Emergency medicine physicians should expect to see an ever greater number of patients with this problem in their daily practice. Therefore, a firm understanding of septic shock is requisite.

Definitions

Sepsis

Sepsis, septic syndrome, and septic shock are distinct terms that require definition (Table 6-1). Sepsis has been defined as "the presence of various pus-forming and other pathogenic organisms, or their toxins, in the blood or tissues [2]." Previous clinical usage of the term *sepsis* often implied that the patient must subsequently have a positive blood or closed space culture; this usage has been modified since it has become clear that, while bacteria are the most common cause of septic shock, some patients may not have a positive blood culture or may have a nonbacterial cause of sepsis. A redefinition of sepsis has recently been proposed: clinical evidence of infection, tachypnea (respiration > 20 breaths/min; if mechanically ventilated, > 10 l/min), tachycardia (heart rate > 90 beats/min), and hyperthermia or hypothermia (core rectal temperature > 38.3°C or < 35.6°C) [3]. Septicemia has been defined as "systemic disease caused by the spread of microorganisms and their toxins in the circulating blood [2]." The imprecision of this term has led one author to advocate its abandonment [3].

Septic Syndrome

The term *septic syndrome* has recently been proposed, primarily to assist in the selection of subjects for clinical studies. Septic syndrome is defined as clinical evidence of infection, fever or hypothermia, tachypnea, tachycardia, impaired organ system function or perfusion as evidenced by altered mentation, hypoxia, oliguria, disseminated intravascular coagulopathy (DIC), or elevated plasma lactate [4]. Septic syndrome has been more fully

Table 6-1. Definitions

Bacteremia
Presence of bacteria in blood
Criterion: positive blood culture

Sepsis
Suspect infection plus systemic response
Criteria:
   Temperature > 38.3°C or < 35.6°C
   Heart rate > 90/min
   Respiratory rate > 20/min or 10 l/min

Septic Syndrome
Sepsis plus inadequate organ perfusion
Criteria (one or more of the following):
   Altered mental status
   Hypoxemia
   Oliguria
   DIC
   Increasing plasma lactate

Septic Shock
Sepsis syndrome plus hypotension
Criterion: blood pressure systolic < 90 mm Hg or
   drop from baseline of 40 mm Hg

Table 6-2. Sepsis syndrome: organ dysfunction

Organ	Dysfunction	Objective data
CNS	Altered mental status	Glasgow coma score
Lung	Hypoxemia	PaO_2 < 75 mm Hg PaO_2/FIO_2 < 280
Kidney	Oliguria	< 30 ml/hr urine
Hematologic	DIC	↓ Plts > 25% and > 20% ↑ PT or ↑ PTT & FSP or ↑ D-dimer
General	Metabolic	> 5 mEq/L lactate

sepsis and septic shock cannot always be made prospectively. The term *bacteremia* should be reserved for patients with invasion of the blood stream by bacteria.

characterized as "sepsis with evidence of altered organ perfusion. It may be expressed as tachycardia, fever or hypothermia, tachypnea, and evidence of inadequate organ perfusion, including one or more of the following: $P_AO_2/FIO_2 \leq 280$ (without other pulmonary or cardiovascular disease as the cause); elevated lactate level (> upper limits of normal for the laboratory); oliguria (documented urine output < 0.5 ml/kg body weight) for at least one hour [3]" (Table 6-2).

Septic Shock

Septic shock is defined as "the sepsis syndrome with hypotension (systolic blood pressure < 90 mm Hg or a decrease from baseline systolic blood pressure > 40 mm Hg) that may respond (nonrefractory) or may not respond (refractory) to intravenous fluids or pharmacologic intervention [3]." Clinicians more typically apply the term *septic shock* to patients with shock (usually defined as hypotension with a systolic blood pressure < 90 mm Hg) caused by one or more microbes (usually bacteria), often accompanied by tachycardia, peripheral vasoconstriction, and oliguria or anuria. Clear distinction between

Etiologies

Septic shock is most frequently caused by bacteria. Of these cases approximately 70% are due to gram-negative bacteria [5]. The remainder are caused by gram-positive, mixed bacterial, fungal, or viral organisms. In the United States parasites rarely cause septic shock. Certain populations and subgroups tend to develop infections with certain organisms [6]. For example, granulocytopenic patients tend to develop *Escherichia coli, Pseudomonas aeruginosa,* or *Klebsiella* infections [7]. Immunocompromised patients acquire unusual septic organisms, for example, *Pneumocystis carinii* or *Toxoplasma gondii.* Patients who are IV drug abusers often have staphylococcal infections [8]. Asplenic patients tend to have *Streptococcus pneumoniae* disease [9, 10]. Elderly patients with decubiti are prone to *Bacteroides fragilis* sepsis [11].

Predisposing Factors

As mentioned earlier, septic shock typically occurs in patients with predisposing factors (Table 6-3) [7, 12–16]. A majority of these factors are found primarily in middle-aged and elderly patients. An exception is AIDS in children and young adults. As

Table 6-3. Factors that are predisposing to septic shock

Alteration in host defenses: immunodeficiency

Severe underlying illnesses: diabetes, cirrhosis, renal failure

Presence of foreign bodies: urinary catheter, intravenous catheter, endotracheal tube, cardiac valve, shunts, prostheses, etc.

Obstructive process: kidney stone, gallstone, bowel obstruction, etc.

Treatment with steroids

Treatment with antimetabolites or cytotoxic agents

Prior antibiotic therapy

---

also mentioned earlier, an increasing percentage of the U.S. population is elderly. Very simply these people are subject to acquiring predisposing factors. For example, America's elderly are increasingly living in nursing homes. Patients in nursing homes commonly are given indwelling urinary catheters. The presence of such a catheter, bypassing normal mucosal and physical barriers, frequently leads to the production of a urinary tract infection [17, 18]. Perhaps one of the most common presentations of sepsis or septic shock in an emergency department is that of a patient with a urinary tract infection as a result of an indwelling Foley catheter (urosepsis) [19]. Similarly cancer is a disease predominantly found in the middle-aged and the elderly. Those patients receiving cancer chemotherapy or radiotherapy are at higher risk for sepsis and septic shock, particularly when their leukocyte count is very low. As can be seen from these examples, emergency medicine specialists must be prepared to see an increasing number of patients with septic shock in their future clinical practices, largely as a result of changing demographics.

Pathophysiology

An abbreviated review of the pathophysiology of sepsis is primarily helpful to the emergency medicine physician in understanding the most promising form of therapy, immunotherapy (discussed below). For an in-depth review of the subject, the reader is referred elsewhere [20–23]. Sepsis initiates

from a nidus of infection, which then results in growth of more organisms, followed by further elaboration of microbial endotoxins and exotoxins. More important the net result of microbial growth and elaboration of toxins is the production of endogenous mediators and interactions with other physiological systems, for example, the complement, kinin, and coagulation systems [24].

Endotoxin from the cell wall of gram-negative bacteria traditionally has been considered the fundamental mediator of sepsis [23]. This substance is a lipopolysaccharide called lipid A. Infusion of lipid A produces many of the manifestations of sepsis in both animals and humans. However, other organisms without endotoxin, such as gram-positive staphylococci, are also able to cause sepsis [8, 25]. While these organisms cause most of their effects by toxic shock syndrome toxin-1, other gram-positive organisms probably produce their effects by their interaction with the host's endogenous systems and cells (macrophages) [26, 27].

The list of endogenous mediators of sepsis has steadily grown and now includes cytokines (tumor necrosis factor and interleukins), platelet-activating factor, humoral defense systems (complement, kinins, coagulation), myocardial depressant substance (MDS), endorphins, histamine, and arachidonic acid metabolites [4, 28, 30]. Tumor necrosis factor (TNF), also known as cachectin, appears to be a major mediator in diverse types of sepsis. Extensive reviews of this most important mediator can be found elsewhere [28, 31–35].

One or more of these mediators, on stimulation, production, or alteration by bacterial toxins, produce profound effects on the peripheral vasculature and the heart [22, 36–38]. In the periphery vasodilatation, vasoconstriction, redistribution of blood flow, and endothelial destruction occur [38–41]. In the myocardium depression of inotropy and dilatation occur [29, 42, 43]. The result of these actions on the peripheral vasculature and the myocardium is the production of cardiovascular insufficiency (i.e., shock), in which the myocardium fails to meet the metabolic needs of the tissues, and the tissues also fail to utilize oxygen [44–46]. Subsequently a decrease in systemic vascular resistance and a depressed cardiac output lead to hypotension and death, often combined with multiple organ system failure [47].

Clinical Manifestations

The clinical manifestations of sepsis, septic syndrome, and septic shock are often subtle or absent. This is probably more true in the elderly [48, 49]. Many of the clinical symptoms and signs are nonspecific and nondiagnostic [50]. Thus, the task of the emergency medicine physician is difficult, particularly in light of the limited time frame in which evaluation occurs. Despite its triteness, "maintaining a high index of suspicion" for this sometimes subtle disease process remains one of the best tools for success. Unlike many benign disease processes encountered in the emergency department, the failure to diagnose sepsis frequently results in profound morbidity or, all too often, mortality.

Symptoms

The symptoms of sepsis, septic syndrome, and septic shock are often overshadowed by the signs. Fundamentally there are no symptoms in this disorder that are specific or pathognomic [50]. Some symptoms may be referable to the organ system primarily involved, cough and chest pain in pneumonia, or flank or low back pain in pyelonephritis. If adult respiratory distress syndrome (ARDS) is present (see below), dyspnea may be present. Other systems may be secondarily involved and produce noticeable symptoms (diarrhea or jaundice). While the jaundiced patient is frequently deemed "another patient with viral hepatitis," the presentation of icterus in a patient with one or more predisposing factors for sepsis should alert the astute clinician to consider this diagnosis [51, 52]. Most patients, however, will have nonspecific constitutional symptoms of malaise, fatigue, and a sense of ill-being or unexplained apprehension or confusion.

Signs

The classical manifestations of septic shock are chills, fever, and hypotension. This classical triad is seen in approximately 30%–40% of all patients subsequently shown to be septic [13]. Fever may not be as common as is widely believed. In one series the patient's maximum rectal temperature ranged from 36.7°C–42.8°C [53]. In the same study the initial temperature was less than 36.4°C in 13% of patients. In another series a temperature greater than 38.3°C was found in 170 out of 173 patients [13].

If by history, physical exam, or laboratory study the physician suspects that the patient should have a fever but does not (when measured in the emergency department), then a number of explanatory possibilities can exist. First, prior to presentation, the patient may have taken an analgesic that is also an antipyretic. It should be remembered that many patients in nursing homes have standing orders for acetaminophen PRN fever and are frequently given this antipyretic prior to their presentation to the emergency department. A careful review of the medication record is required to assist the clinician. A second possibility is that the medication history may be incorrect, often because when asked if they are taking any medication, patients deny any such ingestion. Patients often do not consider aspirin or acetaminophen to be "medication," (i.e., only a prescription item is a "medication" to them). Patients must be specifically questioned using the words "aspirin" and "Tylenol." A third possibility is that the temperature reading provided to the physician is inaccurate, particularly if it was taken orally. Temperatures fluctuate, and repeat temperatures may vary substantially from those obtained initially.

Hypotension may be seen in up to 40%–50% of septic patients [13, 53]. Hypotension is often defined clinically as a systolic blood pressure less than 90 mm Hg or a drop from baseline greater than 40 mm Hg. The patient's blood pressure on cursory initial review may seem normal. Unfortunately the busy emergency medicine physician may fail to ascertain the patient's baseline blood pressure. As is well known, isolated systolic hypertension is common in the elderly, and a seemingly "normal" systolic blood pressure of 120 mm Hg may actually represent a significant decline from the patient's norm.

Tachypnea and respiratory alkalosis may be one of the earliest and most subtle signs of sepsis [54]. The tachypnea may be an attempt to produce a compensatory respiratory alkalosis for the ongoing metabolic acidosis of sepsis. The central respiratory drive may be increased by microbial constituents (e.g., endotoxin) or by mediators released in response to those microbes. Therefore, if a patient has normal vital signs, with the exception of an elevated respiratory rate, early sepsis should be considered.

Another subtle sign is a change in mentation. Patients may exhibit apprehension, agitation, withdrawal, confusion, dementia, or stupor [55]. Patients may be brought to the emergency department because they "just aren't acting right," with subtle changes in their baseline mental activity.

Frequently patients are referred from a nursing home because of a history of oliguria or anuria. While an obstructed indwelling catheter may be the cause, it is important to consider the possibility of sepsis [56, 57].

An organ system that is occasionally key to the diagnosis of sepsis is the skin [58]. Cutaneous manifestations of sepsis include petechia, purpura, cellulitis, acrocyanosis, necrosis of distal phalanges, and ecthyma gangrenosum [59]. Ecthyma gangrenosum may start as macular red or purplish lesions, which progress to round or oval lesions 1–5 cm in diameter with a raised rim of erythema and induration surrounding a flat or vesicular or necrotic ulcerated central area. These are classically associated with *P. aeruginosa* infections, although other organisms have been implicated [59]. (See Chap. 9 and Color Plate 4.)

Laboratory Findings

As with the history and the physical examination, laboratory studies may be neither very sensitive nor specific. While many patients have a leukocytosis, leukopenia (even in the absence of cytotoxic chemotherapy or AIDS) may also be present. In one series the mean WBC count was 18,900, with a range of 3,600–57,000 [13]. The differential count is sometimes helpful if it shows a left shift, with a predominance of bands or simply a predominance of segmented polymorphonuclear (PMN) leukocytes. In the same study the mean PMN percentage was 78%, with a range of 35%–92% [13]. Other CBC findings can include toxic granulations, Dohle bodies, and vacuolization, none of which are highly specific. Bacteria are rarely seen in the leukocytes on peripheral blood or buffy coat smears or, in the case of overwhelming sepsis, outside the leukocytes. Significant changes in the red cell series are not usually seen, and the hemoglobin and he-

matocrit are often normal [13]. The platelets are sometimes decreased. A platelet count less than 150,000 was seen in 56% of patients in one series [53]. DIC, as defined by the presence of thrombocytopenia, elevated fibrin split products, decreased fibrinogen, factor V, and factor VIII, was seen in 11% of patients [53]. However, DIC sufficient to cause clinical bleeding occurred in only 3% of all the patients [53]. As mentioned earlier, respiratory alkalosis may be found on arterial blood gas analysis. In one series the average pH was 7.4, with a range of 7.09–7.69, while the mean carbon dioxide tension was 32 mm Hg (range 21–50) [60]. Serum electrolytes are frequently normal. The presence of dehydration can of course lead to an elevation of the BUN, and metabolic acidosis can result in a decrease in serum bicarbonate.

Adult Respiratory Distress Syndrome

The frequent occurrence of adult respiratory distress syndrome (ARDS) in patients with sepsis deserves special mention [61–63]. It has been estimated that 30%–40% of patients with sepsis or septic syndrome develop ARDS [64, 65]. ARDS is usually defined as an arterial oxygen tension less than 65 mm Hg while breathing at least 40% oxygen or a ratio of arterial oxygen tension to alveolar oxygen tension less than or equal to 0.3, bilateral diffuse infiltrates on chest x-ray that are compatible with pulmonary edema, and a pulmonary artery wedge pressure less than or equal to 18 mm Hg [65]. An alternative "lung scoring system" using the parameters of chest x-ray, PaO_2/FIO_2, respiratory compliance, and positive end-expiratory pressure has also been advocated [66]. Given the frequent occurrence of ARDS in patients with sepsis, it is incumbent on the emergency medicine physician to both recognize and initially manage this condition. It is almost a universal necessity to obtain an arterial blood gas determination and a chest x-ray on all patients with sepsis or septic shock. Any patient with radiographic findings suggestive of pulmonary edema must be considered a possible ARDS victim. Unfortunately the pulmonary artery wedge pressure is rarely if ever obtained in the emergency department, since such invasive monitoring is usually reserved for intensive care units.

Differential Diagnosis

As can be seen from the section on clinical manifestations and laboratory findings, sepsis and septic shock can be subtle or obvious. It is the subtle condition that poses most of the problems for the emergency medicine specialist. Starting with the simplest clinical usage of the term *shock* (i.e., a systolic blood pressure less than 90 mm Hg), the physician must keep in mind the basic differential diagnosis for shock: cardiogenic, oligemic, extracardiac obstructive, and distributive (Table 6-4). Most patients have only a single cause for shock, not two.

To distinguish septic shock from other causes of shock, close attention must be given to the history. Patients with septic shock frequently have one or more predisposing factors for microbial attack, and the onset is usually gradual, unlike the sudden onset of cardiogenic shock from infarction. The patient

Table 6-4. Types of shock

Distributive
Septic shock
Anaphylaxis
Toxicological (overdose)
Neurogenic
Endocrinologic shock

Oligemic Shock
Hemorrhage
Fluid depletion

Cardiogenic
Myopathic (reduced systolic function)
  Acute myocardial infarction
  Dilated cardiomyopathy
  Myocardial depression in septic shock
Mechanical
  Mitral regurgitation
  Ventricular septal defect
  Left ventricular outflow obstruction
  Aortic stenosis
  Hypertrophic cardiomyopathy
Arrhythmic

Extracardiac Obstructive Shock
Pericardial tamponade
Constrictive pericarditis
Pulmonary embolism (massive)
Aortic coarctation
Severe pulmonary hypertension

Adapted with permission from Ref. 22.

with anaphylactic hypotension similarly has an abrupt change in condition. The activities of the patient just prior to the onset of the presentation are of crucial importance. Patients with septic shock frequently are noted to have had an antecedent low-grade illness (e.g., a cough or an upper respiratory tract infection), or they have had a recent anatomical factor (e.g., placement of an indwelling urinary catheter or intravenous line). Patients with hemorrhagic shock usually have antecedent trauma, although occult hemorrhage may initially elude the unsuspecting physician. A history of recent ingestion of or exposure to new products must be ascertained. In some patients their age, sex, or associated conditions might suggest the diagnosis: a ruptured ectopic pregnancy in a female of childbearing age; a dissecting aorta in a patient with a history of hypertension; adrenal insufficiency in a noncompliant steroid dependent patient, and so on.

The critical nature of hypotension in the patient with septic shock generally produces a sense of profound urgency in the physician. However, it is in the septic patient without shock that the physician frequently is lulled into a false sense of complacency. The patient may appear relatively well or manifest only apprehension, tachypnea, or tachycardia. There may be no profound evidence of toxicity. While on the surface all is fine, microbial attack is ongoing and if not recognized early may shortly lead to shock and later death. The physician must particularly place sepsis in the differential diagnosis of an increasingly elderly patient population. The lack of gross physical findings (even a fever) should never sway one's opinion. It is precisely these patients (i.e., the elderly) who not only are most at risk for sepsis, but who also frequently lack concrete findings to support the diagnosis of sepsis [49]. The absence of a fever does not rule out sepsis; neither does a normal leukocyte count. It will be necessary to use sepsis as a working diagnosis in many patients without the benefit of confirmation of this diagnosis or identification of a source.

Outcome

Studies by McCabe et al. and Kreger et al. have shown that the primary determinant of a patient's outcome from sepsis or septic shock is the severity of the patient's underlying disease [5, 12, 13, 53]. These underlying diseases were arbitrarily categorized into: rapidly fatal, diseases estimated to be fatal within one year (e.g., acute leukemia or blastic crisis); ultimately fatal, diseases estimated to be fatal within 4 years (e.g., metastatic carcinoma, lupus nephritis, cirrhosis with hepatic coma or bleeding varices, chronic renal failure with BUN > 70), and nonfatal diseases (e.g., diabetes). In one study the mortality in these three patient groups was, respectively, 40%, 31%, and 15% [5]. Various other factors have been linked with worse survival outcomes, including age greater than 60, neutropenia (leukocyte count < 1500/μl, nosocomial infections, presence of shock, source of infection, degree of bacteremia, maximum temperature < 38.3°C on the day of bacteremia, interval to initiation of treatment, and appropriateness of initial antibiotic therapy [5, 67]. In Kreger's series if appropriate antibiotics were given, the mortality in the three broad groups mentioned initially was 29%, 26%, and 11%, respectively [5]. In the same series if inappropriate antibiotics were given, the mortality was 77%, 38%, and 29%, respectively (all significantly different from the groups receiving appropriate antibiotic therapy) [5]. It does not appear that the causative organism, for example, gram-negative bacteria or gram-positive bacteria, is clearly a factor in outcome. Sepsis and septic shock, whatever the inciting microbes, carry uniformly poor outcomes.

Therapy

Management Steps

Because of the inability to definitively diagnose sepsis, septic syndrome, or septic shock, the emergency medicine physician must start empiric or presumptive therapy in a rapid fashion. Absolute confirmation of the diagnosis is often obtained only retrospectively. If therapy is delayed until the diagnosis is established, the patient will almost assuredly expire prior to that time. Optimal management ideally would include seven steps:

1. initial provision of advanced life support, (i.e., attention to airway, breathing, and circulation)
2. recognition of sepsis
3. identification of its source

4. identification of the causative agent and its antibiotic susceptibility
5. immediate provision of the appropriate antibiotic in an effective dose
6. relief of any obstructive process, removal of foreign bodies, and drainage of any closed-space infection
7. management and prevention of complications

Frequently these steps cannot be so easily separated in time and sequence, and it is often necessary for the emergency medicine physician to carry out several of these steps simultaneously.

Fluids

Obviously the first management step, initial advanced cardiac life support measures, takes precedence over all other steps. The physician must establish an airway, assist ventilation as needed, and finally support circulation, primarily with fluids [68, 69]. Fluid resuscitation is often performed suboptimally. The patient with sepsis may have a profound relative vascular volume depletion, decline in systemic vascular resistance index, and a decrease in cardiac output [21, 43]. A decrease in cardiac output is thought to be due at least in part to the negative inotropy of a putative myocardial depressant factor or substance [29, 43]. Therefore, the patient should initially receive an intravenous fluid bolus of at least 200–500 ml at a wide open rate; this fluid challenge should be repeated until the systolic blood pressure is equal to or greater than 90 mm Hg or until approximately 2–3 liters of fluid have been infused. In some cases the patient may require 5 or more liters of fluid. The type of fluid to administer remains controversial [70, 71]. The debate between crystalloid and colloid solutions has not been resolved. It has been suggested that crystalloids may be the best fluid in early sepsis, while colloids are best in late sepsis [70]. Unfortunately the emergency medicine physician cannot easily distinguish between these two states. In addition differences in outcome using one or the other fluid have not been consistently demonstrated in relevant studies of human sepsis. Until such improved outcome has been shown, given the cost of colloid, crystalloid solution, particularly normal saline, remains the most reasonable choice. It must be emphasized that patients in septic shock may require very large amounts of intravenous fluids before their blood pressure rises. The goal is to increase the left ventricular preload and increase the pulmonary artery wedge pressure to a level that maximizes cardiac output. In the absence of a pulmonary artery catheter or central venous pressure monitoring catheter, the clinician simply may need to give up to 3 liters of saline empirically. Assessment of parameters such as jugular veins, pulmonary auscultation, mentation, peripheral skin appearance, and urine output (by indwelling catheter) may be helpful.

Following the infusion of 2–3 liters of fluids, if the patient remains hypotensive, consideration must be given to intravascular monitoring. Although a pulmonary artery catheter offers major advantages, this monitoring capability is not usually available or appropriate in most emergency department settings [72, 73]. Therefore, insertion of a central venous line for measurement of central venous pressure (CVP) is the typical measure taken in the emergency department. While CVP monitoring has multiple limitations and is perhaps useful only when assessed serially, in the absence of a more definitive and accurate pulmonary arterial catheter, the CVP provides a general monitor of fluid status [74]. If the CVP is low (below 10 cm), it is reasonably safe to continue large amounts of crystalloid.

Attention must be paid to the possibility that large fluid infusions can result in a decline in the hemoglobin content of the blood. This would produce a decrease in the oxygen-carrying capacity of each milliliter of blood perfusing the vital organs as well as the periphery. Therefore, reassessment of the hematocrit should be performed if large amounts of fluid are given. Red blood cell transfusion should be considered in patients with a hemoglobin less than 12 g, rather than the often mentioned level of 10 g [75].

Vasopressors

If the patient remains hypotensive after approximately 3 liters of saline have been infused, and if a CVP line is present and demonstrates a CVP of approximately 15–18 cm, then the patient should receive a vasopressor (Table 6-5) [76, 77]. A common mistake prior to this point is the initiation of vasopressor therapy before "the tank is filled" (i.e.,

Table 6-5. Vasopressor drugs useful in septic shock

Drug	Dosage (IV)
Dopamine	2–25 μg/kg/min.
Dobutamine	2–25 μg/kg/min.
Norepinephrine	0.01–1.5 μg/kg/min.
Phenylephrine	40–180 μg/min.
Epinephrine	1–8 μg/min.

before the intravascular volume and preload are optimized). Failure to provide an adequate preload followed by vasopressor therapy can result in premature worsening of a peripheral lactic acidosis. Once the "tank is full" then and only then should a vasopressor be added to improve hemodynamic parameters. The vasopressor traditionally used in this setting is dopamine. Initial doses, even in the so-called renal vasodilatory low-dose range, may provide surprisingly good increases in systolic blood pressure above 90 mm Hg. An initial dose of 2 μg/kg/min should be started, with subsequent elevation to 25 μg/kg/min, titrating to a mean BP of 60 mm Hg or a systolic BP of 90 mm Hg. If the blood pressure remains below this, then another agent should be added. Recent work suggests that septic patients may have an intrinsic decrease in myocardial performance that is not due simply to changes in preload or afterload [22, 38]. Therefore dobutamine, a positive inotropic agent, when combined with higher doses of dopamine (vasoconstrictor doses), may offer benefit as the second agent. Dobutamine may have slight peripheral vasodilatory effects. However, when combined with higher vasoconstricting doses of dopamine, the systemic vascular resistance may not be clearly decreased by the dobutamine. Dobutamine should be started in a dose of 1–2 μg/kg/min and increased up to 25 μ/kg/min. If the patient still remains hypotensive, recent work suggests that the almost pure alpha agonist norepinephrine (in low doses of 0.01–1.50 μg/kg/min) may provide a significant elevation of the blood pressure, particularly in situations where dopamine and dobutamine have failed [78–80]. Recently norepinephrine has been advocated as the second drug of choice, to be used immediately after fluid and dopamine have failed to adequately elevate the blood pressure [68].

Identification of Organism

While the first management step is being accomplished, the second, third, and fourth steps (recognition of sepsis, identification of its source, and identification of causative agent and its antibiotic susceptibility) are often ongoing as well. Definitive isolation of the causative agent is usually not accomplished by the emergency medicine specialist, given the inherent time limitations of the practice. Nevertheless, there are a few steps that can be taken to identify the precise etiological agent in some cases. One of the simplest tools available is that of the Gram's stain. If positive (i.e., if it shows a predominance of one organism), it can rapidly provide a moderately accurate diagnosis in the emergency department. For instance, a Gram's stain of purulent sputum that shows numerous PMN leukocytes with gram-positive diplococci can reliably provide the diagnosis of pneumococcus as the agent of sepsis. The Gram's stain of cerebrospinal fluid (CSF) that shows gram-negative diplococci favors the diagnosis of *Neisseria meningitides*.

Other tests that can rapidly identify bacterial species, for example, counterimmune electrophoresis (CIE), can be helpful if positive. CIE, latex agglutination, and enzyme-linked immunoabsorbent assay are techniques that identify antigenic constituents of microbes or antibodies directed against them [81, 82]. These tests are particularly helpful in patients with partially treated infections (i.e., those patients whose etiologic agent is masked or obscured). CSF from a patient with partially treated meningitis provides excellent specimens for these tests. Unfortunately these tests are not infallible, and a negative CIE does not rule out infection with such species as *N. meningitides* or *Haemophilus influenzae* [83]. In addition some of these tests often are unavailable or in very limited clinical use (see Chap. 3).

To properly accomplish the fifth management step, prompt delivery of antibiotics, the emergency medicine physician must first obtain appropriate samples for culture and antibiotic-sensitivity testing. As a minimum both urine and blood cultures must be obtained on every septic patient prior to the initiation of antibiotic therapy. In addition other cultures of pertinent sites must be obtained as needed. For instance, if a pneumonia is suspected,

then sputum or an endotracheal aspirate must be obtained. Similarly cultures of any wounds, decubiti, skin lesions, catheter tips, and so on, must be obtained. If a patient has suspected meningitis, a lumbar puncture must be performed expeditiously. However, a lumbar puncture must not be performed if the patient is suspected of having elevated intracranial pressure. In those cases a CT scan should be done prior to the lumbar puncture. In the interim, prior to the lumbar puncture, the patient should receive a first dose of antibiotics, since deferral of antibiotic therapy until after a CT scan and lumbar puncture are completed may result in unacceptable delays in antibiotic therapy [84]. The first dose of antibiotic therapy can affect the subsequent yield of the CSF Gram's stain or cultures; however, the presence of meningitis, for example, by identification of CSF pleocytosis, probably will not be significantly affected [84]. Nevertheless CSF cultures may return positive even if the patient has received a single dose of antibiotic [84] (see Chap. 31).

Blood cultures must be obtained in the correct number and fashion (see Chap. 3) [85]. Three blood culture sets are recommended as optimal for the detection of bacteremia [86]. There probably is not a distinct advantage of waiting any period of time between obtaining each culture. Each culture should be obtained from a different site. Obviously careful skin preparation is important. The optimal amount of blood per culture bottle must be obtained, and this amount can be determined by consultation with the pathologist or microbiologist. Too little or too much blood in the culture bottle can reduce the accuracy and yield of the culture. Finally it must be remembered that once collected all cultures must be rapidly processed in the laboratory. Blood cultures that are not promptly incubated and other cultures that are not promptly processed and plated may be essentially worthless.

Antibiotics

All cultures must be obtained expeditiously and antibiotics started immediately thereafter [87]. Sepsis is a medical emergency, and despite the relatively benign appearance of some septic patients, they have septic shock in waiting. The shock state might be prevented by the prompt administration of appropriate antibiotics [53]. An interesting contrast is between the promptness of care received by cardiac arrest victims (a disorder with uniformly abysmal outcomes) compared to the almost leisurely approach received by septic patients, who probably have a greater chance of hospital discharge, particularly if treated prior to the onset of shock. The concept of a "code yellow" for sepsis is very reasonable.

In the absence of an accurate microbial identification, the clinician is left with seemingly little help in the selection of antibiotic therapy. This bleak outlook is modified by the realization that if a probable site of origin is identified, then the probable bacterial agent may also be predicted, based on previous clinical studies. Identification of the site is based on the history, the physical examination, and simple laboratory or radiographic tests. Careful attention to precipitating events must be made. The urinary tract may be the source if an indwelling catheter, instrumentation, or obstruction is present. The bowel as the primary site of infection is suggested by the presence of obstruction, perforation, abscess, neoplasia, or diverticula. The biliary tract may be the site if the patient has a history of gall stones or recent instrumentation, or surgery. The vascular system may be suspected as the infection site if an intravenous catheter or pacemaker was placed or another vascular surgical procedure has occurred.

Once a probable site has been identified, then

the probable microbe may be predicted. The simplest example is that of the urinary tract. If this system is identified as the source, then previous studies have shown that the most frequent etiologic agents are *E. coli*, *Klebsiella-Enterobacter-Serratia* organisms, *Proteus* species, and *P. aeruginosa*. Similarly if the probable site of infection is that of the bowel, then it is likely that the causative bacteria include *Bacteroides* species, *E. coli*, *Klebsiella-Enterobacter-Serratia* organisms, and salmonella. An outline of findings from one large study is shown in Table 6-6. While this table provides some guidance, it also demonstrates that there is a wide range of bacteria subsequently identified as the predominant microbe derived from a single anatomic site. Therefore, antibiotic therapy cannot be limited to that which is effective against a single bacterial species. The clinician can rarely be sure of the exact organism that must be treated initially. Patients can also have polymicrobial infections. The clinical appearance of a patient in septic shock from a gram-negative rod cannot be reliably distinguished from that due to gram-positive cocci [60, 88, 89]. In most cases initial antibiotic therapy must include drugs effective against both types of bacteria [90, 91].

Most recommended antibiotic regimens classify patients into distinct groups, with different regimens for each group. These classifications are based on the retrospective identification of causa-

Table 6-6. Relation of etiologic agents to site of origin of gram-negative bacteremia

Organism	Site of origin								
	Unknown	Urinary	Respiratory	GI	Biliary	Other	Skin	Reproductive	Total
E. coli	47	97	8	19	6	4	9	2	189
Klebsiella	23	26	12	7	1	3	1	1	74
Enterobacter	20	13	4	3	3	1	3	0	47
Serratia	2	3	3	1	0	2	0	0	11
Pseudomonas	13	18	15	2	0	3	8	1	60
Proteus and Providencia	10	31	0	1	0	3	4	0	49
Bacteroides	13	0	0	24	0	0	2	2	41
Other	20	1	4	8	1	1	0	1	36
Mixed	33	23	9	21	1	3	13	2	105
Total	181	209	55	86	12	20	40	9	612

Adapted with permission from Ref. 5.

tive agents within each group of septic patients. For instance, compromised hosts are prone to infections with a wide variety of microbes [87]. Of the several bacteria that have been shown usually to cause sepsis in neutropenic patients, *P. aeruginosa* is notable [92, 93]. This organism, however, is rarely the cause of sepsis in a normal host with a community acquired infection. Therefore, empiric antibiotic therapy for a neutropenic patient must provide antibiotic coverage for *P. aeruginosa*, while antibiotic therapy for a nonneutropenic patient with a community acquired infection does not need to include agents effective against *Pseudomonas* organisms [6, 94]. Included in most broad recommendations is the categorization of patients with either community acquired or hospital acquired infections [95]. This is again based on retrospective profiling of causative agents in these patients. Patients who reside in nursing homes are considered to be microbiologically equivalent to hospitalized patients (i.e., their infections are not "community" acquired). In addition the physician must be aware of local patterns of resistance. At certain hospitals gram-negative bacterial isolates frequently are resistant to the classical aminoglycosides gentamicin and tobramycin. In those cases the bacteria usually are sensitive to amikacin, which must be used in place of the older aminoglycosides as initial empiric therapy. Another example is that of *E. coli*. If the *E. coli* (isolated from the urinary tract of patients presenting to a single hospital) are shown to be frequently resistant to ampicillin, obviously that drug must be replaced by another in the empiric regimen for patients with urosepsis.

A simple regimen for patients with sepsis is outlined in Table 6-7. While more tailored regimens may be suggested by identification of a particular site or probable organism, initial therapy is best kept in a broad spectrum because of the problems mentioned above. Subsequent deletion of an antibiotic in the later hospital course is clearly preferable to the realization that a necessary drug was not started initially. Combinations of at least two agents are strongly recommended as standard therapy [23, 96]. While monotherapy with newer agents such as imipenem theoretically may seem advantageous and promising, such monotherapy is not recommended at this time [87, 96, 97]. In addition to the regimens in Tables 6-7 and 6-8,

Table 6-7. Recommended antimicrobial regimens of empiric (presumptive) therapy for gram-negative bacteremia

1. Community-acquired infection in the nonneutropenic patient (neutrophil count $\geq 1000/\mu l$)
   Suspected urinary tract source: ampicillin and an aminoglycoside
   Nonurinary tract source: a third-generation cephalosporin with or without an aminoglycoside
2. Hospital acquired infection, nonneutropenic patient
   A third-generation cephalosporin plus an aminoglycoside
3. Neutropenic patient with hospital-acquired infection
   Antipseudomonal penicillin (e.g., ticarcillin or piperacillin) plus an aminoglycoside
4. Thermal injury > 20% body surface area
   Same as No. 3
5. Pulmonary source associated with inhalation therapy equipment
   Same as No. 3
6. Established or suspected gentamicin resistance
   Amikacin
7. Nosocomial infection in the setting of resistance to penicillins and cephalosporins
   Imipenem with or without an aminoglycoside
8. History of IVDA or indwelling catheter
   Nafcillin and aminoglycoside
9. Penicillin-allergic patient
   Cephalosporins, vancomycin, or chloramphenicol replace penicillin for gram-positive coverage, aztreonam for gram-negative coverage.

Adapted with permission from Ref. 23.

close consultation with both the infectious disease subspecialist and the microbiology laboratory is helpful. (For greater detail on broad antibiotic therapeutic principles, see Chap. 4.)

As mentioned earlier the vast majority of patients with sepsis, septic shock, or septic syndrome have a bacterial, usually gram-negative, etiology. Only occasionally do patients have fungal or parasitic sepsis. Patients with dysfunction of cellular immunity are particularly prone to fungal infections, for example, *Candida* species, *Crytococcus neoformans*, and *Histoplasma capsulatum* (see Chap. 16). These patients also develop infections from other unusual microbes more frequently, for exam-

Table 6-8. Recommended antibiotic adult dosages for sepsis

Antibiotic	Dosage
Aminoglycosides	
Gentamicin (Garamycin and generic)	1.5–2.0 mg/kg IV loading dose (subsequent maintenance doses determined by renal function and antibiotic levels)
Tobramycin (Nebcin)	1.5–2.0 mg/kg IV loading dose
Amikacin (Amikin)	5.0 mg/kg IV loading dose
Cephalosporins	
Third Generation	
Ceftazidime (Fortaz, Tazicef, Tazidime)	1.0–2.0 g IV q8h
Cefotaxime (Claforan)	1.0–3.0 g IV q6h
Ceftriaxone (Rocephin)	1.0–2.0 g IV q12h
Cefoperazone (Cefobid)	2.0 g IV q8h
Ceftizoxime (Cefizox)	1.0–4.0 g IV q8h
Antipseudomonal Penicillins	
Carbenicillin (Geopen)	5.0 g IV q4h
Ticarcillin (Ticar)	3.0 g IV q4h
Mezlocillin (Mezlin)	3.0 g IV q4h
Azlocillin (Azlin)	3.0 g IV q4h
Piperacillin (Pipracil)	3.0 g IV q4h
Drugs Useful in Penicillin Allergy	
Vancomycin (Vancocin)	500 mg IV q6h
Chloramphenicol (Chloromycetin and generic)	12.5–25 mg/kg IV q6h
Aztreonam (Azactam)	2.0 g IV q6–8h
Drugs Useful in Anaerobic Infections	
Metronidazole (Flagyl & generic)	15 mg/kg IV loading dose
Clindamycin (Cleocin)	600–900 mg IV q8h
Drugs Useful in Staphylococcal Infections	
Nafcillin (Unipen, Nallpen, Nafcil, generic)	1.5 g IV q4h
Oxacillin (Prostaphlin, Bactocil)	2.0 g IV q4h
Methicillin (Staphcillin)	2.0 g IV q4h
Vancomycin	500 mg IV q6h
Miscellaneous	
Ampicillin (Omnipen, Polycillin, Totacillin, generic)	1.0–3.0 g IV q6h
Ampicillin/sulbactam (Unasyn)	1.5–3.0 g IV q6h
Imipenem/cilastin (Primaxin)	0.5–1.0 g IV q6h
Ticarcillin/clavulanate (Timentin)	3.1–6.2 g IV q6h

ple, *Listeria monocytogenes, T. gondii,* cytomegalovirus, varicella and herpes simplex viruses. Patients with AIDS are prone to infection with similar unusual organisms, particularly *P. carinii* (see Chap. 17).

Should immunocompromised patients, for example, renal transplant patients or patients with AIDS, receive empiric antifungal or antiparasitic therapy if they present with sepsis [98]? Currently most of these patients do not receive immediate empiric antifungal or antiparasitic therapy in the emergency department unless there is more identifying or suggestive information [87, 99, 100]. For instance, in a patient with AIDS and sepsis, the presence of a diffuse interstitial infiltrate on chest x-ray is highly suggestive of *P. carinii* pneumonia, and initiation of antipneumocystis therapy clearly would be indicated. Unfortunately the situation with fungi is rarely so simple [100]. *Candida* species are not usually identified in the initial evaluation of an immunocompromised patient. At present the majority of septic immunocompromised patients are not initially given antifungal therapy in the emergency department. Failure to respond to antibacterial therapy in the subsequent hospital course is an indication for starting antifungal therapy.

Third-generation cephalosporins include ceftazidime, cefoperazone, cefotaxime, ceftizoxime, ceftriaxone, and moxalactam [101, 102]. Ceftazidime or cefotaxime are frequently chosen. Aminoglycosides include gentamicin, tobramycin, and amikacin. Antipseudomonal penicillins include carbenicillin, ticarcillin, mezlocillin, azlocillin, and piperacillin. Suggested initial antibiotic doses are listed in Table 6-8. Antibiotics should be given in the upper end of their dosing range [103, 104]. It is also important to remember that in patients with renal insufficiency or renal failure, an aminoglycoside should be given in its *full* loading dose as the initial dose [105]. It is only the subsequent (maintenance) doses of aminoglycosides that may require reduction in the presence of renal failure [106]. The first dose of an aminoglycoside should not be reduced because of renal disease or concern about nephrotoxicity.

Mention should be made of special situations. For example, in the penicillin-allergic patient, it is important to determine the precise allergic reaction, if any, that the patient previously has experienced with penicillin. Many infectious disease specialists recommend that cephalosporins can be given to a penicillin-allergic patient if the patient has a history of only a minor allergic reaction (minor urticaria) without any major anaphylactic reaction with bronchospasm or hypotension. Although it is estimated that 2% of penicillin-allergic patients will be allergic to cephalosporins, in clinical practice the majority of patients with a history of allergy to penicillin receive cephalosporins without any adverse reaction. As a general rule in cases of sepsis where this allergic issue arises, and the clinician wants to avoid a B-lactam antibiotic (penicillins or cephalosporins) for gram-positive coverage, then vancomycin is the antibiotic most frequently recommended as a substitute [110]. Chloramphenicol has also been used in situations where a pneumococcal or meningococcal infection is present in a penicillin-allergic patient [111]. Aztreonam is another alternative for patients with penicillin allergy [112]; however, it is not effective against grampositive bacteria and anaerobes.

Other situations that require modification of the above recommendations are cases of possible anaerobic bacterial infection [113, 114]. These cases include aspiration pneumonia and below-the-diaphragm infections, such as bowel obstruction or female genital tract infections. In those cases metronidazole, clindamycin, imipenem-cilastin, ampicillin-sulbactam, or ticarcillin-clavulanate should be used [115, 116].

Patients prone to staphylococcal infections also deserve special mention. It is well established that septic patients who use intravenous drugs and patients who have indwelling intravenous catheters have a high incidence of coagulase-negative staphylococci or *S. aureus* infections [8, 117]. In those cases effective antistaphylococcal coverage must be ensured. Typical antistaphylococcal antibiotics are the penicillinase-resistant penicillins (oxacillin, nafcillin, methicillin), and vancomycin [110, 118].

Another group that may develop infections from predictable organisms is surgically splenectomized or effectively splenectomized patients (e.g., patients with sickle cell disease). Their defect in humoral immunity results in frequent infections from *S. pneumoniae* and occasionally *H. influenzae* or *N. meningitides* [10].

The septic patient who recently has been exposed to organisms with multiple antibiotic resistances or who is at high risk for polymicrobial infection should probably receive a combination of amikacin and imipenem-cilastin [119]. In some centers ampicillin-sulbactam or ticarcillin–clavulanic acid are substituted for the third-generation cephalosporins or imipenam, as recommended in Table 6-7 [120].

Management of Complications

The many organ systems that sepsis can affect are listed in Table 6-9. The major complication of sepsis is ARDS, and a large number of septic pa-

Table 6-9. Sepsis syndrome: end organ effect

System	Dysfunction/manifestation
Cardiac	Decreased myocardial contractility
	Vascular vasoconstriction
Vascular	Smooth muscle constriction
	Enhanced vascular permeability
	Vasodilation
	Endothelial destruction
	Redistribution of blood flow
Hematologic	Platelet aggregation
	Leukocyte degranulation
	Leukocyte adhesion
	DIC
Pulmonary	ARDS
	Vascular vasoconstriction
	Hypoxemia
Hepatic	Jaundice
	Liver function test abnormalities
Renal	Oliguria, azotemia
	Acute tubular necrosis
	Acidosis
	Proteinuria
Gastrointestinal	Adynamic ileus
	Diarrhea
	Gastrointestinal bleeding

tients develop this complication. If ARDS is present, then the task of the emergency medicine physician is relatively straightforward. Besides treatment of the underlying etiology, patients with ARDS are primarily given only supportive therapy with increasing doses of oxygen to keep the arterial oxygen tension above 60 mm Hg or the oxyhemoglobin saturation greater than 90%. Endotracheal intubation and mechanical ventilation are performed if necessary to achieve this goal [121]. Adjunctive therapy, for example, with steroids, has not been shown to be effective and is not recommended [122–124]. Beyond the basic management steps for any patient in sepsis, these few recommendations are the only aspects of ARDS treatment that the emergency medicine physician realistically can be expected to perform. In cases of ARDS treatment of the underlying etiology (i.e., sepsis) and supportive care are the main goals in the emergency department.

New Controversial Therapies
STEROIDS
Steroid therapy for sepsis and septic shock has been used for many years [125–127]. A body of experimental work in animals, as well as one widely quoted study in humans, forms the foundation for this practice [128–130]. However, the study in humans contained several methodological flaws, and the animal studies did not closely emulate the clinical situation of human sepsis. Therefore, in the 1980s several human trials of steroid therapy were conducted [1, 131, 132]. The largest were prospective, randomized, double-blind, placebo-controlled, multicenter studies. In one study the use of steroids (methylprednisolone 30 mg/kg or dexamethasone 6 mg/kg) was associated with a significant reversal of the shock state and improved survival at 5 days [131]. Unfortunately this result did not translate into an improved overall outcome, and the ultimate mortality of the steroid- and non-steroid-treated groups was not significantly different. Subsequently another study reported that the use of steroids (methylprednisolone 30 mg/kg q6h for four days) did not result in the prevention of shock, the reversal of shock, or improved overall mortality [1]. In that study a subgroup of steroid-treated patients with elevated initial serum creatinine levels had a significantly increased mortality at 14 days when compared to the placebo group. Finally these findings were replicated by another large high-quality study (treating early sepsis with methylprednisolone 30 mg/kg followed by an infusion of 5 mg/kg for 9h).[132] The study found no difference in the 14-day mortality between the steroid group and the placebo group. Given the type and the quality of these more recent human studies, the use of steroids in human sepsis, septic shock, or septic syndrome is no longer recommended [124]. It must be emphasized that the emergency medicine specialist should adhere to these current recommendations, which are based on sound scientific human research rather than on anecdote or the historical use of a drug. While certain subsets of patients may benefit from the use of steroids, these subsets have not yet been identified. In addition the efficacy of steroids to prevent the development of ARDS or to decrease the morbidity or mortality of ARDS has not been demonstrated [122–124].

NALOXONE

Exogenous and endogenous opiates (endorphins) can produce hypotension, and endogenous opioid secretion is elevated during stress. Adrenocorticotropin and beta-endorphin are secreted by the pituitary gland [133]. Naloxone reverses the depressant effects of opiates. Therefore, this compound has been examined in the hypotensive stress state of sepsis. It has been assumed that the reversal of shock by naloxone supports a pathophysiological role of opiates, but this assumption may be overly simplistic or erroneous [134, 135]. Naloxone has been studied primarily in animal models of sepsis [136, 137]. Hypotension induced by *E. coli* infusion was reversed by naloxone, in a dose-related, stereospecific manner [138]. The exact mechanism of this reversal is unclear, but endogenous opiates, CNS effects, and an intact adrenal medulla all appear to be involved [135, 138, 139]. Naloxone improved mean arterial pressure in one model; however, it did not improve survival [140]. Anecdotal reports in humans suggest that naloxone could improve blood pressure [141], so small prospective trials of naloxone in human sepsis have been performed. A study of 13 patients treated with 0.4–1.2 mg/kg naloxone bolus found an increase in systolic blood pressure within minutes after treatment [142]. Another study of 13 patients found a significant increase of mean arterial pressure in patients treated with 0.03 mg/kg naloxone bolus and 0.2 mg/kg per hour continuous infusion for 1 hour [143]. Only 1 of the 13 patients survived [143]. A randomized placebo-controlled study in 28 patients found no improvement in blood pressure or survival rates using a 0.4–1.2 mg/kg bolus [144]. Another similar study more recently found a significant increase in mean arterial pressure in 5 of 11 patients within 20 minutes of naloxone treatment [145]. Again, however, there was no significant difference in overall survival between the treated and the untreated groups. Another randomized placebo-controlled trial of 0.03 mg/kg bolus and 0.03 mg/kg per hour continuous infusion found a decrease in vasopressor requirements in the naloxone group [146]. Mortality was less in the treated group, but this study was extremely small.

Naloxone may provide temporary improvements in blood pressure during septic shock [147]. Unfortunately, at least in initial studies, this gain has not translated into improved overall survival. Larger trials may be needed to delineate what future role, if any, naloxone will play in the treatment of septic shock.

NONSTEROIDAL ANTI-INFLAMMATORY AGENTS

Sepsis is frequently accompanied by the generation and release of arachidonic acid metabolites [148, 149]. These metabolites produce many cardiovascular and pulmonary effects. During sepsis free arachidonic acid is released from membrane phospholipids as a result of multiple stimuli: endotoxin (lipid A), the complement system, platelet aggregation, other leukocyte inflammatory mediators, and so on. Arachidonic acid is transformed into prostaglandin endoperoxidases by cyclo-oxygenase [150]. The endoperoxides are converted to prostacyclin (PGI_2) and metabolized by thromboxane synthetase to thromboxane (A_2) [150]. PGI_2 relaxes vascular smooth muscle [151]. There are a multitude of interactions and pathways of chemical reactions in the metabolism of arachidonic acid, and this brief summary must suffice here [152]. Because of the known effects of these metabolites, it has been hypothesized that interference with the arachidonic acid metabolism may decrease the injury of sepsis. Several compounds inhibit cyclo-oxygenase and therefore decrease the formation of cyclic endoperoxides, prostaglandins, and thromboxanes. Aspirin, indomethacin, and ibuprofen are several cyclo-oxygenase inhibitors that have been studied [153, 154]. Ibuprofen has received more attention [155]. Unfortunately many of the studies have involved pretreatment of experimental animals, a model very dissimilar to typical clinical scenarios. One model that treated animals 5 minutes after an *E. coli* endotoxin challenge found an improvement in blood pressure and cardiac index after endotoxin injection [156]. While nonsteroidal anti-inflammatory therapy offers a theoretical advantage, its actual clinical efficacy, if any, has not been determined.

HEMOFILTRATION

As has been increasingly evident in recent years, sepsis is mediated by a host of endogenous and exogenous substances. Recently it has been reasoned that filtration of the blood and removal of one or more of these mediators may be beneficial. A limited number of studies have been reported [157–159]. Using a polystyrene polymyxin B filter to hemoperfuse serum, removal of both endotoxin and TNF occurs [157, 159]. In a canine model some improvements in blood pressure and survival rate were noted [158, 159]. One patient with gram-negative sepsis showed hematological and hemodynamic improvement with hemoperfusion [157]. In another animal model hemofiltration removed arachidonic acid metabolites in the treated group; however, survival times were not improved [160]. This novel approach to sepsis holds some promise, but it must be remembered that once certain "cascades" of the septic process are set in motion, it may not be that helpful to subsequently remove the inciting substance(s).

IMMUNOTHERAPY

The most promising form of therapy for sepsis appears to be immunological. Immunotherapy is based on an understanding of the pathophysiology of sepsis. As briefly outlined earlier, the organisms that cause sepsis do so by production of toxins, for example, by growth of organisms that have endotoxin as a component of their cell wall (e.g., gram-negative bacteria) or by the release of exotoxins (e.g., toxic shock syndrome toxin-1 by staphylococci). These initiating toxins are thought to interact with (increase or modify) endogenous mediators. The best example of such a mediator is the cytokine TNF. These endogenous mediators then produce the more familiar effects on the peripheral vasculature, the myocardium, and other organs. Immunotherapy revolves around immunologically attacking the organisms themselves, constituents of the organisms (the endotoxin component of gram-negative cell walls), or the endogenous mediators.

Bacterial lipopolysaccharides (LPS) are composed of three portions: lipid A, the core polysaccharide, and the oligosaccharide side chains [23, 162]. Lipid A is thought to be the primary toxic component. Initial studies of immunotherapy used a bacterium, E. coli J5. This bacterium does not have oligosaccharides attached to the cell wall LPS. Therefore, the bacteria present the core polysac-

charide-lipid A complex on their surface. The presentation of this glycolipid is immunogenic (it results in the production of antibodies directed against the core glycolipid). Starting in the early 1970s volunteers were immunized with boiled whole-cell E. coli J5 vaccine, and the antiserum they developed (i.e., antibodies to E. coli J5) was harvested. This antiserum was then used to passively immunize patients with severe gram-negative bacteremia and shock. In a randomized double-blind study mortality in the treatment group was significantly lower than in the untreated control group [163]. In a later study this antiserum was used in an attempt to prevent gram-negative shock and death in surgical patients [164]. As expected, the incidence of shock, as well as mortality, was significantly lower in the treated group. However, some studies have not shown consistent improvement when anti-LPS antibodies were used [165, 166].

Monoclonal antibodies to lipid A have been developed [167]. Two large, multicentered, randomized, double-blind, controlled trials using anti-endotoxin monoclonal antibodies have been published. Direct comparison of the efficacy of the two products, E5 and HA-1A, is difficult because of differences in their design, their definitions of shock, and their methods of subgroup analysis. Both antibodies, however, have shown efficacy in improving survival and resolution of major morbidities in patients with gram-negative sepsis but no reduction in mortality in those patients with refractory shock [168]. The second study using HA-1A revealed similar efficacy in all gram-negative bacteremic patients with or without shock [169]. Based on results such as these, it is clear that antiendotoxin monoclonal antibodies will have an important role in therapy of gram-negative sepsis.

As briefly discussed in the section on pathophysiology, sepsis is probably mediated by one or more intermediating substances, forming a common pathway. As also discussed previously, the substance that seems to be the single most important endogenous mediator is the cytokine TNF [28, 32, 35]. While an extensive discussion of TNF is beyond our scope here, a minimal understanding of it will assist the clinician. TNF is a polypeptide that has several forms. The alpha form is also called cachectin [32]. TNF is produced by macrophages

[33, 170]. Infusion of LPS to humans results in the liberation of TNF [171, 172]. TNF mimics virtually all the changes seen in gram-negative sepsis. Fever, tachycardia, capillary leak syndrome, shock, respiratory arrest, hemorrhagic necrosis, acute tubular necrosis, lactic acidosis, stress hormone release, hyperglycemia, hypoglycemia, and cytotoxicity are produced by TNF [32]. TNF also stimulates or modulates other cytokines and intermediating substances, including interleukins, eicosanoids (prostaglandins, leukotrienes, platelet-activating factor), and bradykinin [173]. TNF is elevated in patients with bacterial as well as parasitic sepsis [174–176].

In light of the promising findings of the monoclonal IgM antiendotoxin antibody studies, it is not surprising that antibodies to TNF are currently receiving a great deal of investigation. The theoretical advantage of this approach is enormous: if the "common pathway" cytokine TNF is removed by immunological attack, it should be possible to abort or prevent any further injury.

Unfortunately the pharmacokinetics of TNF cast some doubt on this simplistic therapeutic approach. TNF is only transiently produced in response to challenge with LPS, and peak levels appear about 1.5 hours later, with a rapid decline thereafter [177, 178]. Septic syndrome thus appears to be initiated by a relatively early outpouring of this endogenous cytokine, and subsequently the full-blown syndrome is propagated by a cascade of other mediators. Therefore, an attack on TNF, unless initiated early in the disease process, may be too late.

Several animal studies using antibodies directed against TNF have found major beneficial effects; human studies are underway. In one study pretreatment with anti-TNF antibodies resulted in the prevention of myocardial depression, shock, multiple-organ injury, and death [179]. A recent study in primates showed that early treatment with anti-TNF antibodies prevented death in all treated animals after *E. coli* infusion [180].

Clearly further work on anti-TNF antibodies holds promise. Further elucidation of the mediators and cascading steps may result in the development of a multipronged attack at different steps of the syndrome. Immunotherapy seems to be the most promising step taken in many years. Conventional therapy with fluids, vasopressors, and antibiotics currently results in abysmal outcomes. Immunotherapy or other advances are clearly needed to improve survival rates.

Emergency medicine specialists have traditionally held a strong clinical approach to medical problems. Nevertheless, advances in basic sciences now prod the clinician to acquire and maintain a greater understanding of one of these areas (i.e. immunology). In the future our armamentarium may include potent and effective immunological weapons against attacking microbes. These types of weapons may also be directed against the endogenous systems, which run amok in our patients following microbial invasion [181].

Miscellaneous

Other new and experimental therapeutic modalities for sepsis include pentoxyfylline, antihistamines, antibradykinins, and antithromboxanes [161]. An extensive discussion of these and other treatments is beyond our present scope. Nevertheless, the reader should not be surprised to learn of these and other treatments in the near future. Focus will most likely be on therapy that attacks or modulates the mediators of sepsis.

As the U.S. populace ages and sepsis becomes ever more frequent, the emergency medicine physician must stay abreast of this important topic. Even one of the seemingly easiest parts of management, antibiotic therapy, requires updating on a regular basis. Whether it is new and exciting advances in immunotherapy or some other area in this broad disease process, it is clear that clinicians must periodically review sepsis in their future continuing education.

References

1. Bone RC et al. A controlled clinical trial of high-dose methylprednisolone in the treatment of severe sepsis and septic shock. *N Engl J Med* 317:853–58, 1987.
2. Stedman TL. *Stedman's Medical Dictionary* (25th ed.). Baltimore: Williams & Wilkins, 1990.

3. Bone RC. Sepsis, the sepsis syndrome, multi-organ failure: a plea for comparable definitions. *Ann Intern Med* 114:332–33, 1991.

4. Balk RA, Bone RC. The septic syndrome. Definitions and clinical implication. *Crit Care Clin* 5:1–8, 1989.

5. Kreger BF et al. Gram-negative bacteremia III. Reassessment of etiology, epidemiology and ecology in 612 patients. *Am J Med* 68:332–43, 1980.

6. Schimpff SC. Infections in the compromised host. In GL Mandell, RG Douglas Jr, JE Bennett (eds.). *Principles and Practice of Infectious Disease* (3rd ed.). New York: Churchill-Livingstone, 1990. Pp. 2257–62.

7. Pizzo PA, Myers J. Infections in the cancer patient. In VT DeVita Jr, S Hellman, SA Rosenberg (eds.). *Cancer: Principles and Practice of Oncology* (3rd ed.). Philadelphia: Lippincott, 1989. Pp. 2088–2133.

8. Crane LR et al. Bacteremia in narcotic addicts at the Detroit Medical Center. *Rev Infect Dis* 8:364–73, 1986.

9. Gopal V, Bisno AL. Fulminant pneumococcal infections in "normal" asplenic hosts. *Arch Intern Med* 137:1526–30, 1977.

10. Septic shock in a young splenectomized man [clinical conference]. *Am J Med* 74:129–43, 1983.

11. Bryan CS, Dew CE, Reynolds KL. Bacteremia associated with decubitus ulcers. *Arch Intern Med* 143:2093–95, 1983.

12. McCabe WR, Jackson GG. Gram-negative bacteremia. I. Etiology and ecology. *Arch Intern Med* 110:847–55, 1962.

13. McCabe WR, Jackson GG. Gram-negative bacteremia. II. Clinical, laboratory, and therapeutic observations. *Arch Intern Med* 110:856–64, 1962.

14. McCabe WR. Gram-negative bacteremia. *Dis Mon* 19:1–38, 1973.

15. McCabe WR, Olans RW. Shock in gram-negative bacteremia: predisposing factors, pathophysiology, and treatment. In JS Remington, MN Swartz (eds.). *Current Clinical Topics in Infectious Diseases* (vol. 2). New York: McGraw-Hill, 1981. Pp. 121–50.

16. Stuck AE, Minder CE, Frey FJ. Risk of infectious complications in patients taking glucocorticosteroids. *Rev Infect Dis* 11:954–63, 1989.

17. Schaeffer AJ. Catheter-associated bacteriuria. *Urol Clin North Am* 13:735–47, 1986.

18. Johnson JR, Stamm WE. Urinary tract infections in women: diagnosis and treatment. *Ann Intern Med* 111:906–17, 1989.

19. Bahnson RR. Urosepsis. *Urol Clin North Am* 13:627–35, 1986.

20. Parker MM, Parillo JE. Concepts in emergency medicine and critical care, hemodynamics and pathogenesis. *JAMA* 250:3324–27, 1983.

21. Parillo JE. Septic shock in humans: clinical evaluation, pathogenesis, and therapeutic approach. In WC Shoemaker et al. (eds.). *Textbook of Critical Care* (2nd ed.). Philadelphia: Saunders, 1989. Pp. 1006–24.

22. Parillo JE et al. Septic shock in humans: advances in the understanding of pathogenesis, cardiovascular dysfunction, and therapy. *Ann Intern Med* 113:227–42, 1990.

23. Young LS. Gram-negative sepsis. In GL Mandell, RG Douglas Jr, JE Bennett (eds.). *Principles and Practice of Infectious Disease* (3rd ed.). New York: Churchill-Livingstone, 1990. Pp. 611–39.

24. Mizock B. Septic shock. A metabolic perespective. *Arch Intern Med* 144:579–85, 1984.

25. Natanson C et al. Role of endotoxemia in cardiovascular dysfunction and mortality. *Escherichia coli* and *Staphylococcus aureus* challenges in a canine model of human shock (published erratum appears in *J Clin Invest* 83:1087, 1989). *J Clin Invest* 83:243–51, 1989.

26. Parsonnet J. Mediators in the pathogenesis of toxic shock syndrome: overview. *Rev Inf Dis* 11 (suppl):S263–69, 1989.

27. Reingold AL. Toxic shock syndrome. In AS Evans, PS Brachman (eds.). *Bacterial Infections of Humans.* New York: Plenum, 1991. Pp. 727–43.

28. Tracey KJ, Lowry SF. The role of cytokine mediators in septic shock. *Adv Surg* 23:21–56, 1990.

29. Reilly JM et al. Circulating myocardial depressant substance is associated with cardiac dysfunction and peripheral hypoperfusion (lactic acidemia) in patients with septic shock. *Chest* 95:1072–80, 1989.

30. Handley DA. Platelet-activating factor as a mediator of endotoxin-related diseases. In DA Handley et al. (eds.). *Platelet-Activating Factor in Endotoxin and Immune Diseases.* New York: Dekker, 1990. Pp. 451–95.

31. Beutler B, Cerami A. Cachectin: more than a tumor necrosis factor. *N Engl J Med* 316:379–85, 1987.

32. Beutler B, Cerami A. The history, properties, and biological effects of cachectin. *Biochemistry* 27:7575–82, 1988.

33. Beutler B. Cachectin in tissue injury, shock, and related states. *Crit Care Clin* 5:353–67, 1989.

34. Beutler B. The tumor necrosis factors: cachectin and lymphotoxin. *Hosp Pract* 25:45–56, 1990.

35. Simpson SQ, Casey LC. Role of tumor necrosis factor in sepsis and acute lung injury. *Crit Care Clin* 5:27–47, 1989.

36. MacLean LD et al. Patterns of septic shock in man—a detailed study of 56 patients. *Ann Surg* 166:543–62, 1967.

37. Cunnion RE, Parrillo JE. Myocardial dysfunction in sepsis. *Crit Care Clin* 5:99–118, 1989.

38. Suffredini AF et al. The cardiovascular response of normal humans to the administration of endotoxin. *N Engl J Med* 321:280–87, 1989.

39. Loeb HS et al. Haemodynamic studies in shock associated with infection. *Br Heart J* 29:883–94, 1967.

40. Gunnar RM et al. Hemodynamic measurements in bacteremia and septic shock in man. *J Infect Dis* 128 (suppl):S295–98, 1973.

41. Coalson JJ. Pathology of sepsis, septic shock, and multiple organ failure. In WJ Sibbald, CL Sprung (eds.). *Perspectives on Sepsis and Septic Shock.* Fullerton, CA: Society of Critical Care Medicine, 1986. Pp. 27–60.

42. Parker MM et al. Profound but reversible myocardial depression in patients with septic shock. *Ann Intern Med* 100:483–90, 1984.

43. Parker MM, Parillo JE. Myocardial function in septic shock. *J Crit Care* 5:47–61, 1990.

44. Abel FL. Does the heart fail in endotoxin shock? *Circ Shock* 30:5–13, 1990.

45. Harkema JM et al. Cellular dysfunction in sepsis. *J Crit Care* 5:62–69, 1990.

46. Dantzker D. Oxygen delivery and utilization in sepsis. *Crit Care Clin* 5:81–98, 1989.

47. Pinsky MR, Matuschak GM. Multiple systems organ failure: failure of host defense homeostasis. *Crit Care Clin* 5:199–220, 1989.

48. Smith IM. Infections in the elderly. In B Isaacs (ed.), *Recent Advances in Geriatric Medicine.* Edinburgh: Churchill-Livingstone, 1982. Pp. 214–39.

49. Fox RA. Atypical presentation of geriatric infections. *Geriatrics* 43:58–68, 1988.

50. Harris RL et al. Manifestations of sepsis. *Arch Intern Med* 147:1895–1906, 1976.

51. Miller DJ et al. Jaundice in severe bacterial infection. *Gastroenterology* 71:94–97, 1976.

52. Sherlock S. The liver in infections. In S Sherlock (ed.), *Diseases of the Liver and Biliary System* (8th ed.). Boston: Blackwell, 1989. Pp. 582–83.

53. Kreger BF, Craven DE, McCabe WR. Gram-negative bacteremia. IV. Reevaluation of clinical features and treatment in 612 patients. *Am J Med* 68:344–55, 1980.

54. Simmons DH, Nicoloff J, Guze LB. Hyperventilation and respiratory alkalosis as signs of gram-negative bacteremia. *JAMA* 174:2196–99, 1960.

55. Esposito AL et al. Community-acquired bacteremia in the elderly: analysis of one hundred con-secutive episodes. *J Am Geriatr Soc* 28:315–19, 1980.

56. Rasmussen HH, Ibels LS. Acute renal failure. *Am J Med* 73:211–18, 1982.

57. Balslov JT, Jorgensen JE. A survey of 499 patients with acute anuric renal insufficiency. Causes, treatment, complications and mortality. *Am J Med* 34:753–64, 1963.

58. Kingston ME, Mackey D. Skin clues in the diagnosis of life-threatening infections. *Rev Infect Dis* 8:1–11, 1986.

59. Musher DM. Cutaneous and soft-tissue manifestations of sepsis due to gram-negative enteric bacilli. *Rev Infect Dis* 2:854–66, 1980.

60. Winslow EJ et al. Hemodynamic studies and results of therapy in 50 patients with bacteremic shock. *Am J Med* 54:421–32, 1973.

61. Fowler AA et al. Adult respiratory distress syndrome: risk with common predispositions. *Ann Intern Med* 98:593–97, 1983.

62. Bersten A, Sibbald WJ. Acute lung injury in septic shock. *Crit Care Clin* 5:49–79, 1989.

63. Niederman MS, Fein AM. Sepsis syndrome, the adult respiratory distress syndrome, and nosocomial pneumonia. *Clin Chest Med* 11:633–56, 1990.

64. Kaplan RL, Sahn SA, Petty TL. Incidence and outcome of the respiratory distress syndrome in gram-negative sepsis. *Arch Intern Med* 139:867–69, 1979.

65. Hyers TH. Adult respiratory distress syndrome: definition, risk factors, and outcome. In WN Zopol, F Lemaire (eds.). *Adult Respiratory Distress Syndrome.* New York: Dekker, 1991. Pp. 24–26.

66. Matthay MA. The adult respiratory distress syndrome definition and prognosis. *Clin Chest Med* 11:575–78, 1971.

67. Bryant RE et al. Factors affecting gram-negative rod bacteremia. *Arch Intern Med* 127:120–28, 1971.

68. Parrillo JE et al. Septic shock in humans: advances in the understanding of pathogenesis, cardiovascular dysfunction, and therapy. *Ann Intern Med* 113:227–42, 1990.

69. Shine KE et al. Aspects of the management of shock. *Ann Intern Med* 93:723–34, 1980.

70. Demling RH. Colloid or crystalloid resuscitation in sepsis. In WJ Sibbald, CL Sprung (eds.). *Perspectives of Sepsis and Septic Shock.* Fullerton, CA: Society of Critical Care Medicine, 1986. Pp. 275–300.

71. Falk JL, Rackow EC, Weil MH. Colloid and crystalloid fluid resuscitation. In WB Shoemaker et al. (eds.). *Textbook of Critical Care.* Philadelphia: Saunders, 1989. Pp. 1055–73.

72. Sprung CL (ed.). *The Pulmonary Artery Catheter:*

Methodology and Clinical Applications. Baltimore: University Park Press, 1983.

73. Matthay MA, Chatterjee K. Bedside catheterization of the pulmonary artery: risks compared with benefits. *Ann Intern Med* 109:826–34, 1988.

74. Shoemaker WC. Physiologic monitoring of the critically ill patient. In WC Shoemaker et al. (eds.). *Textbook of Critical Care.* Philadelphia: Saunders, 1989. P. 150.

75. Iverson RL. Septic shock: a clinical perspective. *Crit Care Clin* 4:215–28, 1988.

76. Higgins TL, Chernow B. Pharmacotherapy of circulatory shock. *Dis Mon* 33:309–61, 1987.

77. Boyd JL III, Stanford GC, Chernow B. The pharmacotherapy of septic shock. *Crit Care Clin* 15:133–50, 1989.

78. Desjars P et al. A reappraisal of norepinephrine therapy in human septic shock. *Crit Care Med* 15:134–37, 1987.

79. Melchior JC et al. Hemodynamic effects of continuous norepinephrine infusion in dogs with and without hyperkinetic endotoxic shock. *Crit Care Med* 15:687–91, 1987.

80. Meadows D et al. Reversal of intractable septic shock with norepinephrine therapy. *Crit Care Med* 16:663–64, 1988.

81. Martin WJ. Rapid and reliable techniques for the laboratory detection of bacterial meningitis. *Am J Med* 75:119–23, 1983.

82. Wilson CB, Smith AL. Rapid tests for the diagnosis of bacterial meningitis. In JS Remington, MN Swartz (eds.). *Current Clinical Topics in Infectious Diseases* (vol. 7). New York: McGraw-Hill, 1986. Pp. 134–56.

83. Kaplan S. Antigen detection in cerebrospinal fluid—pros and cons. *Am J Med* 75:109–18, 1983.

84. Greenlee JE. Approach to diagnosis of meningitis. Cerebrospinal fluid evaluation. *Infect Dis Clin North Am* 4:583–98, 1990.

85. Strand CL, Shulman JA. *Bloodstream Infections.* Chicago: American Society of Clinical Pathologists Press, 1988.

86. Young LS et al. Gram-negative rod bacteremia: microbiologic, immunologic, and therapeutic considerations. *Am Intern Med* 86:456–71, 1977.

87. Young LS. Fever and septicemia. In RH Rubin, LS Young (eds.), *Clinical Approach to Infection in the Compromised Host* (2nd ed.). New York: Plenum, 1988. Pp. 75–114.

88. Shine KI et al. Aspects of the management of shock. *Ann Intern Med* 93:723–34, 1980.

89. Wiles JB et al. The systemic septic response: does the organism matter? *Crit Care Med* 8:55–60, 1980.

90. Bush LM, Levison ME. Antibiotic selection and pharmacokinetics in the critically ill. *Crit Care Med* 4:299–324, 1988.

91. Wilkowskey CJ, Hermans PE. General principles of antimicrobial therapy. *Mayo Clin Proc* 62:789–98, 1987.

92. Tapper MC, Armstrong C. Bacteremia due to *Pseudomonas aeruginosa* complicating neoplastic disease: a progress report. *Infect Dis* 130(suppl): S14–23, 1974.

93. Schimpff SC et al. Significance of *Pseudomonas aeruginosa* in the patient with leukemia or lymphoma. *J Infect Dis* 130(suppl):S24–31, 1974.

94. Young LS. Empiric antimicrobial therapy in the neutropenic host [editorial]. *N Engl J Med* 315: 580–81, 1986.

95. Maki DG. Nosocomial bacteremia. An epidemiologic overview. *Am J Med* 70:719–32, 1981.

96. Hughes WT et al. Guidelines for the use of antimicrobial agents in neutropenic patients with unexplained fever (published erratum appears in *J Infect Dis* 161:1316, 1990). *J Infect Dis* 161: 381–96, 1990.

97. Young LS. Combination or single drug therapy for gram-negative sepsis. In JS Remington, MN Swartz (eds.). *Current Clinical Topics in Infectious Diseases* (vol. 3). New York: McGraw-Hill, 1982. Pp. 177–205.

98. Terrell CL, Hermans PE. Antifungal agents used for deep-seated mycotic infections. *Mayo Clin Proc* 62:1116–28, 1987.

99. Ruskin J. Parasitic diseases in the compromised host. In RH Rubin, LS Young (eds.). *Clinical Approach to Infection in the Compromised Host* (2nd ed.). New York: Plenum, 1988. Pp. 253–304.

100. Meunier F. Fungal infections in the compromised host. In RH Rubin, LS Young (eds.). *Clinical Approach to Infection in the Compromised Host* (2nd ed.). New York: Plenum, 1988. Pp. 193–220.

101. Donowitz GR, Mandell GL. Beta lactam antibiotics. *N Engl J Med* 318:490–500, 1988.

102. Donowitz GR. Third generation cephalosporins. *Infect Dis Clin North Am* 3:595–612, 1989.

103. Moore RD, Smith CR, Lietman PS. The association of aminoglycoside plasma levels with mortality in patients with gram-negative bacteremia. *J Infect Dis* 149:443–48, 1984.

104. Moore RD, Smith CR, Lietman PS. Association of aminoglycoside plasma levels with therapeutic outcome in gram-negative pneumonia. *Am J Med* 77:657–62, 1984.

105. Van Scoy RE, Wilson WR. Antimicrobial agents in adult patients with renal insufficiency: initial dos-

age and general recommendations. *Mayo Clin Proc* 62:1142–45, 1987.

106. Gilbert DN, Bennett WM. Use of antimicrobial agents in renal failure. *Infect Dis Clin North Am* 3:517–31, 1989.

107. Saxon A et al. Immediate hypersensitivity reactions to beta-lactam antibiotics. *Ann Intern Med* 197:204–15, 1987.

108. Weiss ME, Adkinson NF. B-lactam allergy. In GL Mandell, RG Douglas Jr. (eds.). *Principles and Practice of Infectious Disease* (3rd ed.). New York: Churchill-Livingstone, 1990. Pp. 264–69.

109. Donowitz GR, Mandell GL. Cephalosporins. In GL Mandell, RG Douglas Jr (eds.). *Principles and Practice of Infectious Disease* (3rd ed.). New York: Churchill-Livingstone, 1990. Pp. 249.

110. Hermans PE, Wilhelm MP. Vancomycin. *Mayo Clin Proc* 62:901–05, 1987.

111. Wilson WR, Cockerill FR III. Tetracyclines, chloramphenicol, erythromycin, and clindamycin. *Mayo Clin Proc* 62:906–15, 1987.

112. Saxon A. Antibiotic choices for the penicillin-allergic patient. *Postgrad Med* 83:135–148, 1988.

113. Finegold SM, George WL (eds.). *Anaerobic Infections in Humans.* New York: Academic Press, 1989.

114. Styrt, Gorbach SL. Recent development in the understanding of the pathogensis and treatment of anaerobic infections. *N Engl J Med* 321:298–302, 1989.

115. Rosenblatt JE. Antimicrobic susceptibility of anaerobic bacteria. In SM Finegold, WL George (eds.). *Anaerobic Infections in Humans.* New York: Academic Press, 1989. Pp. 731–54.

116. Finegold SM. Therapy of anaerobic infections. In SM Finegold, WL George (eds.), *Anaerobic Infections in Humans.* New York: Academic Press, 1989. Pp. 793–818.

117. Corona ML et al. Infections related to central venous catheters. *Mayo Clin Proc* 65:979–86, 1990.

118. Wright AJ, Wilkowske CJ. The penicillins. *Mayo Clin Proc* 62:806–20, 1987.

119. Sobel JD. Imipenem and aztreonam. *Infect Dis Clin North Am* 3:613–24, 1989.

120. Bush LM, Calmon J, Johnson LL. Newer penicillins and beta-lactamase inhibitors. *Infect Dis Clin North Am* 3:571–94, 1989.

121. Lee RM, Balk RA, Bone RC. Ventilatory support in the management of septic patients. *Crit Care Clin* 5:157–75, 1989.

122. Bernard GR et al. High dose corticosteroids in patients with the adult respiratory distress syndrome. *N Engl J Med* 317:1565–70, 1987.

123. Luce JM et al. Ineffectiveness of high-dose methylprednisolone in preventing parenchymal lung injury and improving mortality in patients with septic shock. *Am Rev Resp Dis* 138:62–68, 1988.

124. Brigham KL. Corticosteroids in adult respiratory distress syndrome. In WM Zapol, F Lemaire (eds.). *Adult Respiratory Distress Syndrome.* New York: Dekker, 1991. Pp. 285–304.

125. Sheagren JN. Septic shock and corticosteroids [editorial]. *N Engl J Med* 305:456–58, 1981.

126. Kass EH. High-dose corticosteroids for septic shock [editorial]. *N Engl J Med* 311:1178–79, 1984.

127. Nicholson DP. Review of corticosteroid treatment in sepsis and septic shock: pro or con. *Crit Care Clin* 5:151–55, 1989.

128. Schumer W. Steroids in the treatment of clinical septic shock. *Ann Surg* 184:333–41, 1976.

129. Hinshaw LB, Beller-Todd BK, Archer LT. Current management of the septic shock patient: experimental basis for treatment. *Circ Shock* 9:543–53, 1982.

130. Ottosson J et al. Experimental septic shock—effects of corticosteroids. *Circ Shock* 9:571–77, 1982.

131. Sprung CL et al. The effects of high dosage corticosteroids in patients with septic shock. A prospective controlled study. *N Engl J Med* 311:1137–43, 1984.

132. Hinshaw L et al. Effect of high-dose glucocorticoid therapy on mortality in patients with clinical signs of systemic sepsis. *N Engl J Med* 317:659–65, 1987.

133. Guillemin R et al. Beta-endorphin and adrenocorticotropin are secreted concomitantly by the pituitary gland. *Science* 197:1367–69, 1977.

134. Holaday JW, Faden AI. Naloxone reversal of endotoxin hypotension suggests role of endorphins in shock. *Nature* 275:450–51, 1978.

135. Holaday JW. Opioid antagonists in septic shock. In RK Root, MA Sande (eds.). *Septic Shock Contemporary Issues in Infectious Disease* (vol. 4). New York: Churchill-Livingstone, 1985. Pp. 117–34.

136. Murray MJ, Offord KP, Yaksh TL. Physiologic and plasma hormone correlates of survival in endotoxic dogs: effect of opiate antagonists. *Crit Care Med* 17:39–47, 1989.

137. Reynolds DG et al. Blockade of opiate receptors with naloxone improves survival and cardiac performance in canine endotoxin shock. *Circ Shock* 7:39–48, 1980.

138. Faden AI, Holaday JW. Experimental endotoxin shock: the pathophysiologic function of endorphins and treatment with opiate antagonists. *J Infect Dis* 142:229–38, 1980.

139. Faden AK, Holaday JW. Naloxone treatment of

endotoxin shock. *J Pharmacol Exp Ther* 212: 441–47, 1980.

140. Hinshaw LB et al. Evaluation of naloxone therapy for *Escherichia coli* sepsis in the baboon. *Arch Surg* 123:700–704, 1988.

141. Tiengo M. Naloxone in irreversible shock [letter]. *Lancet* 2:680, 1980.

142. Peters WP, Johnson MW, Friedman PA. Vasopressor effect of naloxone in septic shock. *Lancet* 1: 529–32, 1981.

143. Hackshaw KV, Parker GA, Roberts JW. Naloxone in septic shock. *Crit Care Med* 18:47–51, 1990.

144. DeMaria A et al. Naloxone versus placebo in treatment of septic shock. *Lancet* 1:1363–65, 1985.

145. Safani M et al. Prospective, controlled, randomized trial of naloxone infusion in early hyperdynamic septic shock. *Crit Care Med* 17:1004–09, 1989.

146. Roberts DE et al. Effects of prolonged naloxone infusion in septic shock. *Lancet* 2:699–702, 1988.

147. Groeger JS, Carlon GC, Howland VS. Naloxone in septic shock. *Crit Care Med* 11:650–54, 1983.

148. Cook JA, Wise WC, Halushka PV. Elevated thromboxane levels in the rat during endotoxic shock. *J Clin Invest* 65:227–30, 1980.

149. Petrak RA, Balk RA, Bone RC. Prostaglandins, cyclo-oxygenase inhibitors, and thromboxane synthetase inhibitors in the pathogenesis of multiple systems organ failure. *Crit Care Clin* 5:303–14, 1989.

150. Simon LS, Mills JA. Drug therapy: non-steroidal anti-inflammatory drugs. *N Engl J Med* 302: 1179–85, 1980.

151. Moncada S, Vane JR. Pharmacology and endogenous roles of prostaglandin endoperoxides, thromboxane A_2 and prostacyclin. *Pharmacol Rev* 30:293–331, 1978.

152. Curtis-Prior PB (ed.). *Prostaglandins: Biology and Chemistry of Prostaglandins and Related Eicosanoids.* New York: Churchill-Livingstone, 1988.

153. Halushka PV, Wise WC, Cook JA. Studies on the beneficial effects of aspirin in endotoxic shock. Relationship to inhibition of arachidonic metabolism. *Am J Med* 74:91–96, 1983.

154. Fletcher JR, Rumwell PW. Modification, by aspirin and indomethacin, of the haemodynamic and prostaglandin releasing effects of *E. coli* endotoxin in the dog. *Br J Pharmacol* 61:175–81, 1977.

155. Rockwell WB, Ehrlich HP. Ibuprofen in acute-care therapy. *Ann Surg* 211:78–83, 1990.

156. Jacobs ER et al. Ibuprofen in canine endotoxin shock. *J Clin Invest* 70:536–41, 1982.

157. Tani T, Hanasawa K, Kodama M. Usefulness of endotoxin removal from the septic blood with di-

rect hemoperfusion using PMX-F. *Nippon Geka Gakkai Sasshi* 90:1370–73, 1989.

158. Hanasawa K, Tani T, Kodama M. New approach to endotoxic and septic shock by means of polymyxin B immobilized fiber. *Surg Gynecol Obstet* 168: 323–31, 1989.

159. Kodama M, Hanasawa K, Tani T. New therapeutic method against septic shock—removal of endotoxin using extracorporeal circulation. *Adv Exp Med Biol* 256:653–64, 1990.

160. Staubach KH et al. Can hemofiltration increase survival time in acute endotoxemic porcine shock model? *Prog Clin Biol Res* 308:821–26, 1989.

161. Waxman K. Pentoxifylline in septic shock [editorial]. *Crit Care Med* 18:243–44, 1990.

162. Young LS. Gram-negative rod bacteremia: microbiologic, immunologic, and therapeutic considerations. *Ann Intern Med* 86:456–71, 1971.

163. Ziegler EJ et al. Treatment of gram-negative bacteremia and shock with human antiserum to a mutant *Escherichia coli*. *N Engl J Med* 307:1225–30, 1982.

164. Baumgartner JD et al. Prevention of gram-negative shock and death in surgical patients by antibody to endotoxin core glycolipid. *Lancet* 2:59–62, 1985.

165. Calandra T et al. Treatment of gram-negative septic shock with human IgG antibody to *Escherichia coli* J5: a prospective, double-blind, randomized trial. *J Infect Dis* 158:312–19, 1988.

166. Baumgartner JD et al. Association between protective efficacy of anti-lipopolysaccharide (LPS) antibodies and suppression of LPS-induced tumor necrosis factor alpha and interleukin-6; comparison of O side chain-specific antibodies with core LPS antibodies. *J Exp Med* 171:889–96, 1990.

167. Fisher CJ et al. Initial evaluation of human monoclonal anti-lipid A antibody (HA-1A) in patients with sepsis syndrome. *Crit Care Med* 18:1311–15, 1990.

168. Greenman RL et al. A controlled clinical trial of E5 murine monoclonal antibody to endotoxin in the treatment of gram-negative sepsis. *JAMA* 226:1097, 1991.

169. Ziegler EJ et al. Treatment of gram-negative bacteremia and septic shock with HA-1A human monoclonal antibody against endotoxin. *N Engl J Med* 324:429–36, 1991.

170. Kunkel SL et al. Mechanisms that regulate the production of effects of tumor necrosis factor-alpha. *Crit Rev Immunol* 9:93–117, 1989.

171. Michie HR et al. Detection of circulating tumor necrosis factor after endotoxin administration. *N Engl J Med* 318:1481–86, 1988.

172. Cannon JG et al. Circulating interleukin-1 and

tumor necrosis factor in septic shock and experimental endotoxin fever. *J Infect Dis* 161:79–84, 1990.

173. Jacobs RF, Tabor DR. Immune cellular interactions during sepsis and septic injury. *Crit Care Clin* 5:9–26, 1989.

174. Damas P et al. Tumor necrosis factor and interleukin-1 serum levels during severe sepsis in humans. *Crit Care Med* 17:975–78, 1989.

175. Calandra T et al. Prognostic values of tumor necrosis factor/cachectin, interleukin-1, interferon-alpha, and interferon-gamma in the serum of patients with septic shock. *J Infect Dis* 161:982–87, 1990.

176. Scuderi P et al. Raised serum level of tumor necrosis factor in parasitic infections. *Lancet* 2:1364–65, 1986.

177. Fromm RE et al. Circulating tumor necrosis factor in normal volunteers receiving endotoxin. *Crit Care Med* 16:397, 1988.

178. Hesse DG et al. Cytokine appearance in human endotoxemia and primate bacteremia. *Surg Gynecol Obstet* 166:147–53, 1988.

179. Tracey KJ et al. Anti-cachectin/TNF monoclonal antibodies prevent septic shock during lethal bacteremia. *Nature* 330:662–64, 1987.

180. Hinshaw LB et al. Survival of primates in LD 100 septic shock following therapy with antibody to tumor necrosis factor (TNF). *Circ Shock* 30:279–92, 1990.

181. Wolf SM. Monoclonal antibodies and the treatment of gram-negative bacteremia and shock [editorial]. *N Engl J Med* 324:486–88, 1991.

7

Infection and Acute Primary Neurologic Disease

RUSSELL D. SNYDER

This chapter discusses neurologic infections that can result in an altered level of consciousness (LOC) or focal disease. Almost all neurologic diseases that involve the brain may present with a spectrum of symptoms from headache to altered LOC to focal neurologic disease, depending on the progression of the disease and the time in the disease course in which the patient presents. Diseases where neurologic symptoms generally predominate are covered in this chapter; diseases usually associated with systemic involvement are discussed in Chap. 8. When alteration of consciousness is present, patient cooperation may be compromised. The recognition of both change in LOC and focal neurologic disease becomes more difficult. A neurologic infection may be focal at onset, but as the disease process extends or swelling occurs around the lesion, the focal aspects become obscured and the signs and symptoms generalized. Likewise, a disease may present with nonfocal symptoms, but with progression focal symptoms may appear. The initial focus may be in a relatively silent area of the brain and not declare itself until the lesion is large enough to produce more generalized signs and symptoms. Some focal infections of the nervous system are multifocal and may appear to the examiner as generalized processes. The absence of focal neurologic findings does not exclude the presence of focal neurologic disease.

Infections of the nervous system, whether focal or generalized, are frequently associated with fever. Fever in the presence of neurologic signs and symptoms must be investigated thoroughly for a neurologic infection. Infection is a far more common cause of fever than is a brain lesion that has disturbed temperature regulation. Also the absence of fever does not rule out a neurologic infection, especially in the debilitated, the very young, and the very old.

Systemic infectious illness can produce secondary neurologic signs and symptoms such as headache, alteration of consciousness, weakness, and fatigue without direct invasion of the nervous system by the organism. Such signs and symptoms are seldom focal. (These illnesses are discussed in Chap. 8.)

A group of neurologic diseases are associated with systemic infection but are not necessarily caused by the invasion of the nervous system by an infecting agent. These diseases are the so-called postinfectious conditions. The precise pathogenic mechanism underlying these diseases is unclear, but presumably it is immune mediated. These illnesses are discussed later in this chapter.

Signs and Symptoms of Neurologic Disease

Historical Features

Most infections of the nervous system have a gradual onset of symptomatology. A sudden onset, over minutes rather than hours or days, is more in keeping with a vascular accident, a seizure, or trauma.

Complete historical information, when available, is often far more helpful in diagnosis than examination. Fever, headache, alteration of consciousness, and weakness, although nonspecific symptoms in themselves, are the hallmarks of intracranial infection. Spinal cord infection is often accompanied by pain localized to the region of spinal cord involvement, weakness, and sensory disturbance below the level of the lesion, and sphincter involvement. Involvement of the peripheral nervous system is suggested by weakness and sensory disturbance in a patient who is alert.

Historical questions for consideration in each case are listed in Table 7-1. Immunocompromised individuals are at significant risk for the development of infections of the nervous system (Table 7-2).

Table 7-1. Historical questions of importance

Fever?
Headache/pain?
Preexisting symptoms of infection?
Ingestion/drugs?
Level of consciousness/responsiveness/cognitive ability?
Visual disturbance/diplopia?
Trouble hearing?
Swallowing difficulty?
Weakness/localization?
Gait difficulty?
Numbness/tingling/paresthesia?
Unsteadiness/tremor?
Sphincter disturbance?
Medication?
History of previous infection/surgery/trauma?
Immunodeficiency?
Past history/family history of similar disturbances?
Travel history?
Unusual foods?

Table 7-2. Focal neurologic infections in immunocompromised individuals

AIDS
Toxoplasmosis
Cryptococcosis
Progressive multifocal leukoencephalopathy
Tuberculosis

Altered States of Consciousness

Altered states of consciousness are seen to varying degrees in most infections that involve the brain. Signs include confusion, depression of consciousness, disorientation, delirium, hyperactivity, amnesia, and unusual or inappropriate behavior. Depressed consciousness and hyperactivity are generally considered indications of a diffuse brain process. Unusual behavior can result from a focal lesion in an area of the brain such as the temporal lobe. Often the precise pathogenesis for the change in LOC is not known. However, the alteration of consciousness is an important clue that a disease process involves the CNS. Specific infections by neurologic symptom are listed in Table 7-3.

Seizures

A first seizure is an event that may cause an individual with an intracranial infection to be brought to the emergency department. Seizures can be a symptom of any brain insult, infectious or otherwise, and are in themselves frequently nonspecific and of little use in determining etiology. However, the presence of a seizure is very important in directing attention to the CNS. The clinical nature of the seizure can be of localizing value in neurologic disease (Table 7-3).

Seizures are frightening occurrences for those afflicted and for caretakers. They should never be ignored, especially in a patient who has not had previous seizures. A seizure, whether focal or generalized, can be an indication of an infection in the CNS. A seizure with a focal onset can spread to become secondarily generalized and, to the observer, appear as a nonfocal seizure.

Although the generalized tonic-clonic seizure is dramatic, seizures can take many forms, including

Table 7-3. Specific infections by neurologic symptom

Ataxia	*Stiff Neck*
Brainstem encephalitis	Cervical adenitis
Guillain-Barré syndrome	Discitis
Labyrinthitis	Encephalitis
Posterior fossa abscess	Meningitis
Postinfectious leukoencephalitis	Pharyngitis
Progressive multifocal leukoencephalopathy	Retropharyngeal abscess
Syndenham's chorea	Rocky Mountain spotted fever
Toxoplasmosis	Vertebral osteomyelitis
	Viral myositis
Coma or Altered LOC	*Seizure*
Encephalitis	Abscess
HIV encephalopathy	Cystercercosis
Meningitis	Encephalitis, herpes
Postinfectious leukoencephalitis	Febrile seizure
Reye's syndrome	Meningitis
Sepsis	Postinfectious leukoencephalitis
Toxoplasmosis	Toxoplasmosis
Vertigo/Dizziness	*Paralysis: Bilateral, Flaccid*
Encephalitis	Botulism
Labyrinthitis	Diphtheria
Mastoiditis	Guillain-Barré syndrome
Posterior fossa abscess	Poliomyelitis
	Tick paralysis
	Transverse myelitis

focal tonic or clonic activity; a state of confusion with automatic acts; a drop attack; multifocal clonic movements; single jerks, which may be focal or generalized; and staring. The relatively common complex partial seizure is considered to have a focal onset, usually in one temporal lobe, with the clinical characteristics of alteration of consciousness without complete loss of consciousness and sometimes semipurposeful motor activity. A careful description of the seizure by a skilled observer can provide clues to focality. Examination of the patient immediately following a seizure may reveal focal deficits that are not easily detected at other times.

Children under the age of 5 years are subject to febrile seizures. Febrile seizures are not epileptic seizures and do not indicate detectable brain pathology. They are brief, lasting less than 10 minutes, and are generalized and not repetitive. A

temperature elevation is present. No focal findings are present on examination, and the interictal EEG is normal. In the emergency department a febrile seizure is a diagnosis by exclusion (see Chap. 14).

A severely damaged nervous system is unable to produce a seizure. The disappearance of seizure activity in a neurologically impaired individual may be a sign that clinical deterioration has taken place rather than a sign of improvement. Likewise, the appearance of seizures in a severely neurologically damaged patient who is recovering may be an indication of improvement in the CNS, which is now able to produce a seizure.

Neurologic Deficits

A carefully performed and documented neurologic examination is essential. The assistance of a neurologist may be desirable in some situations. The nature of the neurologic lesion is often determined by history and the location of the lesion by examination.

Focal neurologic signs and symptoms will usually be found at some time in the evolution of the conditions discussed in this chapter. The focal nature of a lesion can be determined in a cooperative individual by comparing function between the right and left sides. Focal signs and symptoms may have disappeared by the time the disease process has progressed to the point where the individual is seen in the emergency department.

In a cooperative, alert patient, brain, spinal cord, and peripheral nerve lesions usually can be distinguished by history and examination. Other symptoms and signs may suggest specific disease processes. Table 7-4 lists signs and symptoms of neurologic disease by anatomic location.

EXAMINATION FOR BRAIN DISEASE
Certain findings on examination, once external trauma has been excluded, will suggest that the process is related to an intracranial lesion. Head-

ache may indicate a neurologic process and, when focal, may have localizing value. Vomiting frequently accompanies acute brain disease. LOC is ascertained by noting response to stimuli, including verbal and painful. The Glascow coma score, although developed for the evaluation of cerebral trauma, is useful in documenting LOC in other diseases. The patient's posture and spontaneous movements and cranial nerve abnormalities are noted. These factors persist in those with structural cerebral damage but may fluctuate in those with metabolic or systemic infectious disorders. Hyperventilation can occur in those with systemic infections. Cheyne-Stokes respirations occur but are unusual.

Problems with vision indicate disease of the orbits, their connections to the brain, or the brain itself. Visual problems include diplopia, visual field defects, abnormalities in eye movement, abnormal pupil responsiveness, and depression of corneal reflexes. Any deviation from symmetrical and vigorous movement of the face suggests a brain process. Speech difficulties, especially in an alert patient,

Table 7-4. Signs and symptoms of neurologic disease by anatomic location

Finding	Brain	Spinal cord	Peripheral nerve	Malingering and hysteria
Altered consciousness	+	−	−	+/−
Headache	+	−	−	+/−
Seizures	+	−	−	+/−
Vomiting	+	−	−	+/−
Visual disturbance	+	−	−	+/−
Speech problem	+	−	−	−
Stiff neck	+/−	+/−	−	−
Weakness	+	+	+	+
Paraplegia	−	+	−	+/−
Sensory disturbance	+/−	+/−	+/−	+
Increased tone/hyperreflexia	+	+/−	−	−
Decreased tone/hyporeflexia	−	+/−	+	−
Ataxia	+	+/−	+/−	−
Clonus	+	+	−	−
Extensor toe	+	+	−	−
Incontinence	+/−	+	+/−	−
Autonomic disturbance	+/−	+/−	+/−	−

+ indicates present; − indicates absent.

suggest brain disease. These difficulties can include speech that is not clear and a problem with word finding. Failure of the gag reflex and swallowing difficulties have similar significance. Trouble with hearing and especially a problem with understanding that is not commensurate with the patient's abilities and background suggest an intracranial process.

There may be an accompanying weakness in the extremities, but this finding can also be present in disease of the spinal cord or peripheral nerve. If the weakness is a hemiparesis, either a brain lesion or a high spinal lesion must be considered. Tone is increased, although after an acute lesion hypotonia may be present for several days or longer. Difficulty with respiration will be encountered if the lesion is extensive, and there may be urinary or anal sphincter disturbances. Discrete sensory disturbances are unusual. The tendon reflexes are usually exaggerated, with ankle clonus and an extensor toe sign at least on the side opposite the affected side of the brain.

EXAMINATION OF THE NECK
Care must be exercised in examination of the neck until neck trauma and primary disease of the cervical vertebrae have been excluded. Cervical disease can sometimes be excluded by history but is probably best excluded by cervical spine roentgenogram. The presence of a stiff neck in the absence of cervical disease suggests irritation of the meninges, as occurs in meningitis. Stiff neck is by no means specific for bacterial meningitis and occurs in subarachnoid hemorrhage, viral neurologic infections, incipient brain herniation, and sometimes even in systemic infections. Resistance to passive flexion of the neck can be noted in all but the most deeply comatose patients.

When cervical disease has been excluded, the "doll's eye" maneuver can provide useful information in a patient with altered LOC who cannot cooperate for eye examination. When consciousness is depressed and the brain stem remains relatively intact, brisk rotation of the head from side to side produces a conjugate contraversive eye deviation. When this response is present, damage to the nerves innervating the extraocular muscles or to the connections between those nerves and the ves-

tibular system is unlikely. The doll's eye maneuver is a vestibulo-ocular reflex.

EXAMINATION FOR SPINAL CORD DISEASE
Spinal cord disease may be difficult to detect if there is concomitant brain disease. When only the spine is involved, the patient will be alert and will not have findings of brain disease. Hemiparesis may be present if the lesion is unilateral in the high cervical region, but disease of the spinal cord more commonly leads to paraplegia or quadriplegia. Tone below the level of the lesion initially may be decreased but then becomes increased. Incontinence, especially of bladder function, will be present with an extensive cord lesion. Pain is common at the level of the lesion. Disturbance in other sensory modalities may be seen, depending on the extent of the lesion. A level below which a sensory disturbance is present can be important in localization. If the spinal roots are involved, the sensory disturbance may be in the distribution of a dermatome. Weakness on one side and loss of pain and temperature on the other side are the classic findings of a hemisection of the cord. Tendon reflexes will be normal above the lesion and frequently depressed below the lesion if the lesion is extensive and acute; they will be hyperactive if the lesion is subacute or chronic. The toe signs will be extensor on one or both sides, depending on the extent and the severity of the lesion, and there may be accompanying ankle clonus. High spinal lesions can compromise respirations and autonomic functions, such as blood pressure and temperature regulation.

EXAMINATION OF THE PERIPHERAL NERVES
Peripheral nerve disease can be motor, sensory, or mixed. Weakness is the hallmark of disease of the motor nerves. Hemiparesis does not occur in peripheral nerve disease. The weakness more commonly involves both lower extremities and later the upper extremities. A monoparesis can occur. Tone is decreased. When sensory nerves are involved, numbness, tingling, and deficits to touch and pain will be found in the distribution of the involved sensory nerve. The tendon reflexes are depressed or absent, and the toe sign flexor is absent. Clonus will not occur. Incontinence is unusual acutely, but urinary retention may occur. In some peripheral

nerve conditions, the cranial nerves can be affected after they leave the brain. Extensive peripheral nerve disease may affect respiration and autonomic functions, such as blood pressure and temperature.

EXAMINATION OF COORDINATION

Coordination is of less localizing value unless it is the only neurologic sign present when it suggests cerebellar involvement. Disturbances of coordination such as ataxia, gait difficulties, and problems with rapidly alternating movements can be found in lesions of the brain, spinal cord, and peripheral nerve and are manifestations of weakness. Disturbances in coordination are mainly of confirmatory value. Drugs are major producers of coordination difficulties.

MALINGERING AND HYSTERICAL SYMPTOMS

The experienced physician in the emergency department will only occasionally have difficulty differentiating an acute neurologic condition from malingering or from a hysterical or conversion reaction. Common hysterical symptoms are headache, blurred vision, a lump in the throat, loss of voice, paresthesia, hemiparesis, and paraplegia [1]. A major neurologic deficit not explicable by a spinal cord or peripheral nerve lesion in a patient who is alert and cooperative suggests hysteria. Indifference to a major loss of neurologic function (*la belle indifferance*) usually indicates hysteria or a conversion reaction.

Urgent Investigation of Neurologic Disease

The appropriateness of laboratory studies, such as lumbar puncture and brain imaging, are considered in the following sections, and generalizations for performance of these tests are discussed.

Lumbar Puncture

The clinical presentation of the entities discussed in this chapter will lead the emergency department physician to consider lumbar puncture (LP) in some situations. The performance of an LP engenders a certain amount of risk, although that risk is small [2]. In situations where intracranial pressure is increased or a spinal block is present, the pressure changes produced by removal of cerebrospinal fluid (CSF) can lead to neurologic deterioration or even herniation. This complication can occur during the LP or several hours later. Risk is highest when the increase in pressure is caused by a focal intracranial mass lesion.

A small-bore LP needle should be used and the CSF pressure measured. Only the amount of CSF necessary for appropriate studies should be removed. The quantity of CSF necessary for laboratory examination varies with the clinical situation and the requirements of the laboratory.

The small risk of an LP should not mitigate against its performance in appropriate circumstances. The entities in which CSF examination is particularly useful are listed in Table 7-5.

Brain Imaging

Brain imaging is indicated in many of the conditions discussed in this chapter. These conditions are rare and will not lead to a significant increase in the amount of brain imaging ordered by the emergency department.

Brain imaging helps exclude situations in which LP is of risk. If the clinical circumstances suggest that increased intracranial pressure is present or if an intracranial or spinal mass lesion is considered possible, the performance of a CT scan or an MRI may be appropriate prior to or instead of the initial LP. Removal of CSF by the lumbar route when intracranial pressure is increased can produce dangerous shifts in intracranial contents, especially when the pressure increase is from a focal intracranial mass. Cerebellar tonsil herniation, an indication of an unstable intracranial pressure situation, can produce a stiff neck indistinguishable from the nuchal rigidity of intracranial infection [3]. Brain imaging will assist in determination of the nature and the degree of increased intracranial pressure. If imaging reveals a shift in midline structures, a unilateral dilated temporal horn (suggesting incipient cerebral herniation), a suggestion of herniation of the cerebellar tonsils, or the obliteration of CSF pathways, then a relative contraindication to LP exists [4].

Table 7-5. Infectious causes of abnormal CSF

	PMNs[a]	Lymphs	Pressure increased	Protein increased	Glucose decreased
Viral meningitis	+[c]	+[b]	+/−	−	−
Viral encephalitis	+[c]	+[b]	+/−	+	−
Herpes simplex encephalitis[d, e]	+[c]	+[b]	+/−	+	−
Bacterial meningitis	+[b]	+[c]	+	+	+
Brain abscess[d]	+	−	+	+	−
Subdural empyema[d]	+	−	+	+	−
Cryptococcal meningitis[f]	−	+	+	+	+/−
Cystercercosis[g]	−	+	−	+	+/−
Toxoplasmosis	−	+/−	+	+	−
Postinfectious leukoencephalitis	−	+/−	+/−	+/−	−
Reye's syndrome	−	+/−	+	−	−
Spinal epidural abscess[d]	+	−	+	+	−
Poliomyelitis	+[c]	+[b]	−	+	−
Acute transverse myelopathy[d]	−	+/−	+/−	+	−
Guillain-Barré syndrome	−	−	−	+	−
Botulism	−	−	−	−	−
Diphtheria	−	−	−	+	−

+ indicates present; − indicates absent.
[a] Polymorphonuclear neutrophil leukocytes.
[b] Late.
[c] Early.
[d] Diagnosis not made by LP.
[e] RBC's present.
[f] Encapsulated yeast on India ink smear (latex agglutination for antigen).
[g] Eosinophils present.

In the situation where an intracranial infection is present, the delay encountered in the performance of an LP when brain imaging is undertaken will not necessarily have an adverse effect on the management of the infection. Blood cultures and specimens for antigen studies should be obtained immediately and initial antibiotics instituted appropriate for the suspected organism. Then imaging can be performed. CSF will remain positive for culture for several hours after institution of antibiotics, and the Gram's stain and antigen studies will remain positive for 24–48 hours. Prior administration of mannitol or a similar osmotic agent will enhance the safety of an LP in the presence of increased intracranial pressure. In situations where imaging appears appropriate but cannot be expeditiously obtained, immediate empirical administration of antibiotics suitable for the suspected etiologic organism should be undertaken with indefinite delay of an LP.

Brain imaging is becoming widely available to the emergency department and is very useful in the diagnosis of focal lesions of the nervous system. The CT scan has been the most frequently used technique, but MRI is now also available at many institutions. A CT scan is superior to an MRI for detection of fresh blood and calcification. A CT scan can display shifts in intracranial contents almost as well as an MRI. An MRI is superior to a CT scan for detecting lesions of brain white matter, brain edema, and spinal cord compression. If an unrevealing, noncontrasted CT scan is performed and the emergency department physician has a strong suspicion of the presence of an intracranial mass,

Table 7-6. Optimal diagnostic radiologic modalities

Disease	Modality
AIDS	MRI
Acute transverse myelopathy	MRI
Brain abscess	CCT, MRI
Cryptococcal meningitis	CT, MRI
Cystercercosis	CT, MRI
Herpes simplex encephalitis	MRI
Postinfectious leukoencephalitis	MRI
Progressive multifocal leukoen-cephalopathy	MRI
Spinal epidural abscess	MRI
Subdural empyema	MRI
Toxoplasmosis	MRI
Viral encephalitis	MRI

MRI = magnetic resonance imaging; CCT = contrasted computed axial tomography; CT = computed axial tomography.

this imaging should be followed by a contrasted CT scan or an MRI. In general the results with a high-field MRI are better than those with a low-field MRI. The optimal imaging modalities for specific diseases are listed in Table 7-6.

Other Studies

Cerebral arteriography in focal infection of the nervous system should be requested from the emergency department only in the most unusual circumstance. A similar statement applies to isotope brain scans. EEGs are seldom requested by the emergency department. A suspicion of nonconvulsive status epilepticus, which would be a possible complication of an intracranial infection, may be such an indication.

Infectious Causes of Acute Neurologic Disease

Brain Involvement

VIRAL INFECTIONS
Viral agents can produce a spectrum of disease, ranging from meningitis to encephalitis. Some viruses such as respiratory virus, enterovirus, and arbovirus cause a small degree of meningoencepha-litis with meningitis symptoms and signs predominating. Other viruses cause more extensive brain inflammation, meningoencephalitis, involving both the meninges and the brain itself. These agents include mumps; equine, St. Louis, and California encephalitis viruses; and lymphocytic choriomeningitis virus. A seasonal incidence is shown by most of these viruses (Fig. 7-1).

Viral Meningitis. Most viral meningitis occurs in July, August, and September, when enterovirus infections are most prevalent. These infections can occur in epidemics and family clusters [5]. The onset of a viral meningitis may be abrupt or follow a flu-like prodrome. The fever is usually between 38°C and 40°C and the headache severe and frontal or retro-orbital. The patient develops a stiff neck, which may not be severe. Kernig's and Brudzinski's signs usually are present. The patient may seem drowsy and mildly confused but oriented. Rarely are there focal neurologic signs. Various rashes occur from enterovirus. Those rashes resembling rubella are most frequent, followed by those similar to roseola and the petechial/purpuric rash of meningococcemia. Concomitant herpangina or pleurodynia suggest a coxsackie virus. Viral meningitis occurs most commonly in children and adults less than 40 years. The rubellaform rash is most common in children and adults less than 40 years. Infants are rarely affected, but when they are, they may suffer from an overwhelming multiorgan system infection.

A number of other viruses that cause meningitis exhibit manifestations similar to the enteroviruses. Mumps is most prevalent in late winter and early spring. The meningitis may precede or follow the parotitis or orchitis, or these may not occur at all. The CSF findings are consistent with a viral meningitis, although the glucose may be lower than with other viral etiologies [6]. A history of full immunization within 10 years rules out mumps.

Although it is said that patients with viral meningitis appear less ill than those with bacterial meningitis, the clinical presentations overlap considerably. One cannot reliably distinguish viral meningitis from early or partially treated bacterial meningitis. These illnesses also may be difficult to distinguish in a stoic patient. Examination of the CSF is mandatory to distinguish these conditions

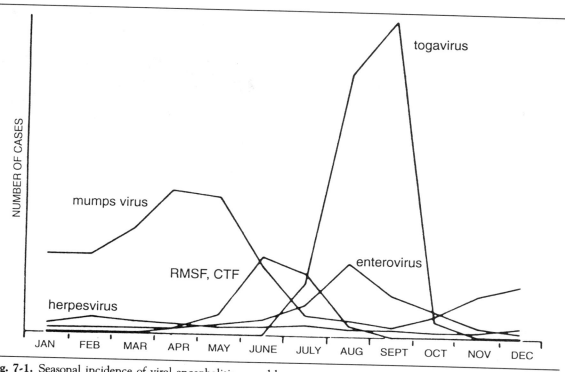

Fig. 7-1. Seasonal incidence of viral encephalitis caused by togaviruses, enteroviruses, mumps virus, herpesvirus, Rocky Mountain spotted fever, and Colorado tick fever. (Reprinted courtesy of DE Griffin, RT Johnson. Encephalitis, myelitis and neuritis. In GL Mandel, RG Douglas, JE Bennett (eds.), *Principles and Practice of Infectious Diseases* (3rd ed.). New York: Churchill-Livingstone, 1990. Pp. 762–69)

(see Table 7-5). Parameningeal infections also can mimic viral meningitis and cause fever, headache, stiff neck, and reactive pleocytosis in the CSF. In viral meningitis the CSF contains 5–500 WBC/μl, with polymorphonuclear neutrophil leukocytes (PMNs) predominating early, changing to about 75% mononuclear cells within 48 hours. The CSF pressure is raised, while protein and glucose are normal [7].

Viral Encephalitis. The onset of encephalitis is abrupt or follows a prodromal illness. In addition to fever, headache, photophobia, retro-orbital pain, nausea, and vomiting, encephalitis is characterized by an altered LOC. Nuchal rigidity may be present but is not as marked as in bacterial meningitis [8]. Drowsiness, confusion, and myalgia are accompanying symptoms. Behavior changes and delirium are present. Seizures often occur, which can be focal or generalized and uncontrollable by usual measures [9]. Pupillary irregularities are found. Papilledema can be seen. The tendon reflexes may be asymmetric and the plantar responses extensor. Hemiparesis or quadriparesis occurs [10, 11]. Viral encephalitis may be mimicked by postinfectious encephalitis; bacterial infections of the CNS, including syphilis, TB meningitis, Rocky Mountain spotted fever, and fungal infections; toxoplasmosis and cysticercosis.

The peripheral WBC can be normal or mildly elevated. The CSF shows a moderate mononuclear pleocytosis with a moderate elevation of protein and normal or slightly low glucose (see Table 7-5). CSF pressure may be elevated. In the acute stage a CT scan and an MRI may show mass effect as well as the presence of a focal lesion.

HERPES SIMPLEX ENCEPHALITIS. When the herpes simplex virus involves the nervous system, it most commonly takes the form of encephalitis, although meningitis, myelitis, and nerve root involvement also occur. Herpes simplex encephalitis can occur at any age and at any time of year.

Infection is commonly unilateral but may be bilateral. The onset is usually abrupt with fever and headache. Altered consciousness is found in 97% of patients as well as clinical features related to the usual sites of infection in the orbital and temporal areas of the brain. The symptoms of involvement of these areas include memory loss, personality change, hallucinations, dysphasia, and hemiparesis. Personality change occurs in 85% of cases and seizures in 38%. The seizures may be focal and suggest temporal lobe involvement. Intracranial pressure may be elevated with papilledema evident. The concomitant finding of a herpetic lesion on the skin or in the mouth has been overemphasized [12]. Conditions that have been confused with herpes simplex encephalitis include other infections, such as tuberculosis; subdural hematoma; cerebrovascular accident; neoplasm; and arteriovenous malformation [13].

An LP should not be performed before imaging. MRI is the investigation of choice and shows focal high-signal lesions in the temporal areas on T2-weighted images [14]. On a CT scan these lesions are seen as low-density areas (Fig. 7-2). The CSF is abnormal in the majority of cases, with increased pressure, moderate elevation of protein, normal or slightly low glucose, and a moderate mononuclear pleocytosis. Red blood cells may be found in the CSF. Brain biopsy at the time of suspicion of herpes simplex encephalitis has become controversial [15, 16].

RABIES ENCEPHALITIS. The incubation period of rabies encephalitis is rarely greater than 1 year, although it can range from days to several years. The initial symptoms are nonspecific and include malaise, headache, fever, cough, and sore throat. Abdominal symptoms include anorexia, nausea, vomiting, and abdominal pain. The only specific feature is pain at the wound site, although it is present in only half of cases. The first neurologic symptoms are those of hyperexitability and include insomnia, irritability, restlessness, and anxiety. These symptoms progress to more overt neurologic symptoms such as delirium, bizarre behavior, seizures, paralysis, and signs of meningismus. Episodes of hyperactivity, which can be triggered by a variety

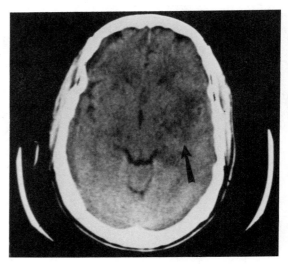

Fig. 7-2. Herpes simplex encephalitis. CT scan of the head without contrast demonstrating focal area of decreased attenuation in the left posterior frontal and temporal lobes (arrow). (Case courtesy of Dr. William Orrison)

of sensory stimuli, alternate with normal periods. Spasm of the larynx and pharynx leads to choking on attempts to drink water, giving rise to the term "hydrophobia." Paralysis progresses and, unless the patient dies from cardiopulmonary arrest, inevitably leads to coma. (Rabies encephalitis is further considered in Chap. 31 and epidemiology in Chap. 12. Rabies postexposure prophylaxis was discussed in Chap. 4.)

Progressive Multifocal Leukoencephalopathy. Progressive multifocal leukoencephalopathy (PML) is a demyelinating disease of older adults that can present as an acute focal neurologic syndrome. The patient is often immunosuppressed or debilitated from a severe systemic disease, such as lymphoma, tuberculosis, or AIDS. Lesions may be found in the cerebral hemispheres, cerebellum, or brain stem. The lesions are multiple, vary in size, and are associated with variable clinical symptomatology.

The neurologic symptoms become manifest over a period of days or weeks. The symptoms usually predominate in one cerebral hemisphere and progress slowly and relentlessly. They include hemiparesis, quadriparesis, field defects, cortical blindness, ataxia, dysphasia, personality change, dementia, and coma. Seizures are rare. Headache is an unusual complaint. Fever is absent unless an intercurrent infection is present [17]. A rapidly progressive multifocal neurologic disease in an immunocompromised individual suggests PML. Other conditions to consider include cryptococcus, toxoplasmosis, and AIDS.

The CT scan may show localized low-density lesions without enhancement. However, these lesions are more evident on MRI, so MRI is the imaging method of choice. The CSF is usually normal.

BACTERIAL INFECTIONS

Bacterial Meningitis. Bacterial meningitis is a medical emergency and must be diagnosed and treated without delay. Most patients will have the acute onset of severe headache, high fever, stiff neck, photophobia, and drowsiness. The typical headache is severe, throbbing, and made worse with movement. It is felt particularly at the back of the head and neck. Nausea, vomiting, and chills may also be present. Neck stiffness, the hallmark of meningeal irritation, usually develops within hours but is not always present [18, 19]. In one report of 86 patients, 25% did not have neck stiffness [20]. The limitation of neck movement is in the sagittal, not coronal, plane. Kernig's and Brudzinski's signs also indicate meningeal irritation and are more common in younger patients. In the patient who appears septic or who has a petechial rash, meningococcemia must be ruled out. An antecedent ear or sinus infection, especially in children, suggests pneumococcus infection.

Although the diagnosis of bacterial meningitis is obvious when the full-blown symptoms are noted, the presentation is often more subtle. The physician must have a high index of suspicion so as not to misdiagnose this virulent entity. The patient may present with any combination of upper respiratory symptoms, fever, malaise, myalgia, headache, and backache, which progress over hours to days to the more typical presentation. Children, the elderly, the immunocompromised, and the chronically ill are more likely to have atypical presentations and may never develop obvious symptoms or signs. The diagnosis should be suspected in those with recent head trauma, neurosurgery, or a CSF shunt.

The differential diagnosis includes sepsis, head trauma, viral or fungal CNS infection, brain abscess, intoxication, AIDS, metabolic derange-

ment, neoplastic meningitis, tetanus, and, in children, a febrile seizure or Reye's syndrome.

CSF will show a polymorphonuclear pleocytosis, elevation of CSF protein, low glucose, and an elevated pressure (see Table 7-5). Because bacterial meningitis can produce increased intracranial pressure, care must be exercised in the performance of an LP. When there is suspicion that intracranial pressure is increased or a focal lesion such as a brain abscess may be present, consideration should be given to the performance of brain imaging prior to an LP. Blood culture and antigen studies on CSF, blood, and urine can be obtained and appropriate antibiotics started prior to the brain imaging.

FOCAL SIGNS. Bacterial meningitis, although generally considered a disease without focal presentation, can present with focal neurologic signs, usually associated with fever and alteration of consciousness. Findings evolve over a period of days or may be fulminant [21]. Perhaps the most common focal sign is a focal seizure. Seizures are found at some time in the course of the illness in 15%–30% of cases, being more common in children. Seizures have been reported as the presenting symptom in 6% of children. Subdural collections can occur, especially in young children, and behave as intracranial masses, either unilateral or bilateral (Fig. 7-3). Hemiparesis, dysphasia, pupillary inequality, and other cranial nerve palsies can all be found [22].

CHILDREN. The infant less than 2 to 3 months of age may demonstrate only extremely subtle manifestations of infection. A change in activity level, poor feeding, increased sleepiness, irritability, or a change in cry may be the only clues of infection. The newborn may be hypo-, hyper- or euthermic. Meningeal signs in the age group are, of course, unreliable. A bulging fontanelle may be masked by dehydration or caused by crying. An LP is mandatory if these abnormalities are noted (see Chapter 14). The symptoms become more specific as the infant develops, although the diagnosis may still be difficult. Meningeal signs are not reliable until 12 to 16 months. The clinical and laboratory data that would mandate an LP in a young child are a frequent subject of debate in the pediatric literature and are discussed in Chap. 14.

THE IMMUNOSUPPRESSED. Bacterial meningitis is more common in the elderly; those with chronic illnesses, such as diabetes mellitus, alcoholism, ma-

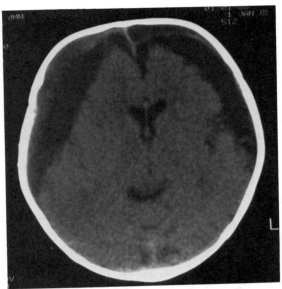

Fig. 7-3. Meningitis. CT scan demonstrating bilateral subdural fluid collections with septation and varying densities. (Case courtesy of Dr. William Orrison)

lignancy, and renal failure; and in the immunosuppressed. The inflammatory response may be blunted, resulting in less dramatic temperature rise (if at all) and meningeal signs. The only clues to diagnosis may be drowsiness, confusion, or dementia. Of 54 patients older than 65 years, 91% were febrile, 43% had headache, 57% had fever, 81% had meningismus, and 89% had altered mental status [20].

Brain Abscess. A bacterial brain abscess is a rare disease. Brain abscess becomes a clinical consideration in the patient with fever and neurologic signs restricted to the brain. Cyanotic congenital heart disease, pulmonary abscesses, infections of the sinuses and ears, penetrating head trauma, and neurosurgical procedures on the head all predispose to brain abscess. The initial infection, which leads to seeding of the brain, may be unnoticed or insignificant. A primary site of infection is not found in 25% of patients [23]. Brain abscess occurs at all ages. Multiple abscesses may be present.

There are seldom clear-cut signs of a brain abscess. Headache may be the initial manifestation. Symptoms are progressive as the lesion expands. As intracranial pressure rises, the headache worsens. It may be localized to the area of the infection, or it may be generalized. It is often worse at night and in the morning or upon lying down. The pain may be intermittent or constant. Nausea and vomiting may occur. Drowsiness and behavioral changes are noted. The scalp overlying the region may be tender. Stiff neck occurs in 25% of patients. Focal neurologic signs vary with the location of the lesion. In studies of 67 and 45 patients with brain abscesses, 80% and 72%, respectively, had headache as their most impressive symptom. In the same studies 33% and 60% were febrile, 50% and 83% had altered mental status, 33% and 49% had meningismus, and 75% and 72% had focal neurologic signs [24, 25]. In another study of 54 patients, focal neurologic signs were present in about half the cases, with fever occurring in about the same proportion [26]. Seizures occur in 30% of the cases and are often focal. As the abscess expands, intracranial pressure continues to increase and signs appear such as third-nerve palsies, stupor, and coma. Papilledema is found in 6% [26].

Brain abscess rarely accompanies bacterial meningitis. Head trauma, neoplasm, and even mild systemic infection can be mistaken for brain abscess. The ability to diagnose this condition depends on the degree of suspicion on the part of the emergency department physician.

The diagnosis of brain abscess is not made by LP. An LP should be avoided because of the increased risk of cerebral herniation secondary to elevated intracranial pressure. Brain imaging, either a contrast-enhanced CT scan or MRI, is in order (Fig. 7-4). On occasions when the CSF is examined, it is usually under increased pressure with a slight pleocytosis, mildly elevated protein, and normal glucose.

Subdural Empyema. Subdural empyema is usually a complication of osseous infection in structures contiguous to the nervous system, such as the sinuses or the middle ear. Subdural empyema leads to fever, headache, nuchal rigidity, lethargy, vomiting, seizures, and papilledema. Headache is present in 65% of cases and focal neurologic signs in 90%. Findings include hemiparesis, visual field defects, and dysphasia. Clinical deterioration is rapid from enlargement of the collection of pus, cerebral

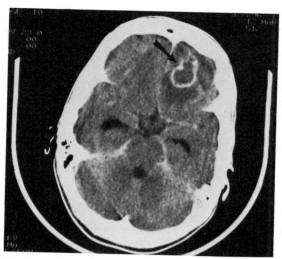

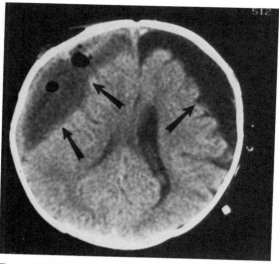

Fig. 7-4. Abscess. Contrast-enhanced CT scan demonstrating ring enhancing mass (arrow) with surrounding decreased attenuation of edema. (Case courtesy of Dr. William Orrison)

Fig. 7-5. Subdural empyema. CT scan of the head without contrast demonstrating extra axial fluid collection on the left of low density consistent with subdural hygroma (arrow) and extra axial fluid collection on the right (double arrows), which is of higher attenuation and contains focal areas of gas accumulation in the subdural empyema. (Case courtesy of Dr. William Orrison)

edema, increased intracranial pressure, and brain herniation.

Many of the signs of subdural empyema are similar to the signs of meningitis, encephalitis, brain abscess, and head trauma. The presence of sinusitis favors the diagnosis of subdural infection.

Brain imaging establishes the presence of a subdural lesion (Fig. 7-5) and may suggest inflammation by reaction of the underlying brain. An LP is contraindicated because of increased pressure. Outcome may be unfavorable [27].

OTHER ETIOLOGIES

Cryptococcal Meningitis. Cryptococcosis is the most common cause of fungal meningitis. Cryptococcal meningitis is a disease of late childhood through middle age. Immunologic difficulties are common in those afflicted. Cryptococcal meningitis becomes a major consideration in an individual with chronic meningitis who is also immunosuppressed. (See Table 8-7 for other causes of chronic meningitis.) The condition produces thickening of the meninges and sometimes obstruction of CSF flow with papilledema. A recent mild respiratory infection may precede the neurologic findings. The patient may have been exposed to pigeon droppings.

Onset is insidious and intermittent. Symptoms fluctuate and may relate to meningitis, vasculitis, intracranial mass, or increased intracranial pressure. Headache, nausea, vomiting, fever, and stiff neck are the usual presenting symptoms. One review, however, noted that 40% of patients were afebrile and 50% were without meningeal signs [28]. Papilledema is a common clinical finding. Cranial nerve palsies may occur, especially of the sixth and seventh cranial nerves. Seizures, either focal or generalized, are often present. In acute cases one or both pupils may be dilated. Impaired consciousness occurs. Hemiparesis is found, presumably secondary to a vasculitis produced by the meningitis. Optic atrophy is a late complication [29]. The course of the disease resembles that of TB meningitis, although it is frequently somewhat slower in evolution except in immunosuppressed individuals, when the course may be rapid.

The peripheral WBC is usually normal. The CSF will commonly be under increased pressure. An India ink preparation of the CSF may reveal the budding yeast forms of *Cryptococcus neoformans* in 60% of patients [30]. A serologic test can be performed on the spinal fluid, which will provide a rapid diagnosis. The CSF glucose is usually low, with a slight elevation of protein and a pleocytosis with mononuclear cells [31] (see Table 7-5). Brain imaging may show cortical inflammation, contrast enhancement of cryptococcus nodules, and hydrocephalus.

Cysticercosis. Neural cysticercosis is the most common parasitic disease of the brain when considered on a worldwide basis. Cerebral infections may be asymptomatic for many years. Symptoms usually occur 2 to 6 years after the initial exposure. In the United States the condition is seen in Hispanics who have lived in Mexico. Young adults are more commonly affected and males more than females [32].

Symptoms depend on the location of cysts and the degree of inflammation they produce. Cysts may be located in the parenchyma or in the subarachnoid space. When cysts are present in the subarachnoid space, chronic meningitis or obstructive hydrocephalus can occur. With the exception of hydrocephalus from a cyst, neurologic findings are focal and depend on the area of the brain affected. Seizures, the most frequent clinical sign, are present in 52% of patients and may be generalized rather than focal [33]. Obstructive hydrocephalus can lead to headache, alteration of consciousness, papilledema, and the need for surgical intervention. Visual disturbances, dysphasia, and hemiparesis may be found [34]. Residence in an area endemic for pork tapeworm increases suspicion of neural cysticercosis in a patient with focal seizures, focal neurologic signs, increased intracranial pressure, or chronic meningitis.

A modest pleocytosis may be present in the CSF with mononuclear cells or eosinophils. The protein may be elevated and the glucose low. About half of the cases of neurocysticercosis will have normal CSF. A serologic test is available on the CSF. A CT scan will show single or multiple lesions with variable calcification, sometimes with surrounding edema (Fig. 7-6), and the cysts can be visualized on an MRI.

Toxoplasmosis. Most infections with toxoplasmosis are asymptomatic. Toxoplasmosis is a serious disease in immunocompromised patients and in

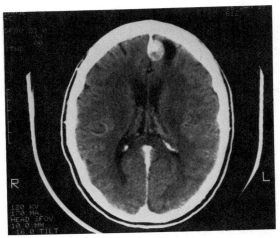

Fig. 7-6. Cysticercosis. Contrast-enhanced CT scan demonstrating a ring enhancing cysticercosis cyst with central calcification adjacent to an area of prior infection identified as a decreased density. (Case courtesy of Dr. William Orrison)

those with congenital infections. Toxoplasmosis has become the most commonly recognized opportunistic infection of the CNS in patients with AIDS, presumably by activation of a latent infection. Organ transplant recipients are another group who contract serious toxoplasmosis encephalitis [35].

The most common presentation is a subacute meningoencephalitis with slowly progressive confusion and depression of consciousness. Chorioretinitis is seen. There may be concurrent signs of meningitis, such as headache and a stiff neck. Seizures, either focal or generalized, may occur. As the disease develops, focal neurologic signs appear, such as hemiparesis, field defects, and aphasia. Symptoms may progress to coma.

Toxoplasmosis in the CNS may also present as a single focus or as multiple foci of infection, which slowly increase in size. The process is equivalent to multiple bacterial brain abscesses, although it may be slower in evolution. The symptoms are those of an expanding intracranial mass with increased intracranial pressure. Severe headache, depression of consciousness, hemiparesis, aphasia, field defects, seizures, and ataxia may be found. Toxoplasmosis should be considered in all immunosuppressed patients with neurologic involvement [36].

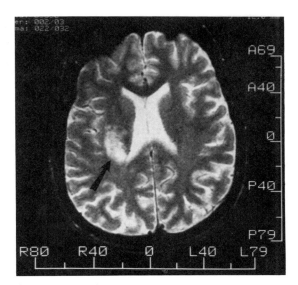

Fig. 7-7. Toxoplasmosis. Axial T2-weighted MR (TR 2500, TE 80) demonstrating focal area of abnormal signal intensity (arrow) with central variable signal intensity. (Case courtesy of Dr. William Orrison)

The CSF shows a moderate mononuclear pleocytosis, slight elevation in protein, and normal glucose (see Table 7-5). Brain imaging will usually be normal in toxoplasmosis meningoencephalitis and abnormal when focal areas of infection and edema are present (Fig. 7-7). Antibodies to toxoplasmosis can be detected except in occasional patients with immunodeficiency.

Amoebic Meningitis. Amoebic meningitis is exceedingly rare (150 cases worldwide) and follows introduction of the organism through the nose while swimming in contaminated water. In addition to fever, headache, and lethargy, nasal symptoms such as rhinitis and decreased sense of smell may be noted.

POSTINFECTIOUS CONDITIONS

Postinfectious conditions are diseases of the nervous system that follow an infection with a virus or bacteria or immunization. The symptoms appear days or months after the clinical infection and are a remote or "allergic" response to the infection. The responsible infectious agent can seldom be isolated at the time the complication develops.

Postinfectious Leukoencephalitis. Postinfectious leukoencephalitis, also known as postinfectious encephalomyelitis, is a rare acute neurologic condition that usually follows an influenza-like or exanthematous viral infection or immunization by a period of 7–10 days. It can occur at any age but is more common in childhood. The condition is considered an immunologic response within the nervous system to the infection. There is no evidence of direct involvement of the nervous system by the infection.

Acute cerebellar ataxia of children is probably a form of postinfectious leukoencephalitis restricted primarily to the cerebellum. The affected individual, over a period of hours or days, develops truncal titubation and ataxia or unsteadiness. The ability to walk is frequently lost. The condition commonly follows an infection with varicella. Brain imaging is usually normal. A mild CSF pleocytosis may be present with the fluid under increased pressure (see Table 7-5).

In the acute demyelinating form of postinfectious leukoencephalitis, onset is abrupt, usually 2–7 days following a viral infection and during a time of improvement from that infection. There is multifocal neurologic involvement with seizures, which can be focal or generalized. Multiple symptoms appear, ranging from confusion to depression of consciousness, optic neuritis, hemiparesis, quadriparesis, dysphasia, and tremor. In the hemorrhagic form onset is very acute and symptomatology more severe. The LOC almost invariably is depressed. These conditions must be differentiated from bacterial or viral meningitis, encephalitis, head trauma, subarachnoid hemorrhage from another cause, and intoxication.

The CSF is normal or shows mild mononuclear pleocytosis and slight elevation of protein [37]. In the hemorrhagic form the CSF will contain red blood cells. An MRI is more sensitive than a CT scan in detecting these lesions and will become abnormal very shortly after onset. Areas of increased signal in the white matter will be present on T2-weighted images [38].

Reye's Syndrome. Reye's syndrome occurs primarily in children [39] but can occasionally occur in adults [39]. Both sexes are involved with equal incidence. Reye's syndrome has been associated with preceding viral infection, particularly with influenza and varicella-zoster viruses. As a consequence the disease tends to peak in winter months during influenza epidemics. In addition to the viral infection, epidemiologic studies have strongly implicated aspirin ingestion during the prodromal illness as increasing the risk of developing Reye's syndrome [40].

Encephalopathy and fatty accumulation in the viscera are the cardinal pathologic manifestations [41, 42]. The brain is usually edematous without inflammation. The liver is enlarged, and microscopic sections show a uniform foaminess of the hepatocyte cytoplasm with an absence of inflammation. The cytoplasmic vacuoles contain lipid.

Reye's syndrome usually presents with a prodromal illness that can be an upper respiratory tract infection, chicken pox, or occasionally gastroenteritis. Usually the prodromal illness is not atypical or severe. As the prodromal illness begins to remit, the child abruptly undergoes a period of severe vomiting. Within 24 hours after the onset of vomiting, an encephalopathy usually develops characterized by irritability, restlessness, spontaneous purposeless movements, and episodes of delirium [42]. The encephalopathy may progress to stupor and coma, coupled with seizures. Hepatomegaly commonly is present, but jaundice is not.

A case of Reye's syndrome is defined by the Centers for Disease Control as the acute onset of a noninflammatory encephalopathy demonstrated by (1) either the presence of less than 8 WBC/μl in the CSF or histologic sections of the brain demonstrating cerebral edema without meningeal or perivascular inflammation; (2) microvesicular fatty metamorphosis of the liver demonstrated by examination of either biopsy or autopsy specimen; (3) aspartate aminotransferase (AST), alanine aminotransferase (ALT), or blood ammonia levels more than three times normal; and (4) no other explanation for the neurologic or hepatic abnormalities [42]. Examination of the CSF is usually normal (see Table 7-5). The CSF opening pressure may be normal or markedly elevated, depending on the stage of the disease. Bilirubin levels are normal. Blood ammonia levels are markedly elevated. Other evidence of liver dysfunction includes hypoglycemia, prolonged prothrombin time, abnormal levels of blood amino acids, elevated serum fatty

acids, and low levels of vitamin K in blood [41]. Metabolic acidosis is followed by a respiratory acidosis. CT and MRI scans may show evidence of cerebral edema.

Treatment of Reye's syndrome is aimed at reducing cerebral edema through judicious use of hyperventilation and mannitol [39]. Treatment is also aimed at correcting liver dysfunctions through administration of vitamin K and glucose. The patient should be hospitalized and placed in the intensive care unit. If coma develops, nasotracheal intubation and respiratory assistance usually are needed.

The illness usually runs its clinical course over approximately 7–10 days. For unknown reasons the encephalopathy may stop at the stage of lethargy or continuously progress to severe coma and death. Overall there is approximately 30% mortality. Morbidity ranges from 12%–24%. Permanent neurologic sequelae include mental retardation, hyperactive behavior, focal neurological deficits, and seizures.

Sydenham's Chorea. Sydenham's chorea is a constellation of acute or subacute involuntary movements that frequently are asymmetrical. The condition has a strong association with rheumatic fever and a preceding group A streptococcal infection. The disease is found in childhood or early adolescence.

Fifty-seven percent of the cases are in females. Choreiform and athetoid movements are present. In 19% of the cases the movements are restricted to one side or are more severe on one side. The movements may be so severe as to prevent walking or getting food to the mouth. Personality change with emotional lability frequently accompanies the condition. Those affected try to hide the movements by converting the involuntary movements into seemingly voluntary movements. Dysarthria is present in 39% of cases and is the most common neurologic sign other than the movement disorder. Confusion, weakness, seizures, and headache occur rarely. The tendon reflexes are "hung up" and sustained grip has a peculiar rhythmic, milking quality. Sustained postures are difficult to maintain. Attacks may be recurrent [43]. The condition progresses for several days, then stabilizes for a period of time, which may be as long as several months. Improvement then occurs in most cases.

The greatest problem in differential diagnosis

concerns a functional or hysterical disturbance. The emergency department physician with experience in Sydenham's chorea will encounter little difficulty. With hemichorea the diagnostic concerns center around brain tumor or brain infarction. Once again clinical experience will make the differential obvious. Chorea can be seen as a complication of pregnancy and occurs in association with hyperthyroidism, lupus, and cerebral palsy.

The antistreptolysin O (ASO) titer will be elevated if a recent group A streptococcal infection has occurred. An EKG should be obtained to rule out an accompanying carditis. The CSF is usually normal. Brain imaging is not revealing.

Optic Neuritis. Optic neuritis can follow several childhood infections, including measles, mumps, pertussis, infectious mononucleosis, and chicken pox [44]. It can also occur following DPT immunization. There is a progressive loss of central vision and decreased visual acuity, with the symptoms being unilateral in about 75% of cases. Retrobulbar pain often is present. In about 50% of patients the optic disk appears normal on initial examination, but in others the disk appears edematous or blurred and the retina may also have flame hemorrhages. The diagnosis is based on the clinical history and examination of the eye. Skull x-rays and a CT scan may be of benefit in ruling out paranasal sinus infection or tumors. The CSF is normal. Most patients have a good recovery, but some are left with a central or paracentral defect in vision. Fewer than 50% of patients with this disorder subsequently develop multiple sclerosis [45].

Deafness and Vertigo. Deafness and vertigo may develop, but only rarely, following bacterial meningitis or infection with mumps, influenza, measles, or varicella-zoster viruses [46]. There is abrupt onset of unilateral hearing loss or severe sensorineural deafness, often accompanied by profound vertigo, nausea, and vomiting. The vertigo resolves slowly, but the partial or complete hearing loss is usually permanent. No therapy is available.

Spinal Cord Involvement

Infection-related lesions of the spinal cord and peripheral nerves and their relation to certain features are listed in Table 7-7.

BACTERIAL INFECTIONS: SPINAL EPIDURAL ABSCESS

Spinal epidural abscess, although rare, is often overlooked and appropriate treatment delayed. The condition occurs in children and adults. Blunt trauma and cutaneous infections are frequent preceding events. The etiologic agent may be bacteria or *Mycobacterium* organisms. Spinal epidural abscess may follow an LP.

Spinal epidural abscess is a painful spinal syndrome [47]. Symptoms are of sudden onset. Pain in

Table 7-7. Infection-related lesions of the spinal cord and peripheral nerves

Features	Spinal epidural abscess	Polio-myelitis	Acute transverse myelopathy	Tetanus	Guillain-Barré syndrome	Botulism	Diphtheria
Acute infection	+	+	−	−	−	−	−
Toxin	−	−	−	+	−	+	+
Postinfectious condition	−	−	+	+	+	+	+
Pain	+	+	+	+	+/−	−	−
Deep tendon reflex	↑	↓	↓	↑	↓	↓	↓
Sensory involvement	+	+/−	+	−	+/−	−	+
Symmetry	+/−	−	+/−	+/−	+	+	+
Ascending paresis	−	−	−	−	+	+	+
Urinary incontinence/ retention	+	+	+	−	−	+	+

+ indicates present; − indicates absent; ↑ indicates increased; ↓ indicates decreased.

a dermatome is the most frequent initial complaint, and pain is present in all cases. Sixty-two percent will have elevated temperature. Headache and nuchal rigidity are uncommon. With increasing size of the lesion, progressive rigid paresis develops below the lesion, as well as sphincter dysfunction. A sensory level may be present. Evolution is usually over several days. The clinical findings are less dramatic when the etiologic agent is *Mycobacterium* [48].

Spinal trauma with or without hematoma formation can mimic a spinal epidural abscess, but with trauma a significant elevation of body temperature is unlikely. Fever usually is absent if the problem is caused by a neoplasm, disk disease, spinal cord thrombosis, or acute back strain. In transverse myelitis the pain is seldom as severe as in spinal epidural abscess, and fever is not as prominent.

Peripheral leukocytosis occurs. Immediate imaging of the spinal canal is indicated [49]. Imaging should precede an LP when spinal epidural abscess is a consideration. MRI is the imaging method of choice. A CT scan or traditional myelography are alternatives. An LP should be performed with caution, if at all. The CSF will be turbid or xanthochromic in 50% of cases, with a polymorphonuclear pleocytosis, elevated protein, normal glucose, and elevated pressure [50]. Osteomyelitis may be present in the region of the abscess.

Viral Infection: Poliomyelitis

Poliomyelitis still occasionally occurs in the United States in spite of extensive vaccination programs. There is also a vaccine-related poliovirus infection that can produce neurologic disease [51]. The incidence of neurologic complications from infection with poliovirus increases with age. Other viral agents, such as coxsackievirus and echovirus, can produce a polio-like illness.

Initial symptoms are those of aseptic meningitis, with fever, malaise, headache, and stiff neck. For many patients these symptoms are the extent of the poliomyelitis infection. In some cases weakness begins several days later in one or more extremities. The affected limbs become painful, stiff, and sensitive to touch. Involvement is usually asymmetric, and the legs may be more involved than the arms. Affected extremities become flaccid and areflexic after an initial brief period of hyperreflexia. Within several days muscular atrophy is noted. Bulbar involvement, which is present in 10%–15% of cases, can result in profound respiratory complications [52]. In an epidemic situation little difficulty should be encountered in recognizing acute poliomyelitis. Polio has been confused with amyotrophic lateral sclerosis, Guillain-Barré syndrome, acute transverse myelopathy, and chemical poisoning.

The CSF will show a mild pleocytosis that is initially polymorphonuclear changing to mononuclear (see Table 7-5). The CSF protein is slightly elevated with a normal glucose.

A slowly progressive, increasing weakness has been noted in muscles that have partially recovered from poliomyelitis. This weakness can occur years after the initial illness [53].

Postinfectious Conditions

Acute Transverse Myelopathy. Acute transverse myelopathy (ATM) is an acute dysfunction of the spinal cord. Patients of any age—between 1 and 80 years—can be affected. The peak incidence is between the ages of 10 and 19 years and after age 40 years [54]. The condition has its onset without any preceding history of neurologic disease. A history of viral infection prior to onset may be reported. Many viruses have been implicated.

The cord may be involved partially or completely, often over a considerable length. The dorsal cord is involved in 68% of cases. The symptoms are either static or rapidly ascending and may be asymmetric. Paresthesia and interscapular pain are the common presenting symptoms. Leg weakness is present in 97% of affected individuals and a sensory level usually can be demonstrated. Urinary retention and overflow incontinence are almost universal findings, occurring in 94% of cases. Maximum deficit is present between 2 hours and 14 days.

Prognosis of ATM depends on the severity and the etiology. Causes include trauma, a postinfectious condition presumed to be immunologic neurologic disease, multiple sclerosis, paraspinous abscess, disk disease, direct infection of the cord by a virus, radiation, neoplasm, vascular malformation of the cord, cord infarction, neuromyelitis optica, syphilis, and vaccine response.

HIV and HTLV-I have been associated with a myelopathy that does not have an acute onset [55]. Spinal syndromes have been reported with cocaine abuse [56]. ATM and Guillain-Barré syndrome are sometimes confused. If urinary incontinence is present in a patient with the acute or subacute development of flaccid lower extremities, ATM should be suspected. The challenge to the emergency department physician is to recognize treatable causes of ATM [57].

Any acute spinal cord lesion demands urgent investigation. A compressive cord lesion, often considered a neurosurgical emergency, must be excluded. An MRI of the affected area of the spine is the best method of investigation. CSF examination should be postponed until after imaging. CSF examination, when performed, may be normal or reveal elevated protein witn pleocytosis.

Tetanus. In the United States tetanus is a rare disease of nonimmunized or partially immunized individuals. It is more common in the newborn and the elderly. Tetanus is of greater significance in some developing countries. Neurologic symptoms, the result of a strychnine-like neurotoxin produced by an infection with *Clostridium tetani* usually remote from the nervous system, occur 1–2 weeks after the primary infection. In newborns the incubation period is shorter, with symptoms present by the second day of life.

The site of the original infection is usually still evident at the time of development of neurologic symptoms. The initial symptoms are nonspecific, with low-grade fever, irritability, and headache. Several days later muscle spasms and rigidity begin. The tetanus can be local, involving the muscles near the infection, or generalized. Muscular rigidity starts in the muscles about the face (risus sardonicus) and neck. The jaws are closed, and there is inability to speak, chew, or swallow (lockjaw). The neonate cannot suck. The body then becomes stiff, and painful spasms occur with movement. Opisthotonos may be pronounced. Periodic increases in truncal rigidity are found (spinal convulsions). Hypoxia may occur from involvement of the respiratory muscles [58]. Early in the course of the illness tetanus may be confused with dental disease, meningitis, other intracranial infections, and hypocalcemia.

No serologic diagnostic test is available. Culture of the organism may be successful from the wound site. The CSF is normal. Brain imaging is normal, unless concomitant hypoxia has produced cerebral edema.

Peripheral Nerve Involvement

GUILLAIN-BARRÉ SYNDROME

Guillain-Barré syndrome (GB) is an acute polyneuropathy. It can occur at any age but is unusual in infancy. An affected individual can progress from normal to being ventilator dependent in 2–3 days, although progression usually continues for 10–12 days followed by a plateau and then gradual recovery. Eighty percent will have undergone maximum progression by 3 weeks into the illness. A stuttering onset occurs in some patients.

Initially dysesthesia of the feet or hands may be found. This is followed by a progressive ascending paresis that usually is relatively symmetrical. Distal or complete loss of tendon reflexes occurs. Sensory findings are mild. Various cranial nerves may be involved, with the face being involved in 50% of the cases. Autonomic dysfunction can increase morbidity, with findings such as tachycardia, cardiac arrhythmias, postural hypotension, or hypertension. Sphincter function usually is not affected. Fever is absent at onset [59, 60]. Patients with GB usually remain alert.

Conditions occasionally confused with GB include ATM, abuse of volatile solvents, acute intermittent porphyria, diphtheric polyneuritis, lead neuropathy, poliomyelitis, botulism, and other toxic neuropathies. The possibility of hysterical paralysis must always be kept in mind, but it will not have the findings on examination of GB. A marked and persistent asymmetry of the weakness, significant bladder or bowel dysfunction, and a sharp sensory level suggest a diagnosis other than GB.

CSF protein is usually elevated after the first week without a significant CSF pleocytosis (see Table 7-5). More than 50 mononuclear cells per microliter in the CSF or the presence of polymorphonuclear cells are against the diagnosis of GB. The CSF pressure is normal.

BOTULISM

The symptoms of botulism usually occur after ingestion of improperly preserved food that contains the neurotoxin, botulinum toxin, produced by *Clostridia botulinum*. Symptoms develop 12–36 hours after exposure to the toxin. An infantile form occurs within the first several months of life and is probably related to production of the toxin in the gut following ingestion of the organism.

The initial symptoms of botulism are nausea, vomiting, dry mouth, dizziness, and blurred vision. These symptoms, which are almost universal, are followed rapidly by weakness of muscles supplied by the cranial nerves, manifesting as dilated pupils; diplopia; dysarthria and dysphagia; generalized weakness; and respiratory paralysis. The tendon reflexes variably are lost [61]. The infantile form presents over a period of several days as constipation, followed by hypotonia, loss of neck control, ptosis, weak cry, and poor suck. Respiratory paralysis can occur in infant botulism [62]. Patients with botulism usually remain alert.

Considerations in differential diagnosis include myasthenia gravis, GB, the Lambert-Eaton syndrome, and diphtheria. In the infant diagnostic concerns include sepsis, meningitis, intoxication, Werdnig-Hoffman disease, congenital myopathy, and infantile myasthenia.

Botulinum toxin can be identified in the serum of an adult or the stool of an infant. An electromyogram shows small compound action potentials, a decremental response with slow repetitive stimulation, and an incremental response with rapid repetitive stimulation. CSF and brain imaging are normal. (See Chap. 31.)

DIPHTHERIA

The neurologic signs of diphtheria follow an oropharyngeal or, less commonly, cutaneous infection with *Corynebacterium diphtheria*, which produces a neurotoxin. Neurologic symptoms are more common in younger patients, as is infection with diphtheria.

Neurologic findings appear 1–2 weeks after the onset of the infection. The first symptoms are in the area of the infection. When the diphtheric infection is a pharyngitis, the initial symptoms are bulbar, especially palatal weakness. As the toxin becomes disseminated, blurred vision and difficulty with accommodation are noted. Then a cranial and somatic polyneuropathy appears, although facial paresis is rare. The polyneuropathy can be mixed motor and sensory. Motor weakness usually begins proximally and spreads distally, although an ascending, predominantly distal polyneuropathy can be found. CNS symptoms occur rarely, manifesting as encephalopathy and hemiparesis. The diph-

theric toxin also affects the heart, producing a myocarditis [63].

The neurologic symptoms of diphtheria may be confused with GB, amyotrophic lateral sclerosis, botulism, or an intoxication affecting the peripheral nerves. A history of nasal voice, dysphagia, blurred vision, and pharyngitis several weeks before the onset of polyneuropathy is strong evidence for diphtheric polyneuritis.

The CSF may be normal or show albuminocytologic dissociation similar to GB. The EKG may be abnormal. The organism can be recovered from the throat even many weeks after the symptoms of pharyngitis.

LEPROSY

Leprosy is an infection with the acid-fast bacillus *Mycobacterium leprae*. Immigration and air travel from endemic areas make it likely that emergency departments in all parts of the world will encounter this problem [64]. Leprosy affects primarily the cooler parts of the body, especially the skin and hence the peripheral nerves. The condition is believed to be the most common cause of peripheral nerve disease in the world [65]. The incubation period varies from several months to several years. The disease is chronic with occasional acute episodes.

The cardinal symptoms of leprosy are loss of sensory perception and local areas of anesthesia. Impairment of pain and temperature sensation can be demonstrated. Painless injury and secondary infection can lead to mutilation and disfigurement. As the disease progresses, the patients complain of pain and paresthesia. The tuberculoid form has small, plaque-like cutaneous anesthetic lesions and easily detected sensory loss. The peripheral nerves are enlarged, especially the greater auricular nerve. In the lepromatous form there is a sensory loss in the hands and feet and a thickening of the facial skin resulting in the "leonine facies."

The diagnosis is usually made by clinical appearance and examination. Residence in an endemic area or contact with infected patients raises the suspicion. Superficial mycoses can cause confusion as can scars, actinic dermatitis, and the many other infections that produce infiltrated lesions of the skin. There is no generally approved serologic test. Acid-fast bacilli can be demonstrated on smears made from scrapings of cutaneous lesions or on skin biopsy. Sensory and motor nerve conduction velocities are slow in areas of lesions [66].

References

1. Purtel JJ, Robins E, Cohen ME. Observations on clinical aspects of hysteria. JAMA 146:902, 1951.
2. Richards PG, Towo-Aghantse E. Dangers of lumbar puncture. Brit Med J 292:605–6, 1986.
3. Glendhill RF. Dangers of lumbar puncture. Brit Med J 292:1986, 1986.
4. Gower DJ et al. Contraindications to lumbar puncture as defined by computed cranial tomography. J Neurol Neurosurg Psychiat 50:1071–74, 1987.
5. Wood M, Anderson M. Neurologic Infections. London: Saunders, 1988. P. 144.
6. Ibid. P. 154.
7. Harter DH, Petersdorf RG. Viral disease of the central nervous system: aseptic meningitis and encephalitis. In JD Wilson et al. (eds.), Harrison's Principles of Internal Medicine (12th ed.). New York: McGraw-Hill, 1991. Pp. 2031–38.
8. David LE. Acute viral meningitis and encephalitis. In PGE Kennedy, RT Johnson (eds.), Infections of the Nervous System. London: Butterworths, 1987. Pp. 155–76.
9. Piatt JH et al. Chronic focal encephalitis (Rasmussen syndrome): six cases. Epilepsia 29:268–79, 1988.
10. Tyler KL. Diagnosis and management of acute viral encephalitis. Sem Neurol 48:480–89, 1984.
11. Whitley RJ. Viral encephalitis. N Engl J Med 323:242–50, 1990.
12. McKendall RR. Herpes simplex. In PJ Vinken et al. (eds.), Handbook of Clinical Neurology. Vol. 56, Viral Disease. Amsterdam: Elsevier, 1989. Pp. 207–27.
13. Whitley RJ et al. Herpes simplex encephalitis: vidarabine therapy and diagnostic problems. N Engl J Med 304:313–18, 1981.
14. Pascual-Leone A, Dhuna A, Langerdorf F. Herpes simplex encephalitis: early magnetic resonance imaging findings in the face of normal electroencephalogram. Ann Neurol 28:280, 1990.
15. Fishman RA. No, brain biopsy need not be done in every patient suspected of having herpes simplex encephalitis. Arch Neurol 44:1291–92, 1987.
16. Wasiewski WW, Fishman MA. Herpes simplex encephalitis: the brain biopsy controversy. J Pediatr 113:575–78, 1988.
17. Walker DL. Progressive multifocal leukoencephalopathy: an opportunistic viral infection of the central nervous system. In PJ Vinken, GW Bruyn (eds.), Handbook of Clinical Neurology (vol. 34). Amsterdam: Elsevier/North-Holland, 1978. Pp. 307–29.
18. Callahan M. Fulminant bacterial meningitis without meningeal signs. Ann Emerg Med 18:90–93, 1989.
19. Geisler PJ, Nelson KE. Bacterial meningitis without clinical signs of meningeal irritation. South J Med 75:448–540, 1982.
20. Gorse GJ et al. Bacterial meningitis in the elderly. Arch Int Med 144:1603–7, 1984.
21. Snyder RD. Bacterial infections of the nervous system. In KF Swaiman (ed.), Pediatric Neurology (vol. 1). St. Louis: Mosby, 1989. Pp. 447–73.
22. Valmari P et al. Childhood bacterial meningitis: initial symptoms and signs related to age, and reasons for consulting a physician. Eur J Pediatr 146:515–18, 1987.
23. Wood M, Anderson M. Neurologic Infections. London: Saunders, 1988. P. 256.
24. Harrison MJG. The clinical presentation of intracranial abscesses. Quart J Med 204:461–68, 1982.
25. Chun CH et al. Brain abscess: a study of 45 consecutive cases. Medicine 65:415–31, 1986.
26. Schliamser SE, Backman K, Norrby SR. Intracranial abscess in adults: an analysis of 54 consecutive cases. Scand J Infect Dis 20:1–9, 1988.
27. Miller ES, Dias PS, Uttley D. Management of subdural empyema: a series of 24 cases. J Neurol Neurosurg Psychiatry 50:1415–18, 1987.
28. Lyons RW, Andriloe VT. Fungal infections in the CNS. Neurol Clin 4:159–70, 1986.
29. Tan CT, Kuan BB. Cryptococcus meningitis, clinical–CT scan considerations. Neuroradiology 29:43–46, 1987.
30. Sabetta JR, Andriole VT. Cryptococcal infections of the nervous system. Med Clin North Am 69:333–34, 1985.
31. Weenink HR, Bruyn GW. Cryptotoccus of the nervous system. In PJ Vinken, GW Bruyn, HL Klawans (eds.), Handbook of Clinical Neurology vol. 35, Infections of the Nervous System. Amsterdam: North-Holland, 1978. Pp. 459–502.
32. Scharf D. Neurocysticercosis: two hundred thirty-eight cases from a California hospital. Arch Neurol 45:777–80, 1988.
33. Sotelo J, Guerrero V, Rubio F. Neurocysticercosis: a new classification based on active and inactive forms: a study of 753 cases. Arch Intern Med. 145:442–45, 1985.

34. Del Brutto OH, Sotelo J. Neurocysticercosis: an update. *Rev Infect Dis.* 10:1075–87, 1988.
35. McCabe R, Remington JS. Toxoplasmosis: the time has come. *New Engl J Med* 318:313–15, 1988.
36. Townsend JJ et al. Acquired toxoplasmosis: a neglected cause of treatable nervous system disease. *Arch Neurol* 32:335–43, 1975.
37. Johnson RT, Griffin DE. Postinfectious encephalomyelitis. In PGE Kennedy, RT Johnson (eds.), *Infections of the Nervous System.* London: Butterworths, 1987. Pp. 209–26.
38. Marks WA et al. Parainflammatory leukoencephalomyelitis: clinical and magnetic resonance imaging findings. *J Child Neurol* 3:205–13, 1988.
39. Davis LE, Kornfeld M. Influenza A virus and Reye's syndrome in adults. *J Neurol Neurosurg Psychiatry* 43:516–21, 1980.
40. Hurwitz ES et al. Public Health Service study of Reye's syndrome and medications: report of the main study. *JAMA* 257:1905–11, 1987.
41. Davis LE. Reye's syndrome. In R McKendall, PJ Vinken, GW Bruyn (eds.), *Handbook of Clinical Neurology.* Vol. 56, *Viral Diseases.* Amsterdam: Elsevier, 1989. Pp. 149–177.
42. Reye RDK, Morgan G, Baral J. Encephalopathy and fatty degeneration of the viscera. A disease entity in childhood. *Lancet* 2:749–52, 1963.
43. Nausieda PA et al. Sydenham chorea: an update. *Neurology* 30:331–34, 1980.
44. Kennedy C, Carroll FD. Optic neuritis in children [trans.]. *Am Acad Ophthalmol Otolaryngol* 64:700–712, 1960.
45. Cohen MM, Lessell S, Wolf PA. A prospective study of the risk of developing multiple sclerosis in uncomplicated optic neuritis. *Neurology* 29:208–13, 1972.
46. Bordley JE, Brookhouser PE, Worthington EL. Viral infections and hearing: a critical review of the literature. 1969–1970. *Laryngoscope* 82:557–77, 1972.
47. Hancock DO. A study of 49 patients with acute spinal extradural abscess. *Paraplegia* 10:285–88, 1973.
48. Del Curling O, Gower DJ, McWhorter JM. Changing concepts in spinal epidural abscess: a report of 29 cases. *Neurosurgery* 27:185–92, 1990.
49. Erntell M et al. Magnetic resonance imaging in the diagnosis of spinal epidural abscess. *Scand J Infect Dis* 20:323–27, 1988.
50. Kaufmann DM, Kaplan JG, Litman N. Infectious agents in spinal epidural abscess. *Neurology* 30: 844–50, 1980.
51. Querfurth H, Swanson PD. Vaccine-associated paralytic poliomyelitis: regional case series and review. *Arch Neurol* 47:541–44, 1990.
52. Davis LE, Reed WP. Infections of the central nervous system. In Rosenberg RN (ed.), *The Clinical Neurosciences* (Vol. 1). New York: Churchill Livingston, 1983. Pp. 351–53.
53. Dalakas MC et al. A long-term follow-up study of patients with post-poliomyelitis neuromuscular symptoms. *N Engl J Med* 314:959–63, 1986.
54. Berman M et al. Acute transverse myelitis: incidence and etiologic considerations. *Neurology* 31:966–71, 1981.
55. Osame M et al. Nationwide survey of HTLV-I-associated myelopathy in Japan: association with blood transfusion. *Ann Neurol* 28:50–56, 1990.
56. Mody CK et al. Neurologic complications of cocaine abuse. *Neurology* 38:1189–93, 1988.
57. Ropper AH, Postkanzer DC. The prognosis of acute and subacute transverse myelopathy based on early signs and symptoms. *Ann Neurol* 4:51–59, 1978.
58. Habermann E. Tetanus. In PJ Vinken, GW Bruyn (eds.), *Handbook of Clinical Neurology.* Vol. 33, *Infections of the Nervous System.* Amsterdam: North-Holland, 1978. Pp. 491–547.
59. Asbury AK, Cornblath DR. Assessment of current diagnostic criteria for Guillain-Barré syndrome. *Ann Neurol* 27(suppl):S21–24, 1990.
60. McKhann GM. Guillain-Barré syndrome: clinical and therapeutic observations. *Ann Neurol* 27 (suppl):S13–S16, 1990.
61. Cherington M. Botulism: ten-year experience. *Arch Neurol* 30:432–37, 1974.
62. Arnon SS, Chin J. The clinical spectrum of infant botulism. *Rev Infect Dis* 1:614–24, 1979.
63. Lupton MD, Klawans HL. Neurological complications of diphtheria. In PJ Vinken, GW Bruyn (eds.), *Handbook of Clinical Neurology.* Vol. 33, *Infections of the Nervous System.* Amsterdam: North-Holland, 1978. Pp. 479–89.
64. Younger B, Michaud M, Fischer M. Leprosy. Our southwest Asian refugee experience. *Arch Dermatol* 118:981–84, 1982.
65. Dastur DK. Leprosy. In PJ Vinken, GW Bruyn (eds.), *Handbook of Clinical Neurology.* Vol. 33, *Infections of the Nervous System.* Amsterdam: North Holland, 1978. Pp. 421–68.
66. Sabin TD, Swift TR. Leprosy. In PJ Dyck et al. (eds.), *Peripheral Neuropathy* (vol. II). Philadelphia: Saunders, 1984. Pp. 1955–87.

Systemic Infections with Headache or Neurologic Signs

Judith C. Brillman

The patient with the acute onset of a fever and a headache or abnormal neurologic signs is one of the most challenging patients an emergency physician will be called on to treat. The illness the patient may have ranges from a self-limiting virus to bacterial meningitis, a medical emergency. Alternatively these symptoms may represent an immunologic or other noninfectious process. It may be difficult or impossible to distinguish among many of these processes while the patient is in the emergency department. The emergency physician must determine if the patient's symptoms are disturbing enough to warrant continued workup and, if they are, to make the appropriate arrangements.

This chapter considers infectious causes of headache, altered level of consciousness (ALOC), and focal neurologic signs that are not primarily neurologic in nature but that may result in these symptoms. Principles of the examination for these symptoms and infectious diseases with primary involvement of the CNS were discussed in Chap. 7. This chapter discusses clues presented by the history and the physical exam that may aid the practitioner in distinguishing among these illnesses.

In the case of headache the emergency physician must determine if the headache results only from the fever, if the headache is significantly predominant to serve as an important clue in the differential diagnosis, or if meningismus truly exists. Many of the entities discussed here are multisystemic, with headache only one part of a constellation of symptoms. In the evaluation of the patient with a stiff neck and a headache, the practitioner must determine early on whether the stiff neck is indeed meningismus or an extension of the myalgias experienced in most febrile illnesses. Tests such as a WBC count and an erythrocyte sedimentation rate (ESR) are rarely helpful in distinguishing one infectious process from another or in differentiating an infectious disease from a noninfectious process (see Chap. 3). The lack of meningismus will lead the practitioner to consider the entities listed in Tables 8-1 and 8-2 as the most likely members of the differential diagnosis. The patient with meningismus must undergo an expeditious but complete neurologic examination to rule out focal neurologic disease. The practitioner must consider the entities listed in Table 8-3. Noninfectious causes of fever and headache that also must be considered are listed in Table 8-4. Symptoms and signs in addition to fever and headache that may help narrow the differential diagnosis considerably are listed in Tables 8-5 and 8-6. Table 8-7 lists diseases that cause meningoencephalitis by the time-course of presentation.

ALOC or focal neurologic signs may represent a

Table 8-1. Systemic infections
with rare neurologic involvement

Bacterial Diseases
Sepsis of any etiology
Ehrliciosis
Legionella
Mycoplasmal pneumonia
Psittacosis
Relapsing fever
Rocky Mountain spotted fever
Shigellosis
Tularemia
Typhoid fever
Typhus

Viral Diseases
Colorado tick fever
Cytomegalovirus
Dengue fever
Infectious mononucleosis
Influenza
Viral hepatitis
Yellow fever

Parasitic Disease
Malaria

Lymphocytic Meningitis Found
Mononucleosis syndrome
Mycoplasmal pneumonia
Psittacosis
Rocky Mountain spotted fever

Table 8-2. Infections of the face that cause headache

Herpes zoster
Mucormycosis
Otitis media
Periorbital/orbital cellulitis
Sinusitis
Tooth abscess

Table 8-3. Infections of multiple organ
systems with direct CNS involvement

Acute Meningitis
Neutrophils predominate
  Focal bacterial infection with CNS seeding
  Strongyloidiasis (gram-negative bacilli)
Lymphocytes predominate
  Enterovirus
  Kawasaki disease
  Leptospirosis
  Lyme disease
  Lymphochoriomenigitis
  Syphilis (secondary)

Chronic Meningitis
Tuberculosis
Coccidiomycosis
Brucellosis
Neurosyphilis (tertiary)

Infections with Common Focal Neurologic Findings
Actinomycosis
Bacterial cerebral abscess
Blastomycosis
Cryptococcosis
Cystercercosis
Herpes encephalitis
Lyme disease
Neurosyphilis (tertiary)
Nocardiosis
Phycomycosis
Progressive multifocal leukoencephalopathy
Subdural empeyema
Toxoplasmosis
Tuberculosis

---

more severe form of any disease that causes headache. Fever, dehydration, and sepsis—all independently can result in ALOC. This is particularly true of the patient who is debilitated or at the extremes of age. Alternatively, direct invasion of the CNS by organisms occurs in many multisystem diseases. This can result in a wide variety of neurologic signs, depending on the extent of illness and the site of involvement. This is the case for all entities listed in Table 8-3. Febrile seizures that occur in children less than 5 years of age may be confused with neurologic disease (see Chap. 14).

Table 8-4. Noninfectious causes of fever
and headache or neurologic signs

Immunologic diseases
  Arteritis
  Systemic lupus erythematosus
  Sarcoidosis
Heat illness
Drugs
Miscellaneous causes
  Malignancy
  Neurogenic fever
  Mollaret's meningitis

Table 8-5. Diseases by symptoms and history

	Symptoms				History	
	Abdominal complaints	Biphasic fever	Nasal symptoms	Sore throat	Animal contact or insect exposure	Travel history/ geographic preference
Blastomycosis						X
Brucellosis	X				X	
Cocciodiomycosis						X
Colorado tick fever	X	X			X	X
Dengue fever		X	X	X	X	X
Ehrlichiosis					X	
Enterovirus	X		X			
Viral hepatitis	X		X	X		
Influenza			X	X		
Kawasaki disease	X					
Legionella	X					
Leptospirosis	X	X		X	X	
Lyme disease	X			X	X	
Malaria					X	X
Meningococcemia			X	X		
Mononucleosis syndrome	X			X		
Mucormycosis	X		X			
Mycoplasma syndrome	X		X	X		
Psittacosis	X				X	
Relapsing fever	X	X			X	X
RMSF	X				X	X
Sepsis	X					
Syphilis	X			X		
Tuberculosis	X					
Tularemia	X				X	
Typhoid fever	X					X
Typhus	X				X	X
Yellow fever	X	X			X	X

Infectious Causes of Headache

Vascular Dilation versus CNS Disease

Patients with fever and headache represent a heterogeneous group of patients. Fever, by causing intracranial vasodilation, results in headache. We are all familiar with this type of headache, which can be frontal, bitemporal, or retro-orbital. It is constant, throbbing, and worsened by movement. It is relieved at least partially by antipyretics.

The overall appearance of a patient with fever and headache depends on the severity of the underlying illness. The patient with a low-grade fever and a minor headache who is alert and has no focal neurologic signs will rarely have a life-threatening illness. As with most statements in medicine, however, this one is not absolute, since the patient may be presenting very early in the course of a disease that may be quite serious. Many diseases may present with a prodrome that is difficult to distinguish from a self-limited viral syndrome. These illnesses include meningococcal meningitis, Colorado tick fever, dengue fever, yellow fever, and tularemia.

Table 8-6. Diseases by sign

	Arthralgia/ arthritis	Bradycardia (relative)	Conjunctivitis (scleral suffusion)	Jaundice	Lymphadenopathy	Pneumonitis	Rash
Blastomycosis						X	X
Brucellosis	X	X			X	X	X
Coccidiomycosis	X				X	X	X
Colorado tick fever			X			X	X
Dengue fever	X		X	X	X		X
Ehrliciosis	X	X					X
Enterovirus							X
Viral hepatitis	X			X			X
Influenza	X		X		X	X	
Kawasaki disease	X		X		X		X
Legionella		X				X	
Leptospirosis		X	X	X	X	X	X
Lyme disease	X		X		X		X
Malaria				X			
Meningococcemia	X					X	X
Mononucleosis syndrome				X	X		X
Mucormycosis						X	X
Mycoplasma syndrome	X				X	X	X
Nocardia						X	
Psittacosis	X	X				X	X
Relapsing fever			X	X		X	X
RMSF			X	X	X	X	X
Sepsis	X			X	X	X	X
Syphilis	X			X	X		X
Tuberculosis	X				X	X	
Tularemia		X		X	X	X	
Typhoid fever	X		X			X	
Typhus		X	X	X	X	X	
Yellow fever	X	X	X				

Diagnosis of a specific syndrome or illness is facilitated by identifying symptoms or signs that point toward a particular diagnosis. The headache and fever of the patient with coryza and nasal congestion probably does result from a simple upper respiratory tract infection. As the patient looks more ill and the headache becomes a more significant component of the symptom complex, the more difficult it is to rule out on clinical grounds an infection involving the CNS. The febrile patient who repeatedly focuses on the headache or neck or back pain may be giving the physician the only clue to the presence of meningitis.

Further complicating the situation is the aforementioned difficulty of distinguishing the stiff neck that is a manifestation of a generalized myalgia from true meningismus. The patient with neck pain from myalgia may actually be able to move the neck with minimal discomfort, while true meningismus elicits more pain. Myalgia may cause pain on neck movement in all directions, while meningismus causes the most pain on movement of the neck in the sagittal plane. The patient with myalgia may report neck stiffness with sagittal movement, but the one with meningismus will actively resist movement in that direction. An important cause of meningismus

Table 8-7. Diseases that cause meningoencephalitis

Acute (<24 hours)	Subacute (1–7 days)	Chronic
Pyogenic bacteria[a]	Pyogenic bacteria[a]	Tuberculosis
Primary amebic meningoencephalitis (*Naegleria*)	Partially treated bacterial meningitis	Fungal infections[a, b, d]
	Listeriosis	Tertiary syphilis
	Viral infection	Lyme disease
	Secondary syphilis	Brucellosis
	Leptospirosis	
	Relapsing fever	
	Lyme disease	
	Cerebral malaria[a, b]	
	Granulomatous amebic encephalitis[a]	
	Toxoplasmosis (*Acanthamoeba*)	
	Strongyloidiasis[c]	
	Tuberculosis	
	Postinfectious leukoencephalitis[a]	

[a] Discussed in Chapter 7.
[b] Clinical course may be accelerated in immunosuppressed individuals.
[c] Hyperinfection syndrome.
[d] Cryptococcosis, coccidioidomycosis, histoplasmosis, blastomycosis, candidiasis, mucormycosis.

that is often overlooked includes infections of the cervical facial spaces. A complete exam of the mouth, pharynx, and neck is necessary to rule out these conditions. (See Chap. 21 and Chap. 36.)

Any symptoms or signs, no matter how subtle, that point to neurologic involvement should be considered seriously. Determining that a patient is alert or has no focal neurologic signs is frequently difficult. For instance, irritability, inattention, apathy, lethargy, or difficulty with concentration, may be secondary only to generalized malaise, or they may be symptoms of severe systemic illness or CNS involvement. Complaints such as blurred vision, "funny vision," diplopia, photophobia, weakness, or unwillingness to get out of bed can indicate serious problems. (See Chap. 7 for a more complete discussion of the examination for altered mental status and focal neurologic signs.)

Infections of the Face or Head

Any infection of the face or head may cause fever and headache (see Table 8-2). The headaches may be acute or chronic, depending on the course of the underlying disease. There may be localized pain or tenderness over the infected area. The headache of sinusitis is a constant pressure sensation (see Chap.

34). Sinusitis may be accompanied by rhinitis or nasal congestion. The headache generally lies over the affected sinus. Tenderness localizing to the underlying sinus aids in diagnosis. The frontal and maxillary sinuses are easy to palpate, thereby facilitating diagnosis. Ethmoid and sphenoid sinusitis present more difficulties. Sphenoid sinusitis, because of its proximity to the CNS and inaccessibility to direct examination, is particularly difficult to diagnose. The headache may be most prominent at the vertex. In a study of 30 patients with fever and headache due to sphenoid sinusitis, the correct diagnosis was made in only 50% [1]. Clues to headache of dental origin may be pain on eating or pain with a change in mouth temperature (see Chap. 36). Periorbital cellulitis may be indicated by swelling and erythema about the eye, while in orbital cellulitis movement of the eye will be painful (see Chap. 35). Otitis media is rarely confused with facial pain of other etiologies (see Chap. 34). The patient with CNS mucormycosis will present with a chronic course. A low-grade fever and dull headache may be noted. Nasal discharge is tinged with blood. There will be a history of underlying illness, such as diabetes mellitus (see Chap. 16).

Herpes zoster (shingles) frequently involves the head. This disease occurs most commonly in people in the sixth to eighth decades of life. Intense pain in the affected dermatome may precede the rash by 2–3 days. The trigeminal nerve is often affected. Also involved may be the sensory branch of the facial nerve, leading to pain in the tongue and ear canal (Ramsay Hunt syndrome). Postherpetic neuralgia may affect over half of patients. CNS involvement can lead to symptoms of meningitis (see Chap. 32).

Systemic Infections

Infections with Rare Direct Neurologic Involvement

Many systemic diseases present with fever and headache. ALOC or neurologic signs can result from these illnesses. These entities include those whose usual presentations are with nonneurologic focal infections or sets of symptoms but that on occasion present with fever and headache or neurologic signs. The symptoms of these diseases can mimic illnesses in which the CNS is directly invaded. The emphasis in this section is on those diseases in which the CNS generally is not directly involved and in which, should an LP be done, the cerebrospinal fluid (CSF) usually is clear (see Table 8-1). In some of these diseases the pathogenic organism occasionally localizes to the CNS.

MECHANISM OF ALOC

Systemic infections can cause ALOC by resulting in hypoxia, hypercapnia, hypotension, hypoglycemia, hypo- and hyperosmolar states, alterations of pH, and electrolyte imbalances. Bacteria and toxins can compete for nutrients or inhibit enzymatic reactions in the brain. Extremes of body temperature (>41°C) cause coma through an alteration of neuronal metabolism. ALOC and fever may be the only signs of severe systemic infections. Systemic infections usually do not cause focal or lateralizing signs. When focal signs are present, they are transient. Brainstem function and brain imaging generally are normal. Residua from previous neurologic disease can also confuse the clinical picture. Infections may magnify underlying neurologic disorders.

Systemic infections, while not so severe as to cause coma, can cause other decreases in mental function. Alertness, attentiveness, and ability to concentrate may be affected first. These may be the first subtle signs of infection, especially in the elderly. Confusion may lead to idleness, as noted by the English phrase referring to the patient who has "taken to his bed." Only automatic acts and verbal responses may be preserved. Reactions may be slow or answers brief and mechanical.

Systemic infections can also result in agitation and irritability. Perceptual disturbances and hallucinations may occur. The patient may be restless and tremulous. Talk may be constant and incoherent. Paranoia results from the misinterpretation of outside stimuli.

SPECIFIC ENTITIES

Generalized Symptoms. The patient with gram-negative or gram-positive sepsis may present with symptoms ranging from headache to ALOC to coma (see Chap. 6). Many patients will appear extremely ill, but the diagnosis is most difficult in those with more subtle presentations. Fever is usual, but the patient may be hypothermic or euthermic. Sepsis should be suspected in any patient with a chronic illness or immunologic compromise. Signs of a focal disease, such as pneumonia or endocarditis, that has disseminated should be sought. A hyperdynamic state characterized by tachycardia out of proportion to the degree of fever, tachypnea, and vasodilation may be noted. If a change in the level of consciousness is significant, an LP will be necessary to rule out the spread of the pathogenic organism to the CNS.

Influenza generally occurs as a pandemic in the winter. It begins abruptly with a fever rising to 38°–39°C over the first day, with chills, myalgia, and malaise. Headache, either generalized or frontal, may be prominent. Respiratory symptoms include dry cough, sore throat, and nasal discharge and obstruction. Physical examination is remarkable only for cervical adenopathy and occasionally scattered rhonchi and wheezing on chest exam. The respiratory symptoms and pandemic nature can help distinguish influenza from other illnesses. The nasal symptoms are usually more pronounced in the common cold and are not present in many other systemic infections. The clinical spectrum of influenza can range from being indistinguishable from the common cold to a severe illness with little coryza. Neurologic complications from influenza are rare but include encephalitis, transverse myelitis, and Guillain-Barré syndrome (see Chap. 7). Reye's syndrome may follow influenza B (see Chap. 7).

Fever, headache, chills, and malaise are also part of the symptom complex of the infectious mononucleosis syndrome caused by the Epstein-Barr virus (EBV) or cytomegalovirus (see Chap. 11). EBV causes a diffuse pharyngitis with exudate and lymphadenopathy in 90% of patients with this syndrome. Fever is present in 90%, is higher in the late afternoon, and ranges from low grade to 40°C. Neurologic complications occur in fewer than 5% of patients and may be found in the absence of other symptoms. These complications include cranial nerve palsies and encephalitis, leading to confusion with herpes simplex encephalitis. Neurologic symptoms may herald the onset of mononucleosis or occur during convalescence. Other complications of mononucleosis can confuse the diagnosis and include cardiac, hematologic, hepatic, splenic, and pulmonary problems. Clinically significant cytomegalovirus disease is more common in the immunocompromised patient. The lungs, liver, gastrointestinal tract, and retina may be involved. Less often CNS involvement is noted, and symptoms are mild and nonspecific.

Respiratory Symptoms. Legionellosis generally presents with pulmonary findings (see Chap. 24). However, in the acute, self-limited manifestation called Pontiac fever, headache, fever, and myalgia may predominate. Clinically it resembles influenza. In those with Legionnaires' disease, headache or neurologic signs may accompany pulmonary findings. In a study of 912 patients, neurologic symptoms occurred in 30%. Mental changes ranging from confusion to coma were most common, while cerebellar ataxia was the most common focal neurologic sign. CSF usually is normal, although pleocytosis may be found in 20% [2].

Mycoplasma pneumoniae, a common cause of respiratory infections and atypical pneumonia, causes neurologic problems in about 0.1% of patients [3]. These problems follow the respiratory symptoms by about 10 days and occur most frequently in males under age 20. Meningoencephalitis, cerebellar ataxia, myelitis, and Guillain-Barré syndrome all have been reported (see Chap. 7). CSF abnormalities are variable but can include a lymphocytic pleocytosis and increased pressure.

Psittacosis, a disease of bird handlers, presents with fever and often a severe headache (see Chap. 23). Myalgia, dry cough, a relative bradycardia, and abnormal chest x-ray are commonly noted. Spasm of the neck and back may be prominent. Meningoencephalitis is uncommon.

Gastrointestinal Symptoms. The initial manifestations of typhoid fever are often severe, generalized headache and fever. The fever may increase in a stepwise pattern until it reaches 40°C in the first week. Abdominal symptoms, a dry cough, and rash (rose spots) may also be noted. The generalized infection may be so severe as to lead to alterations in mental status. The bacteria may localize in any body tissue, including the CNS. Typhoid fever is also a disease of travel.

Shigellosis, while primarily a cause of gastroenteritis, may have extraintestinal manifestations, including seizures (see Chap. 25). These are most common in children under age 5 and may not be accompanied by a high fever. Transient peripheral neuropathies and Guillain-Barré syndrome may occur rarely.

Any viral hepatitis that leads to fulminant hepatic failure causes mental status changes, beginning with lethargy, somnolence, and personality change. Agitation, confusion, or aggressiveness may be noted. More severe hepatic failure leads to stupor and coma.

Tick-Borne Illness. Rickettsial diseases (see Chap. 11), such as Rocky Mountain spotted fever (see Chap. 9) and murine typhus, manifest initially by abrupt onset of headache and fever, which may rise to 40°C. The headache is excruciating and can be generalized or frontal. The characteristic rash may not appear until the fourth or fifth day. Rigors, nausea, vomiting, and myalgias are also present [4]. Neurologic manifestations are common, beginning with headache, restlessness, neck and back stiffness, and photophobia. These may progress to muscular rigidity, coma, seizures, and deafness. In moderate to severe disease it may be necessary to perform an LP to rule out meningitis. The CSF findings will be normal or may contain a few lymphocytes or mildly elevated protein [5]. At least half the cases of Rocky Mountain spotted fever occur in the southern Atlantic and southern central states. The geographic history, a history of tick bite, or occurrence during seasons of tick activity help support the diagnosis of Rocky Mountain spotted fever. The manifestations of typhus are generally milder than those of Rocky Mountain spotted fever. Typhus is most common in the southeastern and Gulf Coast states and is transmitted by fleas.

An unusual rickettsial disease spread by ticks is ehrlichiosis. A prodrome of malaise, low back pain, and nausea occurs. Headache, high fever, and a relative bradycardia follow. Unlike RMSF a rash is rare. The illness is most common in those persons exposed to dogs that harbor ticks in the southeastern and southern central areas of the United States.

Animal contact or tick bite supports the diagnosis of tularemia (see Chap. 11). The patient will usually have a papule or ulcer at the site of entry. Fever, headache, chills, myalgias, and malaise occur. The eyes, pharynx, GI tract, or lungs may be involved. Meningitis has been reported.

Relapsing fever, caused by *Borrelia* spirochetes, is either louse- or tick-borne and can be a disease of travel. The patient may have the acute onset of fever to 40°C, headache, myalgia, cough, and abdominal symptoms. Meningismus occurs in 40% of patients [6]. Hepatic and splenic tenderness, jaundice, and bleeding also are common. Cerebral hemorrhage may occur. Crisis occurs either with resolution of the fever or antibiotic treatment. One or more relapses are also noted.

Colorado tick fever, an arbovirus infection, usually occurs in persons with extensive outdoor exposure in late May to July. The clinical symptoms are similar to those of dengue fever. Aseptic meningitis and encephalitis have been reported with this disease.

Diseases of Travel. Diseases encountered by travelers may cause fever, headache, and neurologic signs (see Chap. 12). This is true of dengue fever and yellow fever. Dengue fever causes a severe headache, fever to 40°C, and excruciating myalgias. Retro-orbital pain, photophobia, ocular soreness, and scleral injection are characteristic. A rash may occur, and a hemorrhagic form exists. CNS symptoms such as seizure and coma are terminal events. Dengue is found in the tropics and subtropics, including Mexico and the Caribbean. Yellow fever is similar to dengue, although the myalgias are not as severe and the ocular symptoms not as prominent. Severe yellow fever results in hemorrhage and CNS manifestations that include agitation, delirium, and coma.

If a patient with malaria (see Chap. 12) presents during a paroxysm, fever up to 41°C and headache will be prominent, and delirium may occur. Myalgia, splenomegaly, and anemia may be noted. The only unique characteristic of this illness is the intermittent nature of the paroxysm, which is not always present. Malaria is endemic in areas of Central and South America, Africa, Asia, and the Pacific basin. Cerebral malaria is the most serious complication and occurs only with *Plasmodium falciparum*. It results in an encephalopathy, signs of which include depressed consciousness, seizures, gaze disturbances, and altered tone and reflexes. CSF findings usually are normal, although pressure may be increased.

Infections with Common Direct Neurologic Involvement

In many systemic diseases direct neurologic involvement commonly occurs. In all the diseases considered in this section, the CNS findings are abnormal. Initially cellular elements may be mostly polymorphonuclear neutrophil leukocytes (PMNs), but as the infection becomes established, a mononuclear pleocytosis is noted. CSF pressure and protein are mildly elevated, while glucose is normal. Table 8-3 lists diseases of multiple organ systems in which the CNS is directly invaded.

SYSTEMIC DISEASES

Any systemic bacterial disease can localize to the CNS, and bacterial meningitis can develop. The diagnosis of a localized infection does not lower the likelihood of meningitis. Headache, neck pain, backache, drowsiness, or apathy should not automatically be attributed to the presence of an infection outside the CNS, unless infection in the CNS has been ruled out. In certain circumstances some bacteria localize to the CNS more often than others. Examples of these include *Haemophilus influenzae* type B in young children and *Neisseria meningitides* and *Streptococcus pneumoniae* in both children and adults. Neonatal meningitis can be caused by group B streptococcus or *Escherichia coli. Listeria monocytogenes* causes meningitis in 70%–80% of cases and occurs in neonates and pregnant, debilitated, and immunosuppressed adults [7]. Gram-negative organisms can result in meningitis in elderly, immunocompromised, and hospitalized patients. A systemic bacterial infection can also result in a cerebral abscess.

Leptospirosis (see Chaps. 11 and 26) is a biphasic illness presenting with the abrupt onset of headache, myalgias, a rising fever to 39°C or greater, and conjunctival suffusion in 33%–85%. In the second, or immune, phase 5%–15% of patients experience meningitis. Delirium and mood disturbances are the most common neurologic symptoms, but cranial nerve palsies and other focal neurologic signs may occur. CSF will have 50–1000 WBC/μl, and lymphocytes will usually, but not always predominate. CSF pressure is usually raised, protein ranges from 0.4–3.0 g/l, and glucose is normal [8–10].

A variety of viruses can invade the CNS, causing some of the usual nonspecific viral symptoms. Enterovirus, particularly coxsackievirus and echovirus, are responsible for more than 50% of acute lymphocytic meningitis in temperate climes [11]. In the preimmunization era, mumps was the most common viral cause of lymphocytic meningitis. (See Chaps. 7 and 31 for a more complete discussion of viral meningitis.)

Lymphocytic choriomeningitis (LCM) virus usually causes a syndrome similar to influenza. The disease almost always is secondary to exposure to small laboratory animals, such as hamsters. Fever, headache (generally retro-orbital), malaise, and myalgias are common, as are mild respiratory and abdominal complaints. These symptoms wax and wane over 1–3 weeks. In those with neurologic involvement, the fever and headache reoccur. Symptoms of meningitis, encephalitis, or focal CNS involvement may be found. In all CNS involvement by these viral agents, the CSF findings are typical of lymphocytic meningitis.

An acute or subacute lymphocytic meningitis occurs in 1%–2% of patients with syphilis (see Chaps. 30 and 31). Neurosyphilis, part of the secondary stage, is more common in males than in females. The number of cases appears to be increasing. It occurs about 6 weeks after the primary infection and resembles a viral CNS infection. The affected individual is usually symptomatic for several weeks with headache, vomiting, irritability, and confusion. Seizures have been noted, as well as cranial nerve palsies. Skin lesions are common.

Meningovascular syphilis, part of the tertiary stage (see Chaps. 30 and 31), occurs within several years of the primary infection and can present with focal neurologic findings. The meningitic form is a granulomatous meningitis with all the features of bacterial meningitis, including fever, headache, confusion, seizures, aphasia, hemiparesis, and cranial nerve involvement, plus the finding of Argyll Robertson pupils (the pupils are small, irregular, and unresponsive to light or mydriatics but responsive to accommodation). Optic atrophy may occur. The meningitis may involve the base of the brain, leading to cranial nerve findings in about 40% of cases. An associated intracranial vasculitis can produce focal neurologic signs such as hemiparesis, basilar artery insufficiency, and hemianopsia. Hemiparesis is present at some time in the illness in about 85% of cases. Vascular involvement is important in the production of symptomatology and can lead to a sudden deficit as well as progressive neurologic symptomatology [12]. Cord infarction can occur. A gumma may mimic a brain neoplasm.

Tabes dorsalis appears 10–25 years after the primary syphilitic infection and leads to sensory deficits that can manifest as loss of joint position sense, loss of vibratory sensation, sensory ataxia, bladder dysfunction, and a wide-based foot-drop gait. Sharp, lancinating pains occur in the legs or abdomen. These pains are sudden and brief, occur in clusters, and are intolerable. The joints may be destroyed by repetitive trauma (Charcot joints). The tendon jerks are lost. Bladder and bowel function become impaired. The Argyll Robertson pupil is present in 70% of the cases of tabes dorsalis [13].

The diagnosis of neurosyphilis is established by an LP with a positive CSF Venereal Disease Research Laboratory (VDRL) test. The CSF will show a mild lymphocytic pleocytosis with elevated protein and normal glucose.

DISEASES WITH RASH

Lyme disease (see Chap. 12) is caused by an infection with the spirochete *Borellia burgdorferi*, which is transmitted to humans by ixodid ticks. Infection with this spirochete appears responsible for an ever increasing number of both acute and chronic neurologic constellations, and Lyme disease has become the great mimicker of other neurologic diseases [14].

In a study of 314 patients 64% had headache, 59% had fever, and 48% had stiff neck as presenting symptoms [15]. Multifocal neurologic manifestations occur in 5%–31% of Lyme disease [15–17], with a median onset of 4 weeks after the onset of erythema chronicum migrans. The triad of neurologic manifestations is made up of meningitis, cranial neuritis, and inflammation of spinal roots. Although sometimes incomplete this triad is considered to be a unique clinical picture. Various cranial neuropathies are present in 50% of those with Lyme meningitis, especially bilateral Bell's palsy. Spinal root involvement occurs in 32% [18]. Focal meningoencephalitis, which may be accompanied by seizures and headache, has been identified on brain imaging [19]. Encephalitis, encephalopathy, and psychiatric disorders have all been recognized. A myelopathy may appear. Neurologic involvement is not present in all cases of Lyme disease.

A mild chronic encephalopathy is a common late neurologic manifestation [20]. The period of latency resembles that in tertiary syphilis. A response to antibiotics supports the role of spirochetal infection. The encephalopathy may not be apparent until many months after the infection and presumably is a remote effect. Eighty-nine percent of the patients with chronic neurologic symptoms have encephalopathy, and 70% have polyneuropathy [21].

The differential diagnosis includes meningitis, encephalitis, vasculitis, Guillain-Barré syndrome, transverse myelitis, Bell's palsy, and multiple sclerosis.

CSF anti–*B. burgdorferi* antibody is a useful indicator of CNS involvement. An MRI may reveal multiple, small white-matter lesions suggestive of a multifocal inflammatory condition. The CSF will show normal opening pressure with elevated protein, normal glucose, and a predominantly mononuclear pleocytosis.

Coccidiomycosis is a disease of the southwest United States. Neurologic manifestations usually follow skin and respiratory manifestations within 3 months. Neurologic disease occurs in 30%–50% of individuals with disseminated disease [22]. Headache, personality change, and symptoms of chronic meningitis predominate, although granulomas may lead to focal CNS signs [23].

Kawasaki disease (see Chap. 14), generally noted for the fever, lymphadenopathy, and exanthem and enanthem it causes in children, may rarely cause a lymphocytic meningitis. Although the agent has not been identified, it may well be infectious.

CHRONIC PRESENTATION

Although the incidence of tuberculosis (TB) has been declining, the association of tuberculosis with the epidemic of HIV infection may lead to an increased incidence of TB [24]. TB can occur within the nervous system as meningitis or as a mass lesion.

TB meningitis begins with listlessness, low-grade fever, anorexia, and headache. Lethargy is an initial finding in 44% of cases. Fever is present in 80% and headache in 62%. Nuchal rigidity is often minimal initially. With time stiff neck and confusion appear, followed by significant depression of consciousness, seizures, and focal neurologic signs. TB meningitis has a special propensity for involvement of the base of the brain and thus interferes with functioning of cranial nerves and the flow of CSF. Hydrocephalus may result. Focal lesions, when present, can occur secondary to panarteritis [25]. Focal deficits from this vasculitis can involve the brain, cranial nerves, or spinal cord [26]. Tremulousness and other involuntary movements may be seen. Seizures can occur at any time in the illness. Focal seizures are more common in adults and generalized seizures more common in children.

Although tuberculomas are relatively rare in the United States, in some parts of the world they represent the most common form of intracranial mass lesion. Tuberculomas, which present as focal intracranial masses, are usually located in the cerebral or cerebellar hemispheres, although occasionally they are found in the brain stem or spinal cord.

Another focal neurologic sign of TB is Pott's paraplegia. This condition is secondary to compression of the spine from TB infection of the vertebrae. The paraplegia can be relatively sudden in onset.

TB is difficult to distinguish from other causes of intracranial mass lesions and other forms of chronic meningitis, such as fungal infection. TB elsewhere in the body, a positive tuberculin skin test, or a close relative with TB is an important finding, but the absence of these findings does not exclude the possibility of TB in the nervous system.

CSF examination shows a moderate mononuclear pleocytosis, an elevated protein, and a low glucose. CSF pressure may be elevated. Culture of the CSF for TB and acid-fast stain is in order. Brain imaging may reveal the presence of a tuberculoma.

Brucellosis (undulant fever) (see Chap. 11) may be found in those with contact with cattle, swine, goats, or sheep or those who drink unpasteurized milk. A toxic course may occur, but an insidious course of low-grade fever, headache, and myalgia may be noted. Localized disease can occur at any of several organ systems. Neurologic involvement includes meningoencephalitis, myelitis, radiculitis, or peripheral neuropathy. Neurologic involvement is more often chronic than acute. CSF changes are characteristic of a chronic meningitis.

Actinomycosis is a chronic bacterial disease characterized by contiguous invasion, usually spreading from the mouth, intestine, or lung. Neurologic involvement takes the form of a brain abscess and is rare.

Blastomycosis is an uncommon fungal infection that rarely may spread from the lungs to the CNS. Chronic meningitis or cerebral abscesses may be found. Skin and bone involvement are common.

IMMUNOCOMPROMISE

Of adults with HIV infection 31%–65% will have neurologic complications (see Chaps. 17 and 31). Symptoms have involved the brain, spinal cord, and peripheral nerves. The earliest abnormalities occurring in 67% of seropositive subclinical neurologic infections are found in nerve conduction velocity or in the EEG [27].

When constitutional symptoms of AIDS develop, mild cognitive impairment may be noted, as well as mononeuritis multiplex or distal symmetric polyneuropathy. After the primary infection an acute aseptic meningitis may appear, with the usual findings of headache, fever, stiff neck, and CSF pleocytosis. Acute Guillain-Barré syndrome or chronic inflammatory demyelinating polyneuropathy may occur. Herpes zoster may be found. Myelopathy and myopathy have been reported.

An AIDS dementia complex has been described in otherwise asymptomatic individuals with HIV infection. The earliest stage manifests as mild cognitive and motor dysfunction without impairment in work capacity or in activities of daily living [28].

In the later stages of symptomatic AIDS, CNS opportunistic infections may appear, such as toxoplasmosis and cryptococcal meningitis as well as progressive multifocal leukoencephalopathy (PML). Primary lymphoma of the brain can occur, with the production of focal findings [29].

An MRI is helpful in the differential diagnosis of CNS lesions in AIDS. The MRI may distinguish among toxoplasmosis, PML, cytomegalovirus infections, and HIV infection [30].

Nocardiosis generally is a disease of the immunocompromised. It begins with pulmonary involvement but can undergo hematogenous dissemination to any organ system. In addition to pulmonary disease, fever, malaise, and weight loss are noted. One-quarter to one-third of those with nocardiosis develop CNS complications [31]. Single or multiple brain abscesses are most common, although meningitis and spinal cord abscesses may occur.

Phycomycosis, in addition to causing rhinocerebral mucormycosis, can cause an acute systemic infection. Pulmonary symptoms are prominent, and the brain may be involved, as well as the liver, kidney, and spleen.

Strongyloidiasis occurs sporadically in the southern United States and Puerto Rico and is endemic in the tropics. The disease can result in rash and various pulmonary and abdominal complaints. Dissemination may occur in the immunocompromised host. The parasite can carry gram-negative bacteria from the GI tract and lead to gram-negative meningitis.

Noninfectious Causes of Fever and Headache

As is the case for infectious diseases noninfectious diseases can cause a spectrum of symptoms from headache to neurologic signs. Noninfectious causes of fever and headache often are overlooked; several of these are listed in Table 8-4. Some of the causes in this category can also cause focal neurologic disease, including seizures in the case of CNS stimulants and sedative hypnotic withdrawal and a depressed sensorium in the case of sedative hypnotics.

Immunologic Diseases

Immunologic disease can sometimes cause both fever and headache or neurologic symptoms. It is crucial that giant cell arteritis be included in this differential since its morbidity is great if untreated. In one study of 27 patients 87% had headache [32]. The headache is intense, throbbing, and constant. Low-grade fever is present in the majority of patients. Patients often note scalp tenderness and jaw claudication. Those affected are generally older than 60, and their ESR exceeds 50. Visual loss and cerebral infarction are the most serious complications of this process. Periarteritis nodosa can cause a similar clinical picture in all ages.

Systemic lupus erythematosus, although often causing fever, generally does not cause headache unless the CNS is directly involved, as it may be in 20%–50% of patients [33]. CNS symptoms vary depending on the degree of CNS involvement. The most common CNS manifestation is mild mental dysfunction. Deficits can occur from involvement of any portion of the brain, meninges, cranial nerves, spinal cord, or peripheral nerves. The CSF demonstrates a lymphocytosis and a slightly increased protein.

Sarcoidosis is a chronic, multisystem disease whose etiology may be immunologic. Acute or subacute sarcoidosis can cause symptoms such as fever, malaise, anorexia, and respiratory complaints. In the form that has an insidious onset, pulmonary symptoms are most prominent. Nervous systems complaints are found in 5% of individuals [34]. Transient facial nerve paralysis is most common, but other cranial nerve abnormalities or a chronic lymphocytic meningitis may be noted.

HEAT ILLNESS

The possibility of heat illness often is neglected if no history of exposure to a heat load is obtained. Heat exhaustion is characterized by headache, weakness, nausea, giddiness, and muscle cramps. Body temperature is usually less than 38°C. The sensorium is clear, and focal neurologic signs are not found. As the body loses its adaptive responses to the heat load, heat stroke occurs. The ability of the hypothalamus to regulate body temperature is lost. Necessary to the diagnosis of heat stroke is an elevated temperature, generally greater than 40°C and CNS dysfunction. Delirium, lethargy, stupor, and coma can occur. The extremities may be flaccid with decreased tendon reflexes. The heat load may be obvious, as in the exertion in the heat of an unacclimated person. It also may develop in patients (especially the urban elderly) exposed to high temperatures and humidity over a period of days who are unable to seek a cooler environment or who lack access to fluids. Patients will have headache, hot skin, and altered mental status. Dehydration alone can cause a fever and headache.

Drugs

In drug fever, an idiosyncratic reaction to therapeutic drug doses, headache occurs in more than 15% of patients. Other features are rigors (53%), myalgias (25%), hypotension (18%), and rash (18%). Fevers from 38°–43°C have been noted [35]. Multiple drugs have been implicated. The onset can range from a week to a month after administration of the drug.

Fever and headache or neurologic signs generally are not the predominant symptoms of any toxic drug interactions. However, because presentations may be atypical, several entities will be mentioned here. Monoamine oxidase inhibitors, when interacting with drugs such as narcotics or sympathomimetics, can cause these symptoms. CNS and peripheral sympathetic stimulation result in fever, headache, hyperreflexia, nausea, tremors, and palpitations. Another drug interaction that causes fever and headache is disulfiram with ethanol. Other symptoms include flushed skin, nausea, palpitations, dyspnea, tachycardia, and hypotension. Table 8-8 lists other drugs that can result in fever and headache.

Miscellaneous Causes

For many illnesses, fever and headache or neurologic signs may not consistently be the initial features, but an individual case may present to the emergency physician in this manner. In lymphoma fever commonly is the principle initial symptom. Acute leukemia may present with a high fever and prostration. Alternatively the fever may be low

Table 8-8. Drugs that can cause fever

Drugs	Comments
Interacting drugs	
MAO inhibitors and narcotics or sympathomimetics	
Disulfiram and ethanol	
Stimulants	Cause increased muscle
Cocaine	and CNS activity
Amphetamines	
LSD	
Sedative-hypnotics	Cause intracranial
Glutethimide	hypertension
Methyprylon	
Withdrawal	
Industrial chemicals (insecticides, refrigerants, propellants)	
Metal fumes	Cause metallic taste
Organochlorine	
Methyl chloride	
Methyl bromide	
Salicylates	Cause increased metabolic rate
Thyroid hormone	Causes increased metabolic rate

grade. In both malignancies headache, neck stiffness, and neurologic symptoms may occur when there is CNS infiltration.

Neurogenic fever results from an inability of the CNS to regulate body temperature. This condition occurs when the anterior hypothalamus is dysfunctional. A variety of other neurologic signs may be noted if the lesion extends from the hypothalamus to other areas of the brain. Fevers may rise to 41°C or be low grade. Tachycardia, tachypnea, cold extremities, and dry skin are noted. Antipyretic agents are ineffective. Other syndromes resulting from hypothalamic damage, such as endocrine and emotional problems, may be noted.

Mollaret's meningitis is an unusual and idiopathic cause of recurrent meningitis. Onset of fever and meningeal signs is abrupt. The CSF during the first day of illness will demonstrate 100–3000 WBC/μl, mostly PMNs and an unidentifiable mononuclear cell. An LP after 24 hours of symptoms will reveal a lymphocytic meningitis. It may reoccur within weeks or months for several years [36].

References

1. Lew D et al. Sphenoid sinusitis, a review of 30 cases. *N Engl J Med* 309:1149–54, 1983.
2. Johnson JD, Raff MJ, Van Arsdall J. Neurologic manifestations of legionaires' disease. *Medicine* 63: 303–10, 1984.
3. Wood M, Anderson M. *Neurologic Infections.* London: Saunders, 1988. P. 563.
4. Helmick CG, Bernard KW, D'Angelo LP. Rocky Mountain spotted fever: clinical, laboratory and epidemiologic features of 262 cases. *J Infect Dis* 150: 480–88, 1984.
5. Woodward T. Rickettsial diseases. In E Braunwald et al. (eds.), *Harrison's Principles of Internal Medicine* (12th ed.). New York: McGraw-Hill, 1991. Pp. 753–63.
6. Perine PL. Relapsing fever. In JD Wilson et al. (eds.), *Harrison's Principles of Internal Medicine* (12th ed.). New York: McGraw-Hill, 1991. Pp. 666–67.
7. Wood M, Anderson M. *Neurologic Infections.* London: Saunders, 1988. P. 108.
8. Sperber SJ, Schleupner CJ. Leptospirosis, a forgotten cause of aseptic meningitis and multisystem febrile illness. *South Med J* 82:1285–88, 1989.
9. Wood M, Anderson M. *Neurologic Infections.* London: Saunders, 1988. P. 161.
10. Sanford JP. Leptospirosis. In E Braunwald et al. (eds.), *Harrison's Principles of Internal Medicine* (12th ed.). New York: McGraw-Hill, 1991. Pp. 652–55.
11. Wood M, Anderson M. *Neurologic Infections.* London: Saunders, 1988. P. 143.
12. Reik L. Spirochaetal infections of the nervous system. In PGE Kennedy, RT Johnson (eds.), *Infections of the Nervous System.* London: Butterworths, 1987. Pp. 43–75.
13. Wolters EC. Neurosyphilis: a changing diagnostic problem? *Eur Neur* 26:23–28, 1987.
14. Halperin JJ et al. Lyme neuroborreliosis: central nervous system manifestations. *Neurology* 39: 753–59, 1989.
15. Steere AC et al. The early clinical manifestations of Lyme disease. *Ann Intern Med* 99:76–82, 1983.
16. Steere AC. Lyme borreliosis. In JD Wilson et al. (eds.), *Harrison's Principles of Internal Medicine* (12th ed.). New York: McGraw-Hill, 1991. Pp. 667–69.
17. Wood M, Anderson M. *Neurologic Infections.* London: Saunders, 1988. P. 141.
18. Pachner AR, Steere AC. The triad of neurologic manifestations of Lyme disease: meningitis, cranial neuritis and radiculoneuritis. *Neurology* 35:47–53, 1989.
19. Feder HM, Zalneraitis EL, Reik L. Lyme disease:

acute focal meningoencephalitis in a child. *Pediatrics* 82:931–34, 1988.

20. Halperin JJ et al. Lyme borreliosis-associated encephalopathy. *Neurology* 40:1340–43, 1990.

21. Logigian EL, Kaplan RF, Steere AC. Chronic neurologic manifestations of Lyme disease. *N Engl J Med* 323:1438–44, 1990.

22. Wood M, Anderson M. *Neurologic Infections.* London: Saunders, 1988. P. 244.

23. Sabetta JR, Andriole VT. Cryptococcal infections of the nervous system. *Med Clin North Am* 69:333–44, 1985.

24. Rieder HL et al. Epidemiology of tuberculosis in the United States. *Epidemiol Rev* 11:79–89, 1989.

25. Ogawa SK et al. Tuberculous meningitis in an urban medical center. *Medicine* 66:317–26, 1987.

26. Kocen RS. Tuberculosis of the nervous system. In PGE Kennedy, RT Johnson (eds.), *Infections of the Nervous System.* London: Butterworths, 1987. Pp. 23–42.

27. Koralnic IJ et al. A controlled study of early neurologic abnormalities in men with asymptomatic human immunodeficiency virus infection. *N Engl J Med* 323:864–70, 1990.

28. Sidtis JJ, Price RW. Early HIV-1 infection and the AIDS dementia complex. *Neurology* 40:323–26, 1990.

29. Human immunodeficiency virus (HIV) infection and the nervous system: report from the American Academy of Neurology AIDS Task Force. *Neurology* 39:119–22, 1989.

30. Jarvic JG et al. Acquired immunodeficiency syndrome: magnetic resonance patterns of brain involvement with pathologic correlation. *Arch Neurol* 45:731–36, 1988.

31. Wood M, Anderson M. *Neurologic Infections.* London: Saunders, 1988. P. 308.

32. Gonzalez EB et al. Giant-cell arteritis in the southern United States. *Arch Intern Med* 149:1561–65, 1989.

33. Hain BH. Systemic lupus erythematosus. In E Braunwald et al. (eds.), *Harrison's Principles of Internal Medicine, ed. 12.* McGraw-Hill Book Co., New York, 1991, Pp. 1418–1423.

34. Crystal RG. Sarcoidosis. In JD Wilson et al. (eds.), *Harrison's Principles of Internal Medicine,* (12th ed.). McGraw-Hill Book Co., New York, 1991, Pp. 1463–69.

35. Mackowiak PA. Southwestern Internal Medicine Conference. Drug fever: mechanisms, maxims and misconceptions. *Am J Med Sci* 294:275–86, 1987.

36. Hermans PE, Goldstein NP, Wellman WW. Mollaret's meningitis and differential diagnosis of recurrent meningitis. *Am J Med* 52:128–40, 1972.

9

Fever and Rash

GEORGE L. STERNBACH

The clinician's initial approach to the patient with rash and fever is identical to that employed with any emergency patient. After ensuring adequate airway exchange and respirations, attention must be directed to circulatory status. If shock is present, immediate intervention follows, with the administration of intravenous fluids and, if indicated, vasopressors.

Although such actions will be necessary in only a small portion of patients presenting with rash, in those instances in which hemodynamic instability is present, initiation of therapy should antecede the acquisition of a detailed history and the performance of strictly diagnostic investigations. In the patient whose clinical presentation is consistent with meningococcal sepsis or septic shock of other origin, the early institution of intravenous antibiotics is an additional priority.

A decision must be made early in the course of management regarding the need for isolation precautions. Isolation is required primarily for patients whose illness is likely to allow airborne transmission of infection. Medical personnel should also apply precautions in their exposure to blood, secretions, and other body fluids. Reverse isolation procedures may be required in the immunocompromised patient.

In obtaining a history the clinician first elicits information regarding the timing and the pattern of development of the rash, as well as its temporal relationship to other symptoms, such as fever, chills, and arthralgia. Attention should be paid to the prevalence of seasonal febrile illness, as well as the presence of current infectious outbreaks in the community. For example, infections with measles, varicella, and rubella are more common in the winter and spring. Rocky Mountain spotted fever has a higher incidence during the summer months. Additional pertinent information includes a history of the following:

- prior medical illness
- recent exposure to individuals with febrile illness
- exposure to rural habitat or animals
- travels outside the local area
- current use of medications
- drug allergy
- parenteral use of illicit drugs
- valvular heart disease
- sexually transmitted disease
- potential for immunosuppression (e.g., on the basis of malignancy, chemotherapy, steroid use, or asplenism)

Evaluation of the nature and the extent of the skin eruption is of primary importance in the physical examination. Prior to this evaluation, however, the general appearance of the patient, the degree of toxicity, and the vital signs are assessed. Important additional physical signs include the presence of genital or mucous membrane lesions, lymphadenopathy, hepatic or splenic enlargement, signs of articular or periarticular inflammation, meningismus, and nuchal rigidity.

Differential Diagnosis

Infections

The presence of a skin eruption in the patient who is acutely ill will frequently direct attention to the possibility of an infectious etiology. Early diagnosis of potentially life-threatening infections, such as meningococcemia and Rocky Mountain spotted fever, can be aided by the presence of distinctive cutaneous lesions. The skin eruption may, consequently, serve as a finding that directly guides appropriate initial therapy. Other diagnoses to immediately consider in the patient appearing toxic with rash include bacterial sepsis, toxic shock syndrome, and typhoid fever.

In many instances the patient suffering from a fulminant infectious process displays high fever, toxicity, and substantial vital sign alterations of tachycardia and hypotension. In such cases there is a wealth of indications of the severity of a particular presentation even prior to a skin eruption being identified. However, such may not be the case in all instances. An example is the debilitated or immunocompromised patient, who may present with a serious infection in the absence of one or more cardinal findings of infection (e.g., fever or leukocytosis). The presence of skin lesions can be valuable indicators of infection in such patients.

In other instances, although the clinical presentation may not be that of an overwhelming infection, a serious process may, nevertheless, be present and accompanied by distinctive skin manifestations. An example is subacute infective endocarditis, which may be difficult to recognize because of the nonspecific nature of many of the presenting findings. Early diagnosis of this entity may prevent subsequent morbidity. Other examples include illnesses caused by other spirochetes (Lyme disease and syphilis being the most obvious examples) that characteristically produce cutaneous manifesta-

tions in their early stages. When such illnesses can be diagnosed and treated during these stages, the substantial visceral damage that occurs in advanced disease can be avoided.

Although the concurrent presence of rash and fever is the hallmark of infectious illness, the presence of fever and rash does not invariably indicate infection, just as the absence of fever does not exclude an infectious process. Drug reaction and toxic epidermal necrolysis are noteworthy examples of noninfectious causes of rash and fever. Historical information, particularly a patient's antecedent use of medications, must always be carefully considered in the diagnostic process. Table 9-1 lists some diagnostic modalities that can be employed in the evaluation of the patient with skin eruption.

A number of serious infectious illnesses can produce petechial or purpuric eruptions. These diseases include meningococcemia, Rocky Mountain spotted fever, disseminated gonococcal infection, ehrlichiosis, dengue fever, typhus, leptospirosis, infectious endocarditis, and pseudomonas septicemia. Early in the course of most of these illnesses, however, the eruptions may be macular or maculopapular before they become petechial.

PETECHIAE

Bacteremia and Endocarditis. *Pseudomonas* septicemia has a tendency to occur in patients who are immunosuppressed and those with burns or ma-

Table 9-1. Diagnostic modalities

Disease	Modality
Dermatophyte	Scraping (KOH or Gram's stain)
Ecthyma gangrenosum	Biopsy
Erythema nodosum	Biopsy
Disseminated gonorrhea	Biopsy
Lesions in immuno-compromised host	Biopsy
Meningococcemia	Biopsy
Rocky Mountain spotted fever	Biopsy
Primary and secondary syphilis	Dark-field microscopy
Varicella zoster	Vesicle culture and Tzanck smear

lignant tumors. Petechiae and purpura on both the skin and the mucous membranes may occur in leptospirosis. There may be localization of the skin eruption to the shins. Physical findings that can be suggestive of this disease include hepatosplenomegaly, jaundice, and lymphadenopathy (see Chap. 25).

Skin eruption is not usually the most prominent aspect of the clinical picture of infective endocarditis. Lesions usually are sparse and have a predilection for the distal areas of the body. These lesions include Janeway's lesions, Osler's nodes, splinter hemorrhage, and petechiae. Associated physical findings (e.g., cardiac murmur, splenomegaly) should be sought. Many cases of native valve endocarditis (with which skin manifestations are most consistently associated) have a subacute onset. Fever is usually present but rarely above 39.4°C. The predominant symptoms (malaise, anorexia, fatigue, and weakness) are nonspecific. Endocarditis related to IV drug abuse is more likely to present as an acute fulminant disease, but skin manifestations are less common in this form of infective endocarditis (see Chap. 24).

Gonococcemia typically produces distal lesions, with involvement of the extremities being most common. There is usually sparing of the scalp, face, trunk, and oral mucous membranes. Lesions occur on the palms, soles, and periarticular areas and tend to be scanty but widely distributed. More cases occur in women than men, and symptoms of urogenital or anorectal gonorrhea may be present. Other associated findings of importance are tenosynovitis and monoarticular or oligoarticular arthritis.

Meningococcemia produces distal lesions mostly on the extremities and the trunk, but there may also be involvement of the head, palms, soles, and mucous membranes. Lesions are macular initially and may become petechial or purpuric, but they are not pustular in appearance, as are lesions of gonococcemia. Associated headache and meningismus should call to mind the possibility of associated meningococcal meningitis.

Travel-Related Infections. Eliciting a travel history is essential in the diagnosis of dengue and other hemorrhagic fevers. Dengue occurs in the eastern Mediterranean, southeast Asia (the Philippines, Vietnam, Thailand, Malaysia, Indonesia), Africa, India, Hawaii, and portions of the Caribbean. Features of the disease include the sudden onset of high fever, chills, fatigue, and myalgia. The rash has a predilection for the face, neck, and chest and may initially be maculopapular, morbilliform, or scarlatiniform. The hemorrhagic form of dengue fever can produce (in addition to a petechial eruption) bleeding gums, epistaxis, hematemesis, melena, hepatomegaly, and shock. (See Chap. 19.)

Bite-Related Infections. A history of bites by lice or ticks is helpful in the diagnosis of typhus, Rocky Mountain spotted fever, and Ehrlichiosis. Epidemic typhus is contracted through infestation with body lice. The eruption initially is pink and macular, beginning on the body and axillary folds and rapidly spreading to the rest of the body but sparing the face, palms, and soles. The macules may become hemorrhagic, and gangrene of the fingers, toes, and nose may occur.

Rocky Mountain spotted fever, unlike typhus, begins on the ankles and the wrists rather than on the trunk, although subsequent spread to the trunk does occur. Involvement of the palms and the soles is characteristic. Ehrlichiosis is a rickettsial disease closely related to Rocky Mountain spotted fever that most commonly occurs in males aged 30 to 60. In this disease an eruption occurs in only about 20% of cases. (See Chap. 12.)

MACULOPAPULAR RASHES
The patient with a maculopapular rash may appear extremely ill. Toxin-induced eruptions, such as staphylococcal scalded skin syndrome and toxic shock syndrome, do not become petechial, nor does the dermatosis of typhoid or Kawasaki syndrome. A number of specific criteria for toxic shock syndrome have been established (see pp. 183–184). In addition, the presence of conjunctival, oropharyngeal, or vaginal erythema and palmar edema may be indicators that toxic shock syndrome is present. Most cases have been described in menstruating women, but it can occur from any *Staphylococcus aureus* infection.

Kawasaki syndrome occurs almost exclusively during childhood. Over 75% of cases occur in children less than 5 years of age [1]. The syndrome does not occur in neonates and is uncommon after age 8. Involvement of the conjunctiva and oral mucosa is the rule, as is erythema of the palms and the soles.

The characteristic skin lesions of typhoid are "rose spots," hyperemic papules 2–4 mm in diameter and tending to occur on the trunk (see Chap. 26). Additional clinical findings that may be present in typhoid include abdominal pain and tenderness and splenomegaly.

Noninfectious Causes of Rash and Fever

DRUG ERUPTIONS

Virtually any type of dermatosis can be a consequence of a drug reaction. Drug eruptions can be exanthematous, urticarial, eczematous, vasculitic, purpuric, or photosensitive. Drugs may be the cause for eruptions of toxic epidermal necrolysis, erythema multiforme, and erythema nodosum. The most difficult differentiation of drug eruption is likely to be from a viral exanthem. Both usually are of abrupt onset, are generalized, and tend to be macular or papular in morphology. Fever may be present in either entity. The distinction requires interpretation of historical information and physical findings.

Drug reactions tend to appear within a week after the drug is taken. Skin lesions, however, may appear even after a drug has been discontinued if that agent or its metabolites persist in the system. Penicillin, sulfonamides, tetracyclines, salicylates and other nonsteroidal anti-inflammatory agents, barbiturates, and phenytoin are important causes of drug eruption.

TOXIC EPIDERMAL NECROLYSIS

Nonstaphylococcal-induced toxic epidermal necrolysis has as its main feature the separation of large sheets of epidermis from underlying dermis. The full thickness of epidermis is involved. The appearance of erythema usually precedes loosening of the epidermis. The onset is usually on the face, and mucous membrane involvement is the rule. Involvement of the eyes may be particularly troublesome, even resulting in permanent injury [2].

In patients with pigmented skin the pigment is entirely removed when the skin desquamates. This is unlike the situation in staphylococcal scalded skin syndrome (which toxic epidermal necrolysis resembles clinically), in which substantial pigment remains.

Toxic epidermal necrolysis is related to the use of drugs, infection, or medical illness, or is idiopathic.

The idiopathic form is associated with a substantial mortality. Drugs are an important cause of toxic epidermal necrolysis. Among those that have been implicated as inciting agents are the long-acting sulfa drugs, penicillin, aspirin, barbiturates, phenylbutazone, phenytoin, and allopurinol. Toxic epidermal necrolysis has followed vaccination and immunization against poliomyelitis, measles, smallpox, diphtheria, and tetanus. It also has been found in association with lymphoma.

The mechanism of production is not known. Treatment includes fluid replacement and the administration of systemic corticosteroids, although the benefit of corticosteroids is controversial.

The Immunocompromised Patient

The presence of a cutaneous eruption in a patient with immune compromise can be an important indicator that an infectious illness is present. By the same token skin eruptions occurring with atypical distributions or in severe forms should call to mind the possibility of an underlying immune system dysfunction. (More detailed discussions of infection in the immunocompromised patient are found in Chap. 16 and Chap. 17). Those infectious illnesses producing cutaneous manifestations most commonly encountered in immunocompromised patients are listed in Table 9-2. In some instances (e.g., herpes simplex, varicella-zoster, candidiasis) such infections undergo diffuse cutaneous or visceral dissemination and may become life threatening [3, 4].

Table 9-2. Infectious eruptions in immune system compromise

Bacterial
Staphylococcus
Pseudomonas
Viral
Herpes simplex
Varicella-zoster
Fungal
Candida
Coccidioides
Cryptococcus
Histoplasma

Lesion Morphology

The categorization of skin lesions traditionally is along morphologic lines. Lesions associated with infection can be macular, papular, maculopapular, vesicular, pustular, nodular, purpuric, or ulcerative. The most common infectious illnesses and the eruptions they produce are listed in Table 9-3. Morphologic identification of skin lesions is often the first step in diagnosing the etiology of a cutaneous eruption.

Most skin lesions have essentially round shapes. Annular lesions are those with a discernible and palpable ring-like border and a centrally normal or

Table 9-3. Morphologic appearances of various common eruptions

Illness	Macular	Papular/ maculopapular	Pustular	Vesicular	Nodular	Petechial/ purpuric	Ulcerative
Cellulitis	X						
Erysipelas	X						
Toxic shock syndrome	X						
Staphylococcal scalded skin syndrome	X						
Lyme disease	X	X					
Scarlet fever	X	X					
Meningococcemia	X	X				X	
Dermatophytosis	X	X					
Cryptococcosis	X	X					X
Infective endocarditis	X	X	X			X	
Syphilis	X	X					X
Rocky Mountain spotted fever	X	X				X	
Typhoid fever	X	X					
Gonococcemia		X	X			X	
Pseudomonas septicemia		X	X				X
Erythema multiforme	X	X		X			
Viral exanthem	X	X		X		X	
Measles		X		X			
Atypical measles				X		X	
Roseola		X					
Rubella		X				X	
Coccidioidomycosis		X	X		X		X
Histoplasmosis		X			X		
Folliculitis			X				
Herpes simplex				X			
Herpes zoster				X			
Varicella				X			
Coxsackievirus		X		X		X	
Erythema nodosum					X		
Candidiasis					X		
Sporotrichosis					X		X
Blastomycosis					X		X

Table 9-4. Annular lesions

Eruption	Etiologic agent	Distribution	Description
Tinea corporis	Dermatophytes	Variable	Scaly, brown
Erythema migrans	*Borrelia burgdorferi*	Variable, often thigh, groin, or axilla	Erythematous or bluish-red; may have central papule or vesicle
Erythema multiforme	Multiple	Variable, but often symmetrical, involving hands and feet	Hallmark is target lesion
Secondary syphilis	*Treponema pallidum*	Face	Circular or gyrate; slightly scaling edges
Urticaria	Multiple	Variable	Red or pink wheals
Bullous impetigo	*Staphylococcus aureus*	Variable, hands and face common	Crusted lesions

less involved area. An annular configuration is not common and should call to mind a number of possible infectious etiologies (Table 9-4).

The distribution of lesions occasionally is helpful in diagnosis. The palms of the hands and the soles of the feet are frequently spared in infectious eruptions. The presence of lesions on the palms and the soles is characteristic of a small number of illnesses (Table 9-5).

Macular Lesions

Macules are lesions characterized by a change in the color of the skin. There is no palpable component to the eruption. In infectious illness macular lesions usually are pink or red (although they may be hyper- or hypopigmented, for example, in cutaneous fungal infection) and usually blanch upon application of pressure, indicating that the erythema is due to vasodilation. Nonblanching erythematous eruptions are likely to be the consequence of extravasation of blood.

The presence of a purely macular eruption in

Table 9-5. Infectious eruptions involving the palms and soles

Erythema multiforme
Hand-foot-and-mouth disease
Infective endocarditis
Kawasaki syndrome
Rocky Mountain spotted fever
Secondary syphilis
Toxic shock syndrome

infectious illness is uncommon. A number of significant infectious illnesses, however, have a transient phase that includes the presence of a macular eruption. These diseases include dengue fever, typhus, typhoid fever, and leptospirosis. The presence of a diffuse macular erythroderma should call to mind a toxin-induced infectious syndrome, such as toxic shock syndrome, scarlet fever, or staphylococcal scalded skin syndrome. The distinction among these conditions must be made on the basis of nondermatologic clinical features. A localized macular eruption suggests a more focal infection, such as cellulitis.

Maculopapular Lesions

Papules are small (less than 1 cm) lesions that are raised above the surface of the skin. A maculopapular rash contains both macular and papular components, which tend to be confluent. A large variety of eruptions, both infectious and noninfectious, are maculopapular or papular. Maculopapular eruptions are characteristic of viral illness. Many viruses (often of childhood) are known to produce exanthems. In a few instances of viral infection the dermatologic features are characteristic, but in most others the eruption itself is not distinguishable from that produced by a variety of other viruses. The diagnosis in such cases is best made on the grounds of the remainder of the clinical picture, the distribution of lesions, and the direction of spread of those lesions. Tables 9-6 and 9-7 list these features for some common infectious illnesses of childhood with maculopapular eruptions (see Chap. 14).

Table 9-6. Characteristics of childhood exanthems

Illness	Area of initial involvement	Areas of subsequent involvement	Other features
Measles	Face or trunk	Extremities	Koplik's spots
Roseola	Trunk	Neck and extremities	High fever
Rubella	Face	Neck, trunk, and extremities	Lymphadenopathy
Scarlet fever	Chest	Head and extremities	Desquamation, pharyngitis
Hand-foot-and-mouth disease	Face or trunk	Extremities	Intraoral ulcerations
Chickenpox	Face or trunk	Extremities	Lesions in crops; lesions of different ages in same location

Table 9-7. Age and appearance of childhood exanthems

Illness	Peak age	Appearance of rash
Measles	3–6 years	Purplish-red maculopapules; confluent on face and neck
Roseola	6 months–3 years	Pink or rose-colored macules or maculopapules 2–3 mm in diameter
Rubella	5–9 years	Pink-red maculopapules that may coalesce
Scarlet fever	2–10 years	Pinhead-sized papules on an erythematous base with a sandpaper texture
Hand-foot-and-mouth disease	1–5 years	Erythematous macules and papules 2–10 mm in diameter that may become vesicular
Chickenpox	<3 years (90%)	Macules progressing to papules to vesicles 2–3 mm in diameter on erythematous base with crust

A number of bacterial and rickettsial infections may present with maculopapular eruptions, including meningococcemia, Rocky Mountain spotted fever, enteric fever due to *Salmonella typhi,* and secondary syphilis. In the instances of meningococcemia and Rocky Mountain spotted fever, the eruption may subsequently evolve to become petechial or purpuric. The lesions of erythema multiforme are characteristically maculopapular, though they may be bullous.

Pustular Lesions

Pustules are focal intradermal accumulations of serum and inflammatory cells (purulent material). The presence of diffuse pustular lesions usually represents a noninfectious dermatologic disease, such as pustular psoriasis, or a cutaneous infection, espe-

cially with staphylococcus or pseudomonas. The presence of focal pustular lesions should also call to mind staphylococcal infection. Gonococcemia and bacterial endocarditis also produce pustular skin lesions; associated clinical features, such as arthralgia, vaginal discharge, and heart murmur, should be sought as clues to the presence of these entities.

Vesicular Lesions

Vesicles are sharply circumscribed elevated lesions that contain clear fluid. Vesicles larger than 1 cm in diameter are called bullae. Vesicular eruptions of infectious etiology usually are the result of viral infection, most commonly herpes simplex and varicella-zoster viruses. Various enteroviruses and coxsackieviruses (most notably coxsackievirus A16, which causes hand-foot-and-mouth disease) can also produce vesicular eruptions. Differentiation is on the basis of lesion appearance and distribution, as discussed next.

Nodular Lesions

Nodules are elevated intradermal lesions that are usually round or elliptical. These are deep lesions, and the skin can be moved over them. Erythema nodosum, a well-recognized focal nodular eruption, may be a reflection of infection, most commonly streptococcal infection. The presence of a disseminated nodular eruption should call to mind a deep fungal infection. Septicemia due to *Candida* species produces an eruption characterized by discrete, firm, raised, nontender nodular lesions. These lesions may have a pale center and, though usually generalized, they may be localized to a small area of the skin. *Candida* sepsis is most likely to be encountered in immunocompromised patients.

Purpuric Lesions

Purpuric lesions result from hemorrhage into the skin. Petechiae are small (<3 mm in diameter) lesions containing hemoglobin or extravasated red blood cells. Larger lesions are called ecchymoses. Such lesions do not blanch with application of pressure. A generalized purpuric eruption is always of concern and should immediately call to mind the possibility of bacterial septicemia, particularly with *Neisseria meningitides*. Janeway's lesions that represent septic emboli occasionally may be purpuric. Such lesions, however, usually develop later in the course of an illness than does purpura due to gram-negative infection, where purpura characteristically appears 1–3 days after the onset of infection. The differential diagnosis of a petechial or purpuric eruption also includes leukemia, idiopathic thrombocytopenic purpura, and Henoch-Schoenlein purpura [5].

Pathology

Skin Host Defenses

A number of characteristics of skin act to prevent infection. Normal skin is colonized by large numbers of organisms that live harmlessly on its surface [6]. The presence of such organisms works to inhibit the growth of more pathogenic species. In addition the dryness of the skin provides insufficient moisture for the growth of various organisms. Intact skin serves as a formidable physical barrier to penetration by microorganisms. The skin is also supplied with a variety of cellular and humoral mediators of inflammation that augment defense against infection [6].

Pathogenesis of Rash in Infection

Infection can produce skin eruptions by a number of mechanisms. Skin rash can result from a local infection when a microbe penetrates the outermost layer of the skin, the stratum corneum. A skin eruption can also be produced by the systemic effects of microorganisms on the skin. Such a cutaneous manifestation of a systemic infection is known as an *exanthem*. A comparable eruption involving the mucous membranes is termed an *enanthem*. Various characteristics of common enanthems are listed in Table 9-8. Release of toxins, instigation of an inflammatory response, and vascular effects are other methods by which microbes produce skin manifestations of infection.

BACTERIAL SEPTICEMIA
Skin lesions associated with bacterial septicemia are produced by five processes [7]:

- Disseminated intravascular coagulation and coagulopathy
- Vascular occlusion by bacteria
- Immune complex formation and immune vasculitis
- Embolism
- The action of toxins

Disseminated Intravascular Coagulation. The skin manifestations of disseminated intravascular coagulation (DIC) are symmetrical peripheral gangrene, localized gangrene, purpura fulminans, acrocyanosis (a nonblanching cyanosis that may involve the legs, lips, nose, earlobes, and genitalia), and bleeding from wounds and venipuncture sites [7].

N. meningitides is the organism that most commonly produces DIC, and the patient presenting to the emergency department with fever and purpura should be assumed to have meningococcal infection

Table 9-8. Features of common enanthems

Enanthem	Features
Endocarditis	Petechiae on palate
Hand-foot-and-mouth disease	Erythematous papules or vesicles that ulcerate, appearing on the anterior pharynx (tongue, anterior buccal mucosa, lips)
Herpangina	Erythematous macules involving the posterior pharynx (soft palate, uvula and tonsillar pillars); no cervical lymphadenopathy
Herpes simplex stomatitis	Vesicles and ulceration occurring anywhere in the mouth, including the tongue and gums; possible tender cervical lymphadenopathy
Kawasaki syndrome	Strawberry tongue; diffuse erythema of the lips, pharynx, and oral mucosa; bulbar conjunctival involvement
Measles	Small red spots with blue-white centers, usually on the buccal mucosa opposite the molar teeth; Koplik's spots
Mononucleosis	Pharyngitis; petechiae at the junction of the hard and soft palates
Oral candidiasis	Mucous membrane erosion underlying a whitish plaque or pseudomembrane; cheilitis at the corners of the mouth may be present.
Scarlet fever	Strawberry tongue; petechiae of the palate
Toxic shock syndrome	Strawberry tongue

and managed accordingly. However, infection with a variety of other microbes can produce purpuric or gangrenous skin lesions. These organisms include *S. aureus*, *Escherichia coli*, *Klebsiella* species, *Aeromonas* species, *Aspergillus* species, and a variety of viruses [8].

Vascular Occlusion. Extensive purpura can occur in the absence of DIC in meningococcal and other infections. Lesions may initially be macular or petechial. These ecchymotic skin lesions are the result of vascular invasion and occlusion by bacteria. Bacteria can be cultured from such lesions, unlike in DIC.

Immunologic Mechanisms. Both meningococcus and gonococcus can produce skin lesions that are immunologically mediated. Such lesions are usually maculopapular, but they can be nodular, pustular, or purpuric. They typically are delayed in their onset, usually appearing several days after the onset of illness. Immune mechanisms may also be responsible for some skin lesions of endocarditis.

Embolism. Embolic lesions can have a number of morphologic appearances, being erythematous, purpuric, or pustular. Although the most widely appreciated association of embolic lesions is with endocarditis, they also can occur in typhoid fever, gonococcemia, and noninfectious illness such as systemic lupus erythematosus [7]. The most common embolic eruptions are Janeway's lesions, which are macular, pustular, or purpuric lesions that appear predominantly on the palms and the soles. Osler's nodes may be similar in distribution and appearance, characteristically being nodular erythematous lesions with pale centers. They are considered to be most pathognomonic of bacterial endocarditis. Osler's nodes are tender, however, a feature that distinguishes them from Janeway's lesions [9].

A variety of other skin manifestations are seen in infective endocarditis. These can be of some diagnostic significance, since the diagnosis may be difficult on the basis of other clinical parameters at the time of initial presentation. Petechiae are the most common lesions, occurring in about half of patients. The conjunctiva and oral mucosa are the most typical areas of involvement. Splinter hemorrhages occasionally occur in patients with endocarditis. Although these and other skin lesions of endocarditis are considered to have an embolic pathogenesis, immune mechanisms may be involved in their production. (Infective endocarditis is discussed in greater detail in Chap. 24.)

Toxins. The skin lesions produced by scarlet fever, toxic shock syndrome, and staphylococcal scalded skin syndrome are examples of dermatologic manifestations due to the effects of toxins. The appearance is generally that of a diffuse blanching erythroderma. Associated mucous membrane lesions may be present.

DIRECT BACTERIAL SKIN INFECTION
Staphylococcal infection produces skin eruptions by a number of pathogenic mechanisms. Cellulitis, folliculitis, and bullous impetigo are produced by direct infection of the skin and subcutaneous tissue. Staphylococcus is a normal skin surface organism, but a number of factors, most notably the impenetrability of the stratum corneum, rapid epithelial cell turnover, and skin pH ordinarily prevent staphylococcal infection [6]. A variety of lesions can be produced by staphylococcal septicemia. These include purpuric, pustular or erythematous lesions, Osler's nodes, and Janeway's lesions.

Group A beta-hemolytic streptococcus is the most frequent cause of bacterial skin infection [10]. All such infections carry with them the risk of poststreptococcal glomerulonephritis.

Diseases caused by spirochetes tend to be characterized by occurrence in stages, with remissions and exacerbations and different clinical manifestations at each stage. The emergency physician is most likely to encounter spirochete diseases in the form of primary or secondary syphilis and stage 1 of Lyme disease.

VIRAL INFECTIONS
A large number of viruses, predominantly the coxsackievirus and echovirus groups, are known to produce a skin eruption as a manifestation of infection. Most viral exanthems are maculopapular, although scarlatiniform, erythematous, urticarial, vesicular, and petechial rashes occasionally are seen. The eruptions are variable in their extent, are nonpuritic, and usually do not desquamate. Oropharyngeal enanthems also may be present.

Since the clinical appearances of various infections are similar, distinguishing among them frequently is difficult. The distinction must often be made on features other than the appearance of the exanthem, such as cough, lymphadenopathy, or mucous membrane lesions. Epidemiologic information regarding the occurrence of illness in the community can aid in suggesting the diagnosis, as may a history of exposure to others with known illness.

Entities by Morphology
Macules
In this section and those that follow, eruptions are discussed under the morphologic appearance that is most characteristic. It should be recognized, however, that a number of diseases may present in a variety of morphologic forms (see Table 9-3).

FOCAL RED MACULES
Cellulitis. Cellulitis is an infection of subcutaneous tissue in which the causative organism is usually a staphylococcus or a group A streptococcus. Erythema, swelling, and local tenderness are usually present. The margins of the lesion are not elevated or sharply defined. (See Chap. 32.)

The appearance of cellulitis in young children should suggest an infection with *Haemophilus influenzae* (see Chap. 14). Patients infected with this organism are usually 6 months to 2 years of age. The area involved is usually the face. A bluish or purpled-red discoloration is accompanied by marked temperature elevation and irritability [11]. Blood cultures are positive for *H. influenzae.*

Erysipelas. Erysipelas is a streptococcal infection of the skin and subcutaneous tissue. The involved area is red, indurated, and edematous. The borders of the lesion are elevated and sharply demarcated. The malar region of the face is the most commonly involved area in adults. Involvement of the abdominal skin is common in neonates. Fever, chills, and systemic toxicity may be present. (See Chap. 32.)

FOCAL BROWN MACULES/DERMATOPHYTOSIS
The dermatophytoses (ringworm) are superficial fungal infections limited to the skin and are characterized by scaling and pruritus. (See Chap. 32). Tinea corporis affects the arms, legs, and trunk and is classically a sharply marginated, annular lesion with raised or vesicular margins and central clearing. Lesions may be single or multiple, the latter occasionally being concentric. Lesions fluoresce green-yellow under long-wave ultraviolet (Wood's lamp) light.

Tinea versicolor is characterized by brown, yellow, or hypopigmented macules that may coalesce to form large irregular patches. The upper trunk, arms, and neck are the areas most commonly involved. The lesions fluoresce yellow or tan under the Wood's lamp.

Dermatophytes generally thrive in an atmosphere of excessive heat and moisture and grow only in the outer (keratin) layer of the skin. Keratin tends to accumulate in the body folds, such as between the toes and in the groin, axilla, and inframammary areas. With the exception of infection of the scalp (tinea capitis) dermatophyte infections are not markedly contagious. Any eruption thought to be a dermatophyte infection should be sampled and examined under the microscope in a potassium hydroxide preparation.

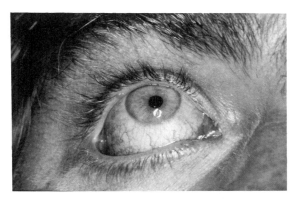

Fig. 9-1. Mucous membrane inflammation in toxic shock syndrome. (Courtesy of Frederick Koster, M.D.)

SCATTERED RED MACULES

Toxic Shock Syndrome. Toxic shock syndrome is an acute febrile illness characterized by the appearance of a rash that is typically a diffuse, blanching, macular erythroderma (sunburn-like rash). The redness may involve the palms, soles, and perineum and be accompanied by generalized nonpitting edema. (See Color Plates 1 and 2.) The rash rarely is vesicular or petechial. Accompanying nonexudative mucous membrane inflammation is common (Fig. 9-1). Pharyngitis, sometimes accompanied by strawberry tongue, conjunctivitis, or vaginitis, may be seen. As a rule the rash fades within 3 days of its appearance. This is followed by a full-thickness desquamation, most commonly involving the hands and the feet.

In addition to rash, toxic shock syndrome is classically composed of high fever, hypotension, and constitutional symptoms. The syndrome is best known as occurring in young women who use tampons, but it also can occur following vaginal or caesarean deliveries; in either sex from an *S. aureus* infection, such as those of the skin, musculoskeletal system, or lungs; or during the postoperative period in men and children. It is linked to culture of exotoxin-producing (TSST-1) *S. aureus*.

The onset and progression of toxic shock syndrome is strikingly rapid. Diagnostic criteria require the presence of (1) fever of at least 38.9°C; (2) hypotension, with a systolic blood pressure of 90 mm Hg or less; (3) skin rash; and (4) involvement of at least three organ systems (Table 9-9). Hypo-

tension is the result of decreased vasomotor tone and nonhydrostatic leakage of fluid from the intravascular to the interstitial space [12].

Systemic involvement can include myalgia, arthralgia, adult respiratory distress syndrome, encephalopathy, renal failure, anemia, disseminated intravascular coagulation, or hepatic or gastrointestinal dysfunction. Headache, muscle or joint pain, alteration of consciousness, vomiting, or diarrhea may be present. Generalized myalgia, muscle tenderness, and weakness are among the earliest and most prolonged manifestations of toxic shock syndrome [13]. Table 9-10 lists the signs, symptoms, and laboratory abnormalities in patients with toxic shock syndrome.

Management of the patient with toxic shock syndrome relies on aggressive fluid management and antibiotic administration. Appropriate cultures (vaginal, cervical, other infectious foci, and blood) are collected. Tampons or other vaginal foreign bodies are removed. Nafcillin (2 g IV q4h) is given. In the penicillin-allergic patient cephalothin (2 g IV q4°), cephazolin (1 g IV q8°), or vancomycin (30 mg/kg per 24 hours divided into 2–4 doses) is given.

Staphylococcal Scalded Skin Syndrome. This syndrome is characterized by acute loosening of large sheets of epidermis from underlying dermis. The illness begins with erythema and crusting around the mouth. A diffuse generalized erythroderma is present that resembles a sunburn. The

Table 9-9. Frequency of signs, symptoms, and laboratory abnormalities in 52 patients with toxic shock syndrome

Clinical signs and symptoms[a]	%	Laboratory findings	%
Diarrhea	98	Elevated serum creatinine	69
Myalgia	96	Thrombocytopenia[b]	59
Vomiting	92	Hypocalcemia[c]	58
Temperature $\geq$ 40°C	87	Azotemia	57
Headache	77	Hyperbilirubinemia	54
Sore throat	75	Elevated hepatic enzymes	50
Conjunctival hyperemia	57	Leukocytosis[d]	48
Decreased sensorium	40	Abnormal urinary sediment[e]	46
Vaginal hyperemia	33	Elevated CPK[f]	41
Vaginal discharge	28	Immature leukocytes $\geq$ 50%	36
Rigors	25		

[a] Rash and shock are omitted since they are part of the definition of toxic shock syndrome.
[b] Platelet count < 100,000/μl.
[c] Serum calcium $\leq$ 7.5 mg/dl.
[d] White blood cell count $\geq$ 15,000/μl.
[e] At least five white blood cells per high-power field, $\geq$ two red blood cells per high-power field, or the presence of red blood cells casts.
[f] Creatine phosphokinase.

Table 9-10. Criteria for the diagnosis of TSS

Temperature > 38.9°C
Systolic blood pressure < 90 mmHg
Rash with subsequent desquamation, especially on palms and soles
Involvement of at least three of the following organ systems:
  Gastrointestinal (vomiting, profuse diarrhea)
  Muscular (severe myalgia, or greater than fivefold increase in CPK)[a]
  Mucous membranes (vagina, conjunctivae, or pharynx): frank hyperemia
  Renal insufficiency (BUN[b] or creatinine at least twice the upper limit of normal, with pyuria in the absence of
    urinary tract infection)
  Liver/hepatitis (bilirubin, SGOT,[c] and SGPT[d] at least twice the upper limit of normal)
  Blood (thrombocytopenia < 100,000 per μl)
  CNS (disorientation without focal neurologic signs)
Negative results of the serologic tests for Rocky Mountain spotted fever, leptospirosis, and measles

[a] Creatine phosphokinase.
[b] Blood urea nitrogen.
[c] Serum glutamic-oxaloacetic transaminase.
[d] Serum glutamate pyruvate transaminase.

erythema then spreads down the body, and bulla formation and desquamation follow. The mucous membranes usually are not involved at all, but minor involvement is seen occasionally. After desquamation occurs, the lesions tend to dry up quickly, and clinical resolution occurs in 3–7 days.

Staphylococcal scalded skin syndrome has an excellent prognosis. Treatment includes anti-staphylococcal antibiotics, fluid replacement, and other supportive measures. It is caused by an infection with phage group 2 exotoxin-producing staphylococci. It is similar in clinical appearance to toxic epidermal necrolysis. The two conditions are histologically distinguishable by skin biopsy.

Staphylococcal scalded skin syndrome generally occurs in children 6 years of age and younger.

Scarlet Fever. The eruption of scarlet fever is caused by elaboration of erythrogenic toxin by group A beta-hemolytic streptococci. The rash consists of a generalized papular eruption overlying a hyperemic base that begins on the upper chest and spreads rapidly to the head and the extremities. It may spare the perioral area. The skin has a rough sandpaper-like texture because of the many punctate lesions. The pharynx is injected, and there may be erythematous lesions or petechiae on the palate. A beefy red "strawberry" tongue may be present. Following the resolution of the symptoms, desquamation of the involved areas occurs and is characteristic of the disease.

The origin of the infection is usually a streptococcal pharyngitis, although surgical wounds infrequently become infected with streptococci and scarlet fever results. Nonsurgical scarlet fever is seen primarily in children 2–10 years old. The illness has an abrupt onset with fever, chills, headache, nausea, malaise, and sore throat followed in 12–48 hours by the rash.

Complications include infection of the lymph nodes, the middle ear, and the respiratory tract. The rash may be confused with that of toxic shock syndrome or Kawasaki disease. Late complications consist of the development of rheumatic fever and acute glomerulonephritis. (For treatment of streptococcal pharyngitis, see Chap. 21.) Therapy is directed toward preventing complications, although it is not clear that glomerulonephritis is preventable with antibiotic therapy.

URTICARIA

Urticaria is among the most common skin lesions seen in the emergency department. Lesions appear as circumscribed raised wheals (hives), which represent localized edema produced by fluid extravasation. Hives may be slightly erythematous and display central clearing. Various mediators, including histamine, bradykinin, kallikrein, and acetylcholine, are thought to play a role in the production of urticaria. Most cases of urticaria seen in emergency medicine relate to allergic reactions or represent drug reactions produced by nonimmunologic mechanisms.

Although infection is a relatively uncommon cause of urticaria, occult infections with *Candida* species, the dermatophytes, bacteria, viruses, and parasites can trigger hives (Table 9-11). Of the bacterial infections, those involving the sinuses, the respiratory tract, and the bladder are most common. Viral infections that may produce urticaria include hepatitis and mononucleosis. Rarely coxsackievirus A9, 16, and B5 and echovirus 11 have been associated with urticarial lesions [14].

OTHER MACULAR ERUPTIONS

Other eruptions that may be macular include meningococcemia, viral exanthems, rubella, erythema marginatum (rheumatic fever), Rocky Mountain spotted fever, measles, roseola, cryptococcosis, secondary syphilis, dengue fever, typhus, typhoid fever, and erythema migrans (Lyme disease).

Papular and Maculopapular Lesions

FOCAL MACULOPAPULES/LYME DISEASE

Rash is the most distinctive clinical feature of Lyme disease, a tick-borne illness caused by the spirochete *B. burgdorferi*. About 86% of patients with

Table 9-11. Infectious causes of urticaria

Bacterial
Cholecystitis
Dental infection
Gastroenteritis
Respiratory tract infection
Sinusitis
Tonsillitis
Urinary tract infection
Fungal
Candidiasis
Dermatophytosis
Parasitic
Amebiasis
Giardiasis
Malaria
Pediculosis
Scabies
Trichomoniasis
Viral
Coxsackievirus
Echovirus
Hepatitis B
Mononucleosis

Lyme disease develop erythema migrans [15] (Fig. 9-2). (See Color Plate 3.) The tick bite usually results in the development of a small red papule, followed several days later by gradual expansion of the redness around the papule and partial central clearing. Lesions in severe cases can be vesicular or necrotic. Approximately 50% of patients develop multiple annular secondary lesions [16]. Though similar in appearance to the initial lesion, these lesions are smaller, lack indurated centers, and tend to migrate less. Subsequent stages of Lyme disease consist of cardiac, neurologic, and joint involvement (see Chap. 7).

The initial stage of the disease may be characterized by fever, headache, photophobia, malaise, fatigue, stiff neck, myalgia, arthralgia, or lymphadenopathy. All these conditions are relatively nonspecific, however, and it is only the dermatologic manifestation that is unique to Lyme disease.

Scattered Maculopapular Lesions
Viral Causes.

VIRAL EXANTHEMS. Infections caused by echovirus type 16 (Boston exanthem) and coxsackievirus B5 can produce a syndrome that resembles roseola infantum. Although children under 8 years of age usually are affected, the syndrome can occur in older children and adults, which is extremely unusual in roseola. (See Tables 9-6 and 9-7.)

Fig. 9-2. Erythema chronicum migrans in Lyme disease: serpiginous lesions of erythema chronicum migranes. (Courtesy of Upjohn Pharmaceuticals)

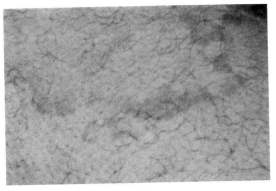

Infections caused by coxsackievirus A16 can cause a distinctive syndrome of vesicular stomatitis and exanthem involving the dorsa of the hands and the lateral borders of the feet (hand-foot-and-mouth disease). The eruption occasionally is associated with other coxsackieviruses and enteroviruses. Involvement is most common in children aged 1–5 years. The oral lesions are the most consistent feature of the illness and consist of erythematous papules 2–8 mm in diameter that go on to ulcerate. The lesions are painful and usually appear on the tongue or buccal mucosa and occasionally on the lips, gums, and palate. The exanthem consists of erythematous macules and papules and occasionally vesicles. Involvement of the hands, feet, and mouth is seen in approximately two-thirds of cases. Less frequently either skin or mucous membrane lesions are present alone [14].

Disease caused by coxsackievirus A9 has been studied extensively. It can be associated with meningoencephalitis or interstitial pneumonia. The rash usually is maculopapular, begins on the face or trunk, and spreads to the extremities. A vesicular eruption resembling varicella may occur [17].

Herpangina is an exanthem produced by a variety of enteroviral serotypes. The illness is characterized by the abrupt onset of fever, myalgia, pharyngitis, and dysphagia. These features may precede the characteristic exanthem, which initially consists of erythematous macules 1–4 mm in diameter and usually involving the soft palate, uvula, and tonsillar pillars. The lesions subsequently undergo central necrosis and ulceration. The oral lesions can persist for up to a week. The appearance of the lesions may be similar to that of hand-foot-and-mouth disease or herpes simplex gingivostomatitis, but the lesions of herpangina tend to be located more posteriorly in the mouth. Herpangina should be suspected in a child who will not eat or drink.

Treatment of children with the exanthems described here is symptomatic. Attention should be paid to the patient's hydration status and to the possibility of superinfection.

RUBEOLA (MEASLES). Rubeola is a highly contagious viral illness, with transmission in susceptible populations approaching 100% by the respiratory route [18, 19]. The incubation period is 9–11 days. The onset of symptoms is with fever and malaise, the fever usually increasing daily in a stepwise fashion until it reaches around 40.5°C on the fifth or sixth day of the illness. Cough, croyza, and conjunctivitis begin within 24 hours of the onset of symptoms.

On the second day of the illness, Koplik's spots appear on the buccal mucosa in approximately 80% of cases [17] and are pathognomonic of the disease. They appear as small, irregular, bright red spots with bluish-white centers. Beginning opposite the molars, Koplik's spots spread to involve a variable extent of the oropharyngeal mucosa.

The cutaneous eruption of rubeola begins on the third to fifth day of the illness. Maculopapular erythematous lesions first involve the forehead and upper neck and spread to involve the face, trunk, arms, and finally the legs and feet. Koplik's spots begin to disappear with the appearance of the rash. By the third day of its presence the rash begins to fade and the fever subsides.

Complications of rubeola include encephalitis, pneumonitis, and otitis media. Otitis media is the most common complication. Measles pneumonia may occur in children, and secondary bacterial pneumonia tends to appear in adults with measles [18]. Rubeola during pregnancy, in contrast to rubella, has not been associated with congenital abnormalities. The illness can be modified or prevented in infants, pregnant women, and the immunocompromised by the intramuscular administration of human immune serum globulin (.25 ml/kg IM; .5 mg/kg IM if immunosuppressed, maximum 15 ml). In other susceptible patients exposed to the disease, measles vaccine may effectively prevent the disease if given within 3 days of exposure.

ATYPICAL MEASLES. The introduction of measles vaccine has resulted in the appearance of an atypical form of measles following exposure to the illness in those who have been vaccinated [19]. The onset of atypical measles is characterized by high fever, cough, headache, and abdominal pain. An eruption appears 2–3 days later, which may be maculopapular, vesicular, or petechial. The rash frequently begins on the palms and the soles and spreads proximally. Pneumonia is a common complication, and leukopenia frequently is present. When the rash is petechial, the atypical measles syndrome requires differentiation from meningococcemia and Rocky Mountain spotted fever.

ROSEOLA INFANTUM. Roseola infantum is an illness characterized by fever, skin eruption, and a paucity of other physical findings. The appearance of the rash coincides with the subsidence of fever. The lesions are discrete pink or rose-colored macules or maculopapules 2–3 mm in diameter. The lesions blanch on pressure and rarely coalesce. The trunk is involved initially, with the eruption typically spreading to the neck and the extremities. Occasionally involvement is limited to the trunk. The rash clears over 1 to 2 days. Conjunctival injection may be seen, as may an enanthem consisting of small macules on the palate.

Human herpesvirus 6 has been implicated as the cause of roseola. Most cases are seen in children under 2 years old. It is estimated that 30% of children develop roseola [20]. The illness does not appear highly contagious, and it is unusual to see more than one child in a family affected [20].

The incubation period is unknown but is estimated to be 10–15 days [21]. The fever typically has an abrupt onset, rising rapidly to 39°–41°C, and is present consistently or intermittently for 3 to 4 days; the temperature then drops precipitously to normal.

Despite the presence of a high fever the infant may not appear particularly ill. The physical findings are entirely nonspecific. The prognosis is uniformly excellent, the most common complication being febrile convulsions. No specific therapy is necessary.

RUBELLA (GERMAN MEASLES). Rubella is a viral illness characterized chiefly by fever, skin eruption, and generalized lymphadenopathy. The rash appears first on the face and spreads rapidly to the neck, trunk, and extremities. The appearance is that of pink and red maculopapules. Lesions on the trunk may coalesce, but those on the extremities typically do not. The rash remains for 1–5 days, classically disappearing at the end of 3 days. The appearance and clearing are much more rapid than in rubeola [21].

Although there has been a marked decrease in the number of cases of rubella since the institution of immunization, higher rates have been noted in older children and adolescents [22]. The incubation period is typically 16–18 days, and the rash heralds the onset of the illness in children. In adults a prodrome consisting of headache, malaise, sore throat, coryza, and a low-grade fever for 1–5 days antecedes the appearance of the rash. These symptoms generally disappear following the appearance of the skin eruption. The incidence of rubella without rash may be as high as 25% [18].

Lymphadenopathy may begin as early as a week before the appearance of the rash. In general, the nodes most apparent in their enlargement are the suboccipital, postauricular, and posterior cervical groups. Palpable adenopathy may be apparent several weeks after the subsidence of other signs.

The major complications of rubella include encephalitis, arthritis, and thrombocytopenia. The most severe complication is fetal damage when rubella occurs during pregnancy (see Chap. 29). A maternal infection can be determined by ascertaining antibody levels acutely and in 2 weeks. A fourfold rise in the titer is diagnostic of rubella infection.

No specific treatment is available for rubella. Immune globulin given to pregnant women does not necessarily prevent viremia. Immune globulin administration may be considered when a pregnant women susceptible to rubella is exposed and refuses abortion if rubella develops.

Bacterial Causes.

ROCKY MOUNTAIN SPOTTED FEVER. Rocky Mountain spotted fever is an acute infection caused by *Rickettsia rickettsii*, an organism harbored by a variety of ticks. The organism is transmitted to humans through the saliva of the tick at the time of a bite or when the tick is crushed while in contact with the host.

The onset of the illness is usually abrupt, with headache, nausea, myalgia, chills, and a fever that spikes to as high as 40°C. Occasionally the onset is more gradual, with progressive anorexia, malaise, and fever. Increased capillary fragility and splenomegaly may be present.

The rash of Rocky Mountain spotted fever develops on the second to fourth (or occasionally as late as the sixth) day of the illness. It begins with erythematous macules that blanch on pressure, appearing first on the wrists and ankles. The lesions spread up the extremities and to the trunk and face in a matter of hours. They may become petechial or hemorrhagic. The presence of lesions on the palms and the soles is particularly characteristic.

SYPHILIS. The causative organism of syphilis is *Treponema pallidum*. The lesion of primary syphilis lasts 3–12 weeks and heals spontaneously. In 6 weeks to 6 months following exposure the disease enters the secondary stage, which may involve a variety of mucocutaneous lesions. These lesions also heal spontaneously in 2–6 weeks. Either a prolonged latent phase or tertiary syphilis follows.

The chancre is the dermatologic manifestation of primary syphilis. Chancres usually appear as single lesions but may be multiple. They appear at the site of spirochete inoculation, usually the mucous membranes of the mouth or genitalia. The chancre begins as a papule and characteristically develops into an ulcer about 1 cm in diameter with a clean base and raised borders. The chancre is painless unless secondarily infected, and it may be accompanied by painless lymphadenopathy.

There are a number of cutaneous manifestations of secondary syphilis. Lesions may be erythematous or pink macules, usually with a generalized symmetric distribution. Pigmented macules and papules classically appear on the palms and the soles. The lesions may be scaly but are rarely pruritic. Papular, annular, and circinate lesions are more common in nonwhites. Generalized lymphadenopathy and malaise accompany the skin lesions. Irregular, patchy alopecia may be seen. Flat, moist, verrucous condyloma lata may appear in the genital area and are highly contagious.

The diagnosis of primary syphilis is made with the identification of spirochetes with dark-field microscopy. Serologic tests for syphilis are invariably positive in cases of secondary syphilis. Such serology should be obtained in any case of a diffuse eruption of uncertain diagnosis. (See Chap. 30 for a more complete discussion of syphilis.)

ERYTHEMA MULTIFORME

Erythema multiforme is characterized by the sudden appearance of skin lesions that are erythematous or violaceous macules, papules, vesicles, or bullae. Their distribution often is symmetric, most characteristically involving the palms and the soles as well as the backs of the hands or feet and the extensor surfaces of the extremities. The hallmark of erythema multiforme is the target lesion, a papule or vesicle surrounded by a zone of normal skin and then by a halo of erythema.

The most common infectious cause of erythema multiforme is herpes simplex infection. There are, in addition, a number of other infectious causes (Table 9-12). The eruption is also associated with noninfectious conditions, most commonly exposure to medications. Various collagen vascular disorders (particularly systemic lupus erythematosus, dermatomyositis, and periarteritis nodosa), pregnancy, and malignancies also have been associated with erythema multiforme. No definite provocative factor can be identified in about 50% of cases.

OTHER PAPULAR MACULOPAPULAR LESIONS

Other eruptions that may be papular or maculopapular include meningococcemia, typhoid, gonococcemia, histoplasmosis, coccidioidomycosis, dengue fever, typhus, infective endocarditis, and scarlet fever.

Nodular Lesions

ERYTHEMA NODOSUM

Erythema nodosum is an inflammatory reaction of the dermis and adipose tissue that consists of painful red to violet nodules that vary in size from less than a centimeter to several centimeters in diameter. The nodules occur most commonly over the anterior tibia but also may be seen on the arms or the trunk.

A number of infectious underlying conditions can produce erythema nodosum (Table 9-13): infections with streptococci, *Yersinia enterocolytica*, and *Chlamydia trachomatis*; tuberculosis; coccidioidomycosis; histoplasmosis; and blastomycosis. In

Table 9-12. Infectious causes of erythema multiforme

Adenovirus 7
Coccidiodomycosis
Coxsackievirus B5, 16
Dermatophytosis
Epstein-Barr virus
Herpes simplex infection
Hepatitis B
Histoplasmosis
Influenza A infection
Mycoplasma infection
Streptococcal infection
Tuberculosis

Table 9-13. Infectious causes of erythema nodosum

Coccidioidomycosis
Histoplasmosis
Lymphogranuloma venereum
Streptococcal infection
Tuberculosis
Yersinia gastroenteritis

addition there are a number of noninfectious etiologies, including sarcoidosis, ulcerative colitis, regional enteritis, systemic lupus erythematosus, pregnancy, and the use of various medications. Oral contraceptive agents are the leading cause of drug-induced cases [23]. Many cases of erythema nodosum are idiopathic.

Histoplasmosis is the most common systemic mycosis in the United States [24]. Symptoms and physical findings generally are nonspecific, and dermatologic findings are not a prominent aspect of the infection. A variety of skin manifestations may, however, be encountered, especially erythema nodosum but also erythema multiforme and maculopapular eruptions.

CANDIDIASIS

Cutaneous findings of systemic candidiasis consist of erythematous macules and papules that may become purpuric or nodular. A nodular eruption is the most characteristic form of disseminated candidiasis. The lesions are firm and nontender and may have a pale center or become hemorrhagic. Lesions can be single or multiple, localized or diffuse [25]. Associated findings include fever and muscular tenderness, especially involving the lower extremities. The diagnosis should be suspected on clinical grounds in the appropriate circumstances. Confirmation is by recovery of *Candida* organisms from blood cultures or skin or muscle biopsy. Candidal dissemination can occur in debilitated or immunosuppressed patients, especially those with indwelling central venous catheters. Candidal-sepsis is a potentially fatal infection in such patients. Gastrointestinal, respiratory, or urogenital infection may result.

There are a number of mucocutaneous manifestations of focal infection with *Candida albicans*, including superficial cutaneous, oral, periungual, perianal, and diaper candidiasis, vulvovaginitis, and balanitis. Areas affected by *Candida* organisms are intensely erythematous with satellite lesions. Mucous membranes of the mouth and the esophagus may demonstrate curd-like white patches. When scraped, these lesions leave a raw surface and microscopically demonstrate hyphae, pseudohyphae, and budding yeast. (See Chap. 32 for a more detailed discussion.)

SPOROTRICHOSIS

Lymphangitis and cutaneous involvement constitute the most common forms of sporotrichosis [26]. (For a more complete discussion of this subject, see Chap. 10 and Chap. 32.) Characteristic lesions are raised erythematous warm and tender nodules that appear along the course of lymphatic drainage. The fungus characteristically gains access to the subcutaneous tissue via a traumatic inoculation, usually in the extremities. Subsequent proximal spread is via the lymphatic channels. Disseminated sporo-

trichosis with involvement of multiple organ systems is rare [27].

OTHER NODULAR ERUPTIONS

Other eruptions that may be nodular include blastomycosis and coccidioidomycosis.

Vesicular Lesions

VARICELLA

Varicella, or chickenpox, is an infection caused by varicella-zoster virus. Following an incubation period of 14–16 days the illness begins with a low-grade fever, headache, and malaise. The rash coincides with these symptoms in children and follows them by 1–2 days in adults.

The skin lesions rapidly progress from macules to papules to vesicles to crusting (Fig. 9-3). Vesicles are 2–3 mm in diameter and surrounded by an

Fig. 9-3. Varicella. Note progression of A, varicella vesicles, to B, varicella pustules, to C, varicella crusts, to D, umbilicated pustules of varicella. (Courtesy of Upjohn Pharmaceuticals)

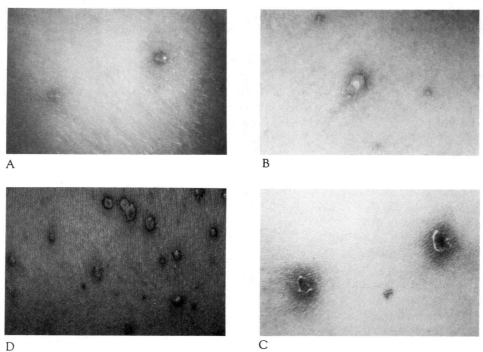

A

B

D

C

erythematous border. Drying of vesicles begins centrally, producing umbilication. The dried scabs fall off in 5–20 days.

Lesions appear in crops on the trunk, scalp, face, and extremities. The hallmark of varicella is the appearance of lesions in all stages of development in one region of the body. Extensive eruptions often are associated with a high and prolonged fever.

Complications include encephalitis, pneumonia, and cellulitis. Varicella pneumonia occurs more commonly in adults than in children. The disease can be transmitted before the diagnosis is clinically evident and is contagious until all vesicles are crusted and dried.

Treatment is supportive, including measures to relieve pruritus and prevent superinfection. Antipruritic drugs can be used along with soaking solutions of aluminum cerate, Burow's solution, or baking soda. Lesions should be kept clean and scratching avoided. The immunocompromised patient or the normal host with visceral involvement may benefit from vidarabine or acyclovir.

HERPES SIMPLEX

(Genital herpes simplex infection is discussed in Chap. 30; herpes simplex is discussed in more detail in Chap. 32.) The hallmark of skin infection with herpes simplex virus (HSV) infection is grouped vesicles on an erythematous base. The lesions are localized in a nondermatome distribution. The mouth is the most common site of nongenital HSV infection (Fig. 9-4). Children are affected more commonly than adults [28]. Small clusters of vesicles appear, but these are soon broken, leaving irregularly shaped crusted erosions. The severity of gingivostomatitis varies from the presence of small ulcers to extensive ulceration of the mouth, tongue, and gums accompanied by fever and cervical lymphadenopathy. Healing typically takes place in 7–14 days, unless secondary bacterial infection occurs.

The eruption may become more generalized in patients with underlying atopic dermatitis and in immune system compromise [29]. The presence of a disseminated HSV eruption in a patient with HIV infection or immune compromise of other etiology constitutes a life-threatening condition. Such patients should be hospitalized for treatment with intravenous acyclovir. (See Chap. 16 and Chap. 17.)

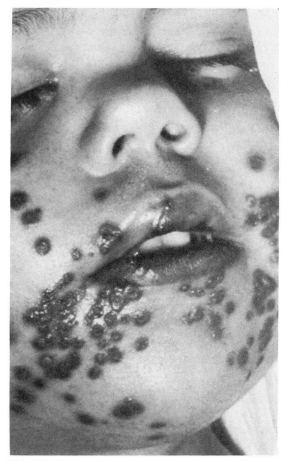

Fig. 9-4. Primary herpetic gingivostomatitis. (Courtesy of Upjohn Pharmaceuticals)

HERPES ZOSTER

Herpes zoster, an infection caused by varicella-zoster virus, occurs exclusively in individuals who have had chickenpox. The rash consists of grouped vesicles on an erythematous base involving one or several dermatomes, usually of the thorax, abdomen, or face. The vesicles initially appear clear, then become cloudy, and ultimately progress to scab and crust formation. Before the appearance of the rash the patient typically develops pain in a dermatomal distribution. The pain is of variable intensity, is sharp, dull, or burning in quality, and precedes the eruption by 1–10 days.

Herpes zoster has a peak incidence in patients 50–70 years of age and is unusual in children.

Although an association with leukemia, Hodgkin's lymphoma, and other malignancies is well known, appearance of the rash rarely antedates the diagnosis of such disease. The majority of cases of herpes zoster occur in healthy individuals.

There is a very low mortality, the condition rarely proving life-threatening even when dissemination to the viscera occurs. However, the condition tends to be more severe in immunosuppressed patients. Cutaneous, visceral, and CNS dissemination occurs more commonly in these patients [29]. Although treatment of herpes zoster with acyclovir rarely is necessary in the general population, high-dosage acyclovir (800 mg 5 times per day), should be instituted in those who are immunosuppressed [30]. (See Chap. 32).

OTHER VESICULAR ERUPTIONS
Other eruptions that may be vesicular include impetigo, atypical measles, erythema multiforme, and coxsackievirus infection.

Pustular Lesions

GONOCOCCEMIA
Disseminated gonococcal disease occurs in about 1%–2% of patients with gonorrhea [31]. Fever and migratory polyarthralgia are common accompaniments to the lesions, although it is the skin findings that often call the diagnosis to attention. The lesions often are multiple and have a predilection for periarticular regions of the distal extremities. The lesions begin as erythematous or hemorrhagic papules that evolve into pustules or vesicles with an erythematous halo. They are tender and may have a gray necrotic or hemorrhagic center. Healing with crust formation usually occurs within 4 days, although recurrent crops of lesions may appear.

PSEUDOMONAS SEPTICEMIA
Skin lesions accompany Pseudomonas aeruginosa infection in only a minority of cases [32]. Although a variety of lesions have been described in conjunction with Pseudomonas bacteremia, the most characteristic lesion is ecthyma gangrenosum [32]. It begins as an erythematous macule that progresses over the course of hours to induration and formation of a hemorrhagic vesicle. (See Color Plate 4.) The presence of lesions surrounded by normal skin

and an erythematous halo is most characteristic. Rupture of the vesicle leaves a punched-out ulcer with a gray-black necrotic base. Although ecthyma gangrenosum usually is due to Pseudomonas septicemia, it occasionally is the consequence of infection with other gram-negative bacteria or Candida [33].

OTHER PUSTULAR ERUPTIONS
Other eruptions that may be pustular include impetigo, folliculitis, infective endocarditis, and coccidioidomycosis.

Purpuric Lesions

MENINGOCOCCEMIA
Of all infectious processes that produce skin findings, meningococcemia most urgently demands prompt diagnosis and early initiation of therapy. Although meningococcemia sometimes constitutes a mild, transient febrile illness, in other instances it can be an acute, fulminant infection capable of being fatal within hours. Purpuric skin lesions have been noted in 80%–90% of patients with fulminant meningococcemia [34].

Various viruses (most notably coxsackieviruses A9 and B3 and echoviruses 4, 9, and 11) also can produce petechial or purpuric eruptions [14]. The clinical syndromes produced by such viral infection may be difficult to distinguish from meningococcemia, especially inasmuch as viral meningitis also may be present.

Lesions of meningococcal sepsis most commonly occur on the trunk and the extremities. Initially the rash may consist of blanching erythematous macular lesions closely resembling a viral exanthem. In fact meningococcemia can be found in patients who have been diagnosed as having a viral upper respiratory infection and exanthem. Such patients may spontaneously recover or go on to develop sepsis or meningitis.

The first petechial lesions frequently are under areas of clothing pressure on the skin and may not be discovered if the patient is not completely undressed. Likewise, all mucosal surfaces must be examined. The lesions, initially 1–2 mm in diameter, coalesce to form larger purpuric lesions. The number of petechiae corresponds with the degree of thrombocytopenia. The number of petechiae should be followed to assess response to initial therapy and the need for additional therapies. Areas of petechiae can be demarcated and the number of lesions within the demarcation counted hourly.

The two major clinical manifestations of meningococcal disease are sepsis and meningitis, which may coexist. (Meningococcal meningitis is discussed in Chap. 31.) The patient with meningococcemia usually quickly appears septic, with malaise, weakness, headache, and hypotension in addition to the rash. Myocarditis may result in congestive heart failure, pulmonary edema, and gallop rhythms. Disseminated intravascular coagulopathy results in increasing numbers of petechiae and oozing from venipuncture sites and mucosal surfaces. Arthritis and pericarditis may also occur.

Meningococci can be recovered from the blood and the cerebrospinal fluid, as well as from aspirates of fresh lesions. Appropriate cultures should be obtained coincident with the initiation of treatment in cases with a suggestive clinical picture. Penicillin (300,000 units/kg/day IV divided q2h, maximum dosage 24 million units/day) is still effective. Chloramphenicol (100 mg/kg/day, maximum dose 4 g/day) can be used in the penicillin-allergic patient. Ceftriaxone and cefotaxime can also be used. Vascular collapse must be anticipated and large-bore IV lines and close monitoring implemented. Volume replacement is essential. After adequate preload is ensured, dopamine can be used for both myocardial stimulation and its vasoconstrictive effects on the peripheral vasculature. Digitalis has been used for myocardial failure. Other drugs used for profound shock include epinephrine and norepinephrine.

Management of disseminated intravascular coagulopathy is problematic and should be done in concert with a hematologist. Heparin use is controversial. Replacement of clotting factors and platelets generally is not recommended.

Complications such as ARDS, metabolic acidosis, and adrenal insufficiency should be anticipated. Close contacts of the index patient require rifampin prophylaxis (see Chap. 5).

OTHER PURPURIC LESIONS

Other eruptions that may be petechial or purpuric include viral exanthems, Rocky Mountain spotted fever, rubella, atypical measles, typhus, pneumococcal septicemia, gonococcemia, infective endocarditis, and gram-negative septicemia.

Ulcerative Lesions

COCCIDIOIDOMYCOSIS

Skin involvement is the most common site of disseminated coccidioidomycosis and can produce papular, pustular, nodular, ulcerative, or verrucous lesions [35]. The verrucous forms are most characteristic. Coccidioidomycosis is endemic in the southwestern United States. Almost all cases involve the respiratory system, extrapulmonary disease being rare. Either erythema nodosum or erythema multiforme can be associated with primary coccidioidomycosis.

CRYPTOCOCCOSIS

Cryptococcosis can have a variety of cutaneous manifestations. Lesions can be papular, pustular, nodular, ulcerative, or purpuric. The most common types of lesions are abscesses and ulcers [36]. Cryptococcal abscesses and cellulitis usually are noninflammatory and seldom painful. Cryptococcal infection exists worldwide, and the organism, Cryptococcus neoformans, has no defined endemic area. Infection most likely is the result of inhalation of organisms. The most common manifestations involve the pulmonary system and the CNS.

The cutaneous lesions of cryptococcosis are nonspecific and may be mistaken for a variety of infections and noninfectious lesions. There is a tendency, however, for widely disseminated disease to occur in patients with immune system compromise [36]. Conditions commonly associated with cryptococcal infection include AIDS, lymphoma, leukemia, carcinoma, collagen-vascular disease, and systemic corticosteroid therapy [37]. Consequently cryptococcosis should be considered in patients known to have these conditions who develop any form of skin lesions.

BLASTOMYCOSIS

Blastomycosis is an uncommon systemic fungal infection. There are two major types of cutaneous lesions, verrucous and ulcerative [38]. Verrucous lesions begin as papulopustules that expand to form crusted, heaped-up gray or violaceous lesions. These lesions usually appear on exposed areas of the body.

Ulcerative lesions form from the initial pustule to produce a superficial ulcer with a bed of granulation tissue that bleeds easily when traumatized. Subcutaneous nodules occasionally are encountered. These nodules constitute noninflammatory abscesses and are seen in conjunction with pulmonary and noncutaneous extrapulmonary disease.

Most cases occur in the states surrounding the Mississippi and Ohio rivers [39]. Blastomycosis begins with inhalation of fungal spores into the lung, and pulmonary involvement is the most common form of the illness. The disease has a variety of extrapulmonary manifestations, however, the most common being cutaneous disease. Skin lesions are usually, though not invariably, seen in patients with active pulmonary disease.

OTHER ULCERATIVE ERUPTIONS

Other eruptions that may be ulcerative include sporotrichosis, ecthyma gangrenosum (*Pseudomonas* septicemia), and primary syphilis.

References

1. Lohr JA, Rheuban KS. Kawasaki syndrome. *Infect Dis Clin North Am* 1(3):559–574, 1987.
2. Rasmussen J. Toxic epidermal necrolysis. *Med Clin North Am* 64:901–20, 1980.
3. Herbst JS, Resnick L. Mucocutaneous manifestations of HIV infection. *Clinics in Dermatology* 7(1):56–64, 1989.
4. Minamoto G, Armstrong D. Fungal infection in AIDS. Histoplasmosis and coccidioidomycosis. *Infect Dis Clin North Am* 2:447, 1988.
5. Valman HB. Common rashes. *Brit Med J* 283:970–71, 1981.
6. Roth RR, James WD. Microbiology of the skin: resident flora, ecology and infection. *J Am Acad Dermatol* 20:367–90, 1989.
7. Kingston ME, Mackey D. Skin clues in the diagnosis of life-threatening infections. *Rev Infect Dis* 8:1–11, 1986.
8. Chu DZJ, Blaisdell FW. Purpura fulminans. *Am J Surg* 143:356–62, 1982.
9. Farrior JB III, Silverman ME. A consideration of the differences between a Janeway lesion and an Osler's node in infective endocarditis. *Chest* 70:239–243, 1976.
10. Scott MA. Bacterial skin infection. *Prim Care* 16:591–602, 1989.
11. Feingold M, Gellis SS. Cellulitis due to *Haemophilus influenzae* type B. *N Engl J Med* 272:788–89, 1965.
12. Chesney PJ. Clinical aspects and spectrum of illness of toxic shock syndrome: overview. *Rev Infect Dis* 11:S1–S7, 1989.
13. Chesney PJ, Davis JP, Purdy WK. Toxic-shock syndrome: management and long-term sequelae. *Ann Intern Med* 96:847–51, 1982.
14. Russo T, Chang T-W. Eruptions associated with respiratory and enteric viruses. *Clinics in Dermatology* 7(1):97–116, 1989.
15. Duffy J. Lyme disease. *Infect Dis Clin North Am* 1(3):511–27, 1987.
16. Steere AC et al. The early clinical manifestations of Lyme disease. *Ann Intern Med* 99:76–82, 1983.
17. Niehart RE, Liu C. Measles. *Clinics in Dermatology* 7(1):1–7, 1989.
18. Moullem M et al. Measles epidemic in young adults. *Arch Intern Med* 147:1111–13, 1987.
19. Nader PR, Horwitz MS, Rousseau J. Atypical exanthem following exposure to natural measles: eleven cases in children previously inoculated with killed vaccine. *J Pediatr* 72:22–28, 1968.
20. Meade RH. Exanthem subitum (roseola infantum). *Clinics in Dermatology* 7(1):92–96, 1989.
21. Bakshi SS, Cooper LZ. Rubella. *Clinics in Dermatology* 7(1):8–18, 1989.
22. Centers for Disease Control. Rubella and congenital rubella syndrome—United States, 1984–1985. *MMWR* 35:129–35, 1986.
23. Sibulkin D. Drug eruptions. *Prim Care* 5:233, 1978.
24. Wheat LJ. Histoplasmosis. *Infect Dis Clin North Am* 2(4):841–59, 1988.
25. DeCastro P, Jorizzo JL. Cutaneous aspects of candidosis. *Semin Dermatol* 4:165–72, 1985.
26. Becker FT, Young HR. Sporotrichosis, a report of 21 cases. *Minn Med* 53:851–53, 1970.
27. Winn RE. Sporotrichosis. *Infect Dis Clin North Am* 2(4):899–911, 1988.
28. Dawkins BJ. Genital herpes simplex infections. *Prim Care* 17:95–113, 1990.
29. Balfour HH Jr. Varicella zoster virus infection in immunocompromised hosts. *Am J Med* 85(suppl. 2A):68–73, 1988.
30. Huff JC et al. Therapy of herpes zoster with oral acyclovir. *Am J Med* 85(suppl.2A):84–89, 1989.
31. Kraus SJ. Complications of gonococcal infection. *Med Clin North Am* 56:1115–25, 1972.
32. Flick MR, Cluff LE. *Pseudomonas bacteremia. Am J Med* 60:501–8, 1976.

33. Fine JD et al. Cutaneous lesions in disseminated candidiasis mimicking ecthyma gangrenosum. *Am J Med* 70:1133–135, 1981.

34. DeVoe IW. The meningococcus and mechanisms of pathogenicity. *Microbiol Rev* 46:162–90, 1982.

35. Knoper SR, Galgiani JN. Coccioidomycosis. *Infect Dis Clin North Am* 2(4):861–75, 1988.

36. Perfect JR. Cryptococcosis. *Infect Dis Clin North Am* 3(1):77–102, 1989.

37. Hay RJ. *Cryptococcus neoformans* and cutaneous cryptococcosis. *Semin Dermatol* 4:252–59, 1985.

38. Witorsch P, Utz JP. North American blastomycosis: a study of 40 patients. *Medicine* 47:169–200, 1968.

39. Bradsher RW. Blastomycosis. *Infect Dis Clin North Am* 2(4):877–98, 1988.

10

Fever and Lymphadenopathy

LOURDES IRIZARRY

The lymphatic system carries fluids from the interstitial space to the blood. It transports lymph, which contains proteins, white cells, and bacteria, away from tissue spaces and serves a filtering-immunologic function in the lymph nodes. Lymphatics draining the entire body coalesce and empty into the venous system via the lymph ducts at the right and left subclavian veins. As bacteria enter lymph nodes located along the lymphatics, they are phagocytized and destroyed by reticulum cells that line the sinuses. Histological changes observed during an inflammatory response are limited but include cellular hyperplasia, dilatation of the lymph sinuses, and swelling of the nodes. Distinctive pathological pictures are observed with certain organisms and infiltrative processes.

History and Physical

Patients presenting with fever and enlarged lymph nodes, either noted by the patients or found during examination, have extensive differential diagnoses (Table 10-1). These diagnoses range from noninfectious entities (such as malignancies, autoimmune disorders, and drug side effects) to an extensive variety of infections. Diagnosis requires a careful history and physical examination and is confirmed by cultures, serology, or biopsy [1].

An extensive history should be obtained, including travel; animal exposure; eating habits; use of alcohol and tobacco; social, family, and occupational background; medications; drugs and chemical exposure; and sexual background. The localization and characteristics of the nodes, such as texture, size, presence or absence of suppuration, and pain, will assist in the working diagnosis.

Cervical lymphadenopathy is usually of infectious etiology. It is commonly seen with viral respiratory tract infections and bacterial—especially of odontogenic origin—or streptococcal pharyngitis. In patients with no respiratory tract symptoms, in whom a dental cause can not be ascribed, concerns about mycobacterial or fungal infections, lymphoma, metastatic carcinoma, or nasopharyngeal cancer have to be raised. In general bilateral adenopathies tend to be infectious, whereas unilateral ones more often are malignant. Infectious adenopathies also tend to be painful and shotty; malignant ones usually are painless, rubbery, often hard and firm. An algorithm, such as the one in Fig. 10-1, is helpful to the clinician in determining the cause.

Supraclavicular nodes are always of concern. Although these nodes may be seen in association with infectious etiologies, especially such fungal infections as coccidiodomycosis and histoplasmosis, they usually represent malignancies of abdominal, pelvic, or pulmonary origin (Fig. 10-2).

Table 10-1. Causes of lymphadenopathy

Infectious diseases
Malignancies
Autoimmune disorders
Drug side effects
Dermopathies

Axillary lymph nodes can be secondary to bacterial infections of the hand or arm and occasionally due to sporotrichosis or cat scratch disease. If these causes are ruled out, malignancy should be suspected, especially lymphoma in a young patient, breast cancer in a female patient, and gastrointestinal and pulmonary malignancies in an elderly person (Fig. 10-3).

Epitrochlear lymph nodes may be seen secondary to hand infections, as well as in people with secondary syphilis and non-Hodgkin's lymphoma.

Inguinal adenopathies tend to be of infectious origin secondary to infections involving the legs, sexually transmitted disease, bubonic plague, or tularemia. Malignant melanomas and lymphoma may be the etiology, if an infectious cause is not found. The workup of inguinal lymphadenopathy can be complex. A systematic approach is described in Fig. 10-4.

In patients with generalized adenopathy the differential diagnosis includes most infectious etiologies, including brucellosis, leptospirosis, listeriosis, and human immunodeficiency virus (HIV) infection, as well as many noninfectious causes, mainly lymphoma, sarcoidosis, collagen vascular disease, immune globulin disorders, myelo- or lymphoproliferative diseases, and drug side effects. The

Fig. 10-1. Algorithm to determine cause of cervical nodes

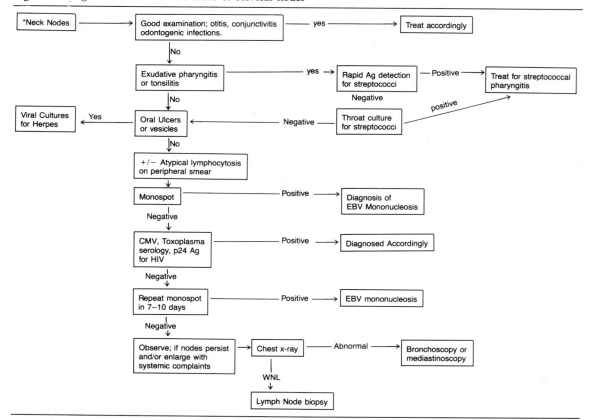

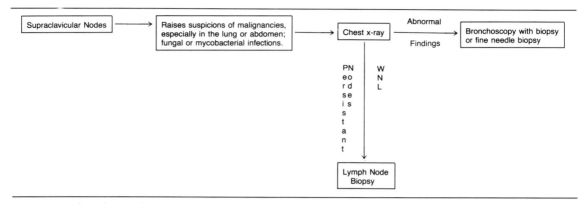

Fig. 10-2. Algorithm to determine cause of supraclavicular nodes

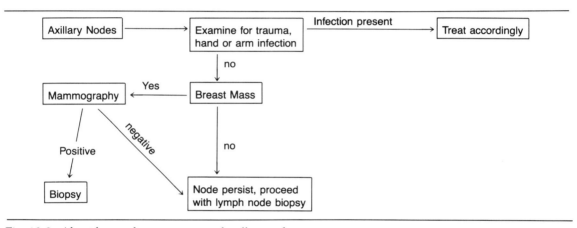

Fig. 10-3. Algorithm to determine cause of axillary nodes

workup is seldom completed in the emergency department, but the initiation of appropriate tests and radiographic studies is the responsibility of the emergency department physician. Figure 10-5 may help direct the clinician. The focused, time-limited approach available in the emergency department setting is the subject of this chapter.

Localized Lymphadenopathy

Moderate enlargement of the cervical and inguinal lymph nodes may be a normal finding, representing residual inflammation from prior infection. However, regional localization of enlarged lymph nodes and their physical characteristics are important clues to the diagnosis. Soft, discrete, mobile lymph nodes are more likely to represent residual inflammation, whereas hard, fixed nodes are more consistent with malignancy. Some infectious diseases have a predilection for lymph node involvement in certain locations (e.g., cervical or inguinal), while others cause adenopathy in any region of the body as determined by the site of the bite or inoculation. Plague, tularemia, and cat scratch disease represent important lymphadenopathic infections that present at any site; they are discussed first.

Regional Lymphadenopathy

PLAGUE

Yersinia pestis, a gram-negative rod, is the etiological agent of bubonic plague. Cases of plague have been reported in China, Burma, Vietnam, Africa, Bra-

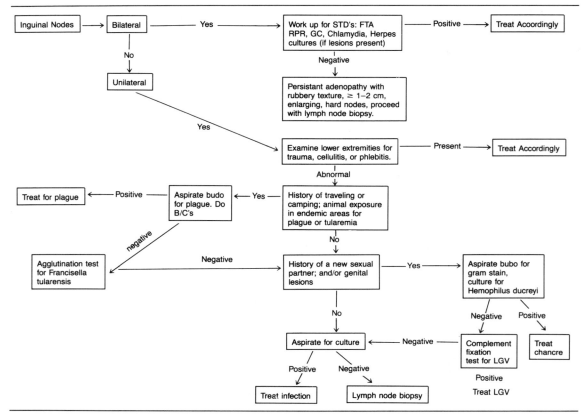

Fig. 10-4. Algorithm to determine cause of inguinal nodes

zil, Ecuador, Peru, Bolivia, and the United States. Although not commonly seen in the United States, every year a few cases are reported from the southwestern states of New Mexico, Arizona, Colorado, Utah, and California [2, 3].

Plague is a summer disease, seen from May to October. Most patients with plague have a history of outdoor exposure in an endemic area, with exposure to fleas, rodents, or rabbits.

Most patients present with fever, chills, and malaise 2–8 days after the exposure. The bubo appears about the same time, usually in the inguinal region, occasionally in the axillary or cervical area (Fig. 10-6). The nodes are very painful, at times limiting motion. They can be rather large, up to 10 cm in diameter in an oval shape. The majority of patients with plague are febrile, with temperatures in the range of 38°–40°C, toxic appearing, lethargic or agitated, with tachycardia and often hypotension.

The liver and the spleen may be tender. The WBC count is elevated with a shift to the left. Leukemoid reactions frequently are seen. The transaminase and bilirubin tend to be elevated. Disseminated intravascular coagulation (DIC) has been reported.

The diagnosis is made by aspirating the bubo for smears and cultures. Caution must be taken when aspirating the node to prevent aerosolization of the organism. A gown and mask should be worn by everyone in the room. Blood cultures also should be drawn. Proper handling of any cultured material from the emergency department to the laboratory must be taken to prevent contamination and aerosolization.

Patients with plague are extremely ill, requiring admission to the intensive care unit, often for adjunctive supportive treatment. Antibiotic therapy should be instituted as soon as all the appropriate cultures are taken. Streptomycin remains the drug

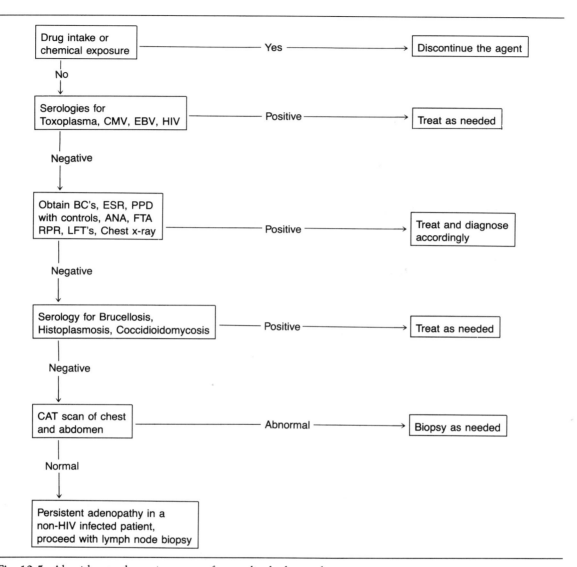

Fig. 10-5. Algorithm to determine cause of generalized adenopathy

of choice for the treatment of plague, although patients usually respond to therapy with other aminoglycosides. The recommended dose of streptomycin is 30 mg/kg per day divided into 2 doses for 10 days. Less acutely ill patients can be treated with tetracycline (2–4 g/day). Tetracycline is contraindicated in pregnant women and children younger than 10 years. Pneumonic plague is very contagious, and patients should be isolated. Contacts of patients with pneumonic plague should receive prophylaxis with tetracycline 2 g/day for 3–5 days. Trimethoprim-sulfamethoxazole is acceptable for prophylaxis of children and pregnant women. Plague is a reportable disease.

TULAREMIA
Francisella tularensis is a small, pleomorphic gram-negative coccobacillus, found primarily in wild mammals and arthropods. *F. tularensis* is distributed through the northern hemisphere. Most cases

reported in the United States originate in Texas, Tennessee, Oklahoma, Missouri, and Arkansas. Most spring and summer cases are tick borne, whereas most winter cases are associated with rabbit exposure, especially in people who skin or eviscerate rabbits [4].

Tularemia is mostly an ulceroglandular disease. After an incubation period of 3–5 days a papule develops at the inoculation site. The papule evolves into an ulcer followed by fever and lymphadenopathy [5].

Most patients present complaining of fever, chills, and fatigue. Skin lesions are present at the entrance site. Most tick-borne cases have tender inguinal adenopathies, while rabbit-associated cases have adenopathies localized to the axillary or epitrochlear regions. The complications of tularemia include pleuropulmonary involvement, peritonitis, pericarditis, and meningitis.

The diagnosis is made on a clinical basis and confirmed by serologies that demonstrate a fourfold increase in titers from acute to convalescent. The organism is rarely seen in Gram's stains or cultured in the laboratory.

As with plague the treatment of choice for tularemia is streptomycin 30 mg/kg per day for 7–14 days. Acceptable modalities of therapy include tetracycline (2–4 g/day) or chloramphenicol (4–8 g/day) for 14 days.

CAT-SCRATCH DISEASE

Cat-scratch disease causes progressive chronic regional lymphadenitis. Caused by a small, pleomorphic gram-negative rod, cat-scratch disease is almost always a diagnosis of exclusion in a patient with a history of cat exposure who has negative cultures and granulomatous changes found at node biopsy. Lymphadenopathy may be generalized but is usually regional, especially axillary, cervical, preauricular, or inguinal. Patients may have accompanying low-grade fevers. Patients with this presentation should have the nodes biopsied; if noncasating granulomes and organisms are found, the diagnosis is probably cat-scratch disease [6]. Recently cat-scratch disease causing granulomatous disease of the liver has been reported in AIDS patients. The diagnoses in those cases were confirmed with biopsies [7]. Until recently no therapy has been available. The organism appears to be

sensitive to ciprofloxacin, which may become the treatment of choice.

Cervical Lymphadenopathy

Causes of cervical lymphadenopathy are listed in Table 10-2.

UNILATERAL PYOGENIC CERVICAL ADENITIS

The most common presentation of enlarged lymph nodes is cervical adenopathy. Unilateral cervical adenitis usually is seen in preschool children. It is usually of pyogenic origin, caused by *Streptococcus*

Table 10-2. Causes of cervical lymphadenopathy

Infectious Causes
Bacterial cervical adenitis (unilateral)
    Staphylococcus
    Streptococcus
Viral respiratory tract infections
    Influenza virus
    Adenovirus
    Rhinovirus
    Coronavirus
    Measles virus
    Herpes simplex virus
    Epstein-Barr virus
    Cytomegalovirus
    HIV (acute)
Pharyngitis
    Streptococcus
    Diphtheria
    Corynebacterium haemolyticum
    Yersinia
Oral and odontogenic infections
    Ludwig's angina
    Vincent's angina
    Lemiere syndrome
Scrofula
Cat-scratch disease
Plaque
Tularemia

Noninfectious Causes
Lymphoma
Lymphoproliferative disorders
Nasopharyngeal cancer
Metastatic carcinoma
Thyroid cancer
Sarcoidosis

pyogenes, Staphylococcus aureus, or sometimes rare organisms such as salmonella. It is accompanied by fever and complaints of sore throat. The face and neck may appear swollen; the lymph nodes are enlarged, warm, fluctuant, and exquisitely tender. An elevated WBC is the rule [8]. Antibiotics directed against streptococci and staphylococci are indicated.

BILATERAL CERVICAL ADENITIS

Bilateral cervical adenitis is seen with an extremely wide range of diseases, including viral pharyngitis, streptococcal pharyngitis, Epstein-Barr virus (EBV), and periodontal infection. Less commonly mycobacteria, HIV, cytomegalovirus, cat scratch disease, sarcoidosis, and lymphoproliferative disorders can cause enlarged neck nodes.

Viral Pharyngitis. Viral pharyngitis commonly is seen during the colder months of the year. Rhinoviruses are seen most frequently during the fall and spring, while coronaviruses are primarily winter diseases. Influenza peaks during the period of December to April. In general viral pharyngitis is associated with minimal systemic complaints. Patients with viral pharyngitis have mild sore throat, a scratchy sensation, or pharyngeal irritation and discomfort. Nasal symptoms are common, but with few exceptions (e.g., influenza) patients do not have high fever, malaise, or prominent myalgia. On examination the pharynx is erythematous without exudate. Cervical lymph nodes, although present, are not tender. Several viral infections need special mention because of their epidemiological implications, differing clinical presentation, or associated mortality. These infections include adenoviral infections, herpes simplex, EBV, influenza, and acute HIV infection.

ADENOVIRUS. Adenoviruses are ubiquitous in nature, have multiple serotypes capable of causing recurrent illness, and can cause acute respiratory infections as well as conjunctivitis, cystitis, infantile diarrhea, intussusception, encephalitis, and meningoencephalitis [9, 10]. Adenoviral pharyngitis differs from other common viral pharyngitis (especially coronaviruses and rhinoviruses) because of prominent systemic complaints. Patients with adenoviral pharyngitis, like those with influenza, complain of general malaise, headache, myalgias,

fever, chills, and dizziness. In addition to pharyngeal erythema and exudate, an associated conjunctivitis is present in approximately 30%–55% of cases. Diagnosis may be suspected during an outbreak; confirmation requires viral culture. There is no specific therapy.

HERPES SIMPLEX PHARYNGITIS. Herpesviruses are distributed worldwide. The primary route of transmission is direct contact with infected secretions. Primary infection with herpes simplex virus (HSV-1) usually is asymptomatic but may be manifested as gingivostomatitis or pharyngitis. Although primary infection tends to occur before the age of 5 years, it may be seen in adults. Patients with herpes pharyngitis have sore throat and fever and may appear toxic, with an erythematous pharynx, fetid breath, and tender cervical adenopathy. Small vesicles that later ulcerate are seen on the oral mucosa and pharynx. Pharyngeal exudates mimicking those seen in streptococcal infection may be present in severe herpetic pharyngitis. The diagnosis is confirmed by culturing the pharyngeal vesicles for HSV. Because therapy with acyclovir is effective, especially in immunocompromised hosts, the cultural confirmation is important. Unlike most viruses culture return is fast (72 hours) and specific. Tzanck smears can assist in making a quick diagnosis in the emergency department. Therapy with acyclovir (5 mg/kg 5 times a day for 5 days) will decrease the severity and duration of acute infection [11].

INFLUENZA. Patients with influenza present with an abrupt onset of fever, chills, headaches, eye pain, severe myalgias (especially of the long muscles of the legs and back), malaise, anorexia, and arthralgias. As the systemic symptoms disappear, upper respiratory symptoms such as nasal obstruction, hoarseness, and sore throat become more prominent. Nonproductive cough usually is present. Most systemic complaints, especially fever, decrease by the third day of illness. On examination patients usually are febrile with red watery eyes, nasal discharge, and erythematous mucous membranes with occasional exudate. Rales and rhonchi may be heard on auscultation of the lungs. Cervical adenopathy, when present, is seen more frequently among children than adults and is nontender. Diagnosis can be made on clinical grounds during an epidemic and by viral culture, throat swab immunofluorescent stain, or serology in sporadic cases.

Therapy with amantadine (100 mg orally twice a day) may be effective if given within the first 24 hours of onset [12].

Bacterial Pharyngitis

STREPTOCOCCAL PHARYNGITIS. Group A streptococcal pharyngitis is among the most common bacterial infections of childhood. All age groups, however, are susceptible, especially young adults who have frequent contact with children. The incubation period is approximately 2–4 days. The illness is characterized by an abrupt onset of sore throat, malaise, fever, and headache. Nausea, vomiting, and abdominal pain are common in children. Fever to 38.3°C or higher accompanies pharyngeal edema and erythema. The tonsils are hyperemic, with a grayish exudate. Enlarged, tender lymph nodes generally are palpable at the angle of the jaw. An elevated WBC is a frequent but nonspecific finding, and specific diagnosis must be made by either throat culture or the rapid antigen detection test. The latter test has a specificity of 95%–99% and a sensitivity of 40%–90% [13–15]. It is the author's opinion that if the Ag detection test is positive treatment is appropriate; if the test is negative, a throat culture should be done. Streptococcal pharyngitis is treated with a single dose of 1.2 million units of benzathine penicillin G. Children weighing 60 pounds or less should receive 600,000 units. An alternative drug is penicillin V 250 mg qid orally for 10 days. Erythromycin is the drug of choice for penicillin-allergic patients.

ANAEROBIC PHARYNGITIS. Most infections that invade the gums and paramandibular spaces are caused by mixed anaerobic bacteria and spirochetes. Patients with anaerobic upper airway infections present with pain and swelling of the neck and face. These patients complain of severe sore throat, dysphagia, and fever. On examination the patient appears toxic and usually is febrile, although the temperature may be only mildly elevated. The patients have a foul breath and purulent pharyngeal exudate.

Rare entities to be considered when evaluating a patient with pharyngeal pain, fever, and enlarged nodes include Ludwig's angina, Lemiére syndrome, and Vincent's angina (the specific features of these syndromes are reviewed in Chap. 36). Equally rare diseases include diphtheria (1–10 cases per year in the United States), Corynebacterium haemolyticum

and yersinial pharyngitis. Diagnosis depends on a high index of suspicion, an epidemic setting, and careful cultures.

SCROFULA
Scrofula, or tuberculous infection of the cervical lymph nodes, is a rare infection caused by Mycobacterium avium intracellulare (MAI) [16] or by Mycobacterium tuberculosis. Scrofula is a chronic disease with an indolent course and minimal systemic complaints (low-grade fever and malaise). It usually is the presence of enlarged, painless, fluctuant nodes that brings the patient to the physician. Biopsy is needed for definitive diagnosis, and therapy consists of prolonged antituberculous chemotherapy and excision and drainage of the nodes.

Preauricular Lymphadenopathy

Preauricular lymphadenopathy is frequently seen in association with conjunctival infections and otitis externa. Causes are listed in Table 10-3.

CONJUNCTIVITIS
Bacteria, viruses, spirochetes, mycobacteria, and fungi can cause conjunctivitis. The term conjunctivitis refers to an inflammation of the conjunctiva, consisting of hyperemia and edema of the

Table 10-3. Preauricular lymphadenopathy

Oculoglandular syndrome (conjunctivitis)
  Viruses
    Adenoviruses (follicular conjunctivitis)
    Papillomaviruses (corneal erosion)
    Picornaviruses (hemorrhagic conjunctivitis)
    Herpes simplex (corneal ulcerations)
    Herpex zoster (corneal ulcerations)
    Measles (rash)
    Mumps (parotitis)
    Influenza (flu-like illness)
  Bacteria
    N. gonorrhea
    F. tularensis
    S. aureus
    S. epidermidis
    S. pneumoniae
    H. influenzae
Mycobacteria
Spirochetes
Cat-scratch disease
Otitis externa

conjunctiva with occasional membrane formation or associated keratitis. A secretion almost always is present. Purulent secretions most commonly are associated with a bacterial infection, whereas a clear discharge most commonly is seen with a viral process. Occasionally preauricular lymphadenopathy occurs secondary to the conjunctivitis. This condition is known as the oculoglandular syndrome and may be due to a variety of organisms.

Streptococcus pneumoniae, S. aureus, Staphylococcus epidermis, and *Hemophilus influenzae* are the etiological agents for most of the bacterial conjunctivitis. Isolated cases of conjunctivitis caused by virtually most pathogenic bacteria have been reported, most of them with the presence of palpable preauricular lymph nodes. Gonococcal conjunctivitis, an infection commonly seen in the past among neonates, is not much of a threat to the newly born any longer, thanks to the implementation of silver nitrate prophylaxis. Still this infection can be seen among adults, who can have a rather indolent course over time, undergoing a prolonged asymptomatic phase, that may eventually lead to corneal ulceration and perforation.

Mycobacteria and spirochetes can cause conjunctivitis. Conjunctivitis due to these organisms tends to be unilateral and to lead to a high rate of ulceration. Prominent preauricular adenopathy usually is found in association with these organisms. Cat-scratch disease, as previously discussed, can also cause a unilateral conjunctivitis with preauricular adenopathy.

Viruses are frequently the cause of epidemic conjunctivitis. Adenoviruses in particular are the single most common cause of epidemic viral conjunctivitis in the United States. The clinical features of this infection include complaints of sore throat with an associated pharyngitis, fever, and conjunctivitis, usually follicular in nature. Keratitis often is present. Papillomaviruses, picornaviruses, and herpes, both simplex and zoster, can cause conjunctivitis. Most of these viruses are associated with preauricular adenopathy. Picornavirus often causes hemorrhagic conjunctivitis, whereas herpetic conjunctivitis is associated with the presence of vesicular lesions of the eyelids and papillomaviruses with corneal erosion.

Most other viruses, including measles, mumps, and influenza, can cause a conjunctivitis concomitant to the clinical illness.

The vast majority of the conjunctivitis have a self-limited course. Topical antibiotics, such as gentamicin, erythromycin, neomycin, and fluoroquinolones, applied every 2–4 hours for 7 days are effective in treating bacterial conjunctivitis.

Gonococcal conjunctivitis requires treatment with topical penicillin. If a penicillinase-producing organism is suspected, systemic therapy with intravenous ceftriaxone is warranted.

OTITIS EXTERNA

Inflammation of the external auditory canal usually is caused by bacteria such as *S. aureus, S. epidermidis,* and *Propionibacterium acnes. Pseudomonas aeruginosa* can cause diffuse otitis externa in swimmers and severe cases of malignant otitis externa among elderly, debilitated, and diabetic patients.

Patients with otitis externa complain of pain and itching of the ear. The skin and the ear canal are erythematous and appear swollen. Palpable lymph nodes in the preauricular region often are present. Malignant otitis externa is characterized by necrosis of the soft tissue and cartilage, pain around the ear, and the presence of a purulent drainage. Patients have severe pain.

Otitis externa responds well to local therapy with topical antibiotics and cleaning. Patients with malignant otitis externa require intravenous therapy with an antipseudomonal agent along with local care.

Axillary Lymphadenopathy

Axillary adenopathy frequently is associated with either malignancy of the lymphatic system or a metastatic solid tumor. Most common is breast cancer with lymph node spread. Axillary adenopathy may also be seen with pyogenic infections of the hand and fingers. More rarely lymphocutaneous sporotrichosis, and cat-scratch disease, plague and tularemia can cause this syndrome. Table 10-4 lists causes of axillary lymphadenopathy.

SPOROTRICHOSIS

Sporothrix schenckii is a dimorphic fungus found in soil and plants. The infection is found most frequently among gardeners, nursery workers, and farmers. The majority of cases of sporothricosis are limited to its cutaneous manifestation, usually presenting with lesions at the inoculation site.

Table 10-4. Causes of axillary
and epitrochlear lymphadenopathy

Axillary Lymphadenopathy
Infectious Causes
   Upper extremity infections (bacterial)
   Sporotrichosis
   Cat-scratch disease
   Plague
   Tularemia
Noninfectious Causes
   Lymphoma
   Breast cancer
   Metastatic carcinoma

Epitrochlear Lymphadenopathy
Infections of hand or forearm
Syphilis (secondary)
Lymphoma

Table 10-5. Causes of inguinal lymphadenopathy

Infectious Causes
Lower extremity infection
Sexually transmitted diseases
Plague
Tularemia
Cat-scratch disease

Noninfectious Causes
Melanoma
Lymphoma
Pelvic malignancy

The lesions consist of purplish-red papules with or without ulcer formation that arise in the extremities where inoculation took place. (See Color Plate 5.) Sporotrichosis usually remains limited to subcutaneous tissue, although inguinal or axillary lymph nodes may be palpable; isolation of the organism from the nodes is not a frequent finding.

Diagnosis of sporotrichosis is made by cultures of the tissue involved. Cutaneous sporotrichosis responds to therapy with potassium iodide. Iatroconazole, still an experimental drug, may be an alternative therapy [17].

Epitrochlear Lymphadenopathy

Epitrochlear lymphadenitis can be found with skin infections of the hand and forearm [18]. The infections usually are due to *S. aureus* or group A strep-

Fig. 10-6. Plague Buboe in axilla

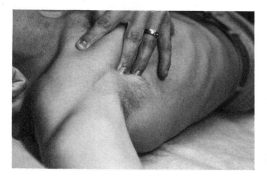

tococci. If untreated, the nodes will continue to enlarge, causing increased pain and edema of the elbow, sometimes difficult to distinguish from cellulitis, bursitis, or septic joint. These infections respond well to treatment with a beta-lactamase–resistant penicillin or a first-generation cephalosporin. Isolated epitrochlear node enlargement in a patient with a nonpruritic rash may be the only clue to secondary syphilis. (See Table 10-4.)

Inguinal Lymphadenopathy

The inguinal nodes receive drainage from the lower abdomen, the perineum, and the lower extremities. Infectious processes in these areas lead to inguinal lymphadenopathy in a fashion similar to epitrochlear and axillary node involvement. Causes of inguinal lymphadenopathy are listed in Table 10-5.

SEXUALLY TRANSMITTED DISEASES
When a sexually active person with inguinal node enlargement is seen, sexually transmitted diseases must be considered along the causative etiologies (see Chap. 30). The genitalia must be examined carefully for evidence of infection and a careful history of sexual exposure taken. Herpes simplex, lymphogranuloma venereum (LGV), syphilis, and chancroid can all cause unilateral or bilateral inguinal adenopathy. Fever, transient genital lesions, and painful or painless adenopathy may be present. Diagnosis of syphilis is made by dark-field microscopic appearance of *Treponema pallidum* obtained by scraping of a chancre or by serology; of herpes simplex by viral tissue culture of the vesicular lesions; of chancroid by culture of needle aspirate of the involved node; and of LGV by serology.

Extremely rare causes of inguinal adenopathy also include bubonic plague, tularemia, and cat-scratch disease.

Generalized Lymphadenopathy

Generalized lymphadenopathy is commonly seen with neoplasms of the immune system, infections, reactive processes, tumors, collagen vascular diseases, and drug reactions, especially to Dilantin, hydralazine, and allopurinol. Causes of generalized lymphadenopathy are listed in Table 10-6. Only the infectious causes are discussed in this section.

Mycobacterial Infections

Miliary tuberculosis can cause fever and lymphadenopathy. Overall the incidence of tuberculosis is higher among blacks, Hispanics, Native Americans

Table 10-6. Causes of generalized lymphadenopathy

Infectious Causes
Brucellosis

Leptospirosis

Listeriosis

Mycobacteria (miliary, MAI)

Fungi (histoplasmosis, coccidiodomycosis)

Syphilis (secondary)

Scrub typhus

Viruses (measles, rubella, EBV, cytomegalovirus, hepatitis B virus, HIV, influenza, dengue fever, Lassa fever, chronic fatigue syndrome)

Protozoa (toxoplasmosis, kala-azar, leishmaniasis, trypanosomiasis)

Helminths (filariasis)

Noninfectious Causes
Lymphoma

Sarcoidosis

Collagen vascular diseases

Hyperthyroidism

Immune globulin disorders

Myeloproliferative disorders

Lymphoproliferative disorders

Metastatic carcinoma

Angioblastic lymphadenopathy

Drug side effects (Dilantin, hydralazine, isoniazid, allopurinol)

and Asiatics. Alcoholism, cirrhosis, and malignancies are frequent underlying conditions found in patients with miliary tuberculosis. Patients with miliary tuberculosis offer vague generalized complaints, including fever, night sweats, weight loss, and fatigue [19]. On physical examination they may have cutaneous sinus tracts, rashes, and adenopathy.

Patients tend to have normal WBC counts, although they may have pancytopenia secondary to marrow involvement. Anemia of chronic disease is common, and patients may have elevated alkaline phosphatase, representing granulomatous disease of the liver. The chest x-ray may show the typical miliary pattern, but some patients present with normal chest x-rays.

The diagnosis can be made by staining and culturing sputum, urine, cerebrospinal fluid (CSF), or bronchoscopic specimens. Diagnosis is often made faster and more efficiently with tissue obtained by biopsy of the liver, bone marrow, or lymph nodes.

Other mycobacterial species can give generalized lymphadenopathy; of special significance is MAI. MAI is not an uncommon finding in patients with AIDS, and when found it is often disseminated. Patients have fever and weight loss, often complain of diarrhea, and have generalized lymphadenopathy. The diagnosis is made with the finding of positive blood cultures, stool cultures, or biopsies of the liver, bone marrow, or lymph nodes.

Fungal Infections

HISTOPLASMOSIS

Histoplasma capsulatum frequently is found at sites where soil has been contaminated with avian or bat excrement. *H. capsulatum* is endemic in the central United States. Histoplasmosis may have an acute self-limited pulmonary presentation. Rarely it is complicated by pericarditis, broncholithiasis, pleural effusions, mediastinal disease, and fistula formation from the mediastinal lymph nodes [20].

H. capsulatum can disseminate, presenting in three different forms: acute disseminated histoplasmosis, most frequently seen in infants; subacute disseminated histoplasmosis; and chronic disseminated histoplasmosis. Patients with chronic disseminated histoplasmosis present with weakness, weight loss, and fevers [21]. On examination they may have generalized lymphadenopathy, oral ulcers, a papular skin rash, and hepatosplenomegaly. Multiple organs may be involved, especially the adrenals (causing Addison's disease), the meninges, and the endocardium.

The diagnosis is made by histopathological demonstration of the organism or by positive cultures of blood or tissue. Disseminated histoplasmosis can be diagnosed by detection of *H. capsulatum* antigen in serum and urine [22]. Amphotericin B is the drug of choice. Ketoconazole also has been shown be be effective [23].

COCCIDIODOMYCOSIS

Coccidiodes immitis is endemic in the southwestern United States [24]. Most of the people infected with coccidiodes have an asymptomatic infection or an illness that resembles an upper respiratory infection. About 0.5% of the population will develop disseminated infection with multiple organ involvement. Disseminated coccidiomycosis presenting in the form of meningitis, cutaneous infection, or musculoskeletal infection or with fever and generalized lymphadenopathy is of special concern in immunocompromised hosts, especially in patients with AIDS. Diagnosis is made by demonstrating the organism in stains and cultures obtained from body fluids or tissue samples.

Brucellosis

Brucellosis is primarily a disease seen in cattle, swine, goats, dogs, and sheep. It is transmitted to humans by direct contact with infected fluids or tissue through the mucous membranes or abraded skin, inhalation of aerozolized infectious material, or ingestion of contaminated meat or dairy products. As a result of aggressive immunization programs for cattle, as well as pasteurization processes, the incidence of brucellosis in the United States has decreased dramatically, with fewer than 200 cases reported over the last decade. Still brucellosis has to be considered in the differential diagnosis of patients presenting with recurring fevers who may or may not have generalized lymphadenopathy.

The incubation period of brucellosis varies from one week to a few months. Some people may have a subclinical presentation, others a mild viral-like syndrome. Patients may have recurrent episodes of brucellosis characterized by sweats, chills, fever, malaise, and headaches. Twenty percent of these patients have splenomegaly on examination. Approximately 20% have adenopathies, especially of the cervical and inguinal areas [25].

A thorough history of animal exposure, occupational background, travel, and ingestion of unpasteurized dairy products is indispensable in these cases. Diagnosis can be made by culturing blood, bone marrow, or other body tissue. Most of the time the diagnosis is confirmed by serological tests, demonstrating either a fourfold increase in the titers of acute and convalescent samples, or a titer equal to or greater than 1:160, using the standard tube agglutination test [26].

A combination of doxycycline plus rifampin for 6 weeks is considered the treatment of choice for brucellosis [27]. Other effective agents include streptomycin, tetracycline, and trimethoprim-sulfamethaxazole.

Leptospirosis

Leptospirosis, caused by spirochetes of the genus *Leptospira*, is a disease primarily seen between summer and fall in persons exposed to infected animal secretions. The most common vehicle of transmission is water or soil contamination with animal urine [28].

The spirochetes penetrate the body through the mucous membranes or broken skin, enter the blood stream, and disseminate. Infected patients may have a subclinical course or present with complaints of influenza-like symptoms. They may have an anicteric phase characterized by myalgias, malaise, fever, headaches, chills, nausea, and vomiting. Abdominal tenderness is found on physical examination, splenomegaly is present in 25% of patients, and conjunctival injection and adenopathy frequently are seen [29]. A more severe form of leptospirosis characterized by jaundice, renal and hepatic insufficiency, bleeding, severe sensorium impairment, and vascular collapse may occur.

Diagnosis of leptospirosis usually is made by demonstrating a fourfold increase in the antibody titer or by isolating the organism from body fluids or tissue. Penicillin G or tetracycline may shorten the duration of the symptoms and reduce the incidence of complications.

Listeriosis

Listeria monocytogenes, a gram-positive aerobic bacillus, is the only member of the genus that has been associated with disease in humans [30, 31]. *L. monocytogenes* can cause anything from a mild to a very severe illness, especially in pregnant women, elderly people, neonates, and immunocompromised hosts. In adults the most common clinical presentation is meningoencephalitis, occasionally cerebritis. The only signs patients may have are fever and personality changes. Focal neurologic signs and coma are seen at a lower frequency.

L. monocytogenes can cause focal infections, including endocarditis, arthritis, osteomyelitis, ocular infections, and brain abscesses. Lymph node infections have been reported. In those cases biopsy specimens are necessary to confirm the diagnosis [32].

Treatment with ampicillin or penicillin appears to be equally effective. Trimethoprim-sulfamethoxazole appears to be effective in the treatment of penicillin-allergic patients.

Syphilis

Two to eight weeks after the appearance of a syphilitic chancre the spirochetes disseminate, and patients present with the usual protean manifestations of secondary syphilis. The most common feature is the presence of maculopapular rash that starts on the trunk and spreads to the extremities, involving the palms and the soles. Persons affected with secondary syphilis often complain of fever, malaise, anorexia, headache, weight loss, and arthralgias. They may have either localized (usually epitrochlear) or generalized adenopathy.

Scrub Typhus

Rickettsia tsutsugamushi is an obligate intracellular bacterium that causes a febrile illness in humans that have been bitten by the larval stage of a trombiculid mite (chigger). Scrub typhus is endemic in Asia, especially Korea, India, and Pakistan, and in Australia.

Patients present with sudden onset of fever, chills, headache, and myalgias 6–18 days after the bite. Initially only tender regional adenopathy at the site of the bite is noticeable. Later a maculopapular rash begins on the trunk and spreads to the extremities. Generalized lymphadenopathy and splenomegaly will be found at this point.

The diagnosis is made by a Weil-Felix agglutination test, indirect microimmunofluorescence, or an immunoperoxidase test.

Therapy with tetracycline or chloramphenicol appears equally effective. Ciprofloxacin may be a good alternative [33].

Viral Illnesses

Many viruses can cause an illness associated with generalized adenopathy and fever. Some have distinctive features that make the diagnosis possible. Among the viral diseases commonly associated with fever and adenopathy are measles, rubella, infectious mononucleosis (EBV and cytomegalovirus), hepatitis B, influenza, dengue fever, Lassa fever, and acute and chronic HIV infection.

EBV MONONUCLEOSIS

Epstein-Barr virus (EBV), an infectious disease mainly of children and young adults, is the most common cause of infectious mononucleosis. In the pre-HIV era, EBV was responsible for 79% of cases, based on positive heterophile-agglutinins [34]. Other infections, notably cytomegalovirus, toxoplasmosis, and acute HIV, as well as rubella, cat scratch disease, and infectious lymphocytosis of infancy and childhood may resemble EBV mononucleosis. Fever, fatigue, sore throat, and cervical or generalized lymphadenopathy, clinically characterize this syndrome.

EBV, a double-stranded DNA virus of the herpesvirus group, is present in saliva during the acute illness and can continue to be intermittently excreted over many months [35]. Spread of the infection is high, with 50%–80% of young adults demonstrating serum antibodies.

Following an asymptomatic incubation period of 14–60 days, a symptomatic viremic prodromal period of 4–7 days occurs, during which time the patient complains of nonspecific symptoms such as headache, malaise, and fatigue. The subsequent clinical course is extremely variable. Some patients, especially young children, may have only a sore throat indistinguishable from group A streptococci or respiratory viruses. Others, especially young adults, develop features described as the "mono syndrome," with tender lymphadenopathy, sore throat, fever, fatigue, and malaise as the key clinical features [36]. Symmetric posterior cervical lymphadenopathy is seen in about 90% of young adults with clinical EBV infection. Anterior cervical node enlargement as well as more generalized adenopathy can be appreciated during the course of the infection. The nodes are 5–25 mm in diameter and are firm, tender, and discreet. After several weeks the lymphadenopathy slowly subsides.

Pharyngitis and tonsillitis occur in about 50% of patients and may be especially severe. Some of the worst cases of exudative tonsillitis in this author's experience have been from EBV mononucleosis. Splenomegaly, found in about 50%–75% of patients, may be tense, tender, and vulnerable to rupture from mild trauma or overly aggressive palpation by the examining physician. The presenting symptom of "mono" may be just left upper quadrant pain due to the splenomegaly. Hepatomegaly is present in only about 10%–50% of cases, but hepatic transaminase abnormalities are uniformly present. Jaundice is unusual and present in only about 5% of cases. Approximately 10% of patients develop a maculopapular, erythematous rash on the trunk and more proximal extremities. Nearly all patients with infectious mononucleosis who are exposed to ampicillin develop this rash, which can be a useful clue to the diagnosis and should be differentiated from the patient who truly has a drug eruption.

Rarely is EBV mononucleosis associated with serious complications. EBV pneumonia, aseptic meningitis, meningoencephalitis, transverse myelitis, acute cerebellar ataxia, Guillain-Barré syndrome, myopericarditis, hemolytic anemia, agranulocytosis, thrombocytopenia, and renal failure have all been reported. Splenic rupture can occur spontaneously or from mild trauma, so the patient should be forewarned. Fatal infectious mononucleosis is rare.

The finding of an absolute lymphocytosis usually with more than 10% of the lymphocytes atypical is present in infectious mononucleosis caused by EBV, *cytomegalovirus, Toxoplasma gondii*, as well as other viral infections. Heterophil antibodies develop as a nonspecific response to EBV infection. The Monospot test measures the heterophil antibody response to EBV mononucleosis with few false-positive reactions. This test is positive in 85%–90% of cases but may be negative in the first 1–2 weeks of the illness. False-positive and false-negative tests are more common in young children [37, 38]. It may remain positive for 3–6 months. The infected patient will also produce several specific antibodies to EBV-associated antigens. Assay of these antibodies are most useful in settings in which false-positive or false-negative results are suspected. The IgM antibody to EBV viral capsid antigen (VCA-IgM) is present in the primary infection and rises after the first week, peaks in 4 weeks, and disappears in 2–6 months. A titer greater than 1:10 is consistent with a recent infection. The anti-EBV IgG antibodies develop more slowly in acute primary infection (after 2–3 weeks) and may persist for life.

When a patient presents to the emergency department with a mono-like illness, a CBC with differential and Monospot test should be obtained. If there is an absolute lymphocytosis with more than 10% atypical lymphocytes and the Monospot test is positive, the diagnosis is substantiated. If the patient has been ill for less than a week, atypical lymphocytes may be few and the Monospot test negative. These simple tests can be repeated in a week. Only 10%–15% of EBV mononucleosis cases will have a persistently negative Monospot test (false-negative), but the IgM anti-EBV serology will still be increased. The liver transaminases will be mildly elevated (two to three times) in nearly all cases, so normal or markedly elevated transaminase suggests another diagnosis.

The management is supportive. Rest, balanced diet, and no physical sports are prescribed during the first 2–3 weeks of the acute illness. Marked tonsillopharyngeal edema with exudates should concern the clinician. A group A beta-hemolytic streptococcus coinfection may be present and require treatment with penicillin. Exudative tonsillitis or pharyngeal or laryngeal edema to such a degree as to obstruct the airway may require corticosteroids (initial dosage of 40–60 mg of prednisone per day for 7–10 days). A tracheostomy rarely is needed. If complications develop, hospitalization for management will be required. Patients seen initially in the emergency department should be referred to a primary care physician for follow-up care.

The prognosis of EBV infectious mononucleosis is excellent for the majority of persons, with symptoms resolving in 2–4 weeks. Chronic EBV infection after the acute primary infection is rare and is characterized by immunologic defects, lymphadenopathy, cytopenia, splenomegaly, pneumonitis, and hepatitis [39]. Another chronic illness, chronic fatigue syndrome, has become popular and describes patients with chronic fatigue, recurring fever, sore throats, lymphadenopathy, myalgia, depression, and disability. Chronic fatigue syndrome was initially ascribed to EBV, but it is now evident that the etiology is much more complex. Chronic fatigue syndrome is discussed in more detail later in this chapter.

Cytomegalovirus Mononucleosis

Cytomegalovirus, a herpesvirus, causes a mono-like syndrome in immunologically normal adults. The pharyngitis and lymphadenopathy are less common and less severe than in EBV mononucleosis, and the disease is seldom definitively diagnosed. Asymptomatic, subclinical infection with seroconversion is the rule. Cytomegalovirus infectious syndromes in newborns and immunoincompetent patients can cause significant morbidity and mortality and are relatively refractory to treatment (see Chap. 14 and Chap. 16).

Infection in the general population is widespread, with a seroprevalence rate in adults of 40%–100% [40]. Transmission of cytomegalovirus in children, youths, and adults occurs in day care centers, in the home, and with sexual activity. Blood transmission has also been documented. The risk of infection is proportional to the number of transfusions and currently is around 3% or less [40, 41].

The clinical manifestations of cytomegalovirus mononucleosis resemble EBV mononucleosis and should be considered in any case of a mono-like illness when the Monospot test is negative. About 50% of patients in the pre-HIV period who were EBV heterophil-negative had cytomegalovirus infection [42,43]. Most patients have fever and mild generalized adenopathy, but tonsillitis or pharyngitis is rare. As with EBV-induced mononucleosis, absolute lymphocytosis with more than 10%–15% atypical cells and clinically insignificant elevation in hepatic transaminases usually are present. Normal hosts can on occasion develop cytomegalovirus complications. Meningoencephalitis, Guillain-Barré syndrome, polyneuritis, myocarditis, hepatitis, pneumonia, hemolytic anemia, and thrombocytopenia have been reported.

The diagnosis requires laboratory confirmation through viral culture, serology, or monoclonal antibody and nucleic acid probes. Several serologic tests are available, and each requires an elevated antibody titer or seroconversion from negative to positive. The complement fixation (CF) test is used by many laboratories, but it is less sensitive and less specific than many of the others [44]. An IgM anti-cytomegalovirus is usually elevated in acute infections, but because false-negative results are known this is not totally reliable. Cytomegalovirus can be cultured from the urine or throat in most patients and from the blood in some infected patients. One should be aware that CMV can be excreted chronically, particularly in the immunosuppressed. The interpretation of the results of any of these tests can be confusing; it usually is best to have them deciphered by an infectious disease specialist. Fortunately it is not necessary for most patients presenting to the emergency department with lymphadenopathy and a mono-like illness to undergo definitive workup for cytomegalovirus but rather to be referred.

Supportive treatment is all that is required for uncomplicated cytomegalovirus mononucleosis. Immunocompromised patients require consultation and referral.

Measles (Rubeola)

Although the introduction of the measles vaccine in 1963 dramatically decreased the incidence of this disease in the United States, approximately two thousand cases a year are still seen.

Measles is caused by a paramyxovirus and spread to susceptible contacts via respiratory secretions. The illness is characterized by malaise, fever, anorexia, cough, coryza, and conjunctivitis appearing 10–14 days after exposure. Later the typical erythematous and maculopapular rash of measles develops. It starts on the face and proceeds down the body. Patients have soft, nontender adenopathy. Koplik's spots (bluish-gray specks on a red base) located in the oral mucosa are felt to be pathognomonic of measles. An atypical presentation of measles has been reported in persons who received the killed measles vaccine in the years 1963–1968. Patients with atypical measles tend to have a shorter prodrome. The rash begins peripherally and may be urticarial, hemorrhagic, maculopapular, or vesicular. The two most worrisome complications of measles include pneumonia and encephalitis.

The diagnosis invariably is done on a clinical basis. Confirmation can be made by isolation of the virus (done mostly in patients in whom a good immunological response may not be expected) and by serologic antibody responses. Treatment is supportive.

RUBELLA (GERMAN MEASLES)

Rubella, caused by a rubivirus, is a common childhood illness characterized by rash, fever, and generalized lymphadenopathy. It is seen more frequently during the spring months. Since the rubella vaccine was marketed in 1969, there has been a significant decrease in the number of cases; nevertheless, a large percentage of the young adult population remain susceptible [45, 46].

Like rubeola, rubella is spread via respiratory secretions; once acquired the immunity is lifelong. The incubation period is 12–23 days. Initial symptoms include fever, malaise, and anorexia. General adenopathy occurs, with predilection for the posterior auricular, posterior cervical, and suboccipital chains. A nonconfluent, maculopapular rash that begins on the face and extends downward develops. Coryza and conjunctivitis usually accompany the rash. Splenomegaly may be present.

Congenital malformations can occur as a result of fetal infection; therefore, any woman of childbearing age susceptible to this disease should be immunized if not pregnant.

Rubella infection acquired postbirth usually is mild, often subclinical, and requires no treatment. The diagnosis is made on clinical grounds using epidemiological information as well as history of exposure. Laboratory tests like WBC counts are not helpful. Leukopenia with atypical lymphocytosis is seen as with many other viral infections. Virus isolation, from nasopharyngeal swabs and urine samples, although difficult and time consuming are feasible. Serological confirmation usually is made using enzyme-linked immunosorbent assay (ELISA) and latex agglutination techniques.

HIV

Acute infection with HIV can resemble infectious mononucleosis, presenting with either localized or generalized lymphadenopathy. A mono-like illness has been described in 55%–92% of persons with acute HIV infection. Because this illness is probably underdiagnosed, the actual incidence is probably higher. The illness begins 1–6 weeks after exposure with complaints of fever, sweats, malaise, myalgia, anorexia, headache, and photophobia [47, 48]. Generalized lymphadenopathy, especially of occipital, cervical, axillary, and inguinal lymph nodes, is found, and an exudative pharyngitis is common [49]. Twenty-five percent of patients have an associated maculopapular rash [50]. Meningismus, peripheral neuropathy [51], oral aphthous ulcers, and candidiasis [52, 53] have been reported with the acute illness. A decreased total lymphocyte count and transaminases and alkaline phosphatase are elevated. Atypical lymphocytes may be seen in the peripheral smear. Patients with neurologic symptoms may have mild lymphocytic pleocytosis in the CSF with normal glucose and protein. Clinical distinction between EBV mononucleosis and acute HIV infection is extremely difficult in the early disease, especially since the HIV antibody (ELISA) remains negative for approximately 2–3 months and false-negative tests for mononucleosis occur in up to 10% of early EBV infections. The only way of confirming the diagnosis at this stage is by obtaining a p24 HIV antigen. No therapy is available other than supportive measurements. Severe cases presenting with meningoencephalitis have been reported to be responsive to therapy with zidovudine [54].

Patients with chronic HIV infection may also have generalized adenopathy, or of infectious origin, due to dissemination of fungal or bacterial infection, especially mycobacterial infection, or secondary to malignancies, such as lymphoma and Kaposi's sarcoma.

Biopsies of lymph nodes may be helpful in making the diagnosis of these conditions, when suspected. Likewise, many of these patients have chronic adenopathy in which the biopsy specimen shows only nonspecific patterns of follicular hyperplasia (with or without fragmentation), follicular involution, or a diffuse pattern with no follicles and lymphocytic depletion [55].

HEPATITIS B

Approximately 200,000 persons in the United States are infected with the hepatitis B virus every year [56]. Transmission occurs by means of sexual contact, exposure to contaminated blood, and vertical transfer from mother to fetus.

Hepatitis B has a fairly long incubation period of 4–28 weeks. Subclinical cases with minimal symptomatology, with or without liver abnormalities, are reported. Most frequently patients present complaining of headaches, malaise, anorexia, nausea, vomiting, fatigue, diarrhea, and arthalgias. Smokers may refer to an aversion toward smoking. Distaste toward food is common. Patients may point out the presence of dark urine and/or light-colored stools.

On examination patients may appear jaundiced with icteric scleraes. Abdominal exam reveals tender hepatomegaly; 10% of patients also have concomitant splenomegaly. Spider angiomas may be appreciated, as well as a faint maculopapular rash. Enlarged lymph nodes are palpable, especially over the posterior cervical region. Some patients may have a serum sickness–like illness characterized by several days of fever, arthralgias, urticaria, and a rash.

Laboratory abnormalities seen in patients with hepatitis include mild anemia, occasional lymphocytosis with the presence of atypical lymphocytes, the presence of urobilinogen and bilirubin in the urine, proteinuria, and elevated bilirubin and transaminases, with serum glutamate pyruvate transaminase (SGPT) (ALT) levels usually higher than those of serum glutamic-oxaloacetic transaminase (SGOT) (AST).

The diagnosis is confirmed with serological tests for hepatitis markers. A positive hepatitis B surface antigen (HB_sAg) is indicative of active disease. In some patients the HB_sAg disappears before clinical symptoms are apparent; in those cases the diagnosis is established by the presence of anti-hepatitis B core IgM (anti-HBC) and subsequently the appearance of anti-HB_s.

CHRONIC FATIGUE SYNDROME

In 1985 reports of a chronic EBV syndrome or chronic mononucleosis were published [57, 58]. The reports consisted of a conglomerate of patients with nonspecific symptoms varying from fatigue and weakness to malaise, fevers, lymphadenopathy, and personality and memory changes, that had no apparent cause. Initial information linked the syndrome with EBV. Subsequent data demonstrated abnormal serologies for cytomegalovirus, herpes simplex, and measles, making the association between EBV and this entity less likely in these patients. Over the following years the name of the syndrome was changed to chronic fatigue syndrome [59].

In 1988 the Centers for Disease Control (CDC) developed a definition for chronic fatigue syndrome (Table 10-7) [60]. This definition is intended to serve as the basis for epidemiologic and clinical studies of chronic fatigue syndrome. Although it may be a useful guide for the evaluation of a patient with a suggestive illness, the definition remains sufficiently nonspecific that it cannot confirm or deny the diagnosis of chronic fatigue syndrome in individual patients. Chronic fatigue syndrome remains a diagnosis of exclusion. Most patients with fatigue have some other organic or psychiatric illness. An extensive workup to find the etiology of a patient's complaints is required. The diagnosis of chronic fatigue syndrome is ascertained only when all other possible causes have been ruled out.

DENGUE FEVER

Dengue fever, which is caused by a flavivirus, is a disease primarily seen in the tropics and occasionally seen in the United States in travelers from endemic areas. It is transmitted by the mosquito *Aedes aegypti* [61].

Patients with dengue fever complain of severe myalgias, headache, retro-orbital pain, and high fevers. On examination they appear toxic, are febrile, and may have generalized adenopathy. Occasionally a maculopapular rash that spares the palms and the soles is present.

There are four different strains of dengue viruses. A hemorrhagic form of dengue is often seen during a second dengue infection, or in persons taking aspirin. Other complications include myocarditis and encephalopathy. The diagnosis can be confirmed by serological testing. The treatment is supportive.

LASSA FEVER

Lassa fever, which is caused by an arenavirus, is a disease seen mainly in west Africa. It differs from

Table 10-7. CDC definition of chronic fatigue syndrome

A case of chronic fatigue syndrome must fulfill the following:
Major criteria: 1 and 2 *plus*
Minor criteria: ≥6 symptom criteria and >1 physical criteria *or* ≥8 symptom criteria

Major Criteria
1. Acute or subacute onset of persistent or relapsing, debilitating fatigue or easy fatiguability in a person who has no previous history of similar symptoms, that does not improve with rest and that is severe enough to reduce or impair average daily activity below 50% of the patient's premorbid activity level for a period of at least 6 months.
2. Reasonable exclusion of other clinical conditions that may produce similar symptoms, based on history, physical examination, and appropriate laboratory findings.

Minor Criteria
A. Symptom criteria (persistence or recurrence ≥6 months)
   1. Mild fever and/or chills (oral temperature 37.4°–38.3°C)
   2. Sore throat
   3. Painful anterior or posterior cervical or axillary lymph nodes
   4. Unexplained generalized muscle weakness
   5. Prolonged (≥24 hours) generalized fatigue following exercise
   6. Generalized headaches
   7. Muscle discomfort/myalgias
   8. Migratory arthralgias without joint swelling or redness
   9. Decreased sexual function
   10. Neuropsychological complaints
   11. Sleep disturbance
B. Physical criteria (documented by a physician on at least two occasions at least one month apart)
   1. Low-grade fever (37.5°–38.3°C oral; 37.8°–38.6°C rectal)
   2. Nonexudative pharyngitis
   3. Palpable and/or tender anterior or posterior cervical or axillary lymphadenopathy

other arenaviruses because person-to-person spread can occur. The disease also can spread by contact with rodents, inoculation of infected fluid, or nosocomial transmission via aerosols [62, 63].

The incubation period is 3–16 days. Most patients complain of chest pain, sore throat, abdominal pain, nausea, and vomiting. Diarrhea and conjunctivitis are seen in approximately 25% of patients. The illness can be complicated by a capillary leak-like syndrome; some patients may develop pericarditis, uveitis, or orchitis.

The virus can be recovered from throat swabs and urine cultures [64]. Serodiagnosis using immunofluorescent antibody IFA or ELISA is fast and sensitive [65]. Ribavirin therapy may be life saving.

Toxoplasmosis

T. gondii, an intracellular protozoan of worldwide distribution, is capable of causing acute or chronic disease of special concern in pregnant women and immunocompromised hosts [66]. Cats appear to be essential for its transmission, although the prevalence of cysts in meat for human consumption, especially pork and lamb, is fairly high (≤ 25%) [67].

Acute toxoplasmosis in the immunocompetent patient presents with adenopathy, primarily involving the cervical chain. The nodes are usually nontender and do not suppurate. Patients may complain of fever, malaise, sweats, and myalgias. On examination they may have hepatosplenomegaly and a maculopapular rash. The course of illness is usually benign. Symptoms resolve within a few months to a year. Clinically it may be difficult to differentiate from infectious mononucleosis, cat scratch disease, mycobacterial and fungal infections, or malignancies. The diagnosis is confirmed either by lymph node biopsy [68] (rarely done in an immunocompetent patient if there is suspicion of toxoplasmosis;) or by the demonstration of increased serological titers with a positive IgM [69].

Acute infection in the immunocompetent host does not require therapy unless there is visceral involvement, in which case treatment with pyrimethamine and sulfadiazine for 2–4 months is indicated. Acute infection in immunocompromised hosts presents mainly as an encephalitis. Chronic CNS infection often is seen in these patients. The diagnoses and therapies for these patients are entirely different (see Chap. 16 and Chap. 31).

Infection acquired during pregnancy represents a major concern, especially if acquired during the third trimester. Treatment of the pregnant woman reduces the chance of fetal infection but does not eliminate it. Pregnant women can be treated with spiramycin during all of gestation or after the first trimester with a combination of pyrimethamine-sulfadiazine [70].

Other protozoal infections that can cause fever and generalized adenopathy include kala-azar, caused by *Leishmania donovani* and seen primarily in South America, China, and east Africa; African trypanosomiasis, or sleeping sickness, caused by *Trypanosoma brucii*; and Chagas' disease, etiological agent *Trypanosoma cruzi*, mainly seen in Central America (including Mexico) and South America.

Helminthic Infections

Lymphatic filariasis, caused by *Wecheria bancrofti* and transmitted by either anophelene or aedes mosquitoes, can cause adenopathy. It is a prevalent disease in South America, Africa, Asia, the Caribbean, and the Pacific. Filariasis caused by *Brugia malayi* is seen mainly in Indonesia, Malaysia, India, China, Korea, Japan, and the Philippines. The most prevalent form of filariasis has a nocturnal periodicity, in which the microfilariae are detected in the peripheral smear only at night. A subperiodic form, most commonly seen in the Pacific, can present with parasitemia at any time.

Patients with filariasis may be asymptomatic, and the diagnosis may be an incidental finding on examination of the peripheral smear. Other patients may have intermittent acute febrile episodes, characterized by lymphangitis and lymphadenitis lasting 3–7 days for 6–10 years. The lymphangitis extends from the draining node toward the periphery. The nodes are painful, and associated thrombophlebitis commonly is seen. An obstructive form, known as elephantiasis and characterized by brawny edema, thickening of subcutaneous tissue, and hyperkeratosis, may be seen.

The diagnosis is made by observing the microfilariae in the peripheral blood smear. Treatment with diethylcarbamazine citrate for 3 weeks reduces the level of microfilariae in the blood [71]. Anti-inflammatory agents may be helpful, and elastic stockings may help to reduce edema.

Noninfectious Etiologies

Neoplasms of the immune system frequently present with adenopathy and fevers. Although they have distinctive features, they share characteristics such as weight loss, night sweats, fatigue, and malaise with many other entities.

Lymphomas, carcinoma, and immunoblastic lymphadenopathy (angioblastic lymphadenopathy) are all characterized by generalized lymphadenopathy, hepatosplenomegaly, and interstitial lung disease. All require lymph node biopsy for histopathological examination to confirm the diagnosis.

Waldenström's macroglobulinemia, multiple myeloma, and monoclonal gammopathies all can present with fever and adenopathies. Diagnosis is confirmed using electrophoresis.

Finally collagen vascular diseases, especially systemic lupus erythematosus, ought to be considered in the differential diagnosis of patients who complain of fatigue, fever, and arthralgias and who may be found to have generalized adenopathy, a malar rash, purpura, splenomegaly, and multisystem disease.

References

1. Abrams D, Foon KA, Gold J. Lymphadenopathy: a diagnostic plan. *Patient Care* April 30:95–112, 1988.
2. Kaufmann AF, Boyce JM, Martene WJ. Trends in human plague in the United States. *J Infect Dis* 141:522–24, 1980.
3. Hull H, Montes JM, Mann JM. Septicemic plague in New Mexico. *J Infect Dis* 155(1):113–18, 1987.
4. Boyce JM. Recent trends in the epidemiology of tularemia in the United States. *J Infect Dis* 131:197–99, 1975.

5. Markowitz LE, Hynes NA, de la Cruz P. Tick borne tularemia. An outbreak of lymphadenopathy in children. JAMA 254:2922–25, 1985.
6. Shinall EA. Cat scratch disease: a review of the literature. *Pediatr Dermatol* 7(1):11–18, 1990.
7. Delahoussaye PM, Osborne BM. Cat scratch disease presenting as abdominal visceral granuloma. *J Infect Dis* 161(1):71–78, 1990.
8. Scobie WG. Acute suppurative adenitis in children. *Scot Med J* 14:352–54, 1969.
9. Fox JP, Hall CE, Cooney M. Observations of adenovirus infections. *Am J Epidemiol* 105:362–86, 1977.
10. Baum S. Adenoviruses. In GL Mandell, RG Douglas Jr, JE Bennett (eds)., *Principles and Practice of Infectious Disease* (3rd ed.). New York: Churchill-Livingstone, 1990. Pp. 1185–90.
11. Shepp DH et al. Oral acyclovir therapy for mucocutaneous herpes simplex virus infections in immunocompromised marrow transplant recipients. *Ann Intern Med* 102:783–85, 1985.
12. Younken SW et al. Reduction of fever and symptoms in young adults with aspirin or amantadine. *Antimicrob Agents Chemo* 23:577–82, 1983.
13. Berkowitz CD et al. Cooperative study of latex agglutination to identify group A streptococcal antigen on throat swabs in patients with acute pharyngitis. *J Pediatr* 107:89–92, 1985.
14. Schwartz RH, Hayden GF, McCoy. Rapid diagnosis of streptococcal pharyngitis in two pediatric offices using a latex agglutination kit. *Pediatr Infect Dis* 4:647–50, 1985.
15. Roddy OF et al. Comparison of a latex agglutination kit and four culture methods for identification of group A streptococci in a pediatric office laboratory. *J Pediatr* 108:347–51, 1986.
16. Spark RP et al. Non-tuberculous mycobacterial adenitis of childhood. The ten year experience at a community hospital. *AJDC* 142:106–81, 1988.
17. Restrepo A et al. Itraconazole therapy in lymphangitis and cutaneous sporotrichosis. *Arch Dermatology* 122:413–17, 1986.
18. Currarno G. Acute epitrochlear lymphadenitis. *Pediatr Radiol* 6:160, 1977.
19. Glasswith J, Robins AG, Snider DE Jr. Tuberculosis in the 1980's. *N Engl J Med* 302:144–50, 1980.
20. Parson RJ, Zarafonites CJD. Histoplasmosis in man. Report of 7 cases and a review of 71 cases. *Arch Intern Med* 75:1–23, 1945.
21. Goodwin R et al. Disseminated histoplasmosis: clinical and pathologic calculations. *Medicine* 59(1):1–33, 1980.
22. Wheat L, Kohler R, Tewari R. Diagnosis of disseminated histoplasmosis by detection of histoplasma capsulatum antigen in serum and urine specimen. *N Engl J Med* 314(2):83–88, 1986.
23. Washburn RG. Reversal of adrenal glucocorticoid dysfunction in a patient with disseminated histoplasmosis. *Ann Intern Med* 110(1):86–87, 1989.
24. Huntington RW. Pathology of coccidiomycosis. In Steven DA (ed.), *Coccidiomycosis: A text*. New York: Plenum, 1980. P. 113.
25. Spink WW. *The Nature of Brucellosis*. Minneapolis: University of Minnesota Press, 1956.
26. Buchanan TM et al. Brucellosis in the United States, 1960–1972. An abattoir-associated disease. *Medicine* 53:415–25, 1974.
27. Joint FAO/WHO Expert Committee on Brucellosis. Brucellosis. Geneva: WHO, 1986.
28. Fergen RD, Anderson NC. Human leptospirosis. *Cit Rev Clin Lab Sec* 5:413, 1975.
29. Heath CW, Alexander AD, Gatton MM. Leptospirosis in the United States: analysis of 483 cases in man 1949–1961. *N Eng J Med* 273:857, 1965.
30. Hoff H, Rocourt J, Marget W (eds.). Listeria and listerosis. *Infection* (suppl 2):16, 1988.
31. Ciesielski CA et al. Listeriosis in the United States: 1980–1982. *Arch Intern Med* 148:1416–19, 1988.
32. Gray ML, Killinger AH. *Listeria monocytogenes* and listeric infections. *Bact Rev* 30:309–82, 1966.
33. McClain JB, Joshi B, Rice R. Chloramphenicol, gentamicin and ciprofloxacin against murine scrub typhus. *Antimicrob Agents Chemo* 32:285–86, 1988.
34. Klemola E et al. Infectious mononucleosis-like diseases with negative heterophil agglutination test. Clinical features in relations to Epstein-Barr virus and cytomegalovirus and antibodies. *J Infect Dis* 121:608–14, 1970.
35. Miller G, Niederman JC, Andrews LL. Prolonged oropharyngeal excretion of Epstein-Barr virus after infectious mononucleosis. *N Engl J Med* 288:229–32, 1973.
36. Evans AS. Infectious mononucleosis and related syndromes. *Am J Med Sci* 276:325–39, 1978.
37. Tamir D et al. Infectious mononucleosis and Epstein-Barr virus in childhood. *Pediatrics* 53:330–35, 1974.
38. Ginsburg GM et al. Infectious mononucleosis in children: evaluation of Epstein-Barr virus-specific serologic data. *JAMA* 237:781–85, 1977.
39. Straus SE. The chronic mononucleosis syndrome. *J Infect Dis* 157:405–12, 1988.
40. Complement-fixing antibodies against cytomegalovirus in different parts of the world. *Bull WHO* 49:103–106, 1973.
41. Preiksaitis JK, Brown L, McKenzie M. The risk of

cytomegalovirus infection in seronegative transfusion recipients not receiving exogenous immunosuppression. *J Infect Dis* 157:523–29, 1988.

42. Armstrong JA et al. Cytomegalovirus infection in children undergoing open-heart surgery. *Yale J Biol Med* 49:83–91, 1976.

43. Horwitz, CA et al. Heterophile negative infectious mononucleosis and mononucleosis-like illness. Laboratory confirmation of 43 cases *Am J Med* 63:947–50, 1977.

44. Betts RF et al. Comparative activity of immunofluorescent antibody and complement-fixing antibody in cytomegalovirus infection. *J Clin Microbiol* 4:151–56, 1976.

45. Banatvala JE, Best JM. Rubella infections. *Lancet* 1:1452, 1973.

46. Preblud SR et al. Rubella vaccination in the United States. A ten year review. *Epidemiol Rev* 2:171–94, 1980.

47. Fox R et al. Clinical manifestations of acute infection with human immunodeficiency virus in a cohort of gay men. *AIDS* 1:35–81, 1987.

48. Lindall B et al. Characteristics of the acute clinical illness associated with human immunodeficiency virus infection. *Arch Intern Med* 148(4)945–49, 1988.

49. Valle SL. Febrile pharyngitis as the primary sigh of human immunodeficiency virus infection in a cluster of cases linked by sexual contact. *Scand J Infect Dis* 19:13–17, 1987.

50. Rustin MHA et al. The acute exanthem associated with seroconversion to human T-cell lymphotropic virus III in a homosexual man. *J Infect Dis* 12:161–63, 1986.

51. Piette AM et al. Acute neuropathy coincident with seroconversion for anti LAV/HTLV III. *Lancet* 1:852, 1986.

52. Pedzamczer D, Casonova A, Santa Maria P. Esophageal candidiasis in the diagnosis of HIV infected patients. *JAMA* 259:1328–29, 1988.

53. Pena JM, Martinez-Lopez M, Arnadich F. Esophageal candidiasis associated with acute infection due to human immunodeficiency virus: a case report and review. *Rev Infect Dis* 13(5):872–75, 1991.

54. Ryan WC et al. *Incidence and nature of severe acute retroviral syndrome during primary human immunodeficiency virus type I infection in 319 seroconverting soldiers.* (abstract 25). Chicago: 31st Interscience Conference on Antimicrobial Agents and Chemotherapy, Sept. 29–Oct. 2, 1991.

55. Ost A et al. Lymphadenopathy in human immunodeficiency virus infection. Histological classification and staging. *APMIS suppl* 8:7–15, 1989.

56. Centers for Disease Control. Inactivated hepatitis B virus vaccine. *MMWR* 31:317–330, 1982.

57. Jones JF et al. Evidence for active Epstein Barr virus infection in patients with persistent, unexplained illnesses: elevated anti-early antigen antibodies. *Ann Intern Med* 102:1–7, 1985.

58. Straus SE et al. Persisting illness and fatigue in adults with evidence of Epstein Barr virus infection. *Ann Intern Med* 102:7–16, 1985.

59. Kamaroff A, Buchwald D. Symptoms and signs of chronic fatigue syndrome. *Rev of Infect Dis* 13(suppl 1):S8–S11, 1991.

60. Holmes GP et al. Chronic fatigue syndrome: a working case definition. *Ann Intern Med* 108:387–89, 1988.

61. Halstead SB. Dengue haemorrhagic fever. A public health problem and a field for research. *Bull WHO* 58:1–21, 1980.

62. Johnson KM et al. Clinical virology of Lassa fever in hospitalized patients. *J Infect Dis* 155:456–64, 1987.

63. Monson MH et al. Pediatric Lassa fever: a review of 33 Liberian cases. *Am J Trop Med Hyg* 36:408–15, 1987.

64. Edmond RTD et al. A case of Lassa fever: clinical and virologic findings. *Br Med J* 285:1001–2, 1982.

65. Jahrlling PB, Niklasson BS, McCormick JB. Early diagnosis of human Lassa fever by ELISA; detection of antigen and antibody. *Lancet* 1:250–52, 1985.

66. Dubey JP. A review of toxoplasmosis in pigs. *Vet Parasitol* 19:181, 1986.

67. Remington JS. Toxoplasmosis in the adult. *Bull NY Acad Med* 50:211–27, 1974.

68. Dorfman RF, Remington JS. Value of lymph node biopsy in the diagnosis of acute acquired toxoplasmosis. *N Engl J Med* 289:878–81, 1973.

69. Welch P et al. Serologic diagnosis of acute lymphadenopathic toxoplasmosis. *J Infect Dis* 142:256–64, 1980.

70. Remington JS, Desmonts G, Kleen J (eds.). *Toxoplasmosis: Infectious Diseases of the Fetus and Newborn Infant.* Philadelphia: Saunders, 1983. P. 143.

71. Ottensen EA. Efficacy of diethylcarbamazine infection with lymphatic dwelling filariae in humans. *Rev Infect Dis* 7:341–56, 1985.

11

Diabetic Foot Infections

RONALD W. QUENZER

Foot infections are one of the most frequent complaints that bring diabetics to the emergency department and one of the most frequent infections that hospitalize the diabetic patient [1]. The average duration of hospitalization for treatment of a diabetic foot infection is 2–4 weeks at a cost of $5000–$10,000 (in this author's experience).

The cost of soft-tissue and bone infections of the foot is greater than $500 million per year in the United States. Approximately 25% of the 12 million diabetics in this country have foot problems, and 1 in 15 of these persons will undergo amputation [2]. There are about 120,000 nontraumatic amputations per year in the United States, of which 50%–70% are in diabetics and most of these are due to foot lesions [3]. After losing one limb, 30%–40% will loose the other within 3 years unless preventive intervention is undertaken [4]. It is estimated that about 50% of the amputations in diabetics could be prevented [5].

Diabetic foot infections represent a spectrum of clinical presentations. Discussed in this chapter are infected penetrating ulcers, cellulitis, necrotizing fasciitis, and septic gangrene. Osteomyelitis and septic arthritis are discussed in detail in Chap. 33.

Pathophysiology

The pathophysiology of diabetic ulcers and skin, soft-tissue, and bone infections in diabetics is complex and multifactorial. It involves neurologic, vascular, musculoskeletal, and selected host-defense abnormalities.

Diabetic Neuropathy

Diabetic neuropathy is the principle factor for diabetic foot infections. Nerve conduction studies reveal an incidence of up to 60% in diabetics [6]. Clinical neuropathy is estimated in 10%–20% of all diabetics, with 50% or more showing clinical evidence after 25 years of diabetes.

Several patterns of diabetic neuropathy are responsible for the varied clinical presentations (Table 11-1) [7]. Peripheral sensorimotor neuropathy is responsible for the majority of foot problems in diabetics. Peripheral sensory neuropathy causes diminished sensation and occasionally insensate feet. Peripheral sensory neuropathy is initially apparent as hypesthesia or occasionally paresthesia in a stocking distribution resulting in an increase in

219

Table 11-1. Diabetic neuropathies

Peripheral sensory
Peripheral motor
Autonomic
Mononeuropathies (focal or multiple)
Cranial

trauma, repetitive mechanical pressure leading to abrasions, ulcerations, and calluses, which can become secondarily infected. The resultant soft-tissue infections represent a focus of infection, which can lead to bacteremia, sepsis, or the development of osteomyelitis in adjacent bones. A totally insensate foot is the end-stage event of the neuropathy. Loss of peripheral motor functions causes atrophy and weakness of the intrinsic muscles of the foot. The classic claw-toe deformity and transfer in weight bearing to metatarsal heads with maldistribution of pressure and shear forces predispose to calluses and ulcerations. Sorbitol and galactitol accumulation and a decline in myoinositol levels in the nerve axons seem to play a major role in the pathogenesis of this metabolic neuropathy and result in a decline in nerve conduction velocity [8–12].

Focal and multifocal mononeuropathies are thought to be due to vascular infarctions as well as direct prolonged pressure on a nerve at a pressure point, such as the peroneal nerve where it passes around the fibular head [13]. The neuropathy can be proximal, distal, or both. In the lower extremities the peroneal nerves and the lateral femoral cutaneous nerves most commonly are involved. Painful paresthesia is the most common symptom. Nerve compression of the peroneal nerve can cause drop foot.

Autonomic neuropathy, which can create a change in blood flow and skin hydration, seldom is present without antecedent peripheral sensorimotor neuropathy. Anhidrosis due to denervation of the sweat glands of the hands and the lower extremities is a common manifestation [14]. Dry, cracking skin predisposes to sores and provides entry sites for bacteria. Sympathetic vascular denervation causes arteriovenous shunting, an increase in capillary pressure, and neuropathic edema [15]. Autonomic temperature control of the skin is lost, and in colder ambient temperatures the feet will be cold to touch. Severe cases of autonomic neuropathy can cause postural hypotension [16]. Multiple factors contribute to this autonomic dysfunction [17, 18].

Peripheral Vascular Disease in the Diabetic

The second important pathophysiologic process in diabetic foot infections is marginal perfusion or limb ischemia due to atherosclerosis in major vessels, including the large-(femoral artery) and medium-sized vessels (tibial and peroneal arteries), as well as microvascular disease. Approximately 15% of diabetics after 10 years of disease and 45% after 20 years have detectable peripheral vascular disease [19]. Atherosclerosis progresses more rapidly in diabetics than in nondiabetics for reasons not understood. Occlusion of the aortoiliac or femoral-popliteal-tibial arteries is responsible for the majority of limb ischemia and in the majority of patients is remedial to revascularization procedures or percutaneous transluminal angioplasty [20–22]. Ischemic tissue is more susceptible to infection, and healing is impaired. The reasons for this condition are not well understood, but nutritional deficiencies, defective inflammatory response, and inadequate local production of growth factors have been proposed.

Musculoskeletal Disease

Diabetic osteoarthropathy, or Charcot's joint, is a noninfectious, destructive, relatively painless neuropathic disorder that results from repeated mechanical trauma to an insensate foot. Joint destruction and subluxation bring about a hyperemic response that causes resorption of normal bone, perpetuating instability and deformity of the foot (Fig. 11-1). Foot deformity leads to pressure sores, calluses, ulcerations, and secondary infections. The end result is a rocker-bottom deformity (collapse of midfoot), often with a midfoot plantar ulceration. Diabetes is the most common cause of Charcot's joint, with an incidence of approximately 1 in 500–750 diabetic patients [23]. The incidence seems to increase with the duration of diabetes. Charcot's joint defect usually is uni-

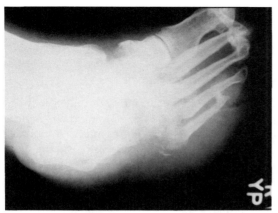

Fig. 11-1. Charcot's foot (neuropathic arthropathy) in a diabetic patient

lateral, and all patients have underlying peripheral sensory neuropathy.

Diabetics develop other deformities of their feet associated with intrinsic muscular wasting as a consequence of neurologic and vascular disease. An anterior equinus foot with hammertoe deformities is common. In the neuropathic foot Fernando et al. demonstrated that the limited joint mobility seen in diabetics leads to abnormal foot pressures and foot ulcerations [24]. Mueller et al. found a significant relationship between the foot deformity and ulcer location [25]. In 7 patients with Charcot's foot 6 showed ulceration at the midfoot; 9 of 18 patients with a compensated forefoot varus showed ulceration at the second, third, or fourth metatarsal head; and 15 of 17 patients with an uncompensated forefoot varus or forefoot valgus showed ulceration at the first or fifth metatarsal.

Digit or partial foot amputation may be definitive treatment for the primary infectious process, but it creates secondary gait and pressure abnormalities, leading to ulcerations and increased potential for diabetic foot infections [26]. For example, amputation of the hallux shifts weight laterally with concentration under the second metatarsal head, whereas loss of a lesser digit has primarily psychological effects. A first-ray amputation encourages excessive pronation, causing medial tarsal collapse and excessive loads borne by the second metatarsal

head. A transmetatarsal amputation often is associated with stump ulcers.

Skin and WBC Host Defenses

Diabetic foot infections respond slowly to treatment. Neutrophil dysfunction, alterations in the skin physiology, and changes in microflora of insulin-dependent diabetic patients are responsible for the diminished host defenses. Polymorphonuclear leukocyte functional changes in diabetics include a decrease in chemotaxis, phagocytosis, and bacteria-killing activities. The clinical significance of these abnormalities in each infectious situation is still unclear.

The skin serves as a barrier to infection of the underlying tissues. Normal skin is resistant to colonization with and invasion by the more pathogenic microorganisms. The intact stratum corneum is the most effective skin barrier. A break in the integrity of this layer or a change in the normal physiologic properties is necessary before most skin infections can occur [27, 28].

Healthy microflora of the healthy foot varies from 10^3 colony-forming units per square centimeter on the dorsum of the foot to 10^7 colony-forming units per square centimeter on the intertriginous toe webs [29–31]. Coagulase-negative staphylococci, micrococci, and diphtheroids represent 99% of the total number of organisms found on healthy clean feet. Although these organisms are not considered to be highly pathogenic or virulent, they do cause foot infections and may be relatively antibiotic resistant.

Patients who are hospitalized or who have insulin-dependent diabetes mellitus, poor hygiene, dermatitis, ischemia, abrasions, lacerations, or ulcerations may develop a change of the normal physiologic status and resident microflora of the skin. Increased colonization of *Staphylococcus aureus* occurs in insulin-dependent diabetes as well as in patients with dermatitis [32–35]. Dermatophytes (e.g., *Candida*, *Trichophyton*, and *Aspergillus* species), various gram-negative bacilli (e.g., *Escherichia coli* and *Pseudomonas* and *Klebsiella* species), and streptococci transiently colonize skin in altered clinical situations. These highly pathogenic organisms usually are responsible for the more serious skin, soft-tissue, bone, and joint infections in diabetics.

Etiology

Most diabetic foot infections are results of minor skin and soft-tissue traumas that allow spread of resident bacteria from the skin surface to deeper structures. The etiology of diabetic foot infections is polymicrobial in approximately 75% of cases [36–39], with a mean of 4.8 species isolated [36, 37]. Aerobic and anaerobic bacteria have been identified in 13%–90% of these infections. The most frequently isolated organisms are S. aureus (30%–50%), coagulase-negative staphylococci, group D enterococci, streptococci, gram-negative bacilli, and anaerobic bacteria (Table 11-2) [40, 41]. Pseudomonas species are responsible for less than 10% of diabetic foot infections [36, 37]. Anaerobes are present in a high percentage of diabetic ulcers, in up to 80% of the patients reported on by Sapico et al. and 57% of patients by Fierer et al. [36, 37]. Bacteroides, anaerobic streptococci, and Clostridium species are the most common anaerobes. Penicillin-resistant Bacteroides fragilis is the single most often isolated anaerobe [37]. Although Candida species may colonize the skin, especially the toe webs of 10%–15% of diabetics, it is an uncommon isolate in foot infections [36].

The organisms responsible for osteomyelitis in diabetics vary only slightly from those isolated from infected ulcers or soft-tissue infections [42]. Osteomyelitis is discussed in detail in Chap. 33.

Clinical Manifestations

The main decisions confronting the emergency department physician are determining the presence, the extent, and the severity of infection in a diabetic with a foot lesion. The severity and the spectrum of diabetic foot infections range from localized superficial infections of the skin or ulcer to deep tissue infections (septic foot) that are limb or life threatening. Patients with long-standing diabetes, sensorimotor neuropathy, peripheral vascular disease, previous foot ulceration, or blindness and the disabled aged are subjects at risk for diabetic foot infections. Gibbons and Eliopoulos have developed a classification system for the severity of diabetic foot infections (Table 11-3) [43]. Emergency department physicians can use this system to determine the need for hospital admission, since there is a tendency to underestimate the severity and the extent of infection in diabetics. Also the rapidity of progress from a localized process to deeper tissue and extremity infection should be appreciated. The morbidity of infections is greater in diabetics than in nondiabetics.

The diabetic presenting to the emergency department with a foot infection requires detailed attention to clinical features to ascertain the extent and the severity of infection. An attempt should be

Table 11-2. Usual pathogens in diabetic foot infections

Aerobes	Anaerobes
Gram positive	Bacteriodes fragilis
S. aureus	Other bacteriodes
Staphylococcus epidermidis	Clostridium species (rare)
Streptococcus pyogenes (group A)	Peptostreptococci
Group B streptococci	Peptococci
Streptococcus viridans	
Group D enterococci	
Gram negative	Fungi
E. coli	Candida species (rare)
Proteus mirabilis	
Klebsiella pneumoniae	
Enterobacter cloacae	
Pseudomonas aeruginosa	

Table 11-3. The Gibbons and Eliopoulos classification system to determine the severity of diabetic foot infections

Group 1	Stable, superficial, uncomplicated ulcers
Group 2	Moderately to severely infected ulcers, threatened limb loss, no signs of systemic toxicity
Group 3	Severely infected ulcers, threatened limb loss, systemic toxicity

made to determine the date that the infection started; history of trauma, puncture, or previous foot surgery; the rate and degree of progression or partial resolution; the presence or absence of systemic response (fever, tachycardia, tachypnea); and recent treatment attempts with antibiotics as well as home remedies. It should be determined if the patient is septic (Chap. 6) and if the infection is responsible for poor diabetic control, diabetic ketoacidosis, dehydration, or renal insufficiency.

Patients may complain of swelling, redness, ulcerations, calluses, wounds, deformity, purulent drainage, fetid odor, or less specific constitutional symptoms of fever or rigors. Seldom does the patient complain of foot pain. Hyperglycemia due to an unrecognized infectious process of the foot may be the only clue to a problem.

The foot and the leg must be examined carefully for ulcerations, sinus tracts, cellulitis, and gangrene. Outlining the margin of cutaneous erythema with indelible ink will later serve as a baseline for evaluation of therapeutic response. The depth and the diameter of ulcers should be determined and recorded. In 1981 Wagner proposed a practical system for grading the diabetic foot, and a modification of this classification has become popular [44]. Subsequently several other classification systems have been devised by various clinical investigators (Table 11-4) [45]. It seems advisable for an emergency department to select one system for regular use. In the modified Wagner system a superficial ulcer is grade I (Fig. 11-2); deep ulcer to bone, joint, or tendon without infection is grade IIA (Fig. 11-3); and an infected deep ulcer is grade IIB (Fig. 11-4). The presence of a deep abscess or osteomyelitis is classified as grade IIIA or IIIB, respectively. Grade IV refers to gangrene of the toe(s) or forefoot, and grade V represents gangrene of the entire foot.

Table 11-4. Classification systems for diabetic foot infections

Wagner (1981)	*Wagner (modified)*
0 Intact skin	0 Intact skin
1 Superficial ulcer	I Superficial ulcer
2 Deep ulcer (to tendon, bone, or joint)	IIA Deep ulcer (to tendon, bone, or joint)
3 Deep ulcer plus abscess or osteomyelitis	IIB Deep ulcer plus infection
4 Gangrene of forefoot	IIIA Deep abscess
5 Gangrene of whole foot	IIIB Osteomyelitis
	IV Gangrene of toes or forefoot
	V Gangrene of whole foot
Calhoun (1988)	*Sims and Cavanagh (1988)*
0 Intact skin plus cellulitis	0 Absent skin lesion
1 Superficial ulcer plus infection	1 Dense callus, no ulcer
2 Septic deep ulcer	2 Preulcerative lesion
3 Deep ulcer plus abscess or osteomyelitis	3 Partial-thickness ulcer
4 Gangrene of forefoot	4 Full-thickness ulcer
5 Gangrene of whole foot	5 Full-thickness ulcer to tendon, bone, joint
	6 Deep ulcer plus abscess; osteomyelitis
	7 Proximal spread of infection
	8 Gangrene of forefoot
	9 Gangrene of whole foot

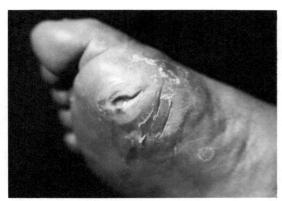

Fig. 11-2. Diabetic patient with a superficial non-infected ulcer in callused skin overlying first MTH—Grade I (modified Wagner system)

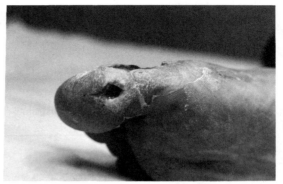

Fig. 11-4. Infected deep ulcer extending to bone on the great toe of a diabetic—Grade IIB (modified Wagner system)

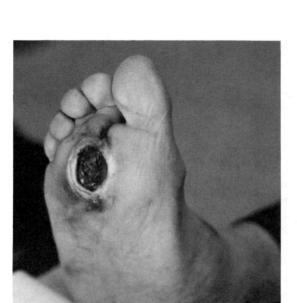

Fig. 11-3. Deep, uninfected neuropathic ulcer on the sole of a diabetic—Grade IIA (modified Wagner system)

Probing ulcers or sinus tracts with a cotton tip applicator or a stiff urethral swab culturette helps the clinician to define the undermining of tissue due to necrosis and the proximity to tendons, bones, and joints. "Probe-to-bone" suggests underlying osteomyelitis. It is good practice for the exam-ining physician to enter a graphic description of the foot infection in the emergency department record.

A thorough evaluation of the neurologic, vascular, musculoskeletal, and dermatologic components of the lower extremity is essential to the diagnosis and therapy of diabetic foot infections (Table 11-5) [46]. Serious foot infections, except for puncture wounds, are uncommon in patients without neuropathy or severe vascular insufficiency. Neuropathic manifestations include decreased or loss of vibratory sense, proprioception, sensation to light touch and pain, or ankle or knee deep tendon reflexes; anhidrosis; or neuropathic edema. Protective sensation of the foot is considered absent if the patient is unable to perceive 10 g of pressure as exerted by a 5.07 Semmes-Weinstein monofilament [47].

Patients with atherosclerotic occlusive disease may notice intermittent claudication, described as pain in the calves when ambulating and relieved with rest. Some patients have rest pain in their feet at night. Vascular abnormalities are best detected at the bedside by the presence of cold feet; loss of hair on the digits; thickening of nails; diminished or absent pedal, popliteal, or femoral pulses; arterial bruits; and gangrene.

Direct visualization of the feet may show significant musculoskeletal complications such as "rocker-bottom" deformity due to neuropathic arthropathy, hammertoes, or cavus feet with claw toes.

Loss of hair on the digits or lower leg, thickening of the nails, shiny skin, chronic tinea infections, keratosis, onychomycosis, and paronychia all support unhealthy skin condition or dermopathy.

Diagnosis

Definitive treatment depends on the type of infectious process. The emergency department physician is challenged to recognize the type of infection in a brief period of evaluation and must recall that the diabetic is susceptible to all the types of skin and soft-tissue infections that are seen in nondiabetics as well, such as paronychia, folliculitis, erysipelas, and infected wounds. However, infected ulcers, cel-

lulitis, necrotizing fasciitis, and gangrenous infections are the most troublesome for diabetics (Table 11.6). Some degree of two or more of these processes may be present simultaneously. Bacteremia is uncommon but, if present, indicates sepsis.

Infected Penetrating Ulcers

The most common foot infection in diabetics, aside from the paronychium, is the infected ulcer. Fortunately most diabetic ulcers are not infected. Unfortunately many infected ulcers are complicated by coexisting deep-space or bone infection. The uninfected ulcer is characteristically painless, 2–25 mm

Table 11-5. Clinical examination of the diabetic foot

Exam	Symptoms	Signs
Neurologic	Numbness, burning, pain, tingling, pruritus, cold feet, weakness	Decreased vibratory sense, decreased position sense, decreased deep tendon reflexes, decreased sensation to touch/pain, weakness, decreased sweating
Vascular	Intermittent claudication, cold feet, rest pain	Atrophy of skin, decreased pulses, femoral bruits, dependent rubor, plantar pallor on elevation, prolonged capillary filling time >3 sec, cyanotic toes, gangrene, lack of hair growth
Musculoskeletal	Bunions, swelling, change in foot shape	Decreased joint mobility, hammertoe deformities, Charcot's foot, cavus feet with claw toes
Dermatologic	Dry skin, nail deformity, shin spots	Dry skin, tinea infections, trophic ulcer, thickened nails, keratoses, paronychia, necrobiosis lipoidica diabeticorum, decreased hair

Adapted from Scardina RJ. Diabetic foot problems: assessment and prevention. *Clin Diabetes* 1:1–7, 1983.

Table 11-6. Clinical diagnosis of the infected diabetic foot

Infection	Signs and symptoms
Penetrating ulcer	Painless ulcer, purulent discharge from ulcer, foul smell of the drainage
Cellulitis	Pain/tenderness (minimal), edema, erythema, bullae, crepitation +/−

Necrotizing fasciitis	Early
	    Fever, first- or second-degree burn appearance to skin, hyperesthesia of overlying skin
	Late
	    Septic patient, grayish discoloration of skin, hypesthesia or anesthesia of overlying skin

Septic gangrene	Crepitation, brawny edema, bullae, purplish-black discoloration, septic patient +/−
Osteoarticular	(See Chapter 33.)
Bacteremia	Septic patient, metabolic and cardiovascular instability

in diameter, 3–6 mm in depth, and surrounded by hyperkeratotic skin. The ulcer that appears clean without exudative drainage, edema, or cellulitis is noninfected. Foul smell, purulent discharge, nonblanching erythema, or cellulitis supports an infectious process (Fig. 11-5). The infection may involve the skin and superficial soft tissue, deep spaces, or bone or joint. If the clinician can probe to the bone through an ulcer or sinus tract with a swab or detect exposed periosteum, osteomyelitis is likely. Deepspace infections are evident with crepitation, wet gangrene, extensive cellulitis, lymphangitis, or systemic toxicity. Foul odor in the presence of an ulcerative lesion implies anaerobes [36].

Cellulitis

The extent of soft tissue infection is particularly difficult to evaluate in the neuropathic and ischemic foot. Pain and tenderness, if present, usually are only mild. Leukocytosis, fever, and other systemic symptoms cannot be relied on to exclude a serious deep-tissue, limb-threatening infection in the diabetic. A deep abscess in the plantar space appears as severe cellulitis, with swelling extending from the sole to the dorsal surface. Marked edema and subcutaneous gas detected as crepitation on physical examination or by x-ray are typical of necrotizing cellulitis (Fig. 11-6). Although anaerobes, especially clostridia and bacteroides are most often associated with tissue gas, several facultative aero-

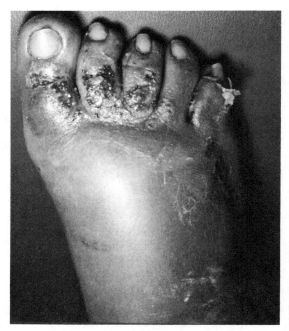

Fig. 11-6. Necrotizing cellulitis of the foot in a diabetic patient. Note gas in soft tissue

bic coliforms and streptococci also can cause gas and a similar infection.

Necrotizing Fasciitis

Necrotizing soft-tissue infections, particularly necrotizing fasciitis, initially may appear rather benign, like a first- or second-degree burn with hyperesthesia of the overlying skin. But within hours cutaneous hypesthesia or anesthesia and edema develop, and the skin turns grayish (Fig. 11-7) [48]. Without early intervention systemic toxicity and sepsis become apparent. The mortality of necrotizing fasciitis in the diabetic is greater than 50% [49].

Septic Gangrene

Gangrene develops when inadequate vascularity and oxygen supply result in ischemic necrosis. Aseptic ("dry") gangrene develops from occlusion of the arteries and is a noninfectious process. Septic ("wet") gangrene develops when microorganisms

Fig. 11-5. Diabetic foot infection with ulcer and cellulitis of the fourth digit

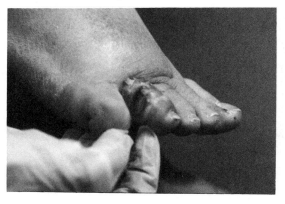

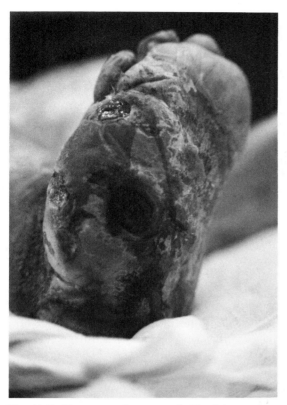

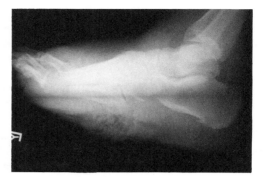

Fig. 11-8. Septic gangrene

Bacteremia

Bacteremia in infected feet of diabetic patients is uncommon but if present usually indicates sepsis. Sapico et al. found that *B. fragilis* and *S. aureus* were the most common isolates in blood cultures [50]. Absence of organisms in the bloodstream should not discount sepsis with its appreciable morbidities and mortality, particularly in the diabetic patient.

Workup in the Emergency Department

Gram's stains, cultures, and radiographs are all helpful in the diagnosis. The Gram's stain can direct more specific initial antibiotic therapy. For example, if large "box-car," gram-positive rods are noted, clostridial infection is evident, and treatment can be specifically selected. Sheets of gram-positive cocci point to streptococci, staphylococci, or both. Gram's stains without organisms or a predominate type indicate the need for broader-spectrum antibiotics. Total concordance of the swab culture of a superficial wound with a deep-tissue culture is unreliable in directing antibiotic therapy. The frequency of total concordance of a curette-specimen culture from the base of the ulcer with a deep-tissue culture is not much better—only 35% in 36 samples in a study by Sapico et al. [36]. However, pus from abscesses or sinus tracts originating from subcutaneous tissue, needle aspirates or biopsy specimens of infected soft tissue, and necrotic tissue samples can yield helpful information.

Fig. 11-7. Necrotizing fasciitis with "fetid foot" of a diabetic patient due to mixed aerobic and anaerobic infections

infect devascularized tissues. Gangrenous infections can be caused by clostridia, other anaerobes, or mixed aerobic-anaerobic organisms that are commonly responsible for diabetic foot infections. Clostridial gangrene is a fulminant, rapidly progressing infection. The patient is septic, anxious, and apprehensive; the foot shows a brawny edema, extensive cellulitis, purplish discoloration, bullae, and crepitation of subcutaneous tissue from gas (Fig. 11-8). Gangrene from other organisms usually progresses more slowly, but if ignored it results in an equally devastating infection. The presence of gangrene signals a poor chance of avoiding some degree of disarticulation. Clues to anaerobic infection are wounds or ulcers with foul smelling discharge, presence of gas in tissue, tissue necrosis, gangrene, and a Gram's stain of exudate that shows several morphologic types of bacteria.

Deep cultures obtained by aspirate or biopsy produce the best etiologic information [51]. Properly collected specimens submitted to the laboratory require precise identification of the source and instruction for Gram's stain, culture (aerobic and anaerobic), and sensitivity. Blood cultures are indicated in patients with any systemic symptoms or signs of infection.

It is good practice to x-ray all infected feet to look for a foreign body, determine the presence of soft-tissue gas, predict the depth of an ulcer, identify any osteoarthropathy, and diagnose osteomyelitis. Bone changes of neuroarthropathy (Charcot's joint) mimic those of osteomyelitis. For comparison prior foot films are invaluable. The diagnosis of osteomyelitis is much more complicated, often requiring bone scintigraphy, MRI, or both. (The radiographic approach is presented in Chap. 33.) Noninvasive vascular testing is indicated in every diabetic patient with signs or symptoms of peripheral vascular disease, but it can be performed following disposition from the emergency department.

Therapy

The task of the emergency department physician is to recognize and determine the seriousness of the infectious process and to initiate therapy to prevent the infection from evolving into a digit-, limb- or life-threatening stage. All patients with diabetic foot infections should be hospitalized. The exception to this is the patient with an infected superficial ulcer.

Treatment should be approached from both medical and surgical points of view. The response to therapy is influenced by the choice of antibiotic, bacteriology, state of circulation, and type of infection [40]. Patients with mixed aerobic and anaerobic infections have a poorer response to therapy than those with monomicrobial infections [37]. Medical management also includes antibiotics, bed rest and elevation of the extremity, diabetic control, and normalization of fluids and electrolytes status.

Infected Ulcers

Infected ulcers require both antibiotics and ulcer débridement (Table 11-7). For infected neuropathic ulcers, ampicillin-sulbactam, ticarcillin-clavulanate, and cefoxitin are all moderately broad-spectrum antibiotics with excellent staphylococcal, streptococcal, and anaerobic activity making them reasonable monotherapeutic choices. The combination of cefazolin and metronidazole gives similar aerobic and anaerobic coverage and is less expensive. Following 5–7 days of parenteral therapy, oral agents can be substituted to complete a therapeutic course of 1–3 weeks. Several ongoing

Table 11-7. Treatment of diabetic foot infections

Disease	Pathogens	Antibiotic	Surgery
Infected ulcer	S. aureus, streptococci, E. coli, bacteroides	Cefazolin plus metronidazole, ampicillin-sulbactam, cefoxitin, ticarcillin-clavulanate	Débridement
Cellulitis	Staphylococci, streptococci, enteric gram-negative bacteria	Nafcillin, cefazolin	None
Necrotizing cellulitis	Staphylococci, streptococci, anaerobes	Ampicillin-sulbactam, cefoxetan, cefoxitin, ticarcillin-clavulanate	Débridement, drainage of abscesses
Necrotizing fasciitis	Streptococci or mixed aerobes/anaerobes	Imipenem, third-generation cephalosporin plus metronidazole or clindamycin	Débridement, wide excision
Septic gangrene	Anaerobes, enteric gram-negative bacteria, staphylococci	Imipenem, third-generation cephalosporin plus metronidazole or clindamycin	Amputation

studies are evaluating the efficacy of oral versus parenteral agents. Infected superficial ulcers can be treated orally. Oral agents such as amoxicillin-clavulanate alone or ciprofloxacin (or ofloxacin) with metronidazole (or clindamycin) provide good spectrum coverage in this situation. Achieving an adequate antibiotic level with oral agents at the site of the foot infection in a diabetic patient is a concern for many physicians.

There is still some interest in topical biological modalities to expedite ulcer healing. These agents include growth factors, cytokines, and polypeptides. Animal studies have been encouraging, but clinical trials are few to date.

Cellulitis

Superficial cellulitis can be treated successfully with antibiotics alone (see Table 11-7). If an abscess is present, then incision and drainage are indicated. A one- to two-week course of antibiotics should be prescribed. Based on the probable pathogens agents active against staphylococci and streptococci usually are quite adequate. Nafcillin 1.5 g IV q4h (or 2 g q6h) or cefazolin 2 g IV q8h is appropriate. As the infection begins to resolve, oral agents can replace parenteral forms of treatment. Dicloxacillin 2–4 g/day, amoxicillin-sulbactam 2 g/day, or cephalexin 2 g/day can be selected, depending on culture results and response to initial therapy. It is prudent to admit these patients to initiate therapy.

Necrotizing Cellulitis/Fasciitis and Gangrenous Infections

Deep necrotizing infections (e.g., fetid foot and septic foot) are medical emergencies. Incision, débridement, and drainage of all infected tissue and abscesses as well as excision of the necrotic tissue within 12–24 hours are essential to improve tissue perfusion, control the infectious process, and lower morbidity and mortality [52, 53]. Necrotizing fasciitis and septic gangrene often require some stage of amputation, if not just extensive excision and débridement of infected and necrotic tissues. In the presence of gangrene surgical intervention is also directed at restoring circulation to ischemic tissue.

Broad-spectrum antimicrobial agents directed at aerobic and anaerobic organisms should be initiated for these infections in the emergency department after blood cultures have been obtained to contain the infectious process and associated bacteremia. Because polymicrobial aerobic-anaerobic etiology can be anticipated, the agent(s) of first choice must be broad spectrum (Table 11-7). Antibiotics with good efficacy in these serious diabetic foot infections due to mixed aerobic and anaerobic bacteria include monotherapy with imipenem or possibly cefoxitin, cefotetan, ampicillin-sulbactam, and ticarcillin-clavulanate. Some clinicians prefer combination therapy with clindamycin plus aztreonam (or aminoglycoside) or metronidazole plus a third-generation cephalosporin (ceftazidime, cefotaxime, ceftriaxone) or aminoglycoside [37, 45, 54–62]. In regions where methicillin-resistant S. aureus (MRSA) is common or methicillin-resistant Staphylococcus epidermidis (MRSE) is cultured, vancomycin (or teicoplanin) becomes necessary. Aminoglycosides can be given to diabetics but should be used with a good deal of caution because of the associated renal toxicity. Serious infections with group D Enterococcus or Pseudomonas organisms generally require one of these agents. Trimethoprim-sulfamethoxazole, with its broad gram-positive and gram-negative coverage, also has a role in these infections, particularly as an oral agent. Likewise, the fluoroquinolones (e.g., ciprofloxacin, ofloxacin, lomafloxacin) are useful as oral agents, particularly against gram-negative pathogens and staphylococci. Streptococci have limited apparent susceptibilities to fluoroquinolones, while anaerobes have none. There is no question that vancomycin (or teicoplanin), aminoglycosides, trimethoprim-sulfamethoxazole, and fluoroquinolones have special utility in diabetic foot infections, but they require the addition of agents active against anaerobes and streptococci for selected circumstances.

Definitive Therapy

Definitive therapy for all foot infections is ultimately determined by the results of blood and deep-tissue cultures and response to empiric therapy. Anaerobes are difficult to isolate, and some laboratories are not adept in anaerobic bacteriology. Therefore, even if an anaerobe is not isolated, the prudent physician still will use antianaerobic antibiotics in situations in which anaerobes are probable. The antibiotics should be continued until all signs of infection have resolved. This requires about two weeks for most cases but several more weeks for more severe infectious processes. Vascular impairment and diminished polymorphonuclear function delay the healing process.

It is preferable in bone and joint infections that the causative organism(s) be definitely identified via bone biopsy or joint aspiration and that bone sequestra and as much infected bone as is structurally possible be removed. In selected situations amputation is necessary. Under ideal circumstances antibiotics should be withheld in patients with osteomyelitis or septic arthritis until after cultures have been obtained by bone biopsy or joint aspiration. However, if the patient has a concomitant infection of the skin and soft tissue (e.g., cellulitis, fetid foot syndrome) or signs of sepsis, then antibiotics should precede any débridement or attempt at bone biopsy or amputation. The histologic, microbiologic, and radiologic diagnoses as well as the medical and surgical therapies for osteoarticular infections are discussed in detail in Chap. 33.

Adjuvant hyperbaric oxygen (HBO) therapy to antibiotics and surgery is useful for some patients with nonhealing hypoxic wounds. Success may approach 65%–70% of those patients who otherwise are candidates for amputation. Wagner recommends HBO in the treatment of grade I–V infections if the transcutaneous oxygen tension (TCO2) is < 30 mmHg. The treatment course is lengthy and expensive, and most facilities do not have HBO capability.

A comprehensive approach to therapy, including control of blood glucose, daily wound care, antibiotics, timely débridement, revascularization when appropriate, and orthotic support, is most successful.

References

1. Whitehouse FW. Infections that hospitalize the diabetic. *Geriatrics* 28:97–99, 1973.
2. Most RS, Sinnock P. The epidemiology of lower extremity amputations in diabetic individuals. *Diabetes Care* 6:87–91, 1983.
3. Rutkow IM. Orthopaedic operations in the United States, 1979 through 1983. *J Bone Joint Surg* 68A:716–19, 1986.
4. Goldner MG. The fate of the second leg in the diabetic amputee. *Diabetes* 9:100–103, 1960.
5. Bild DE et al. Lower-extremity amputation in people with diabetes: epidemiology and prevention. *Diabetes Care* 12:24–31, 1989.
6. Asbury AK, Brown MJ. Clinical and pathological studies of diabetic neuropathies. In Y Goto, A Horiuchi, K Kogure (eds.), *Diabetic Neuropathy. Proceedings of the International Symposium on Diabetic Neuropathy and Its Treatment.* Amsterdam: Excerpta Medica, 1982. P. 50.
7. Boulton AJM. Diabetic neuropathy. In RG Frykberg (ed.), *The High Risk Foot in Diabetes Mellitus.* New York: Churchill-Livingstone, 1991. Pp. 48–59.
8. Brown MJ et al. Nerve lipid abnormalities in human diabetic neuropathy: a correlative study. *Ann Neurol* 5:245–52, 1979.
9. Cogan DG et al. Aldose reductase and complications of diabetes. *Ann Intern Med* 101:82–91, 1984.
10. Simmons DA, Winegrad AI, Martin DB. Significance of tissue myo-inositol concentrations in metabolic regulation in nerve. *Science* 217:848–51, 1982.
11. Finegold D et al. Polyol pathway activity and myo-inositol metabolism. A suggested relationship in the pathogenesis of diabetic neuropathy. *Diabetes* 32:988–92, 1983.
12. Yue DK et al. The effects of aldose reductase inhibition on nerve sorbitol and myoinositol concentrations in diabetic and galactosemic rats. *Metabolism* 33:1119–22, 1984.
13. Ellenberg M. Diabetic neuropathy. In M Ellenberg, H Rifkin (eds.), *Diabetes Mellitus: Theory and Practice* (3rd ed.). Garden City, NY: Medical Examination, 1983. P. 777.
14. Goodman JL. Diabetic anhidrosis. *Am J Med* 41:831–35, 1966.
15. Edmonds ME, Roberts VC, Watkins PJ. Blood flow in the diabetic neuropathic foot. *Diabetologia* 22:9–15, 1982.
16. Hilsted J. Decreased sympathetic vasomotor tone in diabetic orthostatic hypotension. *Diabetes* 28:970–73, 1979.
17. Duchewn LW et al. Pathology of autonomic neuropathy in diabetes mellitus. *Ann Intern Med* 92:301–3, 1980.
18. Williams JG. Autonomic neuropathy in diabetics: a review. *J R Soc Med* 76:502–7, 1983.
19. Janka HU, Standl E, Mehnert H. Peripheral vascular disease in diabetes mellitus and its relation to cardiovascular risk factors: screening with the Dopp-

ler ultrasonic technique. *Diabetes Care* 3:207–13, 1980.

20. Jones AF, Kempczinski RF. Aortofemoral bypass grafting: a reappraisal. *Arch Surg* 116:301–5, 1981.

21. Lally ME, Johnston KW, Andrews D. Percutaneous transluminal dilatation of peripheral arteries: an analysis of factors predicting early success. *J Vasc Surg* 1:704–9, 1984.

22. Chang JB. Popliteal and tibial artery revascularization. In JB Chang (ed.), *Vascular Surgery*. New York: Spectrum, 1985. Pp. 194–229.

23. Sinha S, Munichoodappa CS, Kozak GP. Neuroarthropathy (Charcot's joints) in diabetes mellitus (clinical study of 101 cases). *Medicine* 51:191–210, 1972.

24. Fernando DJS et al. Relationship of limited joint mobility to abnormal foot pressures and diabetic foot ulceration. *Diabetes Care* 14(1):8–11, 1991.

25. Mueller MJ et al. Relationship of foot deformity to ulcer location in patients with diabetes mellitus. *Phys Ther* 70:356–62, 1990.

26. Mann RA, Poppen NK, O'Konski M. Amputation of the great toe: a clinical and biomechanical study. *Clin Orthop* 226:192–205, 1988.

27. Kinsman OS. Attachment to the host as a preliminary to infection. *Semin Dermatol* 1:127–36, 1982.

28. Elias PM. Lipids and the epidermal permeability barrier. *Arch Dermatol Res* 270:95–177, 1982.

29. Aly R, Maibach HI. Aerobic microbial flora of intertriginous skin. *Appl Environ Microbiol* 33:97–100, 1977.

30. Marshall J, Leeming JP, Holland KT. The cutaneous microbiology of normal feet. *J Appl Bacteriol* 62:139–46, 1987.

31. Roth RR, James WD. Microbiology of the skin: resident flora, ecology, infection. *J Am Acad Dermatol* 20:367–90, 1989.

32. Berman DS et al. *Staphylococcus aureus* colonization in intravenous drug abusers, dialysis patients, and diabetics [letter]. *J Infect Dis* 155:829–31, 1987.

33. Hanifin JM, Homburger HA. Staphylococcal colonization, infection, and atopic dermatitis association no etiology [editorial]. *J Allergy Clin Immunol* 78:563–65, 1986.

34. White MI, Noble WC. Consequences of colonization and infection by *Staphylococcus aureus* in atopic dermatitis. *Clin Exp Dermatol* 11:34–40, 1986.

35. Terleckyj B, Abramson C. Microbial ecology of the foot and ankle. In C Abramson, DJ McCarthy, MJ Rupp (eds.), *Infectious Diseases of the Lower Extremities*. Baltimore: Williams & Wilkins, 1991. Pp. 3–16.

36. Sapico FL et al. The infected foot of the diabetic patient: quantitative microbiology and analysis of clinical features. *Rev Infect Dis* 6(suppl 1):S171–76, 1984.

37. Fierer J, Daniel D, Davis C. The fetid foot: lower extremity infections in patients with diabetes mellitus. *Rev Infect Dis* 1:210–17, 1979.

38. Louie TJ et al. Aerobic and anaerobic bacteria in diabetic foot ulcers. *Ann Intern Med* 85:461–63, 1976.

39. Wheat JL et al. Diabetic foot infections. Bacteriologic analysis. *Arch Intern Med* 146:1935–40, 1986.

40. Williams HTC, Hutchinson KJ, Brown GD. Gangrene of the feet in diabetics. *Arch Surg* 108:609–11, 1974.

41. Kahn O, Wagner W, Bessman AN. Mortality of diabetic patients treated surgically for lower limb infection and/or gangrene. *Diabetes* 23:287–92, 1974.

42. Lipsky BA, Pecoraro RE, Wheat LJ. The diabetic foot, soft tissue and bone infection. *Infect Dis Clin North Am* 4:409–32, 1990.

43. Gibbons GW, Eliopoulos GM. Infection of the diabetic foot. In Joslin Clinic and New England Deaconess Hospital, *Management of Diabetic Foot Problems*. Boston: Saunders, 1984. Pp. 97–102.

44. Wagner FW Jr. Algorithms of diabetic foot care. In ME Levin, LW O'Neal (eds.), *The Diabetic Foot* (3rd ed.). St. Louis: Mosby, 1983.

45. Calhoun JH et al. Treatment of diabetic foot infections: Wagner classification, therapy, and outcome. *Foot Ankle* 9:101–6, 1988.

46. Scardina RJ. Diabetic foot problems: assessment and prevention. *Clin Diabetes* 1:1–7, 1983.

47. Holewski JJ et al. Aesthesiometry: quantification of cutaneous pressure sensation in diabetic peripheral neuropathy. *J Rehab Res Dev* 25:1–9, 1988.

48. Sabacinski KA et al. Necrotizing fasciitis. *J Foot Surg* 28:106–11, 1989.

49. Sanders LJ, Murray-Leisure KA. Infections of the diabetic foot. In C Abramson, DJ McCarthy, MJ Rupp (eds.), *Infectious Diseases of the Lower Extremities*. Baltimore: Williams & Wilkins, 1991. Pp. 193–212.

50. Sapico FL, Bessman AN, Canawati HN. Bacteremia in diabetic patients with infected lower extremities. *Diabetes Care* 5:101–4, 1982.

51. Uman SJ, Kunin CM. Needle aspiration in the diagnosis of soft tissue infections. *Arch Intern Med* 135:959–61, 1975.

52. Stamenkovic I, Lew PD. Early recognition of poten-

tially fatal necrotizing fasciitis. *N Engl J Med* 310: 1689–93, 1984.

53. Sudarsky LA et al. Improved results from a standardized approach in treating patients with necrotizing fasciitis. *Ann Surg* 206:661–65, 1987.

54. Barry AL, Jones RN. Cross susceptibility and absence of cross resistance to cefotetan and cefoxitin. *J Clin Microbiol* 25:1570–71, 1987.

55. Cuchural GJ et al. Susceptibility of the *Bacteroides fragilis* group in the United States: analysis by site of isolation. *Antimicrob Agents Chemother* 32:717–22, 1988.

56. Peterson LR et al. Therapy of lower extremity infections with ciprofloxacin in patients with diabetes mellitus, peripheral vascular disease, or both. *Am J Med* 86:801–8, 1989.

57. Hughes CE et al. Treatment and long-term follow-up of foot infections in patients with diabetes or isch-emia: a randomized, prospective, double-blind comparison of cefoxitin and ceftizoxime. *Clin Ther* 10 (suppl A):36–49, 1987.

58. Anania WC et al. A selective clinical trial of ceftizoxime. *J Am Podiatr Med Assoc* 77:648–52, 1987.

59. Le Frock JL et al. Cefoxitin in the treatment of diabetic patients with lower extremity infections. *Infect Surg* May:361–74, 1983.

60. Tan JS, File TM Jr. Diagnosis and treatment of diabetic foot infections. *Compr Ther* 14:57–62, 1988.

61. Rolston KV. Infections involving the skin and soft tissues of the lower extremities. *J Foot Surg* 26:S25, 1987.

62. LeFrock JL et al. Non comparative trial of ticarcillin plus clavulanic acid in skin and soft tissue infections in diabetics. *Am J Med* 79 (S):122–24, 1985.

12

Infection in the Patient with Animal or Insect Contact

GARY L. SIMPSON

Over two hundred infections and syndromes specifically associated with animals or insects have been described in the medical literature. Although the definition is etymologically imprecise,* *zoonoses* is the term generally applied to these diseases. The incidence and prevalence of individual zoonoses in North America may be relatively low, but collectively they produce significant morbidity and mortality. In a recent review of pet-associated illnesses, it was estimated that over four million people are infected with zoonoses annually in the United States, with resulting economic costs measured in the hundreds of millions of dollars per year (Table 12-1†).

For the emergency medicine physician zoonotic infections can present formidable diagnostic challenges. In addition to the daunting array of clinical syndromes, zoonotic infections can be rare but highly lethal, or prevalent but geographically or occupationally restricted. Assessing the relative risk of infection in a given patient requires knowl-

edge of complex vector-host relationships and seasonal variations of disease transmission. Finally the clinical experience of an individual physician in diagnosing and treating these infections may be limited. The purpose of this chapter is to present a conceptual approach to the evaluation of infections that may be animal- or insect-associated, and to describe some clinical settings in which the possibility of infection of zoonotic origin is increased.

Exposure History

Knowledge of certain specific exposures can either increase the likelihood of or virtually eliminate the possibility of many animal- and insect-associated infections. Zoonotic infections can be transmitted to humans by direct contact with infected animals or tissue, by common vehicle (most frequently ingestion of contaminated foodstuffs or liquids), by inhalation of infectious aerosols, or by contact with a variety of insect vectors (Table 12-2). The potential risk for contact and transmission of these infections is related in large part to occupation and avocation, lifestyle, place of residence, and travel.

A preliminary exposure history can be distilled into a brief checklist that should be reviewed with patients who present with any of the clinical

---

* The World Health Organization's definition of zoonoses is "those diseases and infections which are naturally transmitted between vertebrate animals and man" (*WHO Report on Zoonoses*, 1967). Some infections that are considered "zoonotic," such as Lyme disease, would not meet this definition.
† The tables in this chapter were compiled from standard texts and from references 1–10, unless otherwise indicated.

233

Table 12-1. Modes of transmission, incidence, and total estimated direct patient costs of zoonotic diseases associated with pet animals in the United States[a]

Disease	Etiologic agent	Mode of transmission to humans from pet-animal hosts	Human infections		
			Annual incidence	Case-fatality rate	Total direct patient cost
Helminths Toxocaral larva migrans (LM)	*Toxocara canis; Toxocara cati*	Ingestion of eggs in soil or fomites contaminated with feces of dogs and cats	Visceral LM: 10,000; Ocular LM: 700[b]	0.0001% 0.0001%	N.A. N.A.
Cutaneous larva migrans	*Ancylostoma braziliense Ancylostoma caninum*	Skin contact with or ingestion of soil contaminated by infected dogs and cats	Unknown		N.A.
Dirofilariasis	*Dirofilaria immitis*	Mosquito bite (dog is reservoir host)	Unknown[c]		N.A.
Hydatid disease	*Echinococcus granulosus Echinococcus multilocularis*	Ingestion of eggs excreted by dogs and, rarely, cats	*E. granulosus:* 200[d] *E. multilocularis:* 3–2	1%–2% 70%	N.A.
Dipylidiasis	*Dipylidium caninum*	Ingestion of infected fleas from dogs and cats	Unknown	0%	N.A.
Protozoal toxo-plasmosis	*Toxoplasma gondii*	Ingestion of oocysts in soil or fomites contaminated with infected cat feces	Congenital: 3,300 Other: 2,300,000	15.0% 0.0001%	$222,000,000[e] N.A.
Bacteria Brucellosis	*Brucella canis*	Direct contact with infected dogs	4[b]	0.5%	$5,700
Leptospirosis	*Leptospira canicola* L. Licterohaemorrhagiae	Direct contact with urine or other secretions of infected dogs	242[b]	3%	$308,000
Salmonellosis	*Salmonella* spp.	Ingestion of organisms by direct contact with or in food contaminated by infected dogs, cats, or turtles	40,000	0.1%	$12,000,000

Campylobacteriosis	*Campylobacter jejuni*	Ingestion of organisms through contact with infected dogs or cats	210,000	0.1%	N.A.
Tularemia	*Francisella tularensis*	Bite or scratch of cats and dogs	4	1%	$7,234
Plague	*Yersinia pestis*	Scratch or bite of infected cat or dog or flea bites	1–5	15.0%	N.A.
Cat-scratch fever	Probable bacterial infection	Scratch, bite, or other exposure to cats	6,000	<0.1%	$2,000,000
Pasteurellosis	*Pasteurella multocida*	Bite of cats and dogs	14,000	0.25%	$3,600,000
Psittacosis	*Chlamydia psittaci*	Inhalation of organism from droppings or secretions of infected psittacine or other birds	518[f]	<1%	$595,700
Fungi Ringworm (Dermatophytoses)	*Microsporum canis*	Direct contact with infected cats and dogs	2,000,000	0.0%	N.A.
Virus Rabies	Rabies virus	Bite of infected dogs, cats, skunks, and raccoons	2	99%	$6,000,000[g]
Arthropods Mites	*Sarcoptes scabei*	Direct contact with infected pet	Unknown	0.0%	N.A.

[a] All estimates from this source unless otherwise designated. Infections resulting from companion animals (if there is more than one source of infection) estimated using total incidence as reported by Bennett and the proportion attributed to pets as noted.

[b] Division of Parasitic Diseases, Center for Infectious Diseases, Centers for Disease Control, 1984, unpublished.

[c] Through 1951 approximately 60 cases of pulmonary nodules due to *Dirofilaria* were reported in medical literature from the United States.

[d] Approximately 95% of cases are imported.

[e] Based on 1975 dollars. Updated to the 1985 consumer price index, the annual cost would approach $430 million.

[f] Proportion of cases secondary to pets.

[g] Cost of postexposure prophylaxis.

Source: Stehr-Green J, Schantz PN, The impact of zoonotic diseases transmitted by pets on human health and the economy. In JR August, AS Loar (eds.), Zoonotic diseases. *Vet Clin North Am* 17(1):1–15, 1987.

Table 12-2. Communication of zoonotic diseases

Disease	Modes of transmission				
	Aerosol	Ingestion	Contact	Animal trauma	Arthropod vector
Anthrax	Spores in hides Spores in raw wool	Spores in contaminated meat	Spores in hides Spores in environment Spores in bone meal fertilizer	—	—
Arbovirus encephalitis	—	—	—	—	Mosquito
Boutonneuse fever	—	—	—	—	Eastern hemisphere ticks
Brucellosis	—	Goat cheese and milk	Animal products and animals	—	—
Campylobacteriosis	—	Contaminated water, fowl	Puppies with diarrhea Hand to mouth	—	—
Erysipeloid	—	—	Fish slime Shellfish Bone and hide	Lobster or crab claw pinch	—
Leptospirosis	—	Water and milk	Contaminated water	—	—
Lyme borreliosis	—	—	—	—	Ixodes ticks
Pasteurellosis	Possibly cats	—	Cat or dog secretions	Feline and dog bites	—

Plague	Human to human; Cat to human	—	Infected animals	Cat scratch	Infected rodent flea
Q fever	Endospores in contaminated soil	—	—	—	Ticks
Rabies	Probably bat caves	—	Corneal transplant	Wild or domestic animal bites	—
Rat-bite fever	—	Infected urine contaminating milk, water	—	Lab and wild rodents	—
Rocky Mountain spotted fever	Laboratory; Possibly from engorged tick	—	Engorged tick; Conjunctival	—	Dermacenter ticks
Salmonellosis	—	Contaminated poultry and other foods	Fecal material of reptiles, amphibians	—	Cockroaches; Bedbugs
Tularemia	Droplet particles; Dead birds, animals	Contaminated food, including meat	Dressing squirrels, muskrats, etc. (winter, spring)	Rare type of transmission—cat bite	Ticks, deerflies (summer)
Yersiniosis	—	Contaminated milk, water	Probably sporadic cases in farm animals	—	—

Source: Weinberg AN. Ecology and epidemiology of zoonotic pathogens. In AN Weinberg, DJ Weber (eds.), Animal-associated infections. *Infect Dis Clin North Am* 5(1):1–6, 1991.

syndromes described in this chapter. The check-list includes occupation, exposures to rural habitats, known exposures to biting insects or animals (wild, domestic, or pet), place of residence and recent travel outside that immediate area, history of ingestion of unpasteurized milk or dairy products, and knowledge of similarly ill individuals. This quick review can either raise the diagnostic possibility or essentially exclude most infections of zoonotic origin.

Occupation and Recreation

Individuals who may be exposed to animal- and insect-associated infections in the workplace or who may be exposed because of professional or recreational activities in rural or wilderness regions constitute a large portion of the at-risk population for these infections. Table 12-3 contains the World Health Organization (WHO) classification for groups at risk for zoonotic infection. Some high-risk occupations are obvious. For instance, abattoir, or slaughterhouse, workers account for a significant proportion of all cases of Q fever, brucellosis, leptospirosis, and erysipeloid occurring in the United States annually. In a literature review of laboratory-acquired infections, Collins [11] found that laboratory-based professionals were also a notable risk group for classical zoonotic infections, both from direct exposure to pathogens and from secondary exposure to laboratory animals (Table 12-4). However, it is the participants in recreational activities in rural, sylvan, and wilderness areas that constitute the largest and ever increasing at-risk population.

Animals

Individuals exposed to domestic animals and pets, wild animals, and marine life are another risk group for infection. Table 12-5 lists selected diseases transmitted from pets to humans. Comprehensive reviews of infections associated with specific types of animals can be found in references 2 and 12–14. The essential issues for the emergency medicine physician are an appreciation of the remarkable array of infections common to both animals and humans, the enormous potential for animal exposure (e.g., over 60% of U.S. households have a dog

Table 12-3. Groups at risk for zoonotic infections

Group I (Agriculture): Farmers or other persons in close contact with livestock and their products

Group II (Animal-product processing and manufacture): All personnel of abattoirs and plants that process animal products or by-products

Group III (Forestry, outdoors): Persons who frequent wild habitats for professional or recreational reasons

Group IV (Recreation): Persons in contact with pets or wild animals in the urban environment

Group V (Clinics, laboratories): Health care personnel who attend patients and health workers (including laboratory personnel) who handle specimens, corpses, or organs.

Professional and social groups defined by the World Health Organization and the Food and Agriculture Organization. *Source:* World Health Organization. *Bacterial and Viral Zoonoses.* Geneva: WHO, 1982. Technical Reprint Series 682.

Table 12-4. The top 10 laboratory acquired infections

Infection	Number of cases	Number of deaths
Brucellosis	426	5
Q fever	280	1
Hepatitis	268	3
Typhoid fever	258	20
Tularemia	225	2
Tuberculosis	194	4
Dermatomycosis	162	0
Venezuelan equine encephalitis	146	1
Psittacosis	116	10
Coccidioidomycosis	93	2
Total	2168	48

Data compiled by R.M. Pike over several years by literature reviews and surveys of clinical laboratories, primarily in the United States, and published in 1978 (Pike RM. Past and present hazards of working with infectious hazards. *Arch Path Lab Med* 102:333–36, 1978.) *Source:* Collins CH. *Laboratory-Acquired Infections.* London: Butterworths, 1983.

or a cat), and the importance of eliciting detailed animal exposure histories, particularly in patients with perplexing febrile illnesses.

Insects

Many of the infections discussed in this chapter are vector borne. Although a wide range of insects can

Table 12-5. Diseases transmitted from pets

Infectious disease	Cats	Dogs	Fowl, birds	Horses	Mice, rats, hamsters	Rabbits	Fish
Anthrax (B. anthracis)	x	x		x			
Brucellosis (Brucella spp.)		x		x			
Campylobacteriosis (Campylobacter spp.)	x	x					
Cat scratch agent	x						
Cryptosporidiosis (Cryptosporidia spp.)	x	x					
Dirofilariasis (D. immitis)		x					
Echinococcosis (Echinococcus spp.)		x					
Erysipeloid (E. rhusiopathiae)			x				x
Glanders (P. mallei)				x			
Histoplasmosis (H. capsulatum)	x	Excreta					
Leptospirosis (Leptospira spp.)		x		x	x		
Listeriosis (L. monocytogenes)		x	x			x	
Murine typhus (R. typhi)					x		
Ornithosis (C. psittaci)			x				
Lymphocytic choriomeningitis					x		
Mycobacterium marinum				x		x	
Pasteurellosis (P. multocida)	x	x					
Plague (Y. pestis)	x				x	x	
Q fever (C. burnetii)	x						
Rabies	x	x		x			
Rat-bite fever (S. moniliformis)					x		
Rocky Mountain spotted fever (R. rickettsii)		x					
Salmonellosis (Salmonella spp.)	x	x	x	x	x	x	x
Toxocariasis (T. canis, T. cati)	x	x					
Toxoplasmosis (T. gondii)	x						
Tularemia (F. tularensis)	x	x	x	x		x	
Vibriosis (Vibrio spp.)							x
Viral encephalitis			x				
Yersiniosis (Yersinia spp.)		x			x		

Source: Goldstein EJC. Household pets and human infections. In AN Weinberg, DJ Weber, Animal-associated human infections. Infect Dis Clin North Am 5(1):117–30, 1991.

serve as arthropod intermediates in disease transmission (see references 15 and 16 for review), mosquitoes and ticks are the principal vectors in North America. Mosquito exposure is seasonal and usually reported by the patient, if asked. By contrast tick exposures may not be obvious. Some tick species are small and not readily apparent, and tick exposures may be secondary (i.e., exposure via carriage of infected ticks by household pets). In Table 12-6 the tick-associated illnesses occurring in North America are listed in descending order of prevalence. A

careful history of possible tick exposure and a skin survey for attached ticks is mandatory in evaluating unusual febrile illnesses, especially in regions where infections such as Lyme disease, ehrlichiosis, and babesiosis are concentrated.

(Removal of an engorged tick can be difficult and requires care. Not only can potentially infective blood be injected into the patient if the tick is compressed, but body parts remaining after tick removal can result in granulomatous formation (tick granuloma) and local reactions. Limited

Table 12-6. Tick-associated illnesses in North America

Condition	Geographic distribution	Approximate annual number of reported cases	Incubation period	History of tick bite/exposure	Rash	Hematologic abnormalities	Comments
Lyme disease (Lyme borreliosis)	Primarily New England but also Minnesota, Wisconsin, Oregon, and California	9,000	3–32 days	Most patients unaware of tick bite	Erythema migrans (see text)	May have elevated erythrocyte sedimentation rate; otherwise, usually normal.	The most important bacterial vector-borne infection in North America (see text).
Rocky Mountain spotted fever	Primarily Virginia, North and South Carolina, but reported throughout the U.S.	650	4–10 days	Only about one-half of patients report history of tick bite	Fine macular rash on extremities, progressing to petechial purpuric (see text)	Anemia in 5%–30%; thrombocytopenia in more severe cases.	One of the most severe infectious diseases endemic to the U.S. (see text).
Ehrlichiosis	Primarily Virginia and surrounding states	>400	2–21 days	Up to 80% of patients report tick exposures	Macular and petechial rashes reported but uncommon	Leukopenia, absolute lymphopenia, thrombocytopenia, and anemia common.	Described clinically as "Rocky Mountain spotted fever without the rash" although generally a less severe disease; elevated hepatic animotransferase levels in up to 80% of cases.
Colorado tick fever	Rocky Mountain states	300–400	3–6 days (range: 0–14 days)	Up to 90% of patients report tick exposure; about	Rash unusual (reported in <5% of patients)	Leukopenia and thrombocytopenia typical.	Wood tick vector restricted to the Rocky Mountains

				55% report tick bite			and western Black Hills at elevations between 4000 and 10,000 feet.
Tularemia	Primarily western, southern, and mid-Atlantic states and Massachusetts	150	1–10 days	Majority of patients report tick exposure, but few recall tick bites	Rash unusual	WBC counts may be mildly elevated.	Infection results in the ulceroglandular form of tularemia in the vast majority of cases; the primary ulcer can be found on the lower extremities or perineal area in approximately 50% of patients and on the trunk in 30%.
Relapsing fever (borreliosis)	Western states	>50	4–18 days (median: approximately 7 days)	Patients rarely report tick bite or exposure	Macular, papular, or petechial rashes in as many as 30% of cases	Leukocytosis and an elevated erythrocyte sedimentation rate are common.	Large number of cases linked to sleeping overnight in mountain log cabins.
Q fever	Reported in all states	>50	2–4 weeks	Not reported	Virtually never a rash during acute infection; palpable purpuric rash reported in 20% of patients with chronic Q fever	Elevated WBC count in only one-third of cases.	Ticks probably rare mode of transmission of human disease; may present as an undifferentiated febrile illness, pneumonia, endo-

Table 12-6. (continued)

Condition	Geographic distribution	Approximate annual number of reported cases	Incubation period	History of tick bite/exposure	Rash	Hematologic abnormalities	Comments
							carditis, hepatitis, or a variety of neurological syndromes.
Babesiosis	Primarily New York (Long Island), Massachusetts, and Connecticut	>50	1–3 weeks (but may be as long as 6 weeks)	Most patients do not recall tick bite	Rash rare	Anemia and thrombocytopenia are common.	Intercurrent Lyme disease may be common; most infections probably subclinical but may produce severe disease, particularly in asplenic patients.
Oklahoma tick fever	Southwestern U.S.	>1 (?)	Probably 3–7 days	All cases have reported tick bite or exposure	None reported	Transient anemia, leukopenia, and/or thrombocytopenia.	Recently described illness apparently clinically similar to Colorado tick fever.
Tick-borne (Powassan) encephalitis	Northern New York state	>1	8–34 days	Rarely reported	None reported	No typical findings reported.	May resemble herpes simplex encephalitis; approximately half of reported cases have suffered permanent

| Tick paralysis | Western states | Rare | Requires prolonged (5–7 days) tick attachment | Tick detected for diagnosis | None | None reported. | Produces a toxin-mediated, symmetric, ascending paralysis that begins in the lower extremities and may progress to involve the trunk, upper extremities, and head in hours; tick most frequently attached to occipital scalp and removal usually results in rapid resolution of symptoms. neurologic deficits (e.g., hemiplegia). |
| Tick granuloma | Continental U.S. | Unknown (not reported) | Usually days to weeks | Not reported | Local reaction at site of tick bite | None reported. | Erythematous papule or nodule (at site of tick bite), which may be extremely puritic. |

studies and anecdotal reports suggest that the best method of tick removal involves applying forceps to the base of the tick and exerting gentle traction. The use of isopropyl alcohol, fingernail polish or petroleum jelly, or the application of heat (e.g., hot matches or heated paperclips) has not been shown to be effective.)

The identification and speciation of insects (especially ticks) can be helpful in narrowing diagnostic possibilities. To preserve insects for subsequent examination, place them in 70% ethyl alcohol and notify the vector control division of the local health department for assistance.

Food-Borne Exposures

Chapter 25 details the evaluation of suspected, acute, food-borne gastrointestinal disease. However, several classical zoonotic infections can result from animal or insect contamination of foodstuffs.

Table 12-7 lists the infections reported to be transmitted by ingestion of unpasteurized milk (cow's or goat's) and dairy products. Consumption of unpasteurized milk and dairy products persists in certain ethnic and cultural groups in the United States, thus defining them as at-risk populations. Implicating a food-borne source of a particular infection in an individual patient almost invariably leads to diagnosis of that infection in more individuals (i.e., an outbreak).

Geography

Many animal- and insect-associated infections are geographically restricted, rurally, regionally, or internationally. The tick-borne diseases noted in Table 12-6 are examples of infections in which the risk of transmission is limited primarily to rural areas of defined regions of the United States. Determination of potential risks must include a review of

Table 12-7. Infections reported to be transmitted by milk (cow's and goat's) and dairy products

Organism	Clinical syndromes	Comments
Bacillus cereus	Gastroenteritis	Can cause short incubation (nausea and vomiting in 1–6 hours) or long incubation (abdominal cramps and diarrhea in 8–16 hours); food-borne, enterotoxin-mediated gastrointestinal disease.
Brucella species, (B. melitensis, B. abortus)	Brucellosis	Milk-borne transmission accounts for estimated 10% of cases of brucellosis in the U.S.; B. melitensis associated with goats, B. abortus with cattle.
Camplylobacter species (particularly C. jejuni)	Gastroenteritis	Milk-borne outbreaks frequently documented.
Corynebacterium diphtheriae	Diphtheria	Rare mode of transmission of this infection.
Corynebacterium pseudotuberculosis	Suppurative granulomatous lymphadenitis	Rare, usually occupational disease associated with cattle and sheep.
Corynebacterium ulcerans	Exudative pharyngitis, diphtheria-like syndrome	Rare, usually seen in rural populations; particularly associated with sheep.
Coxiella burnetii	Q fever	Unusual but well-documented mode of transmission of Q fever.
Escherichia coli	Gastroenteritis	Outbreaks due to cheese-borne, enterotoxigenic strains of E. coli have been reported.
Listeria monocytogenes	Listerial clinical syndromes, particularly septicemia and meningoencephalitis	Milk- and cheese-borne outbreaks have been reported frequently; probably the leading fatal, food-borne infection in U.S.
Mycobacterium bovis	Extrapulmonary and pulmonary tuberculosis	Rare; usually seen in abattoir workers and cattle herders.

Table 12-7. (*continued*)

Organism	Clinical syndromes	Comments
Salmonella species (including *S. dublin, S. typhi, S. schott-muelleri,* and *S. typhimurium*)	Gastroenteritis, typhoid/enteric fever	Dairy products account for approximately 4% of reported outbreaks.
Shigella species	Bacillary dysentery	Transmission by contaminated food or drink is less common than person-to-person transmission.
Staphylococcus aureus	Acute, toxin-mediated gastroenteritis	Staphylococcal food poisoning is the second most commonly reported cause of acute food poisoning in the U.S.; accounts for approximately 20% of annual outbreaks associated with contaminated food.
Streptobacillus moniliformis	Streptobacillary rat-bite fever (Haverhill fever)	75% of patients have morbilliform, petechial rash (commonly involving the extensor surfaces of limbs near joints); 40% have polyarthritis.
Streptococcus species (*S. pyogenes, S. zooepidemicus*—group A and C streptococci)	Exudative pharyngitis, acute post-streptococcal glomerulonephritis	Rare, although a number of outbreaks have been reported.
Yersinia enterocolitica	Enterocolitis, exudative pharyngitis	Food-borne outbreaks of enterocolitis documented mostly in children. Exudative pharyngitis without abdominal discomfort seen almost exclusively in adults.
Tickborne encephalitis virus (group B arbovirus/Genus: *Flavivirus*)*	Encephalitis	Well-documented outbreaks in eastern and western Europe; case-fatality rates reported as high as 30%.
Toxoplasma gondii	Usually asymptomatic but can cause cervical lymphadenopathy, a mononucleosis syndrome, and chorioretinitis	Only 10%–20% of *Toxoplasma* infections are symptomatic in immunocompetent individuals; however, in certain regions of the U.S. up to 70% of adults are seropositive for antibodies to *T. gondii*.

* Although not reported, transmission of the related Powassan virus is a possibility (see Table 12-16).

places of residence and work, as well as travel outside the immediate area. Infections in international travelers are discussed in Chap. 19.

Seasons

The peak acquisition periods of vector-borne infections range between spring and early fall. However, environmental factors such as increased rainfall or mild temperatures can extend those periods considerably. A small number of animal- and insect-associated infections have unique incidence curves. For example, tularemia has a bimodal distribution of incidence, with apparent tick-borne infections being acquired during spring and summer and direct-contact transmission occurring in winter, particularly during hunting seasons.

High-Risk Pathogens

Before considering specific clinical syndromes associated with animal or insect contact, this section focuses on a limited number of lethal and hazardous infectious diseases in which the emergency medicine physician may perform the pivotal patient evaluation and intervention. These infections were chosen because each one can present as an undifferentiated febrile illness, especially early in the clinical course, and each one can be rapidly fatal. Appropriate and timely chemotherapeutic intervention can be lifesaving in several of the infections, and all require specific travel and exposure histories either to suspect or to exclude their diagnoses. Considerable hazardous risk (particularly to medical personnel) may be associated with exposure to patients infected with these agents, and appropriate management of each infection requires the active participation of local, state, and possibly national public health organizations. Finally, in each of these infectious processes, mortality and infectious risk to secondarily exposed individuals are related directly to delay in diagnosis.

Malaria

Malaria probably is the most important disease of humankind. A protozoan disease transmitted by the bite of female *Anopheles* mosquitoes, malaria annually afflicts 100 million to 200 million persons worldwide. As many as 1 million to 2 million deaths occur in children under the age of 5 years in sub-Saharan Africa alone. Any of the four plasmodial species primarily infecting humans can produce clinically severe illness. The most virulent infections (especially in nonimmune individuals), however, are caused by *Plasmodium falciparum*. Malarious areas are distributed worldwide but notably so in Central and South America, Africa, Southeast Asia, the Middle East, the Indian subcontinent, and Oceania. Malaria's reputation as the "virtuoso performer . . . in the medical theater of disease mimicry" [17] is evidenced by a study by Hyman [18] of a series of 100 mistaken diagnoses that were determined subsequently to be malaria. Historically the prevalence of malaria in the United States has paralleled U.S. military involvement abroad; however, the number of cases in the civilian population has been increasing steadily since the early 1980s. Falciparum malaria is a lethal disease that, without appropriate chemotherapeutic interventions, can kill as many as 25% of nonimmune individuals (i.e., persons not living in endemic areas) within 2 weeks of primary attack [19]. Increasing morbidity and mortality rates are correlated with delay in diagnosis. During the peak Vietnam War era (1963–1972), the case-fatality rate for falciparum malaria in civilian hospitals and medical centers was 24 times greater than in military and Veterans Administration hospitals, where stained blood smears for malaria were obtained routinely on febrile patients [20]. Finally the rapid spread of drug resistance (particularly to chloroquine) in falciparum malaria (see Chap. 19) has further complicated the management of this serious illness.

INITIAL EVALUATION

Any patient with fever who has traveled recently (within the previous 12 months) to an endemic area should be suspected as having malaria until proved otherwise. Clinically malaria presents initially as an undifferentiated febrile illness and is most commonly misdiagnosed as a flu-like or viral syndrome. After a prodromal period lasting 1 to several days, the onset of acute illness is heralded by the malarial paroxysm (sudden onset of fever, chills, and rigor). Nonspecific, generalized complaints (fever, headache, chills, and myalgia) predominate the symptom presentation. Classic periodic fevers are seen in less than one-third of patients. Nausea, vomiting, and diarrhea are reported in 40%–50% of individuals subsequently diagnosed with falciparum malaria. Physical examination frequently reveals tender hepatomegaly and splenomegaly. (It should be noted that vigorous palpation of an enlarging spleen in the setting of acute malaria can result in catastrophic splenic rupture). Lymphadenopathy does not occur in malaria.

Patient history should include a detailed travel itinerary in malaria-endemic areas. Even brief airport stopovers can provide sufficient exposure. In addition histories of blood transfusions or intravenous drug use in endemic regions should be obtained. (Induced malaria acquired by intravenous routes can be particularly virulent). A complete review of prior medication usage is mandatory, especially use of any antimicrobial agents. A history of antimalarial chemoprophylaxis does not exclude the diagnosis of malaria. Moreover, the frequent use by international travelers of common antimicrobial agents with antimalarial activity (e.g., the tetracyclines, trimethoprim-sulfamethoxazole) can complicate and delay definitive diagnosis.

Factors that increase the likelihood of malaria in patients recently returned from malarious areas include failure to maintain appropriate chemoprophylaxis, travel to rural areas of endemic countries, especially during evening hours, history of multiple mosquito bites, and the proximity of return date to the United States from endemic areas to onset of illness (approximately 90% of falciparum malaria cases in the United States present within 1 month of date of entry, but onset of illness can be delayed as long as a year by factors such as chemosuppression).

DIAGNOSIS AND ASSESSMENT OF SEVERITY

Diagnosis and treatment of individual types of malarial infections and their complications are detailed in Chap. 19, but certain points deserve emphasis. In the acute setting malaria is diagnosed only by the demonstration of parasites in stained peripheral blood smears. Examination should be performed by an experienced technician or observer, especially for species differentiation. The diagnosis of malaria can be excluded effectively by several negative smears obtained twice daily (ideally during febrile periods) over successive days. (The increased use of automated hematologic screening of peripheral blood smears may also contribute to a delay in diagnosis of malarial infection. The serendipitous diagnosis of malaria by laboratory technicians examining peripheral blood smears once was common. Patients presenting with even life-threatening malarial infections may have normal hematologic profiles by automated screening.)

The evaluation of the clinical severity of malarial infection caused by *P. falciparum* can be difficult. Patients can progress from clinically stable illness to coma, shock, and death within hours [9]. The major complications of falciparum malaria are well described (see Chap. 19) and include neurologic, pulmonary, renal, hematologic, and metabolic syndromes. The term *cerebral malaria* encompasses several central nervous system syndromes of impaired consciousness [21] and is a particularly lethal complication. Frequent formal mental status testing is mandatory in patients with suspected or proven falciparum malaria.

In the absence of a recognized pernicious syndrome, the density of parasitemia can identify those patients requiring emergency treatment. Parasitemias greater than 5% (250,000 parasites per milliliter of blood) or *P. falciparum* schizonts in peripheral blood smears are indicators of severe infection. Parasite counts above 500,000 per milliliter are associated with greater than 50% mortality [21]. Although high-density parasitemias correlate with severity, the reverse is not invariably true, especially in nonimmune individuals. Because *P. falciparum* parasites are peripherally sequestered during maturation, there may be periods during the course of the infection in which parasites are difficult to detect in blood smears, even in potentially serious infections. Furthermore *P. falciparum* infec-

tions can cycle synchronously with progressively greater numbers of parasites released into the bloodstream with each cycle; hence the previously noted recommendation of obtaining blood smears at least twice daily (ideally during febrile periods) for diagnosis and for monitoring subsequent response to therapy.

Until competent review of stained blood specimens, a presumptive diagnosis of malaria should also be a presumptive diagnosis of falciparum malaria; if there is suspicion of travel to areas of drug resistance, the presumptive diagnosis should be drug-resistant falciparum malaria. Chemotherapy of suspected falciparum malaria, particularly if any of the described complications is present or if drug resistance is possible, should be managed in the hospital (preferably with intensive care capabilities) by an experienced clinician. Clinical consultation with the Malaria Branch of the Centers for Disease Control (CDC) is available on a 24-hour basis (telephone number 404-488-4046). Empiric use of broad-spectrum antimicrobial agents in a febrile patient in whom malaria is in the differential diagnosis can delay the definitive diagnosis and increase the possibility of serious complications. Current treatment guidelines and the identification and management of complications of acute malarial infection are discussed in Chap. 19.

Viral Hemorrhagic Fever

Viral hemorrhagic fever (VHF) is a syndrome that encompasses a number of clinically similar infections, characterized in their early phase by an undifferentiated febrile illness and in their extreme forms by fever, shock, and hemorrhage. VHF is caused by 27 members of 4 distinct families of viruses (arenaviruses, filoviruses, bunyaviruses, and flaviviruses), each geographically restricted by the distribution of their respective animal reservoir or arthropod vector. The spectrum of VHF syndromes is summarized in Table 12-8, but four deserve special consideration: Lassa fever, Ebola and Marburg hemorrhagic fevers, and Crimean-Congo hemorrhagic fever. As a group these illnesses are notable for their potentially extreme severity and high mortality. Each illness has been implicated in significant outbreaks, with documented person-to-person transmission. Because they appear to originate from

Table 12-8. Viral hemorrhagic fevers

Disease[a]	Geographic distribution	Estimated yearly prevalence	Reservoirs	Transmission	Incubation period	Petechiae	Reported case fatality (%)	Comments
Crimean-Congo hemorrhagic fever	Former USSR, eastern Europe, central and western Asia, Africa	50–200 cases	Many wild and domestic mammals	Tick-borne[b]	3–12 days	Yes (common in severe cases)	As high as 88% but as low as 15% for patients treated in hospital	Most commonly seen in agricultural workers; ribavirin has demonstrated *in vitro* activity (see text).
Dengue hemorrhagic fever (Dengue shock syndrome)	Southeast Asia, Caribbean, Oceania, tropical Americas	Tens of thousands of cases	Monkeys	Mosquito-borne	5–8 days	Yes (common)	1%–5%	Most frequently reported in children (<15 years of age) in Southeast Asian countries.
Ebola hemorrhagic fever	Africa	Hundreds of cases during outbreaks	Unknown	Unknown[b]	2–21 days	Yes	Varies with viral biotype; as high as 90%	Sore throat and gastrointestinal symptoms (abdominal pain, vomiting, diarrhea) may be prominent.
Hemorrhagic fever with renal syndrome (Korean hemorrhagic fever, Hantaan hemorrhagic fever, nephropathia epidemica)	Asia, eastern Europe	100,000 cases	Rodents	Rodent-to-human via urine; airborne	9–35 days	Yes	1%–15%	Severity of illness varies regionally (Asian cases frequently are more severe); ribavirin treatment may be effective.

Disease	Geographic location	Number of cases	Reservoir	Transmission	Incubation	Person-to-person	Mortality	Comments
Kyasanur Forest hemorrhagic fever	India	400–500 cases	Rodents, monkeys	Tick-borne	2–7 days	No	8%–10%	Papulovesicular lesions on the soft palate nearly a constant physical finding.
Lassa fever	Africa	250,000–300,000 cases	Rodents	Rodent-to-human via urine[b]	6–21 days	Yes	20% in hospitalized patients	Treatment with ribavirin within the first 8 days of illness can lower case-fatality rate to 1% (see text).
Marburg hemorrhagic fever	Africa	Sporadic cases	Unknown	Unknown[b]	3–9 days	Yes	Approximately 25%	Leukopenia and thrombocytopenia almost uniformly present; most cases laboratory acquired.
Omsk hemorrhagic fever	Former USSR (Siberia)	Zero to several hundred cases	Rodents, muskrats	Tick-borne	2–4 days	No	1%–3%	Outbreaks reported in individuals with direct exposure to sick muskrats.
Rift Valley hemorrhagic fever	Africa	50,000–100,000 cases	Many wild and domestic animals	Mosquito-borne; animal-to-human via blood	3–5 days	Yes	5%–15% in hospitalized patients	Highest risk in workers exposed to infected animals (farmers and shepherds) and carcasses (abattoir workers and butchers).

Table 12-8. (*continued*)

Disease[a]	Geographic distribution	Estimated yearly prevalence	Reservoirs	Transmission	Incubation period	Petechiae	Reported case fatality (%)	Comments
South American hemorrhagic fevers:								
Argentine hemorrhagic fever (Junin hemorrhagic fever)	Argentina	200–2000 cases	Rodents	Rodent-to-human via urine	5–19 days	Yes	10%–20%	Treatment with convalescent-phase plasma within the first 8 days of illness can lower case-fatality rate to 1%.
Bolivian hemorrhagic fever (Machupo hemorrhagic fever)	Bolivia	Limited outbreaks in villages	Rodents	Rodent-to-human via urine	5–19 days	Yes	10%–15%	Both ribavirin and convalescent-phase plasma have been demonstrated effective in primate models, but clinical trials have not been reported.
Yellow fever	Africa, South America	1,000–200,000 cases	New and Old World monkeys	Mosquito-borne	3–6 days	No	20%–50% (in patients with jaundice)	Unique among the viral hemorrhagic fevers for the severity of hepatic impairment.

[a]Three additional viral hemorrhagic fever syndromes (Uruma fever, hemorrhagic exanthema of Bolivia, and Yungas HF) have been reported (all from Bolivia) but have yet to be clearly defined, clinically or virologically.
[b]Documented person-to-person transmission, usually from direct contact with infected tissue, blood, or secretions (see text).

limited geographic foci, detailed travel histories can rapidly exclude these infections from the differential diagnosis of an acutely ill febrile patient. Although each illness can follow a rapidly fatal clinical course, Lassa fever (and possibly Crimean-Congo hemorrhagic fever) may respond to timely antiviral therapy. All four viral agents pose extremely hazardous risks to secondary contacts, especially medical personnel caring for infected patients.

Lassa Fever

Lassa fever is a prevalent disease endemic in much of western Africa. As many as 300,000 human infections, with up to 5,000 deaths, occur annually [22] in the region from Guinea to Central Africa (especially Nigeria, Sierra Leone, and Liberia). Humans are infected by contact with either the natural host (a ubiquitous African rat, *Mastomys natalensis*) or its excreta, by close personal contact with an infected individual, or by direct contact with infected blood, tissue, excretions, or secretions. The clinical spectrum of Lassa fever is broad, but most frequently it presents with an insidious onset of fever, sore throat, and malaise, with progression to severe illness over 3–5 days. Characteristically the pharyngitis is extremely painful, and severe disease is associated with facial edema (without peripheral edema) and neurologic manifestations (including encephalopathies and deafness). Although Lassa fever is grouped with the VHFs, petechiae and ecchymoses are not seen, and only 15%–20% of patients have overt bleeding from mucosal surfaces [23]. The case-fatality rate of hospitalized patients may reach 25%. Poor prognostic indicators include high viral concentrations in blood and the magnitude of serum glutamic oxalic transaminase (SGOT) elevations [24, 25]. Ribavirin chemotherapy can significantly decrease mortality, especially if initiated within 1 week of onset of illness [25]. Prophylaxis with ribavirin should be administered to all high-risk contacts (see reference [26] for definitions of risk groups).

Ebola and Marburg
Hemorrhagic Fevers

Ebola and Marburg hemorrhagic fevers are caused by morphologically identical but antigenically distinct viruses of the family *Filoviridae*. Although there is serological evidence suggesting that the Ebola virus may be endemic in many areas of East Africa, significant epidemics have been reported thus far only for Zaire and Sudan. Limited outbreaks and sporadic cases of Marburg virus infection have been reported from eastern and southern Africa (especially Kenya and South Africa). The epidemiology and the natural mode of transmission of these lethal infections remain unknown. However, person-to-person transmission is well documented, usually in a nosocomial setting after direct exposure to infected blood, tissue, excretions, or secretions. Case-fatality rates for the reported outbreaks have ranged from approximately 25% for the Marburg virus [27], to 70%–90% for the Zaire-variant Ebola virus [28]. The relative virulence of these infections appears to be specific to the filovirus biotypes (biotype or strain variation was also at issue when monkeys imported into the United States from the Philippines were found recently to be infected with an Ebola-like virus [29] that was apparently nonpathogenic for humans). Clinically both Ebola and Marburg virus infections can present early in their course as undifferentiated febrile illnesses. Although the onset of these infections may be insidious, most commonly the onset is abrupt with fever, headache, sore throat, and myalgia. A maculopapular rash is seen in the majority of patients. The clinical course progresses rapidly to include nausea, vomiting, diarrhea, and laboratory evidence of marrow suppression (leukopenia and thrombocytopenia) and hepatic involvement (elevated liver transaminase). Mucosal or gastrointestinal hemorrhage is a grave prognostic sign and generally precedes shock and death. Specific diagnosis and clinical management are discussed in Chap. 19. Treatment is supportive and clearly may require intensive care facilities.

Crimean-Congo Hemorrhagic Fever

Crimean-Congo hemorrhagic fever (CCHF) is an ancient and clinically well described illness endemic to eastern Europe (especially the former USSR), central Asia, and Africa. Although this bunyavirus can infect a wide variety of wild and domestic animals, cattle, sheep, and goats are important reservoirs. Human disease results primarily from the bites of infected ixodid (hard) ticks. Person-to-person transmission has been documented in a series of nosocomial outbreaks [30–33] and appears to be related to direct contact with infected blood or other bodily fluids. The epidemiology of disease transmission varies seasonally and regionally and is largely determined by the ecology of the principal tick species involved (at least 27 species of ticks are known to harbor the virus) [34]. For instance, in the former USSR, CCHF is an occupational disease of dairy farmers and their families.

After an incubation period of 3–12 days, CCHF presents with sudden onset of fever, chills, headache, arthralgia, myalgia (especially of the lower back), and abdominal pain. Although palatal petechiae frequently are seen early, hemorrhagic complications typically appear 3–5 days after onset. Mucosal bleeding, epistaxis, and large ecchymoses are common. Other frequent manifestations include acute icteric hepatitis and laboratory evidence of profound leukopenia and impairments of coagulation function. Poor prognosis is associated with hematuria, proteinuria, and azotemia. Pulmonary edema and shock usually are premorbid events. The case-fatality rate varies widely but ranges as high as 35%–50%, with nosocomial rates even higher [31]. Ribavirin has in vitro efficacy against CCHF virus and is the recommended treatment in the current absence of clinical trials. Diagnosis and clinical management of CCHF are discussed in Chap. 19.

Approach to Patients with Suspected VHF

Detailed guidelines concerning the management of patients with suspected VHF have been published by the CDC [35]. Some general points, however, deserve note. The presenting symptoms of the VHF syndromes are of a nonspecific febrile illness, followed by abdominal pain, nausea and vomiting, and/or diarrhea. Hemorrhage and shock occur relatively late in the clinical courses and are frequently premorbid manifestations. The critical factor for the emergency medicine physician is a high index of suspicion, prompted by the patient's recent travel to the particularly rural areas of the above-mentioned regions. Because of the incubation periods of these illnesses (see Table 12-8), an interval of greater than 3 weeks between the time of possible exposure and the onset of symptoms essentially excludes the diagnosis of the VHF syndrome.

As noted previously all febrile patients recently returned from these regions (particularly sub-Saharan Africa) must be presumed to have malaria until the diagnosis is excluded by thin-smear examination of peripheral blood. If VHF caused by one of these viral agents is suspected, three actions should be taken immediately:

1. Blood cultures for viral isolation should be obtained by closed system, with special care reserved for hazardous pathogens (e.g., HIV).
2. The patient should be isolated under universal barrier precautions and strict barrier-nursing techniques adhered to (sharps exposures probably represent the greatest risks to medical personnel).
3. Local and state health departments should be notified immediately, as well as the Special Pathogens Branch of the CDC (see Chap. 1).

Timely notification of public health offices and professionals offers the emergency medicine physician a number of immediate resources of practical significance:

1. Direct access to experienced physicians who can assist in the clinical management of the infected patient
2. Assistance in handling, transporting, and processing laboratory specimens (a mobile laboratory can be dispatched from the CDC to anywhere in the United States on a 24-hour basis)
3. Assistance in the identification, management, and surveillance of individuals exposed to the index-infected patient
4. Assistance in addressing the concerns and demands of the public and the press (as well as medical staff concerns) regarding the presence of lethal pathogens in the community or the hospital.

This type of technical and logistical support can be critical in an exotic syndrome such as VHF but it can also be helpful in the evaluation and management of most infections and syndromes discussed in this chapter.

Plague

Plague is a historic disease caused by the gram-negative bacillus *Yersinia pestis* which continues to produce misery and death worldwide. Human infection results primarily from the bites of infected rodent fleas. The incubation period is 2–8 days following the flea bite, and the clinical course can be rapidly fatal without prompt, appropriate antimicrobial chemotherapy. Although plague is endemic in many areas of the world, especially Asia and Africa (see Chap. 19), it is regionally restricted in North America to the southwestern United States. The ecology and the epidemiology of plague transmission are complex and differ for the epidemic urban form and the sporadic sylvatic form of disease transmission.

In the United States plague is a seasonal zoonotic infection concentrated in endemic foci throughout the Southwest, with ground squirrels, prairie dogs, and wood rats being important natural reservoirs [36]. Although human infection rarely results from direct contact with infected wild rodents or hares, approximately 85% of human infections are associated with bites of infected rodent fleas. Obvious groups at higher risk of exposure include hikers, hunters, and campers, but domestic pets can provide exposure risks by returning infected rodents or infected fleas to their owners, or by becoming infectious risks themselves (e.g., pharyngeal plague in domestic cats).

Plague can present as any one or combination of the following syndromes. Classic *bubonic plague* is described by sudden onset of fever, headache, and malaise, followed shortly by the appearance of extremely painful, localized lymphadenitis (bubo), usually in the groin (see Chap. 10). Gastrointestinal symptoms (including nausea, vomiting, abdominal pain, and diarrhea) are common. Bubonic plague can progress from first onset of symptoms to rapid clinical deterioration and death in 2–4 days. In *septicemic plague* plague bacilli disseminate rapidly from the initial focus of infection, resulting in the syndrome of septicemic plague. Plague bacillus may be seen on the blood smear (Fig. 12-1). By definition, septicemic plague presents with fever and hypotension but without a bubo (in contrast to bubonic plague with septicemia). The importance of this distinction is highlighted by the report of Hull et al. [37], in which 25% of all cases of plague occurring in over a 5-year period in New Mexico (a state with a high prevalence of plague) were, in fact, the septicemic form. The case-fatality rate was 33%, even in a region where physicians are unusu-

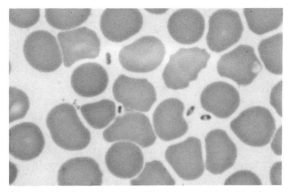

Fig. 12-1. Plague bacillus (*Yersinia pestis*) on blood smear

ally sensitized to the possibility of human plague infections. A remarkable feature of plague sepsis is high-density bacteremia, which premorbidly can reach concentrations of thousands of bacilli per milliliter of blood. Hematogenous dissemination of organisms to the lung with resultant secondary pneumonia (*pneumonic plague*) is associated with mortality in excess of 75% [38]. Plague transmitted by aerosols is highly contagious. Individuals exposed to the pneumonic form reportedly have become ill and died of primary inhalation plague pneumonia, all in a single day [39]. Unusual presentations of plague infections include vesicular eruptions, eschar or ecthyma gangrenosum associated with a bubo, and a meningeal form usually seen as a late complication of inadequately treated bubonic plague. Risk of transmission of plague to close contacts (family, medical personnel, etc.) is related to exposure to respiratory aerosols from patients with pneumonia and to blood (through needlesticks or aerosols) in patients with high-density bacteremia.

From this discussion it follows that the emergency medicine physician must consider the diagnosis of plague in certain clinical settings. If a patient has been in a plague endemic region (New Mexico, Arizona, Utah, Colorado, or California) in the previous 10–14 days (during the seasonal period of March–November), plague must be included in the differential diagnosis of the following clinical presentations:

- Sudden onset of fever and painful, localized unilateral lymphadenitis
- Clinical sepsis in an individual without obvious

focus of infection or without underlying conditions predisposing to sepsis
- Any community-acquired, gram-negative pneumonia

The diagnosis of plague and the treatment of its various syndromes are discussed in Chap. 19. It should be emphasized that patients suspected of having plague with any evidence of pulmonary involvement should be placed in strict respiratory isolation. Local and state health offices should be notified immediately to establish a contact surveillance system and to manage the chemoprophylaxis of possible contacts.

Simian Herpes B Virus Infection

Infection with simian herpes B virus (*Herpesvirus simiae*) is widely prevalent in Old World monkeys. As many as 25% of macaques (primarily rhesus and cynomolgus monkeys) have detectable antibodies to simian herpes B virus. Human infection is rare (fewer than 50 reported cases) but highly lethal (mortality approximately 70%). Virtually all instances of human infection have been in monkey handlers, following a monkey bite or scratch, or in laboratory workers exposed to the virus. Person-to-person transmission by direct contact has been documented [40]. The onset of clinical illness generally has been within one month of exposure. It has been characterized by progressive mucocutaneous disease originating from the site of inoculation and usually progressing to fatal encephalitis. Both in vitro and in vivo efficacy of acyclovir against simian herpes B virus has been demonstrated, and this antiviral agent is the treatment of choice. Detailed guidelines for the management of simian herpes B virus exposures (including wound care of bites and scratches) have been published by the CDC [41]. Medical consultation and laboratory support can be obtained from the Viral Exanthems and Herpes Virus Branch, Division of Viral Diseases, CDC (see Chap. 1).

Rabies and Rabies-Related Viruses

Rabies is a uniformly fatal but preventable viral infection in humans. The clinical presentation, prevention, risk assessment, and guidelines for immunoprophylaxis are detailed in Chap. 5 and Chap. 31. Rabies is included in this section to emphasize the range of animals that can be associated with rabies risk. Rabies is primarily a disease of animals; in the United States skunks, bats, and raccoons are those animals most frequently infected. Wild carnivores highly susceptible to rabies infection include coyotes, wolves, and foxes. Rabies-control programs in the United States have dramatically limited rabies in dog and cat populations, but dogs and cats are still responsible for most bites of humans that require immunoprophylactic decisions. Pets, such as skunks, raccoons, and ferrets, and domestic farm animals, such as cattle, horses, and sheep, can develop rabies and must be considered potential sources of human infection. Detailed information concerning the regional prevalence of rabies in various animals can be obtained from state health departments or offices of epidemiology.

In the United States most human cases of rabies are in individuals bitten by dogs from outside the country, bitten by wild animals, or with unknown exposure history. The difficulty of determining exposure history is illustrated by a recent virological study of fatal rabies cases in U.S. immigrants that suggested that their infections were acquired in their countries of origin up to 7 years prior to onset of illness [42]. Although incubation or latent periods for human rabies infections of up to 19 years have been reported [43], over 95% of cases present within 1 year of exposure.

Five rabies-related, rhabdoviruses have been reported that are morphologically similar but antigenically distinct from rabies virus. Of these only Mokota virus and Duvenhage virus are known to cause disease in humans. Although all rabies-related viruses were previously thought to be restricted to sub-Saharan Africa, recent studies have found a variant of Duvenhage virus to be enzootic in European bats. The practical significance of these newly described viral agents is that they should be included in the differential diagnosis of patients with suspected rabies that may have originated in Africa or Europe. Animal studies of rabies vaccines have demonstrated marginal to nonexistent protection against challenge with rabies-related viruses.

Cutaneous Infections

The skin is a common site for both the introduction and the manifestations of infections associated with animals or insects. Common pyodermas such as impetigo, ecthyma, and cellulitis can be caused by organisms of zoonotic origin (e.g., certain viridans streptococci and β-hemolytic, pyogenes-like streptococci). However, knowledge of an animal source of these infections would be unlikely to aid or affect their evaluation, diagnosis, or treatment. Although not discussed in detail in this chapter, ectoparasites are significant causes of human disease. Common animal-associated syndromes in humans include infestations by canine and feline scabies, otodectic mange (ear mites), cheyletiellosis (mites), three pediculosis (lice) syndromes, flea-bite hypersensitivities, and, rarely, myiasis (maggots). The primary parasitic diseases of skin (e.g., cutaneous larva migrans and cutaneous leishmaniasis) are reviewed in references 44–46.

Diagnostic Approach

The general approach to the diagnosis of cutaneous lesions and infections is detailed in Chap. 9 and Chap. 32. Aspects of cutaneous presentations that should invite scrutiny into possible zoonotic etiologies include the following six factors:

1. *Site.* Inflammation or lesions involving the hands or forearms may reflect direct inoculation syndromes, resulting from occupational (food processing, veterinary medicine, laboratory sciences, etc.) or recreational (hunting, camping, pets, etc.) exposures.
2. *Type of lesion.* Certain types of cutaneous lesions are more frequently associated with zoonotic infections, including nodular lesions, vesicular or papular lesions limited to the hands and forearms, and chancriform lesions.
3. *History of trauma.* Previous trauma (including bites, stings, scratches, and abrasions) at the site of inflammation should prompt a careful review of direct or indirect animal or insect exposure.
4. *Occupation.* Some zoonotic skin infections are largely limited to known high-risk groups. Patients involved in food processing (e.g., abattoir workers, butchers, and fishmongers), veterinary

care (e.g., veterinarians, ranchers, and farmers), wilderness professionals (e.g., guides, hunters, and trappers), and laboratory-based occupations deserve special evaluation for animal- and insect-associated infections.
5. *Travel history.* Several infections described in this section are geographically restricted to limited regions of the United States (or to limited regions of the world). Recent travel outside the patient's local area can extend considerably the differential diagnosis of cutaneous infection.
6. *Clinical course.* The majority of infections listed in this section present as acute syndromes. Of note, however, are chronic cutaneous syndromes (especially if empiric, antimicrobial therapy directed toward staphylococcal and streptococcal organisms has failed), which are more likely to be infections of zoonotic origin.

Some points regarding the modes of diagnosis of zoonotic skin infections should be emphasized. For most infections, scrapings and swabs of superficial cutaneous lesions and aspirates of vesicular and pustular lesions will provide sufficient specimens for diagnostic culture and microscopic examination. However, for many syndromes noted in this section (e.g., the chancriform syndromes), skin biopsy will be the diagnostic procedure of choice. Punch biopsies can be performed quickly in the emergency department setting and frequently prove to be the definitive diagnostic procedure for many zoonotic infections.

To optimize the diagnostic yield of punch biopsies, the procedure should be performed under sterile conditions with barrier precautions, and the resulting cylindrical specimen divided along its vertical axis. One portion of the specimen should be placed directly into a sterile container for culture (bacterial, mycobacterial, fungal, etc.). The other portion should be used first to produce "touch preps" and then placed in formalin for subsequent histologic examination. Touch preps are prepared by securing the tissue specimen with forceps and applying the tissue to a series of glass slides. The slides are allowed to air-dry and then sent to the clinical laboratory for appropriate staining and microscopic examination. Generally organisms are more easily and reliably visualized by this technique than by standard tissue preparations.

Dermatophytoses

Dermatophytoses (tinea, dermatomycosis, ringworm) are common superficial fungal infections of humans and animals. They are caused by members of three genera of pathogenic fungi: *Trichotophyton*, *Microsporum*, and *Epidermophyton*. Diagnosis is suspected clinically by the nature and the location of the cutaneous lesions. Although dermatophytotic skin changes can vary widely, the prototypic presentation is of an expanding annular patch, with scaling and crusting, central clearing, and variable inflammation. The infection usually is localized to an anatomic region: tinea capitis, tinea faciei, tinea corporis, tinea imbricata, tinea cruris, tinea mannum, and tinea unguium (onychomycosis). The range of cutaneous lesions, the clinical syndromes, the diagnostic approach, and treatment are discussed in Chap. 9 and Chap. 32.

In the United States *Trichotophyton verrucosum* (cattle) and *Microsporum canis* (dogs and cats) probably account for most zoophilic dermatophyte infections of humans, although 20 different dermatophytes have been reported to cause human disease [47]. Besides cattle, dogs, and cats other reservoirs for these infections include horses, swine, voles, rabbits, rodents, and poultry.

The importance of considering a zoophilic source of dermatophytosis by an emergency medicine physician is *prevalence* (an estimated 15% of all human dermatophytoses are caused by *M. canis* [48]), *severity* (zoophilic dermatophytes often evoke severe inflammatory responses, which can progress to granulating lesions with pustular folliculitis, or kerions [47, 49]), and *recurrence* (an unrecognized animal reservoir can lead to repeated episodes of infection). It should also be noted that dogs and cats can be asymptomatic carriers of dermatophytal organisms [48, 50].

Chancriform Syndromes

In several cutaneous infections (caused by bacterial, mycobacterial, viral, and fungal organisms), the etiologic agent is inoculated into the skin by direct contact with infected animals, tissues, or bodily fluids. The result is a primary cutaneous lesion, accompanied by varying degrees of local inflammation, lymphangitic spread, and regional lymphadenopathy. Collectively termed *chancriform*, or primary inoculation, syndromes, these infections frequently are associated with specific occupational or recreational exposures. Table 12-9 lists the animal-associated chancriform syndromes reported in North America. The lesions typically originate at sites of trauma (commonly on the hands or forearms) and begin as papules, vesicles, or nodules that subsequently ulcerate. These syndromes may be clinically indistinguishable and generally require biopsy for diagnosis. Sporotrichoid lesions represent a variant of this syndrome (Table 12-10) and are evaluated similarly.

Local Cutaneous Viral Infections

Table 12-11 lists a number of localized, viral skin infections that are confined almost exclusively to certain occupations and avocations. The infections result from direct contact with infected animals and produce lesions generally occurring on the hands and forearms. As a group they are characterized by a confusing historical nomenclature and by a self-limited, benign clinical course with spontaneous resolution (with the exception of rare infections in immunocompromised patients). The major importance of these infections is their differentiation from more serious occupationally related diseases (chancriform syndromes) and from squamous cell carcinomas.

Primary Annular Erythema (Lyme Disease)

Erythema chronicum migrans (ECM) is a primary annular erythematous lesion that is a clinically unique manifestation of Lyme borreliosis. It occurs from 3–32 days after the bite of *ixodid* ticks infected with *Borrelia burgdorferi* and is observed in 50%–75% of individuals subsequently diagnosed with Lyme disease. The lesion originates as a macule or papule at the site of the tick bite and evolves as an expanding, annular erythematous plaque with central clearing. The most common sites are axillae, groin, and thigh. Within days of onset of ECM as many as half of patients develop secondary lesions that resemble but generally are smaller than the primary lesion. Even without specific antimicrobial

Table 12-9. Animal-associated chancriform syndromes in North America

Organism (disease)	Incubation period	Animal exposure	Populations at risk	Comments
Bacterial				
Bacillus anthracis (anthrax; also called malignant carbuncle, charbon, malignant pustule, malignant edema, splenic fever)	2–5 days	Infected livestock (usually carcasses); contaminated wool, hides, pelts, and fur	Industrial: workers involved in processing animals or animal by-products Agricultural: ranchers, farmers, veterinarians	Endemic foci of infections have been virtually eliminated in U.S.; however, sporadic cases continue to occur in select industrial environments handling raw animal products imported from the Middle and Near East and Africa; case-fatality rate in untreated individuals is 5%–20%.
Cat-scratch disease bacterium[a] (cat-scratch disease; also called cat-scratch fever, benign lymphoreticulosis, inoculation lymphoreticulosis, regional lymphadenitis, *la maladie des griffes de chat*)	3–14 days	Scratches or exposure to cats (90% of cases)	Cat owners, veterinarians	Regional lymphadenitis usually develops 2 weeks after the primary inoculation papule and may be associated with a variety of protean constitutional symptoms (fever, malaise, fatigue, etc.).
Corynebacterium pseudotuberculosis and *Corynebacterium ulcerans*	Unknown	Cattle, sheep, horses	Livestock workers	Rare cause of chancriform syndrome but reported in sheep shearers and ranchers.
Dermatophilus congolensis (dermatophilosis; also called streptotrichosis, epidemic eczema, lumpy wool, strawberry foot rot, contagious dermatitis)	Unknown	Cattle and sheep primarily, but has been reported in most domestic and wild animals	Livestock workers, animal handlers	Rare disease with spontaneous resolution and healing in approximately 14 days.
Erysipelothrix rhusiopathiae (erysipeloid; also called erythema migrans, Rosenbach's erysipeloid, sealer's finger, whale finger, blubber finger, fish hand, fish handler's disease, speck	2–7 days	Many species of wild and domestic birds, animals, and sea life	Workers in slaughterhouses, poultry, fish, and shellfish-processing plants, commercial fishermen, aquatic animal handlers, veterinarians	Lesion characterized by raised area of violaceous erythema, which spreads peripherally from the site of injury and fades centrally; pain and local swelling may be out of propor-

Table 12-9. (continued)

Organism (disease)	Incubation period	Animal exposure	Populations at risk	Comments
finger, pork finger, erythema serpens, *rouget du porc, mal rossius, schweinrotpauf, erysipela del cerdo*)				tion to the observed lesion; secondary septicemia and endocarditis are well-described complications.
Francisella tularensis (ulceroglandular tularemia; also called Francis' disease, deer-fly fever, rabbit fever, O'Hara's disease)	2–10 days	Large number of vertebrate and invertebrate species; in U.S. most important exposures are rabbits and ticks (disease transmitted by direct contact and by arthropods)	Trappers, hunters, rural dwellers	Approximately 300 cases reported annually throughout continental U.S.; cutaneous ulcer with eschar formation typically seen on hands or forearms of individuals exposed to rabbits or small game during winter months, or on head, neck, legs, groin, or axillary regions during summer months, when arthropod-borne disease is more common; other described tularemia syndromes, including oculoglandular and pharyngeal, typhoidal (or septicemic), and pneumonic, account for fewer than 10% of all reported cases.
Listeria monocytogenes (listeriosis; also called listerellosis, Tiger River disease, circling disease, silage disease)	Uncertain but probably a few days	Cattle, particularly bovine fetuses	Ranchers, veterinarians	Originally described as papular or pustular eruption on hands and forearms of veterinarians handling aborted bovine fetuses.
Mycobacterium marinum[b]	2–8 weeks	Fish (especially tropical varieties)	Aquarium workers, fishermen	Typically begins as papule with purplish hue, followed by ulceration and lymphatic spread; sporotrichoid presentations are well described.

Pseudomonas mallei (glanders; also called farcy, equinia, equine nasal phthisis, malleus, maliasmus)	1–14 days	Horses, mules, donkeys	Stable workers, veterinarians	Although once worldwide, infection has been eradicated in U.S. and Europe; residual foci of disease persist in some African and Asian countries.
Fungal				
Blastomyces dermatitides (cutaneous blastomycosis; also called North American blastomycosis, Chicago disease, Gilchrist's disease)	Unknown, probably weeks to months	Canines	Dog owners and handlers, veterinarians	Cutaneous manifestations of systemic blastomycosis usually can be distinguished from a primary inoculation syndrome by the absence of regional lymphadenitis; disease has been reported after dog bite.
Sporothrix schenckii (sporotrichosis)	3 weeks to 3 months	Cats, dogs, horses	Pet owners, veterinarians, farmers	Can present as single lesion or as ascending subcutaneous nodules (± ulcerations) along lymph ducts; disseminated disease rare.

[a] As yet unnamed bacterium.
[b] M. marinum is the most frequent mycobacterial cause of the chancriform syndrome, but Mycobacterium fortuitum, Mycobacterium chelonae, Mycobacterium kansasii, Mycobacterium avium-intracellulare, Mycobacterium tuberculous, and Mycobacterium bovis have all been reported as etiologies.

Table 12-10. Differential diagnosis
of sporotrichoid cutaneous lesions

Sporotrichosis*
Cutaneous leishmaniasis* (*Leishmania brasiliensis*)
Cutaneous mycobacterial infection (*M. marinum,*
   M. avium-intracellulare, *M. kansasii,* *M. bovis,*
   M. tuberculosis)
Cutaneous nocardial infection (*Nocardia brasiliensis,*
   Nocardia asteroides)
Cat-scratch disease*
Anthrax*
Tularemia*
Primary inoculation syndromes of histoplasmosis,*
   coccidioidomycosis, and North American
   blastomycosis*
Furunculosis (*Staphylococcus aureus*)
Syphilis

* Zoonotic sources reported.

therapy ECM and the secondary lesions fade in 3–4 weeks (range: 1 day to 14 months).

By convention the manifestations of Lyme borreliosis have been divided clinically into three stages: early localized infection (stage 1), early disseminated infection (stage 2), and late persistent infection (stage 3). However, the progression and the clinical expressions of Lyme disease are highly variable. ECM represents early, localized (stage 1) infection, but widespread hematogenous dissemination can occur within days of onset and frequently is associated with an undifferentiated febrile illness syndrome, with varying and intermittent systemic symptoms (Table 12-12).

Weeks to months after onset of disease a second phase of illness may ensue, which can involve the central and peripheral nervous systems (15%–20% of patients will have frank neurologic abnormalities, including meningoencephalitis with superimposed cranial or peripheral neuropathy); the cardiovascular system (approximately 8% of patients will have cardiac abnormalities, most commonly fluctuating degrees of atrioventricular block); or the musculoskeletal system (about 60% of patients will suffer brief attacks of asymmetric, oligioarticular arthritis, primarily affecting the large joints, particularly the knee). Symptoms can persist for weeks to months and may resolve even without specific antimicrobial therapy.

Late persistent infections (stage 3), which can

occur years after primary inoculation and ECM, may be associated with chronic arthritis (typically only one or a few large joints), chronic skin lesions (e.g., acrodermatitis chronica atrophicans), or uncommon, chronic neurologic syndromes (including demyelinating encephalopathy). The specific syndromes of Lyme disease, and the diagnosis and treatment of these syndromes, are discussed in Chaps. 8, 9, 31, and 33; see also references 51 and 52.

Respiratory Tract Infections

Pharyngitis

Pharyngitis is a common illness that accounts for over 40 million physician visits annually in the United States [53]. The general clinical approach and differential diagnosis of ulcerative-exudative pharyngitis is presented in Chap. 21. Table 12-13 lists some unusual causes of this syndrome that are animal associated. A review of Table 12-13 suggests two clinical settings in which animal sources of organisms that cause exudative pharyngitis should be considered:

1. When recurrent episodes of culture-proven, streptococcal pharyngitis have occurred in a family or a group, particularly if simultaneous antimicrobial treatment of all family or group members has failed to eliminate the recurrences.
2. When patients present with one or more of the following conditions: a prolonged pharyngeal syndrome, especially with leukocytosis and systemic toxicity; absence of a positive culture for group A streptococcus or failure of standard penicillin-erythromycin empiric treatment; and history of relevant animal exposure.

Besides harboring pathogens that can cause serious, potentially fatal infections, the patient may represent the index case of a larger disease outbreak. A suspicion of animal-associated, exudative pharyngitis should be followed by notification of local public health offices.

Lower Respiratory Tract Infections

The clinical diagnosis of acute pneumonia is relatively straightforward (see Chap. 23). The signs

Table 12-11. Cutaneous viral infections associated with occupational exposure to animals

Infection*	Causative agent (poxviridae) viral genus	Animal exposure	Incubation period	Clinical description	Prevalence in humans	Geographic distribution	Occupations at risk
Pseudocowpox (also called milkers' nodules, pseudovaccinia, paravaccinia, milker's node)	Parapoxvirus	Cattle	5–7 days	Erythematous papules evolve to firm, brownish nodules over 4–6 weeks.	Common	Worldwide	Dairy workers, veterinarians
Orf (also called contagious ecthyma of sheep, contagious pustular dermatitis, sore mouth, sheep pox, ecthyma contagiosum, infectious labial dermatitis)	Parapoxvirus	Sheep, goats	3–7 days	Usually a single lesion, beginning as a papule and progressing through a vesicular stage to a red, weeping nodule; resolves in 2–4 weeks.	Unusual	Worldwide	Herders, shearers, butchers, veterinarians
Bovine papular stomatitis (also called bovine pustular stomatitis, stomatitis papulosa, granular stomatitis, proliferating stomatitis, muzzle disease, ulcerative/erosive stomatitis, paratidostomatitis)	Parapoxvirus	Cattle	3–8 days	Red nodules, often with white borders; resolves in 2–4 weeks.	Rare	Worldwide	Ranchers, veterinarians

Table 12-11. (*continued*)

Infection [*]	Causative agent (poxviridae) viral genus	Animal exposure	Incubation period	Clinical description	Prevalence in humans	Geographic distribution	Occupations at risk
Sealpox	Parapoxvirus	Seals	Probably 5–7 days	Identical to pseudo-cowpox.	Rare	Worldwide	Seal handlers
Cowpox	Orthopoxvirus	Cattle	3–6 days	Inflammatory vesicles become purulent, with central umbilication.	Rare	Great Britain, western Europe	Dairy workers, veterinarians
Buffalopox	Orthopoxvirus	Domesticated buffalo	Probably 3–7 days	Papules evolve to vesicles, to umbilicated pustules, to scab formation in 12–16 days.	Common	India, Middle East, former U.S.S.R.	Milkers
Goatpox (variola caprina)	Capripoxvirus	Goats	Probably 3–7 days	Progress from vesicles to scab formation in 10–15 days.	Rare	Africa, Middle East, India	Shepherds, shearers, veterinarians

[*] Although once common, horsepox and classical vaccinia infections have probably ceased to exist as clinically discrete infections.
Source: Nomenclature standards were derived from Robinson AJ, Lyttle DJ. Parapoxviruses: their biology and potential as recombinant vaccines. In M Bims, G Smith (eds.), *Poxvirus as Vaccine Vectors.* Boca Raton, FL: CRC Press. In press.

Table 12-12. Early symptoms and signs of Lyme disease[*]

Symptoms	Percentage of cases	Signs	Percentage of cases
Malaise, fatigue, and lethargy	80	Erythema chronicum migrans	100[*]
Headache	64	Multiple annular lesions	48
Fever and chills	59	Lymphadenopathy	
Stiff neck	48	Regional	41
Arthralgias	48	Generalized	20
Myalgias	43	Pain on neck flexion	17
Backache	26	Malar rash	13
Anorexia	23	Erythematous throat	12
Sore throat	17	Conjunctivitis	11
Nausea	17	Right upper quadrant	
Dysesthesia	11	tenderness	8
Vomiting	10	Splenomegaly	6
Abdominal pain	8	Hepatomegaly	5
Photophobia	6	Muscle tenderness	4
Hand stiffness	5	Periorbital edema	3
Dizziness	5	Evanescent skin lesions	3
Cough	5	Abdominal tenderness	2
Chest pain	4	Testicular swelling	1
Ear pain	4		
Diarrhea	2		

[*] Erythema chronicum migrans was required for inclusion in this study.
Source: Rahn DW, Malawista SE. Lyme disease. *West J Med* 154:706–14, 1991.

and symptoms are well described, and a normal chest examination excludes the presence of the illness in 95% of cases [54]. Since the causative agent will mandate the choice of antimicrobial therapy and influence the decision to admit the patient to the hospital, determining etiology is the challenge for the emergency medicine physician. Organisms associated with animal or insect exposure are unusual causes of community acquired pneumonia. However, delayed diagnosis of several of the syndromes noted in this section, such as pneumonic plague, can result in fatal outcomes.

Table 12-14 lists the characteristics of a number of animal- and insect-associated acute pulmonary infection syndromes (see reference 55 for a detailed discussion). As with the exudative pharyngeal syndromes discussed previously, a review of Table 12-14 suggests two clinical settings in which a respiratory tract infection of zoonotic origin should be considered. The first is a gram-negative, community-acquired pneumonia, especially in patients

without underlying conditions that might predispose to infection. Current reviews [54, 56] report that gram-negative organisms account for only 2%–8% of all community-acquired pneumonia, with the majority of these cases in patients with known predisposing illnesses. The presentation of gram-negative pneumonia in the emergency room should prompt a complete review of possible high-risk, zoonotic exposures. In addition, because of the serious nature of gram-negative pulmonary infections, such as plague and tularemia, all patients should be admitted to the hospital, and transtracheal aspiration for diagnostic culture should be considered.

The second clinical setting in which to query a zoonotic source of lower respiratory tract infection is that of the atypical pneumonia syndrome. Traditionally the syndrome has described a moderately toxic-appearing patient, without chronic underlying disease, presenting with fever, cough with scant mucoid sputum (Gram's stain without predominant

Table 12-13. Pharyngitis associated with animals

Organism (disease)	Reservoirs	Mode of transmission	Comments
Bordetella bronchicanis	Many wild and domestic animals	Close contact	Produces a pertussis syndrome in children.
Chlamydia psittaci (psittacosis, ornithosis, parrot fever)	Psittacine birds are the major reservoir but can be associated with virtually any species of bird	Close contact	Associated with atypical pneumonia syndrome.
Corynebacterium ulcerans	Horses, cattle	Close contact, ingestion (milk)	Produces a diphtheria-like syndrome.
Francisella tularensis (oropharyngeal tularemia)	Most wild animals, especially rabbits (ticks)	Close contact, ingestion, hand-to-mouth (crushing ticks with fingers)	Frequently associated with cervical lymphadenopathy and usually seen in children.
Streptobacillus moniliformis (rat-bite fever, Haverhill fever, erythema arthriticum epidemicum)	Rodents, squirrels, carnivores that prey on infected rodents	Ingestion of contaminated foods or liquids (particularly milk)	Characterized by a systemic febrile illness, erythematous rash (most prominent on hands or feet), and arthralgias; usually occurs in outbreaks.
Streptococcus species, groups A, C, D, G (streptococcal pharyngitis)	Cattle, dogs	Close contact (group C: milk-borne outbreaks)	Pets have been implicated as the source of recurrent streptococcal pharyngitis in families and in sporadic outbreaks of poststreptococcal glomerulonephritis.
Yersinia enterocolitica	Cattle, sheep, dogs, swine	Close contact, ingestion of contaminated foods or liquids (particularly milk)	Rare cause of exudative pharyngitis, which may present with or without abdominal symptoms or enterocolitis; can progress to fatal septicemia; usually associated with outbreaks.
Yersinia pestis (plague, pharyngeal plague)	Rodents, cats	Close contact	Usually associated with anterior cervical lymphadenopathy (cervical bubo).
Vesicular stomatitis virus (vesicular stomatitis)	Cattle, horses, swine	Close contact	Occupational hazard of farm workers and veterinarians; vesicular lesions may be seen in oral cavity.

Table 12-14. Pulmonary infections associated with animals and insects

Infection	Organism	Reservoirs	Exposure	Incubation period	Comments
Anthrax[a]; also called inhalation anthrax, woolsorters disease, malignant pustule, charbon, splenic fever, malignant edema	Bacillus anthracis	Domestic livestock	Inhalation (of spores)	1–10 days	Extremely rare but case-fatality rates can be high; pulmonary lesions usually minimal radiographically; primarily an occupational disease of workers who process imported animal hides, raw wool, etc.
Borreliosis[a]; also called tick-borne relapsing fever, febris recurrens, spirochetal fever, vagabond fever, famine fever, fievre recurrens (French), fiebre raomente (Spanish), Ruckfallfieber (German), bilious typhoid (Egypt), carapata (Bantu), gorgoya (South American Indian), gharibgez (Iran), fowl-nest fever (China)	Borrelia recurrentis	Many wild animal species	Tick bite	1–15 days	Respiratory symptoms occur in about 15% of cases; pneumonia is well-described but unusual complication of tick-borne relapsing fever.
Bovine tuberculosis	Mycobacterium bovis	Primarily cattle but also horses, swine, cats, dogs	Ingestion (especially milk-borne)	Presumably most human disease represents reactivation of chronic (latent) infection.	Unusual cause of tuberculous disease but well described in ranchers and abattoir workers.

Table 12-14. (*continued*)

Infection	Organism	Reservoirs	Exposure	Incubation period	Comments
Brucellosis[a]; also called undulant fever, Mediterranean fever, Malta fever	*Brucella species:* B. *suis,* B. *abortus,* B. *melitensis,* B. *canis*	Swine, cattle, goats, dogs	Inhalation, ingestion, direct contact with infected animals	1–6 weeks but variable	Cough and wheezing may be prominent symptoms of acute infection, but infiltrates usually are not seen radiographically; generally an occupational disease of abattoir workers, farmers, veterinarians.
Colorado tick fever[a]; also called mountain fever	Colorado tick fever virus (orbivirus)	Ground squirrels, chipmunks	Tick bite	3–6 days	Pneumonitis is an unusual manifestation of Colorado tick fever (see Table 12-6).
Glanders; also called farcy, equinia, malleus, maliasmus, equine nasal phthisis	*Pseudomonas mallei*	Primarily horses, mules, donkeys	Inhalation	1–14 days, but reactivation of latent infection can occur years after primary exposure.	Endemic foci in animals in Asia, Africa, South America; ulcerative lesions typically appear in the nostrils; mortality high with acute clinical pulmonary infection.
Histoplasmosis[a]; also called Darling's disease, reticuloendothelial cytomycosis, cavern disease	*Histoplasma capsulatum*	Environmental; many species of wild and domestic animals	Exposure to bat or bird droppings or to contaminated soil (especially in caves and abandoned mines)	5–18 days	Most infections are asymptomatic, but three clinical forms can be distinguished: acute pulmonary, chronic cavitary pulmonary, and disseminated; acute pulmonary form with flu-like

					illness is most common clinical expression of infection; hilar and mediastinal lymphadenopathy may be prominent radiographically; major foci of infections in U.S. are concentrated in the Mississippi, Missouri, and Ohio river valleys.
Leptospirosis[a]; also called Weil's disease, cane cutter's disease, rice field worker's disease, haymaker's disease, peapicker's disease, swineherd's disease, fishhandler disease, Stuttgart disease, enzootic jaundice, hemorrhagic jaundice, infectious jaundice, "yellows," red water, seven-day fever, Japanese autumnal fever, mouse fever, Fort Bragg fever, pretibial fever, canicola fever, marsh fever, swamp fever, mud fever, field fever, waterfield fever, harvest fever, dairy worker fever	*Leptospira* species: *L. australis, L. autumnalis, L. ballum, L. canicola, L. grippotyphosa, L. hebdomidis, L. icterohaemorrhagiae, L. pomona*	Wild rodents, dogs, cats, livestock	Indirect contact with contaminated water or soil; direct contact with infected animals	7–12 days	Pulmonary manifestations common but usually mild; acute alveolar hemorrhage and acute respiratory distress syndrome have been reported; most frequently disease is occupationally related (slaughterhouse workers, animal caretakers, veterinarians).

Table 12-14. (*continued*)

Infection	Organism	Reservoirs	Exposure	Incubation period	Comments
Melioidosis; also called Whitmore's disease, rodent glanders	*Pseudomonas pseudomallei*	Rodents	Direct contact with contaminated soil or water in endemic areas	Likely a few days but most clinical disease probably represents reactivation of chronic (latent) infection	Endemic areas are concentrated in Asia (particularly Southeast Asia), Oceania, and South America; up to 20% of Vietnam War veterans have serological evidence of infection; clinical disease has been documented years after primary exposure to endemic regions.
Pasteurellosis; also called shipping fever, transport fever, hemorrhagic septicemia	*Pasteurella multocida*	Cats, dogs	Animal bite, close contact	Days to months after bite exposures	Pneumonia usually occurs in patients with underlying pulmonary disease; associated with bacteremia in approximately 25% of cases.
Plague; also called pulmonary plague, pneumonic plague, black death, pestilential fever	*Yersinia pestis*	Wild rodents	Inhalation, flea bite, direct contact	2–6 days	Can be primary infection or secondary to septicemia; highly contagious (see text); infected domestic cats can also transmit plague by aerosol, scratch, or bite.
Psittacosis[a]; also called ornithosis, parrot fever, human chlamydiosis	*Chlamydia psittaci*	Primarily psittacine birds (parrots) but almost any avian species	Inhalation, direct contact with infected bird or secretions, bite wounds	Usually 4–15 days but as long as 1 month	Usually related to occupational or avocational exposures (pet and pet shop owners, vet-

Disease	Organism	Reservoir	Transmission	Incubation period	Comments
Q fever[a]; also called abattoir fever, query fever, Balkan grippe/influenza, pneumorickettsiosis	Coxiella burnetii	Wild and domestic mammals, particularly sheep, goats, cattle	Inhalation, direct contact, tick bite	2–4 weeks	erinarians, turkey farmers); patients may have relative bradycardia with temperature elevations. Pneumonitis can be a frequent manifestation of acute Q fever; most commonly an occupational disease of workers exposed to domestic livestock or in meat processing.
Rhodococcal (corynebacterial) pneumonia	Rhodococcus (Corynebacterium) equi	Horses; also cattle, sheep, swine, cats	Inhalation	Unknown	Uncommon; seen almost exclusively in patients with diminished T-cell immunity and with animal exposure history; typically a necrotizing pneumonia resembling tuberculosis.
Rocky Mountain spotted fever[a]; also called spotted fever, petechial fever, macular fever, tick-borne typhus, pinta fever, choix fever, New World spotted fever	Rickettsia rickettsii	Wild rodents, rabbits, ticks	Tick bite	2–14 days	Pneumonitis seen in approximately 15% of cases; rash typically develops between third and fifth day of illness (see text).
Streptobacillary rat-bite fever; also called Haverhill fever, erythema arthriticum epidemicum	Streptobacillus moniliformis	Wild rats	Ingestion, rat bite	3–10 days	Pneumonia rare and usually associated with arthritis and endocarditis.

Table 12-14. (*continued*)

Infection	Organism	Reservoirs	Exposure	Incubation period	Comments
Streptococcal pneumonia	Group C streptococci, e.g., *Streptococcus zooepidemicus*, *Streptococcus equisimilis*	Horses; also cattle, swine	Inhalation	Unknown	Uncommon but associated with significant morbidity.
Tularemia[a]; also called pulmonary tularemia, Francis' disease, deer-fly fever, rabbit fever, O'Hara's disease	*Francisella tularensis*	Wild animals, especially rabbits	Inhalation, direct contact, tick or deer-fly bite	1–10 days	Can be primary infection or secondary to septicemia; can be associated with pharyngeal tularemia; significant risk for transmission in unsuspecting laboratory personnel.
Toxoplasmosis[b]	*Toxoplasma gondii*	Wild animals, domestic livestock, pets (particularly cats)	Ingestion of cysts	Disease in adults usually represents reactivation of chronic (latent) infection but can be newly acquired	One of the organisms in the differential diagnosis of pulmonary infiltrates in the immunocompromised host; frequently associated with CNS infection.

[a] Presentation consistent with the clinical description of atypical pneumonia syndrome has been reported.
[b] Other parasitic zoonoses that may have prominent pulmonary syndromes include ascariasis, capillariasis (due to *Capillaria aerophila*), schistosomiasis, stongyloides, and toxocariasis.

organisms), and minimal pulmonary findings on physical examination. Chest roentgenogram reveals non–pleural-based infiltrates, seemingly out of proportion to the paucity of physical findings. Frequently the patient has failed to respond to empiric penicillin or cephalosporin therapy. Although one recent study [47] questions the clinical uniqueness of this syndrome, the medical literature has historically applied this term to the "classic" presentation of pulmonary infections due to *Mycoplasma pneumoniae, Chlamydia* species, and viruses, which collectively account for as many as 30% of community-acquired pneumonias [45]. Although uncommon, several potentially lethal and clinically indistinguishable infections of zoonotic origin can present as atypical pneumonias, particularly in adults (see Table 12-14). The responsibilities of the emergency medicine physician in this setting include being aware that very serious infections may be in the differential diagnosis of the atypical pneumonia syndrome; reviewing obvious animal/insect or occupational exposures (e.g., psitticine birds, ticks, abattoir workers); being sensitive to the clinical features of the patient's presentation that might signal infrequent causes of the syndrome (splenomegaly, as in tularemia and Q fever; elevated liver enzymes, as in Q fever and psittacosis; cardiac murmur and possible endocarditis, as in Q fever and streptobacillary rat-bite fever, etc.); and, if the patient is to be discharged from the emergency department, scheduling appropriate follow-up visits, either to continue the diagnostic evaluation or to monitor response to empiric antimicrobial therapy.

Gastrointestinal Infections (Enteric Fever Syndrome)

Most bacterial and parasitic causes of acute enterocolitis are either zoonotic or infections common to both animals and humans. The evaluation of acute diarrheal syndromes is described in Chap. 25, and detailed reviews of animal exposures do not appreciably alter the diagnostic approach to these infections. However, the relatively common presentation of fever, abdominal pain (particularly in the right lower quadrant), and gastrointestinal symptoms (constipation or diarrhea) should at least raise the possibility of abdominal

syndromes other than acute appendicitis and acute gastroenteritis. Three such syndromes may be animal or insect associated [57].

The most serious and potentially the most diagnostically challenging of these conditions is the enteric fever syndrome. This syndrome is characterized by sudden onset of fever, headache, and abdominal pain, either diffuse or localized, most frequently in the right lower quadrant. The patient may complain of either constipation or diarrhea. The prototypic illness of this syndrome is typhoid fever, and the presence of rash (especially rose spots, seen in fewer than half of patients), splenomegaly (23%–65% of reported cases [57]), and relative bradycardia may strongly suggest this diagnosis. Table 12-15 summarizes the remarkable array of conditions that can cause or mimic the enteric fever syndrome. Most are zoonotic and unusual but should be considered in patients with this syndrome who have recent, relevant travel histories, noted occupational exposures, or who are older adults.

Other conditions that must be considered in the differential diagnosis of fever and abdominal pain include mesenteric adenitis (most frequently associated with *Yersinia enterocolitica* and *Yersinia pseudotuberculosis*) and the syndrome of abdominal pain and eosinophilia, which can be caused by a number of intestinal parasites. Both conditions can be zoonotic in origin, and both are discussed in Chap. 25.

Acute Undifferentiated Febrile Illness

"Flu-like" illness, or nonspecific viral syndrome, is one of the most common clinical presentations to emergency departments. It is characterized by sudden onset of fever and headache and is associated with generalized constitutional symptoms of malaise, myalgia, weakness, and lethargy. It is the relative severity of the associated systemic symptoms that distinguishes the classical influenza syndrome from the leading cause of morbidity and physician visits in the United States, namely the common cold. Typically the influenza syndrome is self-limited, requiring only symptomatic treatment, with an average duration of 5–7 days. Table 12-16 describes a number of illnesses that can be indistinguishable (especially early in their clinical

Table 12-15. Clinical, epidemiologic, and laboratory clues to the causes of enteric fever and conditions that may mimic enteric fever

Etiologic agent or disease	Clinical clues	Epidemiologic clues	Laboratory clues
Causes of Enteric Fever			
Salmonella typhi	Relative bradycardia, splenomegaly, rose spots, conjunctivitis	Young adults, travel,[a] exposure to known carrier	Cultures (B, BM, U, F), leukopenia
Salmonella paratyphi A, B			
Salmonella choleraesuis			
Yersinia enterocolitica	Stigmata of chronic liver disease, arthritis, erythema nodosum	Older adults ± pet exposure	Cultures (B, F, J), serology
Yersinia pseudotuberculosis			
Campylobacter fetus	Stigmata or chronic liver disease	Older adults, ± farm or small animal contact	Cultures (B, F), serology
Acute brucellosis	Paucity of physical findings	Occupation (abattoir employee, butcher), animal contact (goats, sheep, cattle), diet (unpasteurized cheese)	Cultures (B, BM), serology, leukopenia
Typhoidal tularemia	Severe prostration, splenomegaly	Animal contact (especially rabbits), vector exposure (ticks)	Serology
Conditions That Mimic Enteric Fever			
Bacterial Infections			
Septicemic plague	Severe prostration	Rodent contact, vector exposure (fleas), travel	Cultures (B), serology
Intestinal anthrax	Severe prostration	Travel,[a] diet (undercooked meat)	Cultures (B, F)
Septicemia melioidosis	Severe prostration, pustular skin lesions	Travel[a]	Cultures (B), serology, chest x-ray
Acute bartonellosis	Severe prostration, renal failure	Travel, vector exposure (sandfly)	Cultures (B), blood smear, acute hemolysis
Leptospirosis	Relative bradycardia, conjunctival suffusion	Occupation (farmers, abattoir and sewer workers, veterinarians), animal contact (especially cattle, dogs), swimming[b]	Cultures (B, CSF, U), serology, hepatorenal dysfunction
Relapsing fever	Fever pattern, conjunctival suffusion, splenomegaly, skin rash	Travel,[a] vector exposure (louse, tick)	Blood smear
Legionellosis	Pneumonia, CNS symptoms	Normal or compromised host	Chest radiogram, purulent sputum, DFA of sputum
Intestinal tuberculosis	Stigmata of tuberculosis	Exposure to known case, ± travel[a] ± diet (unpasteurized	Cultures (S, G, BM, L), x-ray (UGI, SBFT)

		milk and milk products, malnourished children	
Abdominal actinomycosis	Abdominal mass, fistula	Adult males	Culture (FD, A), radiograph (UGI, SBFT)
Intra-abdominal abscess	Spiking daily fever, reduced diaphragmatic excursion, intra-abdominal or diaphragmatic pain	Previous surgery, bowel, or biliary tract disease	Leukocytosis, computed tomography, gallium scan, sonography, fluoroscopy
Viral Infections			
Hepatitis	Jaundice, arthritis (with hepatitis B)	Exposure to known case, drug abuse, travel[a]	Liver dysfunction, antigen detection
Dengue	Relative bradycardia, conjunctival suffusion, rash, lymphadenopathy	Travel,[a] vector exposure (mosquito)	Culture (B), serology, leukopenia
Infectious mononucleosis	Pharyngitis, lymphadenopathy, splenomegaly, rash	Young adults	Serology, lymphocyte morphology
Rickettsial Infections			
Epidemic typhus	Conjunctival suffusion, rash, severe prostration	Travel,[a] vector exposure (louse)	Serology
Brill-Zinsser disease	Rash	Older adults, remote travel[a] history	Serology
Endemic typhus	Conjunctival suffusion, rash, splenomegaly	Rat contact, vector exposure (flea)	Serology
Scrub typhus	Conjunctival suffusion, rash, lymphadenopathy	Travel,[a] vector exposure (mites)	Serology
Q fever	Pneumonia, hepatitis	Animal contact (especially livestock), ± travel, ± diet (especially unpasteurized milk)	Serology, chest radiograph, liver dysfunction
Mycotic Infection			
Disseminated histoplasmosis	Mucocutaneous lesions, adrenal insufficiency	Travel,[a] animal contact (chicken, birds, bats), hobby (cave exploration)	Culture (B, BM, L, MM), biopsy (BM, L, MM), chest radiograph
Parasitic Infections			
Malaria	Fever pattern, splenomegaly	Travel,[a] vector exposure (mosquito)	Blood smear
Amebiasis	Colitis, liver abscess	Travel[a]	Stool examination, serology, liver scan, sonography, computed tomography, colon biopsy
Babesiosis	Paucity of physical findings	Travel,[a] vector exposure (tick)	Blood smear, serology
Toxoplasmosis	Lymphadenopathy	Animal contact (cat); diet (undercooked pork)	Serology, biopsy (lymph node), lymphocyte morphology

Table 12-15. (continued)

Etiologic agent or disease	Clinical clues	Epidemiologic clues	Laboratory clues
Trichinosis	Periorbital edema, muscle tenderness	Diet (undercooked pork or bear meat)	Serology, eosinophilia, biopsy (muscle)
Katayama fever (acute schistosomiasis)	Urticaria, lymphadenopathy	Travel,[a] swimming	Eosinophilia
Visceral larva migrans	Hepatosplenomegaly, rash, bronchospasm, ocular lesions	Young children with history of pica, animal contact (dog, cat)	Serology, biopsy (L), eosinophilia
Noninfectious Causes			
Malignancy	Adenopathy, anergy, weight loss	Family history or prior malignancy	Sonography, computed tomography, gallium scan, lymphangiography
Hematologic, intra-abdominal	Skin lesions, arthritis, serositis	Family history	Biopsy of involved tissue, serology (ANA, C), exclusion of other causes
Vasculitic or granulomatous disease (e.g., sarcoidosis, granulomatous hepatitis, Crohn's disease, Still's disease)			

Abbreviations for cultures: B = blood; BM = bone marrow; U = urine; F = feces; J = joint fluid; S = sputum; CSF = cerebrospinal fluid; G = gastric aspirate; L = liver; FD = fistula drainage; A = abscess; T = throat; N = nasal; MM = mucous membrane.
Abbreviations for x-rays: UGI, SBFT = upper gastrointestinal tract with small bowel follow-through.
Abbreviations for serology: ANA = antinuclear antibody; C = complement; DFA = direct fluorescent antibody test.
[a] Travel to endemic areas, either domestic or foreign.
[b] Swimming in contaminated surface water.
Source: Pearson RD and Guerrant RL Enteric fever and other causes of abdominal symptoms with fever. In GL Mandel, RG Douglas, JE Bennett (eds.), Principles and Practice of Infectious Diseases (3rd ed.) New York: Churchill-Livingstone, 1990. Pp. 881–2.

Table 12-16. Undifferentiated febrile illnesses associated with animals and insects in North America

Organism	Principal vector	Principal reservoirs/hosts	Comments
Viral			
California encephalitis virus	Mosquitoes	Squirrels	Most infections subclinical but the virus can cause UFI* and rarely encephalitis; prevalent in farm workers in the coastal western U.S.
Colorado tick fever virus	Ticks	Rodents	Meningoencephalitis can occur; about 50% of patients will have a classic biphasic fever curve (see Table 12-6).
Dengue (1–4) virus	Mosquitoes	Humans	Autochthonous transmission of dengue has been documented along the Texas-Mexican border.
Jamestown Canyon virus	Mosquitoes	Deer	Sporadic cases throughout U.S.; respiratory symptoms may be prominent with the UFI; virus can cause meningitis and encephalitis.
LaCrosse virus	Mosquitoes	Mosquitoes, rodents	Most cases subclinical; <300 cases annually; besides UFI encephalitis and, more commonly, aseptic meningitis can result.
Lymphocytic choriomeningitis virus	None	Mice	Approximately 15% of cases develop meningoencephalitis; may be laboratory acquired.
Oklahoma tick fever virus	Ticks	Unknown	Clinically similar to Colorado tick fever (see Table 12-6).
Rio Bravo virus	None reported	Bats	Rare; most cases reported in U.S. are laboratory acquired; can cause encephalitis.
Snowshoe hare virus	Mosquitoes	Hares, squirrels	Rare; sporadic cases in northern U.S. and Canada; in addition to UFI the virus can cause meningitis and encephalitis.

Table 12-16. (*continued*)

Organism	Principal vector	Principal reservoirs/hosts	Comments
St. Louis encephalitis virus	Mosquitoes	Birds	Most infections subclinical or produce a UFI; however, St. Louis encephalitis is the most prevalent viral encephalitis in the U.S.; infections particularly severe in elderly patients.
Travittatus virus	Mosquitoes	Rabbits	Sporadic cases in the midwestern and eastern U.S.; clinically similar to infections caused by Jamestown Canyon virus.
Vesicular stomatitis virus	Sandflies, midges, black flies	Horses, cattle	Frequently related to occupational exposure to livestock; vesicular lesions may be seen on pharynx, tongue, or buccal mucosa.
Western equine encephalitis virus	Mosquitoes	Birds, horses	Fewer than 20 cases reported annually; clinical illness can range from UFI to meningitis and encephalitis.
Spirochetal and Rickettsial *Borrelia* species B. *burgdorferi* (Lyme disease)	Ticks	White-footed mice	25%–50% of patients with subsequently diagnosed Lyme disease present initially without the characteristic cutaneous manifestation, erythema migrans (see text).
B. *recurrentis* (relapsing fever)	Ticks	Many wild animals	Although B. *recurrentis* can be louse borne, only tick-borne relapsing fever is endemic to North America (see Table 12-6); multiple relapses of febrile illness are characteristic of tick-borne relapsing fever.

Organism	Animal reservoir	Vector	Comments
Brucella species (brucellosis)			Fewer than 200 cases reported annually in U.S., with over half occurring in Texas, California, Virginia, and Florida.
B. melitensis	Goats	None	Generally associated with ingestion of unpasteurized goat's-milk cheese.
B. abortus *B. suis*	Cattle, swine	None	Majority of animal cases in U.S. seen in individuals involved with meat processing, livestock industry, or veterinary services (abattoir workers highest risk group).
B. canis	Dogs	None	Rare
Coxiella burnetti (Q fever)	Cattle, sheep, goats; also cats, wild rabbits	Ticks (although primary mode of transmission is inhalation of small particle aerosols)	Most cases occupationally related (farmers, abattoir workers, veterinarians).
Ehrlichia species (ehrlichiosis)	Unknown	Ticks	Disease is as prevalent as, and clinically similar to, Rocky Mountain spotted fever.
Leptospira species (leptospirosis): *L. australis, L. autumnalis, L. ballum, L. canicola, L. grippotyphosa, L. hebdomidis, L. icterohaemorrhagiae, L. pomona*	Dogs, livestock, rodents and other wild mammals, cats	None	Most infections are secondary to occupational (farmers, abattoir workers, and veterinarians) or recreational (pet handlers, campers) exposures.
Rickettsia rickettsii (Rocky Mountain spotted fever)	Small mammals	Ticks	As many as 86% of cases with ultimately fatal outcomes do not have a rash when initially seen by a physician (see text).

Table 12-16. (continued)

Organism	Principal vector	Principal reservoirs/hosts	Comments
Protozoal			
Babesia microti (babesiosis)	Ticks	White-footed mice	Coinfections with *B. burgdorferi* (Lyme disease) may be common (both infections share the same tick vector and share similar geographic distributions; see Table 12-6); parasites may be confused with *Plasmodium falciparum* on microscopic examination of Giemsa- or Wright-stained blood smears.
Plasmodium vivax (malaria)	Mosquitoes	Humans	Autochthonous infections confined to an isolated focus in southern California.
Toxoplasma gondii (toxoplasmosis)	None	Many wild and domestic mammals, especially cats	Responsible for about 1% of mononucleosis syndromes in immunocompetent patients.
Trypanosoma cruzi (American trypanosomiasis, Chagas' disease)	Reduviid bugs	Many wild and domestic mammals	Rare; reported autochthonous infections in southern Texas and California.

* Undifferentiated febrile illness.

course) from influenza by physical examination and preliminary laboratory evaluation, but that may require specific therapeutic intervention to prevent significant morbidity and potential mortality. In addition, certain septicemic zoonoses, including septicemic plague and tularemia, listeriosis, and the septicemic forms of erysipeloid and *Pasteurella multocida* infections, can present as acute, undifferentiated febrile illnesses. Finally, endocarditis should always be included in the differential diagnosis of the undifferentiated febrile illness syndrome (Table 12-17 lists animal- and insect-associated organisms that cause endocarditis).

The dilemma for the emergency medicine physician is when to suspect an unusual cause for a flu-like syndrome and how to minimize the delay in diagnosis of a potentially treatable condition. A review of Table 12-16 can be helpful. Most of the zoonotic infections in North America have their peak incidence in the spring and summer months, unlike influenza, which occurs almost exclusively in the winter (December–April); most require obvious exposures to mosquitoes, ticks, livestock, etc.; many are geographically restricted to limited regions; and many, particularly viral infections, may occur in outbreaks. From these observations some general statements about the evaluation of the acutely ill, febrile patient with nonspecific constitutional symptoms (especially during the spring and summer months) can be made. First, patients presenting with this syndrome are usually quite ill (the prototypical infection—influenza—is not a trivial disease). Second, certain questions should always be part of the patient evaluation. Besides a general assessment of immune status (by history) and inquiries about valvular heart disease, current medications, and recent contact with similarly ill individuals, patients routinely should be asked about occupational or recreational exposures and exposures to rural habitats, biting insects, and animals (wild, domestic, or pet) that might place them at increased risk for a zoonotic infection. Recent travel history (both outside the United States, as well as outside the patient's local area) should also be obtained. Acute undifferentiated febrile illness in the recently returned international traveler (see Chap. 19) may expand the diagnostic possibilities of this syndrome dramatically. Over 80 arboviral infections alone have been reported to present initially as a flu-like or dengue-like illness. (See reference 58 for a review of arboviral infections in the United States.) A brief review of exposure history (if negative) will virtually exclude the animal- and insect-associated infections caused by the high-risk pathogens discussed previously.

Initial laboratory evaluation of flu-like syndrome may include a complete blood count, a liver aminotransferase determination, and urinalysis. Additional studies would include a Giemsa-stained, peripheral blood smear if malaria is suspected and blood cultures if a cardiac murmur is detected or there is any suspicion of septicemia.

Because some CNS infections, VHFs, Rocky Mountain spotted fever, and other infections may present early in their clinical course as a flu-like illness, patients with this syndrome who are to be discharged from the emergency department should be given careful instructions (preferably written) regarding signs and symptoms that should prompt their immediate return for evaluation. These symptoms would include development of a new rash, petechiae, or other skin lesions; bleeding from any mucosal surface; altered consciousness or confusion; shortness of breath or increasing sputum production; and significant worsening or prolonged duration (more than 1 week) of symptoms.

Fever and Hemorrhagic Cutaneous Lesions

An acutely ill febrile patient who presents with petechial or purpuric skin lesions will always invite aggressive evaluation. Table 12-18 lists a variety of systemic infections in which cutaneous manifestations are frequently prominent. As can be seen, many are classical zoonotic diseases. Of those zoonoses associated with petechial purpuric eruptions, the most prevalent ones endemic to North America are the rickettsial infections; of those, the most prevalent and severe is Rocky Mountain spotted fever [59].

Rocky Mountain Spotted Fever

The etiologic agent of Rocky Mountain spotted fever is *Rickettsia rickettsii*, and the major vectors responsible for disease transmission in North Amer-

Table 12-17. Animal-associated bacteria that cause endocarditis

Organism	Reservoirs	Comments
Brucella species	Swine, cattle, goats, dogs[a]	Endocarditis occurs in <2% of all cases of brucellosis, but is associated with as many as 80% of deaths.
Capnocytophaga canimorsus	Dogs, cats (>50% of infections have followed dog bites)	A gram-negative organism that is penicillin-sensitive but resistant to aminoglycosides.
Chlamydia psittaci	Primarily psittacine birds (parrots) but almost any avian species	Endocarditis is a rare but serious complication of psittacosis.
Coxiella burnetti	Wild and domestic animals[a]	Endocarditis is essentially synonymous with the diagnosis of chronic Q fever.
DF-2 (CDC group)[b]	Dogs, cats (>50% of infections have followed dog bites)	A gram-negative organism that is penicillin-sensitive but may be resistant to aminoglycosides.
Erysipelothrix rhusiopathiae	Many species of wild and domestic birds, animals, and sealife	Endocarditis usually is associated with the septicemic form of E. rhusiopathiae infection; fewer than 20% of patients present with concurrent, typical erysipeloid cutaneous lesions.
Listeria monocytogenes	Most species of wild and domestic birds, animals, and sealife[a]	Endocarditis is an unusual but well-documented clinical listerial syndrome.
Pasteurella multocida	Many wild and domestic animals and birds, particularly cats, dogs, and swine (animal bites account for the majority of infections)	Endocarditis is a rare complication of P. multocida septicemia.
Pasteurella haemolytica	Domestic livestock and fowl	Human infection by P. haemolytica is rare, but endocarditis has been reported.
Salmonella species	Essentially all animal species	Endocarditis is rare; most patients have pre-existing valvular heart disease.
Spirillum minor	Rats (rat bites)	S. minor is a major cause of rat-bite fever in Asia; endocarditis is a complication of untreated rat-bite fever and occurs in the setting of pre-existing valvular heart disease.
Streptobacillus moniliformis	Rats and other small rodents (rat bite)[a]	Rat-bite fever in the U.S. is a rare infection, with most reported cases in animal laboratory staff; endocarditis is a well-recognized complication of untreated disease.
Streptococcus species, e.g., S. canis, S. equi zoo-epidermicus, etc.)	Many domestic animals[a]	The pyogenes-like streptococci (particularly groups C and G) account for 8%–10% of all β-hemolytic streptococcal endocarditis; associated morbidity and mortality are over 30%.
Yersinia enterocolitica	Many domestic animals[a]	Endocarditis is a rare complication of Y. enterocolitica bacteremia.

[a] Transmission of disease by contaminated dairy products has been reported (see Table 12-7).
[b] Centers for Disease Control classification.

Table 12-18. Systemic infection with prominent cutaneous manifestations

Organism (disease)	Macules, papules	Petechia, purpura
Viruses		
Human immunodeficiency (HIV-1) virus	Yes	No
Echoviruses	Yes	Yes
Coxsackieviruses	Yes	Yes
Rubeola (measles)	Yes	No
Atypical measles	Yes	Yes
Adenovirus	Yes	Yes
Lymphocytic choriomeningitis virus	Yes	No
Dengue virus	Yes	Yes
Viral hemorrhagic fevers	No	Yes
Rubella (German measles)	Yes	Yes
Arboviruses	Yes	No
Colorado tick fever	Yes	No
Yellow fever	No	Yes
Vaccinia	No	Yes
Cytomegalovirus	Yes	No
Congenital cytomegalovirus	No	No
Epstein-Barr virus	Yes	Yes
Hepatitis B	Yes	Yes
Parvovirus (erythema infectiosum)	Yes	No
Bacteria		
Chlamydia psittaci	Yes	No
Mycoplasma pneumoniae	Yes	Yes
Rickettsia		
R. rickettsii (Rocky Mountain spotted fever)	Yes	Yes
R. akari (rickettsialpox)	Yes	Yes
R. prowazekii (epidemic/louse-borne typhus)	Yes	Yes
R. typhi (endemic/murine typhus)	Yes	No
R. tsutsugamushi (scrub typhus)	Yes	No
Salmonella typhi	Yes	No
Francisella tularensis	Yes	No
Streptobacillus moniliformis (rat-bite fever)	Yes	Yes
Treponema pallidum (secondary)	Yes	No
Neisseria gonorrhoeae	No	Yes
Neisseria meningitidis	No	Yes
Leptospira sp	Yes	No
Borrelia sp (relapsing fever)	Yes	Yes
Borrelia burgdorferi (Lyme disease)	Yes (annular)	No
Spirillum minor (rat-bite fever)	Yes	No
Staphylococcus aureus	Yes	Yes
Streptococci, group A (scarlet fever)	Yes	No
Fungi (disseminated)		
Candida sp	Yes	No
Cryptococcus neoformans	Yes	No
Histoplasma capsulatum	Yes	No
Blastomyces dermatitidis	Yes	No
Coccidioidomycosis immitis	Yes	No
Protozoal		
Toxoplasma gondii	Yes	No
Plasmodium falciparum (malaria)	No	Yes

Adapted from Weber DJ, Gammon WR, Cohen MS. The acutely ill patient with fever and rash. *In* GL Mandell, RG Douglas, JE Bennett (eds.), *Principles and Practices of Infectious Diseases*, (3rd ed.). New York: Churchill-Livingstone, 1990. P. 480.

ica are the wood tick (in the Rocky Mountain states) and the dog tick (in the eastern and southern United States). Although reported from nearly all states, the highest prevalence of disease in recent years has been in Oklahoma and the Carolinas. Essentially all patients with Rocky Mountain spotted fever present in the spring and summer months, and the highest age-specific incidence occurs in children (age: 5–10 years).

After an incubation period of 4–10 days (median is 7 days), Rocky Mountain spotted fever begins initially as an undifferentiated febrile illness, with myalgias and headache, which may be severe. Associated signs and symptoms are protean (Table 12-19), and gastrointestinal symptoms (nausea, vomiting, abdominal pain, and/or diarrhea) may be prominent. Rash is the major diagnostic sign. Typically it begins as a delicate macular eruption on extremities (particularly around the wrists and ankles) and spreads toward the trunk. As the disease progresses, the lesions involve the palms or the soles

Table 12-19. Symptoms and signs of Rocky Mountain spotted fever

Symptom or sign	Hazard (n = 13)	Sexton (n = 75)	Hattwick (n = 778)	Kaplowitz (n = 131)	Helmick (n = 262)	Kirk (n = 48)
Constitutional						
Fever (38°–39°C)	—[a]	—	—	100	99 (73)[b]	—
Fever (>39°C)	—	—	—	88	90 (63)	—
Fever (unspecified)	100	100	99	—	—	100
Shock	—	—	5	17	7 (<1)	—
Death	—	—	9	8	4 (<1)	2
Triad: fever/rash/tick exposure	—	—	—	—	67(3)	—
Cutaneous						
Any rash	100	100	—	90	88 (49)	96
Maculopapular	—	—	91	—	82 (46)	75
Palms/soles	—	80	—	82	74 (28)	—
Petechial, hemorrhagic	—	45	54	—	49 (13)	52
Gastrointestinal						
Nausea/vomiting	—	39	—	56	60 (38)	48
Abdominal pain	—	33	—	34	52 (30)	31
Splenomegaly	15	17	29	14	16 (3)	27
Hepatomegaly	15	—	—	15	12 (2)	27
Jaundice	—	—	—	8	9 (2)	—
Diarrhea	—	—	—	20	19 (9)	19

Neurologic						
Any headache	100	92	92	79	—	64
Headache, mild–moderate	—	—	—	—	91 (71)	—
Headache, severe	—	—	—	—	52 (40)	—
Ataxia	—	—	—	5	18 (7)	—
Myalgias	—	61	83	72	47 (25)	31
Meningismus	24	13	37	—	18 (5)	29
Stupor	77	—	13	21	26 (6)	40
Coma	—	—	—	10	9 (1)	17
Seizures	—	—	—	8	8 (2)	10
Decreased hearing	—	—	—	—	7 (1)	—
Miscellaneous						
Conjunctivitis	60	15	—	30	30 (13)	—
Lymphadenopathy	0	—	—	—	27 (13)	25
Edema/periorbital edema	—	—	—	20	18 (3)	—
Pneumonitis	—	—	13	17	12 (2)	—
Arrhythmia	—	—	—	8	7 (1)	—
Mycarditis	—	—	—	26	5 (0)	—
Parotitis	—	—	—	—	4 (<1)	—
Arthralgias	—	17	—	—	—	10
Clinical bleeding	—	—	—	15	—	—
Gangrene	—	—	—	4	—	2

[a] —means data not recorded.
[b] ( ) refers to frequency symptom present in first 72 hours of illness.

Source: Weber DJ, Walker DH. Rocky Mountain spotted fever. In AN Weinberg, DJ Weber (eds.), Animal-associated human infections. *Infect Dis Clin North Am* 5(1):19–35, 1991.

Table 12-20. Synopsis of certain epidemiologic and clinical features of selected rickettsioses

Disease	Organism	Geographic area	Hosts		Rash distribution	Eschar
			Arthropods	Vertebrates		
Spotted Fever Group						
Rocky Mountain spotted fever	*Rickettsia rickettsii*	Western hemisphere	Ticks	Wild rodents, dogs	Extremities to trunk	No
Boutonneuse	*Rickettsia conorii*	Africa, Mediterranean, India	Ticks	Wild rodents, dogs	Trunk, extremities, face	Yes
Queensland tick typhus	*Rickettsia australis*	Australia	Ticks	Wild rodents, marsupials	Trunk, extremities, face	Yes
North Asian tick typhus	*Rickettsia sibirica*	Siberia, Mongolia	Ticks	Wild rodents	Trunk, extremities, face	Yes
Rickettsialpox	*Rickettsia akari*	USA, USSR, Korea, Africa	Mites	Mice	Vesicular: trunk, extremities, face	Yes
Typhus Group						
Epidemic typhus	*Rickettsia prowazekii*	Highland areas of South America, Africa, Asia, ?USA	Body lice	Humans, flying squirrels	Trunk to extremities	No
Brill-Zinsser	*Rickettsia prowazekii*	Worldwide based upon immigration	None	Humans (recurrence years after primary attack)	Trunk to extremities (may be absent)	No
Murine typhus	*Rickettsia typhi*	Worldwide in pockets	Fleas	Small rodents	Trunk to extremities	No
Scrub typhus	*Rickettsia tsutsugamushi*	South Pacific, Asia, Australia	Mites	Wild rodents	Trunk to extremities	Yes
Others						
Q fever	*Coxiella burnetii*	Worldwide	Ticks (?)	Cattle, sheep, goats (inhalation of organism)	None	No
Trench fever	*Rochalimaea quintana*	Highly focal	Lice	Humans	Transient or none	No

Source: Saah AJ. Rickettsiosis. In GL Mandel, RG Douglas, JE Bennett (eds.), *Principles and Practice of Infectious Diseases* (3rd ed.). New York: Churchill-Livingstone, 1990. P. 1464.

and become petechial and eventually purpuric. Of note, at least 10% of patients with Rocky Mountain spotted fever have been reported to have no rash, and in approximately 50% of patients the rash does not occur within the first 3 days of illness [60]. Most important as many as 86% of patients with ultimately fatal outcomes do not have a rash when seen initially by a physician [61].

Development of hemorrhagic skin lesions is usually a sentinel event in the clinical course of Rocky Mountain spotted fever and may be associated with significant neurologic, pulmonary, or renal complications. Severe neurologic syndromes (including encephalopathy, seizures, and paresis) have been reported in about 40% of patients [62] and may dominate the clinical presentation after the third day of illness. Pneumonitis is common (see Table 12-14) and potentially life threatening [59]. Renal insufficiency may be seen in 10–15% of cases [60].

The morbidity and the mortality of Rocky Mountain spotted fever are significant. The rate of clinical complications is approximately 40%, and the mortality rate in patients treated with inappropriate antimicrobial agents may be as high as 20% [63]. Both the morbidity and the mortality of Rocky Mountain spotted fever are increased significantly by delay in both diagnosis and institution of specific antimicrobial therapy. As with other potentially lethal infections that may present as an undifferentiated febrile illness, the presumptive diagnosis of Rocky Mountain spotted fever is predicated on an index of suspicion. Acutely ill febrile patients presenting in spring and summer months should have appropriate travel, recreational, and occupational histories reviewed and should be specifically queried about tick exposure. A careful skin survey may detect the early-onset rash. For febrile patients with hemorrhagic skin lesions who clearly will be admitted to the hospital, Rocky Mountain spotted fever should be considered in the design of an empiric antimicrobial regimen. The diagnosis and treatment of Rocky Mountain spotted fever are discussed in Chap. 9.

General Approach to Patients with Fever and Hemorrhagic Lesions

In addition to the clinical approach outlined in Chap. 9 the general evaluation of an acutely febrile patient with hemorrhagic cutaneous lesions should include a complete review of possible occupational and recreational exposures, animal and insect (particularly tick) exposures, travel history outside the patient's immediate area of residence, and a detailed skin survey for eschars (Table 12-20). Recent international travel should prompt consideration of common, life-threatening infections (such as falciparum malaria), as well as rare, life-threatening infections (such as VHFs). In all instances subsequent clinical investigation should be conducted in the hospital; multiple blood cultures are mandatory, and any empiric antimicrobial regimen should include agents specific to each reasonable diagnostic possibility.

References

1. van der Hoeden J (ed.). *Zoonoses*. Amsterdam: Elsevier, 1964.
2. Steele JH (ed.). *CRC Handbook Series in Zoonoses*. Boca Raton, FL: CRC Press, 1981.
3. Acha PN, Szyfres B. *Zoonoses & Communicable Diseases Common to Man & Animals* (2nd ed.). Scientific Publication no. 503, PAHO, 1987.
4. August JR, Loar AS. Zoonotic diseases. *Vet Clin North Am* 17(1):1987.
5. Bell JC, Palmer SR, Payne JM. *The Zoonoses*. London: Edward Arnold, 1988.
6. Blood DC, Radostits OM. *Veterinary Medicine* (7th ed.). London: Bailliere & Tindall, 1989.
7. Mandell GL, Douglas RG Jr, Bennett JE (eds.). *Principles and Practice of Infectious Diseases* (3rd ed.). New York: Churchill-Livingstone, 1990.
8. Warren KS, Mahmond AAF (eds.). *Tropical and Geographic Medicine* (2nd ed.). New York: McGraw-Hill, 1990.
9. Weinberg AN, Weber DJ (eds.). Animal-associated human infections. *Infect Dis Clin North Am* 5(1):1991.
10. Strickland GT (ed.). *Hunter's Tropical Medicine* (7th ed.). Philadelphia: Saunders, 1991.
11. Collins CH. *Laboratory-Acquired Infections*. London: Butterworths, 1983.
12. Bisseru B. *Diseases of Man Acquired from His Pets*. London: Heinemann Medical Books, 1967.
13. Graham-Jones O (ed.). *Some Diseases of Animals Communicable to Man in Britain*. Oxford: Pergamon, 1968.
14. Hubbert WT, McCulloch WF, Schnurrenberger PR (eds.). *Diseases Transmitted from Animals to Man*

(6th ed.). Springfield, IL: Charles C. Thomas, 1975.

15. Snow KR. *Insects and Disease*. New York: Wiley, 1974.

16. Busvine JR *Insects and Hygiene* (3rd ed.). London: Chapman & Hall, 1980.

17. Kean BH, Reilly PC. Malaria—the mime. *Am J Med* 61:159–64, 1976.

18. Hyman AS. Clinical masquerades of malaria. *Naval Med Bull* 45:287–303, 1945.

19. Strickland GT. Malaria. In GT Strickland (ed.), *Hunter's Tropical Medicine* (7th ed.). Philadelphia: Saunders, 1991. Pp. 586–614.

20. Walzer PD, Gibson JJ, Schultz MG. Malaria fatalities in the United States. *Am J Trop Med Hyg* 23:328–32, 1974.

21. World Health Organization Malaria Action Programme. Severe and complicated malaria. *Trans R Soc Trop Med Hyg* 80(suppl):1–50, 1986.

22. McCormick JB et al. A prospective study of the epidemiology and ecology of Lassa fever. *J Infect Dis* 155:437–44, 1987.

23. Fisher-Hoch SP. Lassa fever. In GT Strickland (ed.), *Hunter's Tropical Medicine* (7th ed.). Philadelphia: Saunders, 1991. Pp. 238–41.

24. McCormick JB et al. A case-control study of the clinical diagnosis and course of Lassa fever. *J Infect Dis* 155:445–55, 1987.

25. McCormick JB et al. Lassa fever. Effective therapy with ribavirin. *N Engl J Med* 314:20–26, 1986.

26. Holmes GP et al. Lassa fever in the United States: investigation of a case and new guidelines for management. *N Engl J Med* 323:1120–23, 1990.

27. Martini GA, Siegert R (eds.). *Marburg Virus Disease*. Berlin: Springer-Verlag, 1971.

28. World Health Organization. Ebola haemorrhagic fever in Zaire, 1976: report of an international commission. *Bull WHO* 56:271–93, 1978.

29. Culliton BJ. Emerging viruses, emerging threat. *Science* 247:279–80, 1980.

30. Burney MI et al. Nosocomial outbreak of viral hemorrhagic fever caused by Crimean hemorrhagic fever-Congo virus in Pakistan. *Am J Trop Med Hyg* 29:941–47, 1980.

31. Al-Tikriti SK et al. Congo/Crimean haemorrhagic fever in Iraq. *Bull WHO* 59:85–90, 1981.

32. Suleiman et al. Congo/Crimean haemorrhagic fever in Dubai. *Lancet* 2:939–41, 1980.

33. Swanepoel R et al. Epidemiologic and clinical features of Crimean-Congo hemorrhagic fever in southern Africa. *Am J Trop Med Hyg* 36:120–32, 1987.

34. Hoogstraal H. The epidemiology of tick-borne Crimean-Congo hemorrhagic fever in Asia, Europe, and Africa. *J Med Entomol* 15:304–417, 1979.

35. Centers for Disease Control. Viral hemorrhagic fever: initial management of suspected and confirmed cases. *Ann Intern Med* 101:73–81, 1984.

36. Butler T. Yersinia species (including plague). In GL Mandell, RG Douglas Jr, JE Bennett (eds.), *Principles and Practice of Infectious Diseases* (3rd ed.). New York: Churchill-Livingstone, 1990. Pp. 1748–52.

37. Hull HF, Montes JM, Mann JM. Septicemic plague in New Mexico. *J Infect Dis* 155:113–18, 1987.

38. Palmer DL. Plague and other Yersinia infections. In JD Wilson et al. (eds.), *Harrison's Principles of Internal Medicine* (12th ed.). New York: McGraw-Hill, 1991. Pp. 629–31.

39. Pollitzer R. *Plague*. World Health Organization Monograph Series, No. 22, 1954.

40. Centers for Disease Control. B virus infections in humans—Pensacola, Florida. *MMWR* 36:289–90, 295–96, 1987.

41. Centers for Disease Control. Guidelines for prevention of herpes virus simiae (B virus) infection in monkey handlers. *MMWR* 36:680–89, 1987.

42. Smith JS et al. Unexplained rabies in three immigrants in the United States. *N Engl J Med* 324:205–11, 1991.

43. Gavrila I, Iurasog G, Luca E. Rabies in man: personal observations of seroprophylaxis, prolonged incubation and therapeutic trials. *Ann Inst Pasteur (Paris)* 112:504–15, 1967.

44. Pettit JHS, Parish LC. *Manual of Tropical Dermatology*. New York: Springer-Verlag, 1984.

45. Sams WM Jr, Lynch PJ (eds.). *Principles and Practice of Dermatology*. New York: Churchill-Livingstone, 1990.

46. Farah FS. Parasitic diseases of the skin. *Hosp Med* Feb:112–24, 1991.

47. Scott DW, Horn RT Jr. Zoonotic dermatoses of dogs and cats. In JR August, AS Loar (eds.), Zoonotic diseases. *Vet Clin North Am* 17:117–44, 1987.

48. Scott DW. Feline dermatology 1900–1978: a monograph. *J Am Anim Hosp Assoc* 16:331–459, 1980.

49. Hay RJ. Dermatophytosis and other superficial mycoses. In GL Mandell, RG Douglas Jr, JE Bennett (eds.), *Principles and Practice of Infectious Diseases* (3rd ed.). New York: Churchill-Livingstone, 1990. Pp. 2017–28.

50. Muller GH, Kirk RW, Scott DW. *Small Animal Dermatology* (3rd ed.). Philadelphia: Saunders, 1983.

51. Steere AC. Lyme disease. *N Engl J Med* 321:586–96, 1989.

52. Rahn DW, Malawista SE. Lyme disease. *West J Med* 154:706–14, 1991.
53. Cypress BK. *Office Visits for Diseases of the Respiratory System*. Hyattsville, MD: U.S. Dept. of Health, Education and Welfare, 1979. USHEW: 18.
54. Rodnick JE. Gude JK. Diagnosis and antibiotic treatment of community-acquired pneumonia. *West J Med* 154:405–09, 1991.
55. Weinberg AN. Respiratory infections transmitted from animals. *Infect Dis Clin North Am* 5(3):649–61, 1991.
56. Fang GD et al. New and emerging etiologies for community-acquired pneumonia with implications for therapy. *Medicine (Baltimore)* 69:307–16, 1990.
57. Pearson RD, Guerrant RL. Enteric fever and other causes of abdominal symptoms with fever. In GL Mandell, RG Douglas Jr, JE Bennett (eds.), *Principles and Practice of Infectious Diseases* (3rd ed.). New York: Churchill-Livingstone, 1990. Pp. 880–93.
58. Tsai TF. Arboviral infections in the United States. In AN Weinberg, DJ Weber (eds.), Animal-associated human infections. *Infect Dis Clin North Am* 5(1):73–102, 1991.
59. Weber DJ Walker DH. Rocky Mountain spotted fever. In AN Weinberg, DJ Weber (eds.), Animal-associated human infections. *Infect Dis Clin North Am* 5(1):19–35, 1991.
60. Helmick CG, Bernard KW, D'Angelo LJ. Rocky Mountain spotted fever: clinical laboratory and epidemiological features of 262 cases. *J Infect Dis* 150: 480–88, 1984.
61. Fischer JJ. Rocky Mountain spotted fever: when and why to consider the diagnosis. *Postgrad Med* 87: 109–18, 1990.
62. Kirk JL et al. Rocky Mountain spotted fever: a clinical review based on 48 confirmed cases, 1943–1986. *Medicine* 69:35–45, 1990.
63. Hattwick MAW, O'Brien RJ, Hanson BF. Rocky Mountain spotted fever: epidemiology of an increasing problem. *Ann Intern Med* 84:732–39, 1967.

13

Infection Following Bites, Wounds, and Burns

DOUGLAS LINDSEY
RONALD W. QUENZER

In medicine the management of wounds is a matter of considerable controversy and is subject to constant revision in the light of new data. Unlike operative surgical incisions, in which the most significant infections are of endogenous origin, the infections that supervene in lacerations, punctures, bites, burns, and abrasions are usually due to exogenous organisms that enter through the wound. Deep abscesses can occur in contused tissue without apparent breaks in the skin [1], and purulent tenosynovitis has been observed without evidence of prior injury [2]. These rare instances and some cases of infection in common wounds presumptively can be attributed to endogenous species. All breaks in the skin and the mucosa of bodily orifices are subject to infection, whether the breach is accidental or the result of deliberate surgical intervention. Except for wounds inflicted under strictly controlled germ-free conditions, a certain incidence of wound infection is inevitable.

The incidence of infections in traumatic wounds reported by emergency physicians covers a broad range. Articles from two comparable institutions report an infection rate of 15% in one and 1.5% in the other. This difference can be explained only by differences in the institutional criteria that define infection.

Signs of Wound Infection

The classical signs of infection are erythema, pain or tenderness, swelling, heat, and pus. Celsus in the first century A.D. interpreted *rubor, dolor, tumor,* and *calor* as signs of inflammation, not infection. A certain amount of inflammation is integral to the process of wound healing, and sterile abscesses can be induced by the injection of irritant agents. Arbitrary limits on the degree of expression of the signs of infection or the disregard of pus if no organisms are cultured from the sample are nothing more than artifice to lower infection rates. A clear "yes" or "no" answer on the presence of infection remains, nevertheless, a difficult determination.

Factors That Influence Infection

The incidence, nature, and severity of infection in a wound depend to some degree on (1) the health of the patient, (2) the time since wounding, (3) the extent and the type of tissue damage, (4) the amount and the character of contamination, and (5) the anatomical site.

289

Health of Patient (Host Factors)

Wounds in persons who have peripheral vascular disease, diabetes mellitus, or an immunocompromised condition are problematic. Age alone does not predispose to wound infection. The decreased resistance to infection in the immunosuppressed is covered in Chap. 16. Diabetes per se probably does not increase the incidence of infection, but hyperglycemia, a controllable variable, decreases leukocytes' chemotactic and phagocytic functions. Wound infections are more difficult to treat if they are complicated by peripheral vascular disease or the neuropathic/angiopathic complications of diabetes.

Age of Wound

The earlier a wound is closed, the less likely that it will become infected. Emergency physicians must do what they can to ensure early wound cleansing and closure. Even in patients with multiple major injuries, simple lacerations often can be closed in the intervals between the inevitable imaging procedures. There is no established finite time limit beyond which a wound must not be closed or cannot be closed. Although 6 hours is endorsed by many clinicians based on the findings in the original paper [3, 4], a recent study marks the "golden period" at 18 hours [5]. In that study 65 of 72 wounds (92.1%) 18 hours old or less were not infected, whereas only 89 of 115 older wounds (80.3%) were not infected.

Mechanism of Injury

In general large or deep wounds and stellate wounds are more prone to infection. The sharper the wounding instrument, the less likely the infection [6, 7]. Puncture is defined as a "hole made by a sharp point." The object is usually a nail, a pin, or a tooth. The precise nature of a narrow hole made through multiple, movable tissue plains prevents adequate drainage, irrigation, and débridement.

Nonviable muscle inflicted by the wounding instrument is frequently a concern. Muscle that is discolored, that does not contract well, and that does not bleed freely is contused but not necessarily nonviable. In most instances the contused muscle will heal, except for a necrotic layer of 2–3 mm around the permanent track. Excision of contused muscle sacrifices viable tissue, which can and does repair and regenerate to perform useful function [8–17].

Amount and Character of Contamination

There is a modest measure of clinical utility in making an initial estimate of the nature of the contamination from the circumstances of the injury. The clinician should always consider *Pasteurella multocida* in an infected cat bite, anaerobes in an infected human bite, and mixed aerobic-anaerobic infection in wounds heavily contaminated with soil and vegetation. *Enterobacter agglomerans* is a common infecting organism in farm-machinery wounds [18]. However, a preinfection culture of the contaminated wound is a poor predictor of the cause of infection that may ensue [19–21]. The initial quantity of organisms may influence the infection rate. The critical bacterial load is usually considered to be 10^5 organisms per gram of tissue. If the Gram's stain shows bacteria, this finding supports a heavy, potentially troublesome inoculum.

Anatomical Site

There is no convincing evidence that susceptibility or resistance to infection varies significantly by anatomical region alone. Specific tissue compartments or planes, such as the tendon sheath of the hand, may have higher infection rates. The mechanism of injury commonly found in a particular region, such as puncture wounds of the foot, may result in higher infection rates (see Chap. 33), but this incidence is related to the unique characteristics of the wounds themselves—tissue planes that cause closed spaces or wounds with retained foreign bodies that cannot be removed or cleaned.

Wound Management

Antisepsis

GOWN, MASK, AND GLOVES

The true value of scrubbing, donning a gown and mask, and pulling on sterile gloves will never be determined. Today universal precautions are practiced in the emergency department for protection against the patient as well as for the patient. No practitioner would think of suturing without gloves. Similarly precautions should be taken when examining wounds or changing dressings.

SCRUBS, PAINTS, SOAKS, LAVAGE, AND SHAVING

The most efficacious manner of cleaning a wound is irrigation with normal saline or water to decrease the bacterial load and remove foreign particle contamination. The prior emphasis on volume ("copious lavage") in the cleansing of wounds is giving way to emphasis on pressure [22–25]. Effective as syringe irrigation is [26], the pressure obtained in the use of a syringe does not reach the higher optimal level, nor can a syringe offer a pulsating jet. For small wounds 20 ml of saline pushed out through a No. 20 needle is adequate; for larger or grossly dirty wounds a pulsating pressure jet lavage with 200–2000 ml of water is recommended.

The value of antiseptic preparation of the site before elective surgical intervention was established long ago. However, if the wound already has been inflicted, the situation is different. First, the detergent in the scrub preparation of povidone iodine is cytotoxic and appropriate for use only on intact skin [27, 28]. If povidone iodine is used, a few caveats are in order [29–32]: (1) sterilization is neither instantaneous nor infallible; (2) it is more effective in killing bacteria on clean, normal skin than it is in a wound containing blood and fat; and (3) it is most effective when diluted 1:100 from the stock solution. Second, nothing is to be gained by soaking wounds. Third, shaving the area around a hairy wound may increase the incidence of infection while clipping may not [33]. Finally, it is unnecessary to tell a patient with a sutured scalp wound not to shampoo for 24 hours [34, 35]. Good clinical trials comparing dry versus moist wound healing are limited [36–40].

Exploration

Clarification of the nature and the extent of deep-tissue damage requires careful evaluation of the history, symptoms, and physical examination and may indicate judicious probing or even further incision. The original meaning of the French term *débridement* is "to relieve constriction by incision."

Then treat what you find: treat the wound, not the weapon [41–43]. Manual removal of foreign bodies and débridement may be required before proceeding with closure. If the injury involves a tendon, joint or bone, nerve, or major vessel, consultation is essential. The wound should be rechecked in 24–48 hours.

Infected Wounds

Infected wounds need additional attention. A plain film x-ray should be done if there is any suspicion of foreign bodies, fracture, or osteomyelitis. The infected wound must be débrided with a blade or curette for smaller wounds. A deep sample of tissue and exudate should be obtained for a Gram's stain and culture, followed by irrigation. A dressing then should be applied to protect the wound from contamination, and the patient should always be instructed in wound care. Empiric antibiotics should be initiated prior to the culture results. If the patient is at risk of limb, is septic, or is immunocompromised, or if there is suggestion of joint or bone penetration or lymphangitis, then parenteral therapy is indicated. Otherwise, most wounds can be treated on an outpatient basis with oral agents or occasionally with initial parenteral agents followed by an oral drug.

Immunoprophylaxis

Tetanus prophylaxis must be considered in all wound cases. Large contaminated necrotic wounds are certainly at risk for tetanus, but so are minor wounds such as lacerations, abrasions, and punctures. Administration of tetanus toxoid and tetanus immune globulin should follow the most current recommendations (see Chap. 5).

Whether a break in the skin from the bite or scratch of a wild animal represents a threat of rabies depends entirely on local geographic and species considerations. Animal control authorities, the state public health agency, or infectious disease specialists can provide the proper course to follow. Aggressive wound cleansing is paramount to the therapeutic regime. Administration of rabies immune globulin (RIG) and human diploid cell rabies vaccine (HDCV) should follow the most current recommendations (see Chap. 5).

Antibiotic Prophylaxis

The surgical specialty has developed drug-specific guidelines for the prophylaxis against infection in controlled surgical incisions [21, 44–46]. Although these guidelines do not specifically cover accidental wounds, they still apply [47]. Few studies address systemic prophylaxis in nonsurgical wounds. Antibiotic prophylaxis in surgery applies to the prevention of postoperative wound infection by administering antibiotics preoperatively to attain adequate tissue concentration prior to bacterial contamination of the incision site. In that sense prophylaxis cannot be provided to accidental wounds. The clinician can, however, empirically prescribe antibiotics prior to clinical evidence of infection in selected situations in which significant bacterial inoculation, contamination, and subsequent infection are predictable. Despite the lack of solid data, to one of the authors (RWQ), the use of systemic antimicrobials in early wound management prior to clinical evidence of infection is appropriate for the following high-risk wounds: (1) heavily contaminated wounds, (2) cat bites, (3) human bites, and (4) wounds in diabetic or immunocompromised patients. The drawbacks to the use of antibiotics in these circumstances are cost, toxicity, possible lack of efficacy, and development of bacterial resistance.

Indications for Admission

Most patients with traumatic wounds can be treated as outpatients. Every wound should be followed up for the presence of infection 24–48 hours after the first visit and at the time of suture removal in 7–10 days [48]. If the physician is not confident that the patient can be safely managed as an outpatient, then the patient should be admitted. Admission is sometimes required for relatively minor injuries if the patient's social or psychologic circumstances so dictate. If there is doubt, the physician should admit the patient and reevaluate the decision in 24 hours.

Complications from Infected Wounds

The complications most commonly associated with wounds are cellulitis and fasciitis (see Chap. 32), tenosynovitis, sepsis (see Chap. 6), septic arthritis, osteochondritis, and osteomyelitis (see Chap. 33). The complication risk is not predictable but depends on many factors: host status, amount of contamination, mechanism and depth of the injury, and appropriate care.

Bite Wounds

Animal Bites and Scratches

It is estimated that domestic animals account for 600–800 bites per 100,000 persons annually in the United States [49, 50]. The majority of the victims are children. Approximately 80% of bites are inflicted by the domestic dog, 5%–19% by cats, and 2%–3% by rodents [51–53].

Dog Bites

Physicians in the United States treat about a million dog bites each year [54]. At least one-half of the dog bites involve children, and approximately 10 people die annually from dog bites; one-third of those deaths occur in infants [54]. Dog bites have been reported to be complicated by infection in 5% of cases [55–58].

The dog's mouth harbors an assortment of potential pathogens, including aerobic *Staphylococcus aureus*, streptococci, *P. multocida*, and anaerobic *Peptostreptococci* and *Bacteriodes*. The bacteriology of infected wounds from dog bites is shown in Table 13-1. The likelihood of *P. multocida* infection in dog bites is less than in cat bites. Kizer reported that *P. multocida* was isolated from dog and cat bites at the rates of 50% and 80%, respectively, in a series of 332 animal bite injuries [55]. More recently dog bites have been implicated in soft-tissue infections,

Table 13-1. Bacteriology of infected bite wounds

Dog and cat bites	Human bites
Staphylococcus aureus	Streptococci
Streptococci	*S. aureus*
Pasteurella multocida	*Eikenella corrodens*
Capnocytophaga canimorsus	*Hemophilus* species
"Bacteriodes"	*Neisseria* species
"Peptostreptococcus"	"Peptostreptococcus"
	"Fusobacterium"
	"Bacteroides"

meningitis, sepsis, and death from *Capnocytophaga canimorsus* (formerly DF-2), a gram-negative bacterium [56–63]. Patients with severe alcoholic liver disease or splenectomy appear to be particularly susceptible (see Chap. 16), but immunocompetent individuals are not exempt. *Capnocytophaga* organisms are sensitive to most antibiotics [59], but resistance to penicillins and cephalosporins has been noted and may contribute to the delayed appearance of the septic stage.

CAT BITES AND SCRATCHES

Cat bites usually do not result in puncture wounds that are undermined or that require sutures, but they may be deep and difficult to cleanse. Scratches from cats can be deep enough to demand repair, particularly if they are on the face of child or a female. Death from a cat bite is rare, but the risk for infection is higher (30%–50%) than in dog bites [55, 58].

The single peculiarity of the bites of felines is the frequency with which *P. multocida* is the prime offender and the rapidity (24–48 hours) with which such infections become clinically manifest [64]. Rarely have cats been implicated in *Capnocytophaga* infections [62]. Outdoor cats like to prey on rodents and thus may transmit unusual infections. For example, patients who developed tularemia from cat bites have been reported [65, 66]. The bacteriology of infected wounds from cat bites is shown in Table 13-1.

Cat-scratch disease occurs in patients who have a history of exposure to cats. The majority of patients will recall a cat scratch or bite within 2 weeks of their symptoms and presentation to the emergency department. Lymphadenopathy with or without fever is the most common clinical feature of cat-scratch disease (see Chap. 10).

NONDOMESTIC ANIMALS

Bites of feral animals and exotic pets are not common in the United States. In those few instances, bites and maulings from bears in the wilderness and zoo animal bites are probably the most common. Wolf, fox, skunk, and badger bites may occur and cause much alarm. Most of these wild beasts are powerful and vicious and can inflict serious injury resulting in torn muscles and tendons and gaping wounds. Surgical referral often is required.

Human Bites

Human bites have a terrible reputation for infection; however, much of the cited literature on the malevolence of human bites is biased [67]—the population studied is not the group of subjects bitten, but that fraction of the bitten group that presents for treatment. A study comparing the incidence of infection in human bite wounds compared to nonbite lacerations determined the infection rate to be 17.7% versus 13.4%, respectively [68]. Serious limb-threatening infections can complicate what appears to be an innocuous human bite.

INTRAORAL WOUNDS

Most often intraoral wounds are self-inflicted bites. Such wounds are always thoroughly contaminated with bacteria-laden saliva. However, one study of 100 children found no benefit to penicillin or erythromycin prophylaxis [69]. Antibiotic prophylaxis is not indicated for intraoral lacerations. For through-and-through lip lacerations, the mucosa and vermilion border should be closed with silk and then the skin with monofilament nylon. Absorbable sutures are not recommended intraorally, since they may lose their tensile strength too quickly.

A one-tooth puncture of the tongue does not require sutures, but a laceration may. Silk sutures usually are preferred and need to be removed in about 14 days.

EXTRAORAL

Seventy-three percent of human bite wounds are associated with assault and battery, with the upper extremity as the site of injury in 61% of cases [70]. Full-thickness bite wounds and clenched-fist injuries are most prone to serious infection. Generally traumatic digit amputation does not become an infectious problem unless the wound is closed prematurely.

MICROBIOLOGY

The density of bacteria in the oral cavity is 10^8 to 10^9 bacteria per ml of saliva with a ratio of anaerobes to aerobes of 1:1. The bacteriology of most infected bite wounds is polymicrobial with mixed aerobes and anaerobes (see Table 13-1). The most common isolates are aerobic streptococci, *S. aureus*, *Eikenella corrodens*, *Hemophilus* species, *Neis-*

seria species, and anaerobic "Peptostreptococcus" and "Bacteroides." Less commonly a variety of gram-negative bacilli are found, such as *Escherichia coli*, *Klebsiella* species, and *Enterobacter* species. All of these organisms may be pathogenic. *E. corrodens*, a virulent aerobic gram-negative bacillus, has been cultured in 7%–29% of human bite infections [71–73].

Management

The emergency department physician should attempt to cleanse all bite wounds. If infection appears to be present, a Gram's stain and a culture should be taken of any exudate. Samples from puncture wounds can best be obtained by probing the puncture with a small, stiff urethral swab after cleansing the skin surface with betadine and sterile saline or water. Noninfected wounds can be closed, but leaving the wound open is the best course to follow if there are already signs of infection.

Studies in the use of prophylactic antibiotics in bite wounds are inconclusive. Common practice is to prescribe antibiotics for all cat and human bites, regardless of the lack of clinical infection, because of their high rates of infection. Oral amoxicillin-clavulanate (Augmentin) at 250–500 mg q8h for 3–5 days is the ideal agent. Penicillin, tetracycline, and erythromycin at usual dosages are reasonable alternatives.

All infected bite wounds require systemic antibiotic treatment for 7–14 days. Mild infections can be treated with oral antibiotics, while moderate to severe infections manifested by the association of a systemic response (fever, tachycardia), cellulitis/lymphangitis, or concern for deep-tissue involvement such as fasciitis require parenteral therapy,

consultation, and hospitalization. The antibiotic should be initiated in the emergency department for patients with serious infections after blood cultures have been obtained.

Initial antibiotic therapy should be guided by the type of bite, the results of a Gram's stain, and clinical factors. Amoxicillin-clavulanate as an oral agent and ampicillin-sulbactam (Unasyn) or ticarcillin-clavulanate (Ticarcillin) as parenteral agents have excellent coverage against the aerobic and anaerobic organisms that cause most bite wound infections and are the agents of choice for initial therapy (Table 13-2). Penicillin, tetracycline, and erythromycin are alternatives. Most *E. corrodens*, *P. multocida*, and "Bacteroides" are sensitive to penicillins and tetracyclines but are moderately resistant to penicillinase-resistant penicillins (i.e., oxacillin) and first-generation cephalosporins (i.e., cephalexin). Several combination antibiotic regimens also would be suitable.

Hand Wounds

It is estimated that hand infections account for about 10% of all hand problems. Because of the risk of the loss of a digit or a limb, the high incidence of temporary or permanent loss of function, and the cost of hospitalization and surgery, the emergency department physician must be exceptionally thorough in the evaluation and management of all hand wounds. Whenever there is doubt, consultation should be requested.

The problem for the emergency department physician when presented with an infected swollen hand is determining if the infectious process is superficial to the tendons (cellulitis), directly in-

Table 13-2. Antibiotic treatment for human and animal bite wounds

PO	Dosage	IV	Dosage
Amoxicillin-clavulanate	500 mg q6h	Ampicillin-sulbactam	1.5–3.0 g q6h
		Ticarcillin-clavulanate	3.1 g q6h
Alternative Agents			
Penicillin V	500 mg q6h	Penicillin G	2 million u q4–6h
Tetracycline	500 mg q6h	Erythromycin	500 mg q6h
Erythromycin	500 mg q6h	Cefotaxime	2 g q8h

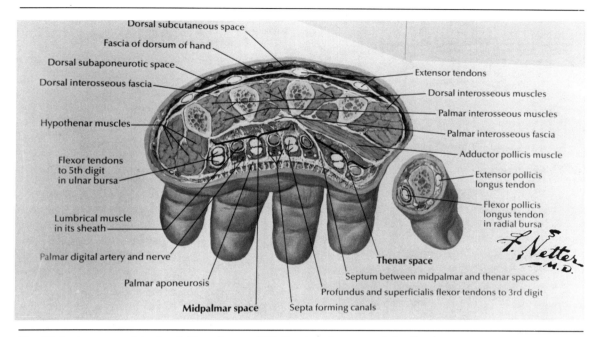

Fig. 13-1. Anatomy of the hand (From Lampe EW. Surgical Anatomy of the Hand. *Clinical Symposia*, Vol. 21, No. 3, Copyright 1969, CIBA Pharmaceutical Company. Illustrated by Frank H. Netter, M.D. from *Clinical Symposia*. Used by permission.

volves the tendons (tenosynovitis), or is in the deeper spaces. Figure 13-1, which displays the anatomy of the hand, can assist the physician in making a correct diagnosis. In many cases even an experienced hand surgeon will have difficulty in defining the process. If there is doubt, the best rule is to assume the worst and explore the hand. Only superficial infections and simple wounds of the hand should be treated on an outpatient basis.

Cellulitis

Cellulitis of the hand presents, as it does in other locations, with swelling, erythema, pain, and tenderness. It begins as a local infection but if untreated often spreads to involve a significant part of the extremity. Initially systemic symptoms and signs are not present, but as the infection progresses, fever, rigors, tachycardia, and tachypnea can develop. Uncomplicated, localized cellulitis without any systemic signs or symptoms can be treated in the outpatient setting. Nearly all cases of hand cellulitis result as a complication of a puncture, bite, or laceration to the hand.

IV drug users are prone to hand infections. The most common sites are the dorsum of the hand, the radial-dorsal area of the wrist, the palmar aspect of the forearm, and the dorsum of the fingers at the proximal interphalangeal (PIP) joint. [74]. These patients usually present 4–5 days after drug injection, when the infection has become painful and clearly evident. Many IV drug users deny drug use, but clues include the location of the wound, sclerotic veins, and needle tracks. Complications are common in this population (see Chap. 18).

Finger Infections

Paronychias and felons account for about one-third of all hand infections.

PARONYCHIA

An infection of the nail fold is known as a paronychia (Fig. 13-2). Fingernail biting and hangnails are common precipitating events. Acute paronychia is recognized by redness, swelling, and pain surrounding the nail. *S. aureus* is the usual pathogen.

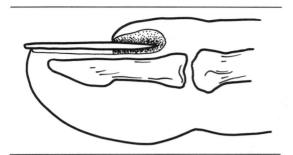

Fig. 13-2. Paronychia

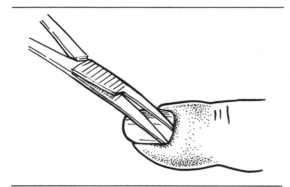

Fig. 13-3. Procedure to drain a paronychia with hemostat

Treatment of a paronychia is straightforward. A simple paronychia usually can be drained by elevating the nail fold with a small hemostat and dissecting along tissue planes into the abscess (Fig. 13-3). A stent (such as Vaseline-impregnated gauze) is placed to allow continued drainage. If that procedure is unsuccessful, once the finger is anesthetized by a digital block and prepped, a No. 11 blade is pressed into the nail sulcus to relieve the pressure of pus in the abscess and then a small instrument is inserted to ensure adequate drainage. A complicated paronychia may require a longitudinal incision parallel to the nail to force adequate drainage, but this measure can deform the nail sulcus and require prolonged healing time. If a simple paronychia is ignored, pus may spread under the nail sulcus to the opposite side, resulting in a "runaround" paronychia. Antibiotic therapy is not required if a simple paronychia can be drained. In cases of a complicated paronychia, the pus should be sent for a Gram's stain and culture, and then an antistaphylococcal antibiotic prescribed for 5–7 days.

Chronic paronychia reflects a chronic inflammatory reaction due to a combination of infection and maceration and obstruction of the proximal nail fold. *Candida albicans* and gram-negative bacilli are the organisms most frequently cultured [75]. A patient with chronic paronychia does not require incision and drainage or antimicrobial administration from an emergency department physician but rather referral to a dermatologist or infectious disease specialist for care.

FELON

Felons are palmar closed-space infections of the distal pad of the finger (Fig. 13-4). Felons are characterized by throbbing pain, marked tenderness, swelling, and redness of the entire pulp. Minor cuts and splinter punctures are common precipitating causes, but usually the patient does not recall the inciting incident. *S. aureus* is the most common pathogen, but gram-negative bacteria and unusual opportunistic organisms may be found in certain situations, particularly in immunocompromised hosts [76, 77]. Antibiotic treatment alone (an antistaphylococcal agent) usually will abort an early felon, but once an abscess is formed, the closed space must be opened to avoid a compartment syndrome of the finger. The treatment usually can

Fig. 13-4. Felon

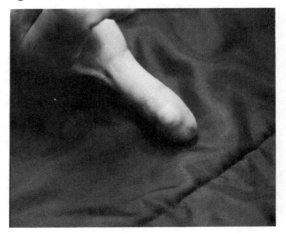

be successfully exercised on an outpatient basis. However, because of the controversy as to the best type of incision and the risk of damaging both digital nerves and vessels, the emergency department physician is best to leave the surgery to an experienced surgeon so that a sensate and painless finger pad can be regained [78].

HERPETIC WHITLOW

Herpesvirus infections can involve any portion of the hand, but herpetic whitlow is the term used to describe a herpes simplex infection of the superficial cutaneous tissue of the finger [79]. The patients are frequently health care workers who are exposed to oral secretions that contain herpes simplex virus (cross-infection) (see Chap. 5). It is also seen in children, patients who have herpes simplex infections at other sites (autoinoculation), and persons whose sexual partners are infected (cross-infection) [80]. The incubation period is 2–14 days, after which the patient presents with minor swelling, intense pain, and one or two clear vesicles with surrounding erythema on the distal digit.

A herpetic whitlow should be differentiated from a bacterial felon or a paronychia. Left untreated a whitlow will resolve in 2–4 weeks, but all patients should receive acyclovir 800–1000 mg/day for 14 days to eradicate the infection more quickly and to diminish secretion of the virus that may put others at risk of infection. Immunocompromised patients may require higher and longer doses of therapy. Prior to treatment the vesicles should be gently unroofed and the fluid sent for viral culture (see Chap. 3). A Tzanck smear (see Chap. 3) is a quick and inexpensive method of diagnosing herpes infections, with a sensitivity of 60%–70% from fresh vesicles [81]. Surgery has no place in the treatment of herpetic whitlows.

Clenched-Fist Injuries

Approximately 40% of human bites are the result of a "fight bite" to the hand associated with assault [70]. A clenched-fist injury also is seen occasionally in athletes, especially basketball players, due to inadvertent contact. The metacarpal-phalangeal (MCP) joint most commonly is involved in a clenched-fist injury (Fig. 13-5). Any puncture or laceration to an MCP joint should be managed as a clenched-fist type of injury. Because of the sharp edge of the front incisors, the wounds frequently appear as minor, clean punctures. The force and the angle of the blow to the victim's mouth determine the depth of the wound. When a tooth strikes the knuckle of a clenched fist and penetrates into the extensor apparatus or into the joint, the wound will not drain when the fingers return to a extended position and the risk of infection increases.

In every case of a clenched-fist injury to a joint area, the wound must be surgically explored. The extensor tendon may be severed and the joint itself penetrated and inoculated with bacteria from the skin and mouth flora, resulting in septic arthritis, tenosynovitis, or osteomyelitis. If the wound is examined only in the open-hand position, natural retraction and realignment of tissue planes will prevent recognition of a partially severed tendon or injury to deeper structures (Fig. 13-6) For the vital structures to be visible to the physician, the wound must be examined in the clenched-fist position. (Hand surgeons who write in German speak of the *Kulissen* effect. A *Kulisse* is a panel of scenery in a theater; when it slides into place, it cuts out the prior scene.) If the tendon is partially or completely severed, the joint is entered, or it is difficult to determine the depth of injury, a surgeon should be consulted.

For superficial wounds clinicians should follow the wound management guidelines and antibiotic therapy recommendations appropriate for other human bites discussed previously in this chapter. Serious clenched-fist injuries require surgery, débridement, cultures, antibiotic therapy, and hospitalization. Parenteral agents should be used initially; ampicillin-clavulanate or ticarcillin-sulbactam in standard dosages is the drug of choice. Alternative agents include trimethoprim-sulfamethoxazole or a second- or third-generation cephalosporin with clindamycin.

Tenosynovitis and Bursitis

A tendon sheath infection can produce serious disability in hand and finger function. Tenosynovitis is a closed-space infection of the tendon(s) contained in the hollow tubular sheaths that are joined at the proximal and distal ends (Fig. 13-7). The thumb flexor sheath connects with the radial bursa,

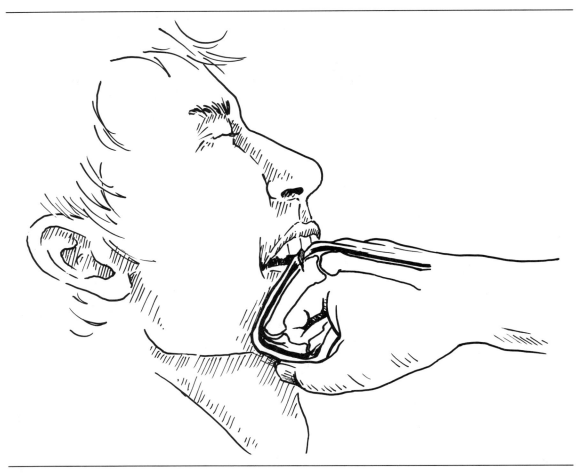

Fig. 13-5. Clenched-fist injury

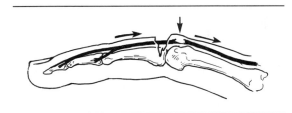

Fig. 13-6. Tendon retraction in open hand position

and the fifth finger flexor sheath has a similar connection with the ulnar bursa; infection of either of these two finger tendons can spread easily into the bursae.

The initiating event to tenosynovitis usually is penetrating trauma. The clinical findings were first described by Kanavel [82]. In the earliest phase of

infection only one sign may be evident, whereas more severe cases will display all four of Kanavel's cardinal signs: (1) uniform swelling of the digit, (2) semiflexed position of the digit, (3) exquisite tenderness along the entire sheath, and (4) marked pain along the entire sheath on passive extension of the digit. Most bacterial infections present in an acute fashion.

S. aureus is the etiologic agent in the majority of tenosynovitis cases, but other organisms, including mycobacteria and fungi, must be considered. Mycobacterial infections of the hand are unusual in the United States, but if a patient presents an insidious course with chronic signs and symptoms of hand infection, then this should be a part of the differential diagnosis. Although mycobacteria can reach structures of the hand by the hematogenous route,

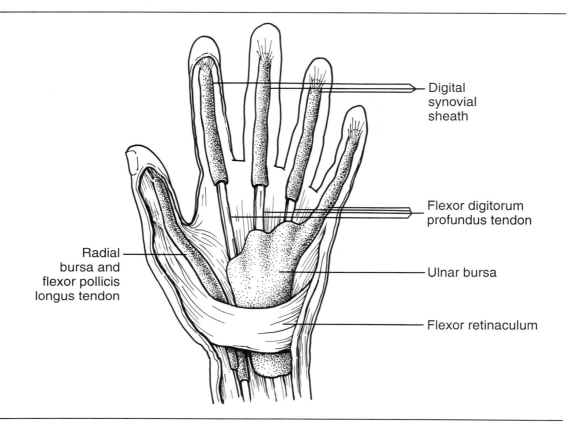

Digital
synovial
sheath

Flexor digitorum
profundus tendon

Ulnar bursa

Flexor retinaculum

Radial
bursa and
flexor pollicis
longus tendon

Fig. 13-7. Tendons and bursae of the hand

the most common mechanism is through direct inoculation. Atypical mycobacteria, particularly *Mycobacterium marinum*, *Mycobacterium fortuitum*, and *Mycobacterium kansasii*, are more common than *Mycobacterium tuberculosis*. Most cases are acquired by a penetrating puncture after exposure to tropical fish tanks or warm fresh-water lakes in the southern and eastern United States. Patients present with chronic swelling, minimal pain, and partial dysfunction of the tendon. Deep-space infections of the hand by mycobacteria are much less common [83]. The clinical diagnosis is made by pursuing detailed exposure and epidemiologic history. Confirmation occurs from histologic and microbiologic findings of granulomata, acid-fast organisms, or mycobacteria species on the culture. Surgery and antimycobacteria agents together are required therapy.

Sporothrix schenckii causes the majority of fungal infections of the hand. Individuals may give a history of working with thorny plants. Sporotrichosis most often presents as a single, painless, chronic,

and indolent papule or ulcer on the hand or extremity (cutaneous sporotrichosis) or as lymphocutaneous sporotrichosis (see Chap. 10). Osteoarticular sporotrichosis can involve the tendon sheath or bursa as well as the bone and joint [84, 85] (see Chap. 33). The hand and the wrist are frequent sites of involvement, but the clinical manifestations of tenosynovitis and bursitis are not unique unless there are associated lymphocutaneous lesions. To make the diagnosis, the surgeon must submit tissue for fungal stain and culture. Iodides usually are not useful for osteoarticular infection. Instead amphotericin B or an imidazole agent is indicated.

Deep-Space Infections

Deep-space infections are serious and managed only on an inpatient basis with surgery and parenteral antibiotics. Failure to make the correct diagnosis and to admit may cost the patient permanent disability or loss of hand. Septic arthritis and osteomyelitis, common complications of deep-space infections, are covered in Chap. 33.

The deep anatomic spaces of the hand are the dorsal subaponeurotic space, the thenar space, the midpalmar space, and the subfascial web space (see Fig. 13-1). The dorsal subaponeurotic space is beneath the extensor tendons over the dorsum of the hand. Patients presenting with swelling of the dorsal surface of the hand may have a cellulitis of the subcutaneous tissue or an actual subaponeurotic-space infection and abscess. If the examining physician is uncertain, a hand surgeon should be consulted. In most cases linear incisions on the dorsum of the hand will be necessary to define the process [86]. If a deep-space infection is identified, the patient will require admission and further care.

The thenar space is dorsal to the flexor tendons of the thumb and the first digit. Infection of this space is evident by the patient complaining of considerable pain and swelling at the thenar eminence and pain with adduction of the thumb to opposition with the fingers. Infection in this space commonly tracks dorsally with swelling on the dorsal-medial aspect of the hand.

Midpalmar-space infections result from a direct perforating injury to the palm. There is both dorsal and palmar swelling of the middle and lateral portion of the hand as well as pain and tenderness.

Infection of the potential subfascial web space usually begins as an infected blister on the palm. The process then spreads in the direction of the least resistance, resulting in swelling of the fingers and the web space dorsally, or what is referred to as a "collar-button abscess."

All deep-space infections of the hand have the potential for serious complications, so consultation in the emergency department with surgery and infectious disease specialists is recommended. A comprehensive plan of management can then be prepared. All deep-space hand infections require surgical exposure, drainage, samples submitted to the microbiology laboratory to identify the cause, and antibiotic therapy. The choice of antibiotics should be determined by the type of injury and results of the Gram's stain and culture, but initial empiric choice should provide coverage against staphylococci and streptococci.

Abrasions

Deep abrasions are best portrayed as "road rashes," whether they are incurred from a road surface or not. Road rashes resemble thermal burns in that the integument from the surface down is damaged or destroyed. They differ from burns, however, in that the surface layers are ablated rather than coagulated. The underlying tissue may be seriously damaged by ablation or contusion, with fascia and muscle sometimes destroyed as well. In hot climates road rashes are a particular problem since they may combine both ablative and thermal injury.

Initially the abrasion should be thoroughly cleansed to remove the burden of bacteria and debris in the wound to ameliorate the risk of infection. This may require detailed scrubbing, but a water jet usually is effective and sufficient. There is no need at this time to obtain superficial wound cultures. The abrasive wound is likely to be contaminated with several ubiquitous and saprophytic microorganisms. If the abrasion appears to include full-thickness loss of dermis, a few well-placed sutures will obliterate or markedly reduce the size of the defect and the extent of invitation to infection. Once the wound is scrubbed or irrigated and sutured, treatment, if indicated, is that of a thermal burn. Most physicians seem to prefer covering the abrasion with some sort of impregnated gauze or membrane. The injury should be reevaluated in 48–72 hours for signs of infection. Once a deep abrasion, burn, or avulsion is covered, adherent material should not be removed or soaked off for follow-up observation. If the eschar or gauze-fiber-reinforced scab is tightly adherent, it is unlikely that there is a wound infection. An estimate of presence of infection can be made by observation of cellulitis around the adherent area as well as lymphangitis extending from the wound border. If infection is present, samples of the exudate and deep-wound surface must be submitted for a Gram's stain and cultures and the wound cleaned and débrided. Antibiotic selection should be guided by the Gram's stain and culture results, but the initial empiric choice should provide coverage against staphylococci and streptococci, for example, oral dicloxacillin or cephalexin at 500 mg qid, parenteral nafcillin at 2 g q6h, or cefazolin at 2 g q8h.

Burns

Only motor vehicle accidents cause more accidental deaths than burns. It is estimated that 2.5 million people seek medical care for thermal injuries each year in the United States. One hundred thousand of these patients require hospitalization, and approximately 12,000 die [87]. Thermal burns differ from chemical and electrical burns [88]. This discussion pertains to thermal burn infections only.

The three most important prognostic variables in burn injuries are the patient's age, the degree of burn injury, and the presence or absence of smoke inhalation [89]. The burn wound, as any other breach of the integument, is susceptible to infection. Infection and cardiopulmonary failure are the two major causes of death in burn victims. Damage to the skin is diffuse and poorly demarcated in surface dimensions and its depth is hard to estimate.

It often is difficult to determine precisely the degree(s) of burn and the percent of body surface area (BSA) affected [88, 90, 91], but this information should be recorded as accurately as possible on a burn wound chart before the patient leaves the emergency department.

Burns are classified as partial thickness (first degree and second degree) or full thickness (third degree). A first-degree burn is limited to the epidermis; the skin is painful and red but without blisters. A superficial second-degree burn involves the uppermost portion of the dermis as well as the epidermis; the skin is painful and red with blisters. A deep second-degree burn extends nearly through the dermis; the skin is pink and less painful. A third-degree burn is a full-thickness injury; the skin is dry, pale, leathery, and nonpainful. To assist in estimating the percent of BSA involved with burns, emergency department physicians use nomograms ("rule of nines" or "rule of palms") or the Lund and Browder chart (Table 13-3).

Table 13-3. Lund and Browder chart

Area	Correspondence of age to percent BSA						2°	3°
	< 1 yr	1–4 yr	5–9 yr	10–14 yr	15 yr	Adult		
Head	19	17	13	11	9	7		
Neck	2	2	2	2	2	2		
Anterior trunk	13	13	13	13	13	13		
Posterior trunk	13	13	13	13	13	13		
R. buttock	2.5	2.5	2.5	2.5	2.5	2.5		
L. buttock	2.5	2.5	2.5	2.5	2.5	2.5		
Genitalia	1	1	1	1	1	1		
R. upper arm	4	4	4	4	4	4		
L. upper arm	4	4	4	4	4	4		
R. lower arm	3	3	3	3	3	3		
L. lower arm	3	3	3	3	3	3		
R. hand	2.5	2.5	2.5	2.5	2.5	2.5		
L. hand	2.5	2.5	2.5	2.5	2.5	2.5		
R. thigh	5.5	6.5	8	8.5	9	9.5		
L. thigh	5.5	6.5	8	8.5	9	9.5		
R. leg	5	5	5.5	6	6.5	7		
L. leg	5	5	5.5	6	6.5	7		
R. foot	3.5	3.5	3.5	3.5	3.5	3.5		
L. foot	3.5	3.5	3.5	3.5	3.5	3.5		
Total								

Management

The initial care of any burn includes cooling a fresh burn by immersion or covering with moist towels. In general, first-degree and superficial second-degree burns heal spontaneously within 2 weeks and present no risk for infections. In contrast, deep second- and third-degree burns require special attention in the emergency department. Cleansing of a burn wound can usually be accomplished by gentle irrigation with saline or tap water. The consensus is to remove any pitch or tar, but some practitioners take issue with this [92, 93]. Foreign bodies in the cornea and conjunctiva must be removed, and an ophthalmic ointment preparation is appropriate [94, 95]. Blisters that are not broken should be left alone, since an intact blister will prevent infection and decrease pain. Broken blisters should be débrided.

Prophylactic systemic antimicrobials are not indicated in acute burn care [91, 96–99]. The role of prophylactic topical agents is less clear. In some hospitals silver sulfadiazine is routine [96, 97], while in others it remains verboten [91]. The cream base of silver sulfadiazine is a superb cover for denuded skin and works as a soothing salve. The agent also has active antimicrobial properties. Other topical antimicrobial agents frequently used include Neosporin, Mycitracin, and Bacitracin ointments. Sulfamylon has the extra advantage of being absorbed well by poorly vascularized tissue. Most infected burn patients need to be admitted for care. S. aureus and Pseudomonas aeruginosa are particularly problematic organisms in this population. Blood cultures and deep-wound cultures should be obtained in these patients prior to antibiotic therapy.

The treatment of serious burn wound infections is beyond the purview of the emergency department. Burn and trauma specialists and infectious disease physicians should be called on to address these problems in the hospital setting. Localized burn infections can be treated in the ambulatory setting, assuming that close follow-up can be arranged with the patient. An oral fluorinated quinolone, such as ciprofloxacin at 500–750 mg q12h is an appropriate initial choice to cover Pseudomonas organisms and staphylococci. Dicloxacillin, a first-generation cephalosporin, and erythromycin lack activity against Pseudomonas organisms and most other gram-negative bacilli but are very active against streptococci and staphylococci and thus are useful in this setting.

Puncture Wounds

Puncture wounds to the feet are common occurrences and are seen frequently by emergency department physicians. Seven to 10% of trauma injuries to the lower extremities are from punctures [100]. Approximately 2–10% of these injuries develop infection, and many of those that do are serious, occasionally limb threatening, and result in protracted disability [101]. Punctures through sneakers (i.e., "sneaker osteomyelitis"), those that occur as barnyard accidents or that are grossly contaminated, or those that involve a lower extremity of a patient with diabetes, severe peripheral vascular disease, or lymphedema are at high risk of becoming infected. In each case the wound must be managed aggressively. Most patients with puncture wounds do not seek medical attention. Those who do do so because infection has become established.

Pathophysiology

The most common sites for puncture wounds to the foot are the metatarsal-phalangeal joints, the metatarsal head, and the plantar fascia [102]. Each location predisposes to selected complications of septic arthritis, osteochondritis or osteomyelitis, and fasciitis or plantar-space abscess, respectively.

A puncture through a sneaker predisposes to Pseudomonas infection due to P. aeruginosa colonizing the inner layers of athletic shoes [103]. When a nail or other sharp object penetrates through these colonized layers, the bacteria are inoculated into the skin, soft tissues, bone, or joint of the foot, thus the popular term "sneaker osteo." Injuries that occur in landfills or barnyards usually are contaminated with vegetable debris or manure and a variety of aerobic and anaerobic microorganisms, including Clostridium tetani, resulting in very serious infections. Diabetics and other patients with vascular insufficiency or lymphatic incompetence rapidly develop serious skin and soft-tissue infections from punctures.

Clinical Features

Initially the uninfected puncture wound appears innocuous and thus may escape thorough attention by the patient or the physician. The actual puncture depth is difficult to estimate and is almost always underestimated. Plain-film x-rays may give added information by detecting a foreign body or bone defect. Because the weight of a person's body impresses a greater depth from a foot puncture, infection of the deep tissue and bone is always a consideration.

Typically infection becomes apparent in the first week following the injury. In the case of punctures associated with *Pseudomonas* infections of soft tissue, bone, or joint, Jacobs et al. found a mean of 6 days with a range of 2–21 days [104]. Osteomyelitis may not be evident for weeks or months. Local pain and tenderness on the sole of the foot brings the patient to the emergency department. Examination usually confirms local tenderness as well as erythema and edema if infection is present. Soft-tissue fluctuation, purulent discharge, cellulitis, and lymphangitis can occur with more delayed presentations. The most common complications are cellulitis, fasciitis, tenosynovitis, sepsis, septic arthritis, osteochondritis, and osteomyelitis.

Therapy and Follow-up Considerations

Thorough exploration, débridement, and irrigation are ideal therapeutic goals. The precise nature of a puncture usually prevents adequate spontaneous drainage and limits the physician's ability to cleanse the wound. In general the principles established for the management of other traumatic wounds are applicable to punctures to the feet, but a few points deserve emphasis. Punctures that are likely to be heavily contaminated with debris and bacteria, those that occur through the sole of a sneaker or to the foot of a diabetic, and those that have evidence of infection require special attention in the emergency department. Such wounds require close inspection, plain-film x-ray, débridement of debris, copious irrigation, and dressing to avoid further contamination. If infection is already established, deep-wound culture obtained with a stiff urethral swab or biopsy is sent to the microbiol-ogy laboratory. Excised necrotic tissue and purulent discharge from abscesses are excellent specimens to submit for a Gram's stain and culture. Wound culturing precedes irrigating to avoid diluting the specimen and decreasing recovery of the organisms.

Although infection may not be clinically apparent, the emergency department physician is advised to initiate a short course of oral antibiotics in high-risk situations in an attempt to decrease the quantity of bacteria inoculated into the tissue with the puncture and to prevent infection. Injuries occurring through the crepe soles of sneakers, work boots, and similar shoes should be empirically treated as if *Pseudomonas* is the predominant contaminate. Ciprofloxacin is active against the majority of pseudomonal strains and for this situation can be administered orally as 500–750mg q12h for 5 days. Note, however, that fluoroquinolones are contraindicated in children and teenagers (see Chap. 4). No other oral agents with activity against *Pseudomonas* are available. Antipseudomonal parenteral agents are not recommended in this situation. Wounds heavily contaminated with organic debris (e.g., a barnyard injury) require anti-aerobic/anaerobic antimicrobials. Amoxicillin-clavulanate 500 mg q8h or cephalexin 500 mg q6h plus metronidazole 500 mg q12h for 5 days are good choices. Punctures to the feet of diabetics also mandate antiaerobic/anaerobic agents such as amoxicillin-clavulanate or cephalexin plus metronidazole. Injuries to nondiabetics with ischemic limbs or lymphedema are likely to result in streptococcal or staphylococcal infection; therefore, oral dicloxacillin 500 mg q6h is a reasonable empiric choice.

Antibiotic selection for infected punctures is determined by the Gram's stain and the nature of the puncture. Oral therapy can be selected for minor localized infections, but parenteral therapy is recommended for high-risk groups or moderate to severe infections. If purulent secretions reveal gram-positive cocci, an antistaphylococcal/antistreptococcal antibiotic should be prescribed, such as dicloxacillin 2 g/day orally for minor local infections or nafcillin 2 g q4–6h IV for serious infections. Infected punctures through crepe soles require ciprofloxacin 400 mg IV q12h or 750 mg po q12h, or ceftazidime 1–2 mg q8h plus an aminoglycoside. Piperacillin or aztreonam are alternatives to ceftazidime. The results of the cultures will guide subsequent antibiotic selection and dosage. Infected barnyard wounds demand parenteral antibiotics and hospitalization. Again, thorough wound care with débridement and irrigation is paramount to a good result. After bacterial and fungal cultures are obtained from the infected puncture site, broad-spectrum antibiotic treatment with ampicillin-sulbactam 1.5–3.0 g q6h or cefazolin 2 g q8h with metronidazole 750 mg q12h can be initiated.

Breaks in the skin integument in diabetics and those with severe vascular insufficiency or lymphedema are always threatened by secondary skin and soft-tissue infections (see Chap. 11 regarding diabetic foot infections). Because of diminished sensation diabetics often present late after the injury and after infection is well established. Infected puncture wounds in this setting require antistaphylococcal/streptococcal agents such as naficillin or cefazolin in the usual dosages plus antianaerobic therapy until culture results are available. Many clinicians prefer to initiate empiric therapy with broader-spectrum agents as is recommended for diabetic foot infections. Ampicillin-sulbactam 1.5–3.0 g q6h or cefoxitin 2 g q6h is an excellent monotherapy choice. A third-generation cephalosporin with metronidazole or clindamycin will provide broader coverage.

Patients with uninfected puncture wounds can be treated as outpatients. In most circumstances infected punctures require hospitalization. The high-risk patients previously described are at greatest threat for complications. All patients for whom follow-up or medication compliance is in question require hospitalization. If complications are present, then hospitalization is also evident. Other patients, after close inspection, cleansing, and radiographic review, can be released. Prior to a patient's being dismissed from the emergency department, the patient or significant other should be instructed about the signs and symptoms of infection. Consideration for tetanus prophylaxis must be individualized (see Chap. 5).

References

1. Heeb MA. Deep soft tissue abscesses secondary to nonpenetrating trauma. *Surgery* 4:550–53, 1971.

2. Fischel DR. Purulent tendon sheath infection [letter]. *Pediatrics* 85:1129, 1990.

3. Friedrich PL. Die aseptische Versorgung frischer Wunden, unter Mittheilung von Thier-Versuchen uber die Auskeimungszeit von Infectionserregern in frischen Wunden. *Arch Klin Chir* 57:288–310, 1898.

4. Schmitt WPL. Friedrich and the problem of wound infection. *Zentralbl Chir* 103:65–69, 1978.

5. Berk WA, Osbourne DD, Taylor DD. Evaluation of the "golden period" for wound repair: 204 cases from a Third World emergency department. *Ann Emerg Med* 17:496–500, 1988.

6. Izmailov GA et al. Evaluation of healing of skin wounds inflicted with steel scalpels with various degrees of sharpness. *Khirurgiia* 6:75–78, 1989.

7. Johnson CD, Serpell JW. Wound infection after abdominal incision with scalpel or diathermy. *Br J Surg* 77:626–27, 1990.

8. Harvey EN. Survival of animals after gunshot wounds. *Mili Med* 203–5, 1948.

9. Dziemian AJ, Mendelson JA, Lindsey D. Comparison of the wounding characteristics of some commonly encountered bullets. *J Trauma* 1:341–53, 1961.

10. Mendelson JA, Glover JL. Sphere and shell fragment wounds of soft tissues: experimental study. *J Trauma* 7:889–914, 1967.

11. Hopkinson DAW, Watts JC. Studies in experimental missile injuries of skeletal muscle. *Proc Roy Soc Med* 56:461–68, 1963.

12. Wang ZB et al. Pathological changes of gunshot wounds at various intervals after wounding. *Acta Chir Scand* No. 508(suppl.):197–210, 1982.

13. Ziervogel JF. A study of muscle damage caused by the 7.62 Nato rifle. *Act Chir Scand* No. 489 (suppl.):131–35, 1979.

14. Fackler ML et al. Openwound drainage versus wound excision in treating the modern assault rifle wound. *Surgery* 105:576–86, 1989.

15. Le Gros Clark WE. An experimental study of the regeneration of mammalian striped muscle. *J Anat* 80:24–36, 1946.

16. Carlson BM, Faulkner JA. The regeneration of skeletal muscle fibers following injury: a review. *Med Sci Sports Exerc* 15:187–98, 1983.

17. Faulkner JA, Carlson BM. Skeletal muscle regeneration: an historical perspective. *Fed Proc* 45:1454–55, 1986.

18. Lindsey D, Hirsch FJ. The infected cat bite. Type case of *Pasteurella multocida* infection. *Ariz Med* 38:623–25, 1976.

19. Becker GD, Welch WD. Quantitative bacteriology

of closed-suction wound drainage in contaminated surgery. *Laryngoscopy* 100:403–06, 1990.

20. Becker GC, Welch WD. Quantitative bacteriology of intraoperative wound tissue in contaminated surgery. *Head Neck* 12:293–97, 1990.

21. Kaiser AB. Antimicrobial prophylaxis in surgery. *N Engl J Med* 315:1129–38, 1986.

22. Bhaskar SN, Cutright DE, Gross A. Effect of water lavage on infected wounds in the rat. *J Periodontol* 40:671–72, 1969.

23. Gross A et al. The effect of antibiotics and pulsating jet lavage on contaminated wounds. *Oral Surg Oral Med Oral Pathol* 31:32–38, 1971.

24. Green VA et al. A comparison of the efficacy of pulsed mechanical lavage with that of rubber-bulb syringe irrigation in removal of debris from avulsive wounds. *Oral Surg Oral Med Oral Pathol* 32:158–64, 1971.

25. Stewart JL et al. The bacteria-removal efficiency of mechanical lavage and rubber-bulb syringe irrigation in contaminated avulsive wounds. *Oral Surg Oral Med Oral Pathol* 31:842–48, 1971.

26. Longmire AW, Broom LA, Burch J. Wound infection following high-pressure syringe and needle irrigation [letter]. *Am J Emerg Med* 5:179–81, 1987.

27. Oberg MS. Povidone-iodine solutions in traumatic wound preparation [correspondence]. *Am J Emerg Med* 5:553–55, 1987.

28. Rothwell KG, Oberg MS. Povidone-iodine solutions in traumatic wound preparation [correspondence]. *Am J Emerg Med* 6:681, 1988.

29. Berkelman RL, Holland BW, Anderson RL. Increased bactericidal activity of dilute preparations of povidone-iodine solutions. *J Clin Microbiol* 15:635–39, 1982.

30. Gottardi W. The influence of the chemical behavior of iodine on the germicidal action of disinfectant solutions containing iodine. *J Hosp Infect* 6(suppl A):1–11, 1985.

31. Zamora JL et al. Inhibition of povidone-iodine's bactericidal activity by common organic substances: an experimental study. *Surgery* 98:25–29, 1985.

32. D'Auria J, Lipson S, Garfield JM. Fatal iodine toxicity following surgical débridement of a hip wound: case report. *J Trauma* 30:353–55, 1990.

33. Alexander JW et al. The influence of hair-removal methods on wound infections. *Arch Surg* 118:347–52, 1983.

34. Noe JM, Keller M. Can stitches get wet? *Plast Reconstr Surg* 81:82–83, 1988.

35. Douglas LG. Stitches and water [letter]. *Plast Reconstr Surg* 82:364, 1988.

36. Mertz PM, Eaglstein WH. The effect of a semiocclusive dressing on the microbial population in superficial wounds. *Arch Surg* 119:287–89, 1984.

37. Mertz PM, Marshall DA, Eaglstein WH. Occlusive wound dressings to prevent bacterial invasion and wound infection. *J Am Acad Dermatol* 12:662–68, 1985.

38. Rodsy M, Clauss L. Cytotoxicity testing of wound dressings using normal human keratinocytes in culture. *J Biomed Mater Res* 24:363–77, 1990.

39. Scein M, Dunn S. What grows beneath op-site surgical wound dressing? *S Afr Med J* 66:752–53, 1984.

40. Falanga V. Occlusive wound dressings: why, when, which? *Arch Dermatol* 124:872–77, 1988.

41. Lindsey D. The idolatry of velocity, or lies, damn lies, and ballistics [editorial]. *J Trauma* 20:1068–69, 1980.

42. Fackler ML. Wound ballistics: a review of common misconceptions. *JAMA* 259:2730–36, 1988.

43. Cooper GJ, Ryan JM. Interaction of penetrating missiles with tissues: some common misapprehensions and implications for wound management. *Br J Surg* 77:606–10, 1990.

44. Polk HC Jr, Lopez-Mayor JF. Postoperative wound infection: a prospective study of determinant factors and prevention. *Surgery* 66:97–103, 1969.

45. Burnakis, TG. Surgical antimicrobial prophylaxis: principles and guidelines. *Pharmacotherapy* 4:248–71, 1984.

46. Chodak GW, Plaut ME. Use of systemic antibiotics for prophylaxis in surgery: a critical review. *Arch Surg* 112:326–34, 1977.

47. Sacks T. Prophylactic antibiotics in traumatic wounds. *J Hosp Infect* 11(suppl A):251–58, 1988.

48. Law DJ, Mishriki SF, Jeffrey PJ. The importance of surveillance after discharge from hospital in the diagnosis of postoperative wound infection. *Ann R Coll Surg Engl* 72:207–9, 1990.

49. Moore RM et al. Surveillance of animal-bite cases in the United States, 1971–1972. *Arch Environ Health* 32:267–70, 1977.

50. Hanna TL, Selby LA. Characteristics of the human and pet populations in animal bite incidents recorded at two Air Force bases. *Public Health Rep* 96:580–84, 1981.

51. Aghababian RV, Conte JE Jr. Mammalian bite wounds. *Ann Emerg Med* 9:79–83, 1980.

52. Strassburg MA et al. Animal bites: patterns of treatment. *Ann Emerg Med* 10:193–97, 1981.

53. Maetz HM. Animal bites, a public health problem in Jefferson County, Alabama. *Public Health Rep* 94:528–34, 1979.

54. Snyder CC. Animal bite wounds. *Hand Clin* 5:571–90, 1989.

55. Kizer KW. Epidemiologic and clinical aspects of animal bite injuries. *JACEP* 8:134–41, 1979.

56. Graham, WP 3d, Calabretta, AM, Miller, SH. Dog bites. *Am Fam Physician* 15:12–137, 1977.

57. Callaham, ML. Treatment of common dog bites: infection risk factors. *JACEP* 7:83–88, 1978.

58. Douglas LG. Bite wounds. *Am Fam Physician* 11:93–99, 1975.

59. Verghese A et al. Susceptibility of dysgonic fermenter-2 to antimicrobial agents in vitro. *Antimicrob Agents Chemother* 32:78–80, 1988.

60. Kalb R et al. Cutaneous infection of a dog bite wound associated with fulminant DF-2 septicemia. *Am J Med* 78:687–90, 1985.

61. Theilade P, Kringsholm B. Death caused by DF-2 following a dog bite. *Forensic Sci Int* 34:255–56, 1987.

62. Carpenter PD, Heppner BT, Gnann JW Jr. DF-2 bacteremia following cat bites. *Am J Med* 82:621–23, 1987.

63. August JR. Dysgonic fermenter-2 infections. *J Am Vet Med Assoc* 193:1506–8, 1988.

64. Feder HM Jr, Shanley JD, Barbera JA. Review of 59 patients hospitalized with animal bites. *Pediatr Infect Dis* 6:24–28, 1987.

65. Quenzer RW, Mostow SR, Emerson JK. Cat-bite tularemia. *JAMA* 238:1845, 1977.

66. Evans ME Tularemia and the tomcat. *JAMA* 246:1343, 1981.

67. Chuinard RG, D'Ambrosia RD. Human bite infections of the hand. *J Bone Joint Surg (Am)* 59:416–18, 1977.

68. Lindsey D et al. Natural course of the human bite wound: incidence of infection and complications in 434 bites and 803 lacerations in the same group of patients. *J Trauma* 27:45–48, 1987.

69. Altieri M, Brasch L, Getson P. Antibiotic prophylaxis in intraoral wounds. *Am J Emerg Med* (6):507–10, 1986.

70. Marr JS, Beck AM, Lugo JA Jr. An epidemiologic study of the human bite. *Public Health Rep* 94:514–21, 1979.

71. Brook I. Microbiology of human and animal bite wounds in children. *Pediatr Infect Dis* 6:29–32, 1987.

72. Goldstein EJ et al. Bacteriology of human and animal bite wounds. *J Clin Microbiol* 8:667–72, 1978.

73. Bilos ZJ, Kucharchuk A, Metzger W. *Eikenella corrodens* in human bites. *Clin Orthop* 134:320–24, 1978.

74. Neviaser RJ, Butterfield WC, Wieche DR. The puffy hand of drug addiction: a study of the pathogenesis. *J Bone Joint Surg (Am)* 54:629–33, 1972.

75. Stone OJ, Mullins JF. Chronic paronychia. *Arch Dermatol* 86:324–27, 1962.

76. Perry AW et al. Fingerstick felons. *Ann Plast Surg* 20:249–51, 1988.

77. Glickel SZ. Hand infections in patients with acquired immunodeficiency syndrome. *J Hand Surg* 13:770–75, 1988.

78. Canales FL, Newmeyer WL. (Mann, RJ. (ed.).) Kilgore ES Jr. The treatment of felons and paronychias. *Hand Clin* 5:515–23, 1989.

79. Stern H et al. Herpetic whitlow: a form of cross-infection in hospitals. *Lancet* 2:871–74, 1959.

80. Gill MJ, Arlette J, Buchan K. Herpes simplex virus infection of the hand. A profile of 79 cases. *Am J Med* 84:89–93, 1988.

81. Solomon AR et al. The Tzanck smear in the diagnosis of cutaneous herpes simplex. *JAMA* 251:633–35, 1984.

82. Kanavel AB. *Infections of the Hand* (7th ed.). Philadelphia: Lea & Febiger, 1939. Pp. 189–220.

83. Crick JC, Vandevelde AG. *Mycobacterium fortuitum* midpalmar space abscess: a case report. *J Hand Surg (Am)* 11:438–40, 1986.

84. Crout JE, Brewer NS, Tompkins RB. Sporotrichosis arthritis: clinical features in seven patients. *Ann Intern Med* 86:294–97, 1977.

85. Wilson DE et al. Clinical features of extracutaneous sporotrichosis medicine. *Medicine* 46:265–79, 1967.

86. Mann RJ. *Infections of the Hand*. Philadelphia: Lea & Febiger, 1988.

87. Deitch EA. Keys to early care of burn patients. *J Crit Illness* 85:1213–22, 1990.

88. Henricks WM. The classification of burns. *J Am Acad Dermatol* 22:838–39, 1990.

89. Zawacki BE et al. Multifactorial probit analysis of mortality in burned patients. *Ann Surg* 189:1–5, 1979.

90. Falcone PA, Edstrom LE. Decision making in the acute thermal hand burn: an algorithm for treatment. *Hand Clin* 6:233–38, 1990.

91. Harrison DH, Parkhouse N. Experience with upper extremity burns: the Mount Vernon experience. *Hand Clin* 6:191–209, 1990.

92. Pruitt BA Jr, Edlich RF. Treatment of bitumen burns [letter]. *Ann Emerg Med* 11:697, 1982.

93. Demling RH, Buerstatte WR, Perea A. Management of hot tar burns. *J Trauma* 20:242, 1980.

94. James NK, Moss AL. Review of burns caused by bitumen and the problems of its removal. *Burns* 16:214–16, 1990.

95. Mathews RC, Sharpnack P. Removal of tar from body parts [letter]. *J Trauma* 20:910, 1980.

96. Lawrence JC. The bacteriology of burns. *J Hosp Infect* 6(suppl B):3–17, 1985.

97. Lawrence JC, Groves AR. Are systemic prophylactic antibiotics necessary for burns? [comment]. *Ann R Coll Surg Engl* 65:279, 1983.

98. McGregor JC. Are systemic prophylactic antibiotics necessary for burns? [letter]. *Ann R Coll Surg Engl* 65:278–79, 1983.

99. Timmons MJ. Are systemic prophylactic antibiotics necessary for burns? *Ann R Coll Surg Engl* 65:80–82, 1983.

100. Brown LL et al. Evaluation of wound irrigation by pulsatile jet and conventional methods. *Ann Surg* 187(2):170–73, 1978.

101. Houston AN, Roy WA, Faust RA. Tetanus prophylaxis in the treatment of puncture wounds of patients in the deep South. *J Trauma* 2:439, 1962.

102. Clinton JE. Puncture wounds by inanimate objects and mammalian bite. In RB Gustilo (ed.), *Orthopaedic Infection, Diagnosis and Treatment.* Philadelphia: Saunders, 1989. Pp. 299–308.

103. Fisher MC, Goldsmith JF, Gilligan PH. Sneakers as a source of *Pseudomonas aeruginosa* in children with osteomyelitis following puncture wounds. *J Pediatr* 106:608–9, 1985.

104. Jacobs RF et al. Management of *Pseudomonas* osteochondritis complicating puncture wounds of the foot. *Pediatrics* 69:432–35, 1982.

14

Infection in the Infant

L. CLARK HANSBARGER

This chapter addresses infections in specific age intervals of infants:

- Birth to 2 weeks
- 2 weeks to 2 months
- 2 months to 6 months
- 6 months to 12 months
- 12 months to 36 months

The reasons for these age intervals are based on the presentation of particular infections, the probability of infection with specific symptoms, and the influence age has on the host response and vulnerability to infections. The infant's symptoms are as variable as the causes and accompany a high anxiety level for both the family and the provider. Since many parents who bring their infant to the emergency department are experiencing their infant's first illness, an additional responsibility rests with the emergency department physician to be comfortable and confident with them.

This chapter does not exhaust the subject of possible infections but covers frequent and challenging illnesses. Many of the infections addressed in the other chapters of this book also apply to infants.

Definition of Infancy

In this chapter the term *infancy* applies to "babyhood." The upper limit is 3 years of age, when the term *preschooler* is used. This time span is arbitrary since infections overlap the age intervals. In addition, these specific age parameters are not universally implemented in the health care community.

Protection

The following principles apply to the protection against infancy infections:

- Breast feeding is a protective strategy against infections, particularly gastrointestinal.
- Immunizations and prior infections of the mother provide a level of passive protection against infections through transplacental gammaglobulins during the infant's first nine months of life.
- Immunizations are an active means of protection for infants if administered in the recommended time sequence.
- Sanitation of the home environment and food preparation minimize infant mortality and morbidity.

Vulnerability

The following medical, social, and behavioral factors affect infant vulnerability to infection:

- Infants simply do not have the degree of immunity that time will bring. It is assumed that every infant shows antibody evidence of at least 7–10 infections per year.
- Gammaglobulin and other defense mechanisms do not function well at birth and may decrease before the infant is 9–12 months of age, thus increasing susceptibility to infection.
- Many infants seen in emergency departments are from economically disadvantaged homes.
- As the care for infants outside the home (e.g., day care centers) increases, infants are exposed more frequently at an earlier age to a variety of communicable diseases.
- With the increase in the survival of high-risk (e.g., premature) infants, a generation of chronically ill children is being seen in the emergency setting because of the threatening or decompensating impact of their infections.
- Some ethnic groups are more vulnerable to infection than others. For example, Native Americans are at jeopardy to encapsulated bacteria such as *Streptococcus pneumoniae* and *Haemophilus influenzae*.
- Dysmorphic, congenital anomalies and genetic problems often are associated with increased vulnerability to specific infections. For example, patients with Down's syndrome often have respiratory problems, and infants with tracheoesophageal fistula are susceptible to pneumonia.
- Infants are not simply small adults, which is evident when surface area, metabolic rate, and respiratory/cardiac rates are compared [1, 2]. Because of relatively increased surface area, respiratory rate, and metabolic needs, all of which contribute to water loss, infants dehydrate more quickly and become acidotic more easily than older children. Because of a more flexible chest wall, limited alveolar surface, and more dead space of the tracheobronchial tree, infants are inefficient breathers under the stress of infection. Since the intestinal mucosa is flatter and immature and the length proportionally longer, infants are more vulnerable to gastrointestinal infections, resulting in profuse loose stools and malabsorption.
- Vulnerable-child syndrome factors must be acknowledged in treating infants brought for emergency care. Anxiety, unfounded concern, prior illnesses, single parenthood, and being an only child are social and behavioral factors that make history taking, interpreting, and planning difficult.
- Children of home birth may not have received appropriate prophylactic measures at birth.

Helpful Hints

The author has collected the following general principles for the treatment of infections over years of patient care.

Communication by telephone is extremely important in three areas: for early, decisive advice for caretakers before they arrive for emergency care; for eliciting additional information from others while evaluating the infant; and for following up the decisions, care, and course of infection after the infant has been sent home [3].

Attention to parents' observations, perceptions, and concerns is invaluable—they know their child. Most mistakes in diagnosis, care decisions, and follow-up are based on underestimating the strengths and weaknesses of the caretakers.

Observations of rashes, asymmetries, and breathing patterns are instrumental in the diagnosis. Infants should be completely undressed for examinations.

Emergency department physicians should follow their instincts, especially when interacting with very young infants and young parents. Infections are extremely threatening in the infant, so overtreatment is good management.

Growth and development charts are very useful [1]. Failure to grow and to develop (i.e., failure to thrive) is a criterion for chronic illnesses such as AIDS and for many disabilities, specifically genetic ones.

The child should remain in the parent's arms or lap as long as possible [4]. General observations such as rash, breathing, CNS status, color (e.g., cyanosis), activity, and motion of extremities are much easier to identify if the child is comfortable. Conducting the physical while the infant is in the parent's arms is particularly important if the child is in respiratory distress.

The following signs and symptoms in infants are different from those in adults:

- Lethargy and irritability are often the only signs or symptoms of infections in infants. The parents feel strongly that the infant is acting differently. The more lethargic and irritable the infant is, the more likely the focus should be on otitis media, meningitis, or bacteremia.
- Vomiting, diarrhea, and anorexia are frequent nonspecific signs and symptoms of infant infections. A complete physical is necessary to find a focus.
- Nasal flaring, respiratory grunts, and a cough followed by crying are serious signs and symptoms of pneumonia.
- Rhonchi, squeaks, and rales are hard to interpret in infants. It is difficult to correlate these findings to specific anatomic diagnoses such as laryngitis, bronchitis, or pneumonia. Distinguishing viral from bacterial etiology is even more laborious. Laboratory and radiologic tests, toxicity assessment, and degree of distress are more dependable mechanisms.

In general an emergency department physician should follow these rules:

- Rectal temperature over 38.2°C in an infant under 2 months indicates sepsis until proved otherwise.
- Meningitis should be considered if an otitis media patient returns within 48 hours and is still symptomatic.
- An infant with a possible infection on the third visit should be admitted to the hospital.
- An infection is assumed to be serious in an infant with genetic, congenital, or dysmorphic features.
- A urine specimen of an infant suspected of having an infection is a wealth of information, in addition to aiding in the treatment decision if the urine is the source of infection. Elements such as ketones, red blood cells, bilirubin, and specific gravity provide information as to the extent of illness (e.g., hydration) as well as the organ systems involved.

With the use of a predictive value index of severity scale, such as the Yale Observation Scale (Table 14-1), a quality physical examination is more thorough and supports intuitive data [5]. The Yale Observation Scale, which was developed by McCarthy et al., is the accepted standard for infants older than 6 months. This scale uses the careful observation of cry, color, hydration, and interaction with parent and provider. Each observation is scored from 1 to 3, with the ranking of 1 being normal. Several observations from experienced users of the scale may be helpful. For any provider a serious illness is more likely to be appreciated if an overall assessment index of the severity scale is used. This scale is not as reliable for infants under 6 months of age and must be coupled with the medical history and laboratory findings [6]. The scale is reliable in defining a less serious illness if the total score is 12 or less. It is accurate in predicting a serious disease if score is 16 or greater. The observation variable *responsiveness* (i.e., playfulness) has the strongest correlation with overall assessment.

A serious illness is suggested by one or more abnormal laboratory results that include bacterial pathogen isolation; x-ray evidence of infection; body fluid pleocytosis or metabolic disturbance; hypoxemia as demonstrated by pulse oximeter of less than 90% oxygen saturation or arterial P_{O_2} 70 mm Hg or less; WBC count of less than 1000/μl or more than 15,000/μl, more than 10,000 neutrophils/μl, more than 500 band forms/μl, and sedimentation rate greater than 30 mm/hr, with rectal temperature 40°C or more [7–9].

Treatment of Fever

A discussion of fever therapy must be based on the answers to four questions:

1. Is it fever?
2. What is wrong with fever?
3. Will the degree of fever or response to additional therapy offer any information?
4. How is fever treated?

In response to the first question, infants under 3 months of age apparently lack sensitization to exogenous pyrogens and have immature thermoregulatory responses; therefore, their ability to mount a febrile response is compromised. Furthermore, like elderly persons, neonates may be hypothermic with significant infection. Any temperature elevation is

Table 14-1. The Yale Observation Scale

Observation item	1 Normal	2 Moderate impairment	3 Severe impairment
Quality of cry	Strong with normal tone *or* content and not crying	Whimpering *or* sobbing	Weak *or* moaning *or* high pitched
Reaction to parent	Cries briefly then stops *or* content and not crying	Cries off and on	Continual cry *or* hardly responds
State variation	If awake stays awake *or* if asleep wakes up quickly when stimulated	Eyes close briefly → awake *or* awakes with prolonged stimulation	Falls to sleep *or* will not rouse
Color	Pink	Pale extremities *or* acrocyanosis	Pale *or* cyanotic *or* mottled *or* ashen
Hydration	Skin normal, eyes normal *and* mucous membranes moist	Skin, eyes normal *and* mouth slightly dry	Skin doughy *or* tented *and* dry mucous membranes *and/or* sunken eyes
Response (talking, smiling) to social overtures	Smiles *or* alerts (≤ 2 mo)	Brief smile *or* alerts briefly (≤ 2 mo)	No smile; face anxious, dull, expressionless *or* no alerting (≤ 2 mo)

Source: McCarthy P. Predictive value of abnormal physical examination findings in ill-appearing and well-appearing febrile children. *Pediatrics* 76(23):167, 1985. Used with permission.

considered significant. An infant under 2 months may be overwrapped, so a temperature of 38°C to 38.5°C should be reevaluated after the infant has been undressed (loosely clothed) for 30 minutes. The accuracy of temperatures taken at home also is subject to criticism if parents are not educated about reliable techniques, although parents in general have a reliable impression of when their infant is hot. A septic workup is not done despite a history of fever at home if the infant does not appear ill, the rectal temperature is less than 38.2°C, and the infant has not had an appropriate dose of antipyretic in the last two hours.

The infrared tympanic membrane thermometer is as reliable as the glass mercury or electronic thermometer for infants over 6 months, but rectal thermometers should be used for confirmation of temperature in very young infants [10, 11].

The second question asks, "What is wrong with fever?" Although there are advantages in the theoretical sense to a fever, an infant is at a disadvantage due to increased metabolic needs resulting in acidosis and increased water loss, poor peripheral autonomic response and thus reduced ability to vasodilate for cooling, and complications of fever, such as seizures, that are more common in children [12, 13].

To the question "Will the degree of temperature or the response to therapy give any further information to the provider?" the answer is generally no in any one patient. A study by Putto et al. stated that viruses produce fevers comparable to severe bacterial infections [14]. Fever is a good indicator of sepsis, however, if it is combined with a significantly high score on the Yale Observation Scale. Even if fever captures a physician's attention, complete information is needed to decide how ill the child is. The response of a fever to antipyretics does not appear to be clinically useful in differentiating the causes of febrile illness in young children [15, 16].

In response to the fourth question, "How is fever treated?" it is therapeutic simply to undress the infant; lightweight clothes are recommended. Warm-water baths offer an immediate evaporation process for cooling. Alcohol baths should not be used since the alcohol is inhaled and is toxic. Alcohol also can create such a cooling effect that the infant proceeds to vasoconstrict rather than to di-

late, as is needed for cooling. Acetaminophen is the drug of choice for fever control in infants. It is highly dependable, less toxic than other drugs, and reasonably well tolerated by infants. The dose is 10–15 mg/kg q4h PO. (See Chap. 2.)

Fever of Unknown Origin

Fever of unknown origin is just what it implies: the inability of the physician to discern on physical examination or by history a specific focus for an infection. If the child does not meet the following criteria, the emergency department physician may simply choose to reassure the parent and arrange an appropriate follow-up. If the infant does meet any one of these criteria, there should be a methodical workup in the emergency department and serious consideration for admission [6, 7]. The criteria are

1. Fever higher than 38.2°C in an infant under 2 months; higher than 39.5°C in an infant 2–6 months; higher than 40.0°C in an infant 6–12 months; higher than 40.5°C in an infant 12–36 months
2. A scale of toxicity (Yale Observation Scale) of 12 or more
3. A WBC count of more than 15,000/μl, more than 10,000 neutrophils/μl and more than 500 band forms/μl
4. Urinary ketones of 3 + or greater

If any of these criteria is met, the infant in question needs a septic workup consisting of the following [7]:

- Lumbar puncture (LP) with cerebrospinal fluid (CSF) cell count, Gram's stain, protein, sugar, and culture
- Urinalysis and culture
- Chest x-ray, posteroanterior (PA) and lateral
- Blood cultures

If these procedures and tests are completed and the child continues to maintain a score on the Yale Observation Scale of less than 16, the 2- to 36-month-old infant is treated as an outpatient with an antibiotic, preferably ceftriaxone IM or IV (50–100 mg/kg) [17]; the infant younger than 2 months and the 2–12-month-old with a score on the Yale Observation Scale of 16 or more are admitted. The child older than one year with a continued score of 16 or more will require careful re-evaluation.

Infants who are discharged should be followed up by telephone or return visit within 24 hours, at which time the results of cultures may clarify the situation. Seldom does the ceftriaxone need to be repeated, so oral antibiotics appropriate for the specific infection (e.g., amoxicillin 40 mg/kg/day ÷ q8h PO) usually can be introduced for the remainder of the treatment.

Admission Rules

Any infection in an infant that meets the following criteria is threatening enough for the emergency department physician to seriously consider admission:

- Fever of known or unknown origin higher than 38.2°C in an infant under 2 months; higher than 39.5°C in an infant 2–6 months; higher than 40°C in an infant 6–24 months; higher than 41°C in a child 24 months or older
- A toxicity/illness rating on the Yale Observation Scale of 16 or more
- A WBC count of less than 1000/μl or more than 15,000/μl, more than 10,000 neutrophils/μl, or more than 500 band forms/μl.

Any or all of these criteria suggest a septic process that should be treated vigorously and in a controlled environment even if a focus as a result of a septic workup started in the emergency department is discovered. In infants the chances of finding a bacterial focus, evidence of dehydration, or exhaustion are much greater using these simple, straightforward criteria. If these rules are applied to a specific diagnosis, such as urinary tract infection (UTI), otitis media, pneumonia, or sepsis, most physicians would agree that the child is quite ill and would meet any quality assurance/utilization review criteria for admission [7].

Infections in Infants up to 2 Weeks Old

Neonatal infections are particularly threatening to patient and provider [16]. The outcome of management depends entirely on the early identification of an infection. Yet recognition is hampered by the characteristics of a neonate (i.e., dependency and uniformity of response to any problem) and the physician's possible unfamiliarity with the normal characteristics of neonates.

The neonate is dependent on the caretaker for observation, communication, and experience to determine the degree of illness. When a caretaker presents to the emergency department with a week-old infant, there is often no available obstetrical or prior medical history. The physician must depend on a high index of suspicion for threatening, potential infection. There is a high probability that an infection acquired in utero or during delivery can become multiorganic and systemic.

A uniformity of symptoms and signs is presented by infants particularly those under 2 weeks of age. The infant's response to any threatening, decompensating system illness is to appear pale, anorexic, tachypneic, tachycardic, febrile, lethargic, and "floppy." In addition to infections these signs and symptoms will occur in a short time with problems such as congenital heart decompensation, congenital endocrine dysfunction, renal failure, child-abuse and head injuries, and metabolic problems.

Unfamiliarity with the infant by young parents as well as the emergency department physician is not an uncommon combination. Examples include the following: (1) the failure to note that infants have nasal stuffiness that is not of infectious origin but a result of small nasal pharynges and nasal mucus; (2) the parents, particularly those who are high risk (e.g., drug abusers), simply do not articulate an adequate medical history; and (3) the patient's medical records fail to include complete information. Sensitivity to high-risk populations, familiarity with newborn-nursery epidemics, and special attention to "infancy disease" training through continuing medical education improve the ability of emergency department physicians to deal with these diseases appropriately.

Vulnerability

The physical changes that occur in an infant in the neonatal period create several unusual situations that produce vulnerability (and identification problems) such that undressing the baby for a physical examination is essential. Newborn care that now includes scalp blood sampling techniques, vacuum forceps, heel sticks, circumcision, tube feeding, and nasal aspirating has created artificial access (vulnerability) for infections.

Familiarity with such transitional physical changes as breast hypertrophy, vaginal-vulva secretions and "withdrawal bleeding," milia, and toxic erythema neonatal skin manifestations enhance the physician's ability to differentiate normalcy from more threatening conditions, such as breast abscesses, vaginitis, and generalized herpes.

The process of transition also includes the umbilical cord separation and umbilical healing process, which creates access by the very nature of its evolution. The cord does not always "dry up and blow away." It may appear exudative, bloody, and granular, but it should not be odorous, erythematous, or purulent. If it is, then umbilicullitis, cellulitis, or fasciolitis must be considered and treated.

Another interesting example of transition and development that creates differential confusion is the lacrimal duct development. For the first 9 months of life, the lacrimal duct may be stenosed. Thus, mild tearing and conjunctivitis are common presenting complaints that must be separated from the more threatening problems of chlamydia conjunctivitis and other infections.

Vulnerability is often a question of congenital abnormality undetected or suspected at birth. Prenatal ultrasonography, comprehensive physicals, and identification of high-risk factors make this less of a problem, but exceptions do occur. Again, the physician must undress and completely examine the baby.

Skin defects that suggest teratomal/dermoid, midline, or ventral closure defects are examples of accesses for infection to the CNS. Dysmorphic features of face and genitalia are highly suggestive of respiratory and urologic infections.

Respiratory symptoms with a history of feeding problems may well be the first hint of tracheoesophageal fistula. The detection of a mass in the abdomen may be the presentation of an unsuspected urologic obstruction as the etiology of infection.

Finally the subject of vulnerability would not be complete without mention of cultural influences. These influences include neonatal ear lobe punctures for earrings, the application of feces to umbilicus, bellybands for umbilical hernia prevention, the stripping back of the prepuce over the uncircumcised glans, social problems such as rat or pet bites, and overwrapping infants, which confuses the temperature issue and macerates the skin.

Specific Infections

Table 14-2 outlines antibiotic therapy for infections common in newborn infants up to 2 weeks old.

SEPSIS

Bacterial Sepsis. Of all the possibilities of infection that an emergency department provider considers in a newborn, septicemia, due to group B streptococcal disease/sepsis (GBS), is the most serious. On a national level GBS has been on the increase in the past decade. The organism is usually acquired from the mother.

The presenting situation most often includes a low-birth-weight infant whose mother was ill during delivery, usually with a premature rupture of membranes or difficult labor. The infant may have had scalp instrumentation for monitoring. Usually the child's newborn nursery care was a normal 24-hour stay with the infant seemingly healthy at discharge. In the 24 hours prior to the emergency department visit, the infant has symptoms of poor eating and is pale, hot, and fussy. In the emergency department setting the child is fussy, floppy, anorexic, pale, tachypneic, tachycardic, and febrile (>38.2°C rectal) and has poor peripheral perfusion.

A septic workup is recommended even if the condition seems better than described or for any infant under 2 months with a temperature higher than 38.2°C. The workup includes an LP when the baby is stable, a blood culture, a urinalysis and culture, and a WBC with differential and erythrocyte sedimentation rate. An option not as helpful is an antigen or antibody screen, such as Bactigen, specific for group B streptococcus. Careful collecting of body fluids and erring in favor of treating a presumptive bacterial infection are emphasized. *Neisseria meningitidis, H. influenzae, S. pneumoniae,* staphylococci, and *Listeria monocytogenes* are frequent pathogens that cause infections similar to GBS and require the same diagnostic and therapeutic urgency.

Table 4-2. Antibiotic therapy for selected infections in infants 0–2 weeks of age

Infection	Antibiotic
Bacterial sepsis	Ampicillin 100 mg/kg/d ÷ q8h IV + gentamicin 7.5 mg/kg/d ÷ q8h IV
If ≥7 days of age at onset	Cefotaxime replace gentamicin with ceftriaxone
Herpes sepsis	Acyclovir 30 mg/kg/d ÷ q8h IV
Meningitis	Ampicillin 200 mg/kg/d q8h IV + gentamicin 7.5 mg/kg/d ÷ q8h IV
If gram-negative bacilli on Gram's stain of CSF	Add cefotaxime 100 mg/kg/d ÷ q12h IV
Pneumonia	Ampicillin 100 mg/kg/d ÷ q8h IV + gentamicin 7.5 mg/kg/d ÷ q8h IV
≥ If 5 days of age at onset	Replace ampicillin with methicillin
Chlamydia conjunctivitis, dacryocystitis	Erythromycin 40 mg/kg/d ÷ q8h PO
Localized macular to bullous lesions (S. aureus)	Erythromycin 40 mg/kg/d ÷ q8h PO
Thrush	Nystatin 1 ml q6h PO
Omphalitis	Methicillin 50–100 mg/kg/d ÷ q12h IV + gentamicin 7.5 mg/kg/d ÷ q8h IV

The rapidity of onset, high mortality, and difficulty in identifying the organism in an emergency visit have led to the early empirical treatment of this problem and hospitalization of the infant. The immediate response is to give oxygen by mask, start a normal saline IV, and give antibiotics (currently ampicillin 100 mg/kg/day ÷ q8h IV and gentamicin 7.5 mg/kg/dose ÷ q8h IV).

Viral Sepsis. A septic, sick baby with jaundice, papular rash, hepatosplenomegaly, and failure to thrive may have a bacterial infection, but it is more likely to have viremia due to herpes, HIV, enterovirus, or cytomegalovirus. The history of exposure, such as genital herpes in the mother, is helpful but often not recognized. A septic workup is in order as soon as the infant is stabilized. The child should be hospitalized. An antiviral agent (acyclovir 30 mg/kg/day ÷ q8h IV) for the most treatable virus (e.g., herpes) should be started as soon as possible.

PNEUMONIA

Respiratory infections during the first 2 weeks of an infant's life are uncommon. But an infant that is discharged, as is common, in the first 24 hours may appear in the emergency department within 72 hours with an aspiration or intrauterine acquired pneumonia. The caregiver's concerns will include difficult feeding, fussiness, and tachypnea. The ob-

servations are tachypnea, mild cyanosis (oxygen saturation <90%), fever, retractions, and rales.

The organisms that cause respiratory infections are similar to those that cause bacterial sepsis, as are the laboratory findings. Again, stabilization of the infant is paramount before proceeding with radiologic studies. Any manipulation or restraint may decompensate the airway enough to produce hypoxemia and shock. The radiologic studies will show patchy hilar and apical opacities (e.g., atelectasis) and occasional pneumothorax.

Antibiotic choice is the same as for sepsis: currently ampicillin 100 mg/kg/day ÷ q8h IV and gentamicin 7.5 mg/kg/day q8h IV.

EYE INFECTIONS

Chlamydial Infection. Chlamydia is acquired from the mother's vagina or cervix during the antepartum period and manifests itself over a period of 2–3 months in a progressive sequence of signs and symptoms that suggests pneumonia. In the first 2 weeks, however, the most likely signs are conjunctivitis and mild nasal stuffiness. The conjunctivitis is manifested by mildly purulent discharge and hyperemia of scleral and conjunctival mucosa.

Because chlamydia is so common and so mild, the effort to differentiate it by culture or immunofluorescence often is deferred and empiric treatment instituted. Treatment is erythromycin (40 mg/kg/day ÷ q8h PO) for at least 14–21 days and referral of the parent for medical evaluation. *Neisseria gonorrheae* and staphylococcus are rarely encountered as conjunctivitis in the emergency department, but the facts that *N. gonorrheae* is increasing nationwide and that home delivery without prophylaxis does occur require physicians to be sensitive to this devastating form of conjunctivitis.

The disease most often confused with neonatal conjunctivitis is lacrimal duct stenosis, which is a common problem of development and which usually clears by the age of 9 months. However, the early development of unilateral or bilateral tearing and purulent discharge is very confusing on the first visit to a health provider. A unilateral conjunctival discharge not associated with nasal discharge suggests lacrimal duct stenosis, so no treatment or at most erythromycin eye ointment is adequate.

Dacryocystitis. Lacrimal duct atresia with dacryocystitis is uncommon. The problem is a red, swollen mass extending from the inner canthus and parallel with the nose. On pressure a purulent discharge emerges from the lower inner canthus lacrimal duct orifice. Fever and irritability commonly result in a septic state if treatment is not initiated. Treatment consists of a systemic antibiotic (erythromycin 40 mg/kg/day ÷ q8h PO) for the most common organism, *Staphylococcus aureus*. If rapid recovery is not apparent, probing of the nasolacrimal duct is necessary.

SKIN

Staphylococcus. Staphylococcal epidemics are dreaded in newborn nurseries. The most frequent manifestation is the rapid onset of generalized macular to bullous lesions, particularly on the trunk and the perineum. The lesions commonly begin by the infant's seventh day of life and eventually result in sepsis. They often infect the breast, the umbilicus, and circumcised areas and cause abscesses of the extremities. Treatment is a systemic antibiotic (erythromycin 40 mg/kg/day q8h PO) to which the organism is sensitive. Nonepidemic staphylococcus dermatitis is also a threat to infants born to health care workers or to women with chronic illness or who recently have been hospitalized.

Candidiasis. Monilia (candida) is the most common fungal infection of infants. It usually is disturbing to parents, so it is commonly seen in children who are brought to the emergency department. The locations of such infections are the mouth (i.e., thrush) and the perineum (i.e., diaper rash). Neither infection site creates many symptoms, although irritability and decreased eating are attributed to such lesions. The mouth lesions are white areas 4–10 mm in diameter on red bases that are not particularly friable. They extend over all of the oral mucosa but are particularly prominent on the buccal mucosa. The perineal lesions are dry, red to purple, confluent, large (4–5 cm in diameter) lesions surrounded by a satellite red, papular rash.

The origin of the fungus and the susceptibility of infants are debatable, but generally it is agreed that candida are everywhere, particularly in the mother's vagina. Hence, the infant is infected at birth. The moisture of the mouth and the perineum then become the media for rapid growth in an infant with no acquired resistance. Treatment is an antifungal agent (Nystatin 1 ml q6h PO) and local Nystatin cream, but for recurrent infections a gentian violet solution is still useful.

Infections in Infants 2 Weeks to 2 Months

The period of time from 2 weeks to 2 months is not one of frequent infections in infants. They do occur, however, and are dramatic as far as the emergency physician is concerned. Most of the infections that occur in the first 2 weeks can extend to 2 months. Table 14-3 summarizes antibiotic therapy for infections commonly found in infants 2 weeks to 2 months old.

Specific Infections

Bacterial Sepsis. Bacterial sepsis is still a threat, so a septic workup is done for any infant under 2 months who presents with a temperature of 38.2°C or more [16]. The baby may be lethargic, irritable, pale, tachycardic, tachypneic, and limp and have vomiting, diarrhea, or poor feeding. The parents

Table 14-3. Antibiotic therapy for selected infections in infants 2 weeks to 2 months of age

Infection	Antibiotic
Bacterial sepsis	Ampicillin 100 mg/kg/d ÷ q8h IV + gentamicin 7.5 mg/kg/d ÷ q8h IV (gentamicin can be replaced by ceftriaxone 50 mg/kg IV qd)
Bacterial meningitis	Ampicillin 200 mg/kg/d ÷ q8h IV + gentamicin 7.5 mg/kg/d ÷ q8h IV (gentamicin can be replaced by ceftriaxone 50 mg/kg IV qd)
Bacterial gastroenteritis	Neomycin 50 mg/kg/d ÷ q6h PO
Chlamydia respiratory infection	Erythromycin 40 mg/kg/d ÷ q8h PO
Pertussis	Erythromycin 40 mg/kg/d ÷ q8h PO
Urinary tract infection	Ampicillin 100 mg/kg/d ÷ q8h IV + gentamicin 7.5 mg/kg/d ÷ q8h IV (gentamicin can be replaced by ceftriaxone 50 mg/kg IV qd)

express their infant's behavior as "He/she just isn't acting right." Such a child should be hospitalized. Treatment of sepsis is ampicillin 100 mg/kg/day q8h IV and gentamicin 7.5 mg/kg/d ÷ q8h IV. An alternative therapy quickly gaining popularity is ceftriaxone 50 mg/kg IV or IM once daily [17].

GASTROENTERITIS/DIARRHEA

Diarrhea in infants is a very common complaint. The most common etiology at this age is enterovirus, but systemic infections, overfeeding, and food intolerance are also frequent causes. The preliminary vital signs and observations made by admitting personnel may be a lifesaving adjunct to the busy emergency department provider. Training admitting personnel to interpret the signs and symptoms of severe dehydration (>10%) is essential to an initiation of appropriate and timely therapy. Because infants are particularly vulnerable to dehydration, the emergency department physician must determine the state of alertness, peripheral perfusion, and metabolic status within minutes of entering the examination room. A lethargic, fuzzy, listless infant is already a victim of shock. An infant or toddler who has hollow eyes, dry skin with poor turgor, and dry mouth and who has not voided in four hours is dehydrated. Obvious tachycardia and delayed capillary refill of more than 2 seconds is evidence of compensation for a hypovolemic state [18]. The infant who is breathing rapidly and deeply with ketotic breath is already seriously acidotic. The hydration status at this age is easily assessed by weighing the infant and comparing it to the most recent weight or the birth weight. A rapid assessment of heart rate, respiratory rate, capillary refill, sensory alertness, and skin elasticity also de-

termines the level of dehydration (<5%, 5%–10%, >10%, >15%) [18, 19]. Table 14-4 outlines the criteria used to determine levels of dehydration.

If the infant is more than 5% but less than 10% dehydrated, an IV or an oral bolus of fluid should be implemented with 20 ml/kg of normal saline. The infant should be checked in 20 minutes and a replacement program instituted over 6 hours in a holding area, if available. If the infant is more than 10% dehydrated, 40 ml/kg of normal saline should be given by IV intracath or intraosseous access. If the infant is less than 5% dehydrated, the parents

Table 14-4. Clinical estimates of fluid deficit in isotonic dehydration

Dehydration (%)	Clinical observations
5	Heart rate (10%–15% above baseline), dry mucous membranes, concentration of the urine, poor tear production*
10	Decreased skin turgor, increased severity of signs for 5% dehydration, oliguria, sunken eyeballs, sunken anterior fontanelle
15	Markedly increased severity of signs for 5% and 10% dehydration, decreased blood pressure, poor tissue perfusion (delayed capillary refill and acidosis)

* In hypotonic dehydration (Na < 130) all manifestations appear at lesser degrees of deficit; in hypertonic dehydration (Na > 150) the circulating volume is relatively preserved at the expense of cellular water, and less circulatory disturbance is seen for a given amount of fluid loss.
Source: Rowe PG. *The Harriet Lane Handbook, Johns Hopkins Hospital* (11th ed.). Baltimore: Year Book Medical Publications, 1987. P. 233. Used with permission.

should be congratulated for keeping up with the loss of fluids and told to continue regular feedings.

A stool examination for polymorphonuclear neutrophils (PMNs) that is positive suggests a bacterial infection, which will require a culture. Neonatal diarrhea complete with mucus and blood and accompanied by mild fever, irritability, and anorexia suggests an enteropathogenic *Escherichia coli.* Treatment with neomycin (50 mg/kg/day q6h PO) is highly effective for a relatively benign but persistent problem.

RESPIRATORY INFECTIONS

Chlamydia. Infants can acquire the usual respiratory infections found in a community, but chlamydia and pertussis are two infections that often confuse physicians. Chlamydia usually is acquired at birth from the mother's vagina or cervix. This infection is insidious in onset and is preceded by upper respiratory cold symptoms, mild fever, and progressive cough. Chlamydia develops over 6–8 weeks from a mild cough and conjunctivitis to a croupy cough, then to pneumonia as demonstrated by physical and radiographic examinations. An eosinophilia is often characteristic of a chlamydial infection. The effective treatment of chlamydia is erythromycin (40 mg/kg/day ÷ q8h PO) for 14–21 days.

Pertussis. Pertussis progresses over several weeks from mild coryza and cough to "whooping" and respiratory distress with very little physical or radiologic evidence of pneumonia. Pertussis is also unique in its ability to produce a marked lymphocytosis. Pertussis is acquired from a respiratory contact endemic source such as family members, day care centers, or nurseries. Most communities have endemic areas and populations with a reservoir of pertussis that infect the respiratory tract of the young infant before immunizations are begun.

Pertussis is modified and its infectiousness effectively reduced with erythromycin (40 mg/kg/day ÷ q8h PO) for 14–21 days. Hospitalization is indicated if there is radiologic evidence of pneumonia, pulse oxygen saturation is less than 90%, and temperature is over 38.2°C.

Viral Infections. Upper respiratory infections at this age often are characterized by nasal stuffiness, cough, tachypnea, and mild fever, with continued appetite, nontoxic appearance, and a score on the Yale Observation Scale of 12 or more. The majority of these infections are viral. The most apparent symptom is noisy, nasal breathing. Upper respiratory infections often are very difficult for parents who want to do something for their infant. The best advice to them is to avoid decongestants and other cold remedies because they make the baby irritable or sleepy. Parents can administer these four steps of treatment: (1) aspirate anterior nostril gently with the rubber nasal aspirator usually given in a discharge package from the newborn nursery; (2) squirt three to four drops of a saline solution (i.e., 3/4 teaspoon salt in 8 oz. water) into each nostril to clear out the midnasal passage; (3) give orally 1/2 oz. water to wash mucus out of oropharynx; and (4) give acetaminophen (dropper 0.4–0.8 ml or 40 mg/dose q4–6h PO) to relieve the discomfort of a cold. Loose clothing on the infant will avoid overheating.

Respiratory syncytial virus (RSV) is characterized by apnea, wheezing, and respiratory distress, which can be frightening for parents to witness. During the winter months RSV exposure is very common, particularly in the day care setting. The symptoms and signs are minimal, with mild coryza and a cough for several days. Fever is rare. Often no symptoms seem apparent to parents until the infant suddenly stops breathing, turns blue, and appears flaccid. These symptoms are quickly reversed by infant stimulation, so the infant appears well when emergency personnel arrive. The infant usually is brought to an emergency department, where symptoms and signs are few or nonexistent, but the parents still are upset. Such an infant should be admitted because the differential is often difficult and the parents are distraught. The differential is seizure or reflux with aspiration, but most often nothing is determined unless a nasal RSV screen and culture are obtained. The RSV screen is an appropriate test to have available on a real-time basis, so that the emergency physician is able to confirm the diagnosis. The etiology of these apnea spells is unknown; the outcome is favorable with usually no more than one or two apnea incidents in the next several days. These cases do not result in SIDS death, so they require no apnea monitors; however, few physicians would discharge a baby with RSV without a monitor.

The bronchiolitis syndrome of wheezing and respiratory distress begins quickly and is prolonged, but mild, for several weeks. Signs of respiratory distress are observed such as cyanosis, nasal flare, respiratory grunt, intercostal retraction, chin pull with respirations, subcostal retraction, and a respiratory rate greater than 40. There is definite expiratory wheezing, marked retractions, and radiologic evidence of hyperinflation and minimal atelectasis. A recent study by Shaw et al. of indicators for serious bronchiolitis emphasizes the importance of the following signs: (1) "ill" or "toxic" appearance; (2) pulse oximetry readings of less than 95%; (3) premature birth at less than 34 weeks; (4) respiratory rate of more than 70 per minute; (5) atelectasis on chest roentgenogram; and (6) age less than 3 months [20]. These infants respond to albuterol (0.02 ml/kg in 2 ml normal saline solution) nebulization. An infant who does not respond to two successive nebulizations, appears fatigued, is dehydrated, and has an oxygen saturation less than 90% should be admitted.

If oxygen saturation is greater than 90% and the baby is feeding well and seems vigorous, ambulatory care that includes albuterol (0.1 mg/kg/d q6–8h PO) will often suffice. Close follow-up every 12 hours is indicated because fatigue and dehydration are serious concerns. Because of the evidence of a close relationship to latent asthma, steroids (prednisone 2 mg/kg/d ÷ q12h PO) are used for more serious cases.

These infants may require hospitalization for vigorous therapy, including endotracheal intubation. Antibiotics are not effective, but ribavirin may be indicated for those at risk or in need of hospitalization.

UTI

The incidence of UTI in neonates is the highest (7+ %) of any age of febrile or septic infants [21]. The reasons range from congenital anomalies to the vulnerability of diaper care. Fever (>38.2°C rectal) may be the only apparent symptom. It is important to apply the rule of septic workup, including an urinalysis and a culture for fever (>38.2°C rectal). Urine collected by "bagging," as long as the perineum is clean and the bag is changed every 2 hours, creates no problems. However, a catheter or suprapubic bladder tap is the recommended method of collection if the emergency department staff are not familiar with bagging techniques. Even if urinalysis is normal, a culture should be obtained because 45% of UTIs at this age may have false negative urinalysis [21].

Because any infant under 8 weeks of age with fever over 38.2°C (rectal) and a suspected UTI is hospitalized, specific urologic workup is deferred by the emergency department. The most common organism is E. coli. The combination of fever and UTI implies that pyelonephritis is present. Although bacteremia is not common in this circumstance, it does occur, so intravenous antibiotics should be used for all patients this age with UTI and fever. Ampicillin (100 mg/kg/d q8h IV) and gentamicin (7.5 mg/kg/d ÷ q8h IV) are started as the appropriate therapy prior to culture and sensitivity results.

ASEPTIC MENINGITIS

The incidence of bacterial meningitis in infants under 2 months is very low, but the incidence of aseptic meningitis in febrile (>38.2°C rectal) infants under 2 months of age is significant [16]. The physical findings are minimal, often only fever. The most common viruses are echovirus and coxsackievirus. The immediate threats of aseptic meningitis are dehydration and seizure. The spinal fluid demonstrates WBCs of more than 5 per μl, predominant lymphocytes, and normal protein and sugar. Because these same findings may be present in early bacterial meningitis in this age group, the infants should be hospitalized and treated for 72 hours with ampicillin (100 mg/kg/d ÷ q8h IV and gentamicin 7.5 mg/kg/d ÷ q8h IV) until cultures are negative.

Infections in Infants 2–6 Months

Infants who are 2 months of age are alert, sociable, and generally healthy looking. They are being exposed to more of the community, are exploring everything they can with their mouths, and are being introduced to a variety of foods. At the same time they are losing their mothers' transplacental immunity and decreasing breast feeding but are not yet immunologically mature. They also must remain dependent on parental decisions affecting their hydration and medication.

The general manifestations of infections are fever, irritability, lethargy, and anorexia, no matter where the infection is. Not eating and irritability are particularly important symptoms of illness in children this age, because generally they eat eagerly and are pleasant, curious, and sociable.

Since infants this age cannot communicate by talking, information about their sensory level is gained by an appreciation of the development of infants at this age such as the hand grasp, response to voice and movement, muscle tone in pulling to a sitting position, and response to medical instruments when offered. Even the knowledge that an infant at this age wets a diaper every 4 hours is an important difference from a child over 2 years of age who can go easily 6–8 hours without urinating.

The examining physician can establish the status of the infant's hydration, toxicity, and seriousness of illness by immediately appraising the level of developmental parameters, respiratory and cardiac rates, capillary refill, and skin turgor [18]. An urgent problem exists if these parameters suggest a decompensating condition.

Immunizations

Since infants 2–6 months old are also receiving their first immunizations, an immunization history is crucial to the evaluation of a febrile illness in this age group. A fever frequently can be attributed to a recent immunization. For example, fever from diphtheria-pertussis-tetanus (DPT) immunization rarely exceeds 39.5°C, usually does not last longer than 48 hours, and usually is not associated with toxicity (Yale Observation Scale >12) or an elevated WBC count. Exceptions are due to three causes: (1) a local reaction usually demonstrated by a red swollen area larger than 2 cm in diameter at the injection site; (2) a hypersensitivity to pertussis vaccine; and (3) rarely a streptococcal abscess at the site of injection as demonstrated by a hot, tender mass.

Protection by immunization is increased with each injection, but if the infant has had only one injection the protection may be little to none, particularly for pertussis.

Specific Infections

Table 14-5 summarizes antibiotic treatment of common infections in infants 2–6 months of age; dosages for antibiotics referred to in this table are listed in Table 14-9.

OTITIS MEDIA

Otitis media is the most common bacterial problem of infancy and early childhood. What is not appreciated is the frequency with which an infant under 6 months is affected. At least a third of infants prone to otitis media have their first episode in the first 6 months of life. The most common organisms are pneumococcus, *H. influenzae*, *Moraxella catarrhalis*, and other streptococci. Pneumococcus is the most prevalent, but the most disturbing is *H. influenzae*, which is resistant to commonly used antibiotics and is more systemically invasive [22].

A typical history for otitis media is two to three days of mild coryza, proceeding to the rapid development of irritability, anorexia, fever, and thick, yellow-green nasal discharge. The infant may pull at the ears, but this action is typical of children this age in their exploratory activities. The physical examination confirms fever, irritability, and upper respiratory signs and symptoms of a cold. The dramatic appearance of a bulging, red tympanic membrane that has no landmarks and is immobile with a pneumatoscope is pathognomonic of suppurative otitis media.

Treatment with antibiotics is indicated because of the incidence of subsequent chronic ear disease, sepsis, and meningitis. Broad-spectrum coverage for *H. influenzae*, pneumococcus, and *M. catarrhalis* is a must at this age. Amoxicillin (40 mg/kg/day ÷ q8h PO for 10 days) is the drug of first choice. If bacterial resistance is suspected—it is present in 12%–25% of *H. influenzae* infections—then Augmentin (i.e., amoxicillin-clavulonic acid) (40 mg/kg/d q8h PO for 10 days) is used.

The diagnosis of otitis media does not preclude the existence of a more serious illness, such as meningitis or occult bacteremia. A septic workup may still be in order for the infant who meets the parameters outlined the section "General Principles," earlier in this chapter. Follow-up in 2 to 3 days is necessary; if there is little improvement, possible complications and resistant organisms must be addressed. Follow-up in 3 weeks ensures completeness of recovery.

RHINITIS

The sinusitis of infancy is persistent rhinitis, often called adenoiditis. Any infant with a persistent yellow-green nasal discharge of more than 5 days' duration is considered a candidate for antibiotic

Table 14-5. Antibiotic therapy of selected infections in children older than 2 months of age*

Infection	Antibiotic
Bacteremia	Ceftriaxone *or* cefotaxime *or* cefuroxime
Bacterial meningitis	Ceftriaxone *or* cefotaxime (alternative: ampicillin + chloramphenicol) *or* dexamethasone
Pneumonia	
Mild	Viral etiology likely
Severe	Methicillin + gentamicin 5 *or* cefuroxime *or* ceftriaxone *or* cefotaxime
In children >5 years	Erythromycin
Epiglottitis	Cefotaxime *or* cefuroxime *or* ceftriaxone (alternative: chloramphenicol)
Urinary tract infection	Amoxicillin *or* trimethoprim-sulfamethoxazole
Osteomyletlitis/septic arthritis	Methicillin + cefotaxime *or* ceftriaxone *or* ceforoxime
Otitis media	Amoxicillin *or* amoxicillin-clavulonic acid *or* erythromycin-sulfisoxazole *or* trimethoprim-sulfamethoxazole
Rhinitis	Amoxicillin *or* amoxicillin-clavulonic acid *or* erythromycin-sulfisoxazole *or* trimethoprim-sulfamethoxazole
Lymphadenitis	Ceftriaxone *or* penicillin G *or* penicillin V
Conjunctivitis	Amoxicillin *or* amoxicillin-clavulonic acid *or* erythromycin-sulfisoxazole *or* trimethoprim-sulfamethoxazole
Periorbital/orbital cellulitis	Cefuroxime *or* amoxicillin-clavulonate
Buccal cellulitis	Cefuroxime *or* amoxicillin-clavulonate
Streptococcal pharyngitis	LA bicillin IM *or* penicillin V
Eccymotic/hemor-rhagic rash	Ceftriaxone + penicillin G
Pustular rash (impetigo)	Penicillin V *or* erythromycin

*Dosages for antibiotics listed in this table will be found in Table 14-9.

therapy (amoxicillin 40 mg/kg/day q8h PO for 10 days). These infants continue to be anorexic, mildly febrile and irritable, and develop a postnasal-drip cough. If not treated, they proceed to develop otitis media or sepsis. At this age the organisms of rhinitis or adenoiditis are the same as for otitis media.

PNEUMONIA

Pneumonia is characterized by fever, tachypnea, anorexia, rales, and a grunting cough. These signs and symptoms often are more alarming in infants than in older children because their airways are relatively small and their chests more flexible. Thus, there is nasal flare, accessory muscle effort, and marked intercostal and substernal retraction, accompanied by cyanosis and fatigued appearance.

A pulse oximeter reading of less than 90% or arterial PO$_2$ of less than 70 mm confirms the severity of the problem and indicates the need for admission.

Those infants who appear to be in respiratory distress and have signs and symptoms typical of pneumonia are easy to diagnose. What is most often problematic is that the seriousness of the illness is underestimated at this age, and the possibility of underlying vulnerability is overlooked. These infants may be manifesting their first episode of an underlying problem such as cystic fibrosis, asthma, tracheoesophageal fistula, reflux, or immunodeficient disease.

The radiologic interpretation of the PA and lateral of the chest greatly assists in distinguishing viral illnesses from bacterial ones. A segmental infiltrate is bacterial while a diffuse, perihilar, and interstitial infiltrate is viral. A WBC count of more than 15,000, more than 10,000 PMNs, and more than 500 bands also suggests a bacterial infection.

The most common bacterial organisms are *H. influenzae* and pneumococcus, which can produce sepsis complications or pulmonary empyema in this age group. Treatment with parenteral broad-spectrum antibiotics (ceftriaxone 50–100 mg/kg/dose qd IM or IV) is an effective immediate treatment [17]. The viral organisms most likely to cause a viral pneumonia are respiratory syncytial, influenza, and parainfluenza viruses.

Infections in Infants 6–12 Months

Most, if not all, of the previous discussions apply to the older infant of 6–12 months as far as etiology and systems are concerned. However, several differences attributable to age are noteworthy. One is the vulnerability to infection as a result of the low point of maternally acquired immunity and before the infant acquires its own immunity. Varicella, rubella, and rubeola become threats, whereas before, with maternal protection, these illnesses were modified or aborted all together.

Another difference is in symptomatology. Older infants can indicate the area of pain and infection. They clearly indicate that they are sick by clinging to their parents or wanting to sleep or not playing or eating. The word *toxic* has meaning in children this age, because objective data, such as the Yale Observation Scale (see Table 14-1) are more dependable [5].

The more typical viral infections common to the community are seen in infants by the age of 9 months. An astute emergency department physician maintains an awareness of the viruses circulating in the community. Infants with viral infections may have higher temperatures than those with bacterial infections [14]. Despite high temperatures, irritability, and tachycardia of 10 beats above normal for each degree of temperature elevation, these infants do not appear toxic.

Several infections appear more often as their incidence increases from this age through 3 years: occult bacteremia, viral enanthems and exanthems

such as herpes, coxsackie, Kawasaki disease, adenovirus, and RSV [23].

Table 14-5 lists antibiotic therapy for the infections discussed in this section.

Specific Infections

OCCULT BACTEREMIA

Nothing is more perplexing than an infant with fever and toxicity but without evidence of focal infection. By all signs and symptoms this child is ill, but there is no radiographic, urologic, neurologic, or other evidence of focal infection. Clearly studies such as a score on the Yale Observation Scale of 12 or more will also suggest a bacterial infection [5]. The first laboratory level of investigation is an LP because these children appear ill enough to make the practitioner worry about meningitis. Only 10% of these taps are positive if the physician's index of suspicion is high, as it should be for meningitis. A blood count then should be ordered and a blood culture collected to save sticking the infant again. The lab results may suggest bacterial infection (i.e., a WBC count >15,000/μl, >10,000 neutrophils/μl, and >500 band forms/μl). The blood culture under these circumstances is positive in up to 10% of cases [24, 25].

Such a case can be handled safely only by parenteral antibiotics at the time of visit and close ambulatory follow-up until blood cultures indicate the status. Even without blood cultures or an elevated WBC count, an infant with a toxicity rating of more than 12 on the Yale Observation Scale, which suggests occult bacteremia, should be treated with parenteral antibiotics until afebrile. Conventional wisdom and experience have shown that those infants who are treated with antibiotics as ambulatory patients have fewer new serious foci, shorter illnesses, and fewer subsequent hospitalizations [26]. The parenteral therapy is done safely with ceftriaxone (50–100 mg/kg/dose IM or IV) every 24 hours on an ambulatory basis. Why be aggressive? The complications of bacteremia such as septic joint, meningitis, and septicemia in this age group, while uncommon, are extremely threatening. However, physicians who have followed infants with positive blood cultures know that many of them are well without therapy several days later [26]. The practitioner should err on the side of treatment with antibiotics, which are discontinued if cultures are negative and infant is well in 72 hours. Outpatient treatment of this syndrome also depends on the availability and the reliability of the parent. A positive blood culture in this situation is tragic if the child does not return for a follow-up visit or the parents cannot be contacted.

UTI

In the workup of a septic appearing child, another body fluid that answers questions is urine. Although the incidence of UTI at this age is small, it must be considered as a diagnosis. If a septic workup is indicated, urine should be collected for analysis and culture. In fact it is best to place a urine bag collector on any infant who appears toxic, septic, or just sick. In addition to ruling out infection by a WBC count of more than 5 on centrifuged urine or positive nitrates and leukocytes on a "dip stick," information about the level of toxicity is reflected by ketones and high specific gravity. The best correlated test with the diagnosis of UTI is bacteria seen in an unspun urine sediment [27].

The threat of a UTI is twofold: any infection of the urinary tract at this age may be initial pyelonephritis, which ultimately will become chronic, and anatomic malformations creating obstructive uropathy amenable to surgery are higher in this age group.

CONJUNCTIVITIS

Purulent conjunctivitis, rhinitis, and otitis media are pathognomonic of an *H. influenzae* infection and often a resistant type B strain. Any infant 6–12 months old with a purulent discharge from the eyes is considered to have a bacterial infection. The exception is if there were known cases in a day care setting or older siblings that suggest adenovirus type 3, 4, or 7.

At this age local ophthalmic antibiotics are not used for three reasons: (1) bacterial infections are more common and often associated with systemic illness; (2) the parent finds it difficult, even traumatic, to administer drops or ointment to the infant's eyes; and (3) there is little, if any, indication for ophthalmic antibiotics in viral conjuncti-

vitis. Systemic use of Augmentin (amoxicillin-clavulonic acid 40 mg/kg ÷ 98h PO) is indicated.

SEPTIC HIP

The septic hip joint is not an easy diagnosis to make, but it is a lot easier if the condition is considered. The common organisms are *H. influenzae* and *S. aureus*. The hip infection begins as a result of a nonfocal minor infection, leading to bacteremia, which then establishes a focus in a joint, usually in the lower extremities. The infant must be undressed for examination.

In an advanced case the infant is toxic and febrile and cries when picked up or moved, such as for a diaper change or an examination. There is pain on motion of the affected joint and often swelling or redness. An earlier case may be far more subtle. Suspect this condition in the febrile child who will not crawl or bear weight on a leg. It may be difficult to isolate the process to a particular joint in an extremity because redness and swelling may not be prominent in deep joints such as the hip. Radiologic evidence of effusion is helpful, but an isotope uptake may be necessary to prove the point. In the meantime a WBC count of more than 15,000/μl, more than 10,000 neutrophils/μl, and more than 500 band forms/μl and a sedimentation rate of more than 30 mm/hr means that an orthopedist or a pediatrician should be called to admit the child. It is imperative to treat with antibiotics (ceftriaxone 50–100 mg/kg/dose q24h IV) and to drain the abscess as soon as possible.

BACTERIAL MENINGITIS

As many as 90% of the LPs performed in the emergency department reveal normal CSF, but in those other 10% of cases where the test is positive treatment is crucial. The infant with meningitis is toxic, lethargic, febrile, very irritable, and inconsolable and cries on movement, particularly when pulling or sitting up. A stiff neck is a classic symptom, but at this age it is difficult to elicit during the early stages of meningitis. A bulging fontanelle is still a presentation, but the fontanelle is also beginning to firm up in late infancy. Furthermore, the dehydration commonly found in the ill infant masks an otherwise bulging fontanelle.

If meningitis is considered, an LP should be performed. Because meningitis is most often due to *H. influenzae* and pneumococcus, suspicion is necessary if an infant has had a cold and fever for several days but is much sicker on the day of the emergency department visit. Any infant who is not responding to treatment of otitis media or sepsis should be tapped. Febrile convulsions are viewed with suspicion if the infant remains lethargic or toxic an hour after the seizure.

Diagnosis is confirmed by CSF that is cloudy, has >5 cell high power field, low glucose, elevated protein, and bacteria on a Gram's stain. The infant should be hospitalized. The recommended therapies are antibiotics (ceftriaxone 100 mg/kg/d IV) and steroid parenterally (dexamethasone 0.15 mg/kg IV $\div$ q6h for 4 days). Currently steroids are recommended to modify the inflammatory cascade system that results from infection and treatment [28]. The most effective use of steroids is intravenous administration before antibiotics. (See Chap. 31 for more discussion on bacterial meningitis.)

WHEEZING AND RSV

It is in this 6–12-month age group that RSV infection, formerly known as bronchiolitis, is most often seen. It is now known that at least 60% of these children will have more typical asthmatic or other allergic problems, but for many years this illness was treated as an isolated incident. Infection was assumed to be part of the problem, but only recently has RSV been identified as the major cause.

At this age the infant is still at a disadvantage of having less alveolar surface for gas exchange relative to height and weight [1, 2]. As a result the increased respiratory rate, coupled with the inefficient flexibility of the chest cage, creates fatigue, retraction, and anxiousness because of marginal oxygenation.

Expiratory wheezing, retraction, and reduced peripheral oxygen saturation with radiologic evidence of hyperventilation are factors for a presumptive diagnosis of RSV-induced bronchial spasm.

Treatment in the emergency department is initiated as soon as possible in the form of a nebulized aerosol of beta-adrenergic bronchodilators (albuterol 0.02 ml/kg in 2 ml normal saline). Response for the majority of cases is perceptible within min-

utes and often sustained for several hours. Continued beta-adrenergic bronchodilators (albuterol 0.1 mg/kg dose q6–8h PO) and corticosteroids (prednisone 2 mg/kg/day $\div$ q12h PO) at home will be sufficient. If the child does not respond, hospitalization is necessary. The child that does not respond to two successive tests of complete doses of nebulized beta-adrenergic bronchodilator or has an oxygen saturation of less than 90% is very likely to require intensive therapy while hospitalized, including intubation because of fatigue, poor ventilation, and protracted respiratory decompensation. As in more typical asthma cases, arterial blood gas values of PO_2 less than 75 torr and PCO_2 greater than 40 torr in these infants indicate need for admission. Normal values, which at an increased respiratory rate suggest rapid decompensation of a previously low CO_2 and pH, are of concern.

ENANTHEMS AND EXANTHEMS

Herpes Simplex Virus and Coxsackievirus. Refusal by an infant to take a bottle or eat and apparent pain in the mouth suggest ulcerative or herpetic lesions of the buccal mucosa, tongue, gingiva, and palate. These infants must have a complete oral examination. Often the whole picture becomes clear with the visualization of a single lesion, which suggests herpes simplex, herpangina, hand-foot-and-mouth disease, or rubeola (e.g., Koplik's spot). Vesicles of herpes simplex are preceded by a generalized prodrome, and involvement of the oral mucosa may be extensive. Vesicles of herpangina are generally on the soft palate, tonsils, and uvula. Vesicles of hand-foot-and-mouth disease can be found on the buccal mucosa and tongue as well as on the hands and feet.

The infant with any of these syndromes has a mild to moderate fever, irritability, and clings to the parents. The extreme possibility is herpes simplex stomatitis, which has been described as "7 days of hell" for the infant and the family because the child is febrile, in pain, and dehydrated (see Fig. 9-4).

By the time the parents have brought the child to the emergency department, the worst may be over and antiviral agents are unlikely to be effective. No local therapy (gum anesthetics) at this age is effective and may even be dangerous because of "-cain" (prelocain, lidocaine, etc.) intoxication and "-cain" methemoglobinemia. Oral or rectal acetaminophen, cold solids and liquids such as ice cream, and bland cool drinks improve the infant's comfort.

Coxsackie infections, of which herpangina and hand-foot-and-mouth disease are instances, are very common as infants approach 1 year of age. A red macular, slightly papular and vesicular generalized rash that blanches on pressure is considered benign. (See Chaps. 9 and 36 for additional information.)

Kawasaki Disease. Kawasaki disease is becoming a common problem among infants 6–12 months of age. In the emergency department the presentation is mostly fever, conjunctivitis, a macular-papular rash, particularly over the extremities, and a generalized lymphadenopathy of nodes larger than 1 cm in diameter. It is accentuated by a toxic appearance of cracked lips, dry skin, irritability, and tachycardia. After at least 1 week of illness the infant's platelet count is more than $500,000/\mu l$.

A history of fever for longer than 5 days with conjunctivitis, adenitis, and macular-papular rash suggests Kawasaki disease rather than the typical virus. The infant should be hospitalized or referred to an appropriate provider to rule out arterial disease, such as coronary aneurysm. Drug therapy, such as gammaglobulin IV or aspirin, is instituted as soon as possible to minimize any complications.

Roseola. Roseola (exanthema subitum) is a herpes virus (HV-6) infection that in children this age can be confusing. Its natural history of several days of high fever and a generalized macular-papular rash over the face, trunk, and extremities creates two problems for the emergency department physician:

1. The fever is high enough in these infants to be worrisome. As a result a septic workup is ordered, and a conclusion of occult bacteremia may be reached. These infants are seldom toxic, their WBC counts most often are normal, even low, and the sedimentation rate is normal. Antibiotics are not necessary.
2. Frequently the infant is treated with antibiotics,

and within several days the rash occurs, resulting in confusion about drug allergy. An experienced physician will be aware of this problem on reviewing the sequence of events.

DIARRHEA

Although enterovirus, adenovirus, and reovirus are causes of infant diarrhea, it is rotavirus that is the most prevalent and problematic. Several days of vomiting and anorexia, followed by prolonged diarrhea for 7–14 days, is highly suggestive of rotavirus. A further history of family and day care or nursery epidemics can confirm this disease.

Emergency department assessment must focus on the hydration status first. Clinical signs and symptoms of dehydration are the same as those described for infants 2 weeks to 2 months old with gastrointestinal complaints (see Table 14-4). Less than 10% dehydration is gauged more by sight in the alert, active child with mild tachycardia (<120 beats per minute), pink and moist skin, and normal breathing. Therapy should be instituted as a bolus (20 ml/kg normal saline), or as an oral solution in a bottle or a nasogastric tube. Because these infants probably will go home, an intensive diagnostic effort is instituted in the emergency department. Parameters that indicate more than 10% dehydration require immediate parenteral access with IV or intraosseous normal saline (40 ml/kg bolus). Final fluid requirement is based on weight, response, chemistries, and urine output. A child with more than 10% dehydration should be admitted for further evaluation and treatment.

A spontaneous stool or rectal swab, which is often odorous, should be examined for PMNs to differentiate viral from bacterial infection. Stool on a slide, mixed with 10% methylene blue, is extremely dependable in identifying PMNs. A count of fewer than 5 PMNs per field is highly suspicious of a noninvasive viral enterocolitis [29]. A confirmation with a rapid rotazyme test, (enzyme-linked immunosorbent assay (ELISA) for rotavirus), of stool settles the matter.

As in any diarrhea situation parents should be advised about feeding therapy and reassured about the course of disease. Otherwise, the child will appear again and again in the emergency department setting. The parents should not deprive the child of food. Unless there is vomiting, the infant should be allowed to stay on formula or milk and eat whatever he/she wants [30]. Rotavirus lasts 7–14 days, long enough so that disaccharide deficiency and food intolerance become more likely if the effect of infection on mucosa (increasing mobility, flattening of mucosa, metabolic derangement, and secretory dysfunction) is enhanced by lack of nutrients and normal stimulation.

The emergency department physician should not predict a short-term cure to the parents. In infants this age even if the diarrhea is not caused by a rotavirus, loose and frequent stools for several weeks are the norm because of immaturity of the gut.

Differential diagnosis includes GI bacterial infections and malabsorption [29]. GI bacterial infections are rare in the infant but if present follow patterns similar to those of the viruses and bacteria discussed in Chap. 25. Malabsorption syndromes appear in infants because of the increased exposure to a variety of foodstuffs, the frequency of antibiotics, and their immature enzyme systems. The stools of these infants are acidic, burn the skin with severe diaper rash, and turn a Chemostix pale yellow. These simple observations, plus failure to thrive, will alert the emergency physician to a more chronic problem.

AIDS

AIDS is characterized in infants by failure to thrive, pneumonia, recurrent or chronic infections, persistent diarrhea, hepatosplenomegaly, and thrombocytopenia. Although the manifestations occur earlier, most become obvious at the age of 6–12 months if the infection was acquired during the perinatal period either from the parent or through transfusion. The index of suspicion is particularly high because much of the at-risk population, for example, children of prostitutes and drug users, frequents the emergency department.

Diagnosis by serologic evidence is discussed elsewhere, but it is difficult. A child with AIDS is admitted because the symptomology suggests severe immunodeficiency. (See Chap. 17 for a detailed discussion of HIV infection.)

Infections in Children 12–36 Months

The toddler stage is an amazing age in children, as they expand their walking, talking, eating, and exploring. Toddlers are not always cooperative, but because they are so curious medical observations and examinations often are completed with the children's assistance. Children's self-esteem is benefitted when physicians talk directly to them, and the value of physicians becomes higher in the eyes of the children and their parents.

The Yale Observation Scale (see Table 14-1) is very useful at this age, as are sedimentation rates and WBC counts [5–8]. A child's temperature is less useful in determining the degree of illness. The safety margin of dehydration, exhaustion, and tolerance for stress in the maturing toddler are much improved over infancy.

Most of those infections mentioned earlier also occur at this age but are less frequent and less threatening. Respiratory, skin, GI infections, and communicable diseases, however, are more frequent.

The caretaker is better able to render care on an ambulatory basis in this age group, but serious consideration for admission for any infection should be based on the following objective findings:

1. A score on the Yale Observation Scale of 16 or higher.
2. Physical findings that suggest decompensation or failure of specific systems: central nervous, cardiac, renal, pulmonary, or hepatic
3. Laboratory data:
   —Sedimentation rate of 30 mm/hr or more
   —A WBC count of 15,000/μl or more, 10,000 or more PMN μl, and 500 or more band forms μl
   —Temperature of 40.5°C or higher
   —Urine ketones and specific gravity 1.030 or greater
   —Bicarbonate 12 or less, sodium less than 130 or greater than 150 meq/L
   —Oxygen 90% or less: less than 74 torr

Any of the above laboratory findings supports the Yale Observation Scale and other physical findings but is not necessarily specific for infection. Poison ingestion, injury, and chronic diseases can mimic infections.

Viral infections are the most frequent infections encountered. In general at least seven to eight such infections can be documented by history and antibody titers every year per child. Such infections are usually mild, but there is fever, irritability, and anorexia. An emergency department physician must be patient and understanding when dealing with a caretaker who is more concerned than the actual illness warrants.

Immunizations

DPT, polio, and H. influenzae immunizations usually are complete by 6 months of age, so protection is assumed even though a booster and a measles-mumps-rubella (MMR) vaccine are given by age 15 months. Not all children, however, have been immunized. Many parents do not immunize their children, delay immunizations, or do not allow pertussis or polio immunization for fear of injury to the child. It is at 15 months that reactions to immunization are again seen, such as to MMR, which can produce an attenuated measles infection after the injection. This reaction is within 10–14 days of immunization and produces fever and often mild coryza and a morbilliform generalized rash.

Abdominal Pain

In the toddler abdominal pain and discomfort are common complaints. The impression of abdominal discomfort often is manifested during any infection. Vomiting and diarrhea are also often present. This systemic response is confusing, even distracting, to an emergency department physician. A complete physical and history are necessary before the illness can be called gastroenteritis. A urinalysis is important to rule out UTI and hepatitis. A three-way radiologic examination that includes an upright and decubitus views of the abdomen, and a PA of the chest should be taken to rule out a significant abdominal problem as well as pneumonia, which is often a cause of abdominal pain.

Febrile Seizure

Febrile seizures are estimated to occur in 4% of children aged 12–36 months. Five percent of these seizures that present to an emergency department

are associated with meningitis [31]. Febrile seizures are a possibility in any infection with fever and are increased if there is a family history of such seizures. They are more likely in a child this age who has had a previous seizure. They are very unlikely to be life threatening or predictive of future seizure disorder. Seizures are frightening to parents and create a more complicated problem for the emergency department physician. Is it meningitis? Table 14-6 is a reliable list of risk factors that indicate the need for an LP. A routine LP may not be warranted if none of these risk factors is present, if a careful history and physical examination have been performed, and if immediate follow-up is available. Febrile seizures seldom are long enough to require anticonvulsants at the time of seizures. The majority of children have already had the seizures before coming to the emergency department and are alert and active on presentation.

The workup for the majority of these situations is to determine the cause of the fever. Any fever-causing infection should be considered, but particular attention should be given to such infections as shigellosis, otitis media, and roseola, which are common inducers of febrile seizures. Hospitalization depends on the cause of the fever, not the seizure itself. Very seldom does a seizure repeat during a particular illness. An antifebrile strategy of cold fluids by mouth, tepid baths, acetaminophen, and lightweight clothes is indicated.

Table 14-6. Risk factors that identify a child with a febrile seizure secondary to meningitis

Visit to a physician in the 48 hours prior to the seizure

Seizure on arrival at the emergency department

Focality to seizure

Suspicious findings on physical examination (rash or petechiae, cyanosis, hypotension, grunting respirations)

Suspicious findings on neurologic exam (stiff neck, increased tone, deviated eyes, ataxia, no response to voice, inability to fix and follow, no response to painful stimuli, positive doll's eye sign, floppy muscle tone, bulging or tense fontanelle)

Source: Joffe A, McCormick M, DeAngelis C. Which children with Febrile seizures need lumbar puncture? AJDC 137: 1153–56, 1983. Used with permission.

Specific Infections

See Table 14-5 for a summary of the antibiotic treatment of the infections discussed in this section.

LYMPHADENOPATHY/ADENITIS

Lymph nodes of under 1 cm are common in infants and children. Those palpable nodes over 1 cm, especially those 4 cm or more, should be taken more seriously by the physician. The most common lymphadenitis is of the cervical lymph chain. These nodes can become infected from hematogenous, oral-nasal-pharyngeal focus and skin. Group A beta-hemolytic streptococcus is the most frequent organism. The infected child will have a unilateral, tender, firm mass in the cervical area, and the overlying skin often will be erythematous and warm to the touch. These nodes are of rapid onset accompanied by fever and mild toxicity. Children with these often are seen in the emergency department because a mass in the neck is frightening to parents. These nodes often will become fluctuant and will eventually drain.

To avoid the need for surgical drainage if the node is not fluctuant, antibiotic treatment is mandatory. The treatment is penicillin (oral or IM 50,000 U/kg, or approximately 60 mg/kg/day ÷ q6h). To ensure that the child is medicated as soon as possible, the first dose should be given in the emergency department. Because coverage is best ensured by a long-acting parenteral antibiotic, ceftriaxone (50 mg/kg/dose IM) is also satisfactory. If the node is fluctuant, surgical intervention will be necessary.

OTITIS MEDIA

Otitis media is still the most frequent focus infection of childhood [22]. The ears must be examined in every child presenting to the emergency department when infection is suspected. A tympanic membrane that has lost recognizable landmarks and is bulging and immobile is diagnostic. A child with otitis media is febrile, irritable, and anorexic, rubs the ear, and has an upper respiratory infection. (See Chap. 34.)

A distressing complication of otitis media at this age is perforation. Often with minimal symptoms, the parent discovers a nonfoul, purulent discharge draining from the ear canal. Perforations heal quickly if they are treated with the same antibiotic program as nonperforated otitis media. Amoxicillin (or Augmentin) (40 mg/kg ÷ q8h PO for 10 days) is used. No local or otic medications are necessary; they only add to treatment costs.

CONJUNCTIVITIS

The red eye is often a perplexing sign because, as suggested previously, *H. influenzae* is a threatening problem during this age. If the discharge is purulent, the coryza purulent, and otitis is present, these children are treated on an outpatient basis with systemic antibiotics (amoxicillin or Augmentin 40 mg/kg/day ÷ q8h PO for 10 days).

On the other hand it is during this age of 12 to 36 months that the true "pink eye" of adenovirus, echovirus, and coxsackievirus begins. These children are seldom ill. No eye treatment is necessary, but "pink eye" is contagious and persists for up to 2 weeks. The exception is adenoid-pharyngeal-conjunctival (APC) fever, which is caused by an adenovirus. Temperature is often higher than 39°C, cervical nodes are 3–4 cm, the pharynx is red, and the sclera are very hyperemic. APC lasts 4–5 days. Fortunately this syndrome is apparent because all the signs and symptoms develop simultaneously within 24 hours of onset. Children with APC have little eye discharge, it is more like tearing, and the scleral erythema is quite pronounced. The patients are not toxic, and treatment is symptomatic.

PERIORBITAL/ORBITAL CELLULITIS

The spectrum of periorbital/orbital cellulitis is serious, and if early infection is not treated, it becomes more complicated. The majority of infants presenting with periorbital swelling and erythema have a preseptal infection. It is distinguished from the more serious orbital cellulitis by the absence of pain, limitation of ocular movement, proptosis, and a score on the Yale Observation Scale of more than 12 (see Table 14-1) [32, 33]. This bacterial inflammation often can be traced to a nasal or sinus infection, but often the infant is febrile and mildly toxic with unilateral swelling and has an erythema of the upper and lower eyelids. The organism that most likely causes periorbital/orbital cellulitis is *H. influenzae* type B, which causes a bluish-purple cellulitis. In the summer months the differential is more difficult because insect bites, trauma, and group A beta-hemolytic streptococcus impetigo are similar. In none of these cases is fever, toxicity, or an elevated WBC count likely. Treatment is ambulatory, unless the score on the Yale Observation Scale is 16 or higher or there is any ocular motion problem, which suggests intraocular involvement. Ceftriaxone should be administered (50 mg/kg IM), with follow-up by telephone or by the patient being seen again in 12 hours. If the child has improved, oral therapy continues with amoxicillin or Augmentin (40 mg/kg ÷ q8h for 10 days). (See Chap. 35 for a discussion of orbital cellulitis.)

BUCCAL CELLULITIS
Buccal cellulitis is a curious infection in toddlers. The complaint is a swollen, red, unilateral buccal area associated with fever and mild to moderate toxicity of a rapid onset. The organism most often responsible is *H. influenzae*. If the infection is not treated vigorously, sepsis and other foci of infection such as meningitis are likely. Because the complication rate is high and the infection difficult to treat, most children with buccal cellulitis are treated as inpatients. But if the child is not toxic (a score on the Yale Observation Scale <12) and only mildly febrile (<39°C), ceftriaxone (50 mg/kg IM/IV) can be used and the child rechecked in 12 hours, at which time another dose of ceftriaxone IM and a prescription for an appropriate oral antibiotic can be given. Continued close follow-up is necessary.

PHARYNGITIS
Pharyngitis is one of the most common infections in childhood. A viral etiology (e.g., coxsackievirus, adenovirus, parainfluenza) is most common in toddlers under 3 years old, but the appearance of group A beta-hemolytic streptococcus becomes more common as the child approaches the age of 3. Although the Epstein-Barr virus and mycoplasma are seen in the infancy and toddler years, they are rare and subject to verification by laboratory confirmation before such diagnoses are made.

Clinically a sore throat is manifested by reluctance to eat, pulling at the neck, and increased salivation. Before the age of 2 years, the sore throat is associated with other respiratory features as coryza, nasal excoriation, cough, mild fever, mild toxicity, and cervical adenopathy, which suggest a generalized infection. After the age of 2, more specific complaints and specific pharyngeal findings are apparent.

In every respiratory, febrile, anorexic situation the pharynx must be examined. If the child does not cooperate, the parent should hold the child in a sitting position with the parent's left arm around the child's abdomen and arms and the parent's right hand holding the child's forehead pressing the head back into the parent's chest. The tongue blade should be positioned quickly by running the blade parallel and along the buccal mucosa. This action stimulates the child's mouth just enough to quickly move the blade parallel with the tongue and then to the back of tongue, where firm pressure elicits a gag and adequate visibility. Hyperemia/erythema usually is all that is seen, but the presence of vesicles suggests coxsackie or herpes as the etiology. A hemorrhagic/petechial enanthem or exudate suggests a bacterial throat infection. If the patient is toxic (a score on the Yale Observation Scale ≥12) and febrile and has tender cervical nodes, a presumptive diagnosis of streptococcus is acceptable in the emergency department. If available a rapid strep test is helpful and a throat culture confirms this diagnosis.

Because many emergency department patients often are poor, have communication or transportation problems, and are at risk for complications, strep throat is treated if there is strong likelihood of its presence based on physical findings, epidemiology, history of exposure, or repeated strep throat, otitis, and the like. The preferred treatment is bicillin LA (300,000 units for a patient under 10 kg, 600,000 units for a patient 10–15 kg, 900,000 units for a patient over 15 kg) in a single dose. (See Chap. 21.)

LOWER RESPIRATORY TRACT INFECTION
In this age group, as in infancy, physical findings are not very specific. A recent study by Cushing confirms the difficulty physicians have in identifying a specific anatomic focus for respiratory symptoms or signs [34]. Respiratory distress is not difficult to determine, but location of the focus is. Nasal flare, accessory muscle pull, intercostal retraction, cyanosis, hyperpnea, and abdominal breathing suggest extraordinary effort to ventilate. Most respiratory infections are viral, systemic, and nonspecific. Even if not complicated by bacteria, these infections create physical signs and symptoms that sug-

gest laryngeal, tracheal, bronchial, and alveolar involvement. RSV, parainfluenza, and influenza are good examples of viral illnesses that are difficult to localize. Bacterial infections, such as epiglottitis and pneumonia, are easier to localize.

Epiglottitis. Epiglottitis is rare, but it is a potentially lethal infection caused by *H. influenzae*. Onset is rapid, and the child is toxic (a score on the Yale Observation Scale >12) and febrile (>39°C). Respiratory distress is classically indicated by a tendency to sit up, lean forward, and concentrate on breathing, as well as salivation and refusal to swallow. The presentation may not always be classic [35].

The most important detail that the practitioner must remember is that a child with epiglottitis is subject to acute laryngospasm and apnea if disturbed. In the emergency department setting the child should be allowed to remain in the parents' care in a comfortable position and given by oxygen mask. The child is then examined as gently as possible by an experienced physician with the assistance of an anesthesiologist or an intensivist prepared to intubate the child and proceed with fluid and antibiotic therapy (ceftriaxone 50 mg/kg dose IV). If an operating room is available expeditiously, it is the best area to examine the child so that maximum resources are available for managing the airway. The child must be hospitalized.

There is a current argument for a less aggressive way to handle such a patient, but caution is necessary [36]. If the infection is seen early or is a laryngotracheal infection, it may be possible to examine the child while he/she is sitting up to rule out a large, swollen, red epiglottis. It is vital that the emergency department physician understand the hazards of epiglottitis. The approach taken in each specific episode is controversial and depends on the experience of the physician and what resources are immediately available to deal with the problem [35–37]. The role of a radiologic confirmation is reserved for the questionable case and to rule out a foreign body. If it appears that only an x-ray is needed, then the condition is not epiglottitis. (See also Chap. 22.)

Croup/Laryngotracheitis. Croup is the common name for laryngotracheitis. Laryngotracheal swelling is a nonspecific response to infection (most

likely parainfluenza or adenovirus) and ambient air problems such as smoking and allergic insult. Affected infants react with a croupy, upper-airway-reactive, respiratory distress sequence often referred to as spasmodic croup. These infants usually become allergic, even asthmatic. For an emergency department provider the difficulty is that this is the first and perhaps only time he or she sees this child, so the approach is more generic.

The infant is brought to the emergency department sometimes having had mild coryza for several days but often with no previous symptoms. The infant often wakes the parents with a crowing, brassy, dry, high-pitched cough associated with irritability, mild distress, and mild toxicity (a score on the Yale Observation Scale <12). Because these symptoms and signs would scare any parent, the emergency department is often the caregiver's first response. The emergency department physician should observe the child for several hours. The symptoms and signs if mild, will decrease or remain stable. Discharge therapy includes fluids, use of a cold humidifier, and a short course of steroids (prednisone 2 mg/kg ÷ q12h PO for 3 days).

The child in moderate distress will be febrile (low grade) and have respiratory distress with hyperpnea, persistent nasal flare, intercostal retractions, tachycardia, but an oxygen saturation of less than 90. Racemic epinephrine nebulization (0.05 ml/kg/dose diluted in 3 ml of saline q2h) should be instituted. A starter dose of steroids and oxygen also should be given. The child should be observed for 6–12 hours in the emergency department observation area or admitted. If the child is in severe distress, treatment is a racemic epinephrine nebulization *with caution*, to prevent laryngospasm and in anticipation of possible intubation. The child then should be admitted to a critical care area. An AP and lateral examination of the neck will confirm the diagnosis of subglottic swelling with the steeple sign and the absence of a foreign body. (See also Chap. 22.)

Retropharyngeal Abscess. The observation of fever (>39.0°C), drooling, hyperextension of neck, toxicity (a score on the Yale Observation Scale >12), and a WBC count greater than 15,000/μl suggests retropharyngeal abscess, which is common during this age [38]. As in epiglottitis and laryngotracheitis a careful examination with preparation for intubation is the rule. The abscess appears on a lateral soft tissue neck radiologic examination as widening of the prevertebral space. Because it is difficult to visualize the abscess by a tongue blade exam, all procedures, including x-ray, should be done by a team comprising an otolaryngologist, an anesthesiologist, and an emergency department physician who is prepared to incise and drain the compromising mass. (See Chap. 21.)

Pneumonia. Fever, respiratory grunt, productive cough, tachypnea, and toxicity (a score on the Yale Observation Scale >12) associated with lower respiratory signs of rales, rhonchi, and chest squeaks suggest an alveolar, pulmonary infection. In children this age it is difficult to differentiate viral from bacterial etiology unless the radiologic exam reveals particulars such as a segmented infiltrate. A familial history of upper respiratory infection or croup and wheezing in the child several days prior to acute onset usually are associated with a viral pneumonia. Pleural effusions, high toxicity rating, and splinting of the chest with respirations suggest bacterial origin. More often than not, the emergency department physician will make the decision of whether the origin is viral or bacterial on the basis of all findings. If the degree of illness mandates hospitalization, the physician should not hesitate to obtain cultures (sputum, blood, and urine) or to start antibiotics.

The most common etiology of bacterial pneumonias is pneumococcus, *H. influenzae*, and *S. aureus*. In children this age all these bacteria are capable of causing sepsis, empyema, and multisystem foci. The etiology of viral pneumonias is RSV, adenovirus, parainfluenza 1, 2, and 3, and influenza A and B.

Hospitalization should be seriously considered if respiratory distress is severe (tachypnea of 40+, splinting with respirations, oxygen saturation of <90%, arterial gases of increased pH, PO_2 less than 74% torr, and PCO_2 greater than 40 torr) and either of the following: (1) toxicity rating on the Yale Observation Scale is 16 or more, or (2) the WBC count is greater than 15,000 μl with 10,000 or more PMN/μl, or more than 500 bands/μl, and the sedimentation rate greater than 30 mm/hr.

If ambulatory care is the decision, but bacterial pneumonia still is highly suspected, parenteral therapy (ceftriaxone 50 mg/kg IM or IV) is encouraged for emergency department patients to ensure adequate therapy in light of their compliance or ability to buy oral medication. Oral antibiotics should be begun within 12 hours (amoxicillin or Augmentin 40 mg/kg ÷ q8h PO for 10 days) with follow-up arrangements in 24 hours. (See Chap. 24.)

Foreign-Body Aspiration Pneumonia. An important differential of pneumonia at this age is foreign-body aspiration pneumonia. Any lower respiratory infection workup should include consideration of this diagnosis. A history of the infant choking on something or persistent coughing as much as a month prior to the acute onset of symptoms should alert the emergency department physician. If such an infection is a possibility, a chest radiologic examination should be performed (right and left decubitus) to observe hyperinflation on the side of the obstructed bronchus. It also should include a hot-light examination for foreign bodies, which are usually radiolucent but may produce suggestible shadows and airway impingement. A highly suspect patient should be referred for a bronchoscopy.

APPENDICITIS

Appendicitis is an infection that usually occurs in childhood or early adulthood. The younger the child the more unusual it is to have a classic presentation. Consequently the perforation rate is high. If the diagnosis is not made or is delayed, perforation is expensive, debilitating, and life threatening and leads to long-term sequelae. If there is doubt, the child should be admitted to an observation ward or monitored for any signs of deterioration by telephone at home.

The symptoms are nonspecific and include vomiting, loose stools, and reluctance to play or to move. The signs of abdominal infection or peritoneal irritation are a mild fever (<38.5°C), moderate toxicity (a score on the Yale Observation Scale >12), anorexia, reluctance to move around, quiet temperament, and abdominal tenderness on examination. The child's abdominal discomfort is not in the classic location of the right lower quadrant (RLQ) unless the child is examined while asleep.

In children of this age group a rectal examination adds little value to the information best obtained by radiologic examination (fecalith and RLQ air stasis) or ultrasound (abscess, fecalith, or fluid/swelling suggestion in RLQ) exams. A rectal exam also is disturbing to the infant and the parents as well. A surgical consultation and subsequent team management toward resolution by surgery is the treatment plan. (See Chap. 27.)

ACUTE GASTROENTERITIS

In this age group, the full assault of gastrointestinal pathogens make acute gastroenteritis (AGE) one of the most common pediatric diseases; indeed, it is the bread and butter of day-to-day practice. Emergency department providers are presented with such a full array and degree of infection that a list of causes (Table 14-7) is appropriate for this group of infections. The discussion here remains more general to some of the causes and to therapy.

Day care, crowding, universal prevalence, and the vulnerability to infections create the situation for such an array and frequency. The tendency for children to react quickly to such infections with vomiting and diarrhea is the reason for parental concern, and the emergency department physician needs to assess dehydration and toxicity as the fundamental problems no matter what the cause. Clinical signs and symptoms of dehydration are described in the discussion of gastrointestinal complaints in infants from 2 weeks to 2 months and in Table 14-4.

For the patient with more than 10% dehydration, parenteral access (either an IV or an interosseous route) is needed immediately. The parenteral treatment for more than 10% dehydration is rapid injection of 20 ml/kg of normal saline and preparation to administer a similar bolus as soon as possible within 20 minutes.

The infant who is mildly (<5%) or moderately (<10%) dehydrated is treated by one of three methods:

1. An intravenous bolus of normal saline 20 ml/kg followed by carefully monitored fluids sufficient to replace lost fluids. This treatment is maintained over 8 hours depending on urine output and recovery until the child is able to sustain oral fluid intake.

2. Nasogastric intubation with fluid administered in a constant rate sufficient to replace calculated fluid loss; maintained over eight hours. The fluid is normal saline 20 ml/kg in the first 20 minutes, then an oral commercial replacement fluid of 50 mg/l sodium, 20 mg/l potassium, and 30 mg/l bicarbonate and a glucose concentration, such as Pedialyte, of 2%–3%.

3. Oral hydration strategy whereby the child takes a bottle or cup of water sufficient to provide 20 ml/kg within the first 20 minutes and then sustains an intake over the next 8 hours to replace loss plus maintenance of a similar solution mentioned in method 2, above.

The preference is to have infants who are less than 10% dehydrated rehydrate themselves and to monitor them closely for oral intake, stool frequency, appearance, and urinary output within the first 4 hours.

Once the patient has been stabilized, further workup leads to reasonable assessment of the etiology. A complete physical exam determines whether there is a focus, such as otitis media or UTI, that has created a diarrhea. The stool should be examined visually for smell, color, blood for a shigella infection, and mucus for a *Campylobacter* infection. A microscopic examination with 10% methylene blue differentiates an invasive, bacterial colitis with WBCs (>5 cells per high-power field) from a noninvasive, viral infection with no WBCs (<5 cells per high-power field) [29]. More specific therapy is determined by etiology (see Table 14-7 and Chap. 25). Fluoroquinolones, which are being used extensively in adults to treat bacterial diarrhea, are not approved in children.

HEPATITIS

Viral hepatitis, whether A or B, is characterized by nonspecific signs and symptoms of anorexia, nausea, vomiting, and abdominal discomfort. The patient is usually anicteric. In general the younger the child the more benign the illness. The diagnosis is possible if the emergency department physician obtains an exposure history, identifies a mildly enlarged and tender liver, and finds no other cause for problems. The habit of obtaining a urine sample for unexplained illnesses will reveal bilirubin and urobilinogen and make the diagnosis possible. Spe-

Table 14-7. Causes, characteristics, and treatment of acute enteritis

Cause	Stool exam	Symptoms	Treatment
Bacterial Salmonella	Liquid, foul, positive for WBCs, positive for gross or occult blood	Fever, abdominal pain	None unless signs of extraintestinal infection or sepsis; ampicillin, amoxicillin, trimethoprim-sulfamethoxazole
Shigella	Small, grossly bloody, frequent	Fever, tenesmus, abdominal pain	None or trimethoprim-sulfamethoxazole
Campylobacter jejuni	Gross blood and mucus in streaks	Few systemic symptoms	None or erythromycin
Yersinia enterocolitica	Liquid, foul, positive for WBCs, positive for gross or occult blood	Fever, abdominal pain	None effective for enteric disease
Aeromonas hydrophila	Watery; mild to moderate	Nausea, vomiting; probably enterotoxin-mediated	Usually self-limited; trimethoprim-sulfamethoxazole
Plesiomonas shigelloides	Watery	Nausea, vomiting; possible enterotoxin	Usually self-limited; trimethoprim-sulfamethoxazole
Escherichia coli Invasive	Small, grossly bloody, positive for WBCs	Abdominal pain, tenesmus	Trimethoprim-sulfamethoxazole; ampicillin; gentamycin
Enterotoxic	Liquid, green, voluminous	Nausea, vomiting; heat labile toxin-mediated	Usually self-limited
Enteropathogenic	Liquid, green, voluminous	Nausea, vomiting; adherence factors important	Usually self-limited
Hemorrhagic serotype 0157:H7	Small, grossly bloody, positive for WBCs	Fever, tenesmus; organism produces shigella-type toxin; may cause hemolytic-uremic syndrome	Trimethoprim-sulfamethoxazole

	Stool	Clinical features	Treatment
Viral			
Rotavirus	Liquid, few WBCs	Vomiting, nausea	None; fluid management
Others: Norwalk, enteric adenovirus, enteroviruses	Liquid, few WBCs	Vomiting, nausea	None; fluid management
Parasitic			
Giardia lamblia	Very foul, liquid, negative for blood, negative for WBCs; cysts present in 30%–60%	Vomiting, nausea, abdominal distension, gas	Furazolidone (5 mg/kg/d for 7 days), metronidazole (15 mg/kg/d for 5 days), or quinacrine (6 mg/kg/d for 5 days)
Entamoeba histolytica	Blood and mucus, trophozoites on fresh stool exam	Abdominal pain, tenesmus	Metronidazole (35–50 mg/kg/d for 10 days)
Cryptosporidium	Watery or bloody, depending on site of infestation	Incidence often in immunodeficient patients but occasionally in healthy children; history of animal exposure	Spiramycin or metronidazole may be tried
Other Toxic Diarrheas			
Clostridium difficile	Bloody, positive for WBCs, cytotoxin present in stool	Abdominal pain, fever; history of prior antibiotic use is typical	Vancomycin (30–40 mg/kg/d for 7 days), metronidazole (25 mg/kg/d for 7 days), oral bacitracin (1500 U/kg/d for 7 days)
Staphylococcus aureus	Explosive, watery, positive for WBCs	Nausea, vomiting, history of group outbreaks	Fluid management
Clostridium perfringens	Explosive, watery, positive for WBCs	Vomiting; abrupt onset; history of meat ingestion	Fluid management

Source: Sondheimer J, Silverman A. In WE Hathaway et al. (eds.), Current Pediatric Diagnosis and Treatment (10th ed.). East Norwalk, CT: Appleton & Lange, 1991. P. 551. Used with permission.

cific liver function tests and antibody titers will clarify the diagnosis.

Hospitalization for hepatitis is seldom necessary for children. Even if dehydration is a problem, it is often mild enough to treat with oral or intravenous fluids in the emergency department. Toxicity is rare, but the Yale Observation Scale is a useful indication for hospitalization. A score on the Yale Observation Scale of 16 or more (see Table 14-1) is reason to hospitalize. *Each case of hepatitis must be reported to the state health department.* (See Chap. 26.)

PYOGENIC AND AMOEBIC LIVER ABSCESS

Although rare two nonviral "hepatitides," pyogenic and amoebic liver abscesses, must be mentioned. Both appear to be on the increase due to immunosuppressive and anti-inflammatory agents and international travel in endemic areas such as Asia and Central America. These liver abscesses are characterized by toxicity (a score on the Yale Observation Scale of 12–16), high fever, and abdominal pain. Laboratory data suggest a septic process, with a WBC count of 15,000 or more with more than 10,000 PMNs µl, a sedimentation rate greater than 30 mm/hr, and ketonuria. An ultrasound can identify definitive lesions, particularly in the right lobe of the liver. Hospitalization for immediate definitive therapy is required for these very threatening, septic conditions. (See Chap. 26.)

UTI

Although not as common in children 12–36 months, UTIs are a threat because there is a tendency to overlook, even discount, the presence of an infection, resulting in recurrent infections caused by undiagnosed anatomical problems. These infections are characterized by fever, abdominal discomfort, nausea, and anorexia. Seldom at this age does the child complain of back pain or dysuria. A child who is toilet trained and who reverts to enuresis or wetting is a suspect for UTI. Parents frequently complain of a smelly urine.

A urinalysis on an otherwise unexplained febrile, toxic (a score on the Yale Observation Scale ≥12) child will confirm the diagnosis. It is possible to obtain a clean-catch urine sample in the older child, but in the younger, untrained infant it is more difficult. Urine obtained by a carefully applied urine bag in place no longer than 2 hours is dependable for culture and definitive findings of WBCs, bacteria, nitrates, and protein. If there is doubt about the urine obtained by a bag or a clean catch, then urine obtained by catheterization or a bladder tap should be used. Once urine has been obtained and cultures are pending, treatment is directed at the most common organism, *E. coli*, with amoxicillin (40 mg/kg/day ÷ q8h) for 10 days. Hospitalization is considered for pyelonephritis if there is toxicity (a score on the Yale Observation Scale ≥16), a WBC count of greater than 15,000/µl, or greater than 10,000 PMNs/µl, fever (≥39.5°C), WBC casts in the urine, and bacteria noted on a microscopic examination of an unspun specimen [27].

The infant with a UTI must have a renal ultrasound. This simple procedure reveals any major anatomical distortion of the renal system and prevents irreversible destruction of renal tissue. The emergency department physician must arrange this ultrasound or ascertain that it will be done by the primary physician.

OSTEOMYELITIS/SEPTIC ARTHRITIS

The two categories of osteomyelitis and septic arthritis are discussed together because they are difficult to differentiate at this age in the emergency department setting and also because they often occur simultaneously. The most frequent infecting organism is *H. influenzae*, but occasionally *S. aureus* and *S. pneumoniae* are responsible in this age group [39]. A child who limps, has pain on movement, doesn't want to bear weight, has a fever, and is irritable and anorexic is a candidate for a diagnosis of septic joint or osteomyelitis. The exact joint, especially a hip or an intervertebral disk, is difficult to determine. An examination that reveals swelling, redness, and warmth will identify the site, but such findings are not apparent when a hip or an intervertebral disk is involved.

Laboratory data of a WBC count of 15,000 or more with 10,000 PMNs µl and a sedimentation rate 30 mm/hr or more are suggestive enough to require an x-ray of all joints on both sides and the vertebrae to detect a joint space swelling, blurred fat-line asymmetry, or frank erosion of bone indicative of infection. A radioisotope scan that reveals hot spots is important in suggesting the location of infection. A febrile, limping child should be scanned. Seldom is trauma or even tenosynovitis a reason for limping or pain on motion in a febrile child with an elevated WBC count and sedimentation rate. Septic joints are destructive in a growing child. Joint aspiration by an experienced physician is diagnostic and necessary when the radiologic picture is questionable and the scan is not immediately available. Hospitalization is absolutely necessary because joint exploration is necessary to relieve pressure by drainage, particularly in the hip. (See Chap. 33.)

EXANTHEMS

Every emergency department physician eventually becomes an expert in exanthems because parents want immediate assistance when they notice a rash. Some of these exanthems are discussed elsewhere in this text (see Chap. 9); others simply must be appreciated by experience and review of Table 14-8.

Ecchymotic/Hemorrhagic Rashes. For an emergency department physician the most important rash to identify is that of *N. meningitides*. This rash is ecchymotic and hemorrhagic and thus does not blanch on pressure. The nonblanching petechial, ecchymotic, or hemorrhagic rash in a febrile, irritable child should be treated quickly to avoid the inevitable disseminated intravascular coagulation so common to meningococcemia. Intravenous access and IV therapy (penicillin G 500–1000U/kg/day ÷ q4–6h) should be followed by hospitalization.

Because *H. influenzae* and occasionally pneumococcus cause a similar rash to meningococcus, ceftriaxone (100 mg/kg/d ÷ q12h) should be added until cultures confirm the infection. (See Chap. 9.)

Red Rashes. Red rashes blanch and offer a fairly reliable sequential history, distribution, and characteristic appearance to allow a differential, as can be seen in Table 14-8. Generally no treatment is necessary. Seldom are these children so toxic that they require hospitalization, except for Kawasaki disease, toxic shock syndrome, leptospirosis, or scarlet fever.

One rash worth more discussion is erythema multiforme. Erythema multiforme is an id reaction associated with infections, usually viral. It is associated with high fevers (>39°C), mild toxicity (a score on the Yale Observation Scale of 12–16), and a perplexing rash that is red, intermittent, and in multiple forms, including target lesions over the whole body. The lesions do not itch and are not the weals and flares of an allergic reaction. For the emergency department physician the rash is particularly aggravating for five reasons: (1) the child seems ill, but no focus is apparent; (2) the rash is so bizarre that the parents are not easily reassured; (3) the swelling of the rash may involve the joints; (4) treatment is not effective in eliminating the rash; and (5) the illness persists for several weeks.

The rash is so classic and complications and bacterial infections are so rare that a comprehensive history, and complete physical examination, and a discussion of the etiology and the course of the rash should be sufficient to reassure the parents. Treatment consists of antifever therapy and an antihistamine, which seems to offer some relief.

Vesicular Rashes. In children 12–36 months vesicular rashes commonly are caused by varicella, herpes zoster, and herpes simplex. Varicella is best recognized as a generalized vesicular rash over the whole body, but it can present as a febrile illness requiring a high index of suspicion. A meticulous examination of the scalp, neck, and oral mucosa can lead to discovery of early lesions. Small, red, papular-vesicular lesions of the skin and herpetic-like lesions of the mucosa herald the more generalized lesions by 24–48 hours. Advice to parents includes reassurance, acetaminophen, frequent baths for skin care, and antihistamines for itching. Aspirin is not given, to avoid Reye's syndrome. If the patient is immunosuppressed, hospitalization and acyclovir treatment are indicated.

Cutaneous herpes simplex and zoster are infrequent infections at this age. When they do occur, the lesions typically are a cluster of vesicular lesions anywhere on the body but most frequently on the face and the trunk.

Pustular Rashes. Pustular, red or often yellow, crusting, weeping lesions suggest group A beta-hemolytic streptococcus impetigo. Most often a summertime infection, it is distributed anywhere on the body and is frequent at this age. Although local antibiotics have been developed for such le-

Table 14-8. Red rashes in children

Disease	Incubation period (days)	Prodrome	Rash	Laboratory test results	Comments, other diagnostic features
Measles	9–14	Cough, rhinitis, conjunctivitis	Maculopapular; face to extremities; lasts 7–10 days; Koplik's spots	Leukopenia	Toxic. Bright red rash becomes confluent, may desquamate.
Rubella	14–21	Usually none	Mild maculopapular; rapid spread face to extremities; gone by day 4	Normal or leukopenia	Postauricular, occipital adenopathy common. Polyarthralgia in some older girls. Mild clinical illness.
Roseola (exanthem subitum)	10–14	Fever (3–4 days)	Pink, macular rash occurs at end of illness; transient	Normal	Fever often high, disappears when rash develops; child appears well. Usually occurs in children 6–24 months of age.
Erythema infectiosum	13–18	None	Erythematous "slapped" cheeks; then reticular rash on extremities, trunk	Normal; (reticulocytopenia)	Rash may reappear over weeks, especially with exposure to heat, sunlight. May cause arthralgia/arthritis, usually in older children or adults. Red cell maturation arrest in children with chronic hemolysis can cause aplastic crisis.
Enterovirus	2–7	Variable fever, chills, myalgia, sore throat	Usually macular, maculopapular on trunk or palms, soles; vesicles; petechiae also seen	Variable	Varied rashes may resemble those of many other infections. Pharyngeal or hand-foot-mouth vesicles with certain coxsackie A types.

Streptococcal scarlet fever	1–7	Fever, abdominal pain, headache, sore throat	Diffuse erythema, "sandpaper" texture; neck, axillae, inguinal areas; spreads to rest of body; desquamates 7–14 days	Leukocytosis; positive group A streptococcus culture of throat or wound	Strawberry tongue, red pharynx with or without exudate. Eyes, perioral area, palms, and soles spared. Pastia's lines. Brief prodrome. Mild variant, scarlatina. Usually occurs in children 2–10 years of age.
Staphylococcal scarlet fever	1–7	Variable fever	Diffuse erythroderma; resembles streptococcal scarlet fever except eyes may be hyperemic, no coated "strawberry" tongue, pharynx spared	Variable leukocytosis if infected	Focal S. aureus infection may be present.
Staph scalded skin	Variable	Irritability, absent to low fever	Painful erythroderma, followed in 1–2 days by dry cracking around eyes, mouth; bullae form with friction (Nikolsky's sign)	Normal if colonized only by staph; leukocytosis and sometimes bacteremia if infected	Normal pharynx. Look for focal staph infection. Usually occurs in infants.
Toxic shock syndrome	Variable	Fever, myalgia headache, diarrhea, vomiting	Nontender erythroderma; red eyes, palms, soles, pharynx, lips	Leukocytosis; abnormal liver enzymes, coagulation tests; proteinuria	S. aureus infection (especially vaginal during menses), multiorgan involvement. Swollen hands, feet. Hypotension or shock.
Erythema multiforme	—	Usually none or related to underlying cause	Discrete, red maculopapular lesions; symmetric, distal, palms and soles; target lesions classic	Normal or eosinophilia	Reaction to drugs (especially sulfas) or infectious agents. Urticaria, arthralgia also seen.

Table 14-8. (continued)

Disease	Incubation period (days)	Prodrome	Rash	Laboratory test results	Comments, other diagnostic features
Stevens-Johnson syndrome	—	Pharyngitis, conjunctivitis, fever, malaise	Bullous erythema multiforme; may slough in large areas; hemorrhagic lips; purulent conjunctivitis	Leukocytosis	Classic precipitants are drugs (especially sulfas); *Mycoplasma pneumoniae* infections. Pneumonitis and urethritis also seen.
Drug allergy	—	No fever or fever, myalgia, pruritus	Macular, maculopapular, urticarial, or erythroderma	Leukopenia, eosinophilia	Rash variable. Severe reactions may resemble measles, scarlet fever; adenopathy, hepatosplenomegaly, marked toxicity possible.
Kawaski syndrome	Unknown	Fever, cervical adenopathy, irritability	Polymorphous (may be erythroderma) on trunk and extremities; red palms and soles, lips, tongue, pharynx	Leukocytosis, thrombocytosis, elevated ESR; negative cultures and streptococcal serology	Swollen hands, feet; prolonged illness; bulbar hyperemia; uveitis; no response to antibiotics. Vasculitis and aneurysms of coronary and other arteries occur.
Leptospirosis	4–19	Fever, myalgia, chills	Variable erythroderma	Leukocytosis; hematuria, proteinuria; hyperbilirubinemia	Conjunctivitis; toxic. Hepatitis, aseptic meningitis may be seen. Rodent, dog contact.

Source: Paisley W, Levin J. Infections viral and rickettsial. In WE Hathaway et al. (eds.). *Current Pediatric Diagnosis and Treatment* (10th ed.). East Norwalk CT: Appleton & Lange, 1991. P. 821. Used with permission.

Table 14-9. Dosages for antibiotic therapy of selected infections in children older than 2 months of age

Antibiotic	Dosages	Special Circumstances
Amoxicillin	40 mg/kg/d ÷ q8 PO/IV	
Ampicillin	200 mg/kg/d ÷ q6h IV	Bacterial meningitis
Amoxicillin-clavulonate	40 mg/kg/d ÷ q8h PO	
Ceftriaxone	100 mg/kg/d ÷ q12h IV	Sepsis, or bacterial meningitis, or ecchymotic/hemorrhagic rash
	50 mg/kg/d q24h IV/IM	Other infections
Cefotaxime	200 mg/kg/d ÷ q6h IV	Bacterial meningitis
	150 mg/kg/d ÷ q6h IV	Other infections
Cefuroxime	100 mg/kg/d ÷ q6h IV	Sepsis or other infections
	75 mg/kg/d ÷ q8h IV	
Chloramphenicol	100 mg/kg ÷ q6h IV	
Dexamethasone	15 mg/kg/d ÷ q6h IV	
Erythromycin	40 mg/kg/d ÷ q6h PO	
Erythromycin-sulfisoxazole	50 mg erythromycin/150 mg sulfisoxazole/kg/d ÷ q6h PO	
Gentamicin	2 mg/kg/d ÷ q8hr IM/IV	
Methicillin	200–300 mg/kg/d ÷ q4–6 hr IM/IV	
Penicillin		
Benzathine penicillin	300,000 units <10 kg, one dose IM	
	600,000 units 10–15 kg, one dose IM	
	900,000 units >15 kg, one dose IM	
Penicillin G	100,000 U/kg 1 ÷ q4–6 h	IV ecchymotic/hemorrhagic rash or other infections
	50,000 U/kg/d ÷ q6h PO or IM	
Penicillin V	50–75 mg/kg/d ÷ q6h PO	
Trimethoprium-sulfamethoxazole	20 mg TMP, 100 mg SMX/kg/d ÷ q12h PO	

sions, systemic penicillin (penicillin V 125–250 mg q6h PO for 10 days) is still the most dependable therapy to avoid lymphadenitis and cellulitis.

References

1. Klugman R. Fetal and neonatal medicine. In R Behrman, R Klugman (eds.), *Nelson Essentials of Pediatrics*. Philadelphia: Saunders, 1990. Pp. 153–206.
2. Smith J. Big differences in little people. *Am J Nurs* 88(2):459, 1988.
3. Schmit BD. *Pediatric Telephone Advice*. Boston: Little, Brown,
4. Smilkstein G. The pediatric lap examination. *J Fam Pract* 4:743, 1977.
5. McCarthy PL et al. Predictive value of abnormal physical examination findings in ill-appearing and well-appearing febrile children. *Pediatrics* 76(2):167, 1985.
6. Baker MD, Avner JR, Bill LM. Failure of infant observation scales in detecting serious illness in febrile, 4–8 week old infants. *Pediatrics*. 85(6):1040, 1990.
7. Cook C, Heidt J. *Assuring Quality Out-Patient Care for Children*. New York: Oxford Univ. Press, 1988. Pp. 39–64.
8. Bedell SE, Bush BT. Erythrocyte sedimentation rate: from folklore to facts. *Am J Med* 78:1001, 1985.
9. McCarthy P, Jekel JF, Dolan TF. Temperature greater than or equal to 40° in children less than 24 months of age: a prospective study. *Pediatrics* 59 (5):663, 1977.
10. Editors: Taking temperatures: the changing state of the art. *Contemp Pediatr* 22, 1985.
11. Kenney RD et al. Evaluation of an infrared tympanic

membrane thermometer in pediatric patients. *Pediatrics* 85(5):854, 1990.

12. Kruse J. Fever in children. *Ann Fam Physician* 37(2):127, 1988.

13. Lorin MI. Is fever a friend or a foe? *Contemp Pediatr* 35, 1986.

14. Putto A, Ruuskanen O, Meurman O. Fever in respiratory virus infections. *AJDC* 140:1159, 1986.

15. Baker MD, Forsarelli PD, Carpenter RD. Childhood fever: correlation of diagnosis with temperature response to acetaminophen. *Pediatrics* 80(3):315, 1987.

16. Berkowitz CD et al. Fever in infants less than two months of age: spectrum of disease and predictors of outcome. *Pediatr Emerg Care* 1(3):131, 1985.

17. Frenkel LD, Multicenter Ceftriaxone Pediatric Study Group. Once-daily administration of ceftriaxone for the treatment of selected serious bacterial infections in children. *Pediatrics* 82(3):486, 1988.

18. Saavedra JM et al. Capillary refilling (skin turgor) in the assessment of dehydration. *AJDC* 145:296, 1991.

19. Rowe PG. *The Harriet Lane Handbook, Johns Hopkins Hospital* (11th ed.). Baltimore: Year Book Medical Publications, 1987. P. 233.

20. Shaw KN, Bell LM, Sherman NH. Outpatient assessment of infants with bronchiolitis. *AJDC* 145:151, 1991.

21. Crain EF, Gershel JC. Urinary tract infections in febrile infants younger than 8 weeks of age. *Pediatrics* 86(3):363, 1990.

22. Bluestone DC, Klein JO. *Otitis Media in Infants and Children*. Philadelphia: Saunders, 1988. Pp. 121–201.

23. Kohl S, Pickering LK. Infectious diseases. In RE Behrman, R Klugman (eds.), *Nelson Essentials of Pediatrics*. Philadelphia: Saunders, 1990. Pp. 284–376.

24. McGowan JE et al. Bacteremia in febrile children seen in a "walk-in" pediatric clinic. *N Engl J Med* 288(25):1309, 1973.

25. Kramer MS, Lane DA, Mills EL. Should blood culture be obtained in the evaluation of young febrile children without evident focus of bacterial infection? A decision analysis of diagnostic management strategies. *Pediatrics* 84(1):18, 1989.

26. Woods ER et al. Bacteremia in an ambulatory setting: improved outcome in children treated with antibiotics. *AJDC* 144:1195, 1990.

27. Pryles CV, Lislik B. Laboratory diagnosis of urinary tract infection, *Pediatr Clin North Am* 18(1):233, 1971.

28. Lebel MH et al. Dexamethasone therapy for bacterial meningitis. *N Engl J Med* 319(15):964, 1988.

29. DeWitt TG, Humphrey KF, McCarthy P. Clinical predictors of acute bacterial diarrhea in young children. *Pediatrics* 76(5):551, 1985.

30. Margolis PA et al. Effects of unrestricted diet on mild infantile diarrhea. *AJDC* 144:162, 1990.

31. Consensus Development Panel: National Institutes of Health. Febrile seizures: long term management of children with fever-associated seizures. *Pediatrics* 66:1009–12, 1980.

32. Smith TF, O'Day D, Wright PF. Clinical implications of preseptal (periorbital) cellulitis in childhood. *Pediatrics* 62(6):1006, 1978.

33. Gellady AM, Shedman SJ, Ayoub EM. Periorbital and orbital cellulitis in children. *Pediatrics* 61(2):272, 1978.

34. Cushing A. Personal communication. 1991.

35. Mauro RD, Poole SR, Lockhart CH. Differentiation of epiglottitis from laryngotracheitis in the child with stridor. *AJDC* 142:679, 1988.

36. Fulginiti VA. Acute supraglottitis (epiglottitis): to look or not? *AJDC* 142:597, 1988.

37. The Pediatric Forum. Oropharyngeal examination for suspected epiglottitis. *AJDC* 142:1261, 1988.

38. McCook TA, Feldman AH. Retropharyngeal masses in the infant and young children. *AJDC* 133:41, 1979.

39. Faden H, Grossi M. Acute osteomyelitis in children, reassessment of etiologic agents and their clinical characteristics. *AJDC* 145:65, 1991.

15

Infection in the Elderly

ROBERT L. RHYNE
RICHARD J. ROCHE

As the population in the United States ages, more health care resources will be devoted to the elderly [1], and emergency departments can expect to see a larger number of acutely ill elderly persons. In 1989 12.5% of the population was 65 or older; by the year 2020 this figure is expected to be 18% [2, 3]. Infections account for a large proportion of the problems that bring elderly people to the emergency department. Pneumonia and influenza are the fifth leading cause of death in people 65 years of age and older [1], and infectious diseases are the leading cause of hospitalization in frail elderly people [4].

Chronic medical conditions and functional debility are also associated with an increased risk of infection in the elderly. The pathophysiology of this increased risk has not been fully explained, but associated factors include multiple comorbid chronic conditions, malnutrition, immobility, institutionalization, and urinary incontinence and catheterization. Infections in institutionalized elderly are often caused by different organisms than community acquired infections and therefore need to be treated as hospital acquired, or nosocomial, infections. Although the usual pathogens associated with a given source of infection usually hold true for the elderly, the risk of aerobic gram-negative bacillary infection is increased [4].

Generalized nonspecific signs and symptoms may be the only clinical findings associated with a serious infection. The presentation may range from a slight change in functional or mental status to obtundation or delirium. Thus, assessment of functional and mental status and determination of functional status prior to the presenting illness become very important in the emergency department. Most elderly people respond to bacterial infections with fever, inflammation, purulence, and leukocytosis, but many have a blunted febrile response and an inability to mount a leukocytosis. This atypical clinical presentation of infectious disease often makes diagnosis and treatment difficult and can lead to misdiagnosis or delays in diagnosis and treatment [1, 4].

Treatment regimens should be based on the likely anatomic source of infection and the associated pathogens. The urinary tract, the lower respiratory tract, and the skin and soft tissue are the most common sources of systemic infections seen in the elderly [4]. Initial treatment often has to be empiric with broad-spectrum antibiotics that cover organisms from these anatomic sources, including anaerobes. Appropriate cultures and other test samples can be collected in the emergency department and subsequently used to guide therapeutic decisions.

The emergency department physician frequently must make treatment decisions for infected elderly patients in the presence of a high degree of uncertainty. Comorbid conditions and institutionalization can lead to infections with atypical pathogens, making those elements of the history very important. The healthy elder with an infection generally presents with clinical findings similar to those of younger adults, but in all elderly, because of age-related declines in organ reserve capacity, infections can quickly become fulminant. This chapter focuses on identifying those clinical uncertainties and quantifying, where possible, the issues related to the unique aspects of infections in elderly people.

Demographics and Epidemiology

The Aging of Our Society

Emergency departments should be interested in the elderly as a specific population because of the future impact this population is likely to have on emergency departments. The size of this population can be anticipated from demographic trends, the so-called "graying of America," and the patterns of illness experienced by this population. The proportion of the population 65 years and older will continue to increase throughout this and most of the twenty-first century as the post–World War II "baby boomers" move through old age. In 1980 those over 65 were 10.8% of the population; in 1989 they were 12.5%. By the year 2000, approximately 35 million, or 13%, of the people in this country will be over the age of 65 [2, 5, 6,], and that proportion is expected to increase to 19% by 2025 [2, 3].

The gain in average human life expectancy thus far in this century, about 26 years, is approximately equal to that seen in the previous 5000 years [7]. In 1900 the life expectancy at birth for the average U.S. citizen was 49 years; in 1988 it was 75.6 years. Likewise, in 1900 a person who lived to be 65 could expect to live approximately 12 more years; in 1987 the life expectancy at 65 was 17 years [8]. The fastest-growing segment of the population in the United States is the age group over 85.

The increasing longevity of our society can be attributed to decreasing infant mortality rates, better medical care, and improved public health mea-

sures. The age-adjusted mortality rates for all ages have been decreasing throughout this century but especially for those over the age of 80 years [3]. Because people are living longer, they are at increased risk for chronic debilitating diseases like arthritis, degenerative joint disease, atherosclerosis, and Alzheimer's dementia. Because of those conditions and increasing frailty with age, elderly people may find that they no longer can care for themselves. Approximately 7% of the U.S. elderly population now reside in long-term-care facilities. Elderly people who have debilitating diseases and who are institutionalized have a higher incidence of infections compared to elders who are healthier and more independent.

Morbidity and Mortality

Although the development of antibiotics to treat infectious diseases in the twentieth century has contributed to increasing longevity in this country [9], the elderly still suffer significant morbidity and mortality from infections [6]. The incidence of acute infections, except pneumonia, is actually lower among healthy, ambulatory, nonhospitalized elderly people than in younger people [1]. However, the elderly are at greater risk for severe complications when they do become infected. Bacterial infections often have a more fulminant course in this population. Their rates of hospitalization and death due to pneumonia are higher than those for younger adults. In 1983 their mortality rate due to pneumonia and influenza was 148 per 100,000 population [1]. Nosocomial infection rates among hospitalized patients are higher in the elderly for all types of infections.

Predisposing Factors

The higher incidence of infections and the resultant mortality rates in certain subgroups of the elderly are not necessarily due to age per se but are associated with decreased reserve capacity and preexisting medical conditions. These risk factors are multifactorial and have not yet been individually quantified [6]. The presence of chronic disease, malnutrition, urinary incontinence, and institutionalization are associated with a higher susceptibility to infections in the elderly [1, 4–7, 10]. The evidence is less convincing that senescence of the immune system by itself predisposes the elderly to infections. This section discusses a number of the more commonly considered conditions thought to predispose elderly people to infections.

Age

A number of changes attributed to the process of aging may result in an increased susceptibility to infection. The function of many organ systems is thought to diminish with age, including the pulmonary, renal, integument, gastrointestinal, and genitourinary organ systems. This decline often is not apparent in routine laboratory testing. As a result the reserve capacity, which normally allows a person or an organ system to handle stressors, diminishes with age, but the corresponding laboratory tests that indicate function remain in the normal range. Convincing evidence is lacking that these declines in function are significant risk factors for infection in the absence of chronic disease or functional impairment. It is more likely that the resultant decline in reserve capacity leads to a more fulminant disease course when the elderly are infected because they cannot react sufficiently to the stress that infections place on their organ systems. There are, however, some age-related processes that are thought to increase susceptibility to infection.

The aging respiratory system is characterized by a decrease in the tidal volume and the number of alveoli and by a diminished chest wall compliance and bronchiolar elasticity [1]. Also the efficiency of the pulmonary mucocillary clearance mechanism decreases with age. These changes, compounded by a diminished gag and cough reflex, impair the normal ability to clear infectious agents and increase the risk of aspiration and subsequent pneumonia.

Skin and subcutaneous tissue, which form an important barrier to infection, undergo numerous changes with aging. There is a decrease in the vasculature, the number of melanocytes, and the quantity of subcutaneous tissue. The susceptibility to injury from toxic and mechanical sources (e.g., ultraviolet light, drying, and cracking) is increased

[1]. The resultant thinning of the integument and the loss of functional capacity of the skin result in slower wound healing and a higher risk of bacterial invasion.

A combination of factors predispose the elderly to infections of the genitourinary tract [11]. Older women have less vaginal glycogen and a higher pH than younger women. Introital colonization, primarily by the gram-negative Enterobacteriaceae pathogens, is thereby increased. Elderly men have a decrease in prostatic secretions and an increased risk for prostatic calculi. There may be impaired bladder emptying secondary to outlet obstruction, drug side effects, or neurologic disorders. The longer time urine stays in the bladder, the higher the risk of infection.

With aging there also is a progressive loss of nephrons and a diminishing glomerular filtration rate (GFR). This decreasing renal function is important in the calculation of dosages of antimicrobial drugs but does not necessarily increase the risk of infection.

Immune Senescence

Older adults are thought to be more susceptible to infection than younger adults because of a decline in host defenses. However, the role of immune senescence contributing to a higher incidence of infections is controversial [12]. Within the immune system cell-mediated immunity appears to diminish more with age than humoral immunity. Some examples of clinical problems thought to reflect immune senescence with aging are the increased incidence of neoplastic processes, the increased incidence of infections, reactivation of viruses (herpes zoster), and the increased incidence of Mycobacterium tuberculosis infections [1].

The impairment in cell-mediated immunity is manifested clinically by skin-test anergy [12, 13]. In a longitudinal 8-year study of 273 healthy elderly volunteers in Albuquerque, New Mexico, 32% were initially anergic. Anergy predicted an increased relative risk in age-adjusted mortality of 1.89 with a 95% confidence interval of 0.94–3.79 [13]. The age-adjusted incidence rates of pneumonia were increased 2.23 times compared to elders who were not anergic (95% confidence interval of 0.64–7.75). The increased mortality rates could have been due to occult cancers and other diseases, but a causal relationship between anergy and infectious disease was not evident. Because anergy is the culmination of several complex immunological steps, it is useful to look at the cellular level of the system to describe where age-related defects might arise.

In the cell-mediated component of the immune system, there is an alteration in the distribution and function of T cells. Although the total number of lymphocytes is normal, only 50% are functionally competent in those over 65 years of age [14, 15]. There is a decreased number of mitogen-sensitive lymphocytes, and those that do respond to mitogen stimulation do not proliferate as vigorously [12]. The mechanism underlying the defect in cell-mediated immunity may be related to a decrease in CD8 suppressor cells and an increase in CD4 helper cells. The ability to secrete lymphokines (e.g., interleukin-II), as well as the generation and function of cytotoxic T cells, is altered [15]. The complement pathway, as well as the function and number of polymorphonuclear leukocytes, however, is normal.

The humoral arm of the immune system is affected to a lesser degree. Immunizations, such as the influenza and pneumococcal vaccines, result in less production of serum antibody in older subjects [5], perhaps because of a decrease in peripheral blood lymphocytes that contain immunoglobulin [16] or a failure of elderly subjects to maintain immunoglobulin levels [12]. The cellular defects in the humoral system may be due to alterations in function of B cells and both helper and suppressor T cells of older adults. Naturally occurring serum bactericidal antibody to *Haemophilus influenzae* declines with age and is lowest in the elderly [5, 16].

Nutrition

Normal changes in aging that affect nutritional state include a slowing of the basal metabolic rate, impaired senses of taste and smell, diminished appetite, and dental problems that make chewing difficult [17]. In healthy elderly volunteers aging is associated with a decreased caloric intake, a decline in lean muscle tissue, and a diminished amount of physical activity. Malnutrition does not occur as a part of the normal aging process.

Malnutrition can develop in the elderly for a variety of reasons that are usually related to disease states [17]. In addition to disease states psychological conditions and economic and social deprivation can also lead to deficiencies of caloric intake, vitamins, and trace minerals. Deficiencies of vitamin B-12, folate, pyridoxine, and zinc are also common. It is thought that these deficiencies lead to a blunting of the optimal immune response, which can contribute to an increased incidence of infections in malnourished elderly people, but a causal relationship has yet to be shown. It is not known if the susceptibility to infections in malnourished elders is due to a blunted immune system or some other condition associated with malnutrition.

Malnutrition is associated, however, with increased morbidity and mortality [17] and can be demonstrated in 35%–65% of hospitalized adults and in at least 50% of nursing home patients [18]. Protein-calorie malnutrition (PCM) leads to low albumin and absolute lymphocyte counts. A serum albumin of less than 2.5 g/dl is considered severe PCM; 2.5–3.0 g/dl, moderate; and 3.0–3.5, mild [18]. Likewise, a total absolute lymphocyte count of less than 800/µm indicates severe PCM; 800–1200/µm, moderate; and 1200–1500/µm, mild. PCM can also result in abnormal liver function tests, but these can also be an indicator of acute infection [19]. A reduced albumin and an elevated alkaline phosphatase have been shown to predict a poor prognosis in acute bacterial infections, but the presence of malnutrition can complicate the interpretation of these tests.

Medications

Medications can play a major role in predisposing elderly persons, who take the greatest number of medications, to infection. Agents with anticholinergic side effects such as antihistamines and some antidepressants [1] diminish secretions, thereby impairing normal clearance mechanisms. Immunosuppressants, like steroids and chemotherapeutic agents, can damage skin barriers, precipitate neutropenia, and impair granulocyte function and cell-mediated immunity. Two very common drugs, tobacco and alcohol, also alter the ability to resist infection [1].

Chronic Diseases and Impaired Functional Status

It has been estimated that more than 85% of elderly patients have one or more chronic diseases or degenerative processes, which increases susceptibility to infection [1]. In general chronic diseases disrupt integumental barriers, impair clearance mechanisms, compromise cellular responses, and decrease mobility. At least one chronic disease, diabetes mellitus, is known to impair the capacity of inflammatory cells to react to microorganisms [5, 20]. Chronic obstructive pulmonary disease (COPD) increases colonization with gram-negative aerobic bacteria and the risk of aspiration [21]. Benign prostatic hypertrophy predisposes men to urinary tract infections. Valvular disease such as aortic sclerosis increases the risk of subacute bacterial endocarditis, and peripheral vascular disease results in skin breakdown and stasis ulcers and renders the host more susceptible to gangrene and cellulitis. Other chronic diseases that are important determinants in causing infections include alcoholism, degenerative joint disease, hypertension, malignancy, ischemic heart disease, and dementia.

It is controversial whether the degree of disability alone correlates with the incidence of infection. A number of studies have shown that dementia, incontinence, and immobility predispose to infectious processes. However, a prospective study by Nicolle et al. demonstrated no correlation between mental status or mobility and the likelihood of infection [22].

Other data show an increased incidence of urinary tract infections (UTIs) among incontinent elderly. Incontinence is present in 5%–20% of elderly people in the community and in 40%–75% of residents of long-term-care facilities [23–25]. Unfortunately it often results in the placement of urinary catheters, both indwelling and condom, which markedly increase the risk of UTI and bacteremia [26, 27].

Immobility from neurologic or musculoskeletal disease, for example, cerebrovascular accident (CVA), increases the risk of infection by contributing to poor personal hygiene, development of decubitus ulcers, decreased cough and gag reflex with subsequent aspiration, and lowered sensitivity to pain [1].

Institutionalization (Nosocomial Infections)

Approximately 7% of the elderly population reside in long-term-care facilities. Elderly patients who live in long-term-care institutions have a higher rate of infection compared to those in the community. In skilled-nursing facilities the prevalence of infection can be as high as 3%–16% [28, 29], and each nursing home resident has an average of one serious infection per year [30]. These infections primarily involve the skin and the respiratory and urinary tracts. There has been a recent rise in the incidence of M. tuberculosis in nursing homes, and any persistent, prolonged, or resistant case of pneumonia is suspect for tuberculosis [31].

There are a number of reasons for the predisposition of infections in institutionalized elderly. Gram-negative bacteria colonize the pharynx and the urinary tract more frequently [32]. A large proportion of residents are bedridden and suffer from chronic underlying diseases. Bacteriuria is a common finding, with 50% of nursing home patients developing this condition within 12 months of admission [33]. Finally infectious episodes can be introduced by staff members, especially viral illnesses like influenza A and respiratory syncytial virus. Pneumonia accounts for 60% of deaths due to nosocomial infection [1].

Patient Presentation

Altered Presentation of Disease

MENTAL STATUS AND FUNCTIONAL CHANGES
Most elderly patients manifest infectious diseases with the classic signs of fever, inflammation, purulence, and leukocytosis that are present in younger patients. But many present with vague diffuse symptoms and fewer focal findings [1]. The only clue that an elderly patient is infected may be a change in behavior or mental status or a failure to

thrive. They often will be unable to communicate their symptoms because of a change in mental status. Therefore, the signs and symptoms of confusion, anorexia, lethargy, tachypnea, and tachycardia may be the only indications of a serious infection.

A delay in diagnosis or a misdiagnosis can result from an altered presentation of disease. Emergency physicians should not, although many often do, assume that elderly debilitated patients are at their baseline mental and functional status when they present to the emergency department. It is not unusual for a normally oriented and intact elderly person to present to the emergency department with delirium secondary to an infection and be assumed to be chronically demented. This is a dangerous assumption because it can falsely lower the therapeutic goals and lead to the withholding or delay of treatment in an otherwise healthy individual. Efforts should be made to establish the patient's baseline mental and functional levels prior to the current illness.

PHYSICAL EXAMINATION

Many elderly people have physical findings that are chronic and may be due to the aging process or other underlying conditions. Examples of these changes include pulmonary crackles that could be secondary to COPD or pulmonary fibrosis, a stiff neck due to arthritis, murmurs that could be due to the normal aging process, suprapubic tenderness, skin erythema, and decreased skin turgor [4, 34, 35].

FEVER RESPONSE

The febrile response of elderly patients with infections can be characterized by two points: (1) the amount of increase in fever is associated with prognosis, and (2) many elderly patients have blunted febrile responses. Infected elderly patients who mount a fever of at least 38.3°C are at greater risk of having a serious or life-threatening infection [36]. Therefore, elderly patients who have fevers must be considered to have serious infections and should be treated aggressively in the emergency department. It is important to note that there may also be a delay in the febrile response that can result in a delay in diagnosis and treatment [36]. No correlation has been shown between the peak of the temperature and the mortality rate [37], but the failure to mount a febrile response in the face of an acute bacterial infection is associated with a higher mortality rate [38].

A normal temperature does not exclude a bacterial infection in an elderly person. Recent literature concludes that most elderly patients with a proven bacterial infection mount a fever [37, 39], although it previously had been thought that the elderly were unable to mount a febrile response to infection. We now know that many, but not all, elderly patients have a blunted fever response to a variety of infections. A blunted or absent febrile response may be due to a defect in the normal thermoregulatory mechanisms [40]. In a study by McAlpine et al. of elderly individuals whose mean age was 81 years, 95% of those with a proven bacterial infection exhibited a temperature greater than 37.2°C on two occasions [39]. The most common sources of infection in this study were the respiratory and the urinary tracts. Another study demonstrated that only 52% of the infected elderly were febrile with a temperature greater than 37.5°C [37]. One study showed that 29% of patients with pneumococcal bacteremia were afebrile [41]. Thus, while there is a high probability that elderly people will mount a febrile response to a bacterial infection, the absence of a fever does not necessarily imply the absence of infection. Indeed, failure to mount a fever in the presence of an infection may signal a higher risk of mortality.

Diagnostic Tests

URINALYSIS

No one test is sufficient to diagnose a UTI in the elderly patient. The high prevalence of asymptomatic bacteriuria makes an isolated urine test of limited value in the absence of symptoms. When a UTI is suspected, the urine should be evaluated for leukocyte esterase, nitrates, and pyuria. In the emergency department a Gram's stain performed on a centrifuged specimen can help identify the type of organism. The specimen should be submitted for culture and sensitivity if indicated.

Care should be taken to use the proper technique to obtain a urine specimen from a catheterized patient. Bacteria isolated from indwelling catheters may not represent true pathogens but rather secondary colonization. Urine from a catheter should be obtained by catheter puncture with a sterile needle, *not* from the drainage bag. The length of time an indwelling catheter has been in place is an important consideration. The two most common organisms recovered from catheters indwelling for more than 30 days are *Enterococcus* species and *Proteus mirabilis*, which may represent colonization of the catheter, not true pathogens [42]. The probability of obtaining false positives is high when specimens are obtained from indwelling catheters [26]. To avoid culturing a contaminant from a catheter specimen, the indwelling catheter should be replaced and a sample taken of the first urine produced after the new sterile catheter is in place.

WBC COUNT AND DIFFERENTIAL

Similar to the febrile response the WBC count has been utilized as a marker of infection, but its reliability has come into question in some instances. In the study by McAlpine regarding the febrile response, only 51% of those with a proven bacterial infection demonstrated a WBC count of greater than 11,000 μl, and 60% had a neutrophil count of greater than 7500 μl [39]. The finding of a left shift, especially bandemia, correlates with the presence of a bacterial infection. Toxic granulation, vacuolization, and Dohle bodies, traditionally used as markers for infection, recently have been shown to have a poor sensitivity [37]. The probability of a bacterial infection is increased when an elderly patient presents to the emergency department with an altered mental status, fever, *and* a left shift (with or without an elevated total WBC count). If all of these signs are absent, the probability of the patient having a bacterial infection is low, less than 6% in one study [37]. Therefore, the presence of an elevated WBC count may indicate the presence of an infection, but a normal WBC count does not necessarily indicate the absence of infection.

The degree of absolute lymphopenia has been correlated with bacterial infection in the aged, which has not been found to occur in younger patients [43]. The degree of lymphopenia can be used as a predictor of outcome or prognosis. As many as 72% of infected elderly with an absolute lymphocyte count of less than 500/μl have a fatal course. Conversely up to 74% who have an absolute lymphocyte count greater than 1500/μl recover.

This parameter can be measured at the time of initial presentation to the emergency department as a prognostic indicator. Subsequent values do not add to the management of the infection because there may be no significant change during the course of the disease. The exact mechanism of lymphopenia during bacterial infection in the elderly has not been determined. It may result from the trapping of cells in immunocompetent areas, lymphocyte destruction, lack of proliferation, or immunosuppression due to stress. Clinically it is important to recognize that the prognosis of bacterial infections in the elderly is closely linked to the severity of absolute lymphocyte depletion.

Another important cause of lymphopenia in chronically ill and institutionalized elderly patients is malnutrition. This factor needs to be considered when a decreased absolute lymphocyte count is demonstrated. An absolute lymphocyte count of less than 1500/μl also has been shown to be associated with PCM [18, 44]. Therefore, in a malnourished elderly individual lymphopenia may not always indicate infection. Albumin and other protein studies may be helpful in differentiating PCM from severe infection.

GRAM'S STAINS AND CULTURES

Gram's stains and cultures of material from likely sources of infection can be useful in selecting the appropriate antibiotics, but only if proper collection techniques according to the sampling sites were used. Properly collected Gram's stains can guide initial therapy until culture and sensitivity results are available. The appropriate sampling techniques are explained in the next section.

Specific Entities

Bacteremia and Sepsis

Bacteremia and sepsis are two distinct entities on an infectious disease continuum. It is possible to have bacteremia without evidence of a systemic infection, which is not considered to be a pathologic or treatable condition. Transient bacteremia occurs with basic procedures, like urethral catherization and dental manipulation. This discussion focuses on bacteremia that is associated with signs of a systemic infection and that therefore is a risk for developing frank sepsis. The specific criteria for the diagnosis of sepsis are covered in Chap. 6.

Sepsis and systemic bacteremia carry a higher mortality rate in the elderly than in younger patients [45]. One study showed the overall survival rate to be 65.8% for community acquired bacteremia, 75% for bacteremia acquired in a nursing home, and 52.8% for hospital acquired bacteremia. The factors correlating with mortality were *Staphylococcus aureus* bacteremia, a lower respiratory tract source, age greater than 85, and a WBC count of less than 5000 μl [45].

Most elderly patients with sepsis present with the classic findings, but the presentation may be atypical. Mental status changes or hypotension may be the only clues. In one study 90% of cases had a temperature greater than 37°C, and 62% had a WBC count of greater than 10,000 μl [45]. The issue of a febrile response is controversial. Studies have shown that up to 13% of patients with bacteremia were afebrile [41].

Blood cultures are essential in making the diagnosis and guiding therapeutic decisions. A focused history and a thorough physical exam with a total skin survey, a chest x-ray, a total WBC with differential count, and a urinalysis should be performed in the initial workup. Appropriate cultures should be obtained if a specific source is apparent. This diagnostic evaluation will help establish an initial treatment plan, which is often empiric and supportive.

In the emergency department many elderly present with systemic infections that are potentially life threatening, but the source may not be obvious. The urinary tract is the most common source of bacteremia and sepsis [5, 45]. In a study by Meyers the sources of bacteremia were urinary tract in 27% of the cases, intra-abdominal in 16%, pulmonary in 12%, skin and soft tissue in 6%, and 21% were indeterminate [45]. Gram-negative organisms are responsible for approximately 60% of episodes of sepsis in the elderly, with *Escherichia coli* and *Klebsiella* species predominating. Gram-positive organisms account for 32%, with *S. aureus* and *Enterococcus faecalis* being the most common. In a study of 100 nursing home patients with bacteremia, polymicrobial sepsis had a mortality rate of 67%, while the overall mortality rate for gram-negative sepsis was 25% [46].

The treatment of suspected bacteremia is most often empiric and should be broad spectrum in nature to cover gram-positive and gram-negative organisms and anaerobes (see Table 15-1). Some practitioners prefer double or triple coverage until culture and sensitivity results are available. Metronidazole can be substituted for clindamycin to cover anaerobes, and aztreonam can be substituted for the aminoglycosides to avoid toxic side effects.

Pneumonia

Bacterial pneumonia is the leading cause of death from infection in the elderly, and influenza is a common predisposing condition that leads to pneumonia [34]. The frail elderly are particularly predisposed to pneumonia because of the multiple chronic diseases present in this population and the increased risk of aspiration. The higher incidence of aspiration pneumonia in the elderly is related to esophageal motility disorders, neoplasms, CVAs, and malnutrition. Other important precipitating factors are decreased clearance of bacteria from the lower respiratory tract and increased colonization with gram-negative organisms. Ambulatory residents of nursing homes have an estimated gram-negative colonization rate of 37%; for bedridden residents the rate is 50% [4]. Other contributing factors to the high mortality rate with pneumonia are bacteremia, empyema, and meningitis [6].

Pneumonia in elderly persons often presents insidiously and without the classic symptoms of fever and productive cough. An elderly patient may not have the classic signs of dullness to percussion, egophony, bronchial breathing, and increased tactile fremitus. Cognitive impairment exhibited as malaise, confusion, or delirium may be the only initial sign of pneumonia and is often associated with tachycardia and tachypnea. The most helpful finding on physical examination may be dullness to percussion [47]. Dehydration, orthostatic hypotension, and falls can also be the presenting complaint and can herald the onset of pneumonia before any other clinical finding is evident. Fever may be absent in 15%–20% of older persons with pneumonia. When a febrile response is present, a pneumococcal infection is most likely.

It is often difficult to obtain an adequate sputum sample in the elderly patient, but it is useful if an acceptable sample can be obtained. A transtracheal aspiration is a viable alternative if the patient is unable to produce an adequate sputum sample. This technique, which was used extensively in the past, fell out of favor for a while, but some authors are again suggesting its use in difficult diagnostic situations. Most patients tolerate a transtracheal aspiration quite well. Indications for this procedure include sputum otherwise not obtainable, severe underlying disease, life-threatening pneumonia, and the likelihood of an anaerobic infection. The respiratory secretions obtained should be Gram stained and sent for culture and sensitivity so that appropriate safe antibiotic therapy can be instituted. Transtracheal aspiration avoids oropharyngeal contamination and increases the validity of the Gram's stain.

Whenever pneumonia is suspected, blood cultures should be obtained from two sites or at different times, as well as a chest radiograph, a total WBC with a differential count, a sputum sample, and an arterial blood gas. Pleural effusions should be tapped to look for empyema.

Radiologic findings of pneumonia may not be evident on initial chest radiographs in the emergency department. This false negative finding is not due to dehydration but is associated with cases of pneumonia in a neutropenic host or an early stage of pneumonia [48]. In the elderly patient with pneumonia, infiltrates may not be evident in the early stages of consolidation. The pattern of consolidation, however, can suggest the etiological agent. Right upper lobe consolidation with a sagging fissure is often seen with *Klebsiella pneumoniae* [10]. Bilateral lower lobe infiltrates with microabscesses and small pleural effusions are suggestive of *Pseudomonas aeruginosa*. Finally necrotizing pneumonia with cavitation is consistent with anaerobic, gram-negative, or *S. aureus* pneumonia.

Streptococcus pneumoniae is still the most common cause of community acquired pneumonia in the elderly [6, 10]. The incidence of *S. aureus* pneumonia increases 10–20 times during influenza epidemics in the older population [21]. Gram-negative organisms are the most common agents causing pneumonia in nursing homes, with *K. pneumoniae* being the most frequent organism isolated [5]. Other important gram-negative agents that cause pneumonia in the aged are nontypable *H. influ-*

enzae, *E. coli*, *Acinetobacter* species, *Branhamella catarrhalis*, *Legionella* species, and *Pseudomonas* species [34].

Initial therapy in the emergency department depends on whether the infection is community or institutionally acquired. Blood cultures should be obtained before antibiotic therapy is begun. Pneumonias in patients from nursing homes should be treated as institutionally acquired. (See Table 15-1 for treatment guidelines.) Second-generation cephalosporins adequately cover gram-negative organisms and *H. influenzae* in community acquired pneumonias. For nosocomial infections *Pseudomonas* and *Klebsiella* species are of concern. Ceftazidime or one of the *Pseudomonas*-sensitive penicillins, for example, piperacillin or ticarcillin, is used in conjunction with an aminoglycoside. Fluoroquinolones are also useful agents in this setting. (Refer to chapter 23 for further diagnostic and therapeutic considerations in pneumonia.)

Meningitis

Meningitis is increasing in the elderly population [34]. In 1978 9.4% of all cases of meningitis occurred in those over age 65 [49]. Meningitis may be secondary to a variety of organisms, including bacteria, viruses, fungi, and mycobacteria. The mortality rate from meningitis in the elderly is 50%–79% [49]. This exceedingly high mortality often results from a delay in diagnosis as well as from underlying debility. The presenting complaint of altered mental status is common in the elderly, and the list of differential diagnoses for this finding is large, usually with meningitis being a less common consideration. It is important that meningitis be considered early in the emergency department evaluation.

As with many other infections in the elderly the presenting symptoms of meningitis can be vague and nonspecific. They may include mental status changes, malaise, anorexia, and headache. When meningitis is suspected on clinical grounds, the diagnosis should be confirmed by lumbar puncture. The cerebral spinal fluid findings in meningitis are similar for all ages and are covered in detail in Chap. 31. Change in mental status also can be attributed to senility, dementia, psychosis, or a CVA. It also can be secondary to meningeal inflam-

Table 15-1. Antibiotic therapy by source and setting

Infection source	Modifying circumstances	Predominant organism	Suggested regimen	Alternative regimen
Systemic infection without obvious source (bacteremia/sepsis)	Adult, nonimmunocompromised	Enterobacteriaceae, group A or D streptococcus, S. pneumoniae, "Bacteroides," Staphylococcus aureus, Coagulase negative staphylococcus, staphylococcus	Cefotaxime ± aminoglycoside or Ampicillin + aminoglycoside + clindamycin or Imipenem	Metronidazole for clindamycin, aztreonam for aminoglycoside
Pneumonia	Community acquired	S. pneumoniae, Haemophilus influenzae, Group A streptococcus, S. aureus, Legionella pneumoniae, mycoplasma	Erythromycin or second-generation cephalosporin or	Ampicillin-sulbactam or trimethoprim-sulfamethoxazole
Pneumonia	Institutionalized (nosocomial)	Klebsiella pneumoniae, Pseudomonas species, Escherichia coli, S. pneumoniae	Ceftazidime or antipseudomonal PCN + aminoglycoside	
Urinary tract (not sepsis)	Institutionalized, indwelling catheter, outlet obstruction	E. coli, Proteus species, Klebsiella species, enterococcus	Trimethoprim-sulfamethoxazole	Ampicillin, ciprofloxacin, or oral first-generation cephalosporin
Urinary tract (not sepsis)		Pseudomonas species	Ciprofloxacin or ceftazidime	Aminoglycoside or aztreonam

Prostatitis	Acute, chronic	Enterobacteriaceae, *Pseudomonas* species	Ciprofloxacin, norfloxacin, or trimethoprim-sulfamethoxazole (for chronic cases treat for 4–6 weeks)	Doxycycline or ampicillin
Skin	Cellulitis/erysipelas	Group A streptococcus, *S. aureus*	Dicloxacillin or nafcillin	Erythromycin or cephalosporin
	Pressure sore	Polymicrobic: anaerobic streptococci, *Enterobacteriaceae*, *Pseudomonas* species, "bacteroides"	Augmentin, cefoxitin + aminoglycoside, imipenem, or ampicillin-sulbactam	Ciprofloxacin and clindamycin
Bronchitis		Virus, *S. pneumoniae*, *H. influenzae*, *S. aureus*, anaerobes	Trimethoprim-sulfamethoxazole or doxycycline	Amoxicillin, Augmentin, cefuroxime, or cefaclor
Influenza	Treat if seen <24–48 hours after onset of illness; prophylaxis after exposure	Influenza A	Amantidine and influenza vaccine (0.5 ml IM)	
Shingles	Treat if seen <72 hours after onset of rash; postherpetic neuralgia	Herpes-zoster virus	Acyclovir 800 mg 5 times a day; Zostrix cream three to four times a day *after* lesions have healed	

mation and edema. The clinical signs of meningitis are less reliable and can be secondary to other chronic conditions. A stiff neck, for example, may mistakenly be attributed to cervical arthritis. Many elderly patients do have neck stiffness without meningitis, but this condition cannot always be attributed to chronic musculoskeletal conditions. When an elderly person presents with signs of an infection without an obvious source and with a stiff neck, a lumbar puncture should be considered.

Of the specific bacterial pathogens pneumococcal meningitis is most common. The incidence is increased when underlying diseases are present [49, 50]. Gram-negative bacteria (e.g., *Neisseria meningitidis*) have been reported to be the etiology of meningitis in up to 20% of geriatric cases [6]. *Listeria monocytogenes*, a gram-positive bacillus and an unusual pathogen, can cause meningitis in the healthy elderly. Gram-negative organisms, including *Pseudomonas* species, the Enterobacteriaceae, and *H. influenzae*, also are responsible for meningitis in this population.

Treatment of bacterial meningitis should be initiated with bactericidal antibiotics. High-dose penicillin G, 2–3 million units IV q4h, is the treatment of choice for pneumococcus and meningococcus. *L. monocytogenes* should be treated with ampicillin, 2 g IV q4h. *H. influenzae* is susceptible to chloramphenicol, 1 g IV q6h, as well as to the third-generation cephalosporins (e.g., ceftriaxone and cefotaxime). Most gram-negative enteric bacilli (Enterobacteriaceae) are susceptible to third-generation cephalosporin. If the organism is unknown, as will most likely be the situation in the emergency department, a third-generation cephalosporin with or without ampicillin should be initiated. Other diagnostic and therapeutic considerations in meningitis and other CNS infections are covered in Chap. 31.

Urinary Tract

URINARY TRACT INFECTIONS

UTIs are covered comprehensively in Chap. 28, but because of their importance and high incidence in the elderly, they deserve special consideration in this chapter.

UTIs are probably the most common bacterial infection in the elderly. The overall occurrence by age 70 is 20% in the community and 30%–50% in

long-term-care institutions [51–53]. In males the incidence of UTI increases dramatically with age, from 2%–4% for those 65–70 years of age to greater than 22% for those over age 81 [54]. The reasons for this increase in elderly men include decreased prostatic secretions and impaired bladder emptying due to prostatic outlet obstruction.

In older persons UTIs may present as an insidious nonspecific deterioration. The classic symptoms of dysuria, frequency, and urgency associated with cystitis usually are absent. UTIs may present solely as a change in mental status or incontinence. In older men the only clue may be urinary hesitancy from prostatic enlargement. Pyelonephritis, even in the aged, usually is associated with fever, anorexia, malaise, and flank pain, but upper UTI may be asymptomatic in more than 50% of cases [55]. Only 50% of the elderly with pyelonephritis have costovertebral angle tenderness [27]. Approximately 20% have pulmonary or gastrointestinal symptoms as a major complaint [27, 52, 56].

UTIs can lead to systemic infections with fever, chills, malaise, and other systemic symptoms. Sepsis also can be a complication of a UTI; the term *urosepsis* should be reserved for the situation where the specific criteria for sepsis are present. The reason for this distinction is important because treatment differs for the two situations. Urosepsis requires hospitalization and intravenous antibiotics, while an uncomplicated UTI often can be treated with oral antibiotics on an outpatient basis. The most frequent complication of a UTI is bacteremia, 26% of which may develop into generalized sepsis [56]. Of those with acute pyelonephritis, 66% will have bacteremia [56, 57]. A rare sequel, vertebral osteomyelitis, should be considered when an elderly patient develops persistent back pain or a fever of unknown origin following a UTI.

The diagnostic evaluation of a suspected urinary tract infection should include urinalysis, a Gram's stain and a culture and sensitivity in every symptomatic patient. The Gram's stain can be performed on a spun or an unspun sample. A spun urine sample with greater than 1 bacterium per oil immersion field has a sensitivity of 98% and specificity of 89% for infection. For an unspun sample with 1 bacterium per oil immersion field, the sensitivity and specificity are 87% and 89%, respectively [58]. Blood cultures should be obtained if systemic infection is present or if pyelonephritis is suspected.

Definitive diagnosis is based on a urine culture of greater than 10^5 colony-forming units (CFU) per milliliter. Other criteria have been proposed but are not widely used. In symptomatic women 10^4 CFU/ml detects 95% of infections [59]. Furthermore, a newer criterion of 10^2 CFU/ml has been suggested when the urine is collected by in-and-out catheterization. It may be difficult for an elderly frail person to collect a clean-catch-midstream specimen, and an in-and-out catheterization often is required because of cognitive impairment or chronic disease.

E. coli is the most common etiologic agent of UTI in the elderly. Other gram-negative organisms are also important. Residents of institutions and individuals with indwelling catheters or outlet obstruction are more likely to have *P. mirabilis* or *Klebsiella, Pseudomonas,* or *Enterococcus* species as the cause of a UTI. Empiric therapy initiated in the emergency department should cover these organisms. Trimethoprim-sulfamethoxazole is a good initial choice except for *Pseudomonas* organisms (see Table 15-1). If an allergy to sulfa is present, then ampicillin can be used, but it should be noted that up to 25% of *E. coli* can be resistant to ampicillin [60]. A fluoroquinolone, (e.g., norfloxacin, ciprofloxacin, ofloxacin, or a cephalosporin) is an appropriate alternative choice. In severe systemic infections ceftazidime or other third-generation cephalosporin and an aminoglycoside can be started until culture results are back. Nitrofurantoin is not used for severe infections because it is a bacteriostatic drug and does not adequately treat blood-borne infections. Therapy should not be delayed until cultures are available, because such delay increases the risk of systemic infection and urosepsis. Adjustment in the therapeutic regime may be necessary when culture results become available.

Different durations of therapy have been studied, and the minimum effective course of therapy remains controversial. Treatment as short as 3 days for an uncomplicated infection and up to 14 days for a complicated infection has been shown to be effective [35, 59, 61]. The authors prefer a course of treatment of 7–14 days. A repeat urine sample can be obtained 4–7 days after completion of therapy to ensure resolution of bacteriuria, especially for those who have complicating factors that increase their risk of infection, for example, catheters, obstruction, or institutionalization. A partially treated infection or a relapse needs to be treated for 2–3 weeks and sometimes longer [59]. If a patient fails to respond to appropriate therapy, a full urologic evaluation is indicated.

ASYMPTOMATIC BACTERIURIA

Asymptomatic bacteriuria (ABU) is common in the elderly and increases with age. In ambulatory populations 18.2% of females and 6% of males may have ABU [62]. The prevalence of ABU in institutionalized elderly increases to 20%–40% [50, 62, 63]. It is not associated with pyuria in at least 50% of the cases, and the source of the bacteriuria can be either the lower or the upper urinary tract. Numerous factors predispose the elderly to ABU compared to the younger population. The elderly suffer more from bladder and sphincter dysfunction and fecal incontinence with perineal soiling and generally have more genitourinary instrumentation. Furthermore, women lose their hormonal protection against introital colonization after menopause. Advanced age in the male is associated with benign prostatic hypertrophy, outlet obstruction, and a paucity of prostatic secretions. All these factors enhance the susceptibility to bacteriuria in the elderly.

Asymptomatic bacteriuria is defined by clinical and laboratory criteria. Patients must be without symptoms of a UTI or a systemic infection. Two urine cultures one week apart containing the same organism and antibiotic sensitivities must be demonstrated. The most commonly isolated organism is *E. coli*, followed by *K. pneumoniae* and *Proteus* and *Pseudomonas* species [62, 63, 64]. Asymptomatic bacteriuria is usually found on an incidental urinalysis.

Multiple studies have shown that treating asymptomatic bacteriuria is ineffective because the condition tends to recur and treatment does not alter the morbidity or mortality. Treatment also increases the risk of developing resistant organisms and drug-related side effects. Therefore, routine screening and treatment for asymptomatic bacteriuria are not suggested [65].

Skin and Soft Tissue

A comprehensive review of infections of the skin and soft tissues is presented in Chap. 32, but cellulitis, pressure sores, and shingles are particular problems for the aged and deserve discussion in this chapter.

CELLULITIS

Numerous changes occur in the skin with aging that predispose the elderly to cellulitis and pressure sores. All layers of the skin become thinner with age, and blood flow diminishes [66]. Eccrine and apocrine gland secretions are diminished, which causes a dryness of the skin and the development of superficial cracks in the epidermis [35, 66]. The number of Langerhans cells, which belong to the mononuclear phagocyte system, is decreased [67], thus increasing the susceptibility of bacterial infection by reducing clearance of invading organisms. As a result of these changes the risk for infection is increased and wound healing is delayed.

Cellulitis is caused by a disruption in the barrier function of the integument and invasion by a pathologic organism. It is usually characterized by a poorly demarcated area of erythema, warmth compared to surrounding skin, hyperemia, and sometimes induration. A *peau d'orange* appearance may be appreciated. Fluctuance and a purulent discharge indicate abscess formation. Unless secondary bacteremia has developed, fever is usually absent. Skin infections are a main source of systemic infection in elderly patients, and a thorough inspection of the skin should be performed in all patients with systemic infections of unknown etiology.

Diagnosis is based primarily on the physical examination. The differential should include burns, insect bites, phlebitis, and deep venous thrombosis. These entities are easily distinguished clinically. Cultures, including the technique of sterile saline injection and withdrawal, are rarely helpful or indicated [68]. A 2–4 mm punch biopsy may lend the etiologic agent.

Staphylococcus spp. and group A *Streptococcus* organisms are the most common etiologic agents. Mixed anaerobic and aerobic infections are associated with underlying diseases (e.g., diabetes) and are more common with infections below the waist. Lymphadenitis, acute lymphangitis, abscess formation, necrotizing fasciitis, and bacteremia with sepsis are all possible complications of cellulitis in the elderly.

The mainstay of therapy is prevention. Elderly patients must be taught skin care and the use of moisturizers. Appropriate therapy for cellulitis includes tepid soaks, débridement as necessary, and antibiotic coverage with an antistaphylococcus (penicillinase resistant) penicillin or a first-generation cephalosporin plus broader coverage when indicated (see Table 15-1).

PRESSURE (DECUBITUS) SORES

Pressure ulcers are an exceedingly common and serious problem in the frail immobilized or institutionalized elderly. They may be present in 15%–20% of nursing home residents [69, 70]. They occur primarily on the following sites: iliac crest, sacrum, trochanter, iliac tuberosity, and lateral malleolus. The risk of mortality is increased fourfold when an ulcer develops and sixfold when healing is delayed [71, 72].

The factors that result in pressure sores are multiple, but the mechanism of injury is always ischemia due to unrelieved pressure. Predisposing factors include malnutrition, shearing forces, friction, moisture from incontinence, and impaired immune function. Although it should not be assumed that all pressure sores are infected, they are generally colonized with bacteria. Secondary infections of pressure sores can develop, especially if perineal soiling from incontinence is present. The infections are generally mixed gram positive, gram negative, aerobic, and anaerobic. The most frequently isolated organisms are the Enterobacteriaceae, *S. aureus*, *Bacteroides fragilis*, *Enterococcus*, and group A *Streptococcus*.

Pressure sores can be classified clinically into four stages [73] (Table 15-2). Stage I sores appear as an area of intact, nonblanchable erythematous skin and can sometimes be indurated. Stage II sores involve skin breakdown limited to the dermis and often look like blisters that have been denuded. Stage III sores are ulcerations that extend into the subcutaneous tissue, down to but not through the fascia. Finally stage IV sores involve penetration of the deep fascia to muscle, periosteum, or bone. Any of these stages can become infected, although infection is more likely when the integrity of the skin has been disrupted, as with stages II, III, and IV. An infection should be suspected when a purulent exudate, a foul odor, fever, surrounding expanding

Table 15-2. Stages and treatment of pressure sores

Stage	Characteristics	General therapy guidelines for all stages
I	Nonblanching erythema, intact skin	1. Relieve pressure.
II	Partial-thickness ulcer limited to dermis	2. Débride wound.
III	Full-thickness ulcer into or through subcutaneous tissue	3. Treat local or systemic infection.
IV	Ulcer extending to muscle or bone	4. Keep clean wound moist.
		5. Provide high calorie diet, including zinc.
		6. Immunize against tetanus.

erythema, or necrotic tissue is present. When examining a stage III or IV pressure sore, the physician should probe the wound with a sterile swab to detect any undermining or tunneling under tissues.

The differential diagnosis includes cellulitis, ischial-rectal abscesses, vasculitides, stasis ulcers, deep mycotic infections, and necrotic malignancies. As with most skin infections, cultures of wound swabs are of limited value and primarily detect colonization. The complications of pressure ulcers include sepsis, osteomyelitis, tetanus, local amyloidosis, and cellulitis. If it is deemed necessary to isolate the offending organism, a tissue biopsy from beneath the ulcer is much more reliable than a swab of the wound.

The treatment of decubitus ulcers varies depending on the stage and the cleanliness of the wound [74]. General principles of therapy include relieving pressure and débridement of nonviable and necrotic tissue. Positioning the patient at a 30–60° oblique angle relieves the most common pressure points and turning every two hours is recommended. Necrotic or fibrinous tissue (eschar) prevents wound healing by inhibiting reepithelialization and the growth of fibroblasts. Healthy granulation tissue appears beefy red and bleeds easily. Débridement can be accomplished with chemical, mechanical, or surgical techniques. Necrotic or dirty wounds without evidence of cellulitis should not be treated with systemic antibiotics but with débridement alone and subsequent close observation. Wet to dry dressings or normal saline washes under pressure can help débride a wound mechanically, but stage III and IV sores often require admission for surgical débridement and flap or graft procedures. Enzyme chemical preparations, such as collagenase, trypsin, and fibrinolysins, can also be used to débride a wound.

After the wound has been cleaned, a variety of dressings or packings can be used, all with the intention of keeping the wound moist. A moist wound heals faster than a dry wound, because a moist environment allows quicker epithelialization. Betadine is cytotoxic and should not be used on pressure sores. Colloid-barrier coverings can help stage I and II sores remain moist and prevent bacterial invasion. Hyperosmolar packing of stage III and IV wounds or moist packings can provide a moist environment and help keep the wound clean.

All infected sores that are thought to be the origin of systemic infections should be treated with broad-spectrum antibiotics directed against aerobic and anaerobic microorganisms. Ampicillin-sulbactam or ticarcillin-clavulanate is an appropriate single agent for initial emperic therapy. Several combination agents also are effective (see Table 15-1).

HERPES ZOSTER

Herpes zoster, commonly known as "shingles," is caused by activation of the varicella-zoster virus. This is a DNA virus that remains dormant or latent in the dorsal root ganglion cells until activated. This entity occurs in approximately 16% of the elderly over age 80 [50]. The most severe and frequent complication of herpes zoster is postherpetic neuralgia, which occurs in 25%–40% of affected patients over the age of 60 [35].

Herpes zoster occurs most often in healthy people 50–70 years old. It can, however, be associated with occult neoplasms, especially lymphoma, and other immunosuppressive conditions. An extensive evaluation for a malignancy is not warranted unless clinical suspicion is high. The presenting symptom is often hyperesthesia or pain in the affected cutaneous dermatomal distribution. This is followed in 3–10 days by a characteristic band of erythematous papules, which progresses to clear vesicles and pustules. Crusting then occurs in 10–12 days and is occasionally associated with scarring. It is customary to have a few vesicles outside the involved dermatome, which should not be confused with dissemination. The most frequently involved dermatomal areas are the thoracic, cervical, and trigeminal distributions. If lesions are found on the tip of the nose, the nasolacrimal branch of the trigeminal nerve is involved, indicating the potential for subclinical ocular involvement even if lesions are not seen in the eye. These patients should be referred to an ophthalmologist.

Diagnosis can be difficult in the preeruptive phase, but once the vesicles appear herpes zoster is easily identified. The virus also can be grown in culture by swabbing the fluid contents of an unroofed vesicle. If the diagnosis is not clear from the clinical presentation and the culture, serology can aid in differentiating the lesions from those of herpes simplex. The differential diagnosis, in addition to herpes simplex, includes pleurisy, trigeminal neuralgia, Bell's palsy, and chickenpox (varicella virus). The initial pain can imitate that of appendicitis, renal colic, cholelithiasis, or colitis, depending on the dermatome involved.

No specific curative treatment for herpes zoster is available. There is some evidence that oral acyclovir therapy, if begun within 72 hours, may shorten the course of the disease and decrease the incidence of postherpetic neuralgia [75]. The dose of acyclovir for herpes zoster is four times that for herpes simplex, or 800 mg 5 times per day for 7–14 days or until all lesions are crusted over. Topical therapy is not beneficial for this condition. Intravenous therapy should be used for disseminated herpes zoster or in patients who are immunocompromised. Some studies have shown that corticosteroids also reduce the course of herpes zoster and the incidence of postherpetic neuralgia, but this treatment is controversial [35, 76, 77]. If treatment with steroids is initiated, the course should consist of a three-week taper starting with a dose of 60 mg per day. As with the acyclovir therapy it must be started early in the course of the disease.

Symptomatic therapy of herpes zoster consists of drying lotions and pain control. Drying lotions such as calamine lotion or Burrow's solution are recommended. The pain from zoster can be relieved with nonsteriodal anti-inflammatory agents, acetaminophen, or aspirin. If those medications are unsuccessful, a tricyclic antidepressant and/or narcotic analgesics should be used. Capsaicin 0.025% (Zostrix), a topical analgesic cream, can be used for postherpetic neuralgia. It should be applied on the affected dermatome three to four times a day. It may require two weeks of application before relief is appreciated. Zostrix should not be used on the initial vesicular or crusted lesions.

Intra-Abdominal Infections

All the intra-abdominal infections discussed in Chap. 27 occur in elderly patients, but appendicitis, cholecystitis, and diverticulitis are particularly problematic in older patients.

APPENDICITIS

Appendicitis is an uncommon disease in the elderly, with only 5% of all cases occurring in this age group [78, 79]. Nonetheless, it must be included in the differential diagnosis of any elderly patient presenting to the emergency department with vague abdominal pain, fever, nausea, and leukocytosis. The diagnosis of appendicitis often is delayed in the geriatric population for a variety of reasons. Nausea and leukocytosis, as well as localization of pain to the right lower quadrant of the abdomen, may not always be present. The patient may be reluctant to seek care, and the medical provider may attribute the complaints to other etiologies, including indigestion, constipation, or gastroenteritis. Consequently there is an increase in morbidity and mortality from appendicitis in the elderly. The mortality rate from appendicitis in the elderly is 2%–14%, and morbid complications occur in 35%–65% of cases [79, 80]. The morbid conditions usually result from a delay in diagnosis and include gangrene, peritonitis, abscess formation, and perforation.

Prompt treatment is essential once the diagnosis has been made, and antibiotic therapy should be instituted while awaiting surgery. *Enterococcus* spp., anaerobes, and the Enterobacteriaceae may be adequately covered with a regimen consisting of an aminoglycoside and ampicillin plus clindamycin or metronidazole. Cefoxitin, ampicillin-sulbactam, or ticarcillin-clavulanate as single agents for community-onset uncomplicated peritonitis are reasonable alternatives.

BILIARY DISEASE

The most common biliary tract disease encountered in the elderly is cholelithiasis. There is a very high rate in the elderly, with one autopsy series demonstrating a prevalence of 30% over the age of 70 [81, 82]. Acute cholecystitis can result from cholelithiasis, but the latter is not always symptomatic. Similar to other infections in the elderly the clinical presentation of cholecystitis is often atypical. The classic manifestations of right upper quadrant pain, fever, chills, and jaundice may be absent. In one series of geriatric patients with acute cholecystitis, 25% did not have abdominal pain and only 41% had peritoneal signs [83]. The diagnosis of acute cholecystitis therefore can be quite challenging in the elderly. When it is suspected, radiological studies should be undertaken to confirm the diagnosis. These include right upper quadrant ultrasound, DECIDA scans, and possibly computerized axial tomography (CAT) scans. There is a 10% incidence of acalculous cholecystitis in the elderly compared to much lower rates in younger populations. Thus, the absence of cholelithiasis on an ultrasound does not exclude the diagnosis.

The complication rate from cholecystitis is extremely high in the elderly, ranging from 15%–40% [79, 83]. These complications include emphysematous gallbladder, gangrenous perforation, and acute suppurative cholangitis, which occurs primarily in the seventh decade. The mortality rate from an episode of acute cholecystitis in the elderly is 7%–10%. Due to this significant rate and the complication rate, early surgical intervention and antibiotic administration are essential. With the advent of the new laparoscopic cholecystectomy technique, operative and postoperative complications and morbidity should be markedly reduced in the future. Antibiotic coverage should include the Enterobacteriaceae and anaerobes such as *B. fragilis*, and *Clostridia* species. The following antibiotic regimens can be employed: an aminoglycoside and metronidazole, ticarcillin-clavulanate, imipenam-cilastatin, or ampicillin-sulbactam.

DIVERTICULITIS

Diverticulitis is primarily a disease of the elderly and has an increased age-specific incidence. Fifty percent of adults will have diverticulosis by the eighth decade, and 10%–25% will experience at least one episode of diverticulitis in their lifetime [84]. The pathological mechanism underlying this disorder involves herniations of the mucosa and submucosa through the colonic muscle at sites where arteries penetrate the muscles. Inspissated fecal material then becomes trapped. The area becomes inflamed and eroded and finally develops microscopic perforations and bleeding. Chap. 27 discusses the pathophysiology of diverticula and diverticulitis in greater detail.

The clinical manifestations of diverticulitis are similar to those exhibited in younger patients. Left lower quadrant abdominal pain, fever, diarrhea or constipation, hematochezia, leukocytosis, and a palpable mass may be present. The differential diagnosis should include irritable bowel syndrome, ischemic colitis, inflammatory bowel disease, appendicitis, angiodysplasia, and adenocarcinoma of the colon.

The diagnosis is based primarily on the appropriate clinical findings. Radiologic studies and endoscopy may support or confirm the diagnosis. Upright plain films of the abdomen should be obtained to look for free air under the diaphragm from a perforation, especially if the patient presents with an acute abdomen. If a barium enema is done, a water-soluble contrast agent, like hypaque, should be used to avoid barium peritonitis. A CAT scan may be most helpful for delineating the presence of pericolonic abscess, obstruction, or fistula formation.

The treatment for the majority of cases is conservative management. Most cases resolve spontaneously, and 70% of the patients will not experience subsequent attacks [85]. Patients may be placed on a high-fiber diet and observed as outpatients. The role of antibiotics for mild cases is controversial, but if utilized tetracycline 500 mg qid or erythromycin 500 mg qid orally are appropriate choices. Metronidazole can be added for better anaerobic coverage.

Indications for admission, parenteral antibiotics, and surgery include failure to respond to a medical regimen, large abscess formation, peritonitis, fistula formation, suspected coexisting carcinoma, and recurrent disease.

HIV AND AIDS IN THE ELDERLY

There is a paucity of systematic information in the literature on AIDS in the elderly [86]. As of April 1990, 3929 cases had been reported to the CDC,

Table 15-3. AIDS deaths by year in persons over 60 years of age

	Year							
	1982	1983	1984	1985	1986	1987	1988	1989
Deaths	2	19	90	230	438	652	769	753

Source: Monthly vital statistics report, NCHS. Used with permission.

but it is clear that the reported cases and the deaths from AIDS have been increasing between 1982 and 1988 [87–89]. The number of deaths from AIDS in those over 60 years of age rose quickly between 1982 and 1988 but decreased in 1989 (Table 15-3). The risk factors for the elderly have been thought to be the same as for younger populations, but if a decline in the number of deaths due to AIDS after 1988 continues, it can be surmised that transfusion was more of a risk factor in the elderly. The decline in 1989 could be consistent with the improved screening of blood products that began in the mid-1980s. This observation may not be a long-term trend, however, and needs more study. The number of reported AIDS cases increased by 23% between 1989 and 1990. Overall 7.3% of the deaths from AIDS have been in those over 55 years of age.

The diagnosis in elderly people may be delayed because they are not generally thought of as a population that experiences AIDS. The presenting signs and symptoms may mimic dementia or other diseases common to the elderly [86]. Studies have shown that survival from diagnosis is markedly reduced in this population, approximately one-third to one-half of that for younger populations. One study from San Francisco showed a median survival of 5.7 months for those over 60 years of age compared to 12.5 months for all patients [90]. As treatment with agents such as AZT is shown to increase survival, people who develop AIDS in younger age groups may live to be elderly, thereby increasing the elderly prevalence and death rates. The treatment for elderly AIDS victims is the same as for younger populations. HIV testing should be considered in elderly patients who present with decline of their functional status, prolonged fever, and recent weight loss and whose diagnosis cannot be established using the conventional approach discussed throughout this chapter. A thorough discussion of HIV infection and the associated illnesses seen in all age groups is found in Chap. 17.

Differential Diagnosis: Noninfectious Imitators

The presentation of infectious and noninfectious diseases in the elderly can be similar. Noninfectious diseases also can cause vague and nonspecific signs and symptoms. Dehydration, fecal impaction, myocardial infarction, congestive heart failure, CVAs, and other diseases can present with altered mental status or functional status. In the authors' experience fever can be the only presenting sign of a myocardial infarction. Certain medications can result in lethargy and changes in mental status. When evaluating an elderly patient in the emergency department, the examining physician must remember that noninfectious conditions can mimic infections.

Pharmacology of Antimicrobials

Initial therapy in the emergency department should be determined by the clinical presentation, the likely source, and a Gram's stain where appropriate (see Table 15-1). In the elderly altered pharmacokinetics also need to be considered.

Elderly patients are more susceptible to toxicity from antimicrobials and may require lower dosages of antibiotics because of declining function of the two main metabolic and excretory organs, the liver and the kidneys. This diminished function is present even though the laboratory tests for serum creatinine and liver functions are usually normal. These organs lose functional reserve capacity with age but usually not enough to alter normal basal functioning. The serum creatinine, therefore, is regarded as a poor measurement of renal function in the elderly. It maintains a normal level despite an inevitable decrease in the creatinine clearance, because there is a concomitant decrease in muscle mass and the volume of distribution with aging. The following Cookcroft-Gault formula can be utilized to estimate the creatinine clearance (CrCl) when calculating dosages in the elderly [4]:

$$CrCl = \frac{(140 - age)(weight \; in \; kg)}{(72kg)(serum \; creatinine)}$$

An adjustment for gender in the equation is not necessary for the older population. To avoid antibiotic toxicity the assessment of renal and hepatic functions may be important because abnormal values may indicate more severe dysfunction.

The incidence of adverse reactions to antibiotics is two to seven times greater in the elderly compared with younger patients [91]. Drug-drug interactions due to polypharmacy contribute to this increased incidence and have implications on how medications are prescribed. Clinicians should use the fewest medications possible to get the appropriate antibiotic coverage, and the dosages should "start low and go slow." The adverse side effects can be reduced by lowering the dose or increasing the dosing interval. The toxicities of commonly used antibiotics must be known and avoided by appropriate administration (Table 15-4). A comprehensive review of all major anti-infectives' adverse effects, indications, and dosing information is contained in Chap. 4.

General Therapeutic Considerations

Providers evaluating elderly patients suspected of having infections should perform a directed history, a physical examination and a limited laboratory examination in an attempt to identify the source of infection. This age group often presents with atypical and nonspecific manifestations of infectious diseases; it is important to evaluate the patient's prior mental and functional status, because return to baseline is the ultimate goal of therapy. After the initial assessment appropriate culture specimens should be obtained prior to initiating antibiotics. Empiric therapy in the emergency department is based on the initial clinical and laboratory assessments. Properly collected cultures will help to identify the infecting organism and will guide the definitive therapy.

Table 15-4. Antibiotic toxicity

Antibiotic	Toxic effect
Aminoglycosides	Nephrotoxicity Ototoxicity
Penicillin (high dose)	Neurotoxicity
Carbenicillin	Volume overload
Isoniazide, tetracycline	Hepatotoxicity
Amantadine, isoniazide	Confusion
Sulfonamides, penicillin, cephalosporins	Hypersensitivity
Erythromycin, acyclovir	Nausea

The decision to admit an elderly patient to the hospital or to discharge to home involves unique considerations. Obviously people who are septic or totally incapacitated require admission. Also, people with concomitant illnesses that might impede recovery (e.g., COPD) and noncompliant patients may benefit from hospitalization. Hypoxemia, dehydration, and the inability to take oral medications are also indications for admission.

An understanding of a person's living situation, functional status, and the availability of community resources can affect significantly the decision to admit or discharge the patient. Important living conditions to consider include whether the patient lives alone, with a caregiver, or in a nursing home. Infected elderly patients who cannot be adequately cared for in their current living situation should be admitted and treated in the hospital. A person often can be discharged to home if a caregiver or a family member is available to administer oral antibiotic therapy, provide supportive care, and monitor specific parameters like temperature, mental status, and hydration. The availability of home care nursing services can be an important adjuvant to the therapeutic and monitoring regimen of the noninstitutionalized elderly. These services also can sometimes provide intramuscular and intravenous administration of antibiotics.

Many services can be provided in nursing homes that are not available in a patient's home, but a nursing home should not be used as a substitute for the hospital. Nursing homes can provide nutrition, hydration, frequent nursing assessment, and sometimes parenteral antibiotic therapy. They usually cannot provide intravenous medication, although more facilities are now moving in that direction. Intramuscular injections usually can be administered and are an attractive alternative if hospitalization is not indicated but oral administration is not an optimal choice of therapy.

When discharging a patient to a nursing home, the emergency department physician should write orders that include specific monitoring parameters to ensure appropriate physician follow-up, for example, vital signs, fluid input and/or output, or glucose levels. These orders should also specify when the antibiotics are to begin and end, because nursing homes have limited formularies and usually need to order the antibiotics from their vendors. The authors have had the experience of writing orders on a Friday afternoon and the medication not being started until Monday morning.

The emergency department physician also needs to assess the patient's functional status prior to making a disposition. The frail elderly are particularly susceptible to dehydration from decreased oral intake and insensible losses. If dehydration is present, admission generally is required for intravenous fluids [47]. Bedbound patients are also a unique category of infected elderly patients. Their reserve capacity usually is diminished from debilitating and chronic disease processes. An infection further decreases this reserve and enhances the risk for developing new morbid conditions, for example, pressure sores. Therefore, infectious diseases need to be treated promptly and adequately in the elderly patient population with regard to their social setting and functional status.

Therapeutic plans at discharge from the emergency department need to include not only antibiotic therapy but also general management considerations. For example, when the source of infection is a pressure sore, the physician should also consider tetanus status, débridement of necrotic tissue, high-caloric intake, and bandaging frequency in the discharge plans. It is essential that the emergency department findings and therapeutic plans be communicated to the patient's primary physician.

Ethical considerations are also an important aspect of treating elderly patients in the emergency department. The self-determination, comfort, and dignity of the patient are primary. The decision to treat needs to be based on the patient's advance directives as well as the underlying quality of life. In the event a patient is not decisionally capable, attention should be focused on what the patient previously has expressed to others in terms of resuscitation, hospitalization, and other therapy. The emergency physician should inquire about a living will and a durable power of attorney, a legal document that establishes the surrogate medical decision maker when a person becomes decisionally incapable.

Primary Prevention: Immunizations

The elderly suffer increased morbidity and mortality from influenza and pneumococcal infections and have the highest incidence of tetanus. All three of these infections are mostly preventable with immunoprophylaxis. Immunoprophylaxis, chemoprophylaxis, and general infection control principles are covered in Chap. 5, but additional emphasis for the elderly seems appropriate here.

Influenza

Influenza results in the greatest number of excess preventable deaths in the elderly from an infectious source. Influenza accounts for 870 of the 100,000 deaths each year of patients with underlying cardiovascular and pulmonary disease [10]. The importance of immunizing the elderly against influenza A and B each year cannot be overemphasized. The vaccination has been shown to afford at least a partial protective effect and to decrease morbidity and mortality in those who become symptomatic. The standard dose is 0.5 ml IM given in late October or early November. Large outbreaks generally occur in the United States in January and February. Protection is conferred about 2 weeks after the injection and lasts 3–6 months [92].

Pneumococcal Pneumonia

A pneumococcal vaccine (Pneumovax) is currently recommended once per lifetime in those 65 years of age and older. There is, however, a great deal of controversy surrounding the vaccine's efficacy and how often it should be given. Studies on immunization with the older 14-valent polysaccharide vaccine showed no evidence that Pneumovax provides any benefit in the reduction, systemic involvement, or mortality from pneumococcal pneumonia in the elderly [5]. The newer 23-valent vaccine may decrease the incidence of bacteremia in the aged [21]. There are few data that demonstrate a protective effect or adequate antibody response, although the vaccine is thought to be 60%–80% effective. Currently it is recommended that the vaccine be given once per lifetime except to COPD and selected immunocompromised patients, to whom it should be administered at least every 5 years.

Tetanus

Many elderly patients have never been immunized against tetanus [93]. Of those who have received tetanus prophylaxis at some point in the past, fewer than 33% in the community and 50% in institutions have protective titers [94, 95]. Thus, it is not surprising that the highest incidence of tetanus is in patients over age 60 [90, 96]. Often there is no implicating wound. Exposure in the elderly most often occurs from gardening injuries in community dwellers and pressure sores in the institutionalized. Tetanus in the elderly is associated with a mortality rate of approximately 76% [97]. It is important, therefore, to immunize the elderly against tetanus. The recommended regimen is a 0.5 ml IM injection of the Td preparation every 10 years or 5 years when there is a contaminated wound injury.

References

1. Garibaldi RA. Infections in the elderly. *Am J Med* 81 (suppl. 1A):53–58, 1986.
2. U.S. Bureau of the Census. *Statistical Abstract of the United States: 1991* (111th ed.). Washington DC, 1991.
3. Cassell CK, Brody JA. Demography, epidemiology and aging. In CK Cassel et al. (eds.), *Geriatric Medicine.* 1990 2nd ed. New York: Springer-Verlag, Pp. 16–27.
4. Jones SR. Infection in frail and vulnerable elderly patients. *Am J Med* 88 (suppl. 3C):30S–33S, 1990.
5. Meyers BR. Serious infections in the elderly. *Mt Sinai J Med* 15(1):18–24, 1987.
6. Berk SL, Alvarez S. Bacterial infections in the el-
derly: special considerations for a special patient population. *Postgrad Med* 77(3):169–79, 1985.
7. Butler RN. Foreword to second edition. In CK Cassel et al. (eds.), *Geriatric Medicine* (2nd ed.). New York: Springer-Verlag, 1990.
8. National Center for Health Statistics. *Vital Statistics of the United States.* In *Life Tables* (vol. II, sec. b). Washington DC: U.S. Public Health Service, 1990.
9. Fries JF. Aging, death and the compression of morbidity. *N Engl J Med* 303:130–35, 1980.
10. Berk SL, Smith JR. Infectious diseases in the elderly. *Med Clin North Am* 67(2):273–93, 1983.
11. Freedman LR. Urinary-tract infections in the elderly [letter]. *N Engl J Med* 309:1451–52, 1983.
12. Burns EA, Goodwin JS. Immunology and infectious disease. In CK Cassel et al. (eds.), *Geriatric Medicine* (2nd ed.). New York: Springer-Verlag, 1990. Pp. 312–29.
13. Wayne SH et al. Cell mediated immunity as predictor of morbidity and mortality in subjects over 60. *J Gerontol* 45:45–48, 1989.
14. Makinodan T et al. Immunologic basis for susceptibility to infection in the aged. *Gerontology* 30:279–89, 1984.
15. Gilles S et al. Immunologic studies of aging: decreased production of a response to T-cell growth factor by lymphocytes from aged humans. *J Clin Invest* 67:937–42, 1981.
16. Phair JP et al. Failure to respond to influenza vaccine in the aged. Correlation with B-cell number and function. *J Lab Clin Med* 92:822–28, 1987.
17. *The Surgeon General's Report on Nutrition and Health.* Chapter 16: Aging. Washington DC: U.S. Public Health Service, 1988. Pp. 595–627.
18. Henderson CT. Nutrition. In CK Cassell et al. (eds.). *Geriatric Medicine* (2nd ed.). New York: Springer-Verlag, 1990. Pp. 535–54.
19. Kenny R. Abnormalities of liver function and the predictive value of liver function tests in infection and outcome of acutely ill elderly patients. *Age and Ageing* 13:224–29, 1984.
20. Tan JS et al. Neutrophil dysfunction in diabetes mellitus. *J Lab Clin Med* 85:26–33, 1975.
21. Mostow SR. Infectious complications in the elderly COPD patient. *Geriatrics* 38(10):42–48, 1983.
22. Nicolle LE et al. Twelve-month surveillance of infections in institutionalized elderly men. *J Am Geriatr Soc* 32:513, 1984.
23. Ouslander JG, Kane RL, Abrass IB. Urinary incontinence in elderly nursing home patients. *JAMA* 248:1194–98, 1982.
24. Thomas TM et al. Prevalence of urinary incontinence. *Br Med J* 281:1243–45, 1980.

25. Yarnell JWG, St. Leger AS. The prevalence, severity and factors associated with urinary incontinence in a random sample of the elderly. *Age and Ageing* 8:81–85, 1979.

26. Carty M, Brocklehurst JC, Carty J. Bacteriuria and its correlates in old age. *Gerontology* 27:72–75, 1981.

27. Gleckman RA. Community acquired urosepsis. In RA Gleckman and NM Gantz (eds.), *Infections in the Elderly*. Boston: Little, Brown, 1983.

28. Cohen ED et al. Nosocomial infections in skilled nursing facilities: a preliminary survey. *Public Health Rep* 94:162–65, 1979.

29. Garibaldi RA, Brodine S, Matsumiyo S. Infections among patients in nursing homes: policies, prevalence and problems. *N Engl J Med* 305:731–35, 1981.

30. Smith PW. Nursing home-acquired infections. *Postgrad Med* 81:55–66, 1987.

31. Stead WW et al. Tuberculosis as an endemic and nosocomial infection among the elderly in nursing homes. *N Engl J Med* 312:1483–87, 1985.

32. Valenti WM, Trudell RG, Bentley DW. Factors predisposing to oropharyngeal colonization with gram-negative bacilli in the aged. *N Engl J Med* 298:1108–11, 1978.

33. Schneider EL. Infectious diseases in the elderly. *Ann Intern Med* 98:395–400, 1983.

34. Musgrave T, Berk SL. Update: infectious diseases in the elderly. *Geriatrics* 14(6):30–37, 1988.

35. Nagami P. Management of common infections in the elderly outpatient. *Geriatrics* 11:67–80, 1986.

36. Keating HJ et al. Effect of aging on the clinical significance of fever in ambulatory adult patients. *JAGS* 32:282–87, 1984.

37. Wasserman M et al. Utility of fever, white blood cells, and differential count in predicting bacterial infections in the elderly. *JAGS* 37(6):536–43, 1989.

38. Finkelstein MS et al. Pneumococcal bacteremia in adults: age-dependent differences in presentation and in outcome. *JAGS* 31:19–27, 1983.

39. McAlpine CH et al. Pyrexia in infection in the elderly. *Age and Ageing* 15:230–34, 1986.

40. Norman DC, Grahn D, Yoshikawa TT. Fever and aging. *JAGS* 33:859–63, 1985.

41. Gleckman R, Hibert D. Afebrile bacteremia. *JAMA* 248:1478–81, 1982.

42. Grahn D et al. Validity of urinary catheter specimens for diagnosis of urinary tract infection in the elderly. *Arch Intern Med* 145:1858–60, 1985.

43. Proust J et al. Lymphopenia induced by acute bacterial infections in the elderly: a sign of age-related immune dysfunction of major prognostic significance. *Gerontology* 31:178–85, 1985.

44. Gross RL, Newborne PM. Role of nutrition in immunologic function. *Physiol Review* 60:188–302, 1980.

45. Myers BR et al. Bloodstream infections in the elderly. *Am J Med* 86:379–84, 1989.

46. Letia U, Serventi I, Lorenz P. Bacteremia in a long-term care facility. Spectrum and mortality. *Arch Intern Med* 144:1633–35, 1984.

47. Bentley D. Diagnosis and management of pneumonia in the elderly patient. *Modern Med* 55:68–82, 1987.

48. Caldwell A et al. The effects of dehydration on the radiologic and pathologic appearance of experimental canine segmental pneumonia. *Am Rev Resp Dis* 112:651–56, 1975.

49. Berk SL. Bacterial meningitis. In R Gleckman, N Gantz (eds.), *Infections in the Elderly*. Boston: Little, Brown, 1983.

50. Roeltgen DP. Infections and the nervous system in the elderly. *Geriatrics* 38(2):105–14, 1983.

51. Dontas AS et al. Bacteriuria and survival in old age. *N Engl J Med* 304:989–1043, 1981.

52. Zilkoski MW, Smucker DR, Mayhew HE. Urinary tract infections in elderly patients. *Postgrad Med* 84(3):191–99, 1988.

53. Bentzen A, Vejlsgaard R. Asymptomatic bacteriuria in elderly subjects. *Danish Med Bull* 27:101–6, 1980.

54. Bertakis KD, Ross JL. Office evaluation of urinary tract infections in elderly women. *J Fam Pract* 24(1):72–75, 1987.

55. Suntharalingam M, Seth V, Moore-Smith B. Site of urinary tract infection in elderly women admitted to an acute geriatric assessment unit. *Age and Ageing* 12:317–22, 1983.

56. Roberts JA. Pyelonephritis, cortical abscess and perinephric abscess. *Urol Clin North Am* 13(4):637–45, 1986.

57. Bohnson R. Urosepsis. *Urol Clin North Am* 13(4):627–35, 1986.

58. Jenkins RD, Fenn JP, Matsen JM. Review of urine microscopy for bacteriuria. *JAMA* 255(24):3397–3403, 1986.

59. Zilkoski MW, Smucker DR. Urinary tract infections in the elderly. *Am Fam Physician* 39:125–34, 1989.

60. Stamm WE, McKevitt M, Counts GW. Acute renal infection in women: treatment with trimethoprim-sulfamethoxazole or ampicillin for two or six weeks. *Ann Intern Med* 106:341–45, 1987.

61. Treatment of UTI. *Medical Letter* 23(589):69, 1981.

62. Boscia JA et al. Epidemiology of bacteriuria in an elderly ambulatory population. *Am J Med* 80:208–14, 1986.

63. Kaye D. Urinary tract infections in the elderly. *Bull NY Acad Med* 56:209–20, 1980.

64. Nicolle L et al. Localization of urinary tract infection in elderly, institutionalized women with asymptomatic bacteriuria. *J Infect Dis* 157(1):65–70, 1988.

65. U.S. Preventive Task Force. Screening for asymptomatic bacteriuria, hematuria and proteinuria. In U.S. Preventive Task Force, *Guide to Clinical Preventive Services*. Baltimore: Williams & Wilkins, 1989.

66. Gilchrest BA. Age-associated changes in the skin. *JAGS* 30:139–43, 1982.

67. Gilchrest BA, Murphy GF, Soter NA. Effect of chronologic aging and ultraviolet irradiation on Langerhans cells in human epidermis. *J Invest Dermatol* 79:85–88, 1982.

68. Nowell PM, Norden CW. Value of needle aspiration in bacteriologic diagnosis of cellulitis in adults. *J Clin Microbiol* 26:401–4, 1988.

69. Cowart V. Pressure ulcers preventable, say many physicians. *JAMA* 257(5):589, 1987.

70. Brandeis GH et al. The epidemiology and natural history of pressure ulcers in elderly nursing home residents. *JAMA* 264:2905–9, 1990.

71. Allman RM et al. Pressure sores among hospitalized patients. *Ann Intern Med* 105(9):337, 1986.

72. Meicher RE, Longe RL, Gelbart AO. Pressure sores in the elderly: a systemic approach to management. *Postgrad Med* 83(1):229, 1988.

73. Yarkony GM et al. Classification of pressure ulcers. *Arch Dermatol* 126:1218–19, 1990.

74. Rousseau P. Pressure ulcers in an aging society. Wounds: A compendium of clinical research and practice. 1(2):135–41, 1989.

75. Goldberg GN. A treatment guide for herpes zoster. *Modern Med* 55:66–76, 1987.

76. Eaglstein WH, Katz R, Brown JA. The effects of early corticosteroid therapy on the skin eruption and pain of herpes zoster. *JAMA* 21:1681–83, 1981.

77. Post BT, Philbrick JT. Do corticosteroids prevent post herpetic neuralgia: a review of the evidence. *J Am Acad Dermatol* 18:605–10, 1988.

78. Yusuf MF, Dunn E. Appendicitis in the elderly: learn to discern the untypical picture. *Geriatrics* 34:73–79, 1979.

79. Norman DC, Yoshikawa TT. Intra-abdominal infection: diagnosis and treatment in the elderly patient. *Gerontology* 30:327–38, 1984.

80. Owens BJ, Hamit HF. Appendicitis in the elderly. *Ann Surg* 187:392–96, 1978.

81. Vartian CV, Septimus EJ. Intra-abdominal infections in the elderly: diagnosis and management. *Geriatrics* 41:51–56, 1986.

82. Amberg JR, Aboralske FF. Gallstones after 70 requiescat in pace. *Geriatrics* 20:539–42, 1965.

83. Morrow DJ, Thompson J, Wilson EE. Acute cholecystitis in the elderly. *Arch Surg* 113:1149–52, 1978.

84. Parks TG. Natural history of diverticular disease of the colon. *Clin Gastroenterol* 4:53–69, 1975.

85. Larson DM, Masters SS, Spiro HM. Medical and surgical therapy in diverticular disease. *Compar Gastroenterol* 71:734–37, 1976.

86. Crystal S, Weiss SH. Diagnosis and treatment of HIV illness in the elderly. *Intern Med Specialist* 11:49–61, 1990.

87. Centers for Disease Control. Update: acquired immunodeficiency syndrome—United States, 1981–1990. *MMWR* 40:358–64, 1991.

88. Centers for Disease Control. Mortality attributable to HIV infection/AIDS—United States, 1981–1990. *MMWR* 40:41–44, 1991.

89. Centers for Disease Control. The HIV/AIDS epidemic: the first 10 years. *MMWR* 40:357–64, 369, 1991.

90. Lemp GF et al. Survival trends for patients with AIDS. *JAMA* 263:402–6, 1990.

91. Gurwitz JH, Avorn J. The ambiguous relation between aging and adverse drug reactions. *Ann Intern Med* 114:956–66, 1991.

92. Influenza Vaccine 1990–91. *Medical Letter* 32(826):86, 1990.

93. Richardson JP, Knight AL. The prevention of tetanus in the elderly. *Arch Intern Med* 151:1712–17, 1991.

94. Crossley TC et al. Tetanus and diphtheria immunity in urban Minnesota adults. *JAMA* 242:2298–2300, 1979.

95. Ruben FL, Nagel J, Fireman P. Antitoxin responses in the elderly to tetanus-diphtheria (td) immunization. *Am J Epidemiol* 108:145–49, 1978.

96. Centers for Disease Control. Tetanus in the United States. *MMWR* 3:602–11, 1985.

97. Laforce RM, Young LS, Bennett JV. Tetanus in the U.S. (1965–1966), epidemiological and clinical features. *N Engl J Med* 280:569–74, 1969.

16

Infection in the Immunocompromised Host

Jonathan S. Serody
Myron S. Cohen

Specific host defenses are individually responsible for different microbial pathogens, making it impossible to generalize about the immunocompromised host. This idea is of critical clinical importance because we now recognize that specific host defense defects lead to predictable kinds of microbial infection; conversely identification of an unusual infectious disease leads to recognition of a defect in host defenses. In addition infections observed in compromised hosts offer tremendous insight into the function and regulation of the immune system.

Patients with defects in host defense generally are managed by subspecialists in infectious diseases, oncology, rheumatology, clinical immunology, and pediatrics. However, such patients invariably enter the health care system through the emergency department. Therefore, an appreciation of the relationship between different host defense defects and infectious complications is critical.

Table 16-1 provides a description of the specific host defenses involved in immune surveillance and their recognized functions. The skin and the mucous membranes are perhaps the most critical defense, and burn injuries represent the prototype limitation to this defense. (The acute care of patients with burns is discussed in Chap. 13.) Compromise to mucous membranes can be observed as part of a more global problem (e.g., the cell-mediated defect in human immunodeficiency virus (HIV) disease) or because of specific tissue or immunoglobulin abnormalities. Phagocytes (including neutrophils and macrophages), immunoglobulin, and complement work in consort. Nevertheless, their separation is made possible by the clinical differences observed in patients in whom these systems are affected. Cytokines, including interleukins, interferons, and tumor necrosis factor, are critical to the function of the immune system. However, specific disease processes or infections related to cytokine deficiency have not yet been clearly defined. Abnormalities in host defense can be inherited or acquired.

Debilitation and chronic disease result in changes in indigenous flora. Colonization of the oropharynx with gram-negative bacilli has been documented in diabetics, alcoholics, and patients with increasing severity of illness. Frequent use of antimicrobial agents also radically alters indigenous flora. The compromised host may also have frequent opportunity for nosocomial exposure. When the compromised hose does become infected, the source often is an unusual pathogen with which the host has been colonized.

Table 16-1. Host defenses and functions in immune surveillance

Immune mediator	Function
Skin	Barrier protection from microorganisms; presentation of antigen
Mucous membranes	Secretion of lysozyme, immunoglobulin, and other compounds with antimicrobial properties
Immunoglobulin	Opsonization of antigen Cell-free lysis of organisms by complement; neutralization of toxins; viral neutralization
Complement	Initiation of inflammatory response; clearance of immune complexes; opsonization of microorganisms; killing certain gram-negative bacteria
Granulocytes	Phagocytosis and killing of microorganisms; inflammatory mediator release at tissue sites
Cytokines (e.g., interleukins 1 and 2, tumor necrosis factor, interferons, colony stimulating factors)	Induction of fever and catabolic state; T- and B-cell proliferation; induction of immunoglobulin synthesis; interference with viral replication; proliferation of stem cell and mature bone marrow cells
Lymphocytes	Immunoglobulin synthesis; enhancement of immunoglobulin synthesis; delayed hypersensitivity; control of immune response; activation of monocytes and macrophages

Patient Isolation

Among the highest priorities for the emergency department physician is immediate isolation of patients with contagious diseases, which commonly occur in compromised hosts (see Chap. 5). Obvious examples include *Mycobacterium tuberculosis*, meningococcemia, and varicella infection, including shingles. Large numbers of hospital personnel are needlessly exposed (and frequently infected) with such organisms because of a lack of sensitivity to the importance of this issue. In addition hospital personnel must employ universal precautions to avoid their exposure to HIV and other contagious viruses, as well as other opportunistic pathogens harbored by these patients. Also, compromised hosts should not be exposed to other patients with infectious diseases. It is obvious that children with leukemia must not be exposed to varicella [1], but it also may be important to prevent compromised hosts from encountering influenza and other common infectious diseases.

Immunoglobulin

Immunoglobulin G Deficiency

Immunoglobulin classes M and G play a vital role in the opsonization and killing of encapsulated bacteria. In addition the subclasses of IgG have received

increased attention, and it appears that IgG subclass 2 is of the greatest importance [2, 3]. Opsonization activities are accomplished when immunoglobulins bind to microbial pathogens through recognition of specific antigenic epitopes. Fc receptors on macrophages and neutrophils bind to the Fc portion of the immunoglobulin, thereby allowing recognition of the microbe and under some circumstances enhanced phagocytosis. Three different types of phagocyte Fc receptors (FcR I–III) have been described [4], and their functions are being dissected. Antibodies also bind to the Fc portion of cytotoxic killer lymphocytes, which may also play a role in defense against some microbial pathogens. Antibodies bound to the surface of a microbe generally will activate the complement cascade, allowing fixation of complement components critical to phagocytosis [5].

IgG is the major immunoglobulin found in serum, although IgA actually is generated in highest concentration on a daily basis [5]. IgG deficiency can be inherited or acquired. Patients with IgG deficiency commonly present with recurrent sinopulmonary infections due to encapsulated bacteria, including *Streptococcus pneumoniae*, *Haemophilus influenzae* type B, and *Staphylococcus aureus*. Infection with these bacteria can be severe in patients with deficiency in IgG. In addition to having bacterial infections children with hereditary IgG deficiency develop chronic enteroviral infections, including meningitis [6]. These children also develop arthritis due to *Mycoplasma hominis* and gastrointestinal infections caused by *Giardia lamblia* and *Campylobacter jejuni* [7, 8].

Patients with multiple myeloma represent the classic example of acquired IgG deficiency in adults. More recently the importance of IgG deficiency in chronic lymphocytic leukemia has been appreciated [9]. Immunoglobulin levels fall with progression of disease, rendering the patient susceptible to infection.

Complex Immunodeficiency Syndromes

Patients with complex immunodeficiency disorders often demonstrate antibody deficiency. In addition to having impaired cellular immunity, patients infected with the HIV virus do not respond appropriately to specific antigens, and infections with encapsulated organisms are common [10]. In the pediatric AIDS population bacterial infections pose a greater threat to patients than do infections caused by *Pneumocystis carinii* [11, 12].

Splenectomy

The spleen clears microorganisms through receptors for the Fc portion of immunoglobulins found on splenic macrophages, as well as serves as a site for the synthesis of antibody. Patients with splenectomy are at increased risk of infection with the encapsulated organisms, especially *S. pneumoniae*, *H. influenzae*, and *Nesseria meningitidis*, which can lead to overwhelming postsplenectomy sepsis. Overwhelming postsplenectomy pneumococcal sepsis is a fulminant, rapidly fatal disease characterized by digital ulceration with necrosis, hypotension, acidosis, disseminated intravascular coagulation (DIC), and shock [13]. A rapid diagnosis of this syndrome can be made by spinning down the blood, isolating the buffy coat, and demonstrating the presence of gram-positive cocci on a Gram's stain [13]. *Capnocytophaga canimorsis* (formerly DF-2), a gram-negative bacteria that is present in the oral flora of dogs, also causes sepsis in splenectomized patients [14]. Infection with *Capnocytophaga* is characterized by hypotension, DIC, skin lesions, and renal failure [15]. In the United States 30% of *Babesia microti* infections are associated with splenectomy [16]. This infection is seen mostly in the states of Massachusetts, Rhode Island, and New York, but it has been reported in the Upper Great Lakes area and California. Babesiosis is transmitted by the *Ixodes dammini* tick. The incubation period after the tick bite is 1–3 weeks before the onset of clinical illness. Malaise, fever, headache, and arthralgias are observed. Hepatomegaly may occur. Hemolytic anemia is seen as a result of parasitization of erythrocytes. Other lab abnormalities include mild elevation in liver enzymes, proteinuria, and hemoglobinuria. Because of the risk of overwhelming postsplenectomy sepsis, all splenectomized patients with fever must be admitted and observed. Empiric treatment for probable source and etiology of infection must be expeditious.

Sickle Cell Anemia

Patients with sickle cell anemia have impaired splenic function because of recurrent autoinfarctions during sickle cell crisis. In addition the serum opsonic activity of these patients may be defective. Patients with sickle cell disease frequently develop infections with encapsulated bacteria, especially pneumococcus [17] and *H. influenzae* but also salmonella, which is the most common cause of osteomyelitis in these patients [18]. Young children with sickle cell disease 6–36 months of age are at several hundreds times the risk of developing sepsis from these organisms than is the normal population. Pneumonia, septic arthritis, osteomyelitis, meningitis, and pyelonephritis are common.

The workup of a febrile patient with sickle cell disease is difficult, because sepsis can masquerade as a trivial infection. The workup of a patient without an obvious source of fever on physical examination should include a chest radiograph, which may demonstrate pneumonia or infarct, a urinalysis, and blood cultures. The patient who looks well, is older than 3 years, and has a minor source of infection, such as otitis media or upper respiratory infection, can be discharged. For children with sickle cell disease who are younger than 3 years and who appear toxic or have a high fever (>40°C) admission should be considered. These factors, along with a left shift or toxic granulations on a WBC count, may correlate with toxicity.

Sepsis, pneumonia, bone and joint infections, pyelonephritis, and meningitis in persons with sickle cell disease must be recognized and treated early. Blood cultures should be obtained if any of these conditions is suspected, as well as cultures of specimens from the individual areas of infection. Bone and joint infections can be difficult to differentiate from infarction. Nuclear bone scans for bone pain or joint aspiration with Gram's stain, cell count, and culture may be necessary. S. aureus, Salmonella species, and enteric organisms are the most common culprits. A lumbar puncture (LP) should be performed in any patient with even subtle neurologic symptoms.

Management of infection in cases of sickle cell diseases requires supplemental oxygen, aggressive hydration, and early antibiotic therapy. Empiric antibiotic therapy with a third-generation cephalosporin, such as ceftriaxone or cefotaxime, is appropriate.

Immunoglobulin A Deficiency

Deficiency of IgA is actually more common than that of IgG. IgA deficiency has been observed with a frequency of 1:328 in a study of healthy blood donors [19]. Most of these patients are asymptomatic, although sinopulmonary and gastrointestinal infections can develop. Patients suspected of having an IgA deficiency disorder should not be transfused with blood products, since they may have IgE antibodies to contaminating IgA, which can induce anaphylaxis.

Patients who present with chronic and recurrent sinopulmonary infections may also suffer from important microcellular defects. For example, Kartagener's syndrome in its complete presentation includes situs inversus, sinopulmonary infection, and infertility. Patients with this disease have a characteristic abnormality in the dynein arms of cellular microtubules, which is observed in more subtle forms of the disease. This microtubular defect prevents normal ciliary function and adversely affects phagocyte chemotaxis [20].

Special Considerations in Emergency Treatment

Treatment of infection in patients with IgG deficiency or prior splenectomy must be emergent. Blood cultures and a buffy coat Gram's stain should be obtained. Most pneumococci in the United States are sensitive to penicillin, although many pneumococci demonstrate intermediate resistance to this agent [21]. Penicillin is not effective against H. influenzae or Salmonella species. We believe ceftriaxone (2–4 g/day) represents optimal therapy. Patients scheduled to undergo elective splenectomy should be given a pneumococcal vaccine before this procedure. Patients with AIDS and neoplasms also should be vaccinated, even though the efficacy of the vaccine in this setting has not been demonstrated. H. influenzae B vaccine is available now, and it can be expected that this vaccine will be used in some new settings in the future.

Evolving Treatment Options

Pooled intravenous immunoglobulin can be used adjunctively in the prevention or treatment of infections in several different disorders [22, 23]. The ability of immunoglobulin to reduce infectious complications in children with hereditary B-cell deficiency has been well documented. A recent study has demonstrated that intravenous immunoglobulin (IVIG) decreases the risk of infection in children with AIDS from 67% to 5% [24, 25]. More recently IVIG (200–400 mg/kg IV q3–4 weeks) has been used successfully in patients with chronic lymphocytic leukemia (CLL) and multiple myeloma [22]. Specific immunoglobulin has been used as prophylaxis and as therapy for hepatitis B, cytomegalovirus (CMV), varicella zoster, and Lassa fever. Penicillin prophylaxis has been successful in children after splenectomy, and current literature indicates that children with sickle cell anemia may also benefit [17].

Complement
Deficiency Disorders

The complement cascade plays a pivotal role in the opsonization and killing of many microbial pathogens [26]. In addition serum complement plays an important role in the intracellular killing of aerobic gram-negative bacteria [26]. Patients with deficiencies in the early cascade protein C1, C2, or C4 rarely present with infection, presumably because the alternative complement pathway allows formation of important terminal complement components. If infections do occur, they are caused by encapsulated organisms such as *S. pneumoniae.* Isolated C4b deficiency has been noted in approximately 2% of white patients and predisposes these patients to infections with *S. pneumoniae, H. influenzae,* and *Neisseria meningitidis.* This same relationship does not appear to be present in black patients [27].

C3 is critical to the function of both the classical and the alternative pathway and is also important as an opsonin; C3 deficiency leads to serious problems in those affected [26]. Approximately 70% of patients with C3 deficiency develop severe and recurrent pneumococcal, *H. influenzae,* and meningococcal infections [28]. Similar problems are encountered in patients that develop antibody against C3 (C3 nephritic factor) and patients with deficiencies in the alternative pathway components H or I.

Deficiencies in the late components of complement, with the exception of C9, lead to a marked increase in disseminated neisserial infections, including *N. meningitidis* and gonorrhea. Meningococcal disease usually occurs in adulthood in affected patients. Meningococcal infection occurs in up to 30% of patients with deficiency in terminal complement components. Surprisingly death from meningococcal disease is rare in patients with deficiency in terminal complement components [28, 29].

Special Considerations in Emergency Treatment

Patients with deficiency in early complement components who present with septicemia should be treated for infection with encapsulated bacteria, as described in the section on immunoglobulin deficiency. Patients with late complement component deficiency should be treated with penicillin 12 million to 24 million units per day adjusted for weight and renal function in six divided doses. Many gonococci and some meningococci are now resistant to penicillin, making ceftriaxone 2 g q12h an acceptable, perhaps preferable, alternative to penicillin. Patients with disseminated neisserial disease require evaluation of the complement system by measurement of total hemolytic complement activity (CH50). Patients with known complement deficiencies who have localized, mild infections do not require hospitalization.

Neutrophil Abnormalities

Qualitative Abnormalities

CHRONIC GRANULOMATOUS DISEASE
Neutrophil abnormalities can be qualitative or quantitative. Qualitative disorders are rare and include defects in attachment (LFA-1 receptor deficiency), chemotaxis, phagocytosis, and microbial killing [30]. Chronic granulomatous disease (CGD) of childhood is the best studied of the disorders of neutrophil function. CGD is an inherited disorder characterized by the inability of neutrophils to generate superoxide. The most common inheritance pattern in this disorder is X linked, although an autosomal recessive inheritance occurs [31]. Patients with this disorder develop recurrent infections during childhood, the most common infectious agent being *S. aureus.* Other organisms that cause infections in these patients include *Serratia marsescens, Nocardia asteroides, Pseudomonas aeruginosa, Salmonella* species, and fungi, including *Aspergillus* and *Candida* species [32]. Patients develop cellulitis, adenitis, and recurrent pneumonias. The diagnosis is made by demonstrating that neutrophils in affected patients will not generate superoxide anions or other reactive oxygen species. It recently has been shown that interferon gamma can reduce the incidence of infection in patients with CGD, although the mechanisms of protection are unknown [33].

Quantitative Abnormalities

Neutropenia is the most common clinical disorder affecting neutrophils. Neutropenia usually is secondary to cancer chemotherapeutic agents, although other drugs such as zidovudine, sulfa compounds, and penicillins can be involved. Rare forms of inherited (cyclic) and acquired neutropenia (e.g., Felty's syndrome) are also observed [30].

The risk of infection during neutropenia is directly related to the absolute neutrophil count and the duration of neutropenia. Infection increases in patients with fewer than 1000 cells per μl and is more common and severe in patients with fewer than 500 cells per μl. The incidence of bacteremia appears to increase in patients with absolute neutrophil counts less than 100 cells per μl compared to counts of 100–500, although this correlation is somewhat controversial.

Infections in neutropenic cancer patients most commonly are caused by enteric aerobic gram-negative rods acquired from the GI tract of the host. Schimpff et al. demonstrated that approximately 80% of the organisms causing infection in the neutropenic host can be isolated from the patient's own flora [34]. Whimbey et al. at the Sloan-Kettering Cancer Center reviewed 158 episodes of septicemia in 117 neutropenic patients. They reported that polymicrobic septicemia was most common (21%), followed by Escherichia coli (16%), Klebsiella species (15%), Pseudomonas species (8%), Candida species (6%), and S. aureus (6%). They also found that several "new" pathogens, including Streptococcus faecalis, Staphylococcus epidermidis, and JK Corynebacterium, were of importance; none of these was present in an earlier study [35]. The emergence of S. epidermidis and JK Corynebacterium most likely is related to the increased use of permanent central venous catheters in these patients. These organisms also can be preferentially selected by treatment of neutropenic patients with antibiotics against gram-negative enteric organisms. It must be emphasized that in the vast majority of febrile neutropenic patients (i.e., 80%) no pathogen will be identified.

The risk of invasive fungal infection appears to increase in proportion to the length of time that the patient is neutropenic [36]. Fungi rarely cause the initial infection in neutropenic patients. However, in patients with persistent neutropenia and on broad-spectrum antibiotics the risk of fungal infection increases. Candida, Aspergillus, Torulopsis, and Mucor species all cause severe infections in neutropenic hosts. Several different clinical complications associated with candidal infection have been described, including skin lesions, pneumonia, meningitis, ophthalmitis, endocarditis, nephritis, and diffuse myositis [37]. A syndrome of hepatic candidiasis has been reported recently [38]. Aspergillus and Mucor species invade blood vessels, causing thrombotic infarcts and necrotizing invasive infection. Necrotizing pulmonary infections can lead to exsanguination from hemoptysis [36].

Special Considerations in Emergency Treatment

Fever in a patient with neutropenia requires emergent intervention. Mortality is highest in patients with cancer chemotherapy in whom mucosal damage from chemotherapeutic drugs can allow access of bowel flora to the bloodstream. Isolator blood cultures should be drawn to improve recovery of fungal organisms. During the physical examination special attention should be given to the following: (1) the skin for possible pustular lesions consistent with Candida infections, ecthyma gangrenosum seen with gram-negative sepsis, or evidence of infection around the site of a central venous catheter; (2) a fundoscopic exam for lesions consistent with candidal endophthalmitis; (3) the oropharynx for evidence of ulcerative lesions; and (4) the rectal area for evidence of a perirectal abscess or cellulitis. Urinalysis with culture, blood cultures, and CXR are essential. A spinal tap should not be performed in the absence of CNS signs or symptoms.

The clinician must recognize that signs and symptoms may be subtle in neutropenic patients, since the inflammatory response is limited [39]. Urinary tract infections (UTIs) may lack pyuria, abscesses are rarely fluctuant or indurated, and pneumonia may be subtle; thus, the lack of inflammation does not rule out infection in the neutropenic patient.

For septicemic patients a source of infection is not documented in 30% of them. This percentage mandates obtaining at least two sets of blood cultures before initiating antibiotic therapy. Single-blood-culture isolates of any gram-negative bacilli, S. aureus, S. pneumoniae, Enterococcus faecalis, or Streptococcus viridans in a patient with oral mucositis should be considered significant. For coagulase-negative Staphylococcus and JK Corynebacterium organisms, two positive cultures are significant. Any positive culture together with a positive culture from another source is also significant.

It is not possible to determine which neutropenic patient has bacteremia, since many bacteriemic patients demonstrate no physical findings of infection beyond fever. Therefore, all neutropenic patients with fever should receive empiric antibiotic therapy.

A consensus panel of the Infectious Disease Society of America (IDSA) has adapted guidelines for the management of neutropenic cancer patients [40]. A summary of these guidelines is provided in algorithm form in Fig. 16-1. Empiric therapy should be initiated rapidly in the emergency department after an initial evaluation. Coverage should be tailored to the infectious agents of local importance. In general an antipseudomonal beta-lactam should be combined with an aminoglycoside (e.g., ceftazidime plus tobramycin). Therapy then can be modified based on culture results and to improve coverage of S. aureus and S. epidermidis (e.g., vancomycin), especially in patients with indwelling central venous catheters. Antibiotic coverage is necessary for patients with necrotizing gingivitis, perirectal infections, and other potential anaerobic infections. Ticarcillin-clavulanate plus an aminoglycoside are ideal therapeutic choices in this situation.

Emerging Concepts

Colonization of neutropenic patients with organisms such as P. aeruginosa and Candida and Aspergillus species increases risk of disease due to these organisms. Prophylactic antibiotics and antifungals can be used to eradicate the carriage of these organisms. Oral trimethoprim-sulfamethoxazole and newer quinolone drugs have been studied extensively [41, 42]. Recent studies have demonstrated that miconazole, an antifungal triazole, can decrease the incidence of candidal fungal sepsis in neutropenic patients when given as initial therapy [43]. Studies are in progress to determine the impact of the prophylactic and therapeutic use of the newer triazole antifungal agents (e.g., fluconazole and itraconazole).

Two important advances that depend on molecular biotechnology deserve emphasis. Colony-stimulating factors (CSFs), including G-CSF (granulocyte CSF) and GM-CSF (granulocyte/monocyte CSF) are available. These drugs reduce the nadir and the duration of neutropenia and the incidence of infection. G-CSF has been approved as an adjunct to cancer chemotherapy. It is likely that a "cocktail" of G-CSF and other cytokines will have an even greater impact.

Gram-negative rod bacteremia has a high mortality in neutropenic patients. The pathogenesis of the disease depends on the effects of lipid A and endotoxin. Two monoclonal antibodies (E5 and HA-1A) are being extensively evaluated for reduction of morbidity and mortality in septic patients [44]. The precise criteria for the usage of these antibodies and the optimal dosage schedule have not been determined (see Chap. 6).

Cell-Mediated Immunity

Cell-mediated immunity is a complex process that involves many different cells of the immune system. Pivotal cells include lymphocytes and macrophages. A simplistic schema of this system is presented in Figure 16-2. In this system the macrophage recognizes and binds to a foreign antigen, which is then presented to a lymphocyte in concert with the macrophage Ia antigen. At the same time the macrophage synthesizes and releases interleukin-1 (IL-1). The complex is presented to the helper subset of lymphocytes, which have a receptor for IL-1 as well as the Ia antigen. Helper (CD4 +) lymphocytes become activated and capable of the production of IL-2, interferon gamma (IFN-gamma) and other cytokines. In addition the activated helper cell is capable of promoting B-cell differentiation and activation and differentiation of CD8 + cells into cytotoxic lymphocytes [45]. Other cytokines, such as IL-4, are required for the transformation of an activated B cell into the immunoglobulin-producing plasma cell. Ultimately lymphocyte-derived interferon gamma acts on the macrophage population to induce cellular activation. Activation of the macrophage by IFN-gamma allows macrophages to kill a variety of intracellular microbes [46].

Many different types of disease impair host cell-mediated immunity, clinically marked as anergy in skin testing. Transient anergy is observed after a variety of viral infections but rarely leads to serious infection. Conversely the anergy observed late in HIV disease leads to a uniformly fatal series of opportunistic infections. Emergency department physicians can expect to encounter patients with all different types of cell-mediated compromise.

Infections in patients with impaired cellular immunity are caused by a much wider variety of microbes than those observed in any other compro-

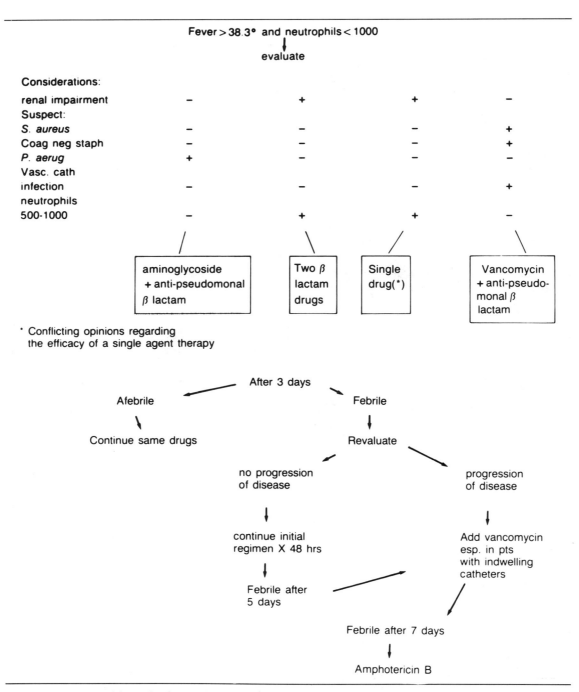

Fig. 16-1. IDSA guidelines for the management of neutropenic cancer patients

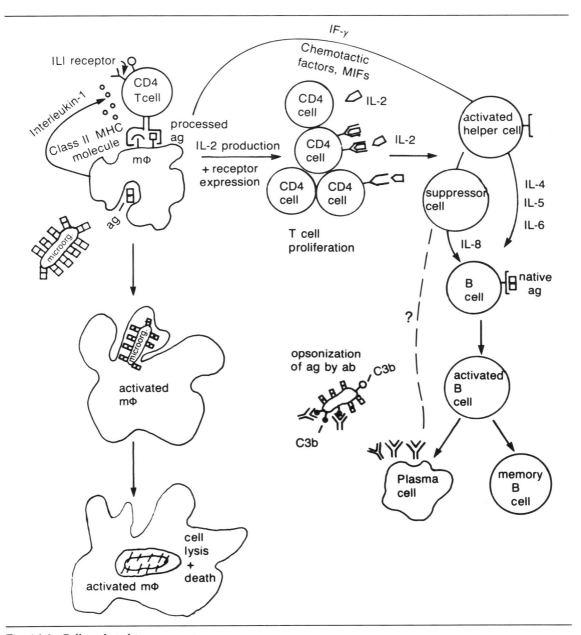

Fig. 16-2. Cell-mediated immune system

mised host. Conversely microbes that cause infection in patients with impaired cellular immunity rarely cause infection in the immunocompetent patient despite their prevalence in the environment. For example, by the age of 4 years 75% of children in the United States have antibodies directed against *Pneumocystis carinii* [47]. The spectrum of infections seen in patients with HIV disease emphasizes the magnitude of the problem. In addition new pathogens heretofore unassociated with human disease have been described at an alarming rate in the patient with HIV disease.

Microbes that cause self-limited infection in the immunocompetent patient lead to life-threatening illness in the immunocompromised patient. CMV, *Toxoplasma gondii*, varicella zoster, and *Candida* infections are examples of this problem.

Acquired Immunodeficiency Syndrome

Infection with HIV ultimately leads to a degree of anergy matched only by the severe immunosuppression associated with bone marrow transplantation. However, patients with HIV disease develop predictable infectious complications during the course of their disease, and so discussion of this problem offers a paradigm appropriate to other patients with defects in cell-mediated immunity.

In HIV disease infectious complications clearly are correlated with the absolute number of CD4+ lymphocytes in the circulation [48]. However, it must be emphasized that the CD4 count will not offer such prognostic information in patients with other types of insults to this system. Furthermore, the correlation of infection with absolute CD4 value is less well understood in children.

Early in HIV disease (>500 CD4+ cells/μl) patients commonly develop herpes simplex or varicella zoster infections. Reactivated herpes infections may present as ulcerative lesions in atypical areas (not just oral or labial areas) and respond relatively poorly to therapy; recurrences after therapy is discontinued are expected [49]. Moreover, patients infected with the HIV virus who have been treated for prolonged periods with acyclovir have developed herpes simplex infections resistant to acyclovir [50]. With a continued fall in the CD4 count, patients develop mucocutaneous candidal infections. Early in the course of HIV infection candidal infection is most commonly found in the oropharynx. As the disease progresses, candidal esophagitis is more frequently encountered [51]. Nonvaginal candidal infection in an otherwise healthy adult strongly suggests HIV disease [52]. It should be emphasized, however, that *Candida* species do not cause disseminated disease in this group of patients in the absence of neutropenia or nosocomial intravenous-line infection.

Finally as the number of CD4+ cells falls below 200/μl, patients infected with HIV develop infections characteristic of AIDS. These include CNS infection with *T. gondii* and *Cryptococcus neoformans*. Pulmonary infections are common and in-

clude infections due to *P. carinii* and mycobacteria (*M. tuberculosis* and *Mycobacterium avium-intracellulare*). *H. capsulatum* and *C. immitus* infections are seen in some parts of the United States. GI tract disease is often due to CMV as well as *Cryptosporidium* organisms, atypical mycobacteria, and occasionally *Strongyloides* and *Giardia* species. Obstructive biliary tract disease can be caused by a number of opportunistic pathogens. As stated previously, patients infected with HIV have not only an impaired cell-mediated immune system but also humoral immune dysfunction. Thus, these patients also have an increased risk of bacterial infection, especially with encapsulated organisms such as *S. pneumoniae* and *H. influenzae* [10]. In addition recurrent salmonella bacteremia has been demonstrated in these patients [53].

SPECIAL CONSIDERATIONS IN EMERGENCY TREATMENT

In patients with defects in cell-mediated immunity signs and symptoms of infection may be less specific because of impaired immune response. For example, only 25%–30% of patients with AIDS caused by cryptococcal meningitis will present with meningismus [54]. Furthermore serologic tests valuable in making the diagnosis of toxoplasmosis and CMV infection have limited value in these patients [55]. For a more complete discussion of HIV-associated infections, an approach to the differential diagnosis, empiric therapy based on the site of infection, specific therapy of the HIV retrovirus, as well as opportunistic infections [56, 57], see Chap. 17.

Transplantation

A detailed description of the infectious complications of transplant patients is beyond the scope of this chapter. However, several points are worth emphasizing. Transplantation of liver, lung, heart, kidney, and bone marrow are now common. In general these patients receive similar antirejection agents (corticosteroids, cyclosporine, azathioprine, and antilymphocyte and antithymocyte globulins) that induce immunosuppression and thus develop infections consistent with defects in cell-mediated immunity. Infectious complications follow the time line demonstrated most clearly in renal transplant patients (Table 16-2). Bacterial infections are

Table 16-2. Infections and renal transplant

Infection site or S	Organisms
1 Month after Transplant	
Wound	Bacteria
Respiratory system	Bacteria
Urinary tract	Bacteria
IV catheters	Bacteria
Liver	HBV, EBV
Skin	HSV
1–6 Months after Transplant	
Respiratory system	TB, *Pneumocystis, Aspergillus,* CMV, Adenovirus (*Histoplasma, Coccidiodes*)
Liver	HCV, NANB
CNS	*Listeria, Aspergillus, Nocardia, Toxoplasma*
Urinary tract	Bacteria, *Candida*
Fever of undetermined origin	CMV, TB
6 Months + after Transplant	
Eye	CMV
CNS	*Listeria, Cryptococcus*
Urinary tract	Bacteria
AIDS syndrome	HIV

an early complication and are the usual cause of infection.

SOLID-ORGAN TRANSPLANTS

Bacterial infections usually are found at the site of transplant. Renal transplant patients often develop cystitis, pyelonephritis, and infected-fluid collections around the transplanted kidney. Lung and heart transplant patients develop pneumonia or bronchitis [58]. Liver transplant patients develop liver, biliary, and other intra-abdominal infections due to enteric bacteria and *Candida* organisms, especially following prolonged use of antibiotics and immunosuppressive agents.

Of the viral infections only herpes simplex occurs within the first month after a transplant. Four to six weeks after the transplantation these patients begin to develop infections because of the severe immune dysfunction caused by chemotherapeutic drugs used to prevent organ rejection.

The most common infectious complication of transplantation is caused by CMV. The frequency

of CMV disease peaks approximately 6 weeks after the transplant, although infectious complications can occur for many months after the transplant. Patients who are CMV negative prior to the transplant and who receive a CMV-positive transplant have the greatest risk of CMV disease. Reactivated CMV infection does not have nearly the risk of disease as does primary infection. Furthermore, CMV infection must be differentiated from CMV disease. Most CMV IgG antibody–positive patients prior to a transplant will have evidence of CMV infection as well as replication after the transplant, as demonstrated by positive cultures in urine, pharynx, and leukocyte buffy coat. Patients with CMV disease have evidence of tissue damage by CMV. CMV infection can cause pneumonitis, hepatitis, gastritis, and colitis. In addition there is evidence that CMV disease increases the risk of rejection of the transplanted organ.

Several unusual infections are associated with specific types of transplantation. Cardiac transplant patients appear to have an increased risk of infections due to *Nocardia species* [59], and *T. gondii* [60], mediastinitis due to *M. hominis* [61], and lymphoproliferative disease due to Epstein-Barr virus (EBV) [62]. Liver transplant patients have an increased incidence of fungal infections due to *Candida* and *Aspergillus* organisms [63]. Other organisms that cause infections in transplant patients include *P. carinii, C. neoformans,* and in certain areas *H. capsulatum* and *C. immitus.*

BONE MARROW TRANSPLANTS

Bone marrow transplants are performed for aplastic anemia, hematologic malignancy, and immunodeficiency diseases. The marrow transplant recipient is at risk for both granulocytopenia and defects in the cell-mediated immunity. Neutropenia occurs in the first 3 weeks following transplant. Graft-versus-host disease and immunosuppressive therapy to treat it result in defects in cell-mediated immunity beginning several weeks after transplant. CMV, interstitial pneumonitis, *Aspergillus* organisms, and *T. gondii* are important infectious agents in the first 100 days after transplant. After 100 days if chronic graft-versus-host disease develops, the patient will be at risk for disease from varicella-zoster virus, *S. pneumoniae,* and endemic and epidemic agents in the locality. If graft-versus-host disease is prevented, the marrow transplant recipient will develop normal immunity.

SPECIAL CONSIDERATIONS
IN EMERGENCY TREATMENT

Despite immunosuppressive therapy most infected transplant patients present with fevers. Patients with respiratory symptoms should have sinus x-rays since sinusitis is common. CXR and sputum Gram's stain and culture in suspected pneumonia are essential. A WBC count and differential, liver function tests, urinalysis and culture, and blood cultures are appropriate. A patient with a persistent temperature above 38.5°C without a clear source should be hospitalized for further evaluation and testing. Any patient with even the most subtle neurologic complaint should undergo a CT scan or MRI and an LP. Viral studies should be obtained only if there is suspicion of a specific viral agent.

The most common infectious causes of a fever in transplant patients are viral syndromes, including CMV and EBV. Toxoplasmosis and CXR-normal P. carinii infection can also present as fevers without a source. Common noninfectious causes of fever include drug reactions (particularly with anti-lymphocyte serums) and rejection (particularly in lung transplants).

Infections of different sites require different approaches. The usual sources of infection are similar to those of nontransplant patients, including the lungs, the urinary tract, and the abdomen. Patients with pulmonary symptoms for fewer than 3 days, purulent sputum, and a focal infiltrate should be admitted and treated for the usual causes of pneumonia. Patients with symptoms for a week or more, a nonproductive cough, and diffuse or nodular lesions on CXR are more likely to have unusual or opportunistic infections. Bronchoalveolar lavage, percutaneous aspiration of peripleural lesion, or lung biopsy may be required for definitive diagnosis. Legionella species and Aspergillus or Nocardia infection also are common in specific areas. Hepatitis is relatively common and can result from hepatitis B or C, CMV, herpes simplex virus, adenovirus, and varicella-zoster. Liver function tests will be abnormal. Definitive diagnosis of these infections requires a biopsy. Fulminant hepatic failure is rare. The highest chance of CNS infection occurs during the first 6 months after transplant. Pyogenic bacteria are unusual; more common pathogens include

Listeria monocytogenes, Aspergillus species, T. gondii, Nocardia species, Mucor species, Candida species, varicella zoster, and progressive multifocal leukoencephalopathy. C. neoformas infection of the CNS occurs later than other infections. CNS infection can have an extremely subtle presentation. Abnormalities of the retina, sinuses, lungs, and skin may help to indicate the etiology of the infection.

Lymphoma and Hodgkin's Disease

Patients with lymphoma, or Hodgkin's disease, are often splenectomized and are at risk for overwhelming postsplenectomy sepsis syndrome, as well as infection from fecal carriage of Salmonella species. Lymphoma can cause urinary obstruction leading to septicemia. Patients with pulmonary symptoms should be evaluated for pneumonia caused by P. carinii and Legionella species. Tuberculosis is also more common in this group of patients. Meningitis with L. monocytogenes, C. neoformans, or tuberculosis may present with only insidious symptoms of headache, fever, or subtle changes in mental status. Cerebral abscesses can be caused by T. gondii, Nocardia species, or M. tuberculosis. Herpes zoster is the major dermatologic problem found in this group. Patients with hematologic malignances are also at risk for acute febrile neutrophilic dermatosis. An acute rise in temperature, skin plaques, and leukocytosis are found in this syndrome, which is responsive to corticosteroids.

There is less degree of urgency in treating febrile patients without neutropenia or splenectomy, so a specific etiology should be established. Patients suspected of infection should be admitted and undergo the appropriate situation-specific diagnostic procedures before initiation of therapy. If the oral temperature is lower than 38.0°C and the patient appears to have a typical upper respiratory infection, the patient may be discharged and followed closely. Patients with temperatures 38.0°C and higher or with evidence of a focal infection require further evaluations.

Other Diseases

There is a wide variety of other diseases that impair cell-mediated immunity. In the United States renal failure, diabetes mellitus, cirrhosis, and steroid or cytotoxic therapy are the etiologies most commonly encountered in clinical practice. Worldwide, malnutrition is the most common cause of impaired cell-mediated immunity. Much rarer forms of impaired cell-mediated immunity are found in congenital diseases such as DiGeorge syndrome, Nezelof syndrome, cartilage hair hypoplasia, severe combined immunodeficiency syndrome, ataxia-telangiectasia syndrome, and Wiskott-Aldrich syndrome. Patients with these conditions who present with infectious illnesses cannot be treated just as normal hosts. The wider range of potential organisms leads to a need for more extensive microbiologic and radiographic testing and a broader spectrum of anti-infectives (e.g., antibacterials, antiparasitics, antivirals, and antifungals). Increased chances of morbidity and mortality mandate admission in most instances.

Miscellaneous

Several different chronic medical conditions are associated with unique infectious complications. These conditions include diabetes mellitus, chronic renal failure, alcoholism with cirrhosis, hemosiderosis, and iron-chelation therapy.

Diabetes Mellitus

Diabetic patients are prone to infections for several different reasons. Autonomic and peripheral neuropathies predispose these patients to repeated trauma of the lower extremity. This leads to an increased incidence of cellulitis and osteomyelitis (see Chap. 11 and Chap. 33). Neurogenic bladder dysfunction allows a large residual volume of urine, which predisposes to UTIs (see Chap. 28). Intrinsic impairment in the host immune system in diabetics also has been demonstrated. Phagocytosis and T-lymphocyte response are impaired [64, 65]. The anergy of diabetic patients is easily appreciated by colonization of the urinary tract of these patients with *Candida albicans*. Particularly serious infections in diabetic patients are rhinocerebral mucormycosis, malignant otitis externa, emphysematous cholecystitis, cellulitis, including necrotizing fasciitis and wound infections, urinary tract infections, and pulmonary infections.

RHINOCEREBRAL MUCORMYCOSIS

Rhinocerebral mucormycosis is caused by fungi of the genus *Rhizopus*. The fungi are widespread in nature, and humans probably acquire them by inhalation of fungal spores. In the normal host *Rhizopus* spores are eliminated by alveolar macrophages. Animal studies have shown that spore germination occurs more readily in the streptozotocin-induced diabetic mouse [66]. Normal human serum inhibits the growth of the fungi, while serum from diabetic patients can actually increases growth [67]. Once these fungi have begun to grow, they have a marked propensity for tissue invasion via blood vessels, leading to thrombosis and infarction.

Patients with rhinocerebral mucormycosis usually are diabetic patients with ketoacidosis. Patients with rhinocerebral mucormycosis develop headache with fever and facial pain. Cranial nerve signs may be present, including ocular findings or fifth- and seventh-nerve palsies. Cavernous sinus and internal carotid artery thrombosis may develop. A necrotic eschar involving the palate and the nasal passages is virtually diagnostic. Bismuth compounds, tetracycline, and other drugs can lead to a coating of the tongue and palate with a fine black coating (of no clinical consequence), which may be mistaken for mucor. Diagnosis of mucormycosis is made by biopsy of the affected area and demonstration of the fungal hyphae by histology. Infectious disease and ear, nose, and throat specialists need to assist with such a patient. Prior to the use of amphotericin B the mortality of this disease was greater than 90%. With aggressive débridement and amphotericin B mortality has been reduced to 15%–50% [68]. Amphotericin B treatment is given at high daily doses of 1 mg/kg to patients with rhinocerebral mucormycosis (see Chap. 31).

MALIGNANT OTITIS EXTERNA

Malignant otitis externa is a condition seen almost exclusively in elderly diabetic patients. The initial description by Chandler referred to 13 patients with deep infections of bone and tissue caused by *P. aeruginosa* [69]. However, other organisms also have been implicated. Affected patients develop ear pain and a purulent drainage from the ear canal. Left untreated the disease will spread into adjacent bone and tissue, causing progressive tissue destruction. Spread of infection into the CNS can cause death. When first described, the disease was usually fatal.

However, aggressive débridement of devitalized tissue combined with a long course of an antipseudomonal penicillin or cephalosporin and aminoglycoside can reduce the mortality to 15% [70].Ceftazidime has been used as a single agent [70]. After initial intravenous therapy long-term outpatient treatment with ciprofloxacin has been effective (see Chap. 34).

EMPHYSEMATOUS CHOLECYSTITIS

Emphysematous cholecystitis is an uncommon manifestation of cholecystitis due to gas-forming organisms, most commonly *Clostridium perfringens*. The pathognomonic finding is the presence of gas roentgenographically in the gallbladder lumen, wall, or elsewhere in the biliary system without an enteric fistula. As of 1975 there were only 161 cases in the literature describing this entity. Emphysematous cholecystitis differs from acute cholecystitis in several ways. Unlike acute cholecystitis due to cholelithiasis, emphysematous cholecystitis appears to have a male preponderance. Gallstones are not seen in this disorder as commonly as in acute cholecystitis. In the review by Mentzer et al. 28% of patients with emphysematous cholecystitis did not have gallstones, compared to only 10% of those with acute cholecystitis [71]. Perforation of the gallbladder is much more common in emphysematous cholecystitis. Diabetes mellitus is commonly associated with emphysematous cholecystitis; it was present in 38% of the patients in the Mentzer review. The mortality of patients less than 60 years of age is significantly increased in emphysematous cholecystitis compared to acute cholecystitis. However, the symptoms and signs of the two forms of cholecystitis are similar; despite the higher mortality patients with emphysematous cholecystitis are no more likely to have peritoneal signs than patients with acute cholecystitis [71]. The key to diagnosing emphysematous cholecystitis is the abdominal roentgenogram showing the presence of gas in the biliary system (see Chap. 27).

CELLULITIS, NECROTIZING FASCIITIS, AND WOUND INFECTIONS

Necrotizing fasciitis and cellulitis are commonly associated with diabetes. In one study 75% of patients with necrotizing cellulitis were diabetics [72]. There also are organisms that are seen more frequently in diabetics compared to a healthy age-matched population. These include group B and group G streptococcal infections.

Because of peripheral nerve damage and its sequelae, diabetics also are prone to traumatic wound infections, especially of the lower extremity. Poor peripheral circulation can lead to gangrene. Skin and soft-tissue infections in diabetics are caused by staphylococci and streptococci, as well as enteric gram-negative organisms and anaerobic organisms. A polymicrobial infection is the rule rather than the exception. Osteomyelitis of underlying bone is a common and serious consequence of these infections. Because of poor arterial circulation, adequate tissue delivery of antibiotics to infected bone can make treatment very difficult (see Chap. 11 and Chap. 33).

Diabetic patients who present with cellulitis need careful examination to exclude necrotizing fasciitis. Bullae, crepitation, and surface hyperesthesia should alert the clinician to the possibility of necrotizing fasciitis. These patients often present with high fever and leukocytosis out of proportion to local complaints. Plain films and a CT scan of the involved area may be required to make the diagnosis. Careful physical examination may be required to find affected tissues. "Silent" infection of the uterus, vagina, thigh, and rectus muscles have all been reported.

Antibiotic treatment of a diabetic with cellulitis should treat enteric gram-negative organisms and anaerobes, as well as staphylococci and streptococci. Imipenem-cilastatin 500 mg IV q6h adjusted for renal function or ticarcillin-clavulanic acid 3.1 g IV q4–q6h or cefoxitin 2 mg IV q6h adjusted for renal function are reasonable choices. Patients with necrotizing fasciitis require an emergent surgical consult for débridement. Early diagnosis of necrotizing fasciitis can decrease mortality from 20%–45% to 10%–15% [73] (see Chap. 32).

UTIs

Clinical experience demonstrates that UTIs in diabetics are more difficult to manage than in normal populations. Neurogenic bladder and glycosuria promote the growth of urinary organisms. Common etiologic agents include coliform organisms, *Pseudomonas* species, group B streptococci, *C. albicans*, and *Torulopsis glabrata*. A UTI can lead to diabetic ketoacidosis, sepsis, perinephric abscess, emphysematous cystitis, emphysematous pyelonephritis and papillary necrosis.

The patient with a lower tract UTI and well-controlled diabetes can be treated as an outpatient with the antibiotics usually used for UTIs (see Chap. 28). These patients, however, require close follow-up. Patients with upper tract or complicated UTIs or metabolic derangements are admitted for intravenous antibiotics; aminoglycosides and contrast dye should be avoided if possible to prevent jeopardizing renal function. Appropriate antibiotics include trimethoprin-sulfamethoxazole, ticarcillin-clavulanate, third-generation cephalosporin, imipenem, and a flouroquinolone. If perinephric abscess is suspected, a CT scan or an ultrasound should be performed. Surgical drainage may be required.

PULMONARY INFECTION

The diabetic may develop pneumonia caused by common community acquired agents as well as gram-negative organisms, S. aureus, and Legionella pneumophilia. Once infected the diabetic is more likely to develop sepsis and metabolic complications, so hospitalization for intravenous antibiotics is necessary. Empiric treatment includes erythromycin for infections caused by S. pneumoniae, Mycoplasma pneumoniae, and L. pneumophilia plus a second- or third-generation cephalosporin for gram-negative coverage.

Renal Failure

Patients with chronic renal failure have an increased incidence of infectious complications, although there is debate as to the specific immune impairment. Studies have demonstrated that neutrophils from renal failure patients have normal bactericidal and phagocytic capacity [74]. Other studies have contradicted this [75]. Patients with chronic renal failure do show evidence of diminished cellular immune response as manifested by anergy to recall antigens.

Renal failure patients are prone to infections with S. aureus. Approximately 60% of patients on hemodialysis are carriers of S. aureus, and this number increases as a function of the amount of time spent on dialysis [76]. In addition these organisms may demonstrate increased virulence. Arteriovenous shunt infections with S. aureus are common and a frequent cause of morbidity in these patients.

Patients on chronic ambulatory peritoneal dialysis (CAPD) have an increased risk of infectious peritonitis. Sixty percent of patients on CAPD will develop peritonitis in the first year [77] and 20%–30% of patients will have recurrent peritonitis, forcing discontinuation of CAPD [78]. Forty percent of patients on CAPD will develop exit-site or tunnel infections. The organisms most commonly isolated are coagulase-negative staphylococci, followed by S. aureus, streptococci, and other skin flora. E. coli and other gram-negative rods and Candida species pose an additional problem.

The diagnosis of peritonitis requires the presence of at least two of the following: (1) symptoms of peritonitis, (2) visibly cloudy fluid with WBCs evident on microscopic examination, and (3) presence of organisms on Gram's stain or culture of the peritoneal dialysate fluid. Abdominal pain and tenderness are seen in approximately 70% of patients, and fever is present in about 50%. Exit-site infections usually present with local purulence or tenderness around the catheter.

Treatment should not be initiated until 50–100 ml of peritoneal dialysate fluid has been obtained for Gram's stain and culture. Two sets of blood culture bottles should be inoculated with this fluid. Several treatment regimens have been subscribed to. Nonseptic patients can be treated by intraperitoneal (IP) administration. Vancomycin 9 mg/kg IP plus tobramycin or gentamicin 0.9 mg/kg IP as initial empiric loading doses can be initiated in the emergency department. The need for IV therapy and modifications of antibiotics will be determined by the patient's status and culture results. Intraperitoneal vancomycin can cause chemical peritonitis, so many physicians prefer giving this agent IV instead of a single initial dose of 100 mg IV. Maintenance therapy is given at reduced doses over 10 days.

Patients with renal failure often have coexisting diseases that will lead to immune impairment, such as diabetes and nephrotic syndrome, or they will be immunosuppressed as a result of the use of oral corticosteroids or cytotoxic therapy. In addition these patients have an intrinsic cell-mediated defect, which leads to an increased incidence of fungal infections due to *C. neoformans* (or in specific areas of the country *Histoplasma* or *Coccidiodes* organisms) and of nocardial and mycobacterial infections. In addition *S. aureus* carriage is common, and *S. aureus* infections are a frequent problem.

Alcoholism and Cirrhosis

Patients with alcoholic cirrhosis have been reported to have defective serum bactericidal activity against *E. coli* [79]. Impaired opsonization by serum from these patients has been described, as has [80] impaired neutrophil chemotaxis [81]. Not surprisingly as a result of these defects, patients with cirrhosis have an increased risk of infection with bacterial organisms (see Chap. 18).

SPONTANEOUS BACTERIAL PERITONITIS

Spontaneous bacterial peritonitis (SBP) is a unique disorder found almost exclusively in patients with ascites secondary to liver disease. The majority of cases of infection in this disorder are felt to be secondary to hematogenous seeding of ascitic fluid [82]. The most common organisms isolated in SBP are enteric gram-negative organisms. In a review of the literature by Wilcox and Dismukes *E. coli* was isolated in 47% of cases, followed by streptococci (26%), *Klebsiella* species (11%), and other gram-negative enteric pathogens (11%). The diagnosis of this entity requires a high index of suspicion in patients with ascites. Fever is the most common presenting feature and is seen in 50%–80% of patients [82]. Abdominal pain is seen in 27%–72% of cases, and series have shown that up to 48% of patients with SBP will have no abdominal complaints [82]. Peripheral blood leukocytosis is common, as are abnormalities in synthetic liver function. Other subtle signs and symptoms include diarrhea, worsening renal insufficiency, refractoriness to diuretics, hypothermia, and unexplained encephalopathy. Up to 33% of patients may be asymptomatic with SBP [83], but appropriately cultured ascitic fluid into blood culture bottles at the bedside will lead to the diagnosis [84]. (The diagnosis and treatment of SBP are covered in Chap. 18 and Chap. 27.)

VIBRIO VULNIFICUS INFECTION

Cirrhotic patients also have a greatly increased risk of developing septicemia due to *Vibrio vulnificus* and *Yersinia* species. *V. vulnificus* is a halophilic marine *Vibrio* species. The onset of infection is typically in the period from March through November. The organism is most commonly found in raw oysters harvested from beds along the coasts of Florida, Louisiana, and Texas. *V. vulnificus* infection can cause several different clinical syndromes, including wound infections, primary septicemia, and GI illness (85).

Wound infections usually occur in patients exposed to water at the time of the wound or just subsequent to the wound occurring. *V. vulnificus* wound infections are characterized by an intense cellulitis with swelling. In a study by Klontz et al. 17% of patients with wound infections had rapid extension of cellulitis and swelling in the extremity with the wound and the development of secondary bullae. In the four patients who died of septicemia secondary to the wound, the median time of sustaining the wound until death was 4.5 days [85]

Primary septicemia with *V. vulnificus* in immunocompromised patients carries a high morbidity and mortality. From 1981–1987 38 cases of primary septicemia with *V. vulnificus* were identified in Florida in which there was no evidence of a preexisting wound infection. These patients presented with fever, hypotension, and/or mental status changes; *V. vulnificus* was isolated from blood or tissue culture in all 38 patients. Sixty-one percent of these patients developed secondary cutaneous lesions characterized by cellulitis, ecchymosis, and bullae; 71% of these patients reported the onset of nausea, vomiting, or diarrhea around the time of their illness [85]. Fifty-five percent of these patients died. Liver disease occurred in 66% of these patients, and other chronic medical diseases were found in 63%, including alcoholism, diabetes mellitus, steroid usage, and cancer [85]. Because of these findings, immunocompromised patients, especially those with cirrhosis, should be instructed not to eat raw seafood, especially raw oysters.

Antibiotic treatment appears to affect the case-fatality rate of infection with *V. vulnificus* especially those with septicemia. Although not statistically significant in the Klontz study, patients who received doxycycline or tetracycline regimens appeared to do better. Patients in whom the physician suspects *V. vulnificus* should have blood cultures drawn and if possible cultures sent of bullae or wounds. We currently recommend treatment with doxycycline 100 mg bid for infections with *V. vulnificus*.

Hemosiderosis and Iron-Chelation Therapy

Patients on iron-chelation therapy have an increased risk of infection, although the specific defect in the immune system in these situations has not been completely elucidated. Disseminated mucormycosis has been described in patients receiving desferoximine for the treatment of iron-overload diseases. Patients with hemachromatosis also have an increased risk of infection due to *Yersinia* species.

References

1. Pinkel D. Chickenpox and leukemia. *J Pediatr* 58:729, 1961.
2. Dagoo-Rynnel B et al. Pneumococcal antibodies of different immunoglobulin subclasses in normal and IgG subclass deficient individuals of various ages. *Acta Otolaryngol* 101:146, 1986.
3. Oxelius V. Chronic infections in a family with hereditary deficiency of IgG 2 and IgG 4. *Clin Exp Immunol* 17:19, 1974.
4. Anderson CL, Loon JR. Human leukocyte IgG Fc receptors. *Immunology Today.* 7:264, 1986.
5. Buckley RH. Humoral immunodeficiency. *Clin Immunol Immunopathol* 40:13, 1986.
6. McKinney RE, Katz SL, Wilfert CM. Chronic enteroviral meningoencephalitis in agammaglobulinemic patients. *Rev Infect Dis* 9:334, 1987.
7. Roifman CM et al. Increased susceptibility to mycoplasma infection in patients with hypogammaglobulinemia. *Am J Med* 80:590, 1986.
8. LaGalbo PR, Sampson HA, Buckley RH. Symptomatic giardiasis in three patients with X-linked agammaglobulinemia. *J Pediat* 101:78, 1982.
9. Robertson TI. Complications and causes of death in B cell chronic lymphocytic leukaemia: a long term study of 105 patients. *Austral N Zeal J Med* 20:44, 1990.
10. Witt DJ, Craven DE, McCabe WR. Bacterial infections in adult patients with the acquired immune deficiency syndrome (AIDS) and AIDS-related complex. *Am J Med* 89:900, 1987.
11. Krasinski K et al. Bacterial infections in human immunodeficiency virus-infected children. *Pediatr Infect Dis* 7:323, 1988.
12. Vernon DD et al. Respiratory failure in children with acquired immunodeficiency syndrome and acquired immunodeficiency syndrome-related complex. *Pediatr* 82:223, 1988.
13. Gopal V, Bisno AL. Fulminant pneumococcal infections in "normal" asplenic hosts. *Arch Intern Med* 137:1526, 1977.
14. Hicklin H, Verghese A, Alvarez S. Dysgonic fermenter-2 septicemia. *Rev Infect Dis* 9:884, 1987.
15. Jobs L et al. Dysgonic fermenter-2: a clinical-epidemiologic review. *J Emerg Med* 7:185, 1989.
16. Dammin GJ et al. The rising incidence of clinical *Babesia microti* infection. *Hum Pathol* 12:398, 1981.
17. Gaston MH, Verter J. Sickle cell anaemia trial. *Statist Med* 9:45, 1990.
18. Cohen JI, Bartlett JA, Corey GR. Extra-intestinal manifestations of *Salmonella* infections. *Medicine (Baltimore)* 66:349, 1987.
19. Clark JA et al. Selective IgA deficiency in blood donors. *Am J Clin Pathol* 80:210, 1983.
20. Eliasson R et al. The immotile-cilia syndrome: a congenital ciliary abnormality as an etiologic factor in chronic airway infections and male sterility. *N Engl J Med* 297:1, 1977.
21. Simberkoff MS et al. Antibiotic-resistant isolates of *Streptococcus pneumoniae* from clinical specimens: a cluster of serotype 19A organisms in Brooklyn, New York. *J Infect Dis* 153:78, 1986.
22. Yap PL. Intravenous immunoglobulin for secondary immunodeficiency. *Blut* 60:8, 1990.
23. Cooperative Group for the Study of Immunoglobulin in Chronic Lymphocytic Leukemia. Intravenous immunoglobulin for the prevention of infection in chronic lymphocytic leukemia. *N Engl J Med* 319:902, 1988.
24. Calvelli TA, Rubinstein A. Intravenous gammaglobulin in infant acquired immunodeficiency syndrome. *Pediatr Infect Dis* 5(supp 1):S207–10, 1986.
25. Fearon DT. Complement. *J Allergy Clin Immunol* 71:520–29, 1983.
26. Fries LF, O'Shea JJ, Frank MM. Inherited deficiencies of complement and complement-related proteins. *Clin Immunol Immunopathol* 40:37, 1986.
27. Bishof NA, Welch TR, Beischel LS. C4B deficiency: a risk factor bacteremia with encapsulated organisms. *J Infect Dis* 162:348, 1990.
28. Ross SC, Densen P. Complement deficiency states

and infection: epidemiology, pathogenesis and consequences of neisserial and other infections in an immune deficiency. *Medicine (Baltimore)* 63:243, 1984.

29. Zimran A, Rudensky B, Kramer MR. Hereditary complement deficiency in survivors of meningococcal disease. High prevalence of C7/C8 deficiency in sephardic Jews. *Q J Med* 63:349, 1987.

30. White CJ, Gallin JI. Phagocyte defects. *Clin Immunol Immunopathol* 40:50, 1986.

31. Curnutte JT. Chronic granulomatous disease: clinical and genetic aspects. In Lehrer RI (mod.), Neutrophils and host defense. *Ann Intern Med* 109:127, 1988.

32. Lazarus GM, Neu HM. Agents responsible for infection in chronic granulomatous disease of childhood. *J Pediat* 86:409, 1975.

33. The International Chronic Granulomatous Disease Cooperative Study Group. Controlled trial of interferon gamma to prevent infection in chronic granulomatous disease. *N Engl J Med* 324:509, 1991.

34. Schimpff SC et al. Origin of infection in acute non-lymphocytic leukemia: significance of hospital acquisition of potential pathogens. *Ann Intern Med* 77:707, 1972.

35. Whimbey E et al. Bacteremia and fungemia in patients with neoplastic disease. *Am J Med* 82:723, 1987.

36. Baker RD. Leukopenia and therapy in leukemia as factors predisposing to fatal mycoses. *Am J Clin Pathol* 37:358, 1962.

37. Jarowski CI et al. Fever, rash, and muscle tenderness: a distinctive clinical presentation of disseminated candidiasis. *Arch Intern Med* 138:544, 1978.

38. Haron E et al. Hepatic candidiasis: an increasing problem in immunocompromised patients. *Am J Med* 83:17, 1988.

39. Pizzo PA et al. Fever in the pediatric and young adult patient with cancer: a prospective study of 1,001 episodes. *Medicine (Baltimore)* 61:153, 1982.

40. Hughes WT et al. From the Infectious Diseases Society of America. Guidelines for the use of antimicrobial agents in neutropenic patients with unexplained fever. *J Infect Dis* 161(6):1316, 1990.

41. Bow EJ, Rayner E, Louie TJ. Comparison of norfloxacin with cotrimoxazole for infection prophylaxis in acute leukemia. *Am J Med* 84:847, 1988.

42. Dekker AW, Rozenberg AM, Verhoef J. Infection prophylaxis in acute leukemia: a comparison of ciprofloxacin with trimethoprim-sulfamethoxazole and colistin. *Ann Intern Med* 106:7, 1987.

43. Wingard JR et al. Prevention of fungal sepsis in patients with prolonged neutropenia: a randomized, double-blind, placebo-controlled trial of intravenous miconazole. *Am J Med* 83:1103, 1987.

44. Ziegler EJ, Fisher CJ, HA-1A Sepsis Group. Treatment of gram-negative bacteremia and septic shock with HA-1A human monoclonal antibody against endotoxin. *N Engl J Med* 324:429, 1991.

45. Royer HD, Reinherz EL. T lymphocytes: ontogeny, function, and relevance to clinical disorders. *N Engl J Med* 317:1136, 1987.

46. Murray HW. Interferon-gamma, the activated macrophage, and the host defense against microbial challenge. *Ann Intern Med* 108:595, 1988.

47. Pifer LL et al. *Pneumocystis carinii* infection: evidence of high prevalence in normal and immunosuppressed children. *Pediatrics* 61:35, 1978.

48. Schnittman SM et al. Increasing viral burden in CD4+ T cells from patients with human immunodeficiency virus (HIV) infection reflects rapidly progressive immunosuppression and clinical disease. *Ann Intern Med* 113:438, 1990.

49. Thiers BH. Acyclovir in the treatment of herpes virus infections. *Dermatol Clin* 8(3):583, 1990.

50. Erlich KS et al. Acyclovir-resistant herpes simplex virus infections in patients with the acquired immunodeficiency syndrome. *N Engl J Med* 320:293, 1989.

51. Wray D, Felix DH, Cummings CG. Alteration of humoral responses to *Candida* in HIV infection. *Br Dent J* 168(8):326, 1990.

52. Imam N et al. Hierarchical pattern of mucosal candida infections in HIV-seropositive women. *Am J Med* 89(2):142, 1990.

53. Glaser JB et al. Recurrent *Salmonella typhimurium* bacteremia associated with the acquired immunodeficiency syndrome. *Ann Intern Med* 102:189, 1985.

54. Zuger A et al. Cryptococcal disease in patients with AIDS. *Ann Intern Med* 104:234, 1986.

55. Wanke C et al. Toxoplasma encephalitis in patients with acquired immune deficiency syndrome: diagnosis and response to therapy. *Am J Trop Med Hyg* 36:509, 1987.

56. Wispelwey B, Scheld WM. Brain abscess. *Rev Clin Neuropharm* 10:483, 1987.

57. Leport C et al. An open study of the pyrimethamine-clindamycin combination in AIDS patients with brain toxoplasmosis [letter]. *J Infect Dis* 160:557, 1990.

58. Ho M et al. Infections in kidney, heart and liver transplant recipients on cyclosporine. *Transplant Proc* 15:2768, 1983.

59. Simpson GL et al. Nocardial infections in the immunocompromised host: a detailed study in a defined population. *Rev Infect Dis* 3:492, 1981.

60. Luft BJ et al. Primary and reactivated toxoplasma infection in patients with cardiac transplants. *Ann Intern Med* 99:27, 1983.

61. Steffenson DO et al. Mycoplasma hominis median sternotomy infections. *Ann Intern Med* 106:204, 1987.

62. Ho M et al. The frequency of Epstein-Barr virus infection and associated lymphoproliferative syndrome after transplantation and its manifestations in children. *Transplantation* 45:719, 1988.

63. Kusne S et al. Infections after liver transplantation. An analysis of 101 consecutive cases. *Medicine* 67:132, 1988.

64. Molenaar DM et al. Leukocyte chemotaxis in diabetic patients and their non-diabetic first degree relatives. *Diabetes* 25:880, 1976.

65. Bagdade JD, Root RK, Bulger RJ. Impaired leukocyte function in patients with poorly controlled diabetes. *Diabetes* 23:9, 1974.

66. Waldorf AR, Ruderman N, Diamond RD. Specific susceptibility to mucormycosis in murine diabetes and bronchoalveolar macrophage defense against *Rhizopus*. *J Clin Invest* 74:150, 1984.

67. Gale GR, Welch A. Studies of opportunistic fungi. I. Inhibition of *R. oryzae* by human sera. *Am J Med Sci* 45:604, 1961.

68. Markevsky AM et al. The changing spectrum of disease, etiology and diagnosis of mucormycosis. *Human Pathol* 11:457, 1980.

69. Chandler J. Malignant external otitis. *Laryngoscope* 78:1257, 1968.

70. Johnson MP, Ramphal R. Malignant external otitis: report on therapy with Ceftazidime and review of therapy and prognosis. *Rev Infect Dis* 12:173, 1990.

71. Mentzer RM et al. A comparative appraisal of emphysematous cholecystitis. *Am J Surg* 129:10, 1975.

72. Stone HH, Martin JD Jr. Synergistic necrotizing cellulitis. *Ann Surg* 175:702, 1972.

73. Sudarsky LA et al. Improved results from a standardized approach in treating patients with necrotizing fasciitis. *Ann Surg* 206:661, 1987.

74. Dobbelstein H. Immune system in uremia. *Nephron* 17:409, 1976.

75. Wierusz-Wysocka B et al. Phagocytosis and neutrophil bactericidal capacity in patients with uremia. *Folia Haematol* 111:589, 1984.

76. Tuazon CU. Skin and skin structure infections in the patient at risk: carrier state of *Staphylococcus aureus*. *Am J Med* 77(suppl):166, 1984.

77. Peterson PK, Matzke GR, Keane WF. Current concepts in the management of peritonitis in continuous ambulatory peritoneal dialysis patients. *Rev Infect Dis* 9:604, 1987.

78. Steinberg SM et al. Report of the national CAPD registry of the National Institutes of Health: characteristics of participants and selected outcome measures for the period January 1, 1981 through August 31, 1984. In National CAPD Registry of the National Institute of Arthritis, Diabetes, and Digestive and Kidney Diseases. Washington, D.C.: U.S. Public Health Services, 1985.

79. Fierer J, Finley F. Deficient serum bactericidal activity against *Escherichia coli* in patients with cirrhosis of the liver. *J Clin Invest* 63:912, 1979.

80. Runyon BA et al. Opsonic activity of human ascitic fluid: a potentially important protective mechanism against spontaneous bacterial peritonitis. *Hepatology* 5:634, 1985.

81. Rajkovic IA, Williams R. Mechanisms of abnormalities in host defenses against bacterial infection in liver disease. *Clin Sci* 68:247, 1985.

82. Wilcox CM, Dismukes WE. Spontaneous bacterial peritonitis. *Medicine (Baltimore)* 66:447, 1987.

83. Correia JP, Conn HO. Spontaneous bacterial peritonitis in cirrhosis: endemic or epidemic. *Med Clin North Am* 59:963, 1975.

84. Runyon BA, Umland ET, Merlin T. Inoculation of blood culture bottles with ascitic fluid: improved detection of spontaneous bacterial peritonitis. *Arch Intern Med* 147:73, 1987.

85. Klontz KC et al. Syndromes of *Vibrio vulnificus* infections: clinical and epidemiologic features in Florida cases 1981–1987. *Ann Intern Med* 109:318, 1988.

17

Infection in the HIV-Positive Patient

FREDERICK T. KOSTER

Since its appearance in 1981 the epidemic of the human immunodeficiency virus type 1 (HIV-1) infection and its uniformly fatal sequel, the acquired immunodeficiency syndrome (AIDS), has become one of the greatest health problems worldwide. Initially in the United States the epidemic was confined to certain urban areas such as New York City, San Francisco, Los Angeles, and Miami, but in 10 years the epidemic has spread to all urban and rural regions. AIDS presents many difficult epidemiologic, social, economical, psychological, legal, and ethical dilemmas, which lie beyond the scope of this chapter. Certain medical problems, which are dealt with here, will be confronted by all emergency department physicians, since all caregivers have an ethical responsibility to care for the HIV-infected patient in emergent or life-threatening medical situations.

Unique Aspects of HIV Infection

The challenges of diagnosing and treating emergent medical problems in the HIV-positive patient are in some ways unique and can be summarized in three areas. First, many patients do not know that they are HIV-positive, they deny their risk of infection, they refuse testing, they do not offer helpful histori-

cal data that would indicate risk of HIV infection, or they refuse to reveal their known HIV-positive status. Knowledge of patients' HIV-positive status is critical to their assessment. Second, HIV-positive patients experience a wide range of immunosuppression that cannot readily be measured in the emergency department. The degree of immunosuppression will increase susceptibility to a multitude of opportunistic and community acquired infections, and the differential diagnosis broadens as the immune status deteriorates. Third, in the setting of HIV infection, many infections have altered or bizarre clinical presentations, multiple infections may present simultaneously, and progression of infection may be extremely rapid.

The challenge has been so great, in fact, that an entire specialty has emerged focused on the medical and psychological care of the HIV-infected patient. It is difficult for the emergency physician, generalist, internist, or surgeon to become familiar with all the infectious, oncologic, and neurologic complications of HIV infection, not to mention the rapidly changing therapies available. Thus, the physician in the emergency department should not hesitate to involve a specialist, when available, early in the emergent care of the HIV-positive patient or to refer the patient for long-term outpatient care.

This chapter covers only the more common complications of HIV infection presenting to the emergency department, and the reader is referred to a number of excellent texts for additional information gency department, and the reader is referred to a number of excellent texts for additional information [1–3]. In addition, a number of electronic databases are available [4]; the most complete bibliographic online database is AIDSLINE through the National Library of Medicine (800-638-8480). The Centers for Disease Control (CDC) in Atlanta, Georgia, maintains the National AIDS Information Clearinghouse, a free service (800-458-5231; international number is 301-217-0023) on HIV-related services, organizations, educational materials, and CDC publications such as *HIV/AIDS Surveillance*.

HIV Transmission and Risk Groups

AIDS is caused by HIV-1; HIV-2, which is rare in the United States, is occasionally imported from western Africa. HIV is a human retrovirus belonging to the lentivirus subfamily and is distinct from another human retrovirus, the human T-cell leukemia/lymphoma virus (HTLV I). HIV can integrate into the DNA of human lymphocytes and can survive in several other cell types such as monocytes and glial cells in the brain, enabling it to establish a persistent latent infection [5]. Transmission can occur at any stage of the infection but is particularly efficient during the first weeks of infection, before the immune response is established, and late in the infection, when immunosuppression is profound.

Blood and semen are the only body fluids that have been shown conclusively to transmit the infection and that contain relatively high titers of virus. Lower concentrations of the virus are found intermittently in cervical and vaginal secretions, and transmission of virus by these fluids occurs. The virus also is found in low concentrations in saliva, tears, breast milk, and amniotic fluid, and transmission likely occurs by the latter two fluids. No epidemiologic evidence has yet indicated transmission by saliva or tears.

There are only three routes of transmission: during sexual intercourse, contact with infected blood or blood products, and in utero from infected mother to fetus [6]. Table 17-1 illustrates the major risk groups in the United States, according to the percentage of AIDS cases reported for each of three categories: adult men, adult women, and children. AIDS is defined as an opportunistic infection or malignancy in someone with HIV infection (Table 17-2). Since HIV infection is not a reportable condition, only crude estimates of the total number of infected individuals are available, and these indicate that there are 1 million to 1.5 million HIV-infected people living in the United States, with over 200,000 cases of AIDS having been reported as of December 31, 1991. Casual contact, including living in the same room, performing a physical examination, and kissing, does not result in risk of transmission [6]. (The risks of occupational contact and transmission are discussed in Chap. 5.)

Diagnosing HIV Infection

Taking the History

Every patient examined for an emergent medical problem should be questioned whether he or she is known to be HIV-infected, has been tested, or is a member of a recognized risk group. Unfortunately few physicians routinely screen their patients for high-risk behaviors, as noted in a recent survey in the Midwest in which only 11% of faculty and physicians in training did so [7]. Questions about a patient's HIV status should be prefaced by a remark that such inquiries are now routine and do not imply prejudicial suspicion of unreported risk. If the patient is unaware of his or her risk, additional questions about sexual history, intravenous needle use, and blood transfusions should be pursued.

Male patients should be asked if they have had "sex with men," rather than whether they are gay or homosexual, since many bisexual men do not consider themselves to be gay. Sexual practices that increase risk of transmission include multiple partners, particularly those among risk groups; receptive anal intercourse or vaginal intercourse accompanied by bleeding from tissue injury; sexually transmitted infections, particularly syphilis, chancroid, and herpes simplex, in which ulcers facilitate the passage of the virus through the mucosal barrier. Nonjudgmental inquiry must be made about drug use with intravenous needles, particularly needle sharing, and include any such habit

Table 17-1. Distribution percentage of AIDS cases by transmission category and year of report, United States, 1981–1988

Category	AIDS cases (%)				
	Before 1985	1985	1986	1987	1988
Adult Males (≥13 Years)					
Homosexual/bisexual only	69	72	71	70	63
IV drug user	15	15	15	14	20
Homosexual and IV drug user	10	8	8	8	7
Hemophilic	1	1	1	1	1
Heterosexual					
Heterosexual contact	<1	<1	1	1	1
Born in Pattern II country[a]	3	1	1	1	1
Transfusion	1	1	2	2	2
Undetermined	2	2	2	3	4[b]
Adult Females (≥13 Years)					
IV drug user	58	53	49	49	53
Coagulation disorder	<1	1	<1	<1	<1
Heterosexual					
Heterosexual contact	16	21	28	27	26
Born in Pattern II country	8	6	6	4	3
Transfusion	8	11	10	13	10
Undetermined	10	9	6	6	8[b]
Children (<13 Years)					
Coagulation disorder	4	6	6	7	7
Transfusion	11	14	13	14	11
Mother with/at risk for AIDS, HIV infection					
IV drug user	45	47	44	41	40
Sex with person at risk	11	17	24	21	21
Born in Pattern II country	22	14	6	7	7
Other	0	2	5	8	9
Undetermined	6	0	2	3	6[b]

[a] Pattern II countries are WHO-designated countries with predominantly heterosexual transmission of HIV.
[b] Of patients initially reported with an undetermined transmission category, 75% are reclassified into known risk categories following investigation. Increases in the proportion of cases with undetermined risk in more recent reporting periods reflect a higher proportion of patients who have not been investigated.
Source: Centers for Disease Control. AIDS and human immunodeficiency virus infection in the United States: 1988 update. *MMWR* 38(S-4), May 1989.

since 1978, sexual activity under the influence of alcohol or drugs, and sex-for-drugs exchange, especially involving crack cocaine.

Serological Testing

Testing for the presence of serum antibody to HIV-1 is highly reliable and sensitive, but false negative and false positive results do occur [8]. The initial test performed is an enzyme immunoassay (EIA), which detects the binding of specific serum antibodies to HIV antigens adherent to a plastic microtiter plate. The reaction takes 2–4 hours, but realistically results are reported 24 hours after collection, since the tests are run as batches by most hospitals and blood centers. If the initial EIA is positive, a second EIA is run on a second sample of blood. If both EIA tests are positive, a confirmatory test, the Western blot (WB), is performed, and results typically are available in 1 week. The EIA

Table 17-2. CDC case definition of AIDS for surveillance purposes

The presence of reliably diagnosed disease that is at least moderately indicative of underlying cellular immunodeficiency, in a person *with no known cause* of immunodeficiency other than HIV infection.[a]

DISEASES DIAGNOSTIC OF AIDS

Bacterial
Extrapulmonary *Mycobacterium tuberculosis*[b]
Disseminated *Mycobacterium avium-intracellulare*
Recurrent *Salmonella* septicemia[b]

Fungal
Candida esophagitis
Cryptococcus neoformans meningitis or other extra-pulmonary form
Disseminated *coccidioidomycosis*[b]
Disseminated *histoplasmosis*[b]

Viral
Cytomegalovirus infection of an organ other than liver, spleen, lymph nodes in a patient >1 month of age
Chronic mucocutaneous *herpes simplex* (lasting >1 month)
Herpes simplex causing bronchitis, pneumonitis, or esophagitis in a patient >1 month of age
Progressive multifocal encephalopathy (*papovavirus*)
HIV "wasting syndrome"[b] (large-volume diarrhea with >10% weight loss)
HIV encephalopathy[b] (also called AIDS dementia)

Protozoal
Pneumocytis carinii pneumonia
Toxoplasma gondii infection of brain in patient >1 month of age
Cryptosporidiosis (diarrhea lasting >1 month)
Isospora belli diarrhea (>1 month)[b]

Malignant
Kaposi's sarcoma in a patient < 60 years of age
Primary lymphoma of the brain in a patient < 60 years of age
Non-Hodgkin's lymphoma[b]

Adapted from *Morbidity and Mortality Weekly Report Supplement* 36: No. 1S, 1987.
[a]1. High dose corticosteroid therapy or other immunosuppressive/cytotoxic therapy ≤3 months before onset of indicator disease
2. Any of the following diagnosed ≤3 months after diagnosis of indicator disease: Hodgkins or non-Hodgkins lymphoma, lymphocytic leukemia, multiple myeloma, other malignancy of lymphoreticular or histocytic tissue
3. A genetic or congenital immunodeficiency syndrome or an acquired immunodeficiency syndrome other than HIV infection, such as hypogammaglobulinemia
[b]With positive HIV serology (regardless of the presence of other causes of immunodeficiency).

has a sensitivity of 97%–100% and a specificity of 99.5%–100% [9]. False negatives occur primarily during the first 4–6 weeks of acute infection prior to the appearance of HIV antibodies, with 95% becoming positive by 3 months, and 98% positive by 6 months. False negatives may also occur with malignancy, intensive chemotherapy, replacement transfusion, bone marrow transplantation, and occasionally with kits that detect primarily antibody to p24 antigen. False positives occur in sera containing various autoantibodies and antibodies against human leucocyte antigen (HLA) class II antigens (multiparous women and multiply transfused patients) and in severe alcoholic liver disease, chronic hepatitis, malaria, hematologic malignancies, acute DNA-viral infections, renal transplants, and Stevens-Johnson syndrome and with passively acquired HIV antibody in hepatitis B immunoglobulin. When populations with a low incidence of true positives are tested, up to 90% of positive EIA tests may be false positives [10], suggesting that indiscriminate screening of all patients visiting the emergency department would be costly and would identify few true positives. False positive WBs occur at a rate of 1 in 20,000 [11] for the same reasons noted for the EIA test.

No patient should be informed of positive results based on the EIA test alone without the confirmatory WB test results. WB positivity depends on the presence of antibody to all three HIV antigens: p24, p41, and gp120/gp160. If only one or two of the bands is present, the WB is reported to be indeterminate. These patients should be retested at intervals of 2–3 months for at least 6 months until the result becomes clearly positive or negative, and a second confirmatory test, such as the indirect immunofluorescent assay, should be performed [12].

Rapid diagnostic tests, which offer results in 30 minutes, would be useful in emergency departments, but they have not yet been tested for sensitivity and specificity in that setting. A rapid latex agglutination test (Cambridge Bioscience) is promising but requires a trained observer for the subjective determination of agglutination [13].

Most state laws mandate informed consent prior to testing, and any pretest and posttest counseling specified by law is an important opportunity to educate patients on risk reduction. Table 17-3 lists the points of discussion that should be included in

Table 17-3. Recommended elements of pretest and posttest counseling for HIV testing

Pretest Counseling

Describe the test as one that detects antibodies, not the virus; positive result indicates HIV infection, not AIDS; the patient is a virus carrier and may infect others.

Tell patient that results are confidential but are entered into the medical record.

Inform patient of availability of anonymous testing and counseling.

Assure patient that there are potential adverse consequences for health-care workers if results are not kept confidential.

Emphasize the importance of reducing the risk of infection by safe and safer sex practices, sterilization of IV drug equipment, treatment of drug addiction, and cessation of IV needle sharing.

Posttest Counseling

Interpret test results, positive or negative.

Reinforce patient's responsibility to reduce risk of infection, whether results are positive or negative.

Refer patient for continued medical, psychological, and social support if results are positive.

Discuss notification of patient's sex partners if results are positive.

pretest and posttest counseling, in sessions that take about 3–5 minutes.

Positive test results can have a profound adverse psychological impact, and immediate referral for counseling may be necessary. Results of a positive test should *never* be given over the telephone or by mail; confidentiality cannot be ensured, and law suits have resulted. It is advisable to give all test results in the office or clinic, in order to answer questions effectively.

If the patient is unconscious or is unable to give consent to be tested, a relative should be sought for consent. If no consent is available and the test result would materially affect the patient's care, the test can be performed, according to most state statutes, but this practice has not been challenged in the courts.

Who Should Be Tested

HIV antibody testing is performed to identify asymptomatic carriers, so that early treatment and reduction of further transmission are possible, and to confirm suspected HIV infection in patients with symptoms suggestive of HIV or its complications, as recommended by the United States Public Health Service [14]. Mandatory testing also is performed when the benefits to public health outweigh the ill effects of testing [15]. Table 17-4 outlines the groups for whom testing is mandatory or recommended due to enhanced risk of undetected HIV infection.

Natural History of HIV Infection

The time course of latency, immune compromise, and symptoms of HIV infection are shown in Table 17-5. Classification of HIV infection stages tends to suggest that there is a linear progression through all stages by each patient [16]. Sequential progression, however, often does not occur, and many patients are therefore unaware of the degree of their immune impairment simply because they are asymptomatic and have not sought medical care for known HIV positivity.

At the time of initial HIV-1 infection, up to 50% of infected persons will experience the acute retroviral syndrome, which is similar to infectious mononucleosis with fever, fatigue, and lymphadenopathy and which may be complicated by aseptic meningitis, hepatitis, splenomegaly, rash, thrombocytopenia, and peripheral neuritis [17]. Resolution of symptoms is followed by seroconversion. During the illness, diagnosis can be made by a positive p24 antigen test, if available. More commonly serologic evidence must await testing during convalescence. Although there is no evidence that zidovudine alters the course of infection, most physicians prescribe zidovudine therapy as soon as the diagnosis is made. The patient is advised to rest, abstain from sex and needle sharing, and seek medical follow-up.

The rate of progression from being asymptomatic to being symptomatic varies considerably among infected individuals, and the reason for this difference is not understood. Progression to AIDS can be predicted by serial tests of immune function. Three tests—CD4 lymphocyte counts, beta-2-microglobulin, and HIV p24 antigen titer—provide optimal information on the degree of immunosuppression and subsequent risk of AIDS [18, 19]. Initial symptoms may be constitutional symptoms that indicate active HIV infection, may be infections that

Table 17-4. Population groups and individuals for whom HIV testing currently is mandatory or recommended

Mandatory
Blood donors
Federal prisoners and inmates of some other correctional institutions
Military recruits and active duty personnel
Job Corps trainees
Foreign service officers
Aliens seeking to immigrate to the United States

Recommended (Consent Required)
Patients in sexually-transmitted-disease (STD) clinics or seeking treatment of an STD
Prostitutes and other individuals who exchange sex for drugs
IV drug users, currently or any time after 1978
Women of childbearing age with recognized risk for HIV infection
Members of high-risk groups (see Table 17-1)
Patients with signs and symptoms indicative of any of the diseases diagnostic of AIDS (refer to Table 17-2)
Patients with signs and symptoms suggestive of HIV infection:
  Asymptomatic lymphadenopathy
  Weight loss without diarrhea
  Unexplained fevers and night sweats
  Mono spot-negative infectious mono-like illness
  Tuberculosis
  Herpes zoster before age 50
  Oral hairy leukoplakia
  Absolute lymphocytopenia < 1000/μl
  Unexplained dementia or cognitive impairment
  High-grade B-cell lymphoma or non-Hodgkin's lymphoma
  Persistent or recurrent candidal infection
  Chronic diarrhea
Anyone who requests the test

indicate immunodeficiency but are not AIDS nor life threatening, or may be diagnostic of AIDS (see Table 17-2 for the CDC definition of AIDS) and are life threatening. In the last group, immunodeficiency is usually profound, with CD4 (T4) counts of less than 200/μl. Once the diagnosis of AIDS has been made (see Table 17-2) [20], survival appears to depend on the individual, the AIDS-diagnostic condition, and the treatment available for both the HIV itself and the accompanying opportunistic infection or malignancy.

Groups of HIV-Positive Patients in the Emergency Department

HIV-positive patients who present for treatment in emergency departments can be characterized by age and by whether their HIV status is known. First are those who are HIV-positive and do not yet know it or who are unwilling to report this status to the emergency department personnel. These patients are challenging, since the history and the physical examination must yield suspicion of HIV infection for the differential diagnosis to be broadened. The second group know they are HIV-positive, but they have not yet experienced symptoms and may or may not have had previous medical care. The third group know they are HIV positive, have had previous HIV-related medical complications, and have varying degrees of medical sophistication. Such patients who have complex medical histories should be instructed to carry with them a problem list and a complete medication list, so any necessary emergency care can be more efficient and targeted. It is also helpful for patients with previous medical care to know their most recent CD4 cell count, since it helps focus the differential diagnosis. CD4 cell counts greater than 500/μl rarely are associated with opportunistic infections. Conversely CD4 cell counts below 200/μl are commonly associated with life-threatening opportunistic infections. (See Table 17-2 for common opportunistic infections and malignancies that complicate HIV infections.) For a discussion of the special group of adult HIV-infected patients who have traveled, consult reference 21.

Children experience the same opportunistic infections and malignancies that adults do, but in addition they suffer from complications that are unique to children or that appear at much greater frequency in infants and children [22], presumably due to their relatively immature immune system. Table 17-6 lists complications that are common in children but uncommon or nonexistent in adults.

Toxicity of Antiretroviral Therapy

Treatment of the HIV infection with zidovudine, dideoxynucleoside analogs, and other experimental therapies is a rapidly changing field that is beyond

Table 17-5. Time course and CDC classification of HIV infection

HIV classification	Time after infection	Event or complication
Acute retroviral syndrome	1–4 weeks 4–24 weeks	Mono-like illness lasting 24–96 hrs Seroconversion
Asymptomatic	2–10 years	CD4 > 600/μl and subtle immu-nodeficiency initially, but CD4 will decrease without symptoms
Persistent generalized lymphadeno-pathy	Intermittently during period of 2–10 years	CD4 > 600/μl and subtle immu-nodeficiency initially, but CD4 will decrease without symptoms
Early symptomatic and constitu-tional disease	Variable: as early as 2 years, as late as 10 + years	Includes thrush, herpes zoster, ITP, some peripheral neuropathies
Advanced HIV disease (AIDS)	Variable: as early as 2 years, as late as 10 + years	Secondary infections, secondary malignancies, neurologic disease

the scope of this chapter and that should not be undertaken in the emergency department. The toxicities of these agents require close monitoring in the outpatient clinic or office. Since well-monitored patients still present to the emergency department for urgent problems, emergency department staff must be aware of the potential toxicities of both approved and experimental agents and be alert to new, unreported side effects of the experimental therapies. Table 17-7 lists the common medications used to treat HIV infection as approved, experimental, or underground therapies. Drug toxicity must be considered in every HIV patient seen in the office or the emergency department.

Table 17-6. Manifestations of HIV infection unique to or more common in children than in adults

Failure to thrive	Developmental delay
Hepatomegaly	Splenomegaly
Chronic, recurrent diarrhea	Parotitis
Atopic skin disease	Herpetic stomatitis
Lymphoid interstitial pneumonitis	Cardiomyopathy
Hepatitis	

Recurrent invasive bacterial infection
  Mild: otitis media, sinusitis, impetigo
  Severe: bacteremia, meningitis, osteomyelitis, septic arthritis, and deep abscesses, usually due to *Staphylococcus aureus*, *Streptococcus pneumoniae*, *Haemophilus influenzae*, or *Salmonella* species

Fever and Other Constitutional Symptoms

Fever

This section discusses fever in the absence of symptoms referable to a specific organ system. Fever can be due to HIV infection alone and is often accompanied by fatigue, night sweats, and intermittent diarrhea. An HIV-seropositive patient has AIDS by definition [20] in the presence of unexplained fever of at least 38.3°C for one month, chronic unexplained weakness, diarrhea, and a loss of more than 10% of baseline body weight. It cannot be assumed, however, that low-grade fever alone or accompanying this group of symptoms is due to HIV without investigations to rule out another infection or a malignancy.

Virtually any infection can present initially as fever without other clues, but several do so commonly. *Pneumocystis carinii* pneumonia (PCP) frequently presents as a febrile prodrome without respiratory symptoms or pulmonary infiltrate. PCP is a life-threatening infection that can rapidly deteriorate, and a diagnostic approach to fever in the emergency department must include a chest x-ray, even in the absence of pulmonary symptoms. Cryptococcosis with fungemia and meningitis can begin as fever without headache, yet develop into life-threatening meningitis in several days. Thus, a serum cryptococcal antigen titer will detect early cases and is an important component of the fever workup. *Mycobacterium avium* complex infection commonly presents only with fever, sweats, and

Table 17-7. Toxicities of AIDS therapies

Drug	Organ system	Signs, symptoms, laboratory
Zidovudine	GI	Nausea, vomiting, acute hepatitis
	Neurologic	Insomnia, headache, Wernicke's encephalopathy, dementia, seizures, lethargy, myalgias, polymyositis, mania, ataxia, nystagmus
	Hematologic	Anemia, macrocytosis, leukopenia, thrombocytosis
	Dermatologic	Nail changes
Dideoxycytidine*	Neurologic	Peripheral neuropathy, dysesthesias
	Dermatologic	Cutaneous eruptions, nail changes, aphthous stomatitis
	GI	Diarrhea
	Miscellaneous	Fever, malaise, peripheral edema
Dideoxyadenosine*	Renal	Acute nephritis, renal failure
Dideoxyinosine*	Neurologic	Peripheral neuropathy, dysesthesias
	GI	Pancreatitis, elevated AST, ALT
	Miscellaneous	Headache, rash, hyperuricemia
Acyclovir	GI	Nausea, vomiting
	Neurologic	Headache, lethargy, confusion, encephalopathy (with rapid infusion)
	Renal	Crystalluria, acute tubular necrosis, renal failure
Ganciclovir	GI	Nausea, vomiting, diarrhea (less common)
	Hepatic	Elevated AST, ALT
	Hematologic	Leukopenia, anemia, thrombocytopenia
	Neurologic	Headache, dizziness, confusion, seizures (less common)
	Renal	Worsening of renal function
Foscarnet*	GI	Nausea, vomiting, diarrhea
	Hematologic	Anemia (rare)
	Renal	Elevated creatinine, nephrogenic diabetes insipidus, renal failure
	Dermatologic	Genital and oral ulcerations, fixed drug eruptions (rare)
	Miscellaneous	Headache, fatigue, malaise, hypercalcemia
Ribavirin	GI	Nausea, vomiting, diarrhea
	Neurologic	Fatigue, headache
	Hematologic	Normochromic, normocytic anemia, bone marrow suppression, aplastic anemia
Dextran sulfate*	GI	Bloating, diarrhea
	Hematologic	Thrombocytopenia, leukopenia, prolonged PT, PTT
Ansamycin*	GI	Nausea, vomiting, diarrhea
	Hepatic	Elevated AST, ALT, alkaline phosphatase
	Hematologic	Neutropenia, thrombocytopenia
Compound Q*	Neurologic	Confusion, disorientation, coma (rare)
	Miscellaneous	Rash, anaphylaxis
Dehydroepiandrosterone (DHEA)*	Hematologic	Glucose-6-phosphate dehydrogenase (G6PD), hemolytic anemia
Interferon	GI	Nausea, vomiting
	Neurologic	Paresthesias, confusion
	Hematologic	Lymphopenia, bone marrow suppression
	Miscellaneous	Fever, malaise, chills
Disulfiram*	Miscellaneous	Metallic taste, abdominal discomfort, flushing, nausea, hypotension (with alcohol)
Imuthiol*	Neurologic	Drowsiness, lethargy, headache (with alcohol)
Isoprinosine*	Miscellaneous	Hyperuricemia
Co-trimoxazole	GI	Nausea, vomiting, diarrhea

Table 17-7. (continued)

Drug	Organ system	Signs, symptoms, laboratory
Sulfadoxine-pyrimethamine	Hematologic	Agranulocytosis, aplastic anemia, leukopenia, thrombocytopenia
Sulfadiazine	Dermatologic	Rash, Stevens-Johnson syndrome, toxic epidermal necrolysis, erythema multiforme
	Neurologic	Headaches, depression, hallucinations, ataxia, tremor (rare)
	Renal	Crystalluria, hematuria, proteinuria
Dapsone	GI	Anorexia, nausea, vomiting
	Neurologic	Headache, nervousness, insomnia, blurred vision, paresthesias, peripheral neuropathy and psychosis
	Hematologic	Methemoglobinemia, hemolytic anemia, agranulocytosis, aplastic anemia, exfoliative dermatitis, toxic epidermal necrolysis, erythema multiforme
	Miscellaneous	Sore throat, fever, pallor, malaise, hepatitis
Trimetrexate*	Hematologic	Leukopenia, thrombocytopenia
	Neurologic	Peripheral neuropathy
	Hepatic	Hepatitis
	Miscellaneous	Rash, azotemia
Pentamidine (intravenous)	Cardiovascular	Hypotension, arrhythmias, phlebitis
	Endocrine	Hyperglycemia and hypoglycemia, hypocalcemia, hypokalemia
	Hematologic	Leukopenia, thrombocytopenia
	Dermatologic	Rash, Stevens-Johnson syndrome
Amphotericin B	Hematologic	Anemia, leukopenia, thrombocytopenia
	Renal	Azotemia, renal tubular acidosis
	Miscellaneous	Fever, chills, rigors, vomiting, headache
Flucytosine	Hematologic	Bone marrow suppression
Ketoconazole	GI	Anorexia, nausea, vomiting
	Miscellaneous	Paresthesias, thrombocytopenia, hepatitis (mild)
Fluconazole	GI	Nausea, vomiting, anorexia
Itraconazole*	Neurologic	Dizziness, headache, delirium, seizures (rare)
	Miscellaneous	Rash, anemia, hepatitis (rare)
Clarithromycin*	GI	Nausea, vomiting, diarrhea
Roxithromycin*	Miscellaneous	Hypoacusis

*Investigational and/or underground therapy; toxicity profile may be incomplete.
Source: Smothers K. Pharmacology and toxicology of AIDS therapies. AIDS Reader 1:29–35, 1991.

fatigue, but it is not life threatening. Infective endocarditis, perhaps more common in HIV-positive than in HIV-negative IV drug users [23], presents with chills, pleuritic chest pain, and arthralgias. Ninety-one percent of HIV-positive patients with endocarditis have a heart murmur, and 53% have vegetations detectable by echocardiography, similar to HIV-negative patients [23].

The history should search for any clue to relate the fever to a specific organ system. The physical exam should look for asymmetric lymphadenopathy, hepatosplenomegaly, petechiae and ecchymoses, perirectal ulceration, asymmetry in the neurologic exam, altered mental status, oral lesions and thrush, rash, pulmonary rales, sinus tenderness, retinal lesions, and abdominal tenderness and masses.

Emergency department physicians should keep in mind, contemplating patient admission, the difficulty in identifying early cases of PCP and cryptococcal infection. Hospitalization is appropriate if the patient is febrile and toxic, neutropenic, bleeding, and thrombocytopenic, or if extended morbidity would ensue with an outpatient evaluation.

Table 17-8. Workup for undifferentiated fever in the HIV-positive patient

In the Emergency Department
Complete blood count
Serum chemistries, including liver function tests
Urinalysis
Blood culture for aerobes, mycobacteria, fungi
Chest x-ray
Serum cryptococcal antigen
HIV serology, if not already documented
Serology for syphilis and toxoplasmosis
Serum hepatitis B antigen
Immediate Follow-up
CD4 cell count
Stool for leukocytes, bacterial enteropathogens, parasites
Optional: serum HIV p24 antigen; serology for histoplasmosis, coccidioidomycosis; gallium scan

Table 17-9. Etiologies of shock with or without ARDS and DIC in HIV-positive patients

Pneumocystis carinii pneumonia
Bacterial sepsis
    Staphylococcus aureus
    Streptococcus pneumoniae
    Clostridium perfringens
    Neisseria meningitidis
    Enterobacteriaceae
    Pseudomonas aeruginosa
Mycobacterium tuberculosis, miliary
Disseminated histoplasmosis

The laboratory exam in the emergency department should include a complete blood count, urinalysis, blood cultures for bacteria and fungi, chemistry panel (electrolytes, glucose, blood urea nitrogen [BUN], creatinine, lactate dehydrogenase [LDH], hepatic transaminases, alkaline phosphatase, amylase, creatine phosphokinase), and serum cryptococcal antigen (Table 17-8). A chest x-ray is important to reveal silent pulmonary infiltrates or hilar lymphadenopathy. The erythrocyte sedimentation rate (ESR) is rarely useful. If the evaluation in the emergency department reveals no clues and hospitalization is not warranted, the patient must be observed every 2 or 3 days, and serologic test results must be reviewed immediately. In this author's experience, important clues usually appear in 7–10 days, pointing to a specific organ system. If symptoms do not abate and a diagnosis is not made, continued vigilance by the outpatient caregivers is necessary.

Shock

HIV-positive patients occasionally present to the emergency department with shock and adult respiratory distress syndrome (ARDS) with multiple organ failure. Severe PCP is the most common cause of this picture, but other etiologies occur in HIV patients (Table 17-9). If disseminated intravascular coagulation (DIC) is present, an etiology other than PCP should be suspected.

Patients who present with shock and fever may have, in addition to bacteremia or fungemia, adrenal insufficiency, which exacerbates the signs of the infection. *Mycobacterium tuberculosis* and cytomegalovirus (CMV) appear to be the primary agents infecting the adrenal glands and causing adrenal crisis. The hypotension, hyperkalemia, and hyponatremia often are not accompanied by hypoglycemia, eosinophilia, and hyperpigmentation [24]. Ketoconazole can exacerbate adrenal insufficiency or even cause it in high doses. Patients who appear depleted of extracellular volume yet fail to respond to IV fluid resuscitation and patients whose serum sodium and potassium suggest hypoadrenalism may benefit from a trial of hydrocortisone, after a random serum cortisol is drawn or an ACTH-stimulation test is performed.

Patients with orthostatic hypotension may suffer from dehydration, an adverse effect of medication (including pentamidine, antidepressants, and narcotics) or from generalized autonomic nervous system dysfunction [25]. In a patient with the latter problem the pulse rate does not increase significantly when changing from a supine to an upright position, while in patients with dehydration the pulse will increase with standing. In the emergency department the patient should be given an IV fluid challenge, and potentially offending medications should be stopped or reduced, with referral to a neurologist if hypotension persists.

Line Sepsis

Bacteremia that originates from an infected permanent venous access device is becoming increasingly common as new IV drugs become available for severe opportunistic infections. This condition is life threatening, since patients with advanced immunodeficiency have compromised antibody production and neutrophil function, and granulocytopenia may be present as well. The syndrome of line sepsis usually has a sudden onset with a shaking chill, followed by high continuous fever and often delirium. Examination of the catheter may reveal no abnormality, an exit-site infection, or a tunnel infection, in which part or all of the overlying skin is tender, red, and swollen with cellulitis. Tunnel infections must be treated with immediate removal of the catheter, even if no other intravenous sites appear available. Subcutaneous reservoirs, such as Portacath or Infusaport, may have only small areas of tenderness, relating to a subcutaneous collection of pus. These abscesses need immediate drainage and removal of the device if the abscess is greater than 2 cm in diameter or cannot be drained completely. Small areas of cellulitis around an exit site, less than 5 cm in diameter, usually can be managed without catheter removal, providing that the tunnel above the cuff of a Hickman, or Groshöng/Broviac catheter is not involved.

The patient should be admitted to the hospital if line sepsis is suspected, blood cultures drawn both through the line and from a peripheral vein, and antibiotics begun immediately. Staphylococci and streptococci represent 90% of the pathogens. Gram-negative coverage for *Escherichia coli* and *Klebsiella* species must be included, since Enterobacteriaceae species have been found in approximately one-third of patients. A third-generation cephalosporin, such as cefotaxime or ceftriaxone, is appropriate.

Lymphadenopathy

Fifty to seventy percent of all HIV-infected patients develop lymphadenopathy, usually in the cervical, submandibular, occipital, and axillary chains and characterized by mobile, rubbery, nontender nodes 1 to 2 cm in size, but occasionally as large as 6 cm. In the emergency department or clinic no diagnostic studies are necessary, unless the lymph-node enlargement is grossly asymmetric, tender, painful, or rapidly enlarging. A fine needle aspiration is sensitive for detecting mycobacterial infections [26]

and can be done in the emergency department for an immediate acid-fast stain. If this study is negative, a subsequent biopsy can be performed later to rule out lymphoma or Kaposi's sarcoma. Cryptococcosis, histoplasmosis, coccidioidomycosis, and toxoplasmosis rarely can be diagnosed by needle biopsy in the HIV-positive patient.

Generalized Weakness

Generalized weakness is a common complaint among HIV-infected individuals and has many causes. Relatively abrupt onset weakness may be due to sepsis, pneumocystis pneumonia, anemia due to bleeding, dehydration, or orthostatic hypotension due to medication. Weakness of insidious onset is more common and may be due to adrenal insufficiency, anemia, polymyositis, orthostatic hypotension due to autonomic nervous system disease, tuberculosis, hepatitis, marked muscle loss due to the wasting syndrome, or the ill-defined weakness and malaise that appears to accompany active HIV infection.

The physical exam must carefully distinguish focal weakness due to neurologic deficits and identify signs of systemic infection and hypotension. Laboratory studies should be directed at detecting electrolyte abnormalities, anemia, neutropenia, hepatitis, hypoxemia, and bacteremia or fungemia. If immediate admission is not indicated, close follow-up care is important, since a diagnosis of wasting syndrome can be made only after other possibilities have been eliminated. It should be noted that since depression and despondency often are associated with marked weakness, the history should inquire whether specific events of daily living have been curtailed. In this author's experience, when the patient has become bedridden due to weakness but makes occasional trips to the market, depression is the major problem and referral to a psychiatrist is appropriate following the medical investigations.

The differential diagnosis of anemia is similar to that of the non–HIV-infected patient, with several exceptions. In general terms, anemia may be due to acute or chronic blood loss, drug toxicity, particularly zidovudine, or azidothymidine (AZT); the anemia of chronic disease; or the apparent effect of HIV on the bone marrow progenitor cells. Less common causes, which are not unique to HIV in-

fection, are infiltration of the bone marrow by inflammation of opportunistic pathogens or malignancy, and intravascular hemolysis due to
thrombotic thrombocytopenia purpura (TTP). In
the emergency department the task is simply to
investigate blood loss in the GI tract and refer the
patient for further workup.

Thrombocytopenia due to idiopathic thrombocytopenic purpura (ITP) is common in HIV infection [27]. The platelet count usually ranges between 20,000 and 120,000/μl, but counts below
20,000 are not uncommon. Major GI or CNS
bleeding is rare, and patients presenting with
counts of 5000/μl may be asymptomatic [author's
personal data]. Some patients present with easy
bruising, petechiae, epistaxis, or bleeding gingiva.
Patients with bleeding and platelet counts below
15,000 should be hospitalized; others should be
referred for bone marrow aspiration and observation. Other common causes of thrombocytopenia
in the HIV-positive patient is thrombocytopenic
purpura in narcotic addicts [28] and drug-induced
thrombocytopenia, most commonly caused by trimethoprim-sulfamethoxazole. A lupus anticoagulant has been described in AIDS [29], usually associated with opportunistic infections, particularly
pneumocystic pneumonia.

Pancytopenia is usually drug induced, but it may
be due to infiltration of the bone marrow with an
opportunistic pathogen or a malignancy, or it may
accompany DIC and ARDS. AZT can cause neutropenia and anemia, but only rarely does it cause
thrombocytopenia.

Pulmonary Syndromes

Pulmonary infections are the most common cause of
acute illness and death in HIV patients.[30] Since
PCP is the most common opportunistic infection in
AIDS and the most common infection defining the
onset of AIDS and still is associated with a mortality of 20%–25%, pulmonary signs and symptoms
must be approached expeditiously and system-
atically in the emergency department. The following discussion is organized around specific symptoms, rather than pathogens, to facilitate the rapid
formation of a differential diagnosis.

Cough

The illnesses that are heralded by cough can be
divided into those associated with insidious onset
and those with abrupt onset. PCP usually begins
with an insidious dry, hacking cough that is worse at
night and that may be associated with substernal
pressure discomfort. The febrile outpatient with a
frequent, spontaneous, dry hacking cough usually
has PCP and deserves diagnostic studies and treatment, even if the chest x-ray does not reveal infiltrates at the time. Figure 17-1 presents an algorithm
for pulmonary complaints. Current use of monthly
or biweekly prophylactic aerosolized pentamidine
or trimethoprin-sulfamethoxozole renders the presenting signs and symptoms of PCP more subtle
[31].

Bronchitis can cause a cough indistinguishable
from that of PCP, although it is more likely to be
productive and unlikely to be progressive or associated with fever. Sinusitis is common among HIV
patients and may present with cough due to postnasal drip, nasal discharge, or headache. In this
author's experience many cases of milder sinusitis
with cough bear few symptoms referable to the
infected sinus, such as maxillary tenderness, and
sinus x-rays may or may not be helpful.

Pulmonary tuberculosis typically presents with
insidious cough, fever, and night sweats and must
be considered in every case of new pulmonary complaints examined in the emergency department. In
the patient with early HIV infection and modest
immune compromise, the picture resembles typical
reactivation disease with apical infiltrates with or
without cavitation, and hilar adenopathy is uncommon. In the advanced stages of HIV infection, the
presentation is typical for progression of primary
infection, even though it is still reactivation of
latent infection, that is, middle- or lower-lobe infiltrates with hilar or mediastinal adenopathy [32]. In
regions with a high incidence of tuberculosis among
HIV patients, such as Florida and New York, all
new HIV patients should be examined for tuberculosis and isolated with a mask in the emergency
department if tuberculosis is suspected. All newly
diagnosed tuberculosis patients should be tested for
HIV infection.

Abrupt onset of productive cough with fever usu-

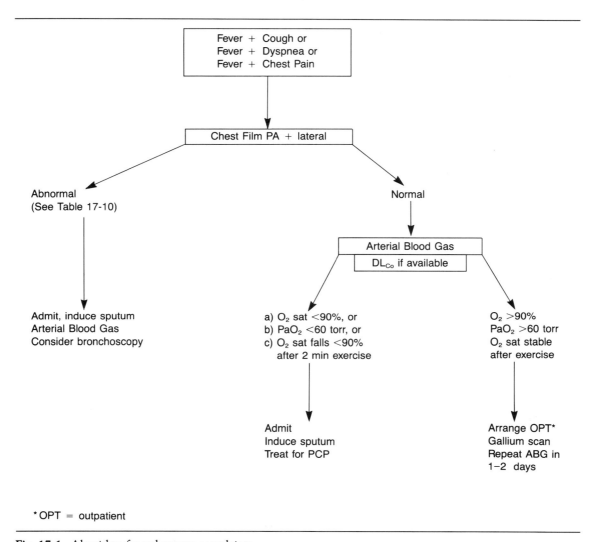

* OPT = outpatient

Fig. 17-1. Algorithm for pulmonary complaints

ally indicates a bacterial pneumonia in HIV-infected patients [33, 34]. The mean time between onset of symptoms and presentation to a physician for bacterial pneumonia is 5 days, compared to 21 days for PCP. Some bacterial pneumonias are not associated with sputum production in HIV-infected patients but rather present with acute chest pain and chills. Pneumococcal bacteremia appears to be increased a hundredfold in HIV-positive individuals, primarily occurring before the onset of the opportunistic infections that define AIDS [35]. The chest x-ray shows a typical lobar or segmental alveolar infiltrate, and a good induced sputum specimen is sufficient to make the bacteriologic diagnosis. The common pathogens occurring in HIV-infected individuals are listed in Table 17-10.

Dyspnea

Shortness of breath with effort is often an early sign of PCP, beginning well before the appearance of pulmonary infiltrates. The combination of fever, dry cough, and dyspnea, or increased A-a oxygen gradient, is sufficient presumptive suspicion to war-

Table 17-10. Pulmonary pathogens causing pneumonitis in HIV-infected patients

Parasites
Pneumocystis carinii (85%)
Toxoplasma gondii (rare)

Bacteria
Streptococcus pneumoniae
Haemophilus influenzae
S. aureus
Moraxella catarrhalis
Legionella pneumophila (1%–4%)

Mycobacteria
Mycobacterium tuberculosis (5%)
Mycobacterium avium-intracellulare (10%–20%)

Fungi
Cryptococcus neoformans (1%)
Coccidioides immitis (rare)
Histoplasma capsulatum
Candida species (rare)

Viruses
Cytomegalovirus (5%–20%, often commensal)
Varicella (rare)
Herpes simplex (rare)

rant a workup for PCP. Dyspnea at rest is even more alarming; if accompanied by tachypnea, it indicates more-advanced PCP. Dyspnea can also suggest bacterial pneumonia, which is commonly accompanied by pleuritic pain in the HIV-positive patient. Advanced pulmonary Kaposi's sarcoma may present with dyspnea, particularly if bleeding into the airway has occurred.

Sudden onset of dyspnea can be due to a pneumothorax, almost always as a complication of active PCP and usually in the patient who has been on prophylactic aerosolized pentamidine and who has a history of prior PCP [36]. In HIV disease the pneumothorax requires admission for chest tube thoracotomy and treatment of the PCP. Sudden dyspnea can also herald pulmonary embolism, pericardial effusion, or asthma. Dyspnea related to pleural effusion and pleuritic pain most commonly is due to bacterial pneumonia.

Hemoptysis

Pulmonary Kaposi's sarcoma is probably the most common cause of hemoptysis in HIV-infected pa-

tients. Bleeding from pulmonary aspergillus infection and tuberculosis also occur. Kaposi's sarcoma is suggested by multiple small round shadows on the chest film, but bronchoscopy is necessary for diagnosis, since bronchial mucosal lesions may be abundant in the absence of chest film signs. Treatment includes oxygen, rest, suppression of cough, transfusion, and correction of coagulopathies and thrombocytopenia.

Approach to Pulmonary Complaints in the Emergency Department

The bedside exam reveals surprisingly little helpful information for pulmonary diseases in the HIV-positive patient. Adventitial sounds such as rales or crackles often are heard in PCP, but commonly the chest exam is normal in spite of hypoxemia and infiltrates.

The chest radiograph is the most useful tool for pulmonary disease in the emergency department, if its limitations are understood [37] (Table 17-11). Physicians ordering chest films should review each one with the radiologist rather than relying on a written report, to achieve an appreciation of the variable clinical correlation between radiograph and final diagnosis. The chest radiograph may be normal or show an interstitial pattern, a focal infiltrate, a cavity, pleural effusion, intrathoracic adenopathy, nodules, or pneumothorax. PCP is associated with interstitial infiltrate, typically in a perihilar distribution, in 80% of cases, with the remainder showing a normal radiograph. Advanced PCP appears as or progresses to a picture similar to ARDS and represents a life-threatening condition. Miliary and focal tuberculosis may be confused with PCP [38, 39]. Lymphocytic pneumonitis, possibly due to HIV, and chronic interstial pneumonitis also present with interstitial patterns and can be distinguished from PCP only by biopsy. Whether CMV can cause infiltrates and significant pulmonary morbidity by itself currently is being debated, although it may accelerate disease due to other pathogens.

Lobar or segmental infiltrates usually indicate bacterial pneumonia, due to *Streptococcus pneumoniae, Haemophilus influenzae, Staphylococcus aureus, Legionella pneumophila,* or *M. tuberculosis.* The presence of cavitation suggests *M. tuberculosis,* but

Table 17-11. Differential diagnosis of pulmonary radiographic findings

Radiographic pattern	Illnesses
Normal	No disease; *P. carinii* pneumonia, disseminated fungal infection, bronchitis
Interstitial infiltrate	*P. carinii* pneumonia, tuberculosis, lymphocytic interstitial pneumonia, nonspecific (HIV?) pneumonitis, pyogenic pneumonia, ARDS, coccidioidomycosis, histoplasmosis
Focal infiltrate	Pyogenic pneumonia, tuberculosis, cryptococcal pneumonia, *Aspergillus* pneumonia,
Nodular infiltrate	Pneumocystis pneumonia, fungal nodule, tuberculosis, Kaposi's sarcoma (usually multiple), lymphoma, carcinoma
Pleural effusion	Kaposi's sarcoma, pyogenic pneumonia, tuberculosis
Mediastinal adenopathy	Tuberculosis, *Mycobacterium avium* complex, lymphoma

the possibility of histoplasmosis and coccidioidomycosis must be entertained if the geographic history is consistent with any prior exposure. Pleural effusion is common in advanced Kaposi's sarcoma but also is often seen in bacterial pneumonia, lymphoma, and tuberculosis. The differential diagnosis of chest radiograph findings is listed in Table 17-11.

Physicians now approach pulmonary complaints with a standard algorithm (see Fig. 17-1). Once the history and the physical exam have suggested pulmonary pathology, the first step in the diagnostic evaluation is a chest film. Since one in five cases of PCP will have a normal chest x-ray on first evaluation, the diagnostic process must continue if the suspicion of PCP remains. In most published algorithms the recommended follow-up study is the diffusing capacity of carbon monoxide. This tests the rate of diffusion of carbon monoxide from inspired air into the blood and is abnormal when inflammation fills the alveoli or interstitial fluid. Ninety-five percent of PCP patients have a diffusing capacity of carbon monoxide of less than 80% predicted value, indicating high sensitivity for PCP, but the test is nonspecific [40]. Diffusing capacities usually are not available in the emergency department, however, so arterial oxygen tension is more useful to screen for PCP. This can be done with an arterial puncture or by the less invasive fingertip hemoglobin oxygen-saturation index. A PaO_2 of less than 60 torr or an oxygen saturation of less than 90% is a presumptive sign of PCP or any other pneumonitis. The sensitivity of the oxygen-saturation test is increased by testing the patient before and after 3 minutes of exercise, either a flight of stairs or repeated steps in the examining room.

Any fall in oxygen saturation of 3% or greater is suggestive of PCP, although the sensitivity of this test is 80%, and the test is inconvenient for an ill patient. More helpful is the observation that when the oxygen saturation rises with exercise, serious pulmonary illness can be ruled out. Regardless of the diagnosis the arterial oxygen saturation assesses the need for supplemental oxygen therapy.

If neither the chest x-ray nor the blood gases yield a clear answer, a gallium scan is useful in indicating early PCP. Gallium scanning is expensive, requires 48 hours before reading, and is nonspecific; therefore, it is reserved for nonemergent outpatient evaluations.

If one of the above tests indicates disease, subsequent evaluation is usually performed on an inpatient basis and includes sputum induction by aerosolized hypertonic saline. If this test is negative twice, bronchoscopy with bronchoalveolar lavage should be performed. These studies have been described and evaluated extensively [41] and will not be elaborated here.

Initiation of treatment should not be delayed pending a definitive diagnosis by induced sputum or bronchoscopy. If PCP is the prime suspect, therapy should be begun immediately with intravenous trimethoprim-sulfamethoxazole 4 mg/kg/q8h, intravenous pentamidine 3 mg/kg/day, or intravenous trimethoprim plus oral dapsone 100 mg/day. Outpatient treatment with aerosolized pentamidine should be reserved only for patients with mild PCP. For patients with rapid deterioration and a PaO_2 of less than 60 torr, immediate therapy with high-dose intravenous corticosteroids should be considered [42].

If a bacterial pneumonia is suggested, therapy should be initiated immediately with intravenous ampicillin-sulbactam combination and the patient admitted. If tuberculosis is suspected, the patient should be isolated in the emergency department with a mask, and treatment recommended on an inpatient basis. Pleural effusions should be sampled by thoracentesis after coagulation studies affirm its safety. If the patient has been recently hospitalized or treated for a pyogenic pneumonia or bacteremia, a relapse with the same pathogen should be suspected and treated, since relapses of bacteremic organisms are common in HIV-infected patients despite adequate conventional therapy. If the patient has an indwelling intravenous catheter or evidence of current intravenous drug use, embolic pneumonia should be suspected, and presumptive therapy with ampicillin-sulbactam should target S. aureus, nonaureus staphylococci, and streptococci, pending the results of blood cultures.

GI Tract Illnesses

Oral Pain

The oral cavity is involved in all stages of HIV infection, from early immunosuppression with hairy leukoplakia and candidiasis to late stages with a number of severe and painful complications. Oral candidiasis (thrush) can present in three forms. The most common pseudomembranous form is characterized by raised cheesy exudate easily scraped off with a tongue blade and usually located on the soft palate and buccal mucosa but found on any mucosal surface. Diagnosis is quick and accurate with a potassium hydroxide preparation or a wet prep stained with a drop of methylene blue, obviating the need for culture. The less commonly diagnosed atrophic candidiasis is manifested by flat erythematous plaques without white exudate, causing discomfort, bleeding, and loss of taste. Hypertrophic candidiasis appears similar to hairy leukoplakia, with a raised nonscrapable white plaque on the palate and lateral tongue. Successful treatment of oral candidiasis depends on the severity of immunodepression. For candidiasis in the early stages, topical nystatin (500,000 units q6h by the swish-and-swallow technique) or clotrimazole troches (10

mg q4h) until the lesions and the discomfort disappear is adequate. In late-stage patients more potent therapy often is required, including ketoconazole 400 mg daily or fluconazole 200 mg daily.

Hairy leukoplakia is unique to HIV infection and is apparently due to epithelial cell infection with Epstein-Barr virus (EBV). Manifested as a raised white plaque along the lateral margins of the tongue and occasionally on the hard palate, hairy leukoplakia is diagnosed clinically by the inability to scrape the exudate off and unresponsiveness to antifungal treatment. In late-stage disease hairy leukoplakia can cause discomfort and dysgeusia and can be treated with oral acyclovir 1.6 g/day.

Gingivitis and periodontitis are common in late-stage disease and can cause severe pain, foul breath, bleeding gums, and loosening of the teeth. Examination reveals a bright red margin of the gums and necrosis of interdental papillae. Treatment of milder cases is successful with topical chlorhexidene (Peridex), but more severe cases may require oral penicillin or metronidazole. This problem can be confused with ulcerative gingivitis caused by gram-negative bacilli and acute Vincent's angina due to anaerobic fusobacterium infection.

Severe aphthous stomatitis, or idiopathic oral ulceration, is probably the most painful and disabling oral disease in HIV infection. It can occur as part of the initial HIV-1 infection (acute retroviral syndrome), or it can occur as a complication of late-stage disease. The etiology is unknown but retroviral-like particles have been seen by electron microscopy in some biopsies. It must be distinguished from herpes simplex stomatitis by viral culture. Treatment is symptomatic with topical anaesthetics such as tessalon pearls. When the pain becomes so severe that all oral intake ceases, some patients require high-dose (100 mg) prednisone for 2 or 3 days, followed by a rapid taper. This therapy is attended by a high risk of exacerbating other infections, such as CMV retinitis, and should be pursued only as a immediate quality-of-life decision. Some patients with idiopathic oral ulcers often have additional ulcers in the esophagus, stomach, and small bowel.

Parotitis is seen in children. In adults a Sjogren's-like syndrome has been described in which parotid gland enlargement is accompanied by xerostomia and conjunctivitis. In the emergency department the history should rule out concomitant tricyclic antidepressant or antihistamine therapy, and the patient should be referred for serologic studies and symptomatic therapy with artificial tears.

Dysphagia

Pain on swallowing, or odynophagia, and dysphagia are common complaints in HIV infection, in contrast to other forms of immunosuppression. Dysphagia can occur during the initial acute retroviral syndrome, can signal the first opportunistic infection defining AIDS, or can occur as a relapsing complication in late-stage disease. *Candida* esophagitis is the most common cause, accounting for 90% of esophagitis in HIV infection. Symptoms of esophageal candidiasis include solid food sticking in the lower neck or midchest, burning pain on passage of any food or liquid, and an aching discomfort in the retrosternal or epigastric region. If fever over 38°C and weight loss accompany the dysphagia, another diagnosis should be entertained. The presence of oral candidiasis usually is accompanied by esophageal involvement in untreated patients, but conversely some patients with esophageal candidiasis do not have visible oral infection due to low doses of antifungal treatment.

In the emergency department the presumptive diagnosis should be obtained from a barium swallow, in which diffuse ulceration and exudates are seen the length of the esophagus. The barium swallow may be insensitive to mild esophagitis. If the barium swallow is negative or if discrete ulcers are seen, the patient should be referred for endoscopy.

Treatment for *Candida* esophagitis can be initiated in the emergency department, based on suggestive symptoms and barium swallow, with ketoconazole 400–600 mg/day or fluconazole 200–400 mg/day. Clinical response is expected in 2–4 days and is more rapid with fluconazole. Lack of a response implies an alternative diagnosis, requiring endoscopy with biopsy. Herpes simplex, CMV, ulcerating hairy leukoplakia, Kaposi's sarcoma, and idiopathic ulceration require histologic confirmation for diagnosis. Treatment of these diseases are discussed elsewhere [43, 44]. Other diseases not associated with HIV infection, such as reflux esophagitis and peptic ulcer disease, are not uncommon in young adults.

Table 17-12. Pathogens responsible for diarrheal syndromes in HIV-infected patients

Syndrome	Pathogens
Acute enterocolitis	*Shigella* species, *Salmonella* species, *Campylobacter* species, *Clostridium difficile* toxin, *Entamoeba histolytica*
Chronic recurrent diarrhea	*Cryptosporidium* species, *Isospora belli, Giardia lamblia, Vibrio* species
Acute proctitis	*Neisseria gonorrhoeae, Chlamydia trachomata, Herpes simplex, Treponema pallidum, Entamoeba histolytica*
Other anorectal diseases	*Lymphogranuloma venereum,* M. *tuberculosis,* cytomegalovirus, Kaposi's sarcoma, squamous-cell carcinoma, papilloma-virus (warts)

Diarrhea

Many enteric pathogens have been implicated in diarrheal illnesses in AJDs patients [45], and the frequency with which any pathogen is found depends largely on the vigor of the investigation. With a few exceptions the treatment is largely symptomatic [46] and is not determined by expensive searches for pathogens. In the emergency department the physician's task is to distinguish the clinical syndromes of acute enterocolitis, chronic recurrent diarrhea, and proctitis and to treat accordingly.

Acute enterocolitis is usually caused by *Shigella* species or *Campylobacter* species, and less commonly by certain *Salmonella* species, *Clostridium difficile,* and *Entamoeba histolytica* (Table 17-12), as in non–HIV-infected individuals (see Chap. 25). The patient presents with fever above 38.3°C, abdominal cramping pain, frequent watery diarrhea, and often severe tenesmus. The patient looks acutely ill and complains of a sudden onset of diarrhea preceded by fever and of increased pain immediately preceding the explosive stool passage. Recent treatment with antibiotics suggests C. *difficile* toxin–mediated colitis. Stool exam for fecal leukocytes should be performed, which will confirm the presence of enteroinvasive infection in most cases, except in granulocytopenic patients. If the digital rectal exam is painful, an anoscopy should be performed, which will confirm the diagnosis of proctitis and permit diagnostic studies appropriate for gay bowel syndrome.

The patient should be admitted to the hospital if dehydration is severe, toxic megacolon is likely, vomiting such that oral intake is impossible, or the patient cannot care for himself or herself. Presumptive treatment of enterocolitis is directed to *Shigella* species, *Salmonella* species, and *Campylobacter* species. Outpatient therapy with ciprofloxacin 500 mg twice a day is convenient and effective. Inpatient therapy for severe dysentery should be intravenous ciprofloxacin or trimethoprim-sulfamethaxazole. Antimotility agents should not be used.

Treatment of dehydration is an important component in the approach to diarrhea in the emergency department. The degree of dehydration can be estimated by change in blood pressure in the recumbent, sitting, and standing positions; if the systolic pressure drops by more than 20 mm Hg from the sitting to the standing position, extracellular water depletion is 5% or greater. Repletion of this loss may require 2–4 l D5^{1}/2N saline, and serum electrolytes should be checked when dehydration is this severe, since acidosis and hypokalemia are common. Even if orthostatic hypotension is not documented, extracellular fluid (ECF) may still be depleted by 1 or 2 liters, and the patient should be instructed in self-care with oral rehydration therapy. Rehydration can be accomplished with commercial preparations such as Pedialyte or Gatorade. The following home preparations also can be effective: one teaspoon of table salt added to a glass of orange juice; a bowl of chicken soup with rice as a source of starch; or ½ cup of rice powder and a teaspoon of salt in a glass of water with cranberry juice for flavor. The patient should be instructed to take 1 cup of oral rehydration fluid for each liquid stool (it is impossible to measure the amount lost) and to observe the frequency and the color of urine to assess the effectiveness of rehydration. All patients who have received IV fluids in the emergency department must be instructed on oral rehydration therapy for later home use.

Chronic recurrent diarrhea not associated with fever is the most common type of diarrhea in HIV infection, is rarely seen in other types of immunosuppression, and can be due to a number of pathogens (see Table 17-12), most of which are not treatable. Antimotility therapy is appropriate and necessary to prevent recurrence of dehydration. Antimotility therapy must be titrated to the severity of the diarrhea and the tolerance of the individual for opiate agents. In general the milder agents with fewer side effects should be used first; if they are unsuccessful in the first 24 hours, more potent agents can be quickly added. There are many empirical regimens; the following regimen is offered as an example. Immodium is used first, taken every 4 hours, up to 5 times per day. If necessary codeine 30 mg is added every 4 hours with the Immodium. If diarrhea volume and frequency continue, paregoric every 2 hours or Lomotil one every 2–4 hours replaces the codeine. If this regimen is unsuccessful with severe voluminous diarrhea, tincture of opium alone should be carefully titrated, beginning with 2–5 drops of concentrated tincture, diluted in juice to obscure the obnoxious taste, and administered every 2 hours until the diarrhea abates or the patient becomes somnolent. The initial use of potent opiates must be supervised by someone other than the patient, to observe for side effects, and driving must be interdicted. Interactions with other drugs also must be considered each time potent opiates are prescribed.

Proctitis

Proctitis has been recognized as part of the gay bowel syndrome in non–HIV-infected men, but its prevalence is higher in HIV-infected men. This group of infections presents with lower-quadrant cramping pain, urgency, tenesmus, small frequent stools often containing mucus and blood, usually minimal diarrhea, and general abdominal complaints. Perirectal ulceration is most commonly due to herpes simplex type 2 infection, although *Treponema pallidum* can produce similar ulcers. Proctitis is most commonly caused by *C. trachomatis*, *Neisseria gonorrhoeae*, and herpes simplex and less commonly by *T. pallidum* and *E. histolytica* (see Table 17-12). (The diagnosis and treatment of these pathogens are discussed in Chap. 30 and reference 47.) Rectal pain also can be caused by prostatic abscess, accompanied by dysuria and urinary retention and requiring admission for ultrasonography and surgical drainage.

GI Hemorrhage

Internal hemorrhage, which is not uncommon in HIV patients, represents a challenge because localization of the bleeding is often difficult and frequently indicates a poor prognosis. In addition to peptic ulcer disease, several causes of hemorrhage are unique to HIV infection. Kaposi's sarcoma is probably the most common cause of hemorrhage, occurring in any segment of the GI tract. Mucosal ulceration due to CMV and M. avium complex can lead to intermittent bleeding from the stomach, small gut, or colon. No specific therapy for these etiologies is helpful at the time of the hemorrhage. Supportive therapy includes admission and red blood cell transfusion as needed, correction of coagulopathies and thrombocytopenia, and endoscopy if peptic symptoms and coffee grounds in the nasogastric tube suggest gastric bleeding. If lower GI bleeding continues for several days, some gastroenterologists elect to perform colonoscopy in an attempt to define and treat single bleeding lesions, and decisions concerning future transfusions should be discussed with the patient and family.

Abdominal Pain

Epigastric pain may be due to esophageal disease, common gastric ailments such as peptic ulcer, gastritis, and gastroesophageal reflux, or problems almost exclusively seen in late-stage AIDS [48–50] (Table 17-13). CMV gastritis, gastric Kaposi's sarcoma, and gastric lymphoma present with isolated pain, nausea, and early satiety. Diagnosis may be suggested by barium contrast studies, but endoscopy with biopsy is required for definitive diagnosis.

Generalized abdominal pain most often accompanies diarrhea or dysentery. Appendicitis remains a common problem in young adults, but its incidence does not appear to be increased in HIV infection. Apparent bowel obstruction from excessive use of opiates for diarrhea, compounding HIV-related autonomic neuropathy, is not uncommon.

Right upper quadrant pain and tenderness, fever, and elevated serum alkaline phosphatase may be due to acalculous cholecystitis or to papillary stenosis and sclerosing cholangitis [51]. Both conditions are associated with infection by Cryptosporidium species or CMV. The presence of postprandial pain

Table 17-13. Differential diagnosis of abdominal pain

Condition	Cause
Stomach	
Gastritis	CMV, *Cryptosporidium* species
Focal ulcer	CMV, *Candida* species
Outlet obstruction	*Cryptosporidium* species, CMV, lymphoma
Small Bowel	
Enteritis	*Cryptosporidium* species, CMV, MAI
Obstruction	Lymphoma, Kaposi's sarcoma
Perforation	CMV, lymphoma
Colon	
Colitis	CMV; herpes simplex virus; *Shigella, Salmonella,*; *Campylobacter* species; *C. difficile*
Obstruction	Lymphoma, Kaposi's sarcoma
Perforation	CMV, lymphoma, herpes simplex virus
Appendicitis	Kaposi's sarcoma, *Cryptosporidium* species
Liver/Spleen	
Infiltration	Lymphoma, CMV, MAI
Biliary Tract	
Cholecystitis	CMV, *Cryptosporidium* species, enterics
Papillary stenosis	CMV, *Cryptosporidium* species, Kaposi's sarcoma
Cholangitis	CMV
Pancreas	
Inflammation	CMV, Kaposi's sarcoma, pentamidine, dideoxyinosine
Peritoneum	
Inflammation	*M. tuberculosis, Vibrio vulnificus*

suggests cholecystitis (see Chap. 27). Papillary stenosis may be accompanied by intrahepatic ductal dilatation on ultrasonography, but hepatobiliary CMV infection without papillary stenosis can have the same findings; referral to a gastroenterologist is appropriate for further studies, including endoscopic retrograde cholangiopancreatography.

Right upper quadrant pain accompanying liver cell injury is common in HIV infection. Hepatomegaly and elevated liver function tests commonly are due to acute viral hepatitis A, B, or non-A/ non-B, alcoholic hepatitis, Kaposi's sarcoma, or M.

avium complex. Less common causes of hepatic cell injury in HIV disease include tuberculosis, lymphoma, CMV, pneumocystosis, leishmaniasis, histoplasmosis, and coccidioidomycosis. In many cases a markedly elevated alkaline phosphatase level is not accompanied by recognizable infection and can be observed. [52]

In the emergency department the approach to abdominal pain is similar to that for non–HIV-infected patients and should include a thoughtful history and examination, blood drawn for liver function tests and amylase, measures to rule out gastrointestinal hemorrhage, anoscopy if tenesmus is present, ultrasonography for right upper quadrant pain, and a review of all medications to rule out toxic hepatitis and pancreatitis. Early use of the abdominal CT scan can identify many unsuspected problems in HIV-infected patients [53]. Serological studies should be submitted for hepatitis markers when appropriate, and stool for *C. difficile* toxin titer submitted when diarrhea and abdominal pain follow antibiotic use. Referral for further diagnostic studies is usually required, since the differential diagnosis is extensive.

Genitourinary Infections

Genital Ulceration

The common genital and sexually transmitted infections caused by herpes simplex virus types 1 and 2, *N. gonorrhoeae*, *Chlamydia* species, and *T. pallidum* are described in Chap. 28–30. In the presence of HIV infection genital ulcers most commonly are due to herpes simplex or syphilis. The differential diagnosis of genital ulcers in HIV-positive patients is the same as for HIV-negative patients. Diagnostic studies must include viral culture for herpes simplex and VDRL plus dark-field exam for *Treponema* organisms. Seroconversion of the VDRL test can be delayed beyond the usual one-month interval and vigorous follow-up testing is required [54], but the clinical presentation usually

Vaginitis

Vaginitis appears to be more frequent, more severe, and more persistent in HIV-infected women. The usual pathogen is *Candida albicans*, with *S. aureus* and undocumented pathogens also common. HIV-positive women are at increased risk of cervical neoplasia. Abnormal pap smears can result from the HIV infection itself, and HPV at least exacerbates the histologic changes in the cervical mucosa [55]. Every woman with HIV infection must be followed carefully with sequential pap smears, and the emergency department is often the only place to alert women and arrange follow-up.

Uremia

AIDS-related pathology of the urogenital tract can be indicated by uremia, pyuria, proteinuria, and infection with a variety of unusual pathogens [56]. Uremia commonly can be due to the following: (1) dehydration from diarrhea or insufficient oral intake; (2) drug-induced nephrotoxicity during treatment with pentamidine, rifampin, dapsone, amphotericin B, or a large number of other agents; and (3) HIV-associated nephropathy, usually associated with nephrotic levels of proteinuria [57, 58]. Referral for renal biopsy is required to distinguish this entity from heroin nephropathy, membranous nephropathy associated with hepatitis B infection, and a variety of other glomerulopathies. Nephrotic syndrome due to syphilis is treatable and reversible. HIV-infected patients also can develop acute renal failure from acute tubular necrosis, acute glomerulonephritis, acute interstitial nephritis, and obstructive uropathy. Fluid and electrolyte abnormalities are common in HIV-infected patients but are no different from those in the non–HIV-infected patient, with the caveat that adrenal insufficiency is not uncommon among patients with AIDS.

Skin Infections

Vesicular Eruptions

Orolabial or facial herpes simplex can be due to type 1 or 2 virus, but typing has little clinical utility. In HIV infection the course of the primary infection is prolonged and recurrences are more frequent and severe [58]. In addition to the usual presentation of isolated painful ulcers on the lips, gums, or buccal mucosa, it can present as satellite lesions distant from mucosal ulceration or as a slowly spreading, weeping, painful ulcer with sharp margins that advances from a parent lesion on the lips or nose. Increasing numbers of herpetic infections treated for months with daily acyclovir do not respond to high doses of oral or intravenous acyclovir, due to resistant strains of herpes [60]. In the author's experience nonhealing sores on the lips and face, often attributed to trauma, constant picking, oxygen cannulas, bite wounds, or malnutrition, are in fact due to herpes simplex and respond to oral acyclovir 200 mg 5 times a day. Topical acyclovir is less effective than oral administration and is reserved for those unable to take or tolerate the oral form.

It is not possible to diagnose reliably a cluster of vesicles as herpes simplex or varicella zoster on the basis of appearance alone; a culture should be performed before treatment on all but the most typical dermatomal zoster lesions, since the prognosis is different. Reactivation of varicella-zoster infection as shingles is often the harbinger of immunosuppression in HIV infection, but it does not have predictive value for the onset of AIDS. With severe immune deficiency repeated attacks of shingles may occur, and chronic zoster attacks may rarely occur. A radicular rash, often involving several adjacent dermatomes, may precede the painful, pruritic vesicular eruption. Cutaneous dissemination, defined as more than 20 vesicles scattered outside the original dermatomes, occurs in some cases and is indistinguishable from primary varicella (chickenpox). Visceral dissemination should be sought in the emergency department as signs and symptoms of pneumonitis, hepatitis, splenitis, pancreatitis, and rarely encephalitis. In asymptomatic HIV patients with CD4 cell counts above 200, zoster confined to one dermatome can be treated for relief of pain with codeine and itching with calamine lotion and benadryl or occasionally with the more expensive topical substance P (Zostrix); many clinicians also would treat with oral acyclovir. In HIV patients with the diagnosis of AIDS, CD4 counts below 200, or other evidence of immunosuppression, dermatomal zoster should be treated with acyclovir [61]. Oral doses required to reach inhibitory serum levels are 600–800 mg 5 times a day. More severe dermatomal disease, ophthalmic zoster, primary varicella, or evidence of cutaneous or visceral dissemination should be treated with intravenous acyclovir 10 mg/kg q8h on an inpatient basis. Steroid therapy to prevent postherpetic neuralgia is controversial and should be avoided in HIV patients due to its immunosuppressive effect. Prophylactic antibiotics to prevent bacterial superinfection in zoster lesions are unnecessary, but vigilance to detect superinfection by culture and Gram's stain is warranted.

Cellulitis, Folliculitis, and Skin Ulcerations

Cellulitis is a relatively uncommon infection in the HIV-positive patient, but it can be caused by unusual pathogens and advance rapidly, necessitating aggressive diagnosis and treatment, especially in the neutropenic patient. In addition to a blood culture, either a punch biopsy or a fine needle aspirate at the leading edge should be performed (see Chap. 32). The cellulitis should be outlined with a nonwatersoluble pen. If the margin of erythema is advancing more than 2.5 cm every 6–8 hours, the cellulitis is painful or larger than 15–25 cm in diameter, the fever is greater than 39°C, or if the patient is neutropenic or has a CD4 cell count less than 200, the patient should be hospitalized, observed for underlying fasciitis, and given an intravenous antibiotic such as ceftriaxone. In the asymptomatic HIV patient mild cellulitis with no fever can be managed on an outpatient basis using an oral antibiotic such as dicloxacillin or erythromycin to target staphylococci and streptococci.

Extensive folliculitis, often accompanied by local cellulitis and covering large areas of the body surface, is commonly called skin sepsis and is not uncommon among HIV-positive patients, particularly those with poor hygiene. Infected follicles may coalesce into a large hidradenitis-like plaque. S. aureus is usually the pathogen, although Pseudomonas aeruginosa can cause severe folliculitis. In the emergency department a culture for bacterial pathogens should be obtained from pus, and deep abscesses underlying ulcers or folliculitis should be incised and drained. Oral dicloxacillin or erythromycin is prescribed for 3–4 weeks. Failures can be treated with ciprofloxacin 500 mg twice a day or a combination of a cephalosporin and rifampin or with topical clindamycin 1% solution. It is impor-

Table 17-14. Differential diagnosis of persistent skin ulcerations in HIV patients

Diagnosis	Comments
Herpes simplex type 1 or 2	Untreated or acyclovir resistant
Secondary syphilis	Lesions teeming with treponemes
S. aureus	Abscess or hidradenitis-like plaque
P. aeruginosa	Chronic ulcer, Ecthyma gangrenosum
Cat-scratch disease	Soft papule, Heralds disseminated disease
Chronic zoster	Verrucous lesions, often acyclovir resistant
M. tuberculosis	Chronic sinus over infected lymph node
M. avium complex	Chronic ulceration
P. carinii	Isolated dermal nodule
Reiter's syndrome	Superficial pustules, keratotic papules
Cryptococcosis	Painless papules, nodules that may ulcerate
Histoplasmosis	Macules, papules, pustules, ulcerations
Coccidioidomycosis	Papules that ulcerate
Sporotrichosis	Subcutaneous nodules and widespread ulcers
Aspergillosis	Necrotic ulcers, often under dressing

tant to instruct the patient to shower daily, to wash the infected area initially with betadine or Hibiclens to reduce infectiousness, and to treat scabies or lice if present. Because recurrences are so common, these patients should be referred to a dermatologist for subsequent care.

Severe forms of seborrheic dermatitis and psoriasis are common in HIV patients, can present as severe atypical forms early in the HIV infection, and may be confused with or complicated by pyogenic skin infections. These two entities should be diagnosed and treated by dermatologists.

Chronic dermal ulcerations, either single or multiple, are not uncommon complaints in HIV pa-tients and present a broad differential diagnosis (Table 17-14). In the emergency department these ulcerations may not be the presenting complaint but rather herald disseminated disease. Thus, their recognition may be the crucial lead to hospitalization and appropriate diagnostic studies. Disseminated cat-scratch disease is not rare in AIDS [62]; the cutaneous form resembles pyogenic granulomas as soft papules or nodules that bleed easily on contact but that may present as plaques or folliculitis or even resemble Kaposi's sarcoma. The gram-negative bacterium can be recognized only on silver-stained biopsies, and the patient needs referral for investigation of dissemination and long-term therapy. Cryptococcosis may present as a painless erythematous papule on the head or neck that then progresses to nodules or ulcers. Disseminated histoplasmosis may present variously as erythematous macules, papules, pustules, ulcerations, and acneiform lesions [63].

Rash and Other Complaints

Extensive maculopapular rash involving the palms and the soles suggests secondary syphilis. In the HIV patient delayed VDRL seroconversion occurs, giving rise to "seronegative" secondary syphilis [54], and repeat serologic testing in 2–4 weeks is important. The initial acute HIV infection is accompanied by a roseola-like rash and may involve the palms and the soles; HIV serology will be negative at the time of the rash. Exfoliative erythroderma is usually due to drug hypersensitivity, although it may complicate psoriasis. Drug reactions due to trimethoprim-sulfamethoxazole are greatly increased in HIV patients with pneumocystis pneumonia [64], while drug eruptions to dapsone, ketoconazole, pyrimethamine, amphotericin B, pentamidine, and zidovudine are not uncommon but are not increased in frequency due to HIV infection.

Molluscum contagiosum and cutaneous papillomavirus (warts) are not problems in the emergency department, but they are significant indicators of severe immunodepression when the lesions are widespread. Kaposi's sarcoma is almost pathognomonic of HIV infection; cutaneous lesions are accompanied by GI lesions in 50% of cases, lymph node involvement in 50%, and pulmonary lesions in 37%.

More detailed discussions of dermatologic involvement in HIV infection can be found in references 65 and 66.

Musculoskeletal Complaints

Myalgias and muscle tenderness, particularly in the large muscle groups of the thigh, can indicate a polymyositis-like syndrome [67]. This syndrome is characterized by proximal muscle weakness, extreme fatigue, and elevated serum muscle enzymes and may be due to the HIV or in some cases to zidovudine [68]. In the emergency department when this clinical presentation is accompanied by elevated creatine phosphokinase (CPK), zidovudine therapy should be stopped and the patient referred for a muscle biopsy.

When muscle tenderness appears localized to the hips and thighs and is accompanied by fever, pyomyositis should be considered. Overlying cellulitis may or may not be present, but unilateral swelling of the thigh is obvious. The patient will not permit a Faber maneuver but will be able to walk. The CT scan is usually positive for attenuation in the fascial planes, but in the author's experience the CT scan can be equivocable early in the disease. Surgical drainage of pus is required, and in some patients more than one procedure may be necessary.

Oligoarticular pain in the large joints has been described [41] as a syndrome unique to HIV-infected patients. The pain may be severe, but it lasts only several hours, migrating to one or more joints during the attack. No etiology is known, and symptomatic treatment with nonsteroidal anti-inflammatory drugs appears helpful. The possibility of other acute syndromes, such as gout and disseminated gonococcal infection, must be entertained. The incidence of Reiter's syndrome may be increased in HIV infection; the complete triad of arthritis, conjunctivitis, and urethritis may or may not be present, but other features can help establish the diagnosis, such as keratoderma blennorrhagicum, dystrophic nails, red plaques in the groin and axillae, circinate balanitis, and a geographic tongue. Arthralgias as part of Sjogren's syndrome has been reported in HIV-infected patients.

Septic arthritis may be more common in HIV infection. In children it is due to encapsulated bacteria, whereas in adults it more likely may be due to disseminated fungal infection.

Joint pain in the feet and legs also appears to accompany the painful distal sensory polyneuropathy, which is unique to advanced HIV infection. In some patients the distal burning and dysesthesias may be less prominent than pain in the joints with movement.

Neurological Complications

Headache

Headache is a difficult symptom to evaluate, since most episodes are benign, but some herald serious life-threatening complications [69]. In the emergency department a careful neurologic exam must be performed to identify any focal deficit, thereby helping to focus the differential diagnosis and, more important, to identify those patients who require admission to the hospital. Any new and persistent headache should be investigated in the emergency department first with a contrast-enhanced CT scan of the head; if no mass lesions are identified (Table 17-15), a lumbar puncture (LP) should be performed. Figure 17-2 is an algorithm for neurologic complaints.

Table 17-15. Causes of intracranial mass lesion in AIDS

Infections
Toxoplasma gondii (multiple ring-enhancing)
Progressive multifocal leukoencephalopathy (JC virus) (diffuse nonenhancing white matter)
M. tuberculosis (single ring-enhancing)
Cryptococcus neoformans
Nocardia asteroides
Pyogenic brain abscess
Histoplasma capsulatum
C. allbicans (rare)
CMV (?)
Herpes simplex encephalitis
Varicella-zoster encephalitis
HIV (demyelination)

Neoplasms
Primary CNS lymphoma
Metastatic lymphoma (rare)
Kaposi's sarcoma (rare)

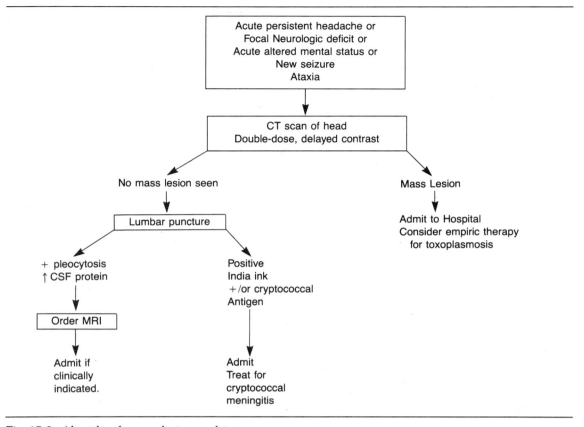

Fig. 17-2. Algorithm for neurologic complaints

Among the etiologies of meningitis cryptococcal meningitis is the most common [70]. Headache and fever almost always are present, but nuchal rigidity is often absent. Cranial nerve palsies and altered mental status are frequent, but the neurologic exam may be entirely normal. Cerebrospinal fluid (CSF) usually shows hypoglycorrhachia, elevated protein, and pleocytosis, but again it may be normal. A cryptococcal antigen titer must be performed on every CSF exam, since either may be the only abnormal result. The CSF exam should also include a VDRL and a bacterial culture. Other rare causes of fungal encephalitis include candidiasis, aspergillosis, coccidioidomycosis, and mucormycosis, in which a biopsy is required for diagnosis.

Aseptic meningitis accompanies the primary HIV meningoencephalitis prior to seroconversion but can also recur. Neurosyphilis may present as a meningitis and may progress more rapidly in the HIV-infected patient. Viral encephalitis due to herpes simplex and herpes zoster is very uncommon but must be included in every differential diagnosis of headache and fever without mass lesion, since acyclovir treatment may be life saving.

Of the three intracranial mass lesions presenting with headache and detected on CT scan or MRI, only cerebral toxoplasmosis commonly presents with fever, although fever is present in fewer than 50% of cases of toxoplasmosis. Clinical presentation of this common complication, which accounts for over 50% of all mass lesions detected by CT scan in AIDS patients, include seizures, hemiparesis, focal neurologic defects, and personality change [71]. The CT scan usually shows multiple ring-enhanced mass lesions and is sufficient evidence to begin presumptive treatment with pyrimethamine and sulfadiazine. Since almost all cases represent reactivation of a latent infection, the serum will contain IgG anti-toxoplasma antibodies.

The other mass lesions that are rarely found in

non-AIDS patients and that can be confused with cerebral toxoplasmosis are primary CNS lymphoma and progressive multifocal leukoencephalopathy (PML). PML presents with progressive dementia, hemiparesis, hemianopsia, ataxia, and other focal deficits [72], making it difficult to clinically distinguish from AIDS dementia complex. PML often can be distinguished as extensive multifocal white-matter lesions on MRI. CNS lymphoma is usually unifocal, but clinically and by CT scan it may be impossible to distinguish from toxoplasmosis. The distinction is usually made with a therapeutic trial of antitoxoplasmosis therapy, reserving brain biopsy for deteriorating patients.

Zidovudine can cause severe headaches, which usually appear during the first week of therapy, quickly resolve on discontinuing the drug, and rapidly recur with resumption of the drug, thus prohibiting its use in fewer than 1% of patients. Other medications that cause headache in AIDS patients include acyclovir, gancyclovir, foscarnet, ribavirin, dapsone, and amphotericin B.

Migraine-like headaches appear to be more frequent and more intense in patients with AIDS dementia complex and a prior history of migraine. In most patients the problem waxes and wanes and in some is clearly related to stress and insomnia. Anxiolytic therapy is helpful after a mass lesion has been ruled out.

Ataxia and Vertigo

Posterior fossa signs and symptoms usually present in the context of other intracranial pathology, with cranial nerve deficits and long tract signs. When brainstem and cerebellar disease are isolated, a mass lesion usually is involved, presenting with cerebellar ataxia, vertigo, diplopia, and headache. The differential diagnosis includes toxoplasmosis, primary CNS lymphoma, PML, and rarely tuberculoma or cryptococcoma. Any cause of meningitis may be associated with posterior fossa signs. As in the approach to headache in the emergency department, a contrasted head CT scan should be performed first, followed by an LP only if meningitis is suggested.

Ataxia is frequently a sign accompanying AIDS subacute dementia complex and the vacuolar myelopathy of AIDS. Since there are no pathognomonic features of these entities, other treatable diseases must be ruled out. Examination should look for spinal cord compression, particularly in patients with acute back pain and deteriorating neurologic deficits. Since prognosis depends on residual function at the time of diagnosis, the spine should be rapidly imaged with a CT scan, and a neurosurgical consultation obtained. Spinal abscesses can be due to toxoplasmosis, tuberculosis, and M. avium complex. Herpes simplex also can cause a temporary transverse myelitis.

Ataxia also can be mimicked by orthostatic hypotension due to dehydration, medications, or autonomic dysfunction. Vertigo can be produced by tricyclic antidepressants and narcotic analgesics, which commonly are taken to excess by HIV-infected patients. Visual disturbances such as diplopia and hemianopsia can imitate ataxia. Posterior column disease due to syphilis may rarely cause ataxia.

Visual Disturbances

The sudden development of visual-field defects, often accompanied by decreased acuity, scotoma, perception of flashes of light and floaters, and pain, almost always represents CMV retinitis in the HIV-positive patient [73]. Immediate referral to an ophthalmologist is the most important course in the emergency department, since complete loss of vision can occur in a few days. CMV retinitis is characterized by fluffy white-to-yellow exudates, often clustering along retinal vessels and accompanied by retinal hemorrhage. Exudate may extend into the vitreous, and retinal detachment is not uncommon. Diagnosis is primarily by typical appearance, although cultures of blood and urine for CMV will support the diagnosis. IV treatment with gancyclovir or foscarnet usually necessitates stopping or reducing the dose of zidovudine.

Early CMV retinitis can be confused with the benign cotton-wool spots, which are the most common retinal lesion of AIDS and appear as superficial fluffy white spots less than one-third of a disk diameter in size. They do not cause visual defects and may fade and reappear, but they need to be followed by an ophthalmologist to identify any new superimposed lesions of CMV retinitis.

Cryptococcus species and Toxoplasma species can cause extensive lesions similar to CMV retinitis, but they usually can be distinguished by an ophthalmologist. Pneumocystis has been found in small numbers of lesions similar to cotton-wool spots, but the general significance of this finding is unclear. Roth's spots due to bacterial endocarditis are few and are surrounded by erythema.

Kaposi's sarcoma commonly involves the eyelids and conjunctiva, appearing as small cherry-red papules or nodules in the upper lid, but rarely causes symptoms and therefore rarely requires treatment.

Seizures

Seizures may accompany any of the CNS disorders discussed here, most commonly mass lesions, encephalitis, and meningitis [74]. Seizures usually occur in the presence of other neurologic findings and should prompt a thorough neurologic exam. An emergent CT scan of the head should be ordered, followed by an LP if no mass lesions are seen.

In the author's experience approximately one-half of the seizures appear to have no apparent cause despite an intensive evaluation, including an MRI and electroencephalogram. Such seizures may be due to the AIDS subacute dementia complex and usually occur in patients with no other acute neurologic findings. They respond to treatment with phenobarbital or phenytoin (Dilantin), with good symptom control, but close observation is required to rule out progression of a life-threatening disorder. Rarely zidovudine, dideoxyinosine (DDI), and itraconazole have caused seizures.

Motor and Sensory Deficits

Motor disorders can be due to long tract intracerebral pathology, spinal cord compression, AIDS vacuolar myelopathy in the cord, profound muscle loss due to generalized wasting, or the inflammatory peripheral neuropathies. Asymmetric weakness suggests intracerebral or spinal cord disease and should prompt a workup in the emergency department. Symmetric weakness with progression over days to months suggests either vacuolar myelopathy or one of the inflammatory neuropathies, mononeuropathy multiplex or inflammatory demyelinating neuropathy, which appear to have an immune basis. Rapid progressive weakness and areflexia may be due to lumbosacral polyradiculopathy, with marked CSF pleocytosis and a poor prognosis. Slow

onset weakness with preservation of ankle jerks, brisk knee jerks, and impaired position sense suggests AIDS vacuolar myelopathy. This condition usually coexists with subacute dementia and peripheral sensory neuropathy and has a poor prognosis.

In the emergency department the task is to narrow the differential diagnosis and to rule out spinal cord compression with a careful neurologic exam and to rule out an intracerebral or posterior fossa mass lesion.

Isolated sensory deficits are common in AIDS patients. One-third of patients suffer from the distal sensory polyneuropathy, which appears as the subacute, often intermittent, development of numbness and tingling in a symmetric, stocking distribution, slowly ascends up the legs over a period of months. This neuropathy may be associated with severe burning pain and has only symptomatic treatment. In the emergency department evidence of toxic neuropathies should be sought in the history, including isoniazid, dapsone, alcohol, vincristine, dideoxyinosine, and dideoxycytidine (DDC).

Changes in Mental Status

Change in an AIDS patient's mental status is a challenging problem for the emergency department, since the distinction must be made between the common AIDS subacute dementia complex and less common presentations of mass lesions, encephalopathies, meningitis, medication side effects, and psychiatric disorders. AIDS dementia complex is seen in at least half of all AIDS patients and is characterized by the insidious onset of loss of recent memory and poor concentration, followed by psychomotor slowing, apathy, social withdrawal, and occasionally paranoid or aggressive behavior. Infections can precipitate the rapid appearance of symptoms, as well as seizures and myoclonus. Physical examination reveals hyperreflexia, Babinski responses, and frontal lobe signs. Mental status testing may reveal loss of ability to recognize objects, draw a symmetric clock, write one's name, remember a list of three objects, and finally loss of orientation to time, place, and person.

In the emergency department a CT scan of the head should be performed, since PML and CNS lymphoma can present only as a change in mental status. Encephalitis due to herpes simplex or toxoplasmosis may initially present with only mental status change during the first day or two, but will rapidly progressive to present other symptoms and signs.

Metabolic encephalopathy in AIDS patients can be due to liver or kidney failure, drug overdose, hypoxia due to pulmonary disease, sepsis, hyponatremia, hypoglycemia secondary to pentamidine therapy, and severe reactions to therapeutic drugs. Zidovudine, intravenous acyclovir, gancyclovir, foscarnet, interferon alpha, and compound Q have been associated with confusion, hallucinations, lethargy, mania, and even coma. Strokes and transient ischemic attacks occur in young HIV-infected patients without apparent reason [75], although marantic endocarditis, vasculitis, and meningovascular syphilis are rare causes.

References

1. Horn J, Yamaguchi E, Chaisson RE. Ambulatory care for the HIV-infected patient. In LR Barker, JR Burton, PD Zieve (eds.), *Principles of Ambulatory Medicine* (3rd ed.). Baltimore: Williams & Wilkins, 1991. Pp. 375–98.
2. Cohen PT, Sande MA, Volberding PA (eds.). The AIDS Knowledge Base. Waltham, Mass.: Massachusetts Medical Society, 1990.
3. Douglas RG et al. Acquired immunodeficiency syndrome. In GL Mandell, RG Douglas, RE Bennett (eds.), *Principles and Practice of Infectious Diseases* (3rd ed.). New York: Churchill-Livingstone, 1990. Pp. 1029–1121.
4. Veenstra RJ, Gluck JC. Access to information about AIDS. *Ann Intern Med* 114:320–24, 1991.
5. Greene WC. The molecular biology of human immunodeficiency virus type 1 infection. *N Engl J Med* 324:308–17, 1991.
5. Centers for Disease Control. Human immunodeficiency virus in the United States. A review of current knowledge. *MMWR* 36:5, 15, 1988.
7. Ferguson KJ, Stapleton JT, Helms CM. Physicians' effectiveness in assessing risk for human immunodeficiency virus infection. *Arch Intern Med* 151: 561–64, 1991.
8. Schleupner CJ. Detection of HIV-1 infection. In GL Mandel, RG Douglas, RE Bennett (eds.), *Principles and Practice of Infectious Diseases* (3rd ed.). New York: Churchill-Livingstone, 1990. Pp. 1092–1101.
9. Reesink HW et al. Evaluation of six enzyme immunoassays for antibody against human immunodeficiency virus. *Lancet* 2:483–86, 1986.
10. Houn HY, Pappas AA, Walker EM Jr. Status of current clinical tests for human immunodeficiency virus (HIV): application and limitations. *Ann Clin Lab Sci* 17:279–85, 1987.
11. Jackson JB, Balfour HH Jr. Practical diagnostic testing for human immunodeficiency virus. *Clin Microbiol Rev* 1:124–38, 1988.
12. Hausler WJ Jr. Report of the Third Consensus Conference on HIV Testing sponsored by the Association of State and Territorial Public Health Laboratory Directors. *Infect Control Hosp Epidemiol* 9: 345–49, 1988.
13. Quinn TC et al. Rapid latex agglutination assay using recombinant envelope polypeptide for the detection of antibody to HIV. *JAMA* 260:510–13, 1988.
14. Centers for Disease Control. Public Health Service guidelines for counselling and antibody testing to prevent HIV infection and AIDS. *MMWR* 36: 509–15, 1987.
15. Centers for Disease Control. AIDS and human immunodeficiency virus infection in the United States: 1988 update. *MMWR* 38 (S-4), May 1989.
16. Moss AR, Bacchetti P. Natural history of HIV infection. *AIDS* 3:55–61, 1989.
17. Kessler HA et al. Diagnosis of human immunodeficiency virus infection in seronegative homosexuals presenting with an acute viral syndrome. *JAMA* 258:1196–99, 1987.
18. Polis MA, Masur H. Predicting the progression to AIDS. *Am J Med* 89:701–5, 1990.
19. Fahey JL et al. The prognostic value of cellular and serologic markers in infection with human immunodeficiency virus type 1. *N Engl J Med* 322:166–72, 1990.
20. Centers for Disease Control: Revision of the CDC surveillance case definition for acquired immunodeficiency syndrome. *MMWR* 36(suppl):1, 1987.
21. Wilson ME, von Reyn F, Fineberg HV. Infections in HIV-infected travelers: risks and prevention. *Ann Intern Med* 114:582–92, 1991.
22. Scott GB. HIV infections in children: clinical features and management. *J AIDS* 4:109–15, 1991.
23. Nahass RG et al. Infective endocarditis in intravenous drug users: a comparison of human immunodeficiency virus type 1-negative and -positive patients. *J Infect Dis* 162:967–70, 1990.
24. Green LW et al. Adrenal insufficiency as a complication of the acquired immunodeficiency syndrome. *Ann Intern Med* 101:497–98, 1984.

25. Cohn JA, Miller L, Polish L. Orthostatic hypotension in human immunodeficiency virus infection may be the result of generalized autonomic nervous system dysfunction. *J AIDS* 4:31–33, 1991.

26. Bottles K, McPhaul LW, Volberding P. Fine needle aspiration biopsy of patients with acquired immunodeficiency syndrome (AIDS): experience in an outpatient clinic. *Ann Intern Med* 108:42–45, 1988.

27. Walsh C et al. Thrombocytopenia in homosexual patients: prognosis, response to therapy, and prevalence of antibody to the retrovirus associated with the acquired immunodeficiency syndrome. *Ann Intern Med* 103:542–45, 1985.

28. Savona S et al. Thrombocytopenic purpura in narcotic addicts. *Ann Intern Med* 102:737–41, 1985.

29. Bloom EJ, Abrams DI, Rodgers GM. Lupus anticoagulant in the acquired immunodeficiency syndrome. *JAMA* 256:491–93, 1986.

30. Murray JF et al. Pulmonary complications of the acquired immunodeficiency syndrome: an update. *Am Rev Respir Dis* 135:504–9, 1987.

31. Jules-Elysee KM et al. Aerosolized pentamidine: effect on diagnosis and presentation of *Pneumocystis carinii* pneumonia. *Ann Intern Med* 112:750–57, 1990.

32. Chaisson RE et al. Tuberculosis in patients with the acquired immunodeficiency syndrome: clinical features, response to therapy, and survival. *Am Rev Respir Dis* 136:570–74, 1987.

33. Polsky B et al. Bacterial pneumonia in patients with the acquired immunodeficiency syndrome. *Ann Intern Med* 104:38–41, 1986.

34. Selwyn PA et al. Increased risk of bacterial pneumonia in HIV-infected intravenous drug users without AIDS. *AIDS* 2:267–72, 1988.

35. Redd SC et al. The role of human immunodeficiency virus infection in pneumococcal bacteremia in San Francisco residents. *J Infect Dis* 162:1012–17, 1990.

36. Sepkowitz KA et al. Pneumothorax in AIDS. *Ann Intern Med* 114:455–59, 1991.

37. Suster B et al. Pulmonary manifestations of AIDS: review of 106 episodes. *Radiology* 161:87–93, 1986.

38. Milligan SA et al. *Pneumocystis carinii* pneumonia radiographically stimulating tuberculosis. *Am Rev Respir Dis* 132:1124–26, 1985.

39. Barrio JL et al. *Pneumocystis carinii* pneumonia presenting as cavitating and noncavitating solitary pulmonary nodules in patients with the acquired immunodeficiency syndrome. *Am Rev Respir Dis* 134:1094–96, 1986.

40. Curtis J, Goodman P, Hopewell PC. Noninvasive tests in the diagnostic evaluation for *P. carinii* pneumonia in patients with or suspected of having AIDS. *Am Rev Resp Dis* 132:A182, 1986.

41. Stover DE et al. Diagnosis of pulmonary disease in acquired immunodeficiency syndrome (AIDS): Role of bronchoscopy and bronchoalveolar lavage. *Am Rev Respir Dis* 102:747–52, 1984.

42. Gagnon S et al. Corticosteroids as adjunctive therapy for severe *Pneumocystis carinii* pneumonia in the acquired immunodeficiency syndrome. *N Engl J Med* 323:1444–50, 1990.

43. Raufman J-P. Odynophagia/dysphagia in AIDS. *Gastroenterol Clin North Am* 17:599–614, 1988.

44. Wall SD et al. Multifocal abnormalities of the gastrointestinal tract in AIDS. *Am J Roentgenol* 146:1–5, 1986.

45. Laughon BE et al. Prevalence of enteric pathogens in homosexual men with and without acquired immunodeficiency syndrome. *Gastroenterology* 94:984–93, 1988.

46. Gazzard BG. Practical advice for the gastroenterologist dealing with symptomatic HIV disease. *Gut* 31:733–35, 1990.

47. Rompalo AM et al. Empirical therapy for the management of acute proctitis in homosexual men. *JAMA* 260:348–53, 1988.

48. Potter DA et al. Evaluation of abdominal pain in the AIDS patient. *Ann Surg* 199:332–39, 1984.

49. Barone JE et al. Abdominal pain in patients with acquired immune deficiency syndrome. *Ann Surg* 204:619–23, 1986.

50. Barone JE et al. Abdominal pain and anorectal disease in AIDS. *Gastroenterol Clin North Am* 17:631–38, 1988.

51. Schneiderman DJ, Cello JP, Laing FC. Papillary stenosis and sclerosing cholangitis in the acquired immunodeficiency syndrome. *Ann Intern Med* 106:546–49, 1987.

52. Payne TH et al. Marked elevations of serum alkaline phosphatase in patients with AIDS. *J AIDS* 4:238–43, 1991.

53. Jeffery RB et al. Abdominal CT in acquired immunodeficiency syndrome. *AJR* 146:7–13, 1986.

54. Hicks CB et al. Seronegative secondary syphilis in a patient infected with the human immunodeficiency virus (HIV) with Kaposi's sarcoma. *Ann Intern Med* 107:492–95, 1987.

55. Maiman M et al. Human immunodeficiency virus and cervical neoplasia. *Gynecol Oncol* 38:377–82, 1990.

56. Kaplan MS, Wechsler M, Benson MC. Urologic manifestations of AIDS. *Urology* 30:441–43, 1987.

57. Humphreys MH, Schoenfeld PY. Renal complications in patients with the acquired immunodeficiency syndrome (AIDS). *Am J Nephrol* 7:107, 1987.

58. Rao TK, Friedman EA, Nicastri AD. The types of

renal disease in the acquired immunodeficiency syndrome. *N Engl J Med* 316:1062–68, 1987.

59. Quinnan GV et al. Herpes virus infection in the acquired immune deficiency syndrome. *JAMA* 252:72–77, 1984.

60. Erlich KS et al. Acyclovir-resistant herpes simplex virus infections in patients with the acquired immunodeficiency syndrome. *N Engl J Med* 320:293–96, 1989.

61. Huff JC et al. Therapy of herpes zoster with oral acyclovir. *Am J Med* 85:84–89, 1988.

62. Koehler JE et al. Cutaneous vascular lesions and disseminated cat-scratch disease in patients with the acquired immunodeficiency syndrome (AIDS) and AIDS-related complex. *Ann Intern Med* 109: 449–55, 1988.

63. Johnson PC et al. Progressive disseminated histoplasmosis in patients with acquired immunodeficiency syndrome. *Am J Med* 85:152–58, 1988.

64. Gordin FM et al. Adverse reactions to trimethoprim-sulfamethoxazole in patients with the acquired immunodeficiency syndrome. *Ann Intern Med* 100:495–99, 1984.

65. Kaplan MH et al. Dermatologic findings and manifestations of acquired immunodeficiency syndrome (AIDS). *J Am Acad Dermatol* 16:485–506, 1987.

66. Berger TG. Dermatologic manifestations of HIV infection. In PT Cohen, MA Sande, PA Volberding (eds.), *The AIDS Knowledge Base*. Waltham, Mass.: Massachusetts Medical Society, 1990.

67. Dalakas MC et al. Polymyositis associated with AIDS retrovirus. *JAMA* 256:2381–83, 1986.

68. Bessen LJ et al. Severe polymyositis-like syndrome associated with zidovudine therapy of AIDS and ARC. *N Engl J Med* 318:708, 1988.

69. Levy RM, Bredesen DE, Rosenblum ML. Neurological manifestations of the acquired immunodeficiency syndrome (AIDS): experience at UCSF and review of the literature. *J Neurosurg* 62:475–95, 1985.

70. Zuger A et al. Cryptococcal disease in patients with the acquired immunodeficiency syndrome. Diagnostic features and outcome of treatment. *Ann Intern Med* 104:234–40, 1986

71. Luft BJ, Remington JS. AIDS commentary. Toxoplasmic encephalitis. *J Infect Dis* 157:1–6, 1988.

72. Berger JR et al. Progressive multifocal leukoencephalopathy associated with human immunodeficiency virus infection. A review of the literature with a report of sixteen cases. *Ann Intern Med* 107:78–87, 1987.

73. Palestine AG et al. Ophthalmic involvement in acquired immune deficiency. *Ophthalmology* 91: 1092–99, 1984.

74. Holtzman DM, Kaku DA, So YT. New onset seizures associated with human immunodeficiency virus infection. Etiology and clinical features in 100 cases. *Am J Med* 87:173–77, 1989.

75. Engstrom JW, Lowenstein DH, Bredesen DE. Cerebral infarctions and transient neurologic deficits associated with acquired immunodeficiency syndrome. *Am J Med* 86:528–32, 1989.

18

Infection in the Substance Abuser (Alcohol and Parenteral Drug Abuse)

SUZANNE M. SHEPHERD
CHARLES K. BROWN

The emergency department is increasingly becoming the portal of entry to health care for many groups of patients, including drug and alcohol abusers. Infectious disease occurs more frequently in these patients than in the general population, ranging from common infections (e.g., cellulitis and pneumonia) through the spectrum of uncommon infections (e.g., endocarditis and tuberculosis) to unusual infections associated with their relatively immunocompromised state (e.g., deep fungal infections and spontaneous bacterial peritonitis) and those infections almost strictly limited to their lifestyle (e.g., mycotic aneurysms and diphtheria).

Because they generally are busy places, emergency departments are not especially conducive to the meticulous history taking and physical examination often necessary to completely evaluate patients with an infectious disease in the differential diagnosis. One thing that is clear, however, is that drug and alcohol abusers have a predilection for infections, and any evidence of such should be aggressively pursued, or the often life-threatening nature of the entire picture will not be uncovered.

The usual patient can describe a symptom or relate a fever or constellation of systemic symptoms that will lead to consideration and appropriate investigation of an infectious illness [1]. This is not necessarily so with the substance-abusing patient. A complete history must be taken and a careful physical examination done to elucidate many signs and symptoms that may indicate infection in the substance abuser. This task can be sometimes difficult and less than pleasant in the irascible, obtunded, or unkempt substance abuser.

When caring for the substance abuser the emergency physician must be a strong patient advocate, often to the patients themselves, to ensure appropriate treatment. The majority of alcoholics with more than minor infections should be admitted for further evaluation, detoxification, and treatment as indicated. In those patients deemed healthy enough for outpatient therapy, close follow-up is mandatory. Patients must be financially and socially capable of purchasing medications or supplies and returning for follow-up to ensure an adequate course of treatment; barring this capability the emergency physician should strive to obtain the involvement of the appropriate ancillary services to help in maintaining the patient's well-being. The information that follows will, when combined with good clinical judgment, provide these patients with excellent care.

Infections in the IV Drug Abuser

Complications of IV drug abuse have assumed dramatic importance medically and economically in the last two decades. Illnesses related to this abuse present a unique and complicated set of diagnostic and treatment dilemmas. Unsterile methods of illicit drug production, adulterants used to cut IV drugs, the types of drugs used, the dissolving of drugs in dirty water or saliva, the practice of filtering drugs through reused fibers, prostitution in "shooting galleries," and other drug-administration rituals and habits contribute to fever and infection in this population [2–11]. The prevalence of human immunodeficiency virus (HIV) and acquired immunodeficiency syndrome (AIDS) in IV drug abusers further adds to the risk of serious and unusual infections. Current estimates of HIV-positive status in IV drug abusers range from 10%–70% [12], making it a wise assumption that a patient's status is positive until proved otherwise.

Fever

INFECTIOUS CAUSES

Fever in the IV drug abuser can be caused by a number of infectious and noninfectious agents. While the frequency of significant infection in IV drug abusers is not known, studies indicate that two-thirds of these patients with fever have a documented infection. A number of studies also have shown that fever may be the only clinical sign of endocarditis and other serious infectious complications of IV drug abuse [3, 4, 7, 13–20]. One to two cases of endocarditis have been estimated to occur per 1,000 IV drug abusers per year [20–24]. Forty-one percent of 180 bacteremic patients studied in Detroit were diagnosed with endocarditis [25]. Prospective studies of febrile IV drug abusers in one New York hospital in 1986 and a Boston hospital in 1988 demonstrated that 13% and 6%, respectively, had endocarditis [15, 26]. The initial emergency department impression has been shown to be an unreliable indicator of final outcome in one prospective study of 238 febrile IV drug abusers [15]. Thus, fever should be considered secondary to a serious illness such as endocarditis until the evaluation is complete. Due to the lack of reliable follow-up and the potential serious morbidity and mortal-

ity related to both effects of local extension, sepsis and embolic involvement with endocarditis, it has become standard practice to hospitalize these patients [7, 13–15, 27].

NONINFECTIOUS CAUSES

Certain illicit drugs can produce fever, including cocaine, phencyclidine, and amphetamines. Drug withdrawal from agents such as the barbiturates also can cause fever. Adulterants used to cut heroin, cocaine, and other drugs can produce pyrogenic reactions [7, 8, 13, 24, 27]. These fevers (of up to 44°C) often occur within minutes of injection, are associated with rigors, hypotension, altered mental status, and leukocytosis, and resolve within 24 hours. In the early 1980s "brown heroin" from Mexico was associated with a complex of fever, paraspinous myalgias, polyarthralgias and tenderness, and inflammation of the involved periarticular structures. Cultures in these patients were negative, and no source for the fevers was identified. Fibers from cotton used to filter drug suspensions or boiled down to extract residual amounts of drug can be injected and have been shown to produce a self-limited febrile syndrome. "Shooting the cottons" is associated with fever, shaking chills, headache, dyspnea, abdominal pain, nausea and vomiting, myalgias, and arthralgias. Physical examination may reveal tachycardia and tachypnea, mild abdominal pain, and inflammatory retinal nodules. Inflammatory pulmonary granulomata may be seen on chest radiograph, and laboratory examination may reveal a significant leukocytosis. It may be clinically impossible to differentiate this syndrome from serious infection in these patients [13, 24, 27, 28].

ORGANISM SOURCE

A number of researchers have attempted to determine the source of the organisms that produce infection in these patients [3, 29, 30]. In 1973 Tuazon and colleagues examined 100 samples of street heroin and 100 samples of injection paraphernalia. The most common isolates were a Bacillus species, Clostridium perfringens, and a coagulase-negative staphylococcus. Heroin samples frequently also yielded Aspergillus species. Staphylococcus aureus was not cultured from any of the samples [31]. Most of these organisms are rarely cultured from documented infections in these patients, but they may produce fever secondary to transient bacteremia. In 1981 Tuazon and associates addressed endotoxin contamination as another potential cause of fever. Only 1 of 38 samples of heroin contained endotoxin, which was present in insufficient quantity to cause fever [32]. Tuazon and coworkers had found, however, that the pharyngeal and skin staphylococcal carriage rate was threefold higher in active drug abusers with staphylococcal endocarditis than in the control population [33]. Furthermore, in most IV drug abusers with staphylococcal endocarditis, the skin was colonized with the same strain of this organism cultured from the blood or valve vegetations [34].

CONFOUNDING FACTORS

Use by IV drug abusers of illicitly obtained antibiotics can further confound the evaluation of fever in this patient population. As many as 60% of IV drug abusers may be concurrently taking antibiotics such as cephalexin, often supplied by the dealer [35], which has contributed significantly to the emergence of resistant organisms such as methicillin-resistant S. aureus. This practice also can ameliorate clinical symptoms and suppress growth in blood cultures [10, 11, 20, 35–38]. Febrile IV drug abusers must be questioned about this practice, and the use of resin bottles for blood cultures should be considered.

Many patients may be reluctant to admit past or present illicit drug use. Persistent nonthreatening questions and careful physical examination are necessary. While the hypertrophic track marks of IV heroin and cocaine abuse are relatively easy to identify, other types of cocaine use can produce very subtle signs [39]. "Skin-popping" sites appear as multiple small skin ulcers in various stages of healing and scarring (Fig. 18-1). Snorting cocaine can result in nasal septal perforation. Any history or evidence of parenteral drug abuse should prompt the examining physician to consider the potentially serious infectious complications discussed next.

Basis of Immunocompromise

A number of studies support immune dysfunction in IV drug abusers separate from those produced by coincidental infection with HIV. IgM and IgG hypergammaglobulinemia and increased opsonin production have been noted. A higher incidence of

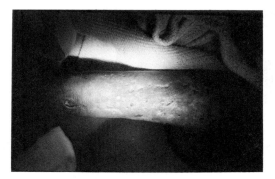

Fig. 18-1. Cutaneous evidence of skin popping

false-positive tests for syphilis, complement fixation tests, and febrile agglutinins have been described. Diminished lymphocyte response to mitogenic stimulation has been demonstrated. Peripheral lymphocytosis and atypical lymphocytosis frequently are noted on blood smears. No apparent correlation between concurrent viral infection or liver disease and these abnormalities has been demonstrated [7, 8, 11, 14].

Specific Infections

Usual organisms and recommended antibiotics for treatment of infection in IV drug abusers are listed in Table 18-1. Antibiotic dosages are listed in Table 18-2.

SKIN AND SOFT-TISSUE INFECTIONS

Skin and soft-tissue infections are the most common presentations of infection in the febrile IV drug user. Increased skin and pharyngeal carriage of staphyloccoci and streptococci, frequent injection of inflammatory materials with nonsterile technique, sharing equipment, and the practice of skin popping in older addicts and women predispose these patients to soft-tissue infections. Cocaine users run additional risk due to their increased frequency of injection, increased use of shooting galleries and shared needles, and the vasoconstrictive properties of the drug [5, 9, 10, 18]. Cellulitis, skin abscesses, septic phlebitis, necrotizing fasciitis, gas gangrene, and pyomyositis commonly are produced [35, 37]. As peripheral veins become obliterated by infection or sclerosis, the IV drug abuser will begin to "shoot" or "pop" larger veins in the neck and groin. Contiguous spread of infection with erosion into an artery, bacteremia, or repeated arterial punctures can

Table 18-1. Common organisms and recommended antibiotic choices in the patient with IV drug abuse

Infection	Pathogens	Antibiotics
Skin		
Superficial infection	S. aureus, group A streptococci	Cephalexin, dicloxacillin, ampicillin clavulanate, erythromycin
Deep, severe, or spreading infection	S. aureus, group A streptococci, gram-negative organisms (including Pseudomonas)	Nafcillin (or tobramycin) plus vancomycin; if pseudomonas suspected, add ticarcillin or ceftazidime
Necrotic infection	C. pefringens, C. tetanus, anaerobes	
Osteomyelitis and septic arthritis	S. aureus, group A streptococci, gram-negative organisms (including P. aeruginosa), N. gonorrhea)	Nafcillin (or tobramycin) plus vancomycin; if pseudomonas suspected, add ticarcillin or ceftazidime
Pneumonia	S. pneumonia, S. aureus, P. aeruginosa	Nafcillin (or tobramycin) plus vancomycin; if pseudomonas suspected, add ticarcillin or ceftazidime
Endocarditis	S. aureus, streptococcal species (including enterococcus), S. viridans), gram-negative organisms (including P. aeruginosa)	Nafcillin (or tobramycin) plus vancomycin; if pseudomonas suspected, add ticarcillin or ceftazidime
Bacterial meningitis	S. aureus, S. pneumonia, N. meningiditis	Ceftriaxone alone or vancomycin plus chloramphenicol

lead to formation of an infected pseudoaneurysm [40–42]. Groin injections also have been associated with Fournier's gangrene, which can be rapidly progressive and life threatening [40, 43].

Bacteriology. Cultures from skin infections in IV drug abusers have yielded multiple organisms. The majority of cases yield staphylococci and streptococci. Bacteremia is common in infection with these organisms and may frequently be associated with metastatic foci of infection. Gram-negative organisms include *Pseudomonas aeruginosa*, *Klebsiella pneumoniae*, *Escherichia coli*, and *Serratia marcescens*. Clostridia and other anaerobes and fungi have been isolated. Mixed infections are not infrequent [27, 31, 44].

Clinical Presentation. Symptoms of soft-tissue infections include pain, swelling, erythema, and fever. Careful examination for fluctuance, crepitance, or evidence of lymphangitis should be performed. Abscesses should be incised and drained, but potential involvement of adjacent blood vessels must be considered. Attempts to manage patients with infected false aneurysms conservatively with antibiotic treatment alone or to aspirate or incise and drain the area can result in a significant hemorrhage [27, 42]. Evidence of deep-tissue involve-

ment, such as crepitus or muscle pain, may require further surgical and medical management. Exploration, débridement, amputation, or use of hyperbaric oxygen may be indicated. If vascular involvement is suspected, expeditious angiography is indicated. Initial evaluation in all patients should include a CBC, a wound Gram's stain, and aerobic and anaerobic cultures. Radiologic evaluation of the affected area is prudent, because extreme tenderness and swelling can mask the signs of gas in the soft tissues. If systemic signs and symptoms are present, a thorough investigation should be made for other potential sites of involvement.

Disposition. IV drug abusers with superficial cellulitis and no evidence of systemic illness can be treated as outpatients. Empiric antibiotic choices should cover staphylococci and streptococci. Choices include cefadroxil (500 mg bid PO), cephalexin (500 mg qid PO), dicloxacillin (500 mg qid PO), ampicillin clavulanate (500 mg tid PO), or erythromycin (500 mg qid PO).

Those patients with potentially severe infections or infections that require extensive wound care should be admitted, because of to the unreliability of follow-up in these patients. Fever, lymphangitis, deep abscesses, and evidence of systemic infection mandate hospitalization. Broad-spectrum intravenous antibiotic coverage should be instituted pending culture results. Antibiotic coverage should include penicillinase-resistant synthetic penicillin (nafcillin 1–2 g q4h) or vancomycin (1 g q12h) plus an antipseudomonal aminoglycoside (tobramycin 3–5 mg/kg/d divided q8h) or an antipseudomonal penicillin (e.g., ticarcillin or piperacillin) or a third-generation cephalosporin (e.g., ceftazidime) [11].

Clostridial Infections. Clostridial species and other anaerobes can produce skin and deep soft-tissue infections. The interconnected abscesses produced by skin popping form an ideal growth media for clostridia. Clostridial infection may not be apparent on examination, and patients are frequently afebrile. An x-ray will demonstrate gas in the soft tissues. Wound botulism, a relatively rare infection in the general population and caused by *Clostridium botulinum*, has been reported in several IV drug abusers. Patients present with nausea and vomiting, hypotension, cranial nerve palsies, and descending paralysis. Diagnosis may be supported by culture results and serum toxin assay. Electromyographic findings, similar to those of Eaton-Lambert syndrome, can provide additional diagnostic information. Treatment includes penicillin G (10 million–30 million U/d) administration, local wound cleansing and débridement, expeditious antitoxin administration, and respiratory support [11, 45].

A second potentially lethal clostridial infection is tetanus, caused by *Clostridium tetani*. Tetanus was first described as a complication of drug abuse in 1876. In 1967 Louria and colleagues reported an average incidence of two IV drug abusers per year admitted to Bellevue with this diagnosis [8]. Even with early recognition the mortality rate remains greater than 50 percent. The incubation period is approximately 2 weeks. Common presenting complaints include jaw pain or stiffness, dysphagia, and often back or abdominal pain. Jaw stiffness progresses to rigidity and trismus, thus the common name "lockjaw." With severe cases generalization of the rigidity may occur, and the patient may present with reflex spasms such as laryngospasm. Fever, diaphoresis, arrhythmias, and autonomic instability may occur. Patients may require ventilatory support; pneumonia and respiratory failure are the leading causes of death. Manifestations generally resolve over 4 weeks. Tetanus is a clinical diagnosis since wound cultures are positive only 20%–40% of the time. These patients should be hospitalized. Wounds must be cleaned and débrided as necessary. Penicillin G is effective against *C. tetani*, but administration of this agent has not been shown to change the disease's course. Human tetanus immune globulin (TIG) (3,000 to 10,000 U IM) should be administered early; it has been found to reduce the fatality rate in mild and moderate cases. Aggressive airway management, occasionally including tracheostomy and respiratory support, may be indicated. Benzodiazepines are a good choice for the symptomatic treatment of muscle spasms. Tetanus immunization status should be inquired about of all IV drug abusers, and immunization should be appropriately updated [11, 27, 46].

SKELETAL AND JOINT INFECTIONS

Skeletal infections in the IV drug abuser most frequently occur via one of two mechanisms: hematogenous spread from a distant site, such as in endocarditis, or contiguous spread from an overlying skin or soft-tissue infection. Primary septic arthritis and osteomyelitis have been found to be more common in this population than previously suspected [27, 47]. Skeletal and joint infections are seen in a healthier, younger population of IV drug abusers than in the general population, where these infections are usually found in the chronically debilitated or immunocompromised patient [27, 47, 48]. These infections are the fourth most common complication of nonalcoholic substance abuse, following skin and soft-tissue infections, hepatitis B, and endocarditis [49].

Skeletal and joint infections are classified traditionally as either pyogenic (bacterial origin) or nonpyogenic (other organisms). Bacterial infections are the most common and can occur in a variety of locations. Clinical features vary depending on the causative organism and site. Symptoms may be subtle. Localized pain and tenderness are often the only clues [11]. (See Chap. 33 for a more detailed discussion of skeletal and joint infections.)

Pyogenic Infections. Pyogenic infections predominate. Eighty-eight percent of the cases reported in one large study were bacterial in origin

[47], with the majority caused by gram-negative organisms. *P. aeruginosa*, alone or in combination, was the pathogen in up to 80% of cases [27, 50–53]. *K. pneumoniae, Enterobacter aerogenes,* and *S. marcescens* were isolated in 10% of cases. Staphylococci and streptococci were isolated in 32% of cases. More recent reports note a predominance of *S. aureus* and groups A and G streptococci; one study reported only an 11% incidence of *P. aeruginosa* [11, 48, 54, 55]. These differences reflect the changing pool of organisms present in any given location at any given time. *Neisseria gonorrheae* has also been reported in septic arthritis in IV drug abusers [48, 56]. In contrast *S. aureus* causes two-thirds of skeletal infections in the general population [56].

Nonpyogenic Infections. Nonpyogenic infections are much less common. *Candida* species were reported to be the causative agents in several cases of hematogenously seeded costochondritis and osteomyelitis [11, 41, 47, 57, 58]. Candidal infections tend to be indolent and slowly progressive. A characteristic presentation of systemic candidiasis has been reported in IV drug abusers. This syndrome includes endopthalmitis, folliculitis, and bony or joint involvement [58]. Roca and Yoshikawa's reported case of thoracic vertebral osteomyelitis produced by *Mycobacterium tuberculosis,* supported earlier case reports of both typical and atypical mycobacterial infections in IV drug abusers. Mycobacterial infection most commonly involves the ribs and the vertebral column [47]. Mycobacterial infections often are acute and associated with significant toxicity, neurologic abnormalities, night sweats, and weight loss. Mycobacterial infections most commonly are associated with coincidental involvement of the lungs, the pelvic organs, and the adrenal glands [47, 59–62].

Osteomyelitis. Osteomyelitis of the vertebral column, especially the lumbar segments, was the most common site of infection (53%) reported in one large study [47]. Eighteen percent of reported infections involved the sternoarticular joint and the pelvic girdle. Seventeen percent of reported infections involved the extremities, especially the hips and the knees. Bones were commonly affected on the left side, probably reflecting the predo-

minance of right-handedness in the general population.

A review by Sapio and Montgomerie of patients with vertebral osteomyelitis noted that patients most often presented with pain and tenderness over the involved bone. A soft-tissue mass might also be palpable. In 78% of patients symptoms were chronic, lasting from 3 weeks to 3 months. Neurologic symptoms, including weakness and sensory deficit, were found not infrequently. Unfortunately fevers were minimal or absent in more than half the patients, and only 35% of patients had a total WBC count of greater than 10,000/µl [50]. The erythrocyte sedimentation rate (ESR) may be elevated [11, 50]. While plain x-ray films are more sensitive in these patients than in those with septic arthritis, they may take 1–12 weeks to demonstrate osteomyelitis [27, 47, 50]. Radioisotope technetium scanning will allow earlier documentation of bony involvement. Computerized tomographic scanning is often helpful in demonstrating infection [63]. MRI also may be useful. Blood cultures are positive in 5%–40% of patients. Pus from contiguous abscesses should be cultured. Biopsy or needle aspiration can be useful methods of obtaining material for culture and sensitivity. Gram's stains should be performed on the materials obtained, but results have not been found to correlate well with culture results [27].

Patients with osteomyelitis merit hospitalization. Unless the patient appears septic or has evidence of endocarditis, antibiotic administration should await culture results. Therapy can be initiated with a penicillinase-resistant penicillin, such as nafcillin (1–2 g q4h IV) or vancomycin (1 g q12h IV) and an aminoglycoside such as gentamicin (3–5 mg/kg/d IV). Methicillin-resistant *S. aureus* has become an increasing problem. Ticarcillin or piperacillin (4 g q4–6h IV) can be added if a *Pseudomonas* species is cultured. Regimens for *M. tuberculosis* include two agents for 2 years. Amphotericin B and flucytosine have been used successfully for candidal infections. The duration of antibiotic treatment is controversial, but 4–6 weeks is recommended by most sources for acute hematogenous pyogenic infections and 6 weeks or longer for subacute or chronic bone infections. Surgical intervention usually does not prove necessary for acute hematogeneous osteomyelitis unless underlying vascular disease or subperiosteal abscess formation is present. Bed rest and splinting may be helpful adjuncts, especially for mycobacterial infections, since mycobacterial lesions are lytic and may lead to significant instability.

Septic Arthritis. Infectious arthritis usually involves the hip or the knee. Sternoclavicular septic arthritis is well described and may be pathognomonic of IV drug abuse. Pain, tenderness, and swelling are usually noted at the involved sites. Range of motion is limited by pain. A history of recent trauma to the area often is elicited, but causal relationship remains unclear. Fever and leukocytosis are more common in these patients than in those with osteomyelitis. The ESR is usually elevated. Plain x-ray films may show surrounding soft-tissue swelling, articular surface erosion, and widened joint spaces, but they can be normal in up to 78% of these patients [49]. Radioisotope technetium scans are usually positive early in the process. Joint fluid should be obtained for cell count, Gram's stain, culture, and sensitivity. Chandresekar and Narula noted that no parameter measured in synovial fluid analysis, except a WBC count greater than 20,000/ml was consistently found [11, 48]. In most cases neutrophils predominate. A gram's stain, if positive, will aid in the choice of antibiotic regimen. IV antibiotic regimens are similar to those for osteomyelitis. Management also includes joint immobilization and physical therapy. Therapeutic arthrocentesis and occasionally open drainage of a septic hip may be required. The orthopedic prognosis in both groups of patients is good.

PULMONARY INFECTIONS

Pneumonia is very common in the IV drug abuser and has become a major cause of death [11, 64, 65]. The reasons are multifactorial and include the following: a decrease in immune function, including that contributed by associated HIV infection, aspiration, and impaired clearance of secretions. Septic thrombophlebitis and pulmonary emboli from endocarditis also contribute to pneumonia and lung abscess. Usual causative organisms include *Streptococcus pneumoniae*, oral flora, *P. aeruginosa*, and *S. aureus*. Emergency department physicians also must consider opportunistic infection with organisms such as *Pneumocystis carinii*, cytomegalovirus (CMV), and atypical mycobacteria in HIV-seropositive patients. Selwyn and colleagues recently showed that approximately 20% of 520 HIV-seropositive and -seronegative IV drug abusers had positive skin tests for tuberculosis on initial screening and that approximately another 12% of each group converted during a 22-month follow-up period. Four percent of HIV-seropositive individuals developed active tuberculosis over that time [61].

These patients usually present with fever, cough, shortness of breath, and chest pain. Admission to the hospital for observation pending culture results is usually advised, due to the frequent occurrence of bacteremia-associated pneumonia in this population and the difficulty in guaranteeing follow-up by these patients. Initial radiographs may show a single infiltrate. Abscess, cavitation, effusion, and multiple foci of infection suggest bacteremic etiology. Blood and sputum cultures, a sputum Gram's stain, and a sputum acid-fast stain are important aids for correct identification of the causative organisms. Echocardiography should be performed promptly if endocarditis is suspected. Empiric therapy with a semisynthetic penicillin (nafcillin) or vancomycin and an aminoglycoside is recommended [11, 27, 65]. (See Chap. 23 for a more detailed discussion of pulmonary infections.)

ENDOCARDITIS

Fever is the cardinal sign of endocarditis in this population [3, 4, 19, 20, 22]. Ten to twenty percent of IV drug abusers with fever have endocarditis [5, 21]. Patients with fever and another obvious source of infection are often bacteremic, but statistically the presence of another source has been found to decrease the likelihood of endocarditis in bacteremic patients [66]. The physician also must suspect endocarditis in an IV drug abuser with positive blood cultures. In one large study the presence or absence of peripheral embolic phenomena or heart murmur could not adequately rule in or rule out endocarditis [15]. Cardiac abnormalities, when present, were due to prior endocarditis or mitral valve prolapse. The criteria used to diagnose endocarditis in the general population are usually absent: IV drug abuser patients are younger and often have no prior history of heart disease [8, 67]. Endocarditis is uncommon in casual and new abusers

[54, 55, 68]. Chambers and colleagues demonstrated a strong association between cocaine use and endocarditis [5]. Several mechanisms may contribute to this. Cocaine users administer drugs more frequently, exposing the valves to frequent high-grade bacteremia and showers of particulate matter. Cocaine does not need to be heated prior to injection [5, 8, 23]. Cocaine users are more likely to share needles or be "shot up" in a shooting gallery [5, 9, 10, 52]. Pharmacologically the vasoconstrictive properties of cocaine may increase the risk of endocarditis [69]. (See Chap. 24 for a more detailed discussion of cardiovascular infections.)

Bacteriology. Despite regional variation in causative organisms, S. aureus is the most common organism (42%–56%) associated with endocarditis in IV drug abusers. The source is usually the drug user himself. S. aureus has been reported to cause up to 80% of right-sided infections [21]. Many of the isolates in several large cities are methicillin resistant [10, 20, 70]. Other commonly isolated organisms reflect those in the external environment and include P. aeruginosa, K. pneumoniae, S. marcescens, and Streptococcus species, including enterococci and Streptococcus viridans [9, 21, 71]. Staphylococcus and Pseudomonas organisms appear to have a predilection for the tricuspid valve [2, 3, 64], while streptococci more commonly infect the left heart. Fungi, primarily Candida species, have been implicated in up to 20% of cases of endocarditis [50, 72], usually involving the left heart. Twenty percent of cases are polymicrobial in origin [3, 73], while some may remain culture negative despite documented valvular pathology.

Pathology. Any valve can be involved; however, right-sided endocarditis is more common [3, 6, 19, 22, 23, 69]. Forty to sixty percent of cases involve the tricuspid valve. One hypothesis that has been suggested to explain this finding is that repeated injection of particulate material may damage the tricuspid endothelium, predisposing it to bacteremic infection [5]. The aortic valve is involved in approximately 20%–35% of cases, and the mitral valve is involved in 15%–20%. The pulmonic valve is involved very infrequently. Multiple valve involvement occurs in 10%–20% of cases [21, 67,

74]. Regional differences in valve location and causative organism are fascinating and may represent differences in drugs used, drug-use rituals, and the prevalence of specific antibiotics on the street in different locations [29]. Four types of valvular lesions can occur: vegetations, cuspal perforation or tear, ring abscess, and ruptured chordae tendineae. Left-sided infections can prove rapidly fatal, and death usually is due to florid pulmonary edema.

Right-Sided Endocarditis. In patients with right-sided endocarditis pulmonary symptoms secondary to septic emboli tend to predominate. These patients most commonly present with pneumonia, empyema, pneumothorax, or multiple pulmonary emboli [20–22, 65]. Progressive infection can lead to pulmonary infarction and life-threatening pulmonary gangrene [65]. Patients may note hemoptysis, cough, shortness of breath, and pleuritic chest pain. Peripheral embolic phenomenon are uncommon. When present embolic phenomena can be manifested as pulmonary hypertension, which can reopen a patent foramen ovale [3, 8, 75]. Systematic embolic phenomena may also be produced by large shunts in the pulmonary circulation [4, 18] or by pulmonary vein thrombosis from septic emboli [18]. The chest radiograph may demonstrate septic pulmonary emboli, seen as scattered wedge-shaped or round densities. Infiltrate or cavitary lesions also may be present [3, 23, 64].

Left-Sided Endocarditis. In left-sided endocarditis symptoms represent local, embolic, and vasculitic phenomena. Insufficiency murmurs are more frequently appreciated (90%) than with tricuspid involvement (30%–50%), although these murmurs may wax and wane [3, 4, 20, 30, 76]. Myocardial abscess formation can extend to the conducting system or pericardial sac [74, 77]. Coronary embolization can lead to sudden death or infarction [64, 78]. Up to 50% of patients will manifest neurologic symptoms and focal signs. Neurologic manifestations include meningitis, toxic encephalopathy, meningoencephalitis, mycotic aneurysm, brain and epidural abscess, subarachnoid hemorrhage, and most commonly cerebrovascular accident [4, 64, 79, 80]. Embolic infarction and mycotic aneurysms most commonly involve the middle cerebral artery [79, 80]. One-quarter of patients with endocarditis will have splenomegaly, depending on the duration of illness, but actual splenic abscess formation is uncommon [2, 4]. Cutaneous manifestations, present in up to 25% of patients, are variable. Although splinter hemorrhages often occur in healthy individuals as a result of minor nail-bed trauma, their presence does support the diagnosis of endocarditis when a large number are present. Tender Osler's nodes and nontender Janeway's lesions, which are manifestations of septic embolization and immune complex deposition, respectively, also support the diagnosis of endocarditis [81–83]. Musculoskeletal manifestations are frequent and include myalgias, arthralgias, and arthritis. Pyuria and hematuria are common findings in IV drug abusers with endocarditis. Renal complications include glomerulonephritis, pyelonephritis, embolic renal infarction, and abscesses [3, 15, 22, 84].

Disposition. All patients suspected of having endocarditis, including any IV drug abuser with fever, should be admitted pending evaluation. This population is notoriously difficult to follow up should outpatient blood cultures prove positive. Marantz and colleagues demonstrated that classical clinical signs of endocarditis, including chest pain, heart murmur, and peripheral emboli, were not statistically associated with this final diagnosis. A past history of endocarditis, rales, leukocytosis, and low serum carbon dioxide were the only findings statistically associated with this final diagnosis. Neither the emergency physician's prediction of significant illness nor the ward physician's decision to begin antibiotics correlated with a final diagnosis of endocarditis [15].

Laboratory Evaluation. Microbiologic evaluation of these patients should include three to five sets of blood cultures and cultures of other potentially infected sites prior to initiation of empiric antibiotic therapy [11, 18, 66]. Blood cultures will be positive in greater than 90% of these patients [2, 21]. Total blood count, ESR, urinalysis, an electrocardiogram, and a set of chest radiographs also should be obtained. Consultants should be contacted early to expedite emergency studies, including echocardiography, arteriography, and computerized axial tomography.

Echocardiography. The use of echocardiography to document valvular vegetations was first described in 1973 [21, 68]. Echocardiography is less sensitive in detecting tricuspid vegetations than left-sided valvular involvement [68]. 2D and M mode echocardiographic findings in endocarditis include valve thickening and shagginess, valve cusp or chordae rupture, and the presence of abscesses [21, 34, 68, 85]. A 2D echocardiograph is slightly more sensitive than an M mode one. A recent study by Daniel and colleagues [86] indicated that transesophageal echocardiography markedly improved abscess identification. Echocardiography is particularly helpful in the patient with negative blood cultures [20, 21, 64, 66, 87].

Therapy. Empiric therapy with a semisynthetic penicillin (nafcillin 1.5–2.0 g q4h) or vancomycin (10–15 mg/kg intravenous q12h, not to exceed 1 g) in the penicillin-sensitive patient, plus an aminoglycoside such as gentamicin (1.5–2.0 mg/kg q8h) is indicated in toxic patients or those with left-sided involvement. In a multicenter prospective, randomized trial, this regimen was found to be superior to treatment with nafcillin or vancomycin alone [21, 38, 74]. A reduced duration of bacteremia and a more rapid defervescence and normalization of the WBC count have been noted with a two-drug regimen in animal studies and clinical trials [66, 88]. Culture results determine further therapy. If a *Pseudomonas* organism is suspected, ticarcillin or piperacillin (4 g q4–6h IV) or an appropriate third-generation cephalosporin (e.g., ceftazidime) can be added to the regimen [27, 66, 18].

Patients who present with cardiac complications merit early consultation by a cardiologist and a cardiovascular surgeon. Early valve replacement should be considered in those patients with significant heart failure, evidence of abscess, recurrent embolization, or infection, such as candida, that is unresponsive to antimicrobial therapy [3, 21, 22, 64, 89–91]. Although IV drug abusers with endocarditis tend to experience less morbidity and mortality than non–drug users with native valve endocarditis, endocarditis can leave these patients with significant residual valvular damage requiring valve replacement or removal. IV drug abusers frequently continue drug abuse postoperatively, significantly increasing their risk of prosthetic valve infection.

NERVOUS SYSTEM INFECTIONS

CNS infections occur as embolic complications of distant infection (such as endocarditis), as primary infections, and as extensions of local vertebral osteomyelitis. Infections include bacterial meningitis, epidural abscesses, and mycotic aneurysms. Signs and symptoms vary, depending on the site of infection. Stroke syndromes, meningitis, and epidural abscess are currently the most commonly reported syndromes. In 1895 Osler first discussed the importance of the triad of heart murmur, fever, and hemiplegia [11]. (See Chap. 31 for a more detailed discussion of nervous system infections.)

Meningitis. Meningitis can be aseptic or bacterial. Symptoms include headache, meningismus, fever, altered mental status, focal neurologic defects, and seizure. Bacterial meningitis can be caused by hematogenously spread *S. aureus, S. pneumoniae,* and *Neisseria meningitidis.* Aseptic meningitis can be coincident to an epidural or brain abscess or a mycotic aneurysm. Aseptic meningitis also can occur as an inflammatory response to bacteremia and microemboli from endocarditis. Cerebrospinal fluid (CSF) analysis may reveal a mononuclear pleocytosis. Cultures are usually negative. Computerized axial tomographic scanning and an MRI are useful adjuncts in defining the type and the extent of lesions. Empiric coverage for bacterial meningitis should include an appropriate third-generation cephalosporin (e.g., ceftriaxone 2 g q12h IV). In the penicillin- or cephalosporin-allergic patient an alternative regimen might include vancomycin and chloramphenicol [4, 22, 27, 64, 79, 80].

Spinal Epidural Abscess. Spinal epidural abscess, uncommon in the general population, has become increasingly frequent in IV drug abusers. This diagnosis is suggested by localized back pain or evidence of nerve root or cord involvement. These patients will subsequently develop weakness and the inability to ambulate. Patients also may develop urinary incontinence [11, 92]. CSF analysis often reveals a mononuclear pleocytosis and increased protein. Myelography, computerized tomography, and an MRI can help to define the extent of infection. *S. aureus* and *P. aeruginosa* are the most commonly reported causative organisms [11, 92]. *M. tuberculosis* also has been reported and may be of particular concern in those patients concurrently positive for HIV. Neurosurgical consultation should be obtained to address drainage and decompression of these lesions [11, 79, 92].

OCULAR INFECTIONS

Endopthalmitis is a well-documented and serious complication of IV drug abuse. Fungal endopthalmitis is most frequently reported, but both bacterial and fungal cases are well described. Both can occur as a result of hematogenous seeding from endocarditis, dermatitis, sinusitis, or septic arthritis or from a primary bacteremia. Ocular manifestations of endocarditis include macular hole formation and Roth's spots [11, 93, 94]. With the rising incidence of AIDS in this population, more cases of toxoplasmosis and CMV retinitis, conjunctival Kaposi's sarcoma, choroidal cryptococcosis, and *Mycobacterium avium-intracellulare* are being seen [11]. (See Chap. 35 for a more detailed discussion of ocular infections.)

Fungal Infection. The most common fungal endopthalmitis is that caused by *Candida* species. Candidal endopthalmitis usually follows an indolent clinical course, progressing over days to weeks. Patients note pain, visual blurring, and decreased visual acuity. Examination of the involved globe most commonly reveals white, cotton-like exudates in the choroid and vitreous haziness. Uveitis, vitritis, or papillitis also may be noted. These eye findings can be subtle. Systemic evidence of candidal infection is rare, and blood cultures are frequently negative. Diagnostic vitrectomy is often necessary. Treatment is controversial and may include intraocular and systemic antifungal therapy and pars plana vitrectomy [93–95].

Aspergillus species are the second most common cause of fungal endophthalmitis. Presenting symptoms are similar to those of candidal infections. Physical examination may reveal conjunctival injection, iritis, vitritis or vitreous fungal mass, hyphema, and retinal detachment. Treatment is similar to that for candidal infection. The prognosis for both of these entities depends on prompt diagnosis and treatment [93, 94]. Infection caused by *Torulopsis*, *Penicillium*, and *Helminthosporium* species also have been reported.

Bacterial Infection. Bacterial endopthalmitis has a more rapidly progressive course. Most cases result from hematogenous seeding, most commonly from endocarditis. Symptoms include injection, pain, decreased vision, and lid and periorbital edema. Inflammation is usually present in both the anterior and the posterior chambers of the involved eye. Roth's spots (white, centered, flame-shaped hemorrhages) and cotton-wool exudates may be noted. Local extension of the infection can result in sinusitis, orbital cellulitis, and meningitis. The most common etiologic agent is S. aureus, followed by Streptococcus species. *Bacillus cereus*, commonly cultured from injection paraphernalia and street drugs, is an important pathogen to recognize, because infection can pursue a rapidly progressive and fulminant course [93, 94]. Early opthalmologic consultation is mandatory. A combined regimen of intraocular, topical, and systemic antibiotics should be employed. Surgery is often required [93–95].

Hepatitis

Hepatitis is common in the IV drug abuser. It is estimated that approximately 80% of addicts have had hepatitis, with 80% of those infections due to hepatitis B. Hepatitis can be contracted after a single episode of IV drug abuse as well as after long-term use. These patients may have hepatitis A, hepatitis B, hepatitis C, or delta agent infection. They frequently progress to chronic active hepatitis, and the mortality in this group is significant. Presenting complaints include fever, malaise, anorexia, nausea and vomiting, arthralgias, right upper quadrant pain, and icterus. Blood obtained should include antigen and antibody screening, transaminase levels, alkaline phosphatase, bilirubin levels, and clotting parameters. The CBC count may be mildly elevated, with a lymphocytic shift. Patients with fever merit a concommitant search for other infections [35, 37, 96–99]. Most patients can be managed as outpatients, unless evidence of significant toxicity, liver compromise (as

evidenced by a prothrombin time >16), or concurrent bacterial infection is present. Appropriate follow-up must be arranged. Patients should be instructed to avoid alcohol and observe body fluid precautions. These patients should be encouraged to inform household contacts and needle and sexual partners. The health department also should be notified. Hepatitis antibody screening and vaccination, as well as HIV screening, should be made available to contacts [27, 98]. (See Chap. 26 for a more detailed discussion of hepatitis).

General Approach to the Febrile Alcoholic

The deleterious effects of alcoholism have been noted for centuries in the United States, as evidenced by Benjamin Rush's tract citing pneumonia, tuberculosis, and yellow fever plus "poverty and misery, crime and infamy, disease and death" as sequelae [100]. With the exception of yellow fever little has changed over 200 years. Alcoholism comes in all shapes and sizes, ranging from the maligned skid row alcoholic to the well-dressed "citizen" to the well-closeted, secretly imbibing elder. Degree of ingestion should be routinely inquired about in all patients, since alcohol influences or causes a wide range of medical, psychiatric, and social illnesses that can affect the emergency department patient.

Life threats, such as airway incompetence, hypoxemia, hypotension, and prolonged seizures, must be immediately and aggressively addressed, with evaluation and treatment occurring simultaneously. Throughout this seemingly disorganized process the physician must persevere in obtaining a history, often from someone other than the patient, such as a relative, and perform a meticulous examination of the unclothed entire patient with an eye toward known common sources of infection in the alcoholic: pneumonia, meningitis, bacteremia, primary peritonitis, cellulitis, and tuberculosis. Ancillary evaluation of the seriously ill patient should be thorough and include a CBC count with differential, chemical profiles, coagulation studies, blood cultures, cultures of all potential sites (including CSF if indicated), and radiologic evaluation of the chest and the tissues underlying any wounds. Even patients with seemingly minor infections need to be viewed with suspicion toward a more severe infectious process. Antibiotic coverage should be broad spectrum (Tables 18-2 and 18-3), as in other immunosuppressed patients, until the source and the pathogen have been isolated.

Host Defenses

The human host has many lines of defense against infection, all of which are influenced by alcohol abuse. Pulmonary mechanical factors, host resistance factors, nutritional factors, and epidemiologic considerations are influenced [101]. Pulmonary mechanical defenses; glottic closure, which is influenced by depressed consciousness; and mucociliary clearance, which is influenced by decreased respiratory excursion are adversely affected. Glottic closure and mucociliary clearance are compromised in animals given nonphysiologic alcohol concentrations but are only suspected in humans [102]. Epidemiologic concerns center around poor hygiene, unsanitary conditions, and high-risk behavior. A variety of metabolic factors influence skin and mucus membrane integrity, bone marrow production of cellular elements, and the functional capacity of leukocytes. The discussion here centers on the immune system as influenced by alcohol.

Alcohol's effects on the immune system are far reaching and generally depressive and have generated many data but few definitive conclusions. The individual roles of liver disease, malnutrition, and alcohol toxicity have not been defined [103]. Leukopenia with hypocellular marrow and maturation arrest has been associated with alcoholism, particularly cirrhosis with hypersplenism [104]. Decreased colony stimulating factor [105] and variable decreases in marrow cellularity with vacuolization of precursors, decreased myeloid-erythroid ratios, and decreased immature granulocytes have been shown to increase rapidly without rebound after 5–9 days of abstinence and adequate nutrition [106].

Defective chemotaxis has been demonstrated in rats [107] but not conclusively in humans. Several authors [108, 109] have found no chemotactic defects using nonphysiologic alcohol concentrations, while others have noted deficits in chemotaxis, mobilization, and adherence with human polymorphonucleocytes (PMNs) [110–112]. Mild to

Table 18-2. Recommended antibiotic dosages

Ampicillin	0.5–1 g q4–6h PO/IM/IV
Aztreonam	1 g q8h–2 gm q6h IV
Cefazolin	.25 g q8h–1.5 g q6h IM/IV
Cefotaxime	1 g q8h–2 g q6h IM/IV
Cefoxitin	1 g q8h–2 g q4h IM/IV
Ceftazidime	1–2 g q8–12h IV
Ceftriaxone	1 g q12h IM/IV
Cefuroxime	0.75–1.5 g q8h IM/IV
Chloramphenicol	50 mg/kg/d divided q6h IV
Clindamycin	150–450 mg q6h PO 150–900 mg q8h IM/IV
Erythromycin	0.5–1 g q6h PO/IV
Gentamicin-tobramycin	1–2 mg/kg q8h IM/IV
Imipenem cilastin	0.5–1 g q6h IM/IV
Metronidazole	15 mg/kg (loading) IV
Nafcillin	1–2 g q4h IM/IV
Penicillin G	20 million units/d IV
Piperacillin or Ticarcillin	q4–6h IV
Rifampin	600 mg/d PO
Tetracycline	0.5–1 g q12h IV
Timentin	3.1 g q4–8h IV
Trimethoprim-sulfamethoxazole	2–2.5 mg/kg TMP divided q6° IV
Unasyn	1.5–3.0 g q6h IM/IV
Vancomycin	1 g q12h IV

moderate and heavy acute intoxication decreased adherence and mobilization, while chronic alcoholism was required for defective chemotaxis [112, 113]. Investigations of adherence causing diapedesis as well as phagocytosis and intracellular killing are inconclusive [105, 114]. Deficient bactericidal activity was transiently noted in normal human volunteers while intoxicated. This did not occur in vitro, leading to conclusions that alcohol or metabolites impair complement production [115]. Other investigators [116, 117] feel that decreased C_3 levels noted in cirrhotics are probably due to decreased hepatic synthesis rather than a direct toxic effect. One study of 27 alcoholics [118] noted normal alternate complement pathway function.

A limited number of studies involving lymphocytes reveal significant changes in both humoral and cell-mediated immunity. Several investigators have noted diffuse increases in immunoglobulins within cirrhotic patients [112, 119–121] and the existence of autoantibodies to testicular, spermatozoal, intestinal, and fibroblastic tissues [112]. This diffuse elevation of immunoglobulins was felt to be secondary to chronic liver disease producing intra- and extrahepatic shunts, thereby preventing access to both Kupffer's cells and the fixed reticuloendothelial system (RES) by the antigenic stimulus [105, 122]. The entire picture is complex, because cell-mediated immunity correlates with liver disease, which often correlates with protein-calorie malnutrition alone, since neither acute intoxication nor well-nourished chronic drinking caused the defects [112]. Much of the investigation has centered around disordered lymphocyte membrane function due to abnormally activated adenyl cyclase and resultant elevated cyclic adenosine monophasphate levels [111, 123, 124]. Lymphocyte mitogenic responses are decreased, but evidence is not conclusive regarding serologic factors [125–127] or malnutrition alone [128]. The lymphopenia returns to normal with abstinence and adequate nutrition [112].

Macrophages originate from identical marrow stem cells as PMNs, and in-vitro human and animal studies have revealed decreased bacterial clearance by fixed-tissue macrophages and mononuclear phagocytic cells [129, 130] in the presence of alcohol [106, 131]. Several investigators have presented an interesting hypothesis [132, 133]. Beta-endorphins from the CNS normally enhance killer-cell activity; since these neurotransmitters are reduced in chronic alcoholism, poor pathogen killing may result. Additionally antiviral immunity requires natural killer cells and antibody-related cytotoxicity, both suppressed by alcohol [134–136].

Many avenues of investigation have been pursued without definitive conclusions. It is likely that both the direct toxic effects of alcohol and the sequelae of malnutrition causing or resulting from liver disease bring about profound detrimental effects in both granulocyte and lymphocyte cell lines with readily discernible clinical implications.

Specific Infections

PULMONARY INFECTIONS

Morbidity and Mortality. Pneumonia is perhaps the most widely discussed infection associated with alcoholism. Morbidity, mortality, bacteriology, and the role of aspiration have been the focus of these discussions. Several large early studies [137, 138] demonstrated age-specific mortality rates of two to three times that for pneumonia within the nonalcoholic general population. A 1972 study of 6,478 male and female alcoholics noted mortalities of three and seven times, respectively, of that expected from pneumonia in the general population [139]. Studies of recurrent pneumonia [140] found a pattern of heavy drinking to precede admission and acute or chronic alcoholism with a 40% incidence to be the most common predisposing factor. Others have corroborated this pattern by noting that 72% of admissions are directly related to alcohol abuse, with 60% of patients inordinately delaying medical attention. Alcohol dependence interfered with treatment in 60% [141]. Two well-designed longitudinal studies [142, 143] compared young and old career Navy alcoholics to their nonalcoholic cohorts, noting that one of four young alcoholic males contracted pneumonia during the first year of service, whereas the older alcoholics had twice the pneumonia rate.

Clinical Presentation and Emergency Department Workup. Clinically alcoholics with pneumonia differ little in their presentation. Fever, chills, cough productive of purulent or bloody sputum, and pleuritic chest pain remain the predominant symptoms. Alcoholics with confusion or depressed consciousness with or without fever must be aggressively evaluated for pulmonary infection, because hypoxia and hypercarbia due to impending respiratory failure can produce the same symptom complex as intoxication alone. Artificial ventilation may be needed, as in any critically ill patient, before further evaluation proceeds. Complete evaluation should be done with an eye toward bacteremia or sepsis, meningitis, and other diseases, particularly gastrointestinal, associated with alcoholism. Laboratory evaluation should include a CBC count with differential, blood and sputum cultures, a sputum Gram's stain (induce if necessary), and arterial blood gas (ABG) analysis. Sputum samples have been shown to correlate with pathogens in only 50% of cases [144, 145]; however, nasotracheal suction or induction may be the most accurate collection method. Pulse oximetry alone can follow trends in oxygenation but gives no actual PO_2 and no indication of PCO_2. Combined with an

Table 18-3. Recommended antibiotic choices in the alcoholic patient

Infection	Pathogens	First choice[*]	Second choice[*]
Lobar pneumonia	Staphylococcus pneumoniae, group A streptococci, Haemophilus influenzae, Klebsiella pneumoniae, Enterobacteriacea, Mycoplasma pneumoniae, Legionella species, Corynebacterium pneumoniae, Staphylococcus aureus	Erythromycin plus any one: ceftriaxone, cefofaxime, cefuroxime, imipenem cilastin, Ticarcillin-clavulonate, Ampicillin-sulbactam	Erythromycin plus Trimethoprim-sulfamethoxazole
Aspiration pneumonia	S. pneumoniae, K. pneumoniae, Enterobacteriacea, bacteroides species, oral anaerobes	Clindamycin plus gentamicin-tobramycin or any one of: cefoxitin, imipenem cilastin, Ticarcillin-clavulonate, Ampicillin-sulbactam, ceftriaxone	Erythromycin plus Trimethoprim-sulfamethoxazole
Lung abscess	Bacteroides, peptostreptococci, fusobacteria	Clindamycin	Cefoxitin, penicillin G, or Ticarcillin-clavulonate
Empyema (drainage required)	S. pneumoniae, group A strep	Penicillin G	Vancomycin
	S. aureus	Nafcillin	Vancomycin
	H. influenzae	Ceftriaxone	Trimethoprim-sulfamethoxazole
	Anaerobic streptococci, Bacteroides species, Enterobacteriaceae	Clindamycin plus gentamicin-tobramycin	Ceftriaxone, cefoxitin, mipenem, cilastin, Ticarcillin-clavulonate or Ampicillin-sulbactam

Condition	Organisms	Drug of choice	Alternative
Spontaneous peritonitis	S. pneumoniae, group A streptococci, Enterobacteriaceae, S. aureus	Ampicillin plus gentamicin-tobramycin or Ticarcillin-clavulonate or Ampicillin-sulbactam	Cefoxitin
Meningitis	Neisseria meningitidis, S. pneumoniae, Listeria monocytogenes, Enterobacteriaceae, Pseudomonas species, H. influenzae	Penicillin G or ampicillin plus ceftriaxone or cefotaxime (ampicillin a must if pathogen is Listeria)	Chloramphenicol[a]
Sepsis (no source)	Enterobacteriaceae, group A or D streptococci, S. pneumoniae, Bacteroides species, S. aureus	Cefoxitin plus gentamicin-tobramycin or ampicillin plus gentamicin-Tobramycin plus clindamycin or Ticarcillin-clavulonate or Ampicillin-sulbactam or imipenem cilastin	Cefoxitin plus aztreonam or gentamicin-tobramycin plus ampicillin plus nafcillin plus metronidazole
Wound sepsis (including necrotizing fasciitis)	Polymicrobial, S. aureus, group A streptococci, anaerobic streptococci, Enterobacteriaceae, Clostridium perfringens, Clostridium tetani, Pseudomonas species	Ampicillin-sulbactam, Ticarcillin-clavulonate or imipenem cilastin	Nafcillin plus gentamicin-tobramycin plus clindamycin
Cellulitis	Group A streptococci, S. aureus	Penicillin G (LD) or nafcillin	Erythromycin or cefazolin
Bullous lesions	Vibrio vulnificus	Tetracycline plus gentamicin-tobramycin	Chloramphenicol
Diphtheria	Corynebacterium diphtheriae	Erythromycin	Penicillin G (LD) or rifampin

*Effects of drugs on fetal development: ceftriaxone—unknown; gentamicin-tobramycin—ototoxicity; chloramphenicol—gray baby syndrome; Trimethoprim-sulfamethoxazole—teratogenic in animals, kernicterus; tetracycline—dental
Severe liver disease requires dosage adjustments of chloramphenicol, clindamycin, erythromycin, metronidazole, nafcillin, vancomycin, and rifampin.
Source: Adapted with permission from Sanford JP. *Guide to Antimicrobial Therapy.* 1990.

initial ABG analysis oximetry provides excellent monitoring, but alone it can be dangerously deceiving. A chest x-ray is usually portable unless the patient is very stable; posteroanterior (PA) and lateral chest x-rays provide the best localization.

Alcoholics with pneumonia should be admitted because of the previously mentioned compromise in host defenses and poor compliance, unless the infection is mild enough and the social situation adequate enough to ensure medication compliance and close follow-up. Empiric antibiotic therapy should be instituted and the appropriate physician contacted for admission.

Etiology. S. *pneumoniae* is the most common pathogen noted in both the general and the alcoholic populations, with little difference in mortality (3% and 4%, respectively) [146, 147] unless severe liver disease or leukopenia is present [148, 149]. Morbidity, however, was notably different in alcoholics, with an increased chance of empyema, longer duration of fever, and slower resolution [147]. Winterbauer [140] noted a subgroup of patients with alcoholism whose only risk factor was having recurrent pneumonia. These patients had 4.2 episodes of pneumonia within an 8-year period. Pneumococcus was pathogenic in 79%, with 21 patients having other single pathogens or combinations of pathogens: K. *pneumoniae* (14), *Haemophilus influenzae* (7), S. *aureus* (6), and group A beta-hemolytic streptococci (3).

A well-recognized relationship among odontogenic disease, aspiration, and pulmonary disease exists. Huxley [150] demonstrated more extensive and frequent aspiration in the alcoholic using indium-chloride 111 tracer. Numerous studies of lung abscesses have noted an incidence of 25%–33% in alcoholics [151–155]. Polymicrobial infection was noted, usually involving mixed aerobic and anaerobic pathogens. The most frequent anaerobes noted were *Fusobacterium nucleatum*, *Bacteroides melaninogenicus*, *Bacteroides fragilis*, and anaerobic cocci. Four basic presentations occur in patients with anaerobic lung disease: lung abscess, necrotizing pneumonitis, pneumonitis, and empyema [152]. Studied patients with a lung abscess presented insidiously with 12 days of symptoms. The dependent portions of the lungs were typically involved, with upper lobe posterior and posteroapical segments and superior and basilar lower lobe

segments being most common. All lung abscesses without empyema resolved medically. Necrotizing pneumonitis, defined as one or more areas of cavitation in one or more segments, carried a higher mortality (5 of 28 cases) and was more symptomatic than lung abscess. The presentation was noted to be either insidious or fulminant. Duration of empyema symptoms ranged from days to weeks and was associated with high fever and marked leukocytosis. Associated parenchymal infection was present in all but one patient. The most important aspect of therapy was adequate drainage. Pneumonitis displayed a relatively acute course, with symptoms lasting fewer than 7 days and a rapid response to therapy. The most useful clinical clues to anaerobic pulmonary infection were putrid sputum or empyema fluid (41%), abscess or empyema (69%), symptoms lasting more than 7 days (57%), and suspected aspiration (72%) [152].

Gram-negative pneumonia is generally uncommon. One study noted a 3.7% incidence [156], and all patients had underlying chronic disease, with 47% having alcoholism alone. Overall mortality was 45%, and 39% of the alcoholics died. Pharyngeal carriage of gram-negative bacteria was felt contributory when combined with aspiration, since 59% of ambulatory alcoholics in this study were carriers versus 14% of the controls. The alcoholics carried larger numbers of organisms, particularly those of the *Klebsiella-Enterobacter* group [157]. The relationship between carrier and invasion is unclear, however, since fewer than 50% of the sputum isolates were corroborated by transtracheal aspiration [144, 145]. In one study of gram-negative pneumonia, all patients had lobar pneumonia, with 50% having multilobar infections, 2 of 12 having lung abscess, and 4 of 12 having empyema. Although gram-negative pneumonia often produces hemoptysis and has lobar consolidation and necrotizing features radiographically, the classic currant-jelly sputum was not observed, and hemoptysis of any sort was noted only with *Klebsiella* and *Proteus* species [156]. Another study [158] noted the characteristic hemoptysis in 50% of patients but no classic radiographic features. Mortality was variable, with 90% mortality accompanying normal or depressed leukocyte counts in one study [158] while another study noted 88% of alcoholics surviving hyperacute infection [159].

H. *influenzae* was noted much less frequently,

with only three studies describing 18 cases with dissimilar outcomes [131, 160, 161]. Conclusions would be difficult to draw from these limited data.

TUBERCULOSIS

Epidemiology. Studies from the United States, Canada, Great Britain, Yugoslavia, and Australia have demonstrated a striking association of tuberculosis (TB), especially pulmonary TB, with chronic alcoholism [162–167]. Alcoholism is closely tied to TB [1, 162, 167–171], and 49% of newly diagnosed TB cases in the 1970s were made in alcoholics [168]. New active TB cases have been shown to be over 50 times more frequent in homeless males than in the general population (22.2 cases per 1000 vs. 0.4 cases/per 1000) [165]. A review of chest radiographs [167] noted jailed chronic alcoholics to have 16 times the evidence of either new or previous TB than those jailed for other reasons. This same population of alcoholics had an 80% positive purified protein derivative (PPD) rate versus 33% for the other inmates. Two studies [162, 166] noted no indirect factors (occupation, smoking history, race, or marital status) to be related to the increased incidence of TB in alcoholics.

A large study of New York City welfare recipients in 1984 developed screening criteria for the substance abuse population. It advocated a cost-effective procedure involving full evaluation of only those patients with both cough and positive PPD. The study noted nine cases of active TB (0.91% incidence), which was 28 times the incidence noted in the general population (0.032%) and cited a 7.2% diagnostic yield when these criteria are used [172].

Clinical Presentation and Emergency Department Workup. Alcoholic patients with TB present with the same subacute symptoms as the general population, cough, malaise, fever, night sweats, and weight loss. No evidence supports an increased incidence of the miliary or extrapulmonary forms of infection over the general population. The key obstacle the emergency physician must overcome is obtaining an accurate history of symptoms or exposure and not attributing the inanition often encountered to the nutritional and social consequences of alcoholism. Patients with suspected TB should be placed in respiratory isolation. Radio-

graphic evaluation should include apical lordotic views to define the upper lobes more completely. Evidence of hilar adenopathy, previous TB, pleural effusion, or pleural thickening should be viewed with suspicion in the clinical setting of alcoholism and pulmonary symptoms. Sputum should be induced or suctioned to obtain reliable specimens, and morning gastric aspirates obtained if possible. Both should be sent for acid-fast stains and culture. Patients should be admitted and treated with two drugs until the acute phase is resolved and outpatient therapy instituted when proper follow-up can be ensured.

Relapse Rates. Several studies [164, 173–175] of inactive TB patients have noted approximate relapse rates of 23% in alcoholics versus 9% of controls, with 42% and 29% of relapses occurring in the first and second year of diagnosis, respectively [175]. Alcoholism interfered with therapy, because patients often were unconvinced of the need for hospitalization, frequently signed out against medical advice, and demonstrated erratic compliance and follow-up [166]. Those alcoholics with TB who comply with the treatment regimen have responses to therapy and relapse rates consistent with nonalcoholics [111, 176–178].

SPONTANEOUS BACTERIAL PERITONITIS

History. Spontaneous bacterial peritonitis, or spontaneous bacteremia, is an unusual occurrence but one closely tied to alcoholism and cirrhosis. One of the earliest reports in 1950 by Whipple and Harris [121] noted two patients with Laënnec's cirrhosis and presumed spontaneous "*Bacillus coli*" bacteremia. Conn [30] reported the first case of spontaneous bacterial peritonitis in 1964, considering ascites the sine qua non of spontaneous bacterial peritonitis, although it can occur without ascites, and coined the term "bacterascites," defining it as a positive culture with under 250 leukocytes/per milliliter of ascites. He further stated that bacterascites precedes spontaneous bacterial peritonitis much as bacteremia precedes sepsis [179].

Pathology. Pathogenic studies center on decreased clearance of organisms by the hepatic RES. Cirrhotics have intra- and extrahepatic shunts, which allow the capillary beds and RES to be bypassed [180], decreasing or eliminating hepatic first-pass removal [179]. Hepatic lymph may contribute to both ascites and infection as the capillary obstruction leads to engorgement of permeable lymphatics, which carry GI bacteria (the most common isolates) leading to bacterascites [179]. Researchers also theorized that retrograde flow through transdiaphragmatic lymphatics or hematogenous spread via toothbrushing, massaging furuncles, or nonoperative genitourinary or GI manipulation were additional portals of bacteremia and spontaneous bacterial peritonitis. Another author theorized that spontaneous bacterial peritonitis results from prolonged bacteremia due to intrahepatic shunting combined with impaired or absent bacterial killing in the transudative ascites [181].

Clinical Presentation. Spontaneous bacterial peritonitis can occur without previous apparent bacteremia, although concomitant GI, pulmonary, or genitourinary infectious sources of bacteremia are commonly described [103, 179, 182, 183]. Alcoholics with abdominal pain are frequently encountered in the authors' practice. Gastritis, pancreatitis, alcoholic hepatitis and the surgical diagnoses, cholecystitis, appendicitis, and diverticulitis are certainly more common than spontaneous bacterial peritonitis, but the alcoholic and especially the cirrhotic with fever and abdominal pain should be strongly considered as having spontaneous bacterial peritonitis. Of note is the high incidence of confusion or encephalopathy in the absence of other symptoms. Fever and leukocytosis are common, but the abdominal pain may be minimal, especially in the obtunded patient, and ascites may not be easily discernible. Conn and Fessel [179] defined spontaneous bacterial peritonitis as the abrupt onset of peritonitis without cause that is frequently associated with enteric bacteria, bacteremia, cirrhosis, and decompensated liver disease. Their series noted fever in 81%, abdominal pain in 78%, and clinical peritonitis in 65%, with 67% clinically silent except for encephalopathy. Impending encephalopathy coincided with peritonitis in 73% of cases and leukocytosis was noted in a large majority. Other studies have described less specific symptoms (Table 18-4) [179, 184–191]. Diagnosis, although difficult because of the low number of bacteria involved early, was typically made 48 hours to 7 days after hospitalization; however, spontaneous bacterial peritonitis could occur at any point in the hospital course.

Paracentesis. Paracentesis is the indicated diagnostic procedure performed in all patients with ascities and an acute febrile illness, abdominal pain, or sudden deterioration in general status. Correction of clotting abnormalities before the procedure is recommended, but infusion of fresh frozen plasma carries the risk of transfusion-associated diseases. The prothrombin time should be corrected to within 3 seconds of normal. The midline approach through the linea alba 2–3 cm below the umbilicus carries the least risk of bleeding. Conn and Fessel noted that paracentesis revealed cloudy fluid in 90% of patients, with leukocyte counts exceeding 300 cells/μl (mostly PMNs). Their criteria for positivity was greater than 250 cells/μl. Although Gram's strains of sediment noted the organism in only 39%, 26 of 31 cultures were positive, with 25 having a single isolate: *E. coli* (36%), *Streptococcus* species (23%), pneumococcus (16%), *Aeromonas* species (8%), and *P. aeruginosa* and *Aerobacter*, *Salmonella*, and *Klebsiella* species (4% each). They noted that blood and ascitic fluid isolated identical organisms in 76% of cases. On reviewing the literature they noted *E. coli* (63%), pneumococcus

Table 18-4. Symptoms and signs associated with spontaneous bacterial peritonitis

Symptoms and signs	Percentage of cases
Leukocytosis	100
Elevated transaminases	100
Jaundice	81
Fever > 38°C	67
Abdominal pain	60
Confusion or encephalopathy	57
Abdominal tenderness	50
Rebound tenderness	42
Decreased or absent bowel sounds	42
Diarrhea	34
Hypotension	27
Hypothermia	11
Neither fever nor abdominal pain	9

(23%), *Streptococcus* species (10%), and entero-cocci and *Candida* species (1% each) [179].

Investigation to increase diagnostic yield from ascitic fluid showed centrifugation improved Gram's stain positivity from 33% to 50%. Conn and Fessel additionally noted that more than a thin film of white sediment after centrifugation indicates positivity to be likely [179, 189]. Inoculating blood culture bottles with ascitic fluid in patients with chronic ambulatory peritoneal dialysis (CAPD) decreased culture negativity more than fivefold [192]. They felt that a 10%-culture-negative rate could be approached with patients with spontaneous bacterial peritonitis instead of the 35%–50% negative rates reported by some laboratories.

The albumin gradient is a reliable indicator of portal hypertension. Portal hypertension exists if the ratio of serum albumin to ascites albumin is less than 1.1. Except for nephrotic syndrome, portal hypertension has the strongest correlation with spontaneous bacterial peritonitis [193, 194]. A Long Beach, California, VA hospital study noted that ascitic fluid in spontaneous bacterial peritonitis had a lower protein value (<0.5 mg/dl) in 50% of patients compared to those with uninfected ascites [190].

Differential Diagnosis. Spontaneous bacterial peritonitis must be differentiated from peritonitis secondary to other causes, including gut perforation, abscess, appendicitis, cholecystitis, and pyelonephritis. Definitions for various forms of peritonitis are given in Table 18-5. Particularly suspect are those patients whose cultures grow multiple organisms, anaerobes, or *Staphylococcus* or *Candida* species as pathogens [179, 184–191, 195, 196]. Other parameters obtained in a more timely fashion than cultures were studied and found helpful [186, 190, 197]. Secondary peritonitis displayed markedly elevated ascitic lactate dehydrogenase (LDH) and lactate levels with markedly decreased ascitic glucose and pH measurements [198–202], whereas cases of spontaneous bacterial peritonitis showed only mildly elevated ascites-serum LDH ratios in 30% of patients and mildly decreased ascites-serum glucose ratios. Ascitic lactate measurements were elevated and pH measurements depressed in only 50% of cases. Other investigators noted no change

Table 18-5. Definitions of various forms of spontaneous bacterial peritonitis

Spontaneous Bacterial Peritonitis
Positive ascitic fluid bacterial culture
Ascitic fluid PMN count greater than 250 cell/μl
No evident intra-abdominal source for the infection

Culture-Negative Neutrocytic Ascites
No growth of ascitic fluid bacterial culture
Ascitic fluid PMN count greater than 500 cells/μl
No recent antibiotic therapy
Absence of an alternative explanation (i.e., a non-infection-related explanation) for an elevated ascitic fluid PMN count, e.g., pancreatitis, hemorrhage into ascites, peritoneal carcinomatosis, or lymphomatosis

Secondary Bacterial Peritonitis
Positive ascitic fluid bacterial culture
Ascitic fluid PMN count greater than 250 cells/μl
An evident intra-abdominal source of infection

Adapted from Runyon BA, Hoefs JC. Ascitic fluid analysis in the differentiation of spontaneous bacterial peritonitis from gastrointestinal tract perforation into ascitic fluid. *Hepatology* 4:447–50, 1984, and from Runyon BA, Hoefs JC. Ascitic fluid chemical analysis before, during and after spontaneous bacterial peritonitis. *Hepatology* 5:257–59, 1985.

in ascitic LDH, glucose, and protein [186, 190, 197], unlike that noted with pleural fluid and CSF. Other authors recommend repeat paracentesis at 48 hours to determine antibiotic efficacy; leukocyte counts less than 50% of initial values indicate appropriate therapy [186, 203].

Disposition and Outcome. Because the sensitivity of tests to evaluate infection of peritoneal fluid is low, all patients with ascites and fever should be admitted until culture results are available. Survival was reported as 78% in 246 patients with spontaneous bacterial peritonitis [179, 184, 186, 189–191]. Leukocytosis, jaundice, and absence of chills were felt to be poor prognosticators for a single episode, while leukocytosis, jaundice, and elevated creatinine implied poor outcome for the hospitalization. A serum bilirubin level greater than 8.0 mg/dl or serum creatinine level greater than 2.1 mg/dl was associated with 90% mortality [186, 190].

Management. The general management of these patients should be similar to those with peritonitis regardless of cause. Intravascular volume support should be appropriate to the patient's need, but caution should be exercised relative to excessive volume administration in the patient with ascites. Urine output becomes a difficult clinical monitor in the patient with ascites, and the Swan-Ganz catheter may be required for volume management.

Antibiotic management is usually started prior to the availability of cultures and requires a certain dependence on the Gram's stain. Penicillin remains appropriate for suspected streptococcal pathogens. vancomycin is usually initiated for suspected staphylococcal pathogens, and drug therapy is then modified if the clinical isolate is found to be sensitive to methicillin. Because of the risk of *Pseudomonas*, aminoglycosides or expanded spectrum cephalosporins can be chosen for gram-negative infections. Because of concerns about nephrotoxicity, aminoglycosides have been discouraged for many of these patients. For suspected polymicrobial infections, broad aerobic and anaerobic coverage is initiated (see Table 18-3). Drug therapy will usually be tailored to cultured pathogens in 48 hours.

BACTERIAL ENDOCARDITIS
Bacterial endocarditis is reported infrequently in cirrhosis and chronic alcoholism, as cited in the classic review by Ratnuff and Patele [204]. They cited Roberts's autopsy study, which found bacterial endocarditis in 6.7% of cirrhotics compared to 3.4% of the normal population. Several more recent studies [205–207] report the incidence ranging from 1%–14% in cirrhotics, whereas another study [208] found pneumococcal endocarditis, pneumococcal meningitis, and pneumococcal pneumonitis "frequent but underemphasized" in chronic alcoholics, noting 9 of 14 with meningitis, 11 of 14 with pneumonia, and 10 of 14 with positive blood cultures for pneumococcus.

Snyder et al. [209] provided one of the few analytical studies of endocarditis and cirrhosis, noting 1.8% of cirrhotics compared to 0.9% of noncirrhotics ($P < .06$) to have endocarditis. A record review of 41,151 live patients with bacterial endocarditis noted a 3.5-fold increased incidence in cirrhotics ($P < .001$) [184, 209]. Their autopsy study noted 50% of cirrhotics as having no underlying valvular disease or only calcific aortic stenosis in 25%, while noncirrhotics had a 46% incidence of rheumatic heart disease. Valvular location was not significantly different from noncirrhotics, but bacterial isolates were; alpha hemolytic streptococci were isolated in 33% of noncirrhotics and 19% of cirrhotics, while gram-negative bacteria were isolated in 19% of cirrhotics and 5% of noncirrhotics. The only mortality-based study noted 11 of 12 cirrhotics with endocarditis dying [110].

BACTERIAL MENINGITIS
Despite the well-known triad of pneumococcal pneumonia, meningitis, and endocarditis, there are no specific existing data of its incidence in alcoholics [101]. Alcoholism and cirrhosis are described as underlying conditions in several series of adult bacterial meningitis, with incidences ranging from 6%–29% [210–212]. Regarding mortality one study noted 47% overall mortality and 48% mortality in alcoholic patients with liver failure and pneumococcal meningitis [213], while another study noted a fourfold increased mortality in pneumococcal meningitis coincident with complicating illness, including alcoholism and liver disease [214].

Listeria monocytogenes causes a wide spectrum of infections, including meningitis, nonmeningitic CNS infections, bacteremia, and endocarditis primarily in immunosuppressed patients, the young, and the elderly. The largest review [215] noted 17 cases of CNS infection in alcoholics, and another study noted 17% with underlying alcoholism [216]. Both studies noted an increase in warmer months and mortality ranging from 40%–65% (identical to nonimmunosuppressed adults). Both meningitic and nonmeningitic CNS listerosis commonly had disturbances of consciousness, coarse tremor, and ataxia, suggesting cerebellar dysfunction in addition to fever. These findings can be easily attributed to alcoholism alone rather than infection. Nuchal rigidity was absent in the nonmeningitic form. Blood and CSF cultures were almost uniformly positive, though slow-growing and often confused with other gram-negative bacteria. Bacteremia with *L. monocytogenes* occurred 13% of the time in alcoholics, equal to the rate in pregnancy [215].

SEPTICEMIA
One study [217] of beta-hemolytic streptococcal septicemia noted alcoholism to predispose to sepsis with particular groups of streptococci. Generally groups A and D were noted with skin entry sites; group C with skin, respiratory, or urinary sources;

group B with urinary sources; and group G most often with malignancy. Alcoholism was significantly more common with group A sepsis and was noted in 32% of group A, 20% of group B, 25% of group C, and 5% of group G streptococci-induced septicemia. No linkage between alcoholism and entry site was explored (although this relation can be inferred). In two studies of pneumococcal bacteremia alcoholism was present in more than 50% of patients under 65 years and was the most common underlying illness [218, 219].

In a study of bacteremic patients with chronic liver disease, skin (28%), pneumonia (23%), unknown (19%), spontaneous bacterial peritonitis (17%) and urinary tract (15%) were noted as sources [212]. Gram-positive bacteria were noted in 69% and gram-negative bacteria in 31%. Soft-tissue infections were streptococcal or staphylococcal, pneumonia was pneumococcal, and spontaneous bacterial peritonitis and urinary tract infection were predominantly gram negative. All patients had a complicated course, with mortality related directly to elevated serum creatinine, marked leukocytosis, and absence of fever. Another study noted mortality to be related to alcoholism and leukopenia but not alcoholism alone [220]. Unsuspected *Salmonella typhimurium* was noted in nearly 50% of septic New York City alcoholics during the customary evaluation for sepsis [221].

In 1979 two distinct syndromes of infection from *Vibrio* species were described [222]. One group of patients, predominantly alcoholics with cirrhosis, developed bacteremia within 24 hours of eating raw oysters, with a mortality of 46%, while another group of nonalcoholics developed wound infections after handling crabs or being exposed to seawater, with negligible mortality. Patients demonstrate bullous, ecchymotic, and necrotic skin lesions. Organisms can be cultured from bullae, blood, necrotic tissue, and rarely stool. Tetracycline is most effective when augmented with débridement, but a wide variety of antibiotics are also effective.

MISCELLANEOUS INFECTIONS

Pancreatic Abscess. Pancreatic abscess is a severe, often life-threatening condition associated with alcoholism. Incidence has been reported at less than 3% of cases of pancreatitis [223, 224]. Several reviews [225–228] describe pancreatic abscess as occurring within 1–4 weeks of the acute episode of pancreatitis. Patients deteriorate during the resolution phase, presenting with nausea, vomiting, fever, abdominal pain, and focal tenderness. Leukocytosis is typical, and over 50% have a palpable mass or fullness. Enteric aerobes and anaerobes require antibiotic coverage, and survival is rare without a drainage procedure. Survival of 67% has been noted with this combination of therapy.

Diphtheria. Pederson et al. [229] discussed 491 cases of diphtheria in indigent adults, of which 16% were nasopharyngeal, 76% cutaneous, and 8% combined. Carriage of *Corynebacterium diptheriae* were noted in 67 patients, with 60% of infections and carriers noted in Seattle's Skid Road area alcoholic population. Poor hygiene and lifestyle enhanced the environmental contamination and person-to-person transmission.

Aeromonas organisms, gram-negative facultative aerobes endemic in soil and water, have been reported as a cause of both spontaneous bacterial peritonitis and bacteremia in adult alcoholics [179, 230]. Sporotrichosis (*Sporothrix schenckii*), a deep mycosis, has been linked to alcoholism since first reported in 1964 [231]. Two subsequent series have noted alcoholism in up to 17% of cases and speculated that an outdoor occupation combined with alcoholism was contributory [232, 233]. Several other rarely reported causes of infection in alcoholics have included *Gardnerella vaginalis* lung abscess [234], *C. perfringens* septicemia [235], and disseminated macronodular cutaneous candidiasis [236].

AIDS

There is no hard evidence of alcohol's role in AIDS except that which supports disinhibition, high-risk sexual behavior, higher-risk substance abuse behavior, increased alcohol use in the drug-using and HIV-positive populations, and alcohol's effects on the human immune system [122]. A review of the sex industry in 1989 [237] noted alcohol and drug use to be high among prostitutes and a high prevalence of HIV positivity in African heterosexual prostitutes. Several authors [238, 239] noted that approximately 44% of drug abusers also abuse alcohol, while other studies have noted that the 30% estimate of alcohol abuse among homosexuals may be conservative [112].

Alcohol has been shown to affect T- and B-lymimmunity increases HIV risk, then alcohol may have an immunological relationship to HIV acquisition and AIDS. Conversely since HIV binds to the T_4 ligand, anything decreasing the number of T_4 lymphocytes or expression of the T_4 antigen on lymphocytes would decrease the rate of HIV acquisition [105]. (See Chap. 17 for a more detailed discussion of AIDS.)

ALCOHOLISM AND HEPATITIS B

Pettigrew and associates [240] first suggested that hepatitis B virus (HBV) and alcoholism interacte to produce liver disease; they found evidence of HBV cell-mediated immunity in HBsAg-negative patients with chronic liver disease. They interpreted this finding to mean that previous or continuing low-grade HBV infection could play a role in the development of chronic alcoholic liver disease. Numerous investigators [241–246] have documented an increased HBV incidence in alcoholics compared to nonalcoholics with detection of both HBsAb and HBsAg, concluding that HBV and alcohol seem to act together to cause liver disease.

Some authors [244] have speculated that portal hypertension allows portosystemic collateral circuphocyte populations, leading to abnormal T-helper and T-suppressor cell function and disordered antibody production [112]. Since it is theoretically possible that anything decreasing cellular and humoral lation, which may allow small quantities of antigenic material from enteric HBV to enter the systemic circulation, but they have found no evidence that a large population harbors HBV in the gut. Other researchers have tested for HBsAb and HBcAb in alcoholic cirrhotics, alcoholics without cirrhosis, and controls with low alcohol consumption, finding prevalence of these HBV markers at 14.8% in cirrhotics, 14.3% in noncirrhotics, and a slight but insignificant increase over controls [247].

Some feel that alcoholics have an increased risk of HBV infection secondary to their social and hygienic circumstances [241], while others feel that alcohol exposure renders the liver liable to injury from hepatotrophic viruses or hepatotoxins, but that the most important factor is probably geographical exposure [246].

FEVER IN THE PATIENT
WITH DELIRIUM TREMENS

Fever in the alcoholic with altered mental status is one of the most complex and challenging problems

Table 18-6. Differential diagnosis in alcoholics with altered mental status

Hypoglycemia
Hypoxia
Carbon dioxide narcosis
Mixed drug and alcohol abuse or withdrawal
Ethylene glycol ingestion
Methanol ingestion
Hepatic encephalopathy
Psychosis
Seizures/postictal state
Hypothermia
Hyperthermia
Intracranial hemorrhage or mass lesion
CNS infection
Anticholinergic poisoning
Thyrotoxicosis
Sedative-hypnotic withdrawal
Electrolyte disturbances
Infection

that any physician can face. Although one initial impression is to attribute any symptoms to alcohol withdrawal, serious and unnecessary morbidity and liability can be caused by the physician who becomes complacent. Many other conditions need consideration in this setting (Table 18-6) [248, 249].

Abrupt reduction or cessation of prolonged alcohol intake causes a withdrawal syndrome consisting of, in decreasing order of frequency, anxiety, insomnia, tremor, tachycardia, systolic hypertension, hyperreflexia, decreased seizure threshold, auditory and visual hallucinations, and finally delirium [250]. True delirium tremens is rare and consists of gross tremor, profound confusion, fever, mydriasis, and frightening visual hallucinations [251]. Fever does not typically occur in alcohol withdrawal and even in the setting of delirium tremens should arouse suspicions of underlying pathology. The question of why the patient stopped drinking should be asked since the answer may provide a point from which to base evaluation. Did the patient become ill, leading to decreased alcohol intake, or vice versa?

Potential infectious sources of altered mental status should be investigated because bacteremia, pneumonia, meningitis, and primary peritonitis occur with increased frequency in the relatively immunocompromised alcoholic patient. The nonmeningitic form of listerosis can mimic cerebellar degeneration and alcohol withdrawal to an extent. Evaluation should include as thorough a history as possible, and the physical examination needs to be meticulous with an eye for manifestations of infection. Nuchal rigidity, Kernig's signs and Brudzinski's signs are not altered with delirium tremens, although they may be difficult to elicit. Mild sedation with lorazepam 1–2 mg IV per dose to relieve agitation may facilitate a better history and physical examination.

Evaluation of infectious causes should include a CBC count with differential, ABG analysis, coagulation studies, chemistry profiles, Gram's stains, and cultures of blood, sputum, urine, wounds, and suspected infectious lesions, in addition to chest radiography. Lumbar puncture may need to be delayed until a cranial CT scan has been performed if focal neurologic findings are present or an adequate fundiscopic examination cannot be performed. Antibiotics should never be withheld until a delayed diagnostic procedure can be performed if clinical suspicions of CNS infection are strong. Coverage should be broad spectrum and appropriate for possible life-threatening infections such as septicemia or meningitis until specific sources and organisms are identified. The emergency physician should approach the febrile alcoholic, whether withdrawing from alcohol or not, with a high index of suspicion for underlying infection.

References

1. American Thoracic Society. Treatment of tuberculosis in alcoholic patients. ATS statement. *Am Rev Respir Dis* 116:559–61, 1977.
2. Cannon NJ Cobbs CG. Infective endocarditis in drug addicts. In D Kaye (ed.), *Infective Endocarditis*. Baltimore: University Park Press, 1976. PP. 111–27.
3. Reisberg RE. Infective endocarditis in the narcotic addict. *Prog Cardiovasc Dis* 22:193–204, 1979.
4. Blanck RR, Ream NW, Deleese JS. Infectious complications of illicit drug use. *Int J Addictions* 19:221–32, 1984.
5. Chambers HF et al. Cocaine use and the risk for endocarditis in intravenous drug users. *Ann Intern Med* 106:833–36, 1987.
6. Cherubin CE. Infectious disease problems of narcotic addicts. *Arch Intern Med* 128:309–13, 1971.
7. Louria DB. Infectious complications of nonalcoholic drug abuse. *Ann Rev Med* 25:219–31, 1974.
8. Louria DB, Hensle T, Rose J. The major medical complications of heroin addiction. *Ann Intern Med* 67:1–22, 1967.
9. Chaisson RE et al. Cocaine use IV infection in intravenous drug users in San Francisco. *JAMA* 261:561–65, 1989.
10. Craven DE et al. Methicillin-resistant *Staphylococcus aureus* bacteremia linked to intravenous drug abusers using a "shooting gallery." *Am J Med* 80:770–76, 1986.
11. Shepherd SM, Whye DW Jr. Infectious diseases in the immunocompromised host. In D Schellinger, A Harwood-Nuss (eds.), *Infections in Emergency Medicine* (vol. I). New York: Churchill-Livingstone, 1989. Pp. 271–80.
12. Centers for Disease Control. Immunodeficiency virus infection. *MMWR* 36:49–801, 1987.
13. Rho YM. Infections as fatal complications of narcotism. *NY State J Med* 72:823–30, 1972.
14. Brown SM et al. Immunologic dysfunction in heroin addicts. *Arch Intern Med* 134:1001, 1974.
15. Marantz PR et al. Inability to predict diagnosis in febrile intravenous drug abusers. *Ann Intern Med* 106:823–28, 1987.
16. Sternbach G, Moran J, Eliastam M. Heroin addiction: acute presentation of medical complications. *Ann Emerg Med* 9:161–69, 1980.
17. White AG. Medical disorders in drug addicts: 200 consecutive admissions. *JAMA* 223:1469–71, 1973.
18. Roberts R, Slovis CM. Endocarditis in intravenous drug abusers. *Emerg Med Clin North Am* 8:665–81, 1990.
19. El-Khatib MR, Wilson FM, Lernes AM. Characteristics of bacterial endocarditis in heroin addicts in Detroit. *Am J Med Sci* 271:197–201, 1976.
20. Levine DP, Crane LR, Zervos MJ. Bacteremia in narcotic addicts at the Detroit Medical Center. *Ann Intern Med* 97:330–38, 1982.
21. Chambers HF, Mills J. Endocarditis associated with intravenous drug abuse. In MA Sande, D Kaye, RK Root (eds.), *Endocarditis*. New York: Churchill-Livingstone, 1984. Pp. 183–200.
22. Banks T, Fletcher R, Ali N. Infective endocarditis in heroin addicts. *Am J Med* 55:444–51, 1973.
23. Jaffe RB, Koschmann EB. Intravenous drug abuse: pulmonary cardiac and vascular complications. *Am J Radiol* 109:107–20, 1970.

24. Harrison DW, Walls RM. Cotton fever: a benign febrile syndrome in intravenous drug abusers. *J Emerg Med* 8:135–39, 1990.

25. Crane RC et al. Bacteremia in narcotic addicts at the Detroit Medical Center: I. Microbiology, epidemiology, risk factors, and empiric therapy. *Rev Infect Dis* 8:364–73, 1986.

26. Somet TH et al. Hospitalization decision in febrile intravenous drug abusers. *Am J Med* 89:53–57, 1990.

27. Shepherd SM, Druckenbrod G, Haywood YC. Other infectious complications in intravenous drug users. *Emerg Med Clin North Am* 8:683–92, 1990.

28. Shragg T. Cotton fever in narcotic addicts. *JACEP* 7:279–82, 1978.

29. Botsford KB et al. Selective survival in pentazocine and tripelennamine of *Pseudomonas aeruginosa* serotype 011 from drug addicts. *J Infect Dis* 151: 209–16, 1985.

30. Tuazon CU, Cardella TA, Sheagren JN. Staphylococcal endocarditis in drug users. *Arch Intern Med* 135:1555–61, 1975.

31. Tuazon CU, Hill R, Sheagren JN. Microbiologic study of street heroin and injection paraphenalia. *J Infect Dis* 129:327–30, 1974.

32. Tuazon CU, Elin RJ. Endotoxin content of street heroin. *Arch Intern Med* 141:1385, 1981.

33. Tuazon CU, Sheagren JN. Increased rate of carriage of *Staphylococcus aureus* among narcotic addicts. *J Infect Dis* 129:725–27, 1974.

34. Tuazon CU, Sheagren JN. Staphylococcal endocarditis in parenteral drug abusers: source of the organism. *Ann Intern Med* 82:788–90, 1975.

35. Schaffer SR, Schaffer SK. Use of prophylactic antibiotics by drug abusers. *JAMA* 252:1410–16, 1984.

36. Novick DM, Ness GL. Abuse of antibiotics by abusers of parenteral heroin or cocaine. *South Med J* 77:302–8, 1984.

37. Pazin GJ, Saul S, Thompson ME. Blood culture positivity: suppression by outpatient antibiotic therapy in patients with bacterial endocarditis. *Arch Intern Med* 142:263–66, 1982.

38. Sheagren JN. *Staphylococcus aureus*, the persistent pathogen. *N Engl J Med* 310:1368–73, 1984.

39. Mittleman RE, Wetli CV. Death caused by recreational cocaine use. *JAMA* 252:1889–93, 1984.

40. Lewis JW et al. Complications of attempted central venous injections performed by drug abusers. *Chest* 78:613–17, 1980.

41. Gimferrer JM. *Candida albicans* costochonditis in heroin addicts. *Ann Thorac Surg* 41:89–92, 1988.

42. O'Leary M. Subclavian artery false aneurysm associated with brachial plexus palsy: a complication of parenteral drug addiction. *Am J Emerg Med* 8:129–133, 1990.

43. Somers WJ, Low FC. Localized gangrene of the scrotum and penis: a complication of heroin injection into the femoral vessels. *J Urol* 136:111, 1986.

44. Biderman P, Hiatt JR. Management of soft tissue infections of the upper extremity in parenteral drug abusers. *Am J Surg* 154:526, 1987.

45. MacDonald KL et al. Botulism and botulism-like illness in chronic drug abusers. *Ann Intern Med* 102:616–18, 1985.

46. Beaty NH. Tetanus. In CW Thorn et al. (eds.), *Harrison's Principles of Internal Medicine*. New York: McGraw-Hill, 1987. Pp. 558–63.

47. Roca RP, Yoshikawa TT. Primary skeletal infections in heroin users: a clinical characterization, diagnosis and therapy. *Clin Orthop* 144:238–42, 1979.

48. Chandrasekar PH, Narula AP. Bone and joint infections in intravenous drug abusers. *Rev Infect Dis* 8:904–10, 1986.

49. Lohr K. Rheumatic manifestations of diseases associated with substance abuse. *Semin Arthritis Rheum* 17:90–98, 1987.

50. Sapio FL, Montgomerie JZ. Vertebral osteomyelitis in intravenous drug abusers: report of three cases and review of the literature. *Rev Infect Dis* 2: 196–203, 1980.

51. Kido D, Bryan D, Hulpern M. Hematogenous osteomyelitis in drug addicts. *Am J Roentgenol Rad Ther Nucl Med* 118:356–61, 1973.

52. McHenry RC et al. Hematogenous osteomyelitis: a changing disease. *Cleveland Clin Q* 42:125–31, 1975.

53. Vollum DI. Skin lesions in drug addicts. *Br Med J* 2:647–52, 1970.

54. Churchill MA, Geraci JE, Hunder GG. Musculoskeletal manifestations of bacterial endocarditis. *Ann Intern Med* 87:754–59, 1977.

55. Ang-Fonte GZ, Rozboril MB, Thompson GR. Changes in nongonococcal septic arthritis: drug abuse and methicillin-resistant *Staphylococcus aureus*. *Arthritis Rheum* 28:210–213, 1985.

56. Waldvogel FA, Vasey H. Osteomyelitis: the past decade. *N Engl J Med* 303:360–68, 1980.

57. Collignon PJ, Sorrell TC. Disseminated candidiasis, evidence of a distinctive syndrome in heroin abusers. *Br Med J* 287:861, 1983.

58. Rowe IF et al. Intervertebral infection due to *Candida albicans* in an intravenous heroin abuser. *Ann Rheum Dis* 47:522, 1988.

59. Forlenza SW, Axelrod JL, Grieco MH. Potts disease in heroin addicts. *JAMA* 241:379–80, 1979.

60. Kaufman DM, Kaplan JG, Litman N. Infectious agents in spinal epidural abscesses. *Neurology* 30: 844, 1980.

61. Selwyn PA et al. A prospective study of the risk of tuberculosis among intravenous drug users with human immunodeficiency virus infection. *N Engl J Med* 320:545–50, 1989.

62. Sunderam G et al. Tuberculosis as a manifestation of the acquired immunodeficiency syndrome (AIDS). *JAMA* 256:362–66, 1986.

63. Buchman AL. *Streptococcus viridans* osteomyelitis with endocarditis presenting as acute onset lower back pain. *J Emerg Med* 8:291–95, 1990.

64. Roberts WC, Buchbinder NA. Right-sided valvular infective endocarditis. *Am J Med* 53:7–19, 1972.

65. Stern WZ, Subbarao K. Pulmonary complications of drug addiction. *Semin Roentgenol* 18:183–97, 1983.

66. Delaney KA. Endocarditis in the emergency department. *Ann Emerg Med* 20:405–14, 1991.

67. Hubbell G, Cheitlin MD, Rapaport E. Presentation, management and follow-up evaluation of infective endocarditis in drug addicts. *Am Heart J* 102:85–95, 1981.

68. Andy JJ et al. Echocardiographic observations in opiate addicts with active infective endocarditis. *Am J Cardiol* 40:17–23, 1977.

69. Robbins MJ et al. Right-sided valvular endocarditis: etiology, diagnosis and an approach to therapy. *Am Heart J* 111:128–35, 1986.

70. Levine DP, Crane LR, and Zervos MJ. Community-acquired methicillin-resistant *Staphylococcus aureus* endocarditis in the Detroit Medical Center. *Ann Intern Med* 97:330–38, 1982.

71. Reiner NE, Gopalakrishna KV, Lerner PI. Enterococcal endocarditis in heroin addicts. *JAMA* 235: 1861–63, 1976.

72. Gombert ME et al. Polymicrobial endocarditis in a drug addict. *NY State J Med* 28:937–39, 1982.

73. Olle-Groig JE, Mildvan D. Possible pathogenic implications of right-sided polymicrobial endocarditis in a heroin abuser. *Eur J Clin Microbiol* 5:449–51, 1987.

74. Robbins MJ, Eisenberg S, Trishman WH. Infective endocarditis: a pathophysiologic approach to therapy. *Cardiol Clin* 5:545–61, 1987.

75. D'Alonza GE, Dantzker DR. Gas exchange alterations following pulmonary thromboembolism. *Clin Chest Med* 5:411–19, 1984.

76. Arnett EN, Roberts WC. Pathology of active infective endocarditis: a necropsy analysis of 192 patients. *Thorac Cardiovasc Surgeon* 30:327–35, 1982.

77. Dinubile MJ et al. Cardiac conduction abnormalities complicating native valve active infective endocarditis. *Am J Cardiol* 58:1213–17, 1986.

78. Pfeifer JF et al. Acute coronary embolism complicating bacterial endocarditis in operative treatment. *Am J Cardiol* 37:920–22, 1976.

79. Lerner PI. Neurologic complications of infective endocarditis. *Med Clin North Am* 69:385–98, 1985.

80. Ziment I. Nervous system complications in bacterial endocarditis. *Am J Med* 47:568–72, 1969.

81. von Reyn CF et al. Infective endocarditis: an analysis based on strict case definitions. *Ann Intern Med* 94:505–18, 1981.

82. Howard EJ. Osler's nodes. *Am Heart J* 59:633–34, 1960.

83. Cross DF, Ellis JG. Occurrence of the Janeway lesions in mycotic aneurysm. *Arch Intern Med* 118:588–91, 1966.

84. Neugarten J, Baldwin DS. Glomerulonephritis in bacterial endocarditis. *Am J Med* 77:297–304, 1984.

85. Lutas EM et al. Relation between the presence of echocardiographic vegetations and the complication rate in infective endocarditis. *Am Heart J* 112:107–13, 1986.

86. Daniel WG et al. Improvement in the diagnosis of abscesses associated with endocarditis by transesophageal echocardiography. *N Engl J Med* 324: 795–800, 1991.

87. Panidis IP et al. Clinical and echocardiographic correlations in right heart endocarditis. *Int J Cardiol* 6:17–31, 1984.

88. Korzeniowski O, Sande MA. Combination antimicrobial therapy for *Staphylococcus aureus* endocarditis in patients addicted to parenteral drugs and in nonaddicts. *Am J Intern Med* 97:496–503, 1982.

89. Alsip SG et al. Indications for cardiac surgery in patients with active endocarditis. *Am J Med* 78: 138–48, 1985.

90. Harris PD et al. Fungal endocarditis secondary to drug addiction. *J Thorac Cardiovasc Surg* 63: 980–85, 1972.

91. Mills SA. Surgical management of endocarditis. *Ann Surg* 195:367–83, 1982.

92. Kuppel BS et al. Epidural spinal infection in intravenous drug abusers. *Arch Neurol* 45:1331, 1988.

93. Kreeger R et al. Endopthalmitis associated with intravenous drug abuse. *Ann Emerg Med* 16: 585–90, 1987.

94. Lederer CM, Sabates FN. Ocular findings in the intravenous drug abuser. *Ann Opthalmol* 14:436, 1982.

95. McLane NJ, Carroll DM. Ocular manifestations of drug abuse. *Surv Opthalmol* 30:305, 1986.

96. Jui J et al. Multicenter HIV and hepatitis B seroprevalence study. *J Emerg Med* 8:243–51, 1990.

97. Fitz JG. Hepatitis C: a new virus for an old disease. *NCMJ* 52:4–8, 1991.

98. Smedile RG et al. Multicentre study of prevalence of HBV-associated delta infection and liver disease in drug addicts. *Lancet* 1:249–51, 1982.

99. DeCock KM et al. Delta hepatitis in the Los Angeles area: a report of 126 cases. *Ann Intern Med* 105:108–14, 1986.

100. Binger C. *Revolutionary Doctor: Benjamin Rush, 1746–1813.* New York: Norton, 1966. P. 200.

101. Adams HG, Jordan C. Infections in the alcoholic. *Med Clin North Am* 68:179–200, 1984.

102. Nungester WJ, Klepser RG. A possible mechanism of lowered resistance to pneumonia. *J Infect Dis* 63:94–102, 1938.

103. Martin WJ et al. Severe liver disease complicated by bacteremia. *Arch Intern Med* 129:555–62, 1962.

104. McFarland W, Libre EP. Abnormal leukocyte response in alcoholism. *Ann Intern Med* 59:865–73, 1963.

105. MacGregor RR. Alcohol and drugs as co-factors for AIDS. *Adv Alcohol Subst Abuse* 7:47–71, 1987.

106. Liu YK. Effects of alcohol on granulocytes and lymphocytes. *Semin Hematol* 17:130–36, 1980.

107. Klepser RG, Nungester WJ. The effect of alcohol upon the chemotactic responses of leukocytes. *J Infect Dis* 65:196–203, 1939.

108. Crowley JP, Abramson N. Effect of ethanol on complement-mediated chemotaxis [abstract]. *Clin Res* 19:415, 1971.

109. Spagnuolo PJ, MacGregor RR. Acute ethanol effect on chemotaxis and other components of host defense. *J Lab Clin Med* 86:24–35, 1975.

110. Brayton RG et al. Effect of alcohol and various diseases on leukocyte mobilization, phagocytosis and intracellular bacterial killing. *N Engl J Med* 282:123–28, 1970.

111. Milne RC. Alcoholism and tuberculosis in Victoria. *Med J Aust* 2:955–60, 1970.

112. Molgaard CA et al. Assessing alcoholism as a risk factor for acquired immunodeficiency syndrome (AIDS). *Soc Sci Med* 27:1147–52, 1988.

113. MacGregor RR, Gluckman SJ, Senior JR. Granulocyte function and levels of immunoglobulins and complement in patients admitted for withdrawal from alcohol. *J Infect Dis* 138:747–58, 1978.

114. Rimland D. Mechanisms of ethanol-induced defects of alveolar macrophage function. *Alcoholism* 8:73–76, 1983.

115. Johnson WD, Stokes P, Kaye D. The effect of intravenous ethanol on the bactericidal activity of human serum. *Yale J Biol Med* 42:71–89, 1969.

116. Grieco MH, Capra JD, Paderon H. Reduced serum beta lc/la globulin levels in extrarenal disease. *Am J Med* 51:340–52, 1971.

117. Petz LD. Variable mechanisms for low serum complement in liver disease [letter]. *Lancet* 2:1033, 1971.

118. Fierer J, Finley F. Deficient bactericidal activity against *Escherichia coli* in patients with cirrhosis of the liver. *J Clin Invest* 63:912–21, 1979.

119. LoGrippo G, Anselm K, and Hayashi H. Serum immunoglobulins and 5 serum proteins in extrahepatic obstructive jaundice and alcoholic cirrhosis. *Am J Gastroenterol* 56:357–66, 1971.

120. Triger DR, Wright R. Hyperglobulinemia in liver disease. *Lancet* 1:1494–97, 1973.

121. Whipple RL, Harris JF. B. coli septicemia in Laennec's cirrhosis of the liver. *Ann Intern Med* 33:462–66, 1950.

122. Stimmel B. AIDS, alcohol and heroin: a particularly deadly combination. *Adv Alcohol Subst Abuse* 6:1–5, 1987.

123. Parker CW, Sullivan TJ, Wedner HJ. Cyclic AMP and the immune response. P Greengard, GA Robison (eds.), *Advances in Cyclic Nucleotide Research, Cyclic AMP and the Immune Response.* New York: Raven, 1974. Pp. 1–79.

124. Wedner HJ, Parker CW. Lymphocyte activation. *Prog Allergy* 21:195–300, 1976.

125. Atkinson JP et al: Stimulation by alcohols of cyclic AMP metabolism in human leukocytes: possible role of cyclic AMP in the anti-inflammatory effects of ethanol. *J Clin Invest* 60:284–94, 1977.

126. Hsu CCS, Leevy CM. Inhibition of PHA-stimulated lymphocyte transformation by plasma from patients with advanced alcoholic cirrhosis. *Clin Exp Immunol* 8:749–57, 1971.

127. Tisman G, Herbert V. In vitro myelosuppression and immuno-suppression by ethanol. *J Clin Invest* 52:1410–14, 1973.

128. Law DK, Dudrick SJ, Obdon NI. Immunocompetence of patients with protein-calorie malnutrition. *Ann Intern Med* 79:545–61, 1973.

129. Guarneri JJ, Laurenzi GA. Effect of alcohol on the mobilization of alveolar macrophages. *J Lab Clin Med* 72:40–51, 1968.

130. Laurenzi GA, Guarneri JJ. A study of the mechanisms of pulmonary resistance to infection: the relationship of bacterial clearance to eiliary and alveolar macrophage function. *Am Rev Respir Dis* 93:134–45, 1966.

131. Kaplan NM, Braude AI. *Hemophilus influenzae* infection in adults. Observations on the immune disturbance. *Arch Intern Med* 101:515–23, 1958.

132. Kay N, Allen J, Morley JE. Endorphins stimulate normal human peripheral blood lymphocyte natural killer activity. *Life Sci* 35:53–59, 1984.

133. Tewari S, Noble EP. Ethanol and brain protein synthesis. *Brain Res* 126:469–79, 1971.

134. MacGregor RR. Alcohol and immune defense. *JAMA* 256:1474–79, 1986.

135. Smith FE, Palmer DL. Alcoholism, infection and altered host defenses: a review of clinical and experimental observations. *J Chron Dis* 29:35–49, 1976.

136. Stacey NH. Inhibition of antibody-dependent cell-mediated cytotoxicity by ethanol. *Immunopharmacology* 8:155–61, 1984.

137. Painton JF, Ulrich HJ. Lobar pneumonia: an analysis of 1,298 cases. *Ann Intern Med* 10:1345–64, 1937.

138. Sundby P. Alcoholism and mortality. Oslo: Universitetsforlaget, National Institute for Alcohol Research. Publ. no. 6, 1967.

139. Schmidt W, deLint J. Causes of death of alcoholics. *Quart J Stud Alc* 33:171–85, 1972.

140. Winterbauer RH, Bedon GA, Ball WC Jr. Recurrent pneumonia. Predisposing illness and clinical patterns in 158 patients. *Ann Intern Med* 70:689–700, 1969.

141. Nolan JP. Alcohol as a factor in the illness of university service patients. *Am J Med Sci* 249:135–42, 1965.

142. Kolb D, Gunderson EKE. A longitudinal study of health risks associated with alcohol abuse in young Navy men. *Drug Alc Depend* 8:131–41, 1981.

143. Kolb D, Gunderson EKE. Alcohol-related morbidity among older career Navy men. *Drug Alc Depend* 9:181–89, 1982.

144. O'Keefe JP et al. A heuristic approach to hospital acquired pneumonia [abstract]. *Clin Res* 24:350A, 1976.

145. Snydman DR, Gorbach SL. Sputum. A diagnostic pitfall in alcoholics. *Arch Intern Med* 138:1778–79, 1978.

146. Tilghman RC, Finland M. Clinical significance of bacteremia in pneumococcic pneumonia. *Arch Intern Med* 59:602–19, 1937.

147. Van Metre TE. Pneumococcal pneumonia treated with antibiotics. *N Engl J Med* 251:1048–52, 1954.

148. Austrian R, Gold J. Pneumococcal bacteremia with especial reference to bacteremic pneumococcal pneumonia. *Ann Intern Med* 60:759–76, 1964.

149. Mufson MA et al. Capsular types and outcome of bacteremic pneumococcal disease in the antibiotic era. *Arch Intern Med* 134:505–10, 1974.

150. Huxley EJ et al: Pharyngeal aspiration in normal adults and patients with depressed consciousness. *Am J Med* 64:564–68, 1978.

151. Barnett TB, Herring CL. Lung abscess. Initial and late results of medical therapy. *Arch Intern Med* 127:217–27, 1971.

152. Bartlett JG, Finegold SM. Anaerobic infections of the lung and pleural space. *Am Rev Respir Dis* 110:56–77, 1974.

153. Kharkar RA, Ayyar VB. Aetiological aspects of lung abscess. *J Postgrad Med* 27:163–66, 1981.

154. Schweppe HI, Knowles JH, Kane L. Lung abscess. An analysis of the Massachusetts General Hospital cases from 1943 through 1956. *N Engl J Med* 265:1039–43, 1961.

155. Shafron RD, Tate CF. Lung abscesses: a five-year evaluation. *Dis Chest* 53:12–18, 1968.

156. Tillotson JR, Lerner AM. Pneumonias caused by gram negative bacilli. *Medicine* 45:65–76, 1966.

157. Bjornboe M et al. Tetanus antitoxin production and gamma globulin levels in patients with cirrhosis of the liver. *Acta Med Scand* 188:541–49, 1970.

158. Limson BM, Romansky MJ, Shea JG. Acute and chronic pulmonary infection with the Friedlander bacillus: a persistent problem in early diagnosis and therapy. *Antibiot Ann* 786–93, 1955–1956.

159. Manfredi F, Daly WJ, Behnte RH. Clinical observations of acute Friedlander pneumonia. *Ann Intern Med* 58:642–53, 1963.

160. Johnson WD, Kaye D, Hook EW. *Hemophilus influenzae* pneumonia in adults. *Am Rev Resp Dis* 97:1112–17, 1968.

161. Levin DC et al. Bacteremic *Hemophilus influenzae* pneumonia in adults. A report of 24 cases and a review of the literature. *Am J Med* 62:219–24, 1977.

162. Brown KE, Campbell AH. Tobacco, alcohol and tuberculosis. *Br J Dis Chest* 55:150–58, 1961.

163. Holmdahl SG. Four population groups with relatively high tuberculosis incidence in Goteborg 1957–1964. *Scand J Respir Dis* 48:308–20, 1967.

164. Hudolin V. Tuberculosis and alcoholism. *Ann NY Acad Sci* 252:353–64, 1975.

165. Jones HW, Roberts J, Brantner J. Incidence of tuberculosis among homeless men. *JAMA* 155:1222–23, 1954.

166. Lewis LG, Chamberlain DA. Alcohol consumption and smoking habits in male patients with pulmonary tuberculosis. *Br J Prev Soc Med* 17:149–52, 1963.

167. Olin JS, Grzybowski S. Tuberculosis and alcoholism. *Can Med Assoc J* 94:999–1001, 1966.
168. Feingold AO. Association of tuberculosis with alcoholism. *South Med J* 69:1136–37, 1976.
169. Feingold AO. Cost effectiveness of screening for tuberculosis in a general medical clinic. *Public Health Rep* 90:544–51, 1975.
170. O'Brien WB, Vindzberg WV, Longo G. Alcohol and tuberculosis, a study of 200 patients admitted to the Dr. V. E. Zambarano Memorial Hospital, Wallum Lake, Rhode Island. *RI Med J* 42:246–48, 1959.
171. Pincock TA. Alcoholism in tuberculosis patients. *Can Med Assoc J* 91:851–54, 1964.
172. Friedman LM et al. Tuberculosis screening in alcoholics and drug addicts. *Am Rev Respir Dis* 136:1188–92, 1987.
173. Christensen O et al. Social problems associated with tuberculosis. *Acta Tuberc Pneumon Scand* 56:39–55, 1963.
174. Kok-Jensen A. The prognosis of pulmonary tuberculosis in patients with abuse of alcohol. *Scand J Respir Dis* 51:42–48, 1970.
175. Segarra F, Sherman DS. Relapses in pulmonary tuberculosis. *Dis Chest* 51:59–63, 1967.
176. Cheung OT: Some difficulties in the treatment of tuberculous alcoholics. *Can J Publ Hlth* 54:281–84, 1965.
177. Kok-Jensen A: Pulmonary tuberculosis in well-treated alcoholics. Long-term prognosis regarding relapses compared with non-alcoholic patients. *Scand J Respir Dis* 53:202–6, 1972.
178. Kok-Johnson A. Insufficiency of primary treatment of pulmonary tuberculosis in relation to marriage and abuse of alcohol. *Scand J Respir Dis* 53:274–79, 1972.
179. Conn HO, Fessel JM. Spontaneous bacterial peritonitis in cirrhosis: variations on a theme. *Medicine* 50:161–97, 1971.
180. Beeson PB, Brannon ES, Warren JV. Observations on the sites of removal of bacteria from the blood in patients with bacterial endocarditis. *J Exp Med* 81:9–23, 1945.
181. Rimola A et al. Reticuloendothelial system phagocytic activity in cirrhosis and its relation to bacterial infections and prognosis. *Hepatology* 4:53–58, 1984.
182. Conn HO. Spontaneous peritonitis and bacteremia in Laennec's cirrhosis caused by enteric organisms. A relatively common but rarely recognized syndrome. *Ann Intern Med* 50:568–80, 1964.
183. Tisdale WA. Spontaneous colon bacillus bacteremia in Laennec's cirrhosis. *Gastroenterology* 40:141–48, 1961.
184. Correia JP, Conn HO. Spontaneous bacterial peritonitis in cirrhosis: endemic or epidemic? *Med Clin North Am* 59:963–81, 1975.
185. Curry N, McCallum RW, Guth PH. Spontaneous peritonitis in cirrhotic ascites. A decade of experience. *Am J Dig Dis* 19:685–92, 1974.
186. Hoefs JC et al. Spontaneous bacterial peritonitis. *Hepatology* 2:399–407, 1982.
187. Kerr DNS, Pearson DT, Read AE. Infection of ascitic fluid in patients with hepatic cirrhosis. *Gut* 4:394–98, 1963.
188. Kline MM, McCallum RW, Guth PH. The clinical value of ascitic fluid culture and leukocyte count studies in alcoholic cirrhosis. *Gastroenterology* 70:408–12, 1976.
189. Pinzello G et al. Spontaneous bacterial peritonitis: a prospective investigation in predominantly nonalcoholic cirrhotic patients. *Hepatology* 3:545–49, 1983.
190. Runyon BA, Hoefs JC. Ascitic fluid analysis in the differentiation of spontaneous bacterial peritonitis from gastrointestinal tract perforation into ascitic fluid. *Hepatology* 4:447–50, 1984.
191. Weinstein MP et al. Spontaneous bacterial peritonitis. A review of 28 cases with emphasis on improved survival and factors influencing prognosis. *Am J Med* 64:592–98, 1978.
192. Luce E et al. Improvement in the bacteriologic diagnosis of peritonitis with the use of blood culture media. *Trans Am Soc Artif Intern Organs* 28:259–61, 1982.
193. Hoefs JC. Serum protein concentration and portal pressure determine the ascitic fluid protein concentration in patients with chronic liver disease. *J Lab Clin Med* 102:260–73, 1983.
194. Pare P, Talbot J, Hoefs JC. Serum-ascites albumin concentration gradient: a physiologic approach to the differential diagnosis of ascites. *Gastroenterology* 85:240–44, 1983.
195. Sheckman P, Onderdonk AB, Bartlett JG. Anaerobes in spontaneous peritonitis. *Lancet* 2:1225, 1977.
196. Targan SR, Chow AW, Guze LB. Role of anaerobic bacteria in spontaneous peritonitis of cirrhosis. Report of two cases and review of the literature. *Am J Med* 62:397–403, 1977.
197. Runyon BA, Hoefs JC. Ascitic fluid chemical analysis before, during and after spontaneous bacterial peritonitis. *Hepatology* 5:257–59, 1985.
198. Brook I et al. Measurement of lactate in ascitic fluid. *Dig Dis Sci* 26:1089–94, 1981.
199. Garcia-Tsao G, Conn HO, Lerner E. The diagnosis of bacterial peritonitis: comparison of pH, lactate

concentration and leukocyte count. *Hepatology* 5(1):91–96, 1985.

200. Gitlin N, Stauffer JC, Silvestri RC. The pH of ascitic fluid in the diagnosis of spontaneous bacterial peritonitis in alcoholic cirrhosis. *Hepatology* 2:408–11, 1982.

201. Kao HW, Reynolds TB. Letter to the editor. *Hepatology* 3:275–76, 1983.

202. Yang CY et al. White count, pH and lactate in ascites in the diagnosis of spontaneous bacterial peritonitis. *Hepatology* 5:85–90, 1985.

203. Cabrera J et al. Aminoglycoside nephrotoxicity in cirrhosis: value of urinary B₂ microglobulin to discriminate functional renal failure from acute tubular damage. *Gastroenterology* 82:97–105, 1982.

204. Ratnoff OD, Patek AJ. The natural history of Lannec's cirrhosis of the liver. *Medicine* 21:207–68, 1942.

205. Lerner PI, Weinstein L. Infective endocarditis in the antibiotic era. *N Engl J Med* 274:259–93, 1966.

206. Pearce ML, Guze LB. Some factors affecting prognosis in bacterial endocarditis. *Ann Int Med* 55:270–82, 1961.

207. Uwaydah MM, Weinberg AN. Bacterial endocarditis—a changing pattern. *N Engl J Med* 273:1231–35, 1965.

208. Buchbinder NA, Roberts WC. Alcoholism. An important but underemphasized factor predisposing to infective endocarditis. *Arch Int Med* 132:689–92, 1973.

209. Snyder N et al. Increased concurrence of cirrhosis and bacterial endocarditis. *Gastroenterology* 73:1107–13, 1977.

210. Carpenter RR, Petersdorf RG. The clinical spectrum of bacterial meningitis. *Am J Med* 33:262–75, 1962.

211. Olsson RA, Kirby JC, Romansky MJ. Pneumococcal meningitis in the adult. Clinical, therapeutic and prognostic aspects in forty-three patients. *Ann Int Med* 55:545–49, 1961.

212. Swartz MN, Dodge PR. Bacterial meningitis—a review of selected aspects. *N Engl J Med* 272:725–31, 779–87, 842–48, 898–902, 954–60, 1003–10, 1965.

213. Richter RW, Brust JCM. Pneumococcal meningitis at Harlem Hospital. *NY State J Med* 71:2747–54, 1971.

214. Weiss W et al. Prognostic factors in pneumococcal meningitis. *Arch Int Med* 120:517–24, 1967.

215. Niemen RE, Lorber B. Listerosis in adults: a changing pattern. Report of eight cases and review of the literature, 1968–1978. *Rev Infect Dis* 2:207–27, 1980.

216. Cherubin CE et al. Listeria and gram-negative bacillary meningitis in New York City, 1972–1979. Frequent causes of meningitis in adults. *Am J Med* 71:199–209, 1981.

217. Skogberg K et al. Beta-haemolytic Group A, B, C, and G streptococcal septicaemia: a clinical study. *Scand J Infect Dis* 20:119–25, 1988.

218. Esposito AL. Community-acquired bacteremic Pneumococcal pneumonia-effect of age on manifestations and outcome. *Arch Intern Med* 144:945–48, 1984.

219. Finkelstein MS et al. Pneumococcal bacteremia in adults: age dependent differences in presentation and in outcome. *J Am Geriatr Soc* 31:19–27, 1988.

220. Perlino CA, Rimland D. Alcoholism, leukopenia and pneumococcal sepsis. *Am Rev Respir Dis* 132:757–60, 1985.

221. Cherubin CE et al. Septicemia with non-typhoid Salmonella. *Medicine* 53:365–76, 1974.

222. Blake PA et al. Disease caused by a marine *Vibrio*. Clinical characteristics and epidemiology. *N Engl J Med* 300:1–5, 1979.

223. Evans FC. Pancreatic abscess. *Am J Surg* 117:537–40, 1969.

224. Kodesch R, Dupont HL. Infectious complications of acute pancreatitis. *Surg Gynecol Obstet* 136:763–68, 1973.

225. Camer SJ et al. Pancreatic abscess. A critical analysis of 113 cases. *Am J Surg* 129:426–31, 1975.

226. Holden JL, Berne TV, Rosoff L Sr. Pancreatic abscess following acute pancreatitis. *Arch Surg* 111:858–61, 1976.

227. Owens BJ, Hamit HF. Pancreatic abscess and pseudocyst. *Arch Surg* 112:42–45, 1977.

228. Warshaw AL. Pancreatic abscess. *N Engl J Med* 287:1234–36, 1972.

229. Pederson AHB et al. Diphtheria on Skid Road, Seattle, Wash. 1972–1975. *Public Health Rep* 92:336–42, 1977.

230. Davis WA II, Kane JG, Garagusi VF. Human *Aeromonas* infections: a review of the literature and a case report of endocarditis. *Medicine* 57:267–77, 1978.

231. Kedes LH, Siemienski J, Braude AI. The syndrome of the alcoholic rose gardener. Sporotrichosis of the radial tendon sheath. *Ann Int Med* 61:1139–41, 1964.

232. Crout JE, Brewer NS, Tompkins RB. Sporotrichosis arthritis. Clinical features in seven patients. *Ann Int Med* 86:294–97, 1977.

233. Lynch PJ, Voorhees JJ, Harrell ER. Systemic sporotrichosis. *Ann Int Med* 73:23–30, 1970.

234. Legrand JC et al. *Gardnerella vaginalis* bacteremia

from pulmonary abscess in a male alcohol abuser. *J Clin Microbiol* 27:1132–34, 1989.

235. Han LK, Lum SK. *Clostridium perfringens* septicaemia associated with liver cirrhosis. *Med J Aust* 2:431–32, 1979.

236. Bardwell A et al. Disseminated macronodular cutaneous candidiasis in chronic alcoholism. *Arch Int Med* 146:385–86, 1986.

237. Plant ML et al. The sex industry, alcohol and illicit drugs: implication for the spread of HIV infection. *Br J Addict* 84:53–59, 1989.

238. Layon J et al. Altered T-lymphocyte subrets in hospitalized intravenous drug abusers. *Arch Intern Med* 144:1376–80, 1984.

239. Small CB et al. Community-acquired opportunistic infections and defective cellular immunity in heterosexual drug abusers and homosexual men. *Am J Med* 74:433–41, 1983.

240. Pettigrew NM et al. Evidence for a role of hepatitis virus B in chronic liver disease. *Lancet* 2:724–25, 1972.

241. Basile A et al. Hepatitis B virus infection in alcoholic cirrhosis. *Br Med J* 282:1705, 1981.

242. Chalmers DM, Bullen AW, Levi AJ. Evidence for previous hepatitis B virus infection in alcohol cirrhosis. *Br Med J* 282:819, 1981.

243. Hislop WS et al. Serological markers of hepatitis B in patients with alcoholic liver disease: a multicentre survey. *J Clin Pathol* 34:1017–19, 1981.

244. Mills PR et al. Hepatitis B antibody in alcoholic cirrhosis. *J Clin Pathol* 32:778–82, 1979.

245. Orholm M et al. Prevalence of hepatitis B virus infection among alcoholic patients with liver disease. *J Clin Pathol* 34:1378–80, 1981.

246. Saunders JB et al. Importance of markers of hepatitis B virus in alcoholic liver disease. *Br Med J* 286:1851–54, 1983.

247. Tabor E et al. Effect of ethanol during hepatitis B virus infection in chimpanzees. *J Med Virol* 2:295–303, 1978.

248. McMicken DB. Alcohol-related disease. In P Rosen (ed.), *Emergency Medicine: Concepts and Clinical Practice* (vol. 2). St. Louis: C. V. Mosby, 1988. Pp. 2065–86.

249. McMicken DB. Alcohol withdrawal syndromes. *Emerg Med Clin North Am* 8:805–19, 1990.

250. Victor M, Adams RD. The effect of alcohol on the nervous system. *Res Publ Assoc Nerv Ment Dis* 32:526, 1953.

251. Victor ML. Treatment of alcoholic intoxication and the withdrawal syndrome: a critical analysis of the use of drugs and other forms of therapy. *Psychosomatics* 28:636, 1966.

19

Infection in the Traveler and Immigrant

DAVID DOEZEMA
MARK HAUSWALD

Diseases that affect travelers and immigrants overlap widely. Because the number of diseases affecting them is enormous, only major syndromes can be covered in this chapter. These diseases are summarized in Table 19-1. Diseases not specifically discussed in this chapter can be suspected if a specific symptom, sign, or laboratory abnormality is noted, and possible causes identified using the tables.

Infection in the Traveler

Since the outbreaks of plague in the Middle Ages, there has been concern about travelers returning with illnesses not present in their home communities [1]. Today illness of travel is usually associated with diseases of developing countries, but earlier European colonization wreaked devastation on indigenous peoples with diseases such as measles, tuberculosis, and syphilis. The number of travelers has increased dramatically in the twentieth century. Roughly 8 million people travel yearly from the United States to developing countries [2, 3]. Air travel now makes it as likely that a traveler will develop symptoms following the return home as during travel, especially with diseases with longer incubation periods. Table 19-1 lists the relative risks of most diseases for travelers.

This section gives the physician an approach for dealing with infections in travelers, immunization and prophylaxis information, and a brief description of important diseases one may encounter in travel to developing countries.

This section also discusses the importance of specific symptoms and signs to the diagnosis of various diseases. A general knowledge of the geographic prevalence of an illness is necessary to trigger the clinician's suspicion, but specific resources may need to be consulted to confirm the diagnosis. Maps showing geographic areas of risk for the major diseases are presented in this chapter.

Risk Factors

The risk of acquiring an illness depends on the geographical area to be visited, the length of stay, and whether the traveler will stay in an urban or rural area. An example of the difference in geographical risk is that fewer Americans visit sub-Saharan Africa than Asia or South America, but 80% of the cases of *Plasmodium falciparum* reported to the Centers for Disease Control (CDC) are from sub-Saharan Africa [4, 5]. The risk of communicable disease to the traveler in North America, northern Europe, and Australia is low; however, even in southern Europe there is an increased risk of GI

Table 19-1. Summary of infectious diseases of travelers and immigrants

Disease	Geographic distribution	History	Physical exam	Laboratory data	Treatment
African trypanosomiasis	Central Africa	Tsetse fly bite; personality change	Painful chancre, intermittent fever, lymphadenopathy, septicemia, CNS dysfunction, myocarditis	Chancre aspirate, lymph node aspirate, blood smears, lumbar puncture	Suramin, pentamidine, melarsoprol; contact CDC
American trypanosomiasis (Chagas' disease)	South America	Reduviid bug bite; common in children; poorly thatched huts	Acute: Erythematous nodule, fever, lymphadenopathy, hepatosplenomegaly, myocarditis, meningitis Chronic: Myocardial dysfunction, megacolon, megaesophagus	Blood smear, serology	Adults: nifurtimox 8–10 mg/kg/d Children: nifurtimox 12.5–20 mg/kg/d Four divided doses for 90–120 D Contact CDC (acute treatment only) Benzonidazole (not available in United States)
Cysticercosis	Central/South America, Africa, India, China	Hogs in contact with human feces; ingestion of undercooked pork	Seizures, meningitis, other CNS findings	Cystic lesions on brain imaging, serology	Praziquantel 50 mg/kg, three divided doses for 14 days; or albendazole plus corticosteroids
Dengue	Tropics of America, Africa, Asia	Mosquito exposure; severe back pain; eye pain	Nausea, vomiting, conjunctival suffusion, macular rash	Viral culture, serology (contact CDC)	Supportive
Hansen's disease (leprosy)	Southeast Asia, sub-Saharan Africa, India, episodic in southwestern United States	Sensation decrease	Hypopigmented, erythematous macules, sharply demarcated macules (tuberculoid); digit loss, nodules in plaques, cool body parts (lepromatous)	Lesion biopsy	Dapsone 50–100 mg/d/PO plus rifampin 300 mg/mo/PO plus clofazimine 50 mg/d/PO; all for 2-year minimum
Leishmaniasis	India, Europe, Asia Africa, South and Central America	Exposure to rodents or dogs, sandfly bite; more com-	Erythematous macule, ulcers, or intermittent fever,	Skin biopsy of ulcer, pancytopenia, bone marrow aspi-	Sodium stibogluconate 20 mg/kg/d- max. 850/mg/d;

	Distribution	Epidemiology/Exposure	Clinical Features	Diagnosis	Treatment
(continued)		mon in children; 3–6 mo. incubation	weight loss, hepatosplenomegaly, petechiae, edema	ration and culture, spleen aspirate, serology	amphotericin or ketoconazole
Malaria	See map Fig. 19-1	Mosquito exposure, paroxysmal fever, inadequate prophylaxis, immigrant with lost immunity	Nonspecific Acute: Possible hepatosplenomegaly Chronic: hepatosplenomegaly, weight loss	Parasites on blood smear serology, anemia/neutropenia	See Table 19-7
Plague	Asia, Africa, South America, sporadic in southwestern United States	Rodent exposure, flea bite	Buboes, pneumonia, septicemia	Blood culture	Streptomycin 30 mg/kg/d IM in two divided doses for 10 d; or tetracycline 2–4 g/d/PO in four divided doses for 10 d; or chloramphenicol IV 2.5 mg/kg loading dose—60 mg/kg/d in four divided doses for 10 d (or hypotension, meningitis); tetracycline 500 mg qid PO (for postexposure prophylaxis)
Schistosomiasis	Caribbean, South America, Africa, Middle East	Acute: Fresh-water exposure, "swimmers itch," serum sickness-like syndrome Chronic: Urinary symptoms	Acute: Nonspecific Chronic: Hematemesis, melena, hepatosplenomegaly, pulmonary hypertension, seizures	Eosinophilia, ova in stool or urine; serology; rectal biopsy	Praziquantel 40–60 mg/kg divided in 2–3 doses for 1 day
Yellow Fever	15° north or south of equator (See Fig. 19-4)	Lack of immunization, mosquito exposure, nonspecific	Nausea, vomiting, biphasic fever; conjunctival infection, hemorrhage, jaundice	Viral culture, serology	Supportive; dialysis

Table 19-2. Considerations for travelers and immigrants: relative risks in developing countries

High: More than 1 case in 10 travelers	Moderate: More than 1 case in 200 travelers but less than 1 case in 10 travelers	Low: More than 1 case in 1,000 travelers but less than 1 case in 200 travelers	Very low: Less than 1 case in 1,000 travelers
Diarrhea	Dengue	Acute hemorrhagic conjunctivitis	Actinomycosis
Upper respiratory infection	Enteroviral infection	Amebiasis	AIDS
	Food poisoning	Ascariasis	Angiostrongyliasis
	Gastroenteritis	Childhood viral infections	Anisakiasis
	Giardiasis	Chickenpox	Anthrax
	Hepatitis A	Measles	Blastomycosis
	Malaria without prophylaxis	Mumps	Boutonneuse fever
	Salmonellosis	Poliomyelitis	Chagas' disease
	Sexually transmitted diseases	Enterobiasis	Chikungunya
	Chlamydial infection	Hepatitis B	Clonorchiasis
	Gonorrhea	Hepatitis: non-A, non-B (epidemic)	Coccidioidomycosis
	Herpes simplex	Leptospirosis	Congo-Crimean hemorrhagic fever
	Nonspecific urethritis	Scabies	Cryptosporidiosis
	Shigellosis	Sexually transmitted diseases	Diphtheria
		Chancroid	Ebola-Marburg hemorrhagic fever
		Syphilis	Echinococcosis
		Strongyloidiasis	Filariasis
		Trichuriasis	Gnathostomiasis
		Tropical sprue	Histoplasmosis
		Tuberculosis	Hookworm
		Typhoid fever	Legionellosis
			Lymphogranuloma venereum
			Malaria with prophylaxis
			Melioidosis
			Paragonimiasis
			Pertussis
			Pinta
			Plague
			Psittacosis
			Q fever
			Rabies
			Relapsing fever
			Schistosomiasis
			Toxocariasis
			Trachoma
			Trichinosis
			Trypanosomiasis
			Typhus
			Yaws
			Yellow fever

Source: Warren KS, Mahmoud AAF. *Tropical and Geographical Medicine* (2nd ed.). New York: McGraw-Hill, 1990. Used with permission.

infection [3]. Business travelers and those staying in urban or resort areas have lower risks of infection because their stay is shorter, and they often are not exposed to insects, contaminated water, or contaminated vegetable produce.

Sources of Information

It is clear that knowledge of disease prevention makes a difference. For example, missionaries with a medical background experience fewer problems than others [3]. A number of excellent sources of information are available to the traveler and the physician. The CDC publishes *Health Information for International Travel*, which is available from the Superintendent of Documents (U.S. Government Printing Office, Washington DC 20402); and the *Morbidity and Mortality Weekly Report* (MMWR), which gives current disease trends. The CDC also has a 24-hour telephone number (404-332-4559) that provides information for international travelers on vaccine requirements and recommendations by geographic area. The World Health Organization (WHO) publishes *Vaccination Certificate Requirement for International Travelers* yearly and *World Health Statistics Quarterly* (available from WHO, 49 Sheridan Ave., Albany, NY 12210).

Why Travelers Get Ill

In spite of effective methods of prevention many travelers become ill. Twenty to 50% of travelers get diarrhea, and up to 50% get some kind of minor illness [2, 3]. Reasons for becoming sick are numerous. Many travelers do not follow advice or take prophylaxis; often the medical advice they receive is inadequate [3]. Many illnesses are not entirely preventable. Vaccines are not completely effective, e.g., cholera vaccine is only 50% effective. Diseases such as malaria have developed widespread resistance to chemotherapeutic agents, and insect vectors are difficult to control. The traveler from a developed country may be more susceptible to certain diseases such as malaria and amebiasis because of insufficient immunity and lack of familiarity with geography, water contamination, or the presence of insect vectors. Animal vectors may not be controlled; for example, dogs are the main reservoir for rabies in developing countries. Unreliable report-

ing methods in some countries limit the accuracy of many recommendations. For these reasons the traveler may return with a disease uncommonly seen by physicians in the United States. Since many patients are otherwise healthy and do not have a personal physician, emergency physicians see a substantial number of travel-related illnesses.

Immunization, Prophylaxis, and Precautions

A few simple precautions and immunizations can make all the difference for the traveler. Polio, measles, mumps, rubella, pertussis, diphtheria, and tetanus are all more common in the developing world; it is imperative that the traveler be current with all routine immunizations. In addition a number of diseases that are risk specific to a given area and situation can be prevented by immunization: rabies, hepatitis A, hepatitis B, typhoid fever, meningococcus, and yellow fever. Other vaccines may be required by a country, so it is important to consult the most recent requirements for a given country (Table 19-3). Travelers should also be aware that there may be discrepancies between officially published immunization requirements and those stated by foreign embassies. Actual practices may also vary over time at ports of entry with different personnel [6].

The CDC's *Health Information for International Travel* has a separate section on geographical distribution of potential health hazards. In addition to immunization, chemoprophylaxis is effective for a number of diseases. Even though resistance to some medications is a worldwide problem, chemoprophylaxis can still prevent most malarial illness. For some people, prophylaxis for traveler's diarrhea may outweigh the risk of side effects. Care with food and water can decrease the risk of diarrheal illness, hepatitis, and typhoid, as well as many parasitic diseases.

Travel tends to loosen the restrictions society places on sexual behavior, and today's tourists are playing a role in spreading sexually transmitted diseases (STDs) formerly played by the military [7]. The physician should emphasize the prevention of STDs, including AIDS and hepatitis B, by advising patients to avoid unsafe sexual contact and to use

Table 19-3. Recommended immunizations for international travel

Vaccine	Type	Route and schedule	Indications	Contraindications	Side effects
Tetanus-diphtheria	Absorbed toxoids	Primary: 2 doses (0.5 ml) IM, 4 weeks apart; third dose 6 to 12 months later. Booster: every 10 years	All adults	First trimester of pregnancy; hypersensitivity or neurologic reaction to previous doses; severe local reaction	Local reactions; occasional fever, systemic symptoms; Arthus-like reactions in persons with multiple previous boosters; rare systemic allergy
Inactivated-bacteria Vaccines					
Cholera	Phenol-killed *Vibrio cholerae* (4×10^9/ml)	Primary: 0.5 ml IM or subcutaneously, or 0.2 ml ID; give 2 doses 1 week to 1 month apart at least 6 days before travel. Booster: 0.5 ml IM or subcutaneously or 0.2 ml ID every 6 months	As required by individual countries (consult CDC); approximately 50% effective	Safety in pregnancy unknown; previous severe local or systemic reaction	Local reaction of pain, erythema, and induration lasting 1 to 2 days; occasional fever, malaise
Haemophilus influenzae type B	N. meningitidis protein conjugate (PRP-OMP)	2–11 mo, 2 doses 2 mo apart 12–14 mo, 1 dose and booster at 15 mo (>2 mo after last dose) >15 mo 1 dose	Children 2 mo to 5 years	None	Fever, local reaction of erythema, swelling, induration
	Diphtheria CRM_{197} protein conjugate (HbOC)	Primary: 3 doses at 2, 4, 6 mo or 2 doses 7–11 mo or 1 dose >12 mo. Booster: after 15 mo if primary series given <12	Children 2 mo to 5 years	None	Fever, local reaction of redness, swelling or warmth
Pneumococcal polysaccharide	23 serotypes	Primary: 1 dose (0.5 ml) subcutaneously or IM	Adults at increased risk of pneumococcal disease	Safety in pregnancy unknown; previous pneumococcal vac-	Approximately 50% of patients have erythema and pain

	Type	Schedule	Indications	Contraindications	Reactions
		Booster: none	and its complications; healthy adults 65 or older	cination	at injection site; fewer than 1% of patients have systemic reaction; Arthus-like reaction with booster doses
Meningococcal polysaccharide	Tetravalent (A, C, Y, W 135)	Primary: 1 dose (0.5 ml) subcutaneously. Booster: unknown	Travelers to areas with epidemic meningococcal disease; required for pilgrims to Mecca, Saudi Arabia	Safety in pregnancy unknown	Infrequent, mild local reactions
Typhoid	Acetone and heat-killed *Salmonella typhi* (10/ml)	Primary: 2 doses (0.5 ml) subcutaneously, given 4 or more weeks apart. Booster: 0.5 ml subcutaneously or 0.1 ml ID every 3 years	Risk for exposure to typhoid fever in many countries of Africa, Asia, Central and South America	Previous severe local or systemic reaction	Local reaction of pain, swelling and induration lasting 1 to 2 days; occasional systemic reaction
	Oral attenuated Ty21a strain *Salmonella typhi*	4 capsules (one every other day) 2 weeks before departure	Risk for exposure to typhoid fever in many countries of Africa, Asia, Central and South America	Antimalarials, antibiotics; safety in immunocompromised patients not known	None known, but new vaccine

Attenuated, Live-virus Vaccines

	Type	Schedule	Indications	Contraindications	Reactions
Measles	Attenuated live viral	Primary: 1 dose subcutaneously, age 12–15 months. Booster: age 4–6 years	Boost previously live-immunized adults born after 1956 without illness; persons given killed measles vaccine or immunized 1963–1967 should receive 2 doses a month apart	Pregnancy; immunocompromised host; history of anaphylaxis to eggs or neomycin	5% to 15% have temperature ≥ 39.4°C 5 to 21 days after vaccination; 5% have transient rash; 4–55% of persons previously immunized with killed vaccine (1963–

Table 19-3. (*continued*)

Vaccine	Type	Route and schedule	Indications	Contraindications	Side effects
					1967) have local reaction
Mumps	Attenuated live viral	Primary: 1 dose subcutaneously Booster: none	Susceptible adults born after 1957, particularly men	Pregnancy; immunocompromised host; history of anaphylaxis to eggs or neomycin	Mild allergic reactions uncommon; rare parotitis
Oral polio vaccine (OPV)	Attenuated live viral, trivalent	1 oral dose	Boost previously immunized persons; complete the series in partially immunized adults; alternative when 2 doses of inactivated polio vaccine cannot be given before travel; not used for primary immunization in persons older than 18 years	Immunocompromised host or immunocompromised contacts of recipients	Rare paralysis (see text)
Rubella	Attenuated live viral	Primary: 1 dose subcutaneously Booster: none	Adults, particularly women of childbearing age, without documented illness or live vaccine on or after first birthday	Pregnancy; immunocompromised host; history of anaphylaxis to neomycin	Up to 40% have joint pains, transient arthralgias beginning 3–25 days after vaccination, persisting 1–11 days; <2% have frank arthritis
Yellow fever	Attenuated live viral	Primary: 1 dose (0.5 ml) subcutaneously 10 days to 10 years before travel Booster: every 10 years	As required by individual countries (see text)	Avoid in pregnant women, unless high-risk travel; immunocompromised host; hypersensitivity to eggs	2%–5% have mild headache, myalgia, fever 5–10 days after vaccination; rare immediate hypersensitivity

Inactivated-virus Vaccines

Vaccine	Composition	Dosage	Indications	Precautions	Side effects
Hepatitis B	Inactivated viral product, purified hepatitis B surface antigen from human plasma	Primary: 2 doses (20 µg/dose) 1 month apart; third dose 5 months after second; IM in deltoid. Booster: not routinely recommended	Health care workers; health care workers in contact with blood; persons residing for >6 months in areas of high endemicity for hepatitis B surface antigen; consider hepatitis B immune globulin + vaccine for high-risk incident (see text); others at risk	Safety to fetus unknown; pregnancy not a contraindication in high-risk persons	Soreness at injection site; rare systemic illness
Hepatitis B	Recombinant-derived hepatitis B surface antigen	Primary: 2 doses (10 µg/dose) 1 month apart; third dose 5 months after second; IM in deltoid. Booster: not routinely recommended	Health care workers; health care workers in contact with blood; persons residing for >6 months in areas of high endemicity for hepatitis B surface antigen; consider hepatitis B immune globulin + vaccine for high-risk incident (see text); others at risk	Safety to fetus unknown; pregnancy not a contraindication in high-risk persons	10%–20% mild local reaction; occasional systemic symptoms of fever, headache, fatigue, and nausea
Inactivated polio vaccine (eIPV)	Killed polio virus, trivalent; enhanced potency	Primary: 2 doses (0.5 ml) subcutaneously at a 4- to 8-week interval; third dose 6 to 12 months after second	Preferred for persons older than 17 years; complete series in partially immunized with OPV or eIPV; give one dose if completely immunized and going to high-risk area	Safety in pregnancy unknown; anaphylactic reactions to streptomycin or neomycin	No serious side effects

Table 19-3. (*continued*)

Vaccine	Type	Route and schedule	Indications	Contraindications	Side effects
Influenza	Inactivated whole and split virus	Annual vaccination with current vaccine	Adults with high-risk conditions (see text); healthy persons more than 65 years old; medical-care personnel	First trimester of pregnancy is relative contraindication; anaphylaxis to eggs	Less than one-third have mild local reactions; occasional systemic reaction of malaise, myalgia, beginning 6–12 hours after vaccination and lasting 1–2 days; rare allergic reaction
Japanese B encephalitis (not available in United States; should seek vaccine abroad; manufactured by Biken, Osaka, Japan)	Inactivated viral	Primary: 3 doses subcutaneously at weekly intervals	Travelers to areas of risk (Southeast Asia, China, India, Japan, Korea, E. USSR) with rural exposure or prolonged residence	Pregnancy; allergy to mice or rodents; immunocompromised host	Local mild reactions lasting 1–3 days
Rabies (human diploid cell vaccine)	Inactivated viral	Preexposure: 1 ml IM in deltoid on days 0, 7, and 28 or 0.1 ml ID on days 0, 7, and 21 to 28 Booster: every 2 years or when antibody titer falls below acceptable level [6, 7]	Travel to areas for >1 month where rabies is a constant threat and for people who explore caves	Allergy to previous doses; may be given in pregnancy if indicated; concurrent chloroquine; ID route should be completed 30 days or more before travel; ID route should not be used with concurrent chloroquine administration	Approximately 25% have local reactions; approximately 20% have mild systemic reactions of headache, nausea, aches, dizziness; rare neurologic illness; occasional immune reactions with booster doses occurring 2–21 days after vaccination
Passive Prophylaxis Immune globulin	Fractionated immunoglobulins (1 ly IgG)	Travel for less than 3 months: 0.02 ml/kg; travel for 4–6 months: 0.06 ml/kg	For prevention of hepatitis A, especially in young children		Local discomfort; rare systemic allergy

Notes:

1. Immunization of children <2 years:

   If possible complete schedule for active immunization of normal infants and children; see Table for *H. influenzae* immunization schedule.

   DTP: Children traveling to endemic area should have received three doses. Two doses may be partially protective against diphtheria and tetanus. Children <7 years who have had fewer than three doses at time of travel to area of risk should complete remaining doses at 4-week intervals.

   Measles: MMR should be given to all children 15 months and older. Age at vaccination should be lowered for children traveling to areas endemic for measles. A second dose should be given at 4–6 years of age.

   Age 12–14 months: MMR prior to departure without need for revaccination until school entry

   Age 6–11 months: 1 dose measles monovalent vaccine with revaccination with two doses MMR at later ages; MMR can be given if measles vaccine unavailable.

   Age <6 months: Protected by maternal antibodies

   Mumps and rubella: Risk of serious illness small, so no reason to give for age <12 months. Parents should be immune in case infant develops illness.

   Polio: Children should receive at least three doses of OPV at 6- to 8-week intervals. Child who has had three doses with >6 weeks since third dose should receive fourth dose. If travel occurs before age 6 weeks, a dose of OPV should be given, but three-dose primary series should be given as before at 4-week intervals after the first dose. If series incomplete at time of travel, complete three-dose series at 4-week intervals. Booster at 4–6 years of age. At least one dose of OPV should be given before travel.

2. Simultaneous and nonsimultaneous administration:

   —In general simultaneous administration of most live and inactivated vaccines has not resulted in impaired antibody response or increased rate of adverse reactions, but vaccines such as cholera, typhoid, and plague if given simultaneously can have accentuated systemic and local reactions.

   —Yellow fever and cholera vaccine should not be given within 3 weeks of each other due to lowered antibody response with simultaneous administration.

   —Live virus vaccines not given on the same day should be given at least 30 days apart.

3. Immune globulin (IG):

   —Live-virus vaccines should not be given for at least 6 weeks and preferably 3 months after IG administration.

   —If live-virus vaccine has been administered, if possible wait at least 14 days before giving IG. If IG must be given earlier than 14 days, the vaccine should be repeated.

4. Patients with altered immunocompetence (leukemia, lymphoma) should not be given live-virus vaccines. Even though live virus vaccines can have increased adverse reactions in HIV-infected individuals and likelihood of successful immune response is reduced, risk-benefit balance usually favors vaccine administration. Inactivated vaccines do not carry increased adverse reactions.

5. Minor febrile illnesses should not defer vaccine administration but moderate to severe febrile illness should postpone vaccination because of possible confusion of superimposed side effects with symptoms of illness.

6. Pregnancy:

   —Because of theoretical risk to fetus, live attenuated virus vaccines should not be given in first trimester of pregnancy, although OPV and yellow fever vaccines can be given if risk of exposure is great.

   —No evidence of congenital rubella syndrome has been seen in infants born to mothers who have received rubella vaccine during pregnancy.

Table 19-4. Summary of health precautions
and prohibitions for travelers

Routine immunizations up to date
Destination-specific immunizations, e.g., yellow fever
Chemoprophylaxis for malaria
Knowledge of risks from food and drink
Water treatment
Insect repellent and mosquito netting
Medical care and emergency sources
Safe bathing and swimming areas
Knowledge of rehydration of infants with diarrhea
Defensive driving and avoidance of nighttime driving
Knowledge of dealing with extremes of temperature
 and altitude
Safe sex

condoms. It is imperative that the physician obtain a sexual history from the traveler.

The risk of the insect-borne diseases—malaria, yellow fever, leishmaniasis, dengue, trypanosomiasis, and others—can be decreased by reducing the chance of being bitten. The most effective insect repellents contain N,N-disthyl-m-toluamide (DEET). A field trial has found a new 35% long-acting cream preparation of DEET to give 99% protection for 8 hours [8]. Mosquito netting, protective clothing, and avoiding exposure during times of insect feeding, usually dusk and dawn, are important additional measures that increase protection. Table 19-4 is a summary of precautions for the traveler.

Initial Approach to the Patient

Many patients volunteer that they have traveled, but it is important that the physician consider the possibility of travel with the presentation of certain symptoms and signs, such as persistent or recurrent fever without localization, diarrhea, or right upper quadrant pain. Travelers and nontravelers present to physicians with similar symptoms, but the act of having traveled can dramatically alter the possibilities. For example, jaundice and right upper quadrant pain might not make a U.S. physician think of amebic liver abscess, but a Mexican physician certainly would consider it. The amount of time that elapsed since return from travel is crucial. Incubation periods are listed in Table 19-5.

In evaluating an ill traveler, the physician must consider exotic diseases, with domestic diseases kept in mind. The history *must* include four areas of information:

1. Travel: route, duration, type
2. Individual risk factors: medical, behavioral
3. Protection: immunizations, chemoprophylaxis, behavior
4. Epidemiology: Are others ill?

As in all patients vital signs must be obtained and the patient assessed for toxicity. General measures to restore vital signs to appropriate levels must be taken at the outset. In performing a complete physical examination, the physician must pay specific attention to the CNS, the respiratory, cardiac, GI, and lymphatic systems, and the skin. Specific areas of attention include the following:

- CNS: delirium, coma, stiff neck, seizures
- Respiratory system: shortness of breath, cough
- Cardiac system: heart size, conduction abnormalities
- GI system: Hepatosplenomegaly, diarrhea, jaundice, right upper quadrant pain
- Lymphatic system: localized or generalized adenopathy, buboes
- Skin: rash, hemorrhage, jaundice, insect bites, other skin breaks

Some general laboratory tests may be appropriate. A complete blood count may reveal eosinophilia or parasites. A dipstick urine examination is an easy screening test. Other laboratory tests of value include the following:

- For febrile illness:
  Thin and thick blood smear for blood-borne parasites such as plasmodia, trypanosomes, and filaria
  Blood cultures
  Liver and renal function tests
- For cases of diarrhea:
  Stool for leukocytes, culture, ova, and parasites
- Serology:
  Spin and save

Table 19-5. Usual incubation periods of selected diseases

Short (≤1 week)	Intermediate (1–4 weeks)	Long (1–6 months)	Very long (2 months to years)
Anthrax	Amebiasis	Ascariasis	AIDS
Boutonneuse fever	Brucellosis	Blastomycosis	Cysticercosis
Chancroid	Chagas' disease	Hepatitis B	Echinococcosis
Chikungunya	Giardiasis	Hepatitis delta	Filariasis
Chlamydial infections	Hemorrhagic fever with renal syndrome	Hepatitis, non-A and non-B (posttransfusion)	Fluke infections
Congo-Crimean hemorrhagic fever	Hepatitis A	Leishmaniasis, cutaneous	Leishmaniasis, visceral
Dengue	Hepatitis, non-A and non-B (epidemic)	Loiasis	Leprosy
Diarrhea, acute	Katayama fever	Malaria	Schistosomiasis
Ebola-Marburg hemorrhagic fever	Lassa fever	Melioidosis	Trypanosomiasis, African (Gambian)
Food poisoning	Leptospirosis	Pinta	
Gonorrhea	Lyme disease	Rabies	
Herpes genitalis	Lymphogranuloma venereum	Taeniasis	
Histoplasmosis	Malaria	Trachoma (scarring)	
Legionellosis	Pertussis	Trichuriasis	
Plague	Q fever	Tropical sprue	
Psittacosis	Strongyloidiasis	Yaws	
Relapsing fever	Syphilis		
Salmonellosis	Trypanosomiasis, African (Rhodesian)		
Tetanus	Typhoid fever		
Trypanosomal chancre	Typhus, louse-borne		
Viral gastroenteritis	Typhus, murine		
Yellow fever	Typhus, scrub		

Source: Warren KS, Mahmoud AAF. *Tropical and Geographical Medicine* (2nd ed.). New York: McGraw-Hill, 1990. Used with permission.

Table 19-6 lists signs, symptoms, and laboratory data that may indicate possible causes.

Diseases in Which Fever Predominates

When presented with a febrile traveler, the physician needs to consider a number of "exotic" diseases. Some of these diseases are, of course, not really exotic but are major world health problems. A number of these diseases are discussed in this chapter; others are covered elsewhere in the book. Some, such as typhoid, brucellosis, rickettsial disease, malaria, visceral leishmaniasis, and acute schistosomiasis, commonly present with fever. Others may add another symptom, such as jaundice, that combined with fever and country of travel will suggest the differential diagnosis. In addition, measles, mumps, rubella, tetanus, diphtheria, hepatitis, tuberculosis, meningococcemia, and rabies need to be considered, depending on the history and immunization status.

MALARIA

The diagnosis of malaria should be considered in every febrile patient from a malaria-endemic area. Physicians working in endemic areas often treat acute febrile illnesses as malaria before confirmation, and travelers in endemic areas are advised to

Table 19-6. Signs and symptoms with possible causes

Signs and symptoms	Possible causes	Signs and symptoms	Possible causes
Systemic Signs and Symptoms		Eosinophilia	Filariasis, fascioliasis, schistosomiasis, strongyloidiasis, toxocariasis, trichinosis
Acute fever	Dengue, Ebola-Marburg hemorrhagic fever, malaria, plague, shigellosis, toxoplasmosis, trichinosis, trypanosomiasis (American), yellow fever		
		Lymphadenopathy	Dengue, filariasis, HIV infection, plague, syphilis, toxoplasmosis, trypanosomiasis (African), trypanosomiasis (American)
Chronic fever	Actinomycosis, AIDS, brucellosis, fascioliasis, histoplasmosis, leishmaniasis (visceral), relapsing fever, toxocariasis, trypanosomiasis (African), tuberculosis, typhoid fever		
		Cardiovascular Signs and Symptoms	
		Heart murmur	Chagas' disease, enteroviral carditis, rheumatic heart disease
Recurring fever	Malaria	Myocarditis	Chagas' disease, rheumatic heart disease, trichinosis, trypanosomiasis (Rhodesian)
Exanthem with fever	Chikungunya, childhood exanthem, dengue, enterovirus exanthems, rickettsioses		
		CNS Signs and Symptoms	
		Altered mentation	Acute psychosis, trypanosomiasis (African)
Fever accompanying hemorrhage or shock	Congo-Crimean hemorrhagic fever, dengue hemorrhagic fever, dengue shock syndrome, Ebola-Marburg hemorrhagic fever, hemorrhagic fever with renal syndrome, Lassa fever, leptospirosis, plague, toxoplasmosis, trypanosomiasis (African), trypanosomiasis (American)	Coma	Cerebral malaria, impending sudden unexplained death of adults, Japanese encephalitis, meningococcal meningitis, rabies, tick-borne encephalitis, trypanosomiasis (African)
		Localizing signs of a neurologic lesion	Angiostrongyliasis, botulism, cryptococcosis, cysticercosis, diphtheria, echinococcosis, gnathostomiasis, Lyme disease, meningococcal meningitis, *Naegleria* infection, poliomyelitis, schistosomiasis, tetanus
Life-threatening signs (e.g., coma, septicemia)	Anthrax, Congo-Crimean hemorrhagic fever, dengue hemorrhagic fever, dengue shock syndrome, Ebola-Marburg hemorrhagic fever, hemorrhagic fever with renal syndrome, impending sudden unexplained death of adults, malaria		
		Dermatologic Signs and Symptoms	
		Analgesia, anal pruritus, pruritus	Leprosy, enterobiasis, onchocerciasis, toxocariasis
Anemia	Diphyllobothriasis, histoplasmosis, hookworm infection, iron deficiency, malaria, tropical sprue, visceral leishmaniasis, vitamin B_{12} deficiency	Rash	Chikungunya fever, childhood exanthems, dengue, enteroviral exanthems, rickettsial diseases
		Swelling or erythematous lesions	Gnathostomiasis, loiasis, Lyme disease, pinta

Table 19-6. (*continued*)

Signs and symptoms	Possible causes	Signs and symptoms	Possible causes
Ulcer, eschar, abscess	Anthrax, Buruli ulcer, Chagas' disease, coccidioidomycosis, cutaneous leishmaniasis, lymphogranuloma venereum, syphilis, scrub typhus, trypanosomiasis (African), yaws	*Genitourinary Signs and Symptoms*	
		Cervicitis	Chlamydial infection, moniliasis, trichomoniasis
		Genital lesions	Chancroid, granuloma inguinale, herpes, lymphogranuloma venereum, syphilis
Gastrointestinal Signs and Symptoms		Hematuria	Schistosomiasis (*S. haematobium*)
Abdominal pain	Amebiasis, anisakiasis, fascioliasis, giardiasis, hymenolepiasis, salmonellosis, shigellosis, strongyloidiasis, taeniasis, typhoid fever	Urethritis	Chlamydial and gonococcal infections
		Ophthalmologic Signs and Symptoms	
Diarrhea, acute	*Bacillus cereus, Campylobacter*, cholera, *Clostridium perfringens, Escherichia coli*, rotavirus, salmonellosis, trichinosis, *Vibrio parahaemolyticus*	Eye pain, swelling, reddening	Chagas' disease (Romana's sign), hemorrhagic conjunctivitis, loiasis, onchocerciasis, trachoma, trichinosis
		Respiratory Signs and Symptoms	
Diarrhea, bloody	Amebic dysentery, *Balantidium coli, Campylobacter*, enteroinvasive *E. coli*, shigellosis	Cough	Ascariasis, bacterial and chlamydial respiratory infections, Lassa fever, paragonimiasis, pertussis, plague, psittacosis, tuberculosis, upper respiratory infections
Diarrhea, chronic	AIDS, clonorchiasis, cryptosporidiosis, giardiasis, strongyloidiasis	Lesions visible on chest x-ray	Blastomycosis, coccidioidomycosis, echinococcosis, histoplasmosis, melioidosis, pneumocystosis, psittacosis, tuberculosis
Hepatomegaly	Amebic liver abscess, Chagas' disease, clonorchiasis, echinococcosis, fascioliasis, histoplasmosis, malaria, opisthorchiasis, schistosomiasis, toxocariasis, typhoid fever, visceral leishmaniasis	Pharyngitis	Diphtheria, streptococcal infections, viral infections
Jaundice	Hepatitis (A, B, delta, non-A non-B; epidemic and transfusion-related), leptospirosis, malaria (*P. falciparum*)	Pneumonia	AIDS, anthrax, ascariasis, blastomycosis, coccidioidomycosis, histoplasmosis, legionellosis, paragonimiasis, plague, pneumococcosis, pneumocystosis, psittacosis, Q fever, scrub typhus, strongyloidiasis, tuberculosis
Splenomegaly	Chagas' disease, malaria, schistosomiasis, typhoid fever, visceral leishmaniasis		
Worms	Ascariasis, enterobiasis, taeniasis		

Source: Warren KS, Mahmoud AAF. *Tropical and Geographical Medicine* (2nd ed.). New York: McGraw-Hill, 1990. Used with permission.

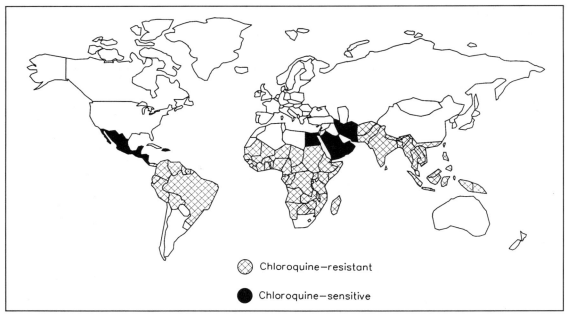

Fig. 19-1. Malarious areas with *Plasmodium falciparum* resistant and sensitive to chloroquine, 1990. Reprinted from Centers for Disease Control. *Health Information for International Travel 1990.* Washington, DC: U.S. Dept. of Health and Human Services, 1990. P. 95. HHS publication no. CDC 90-8280.

self-administer pyrimethamine-sulfadoxine if they develop fever in an endemic area [5]. Since the symptoms of malaria are nonspecific and there is a high misdiagnosis rate, it is especially important to get a complete travel history.

Incidence and Geographic Considerations. There has been a worldwide resurgence of malaria cases after a period in the 1950s and 1960s of success in controlling malaria [9]. Over 60 million cases occur worldwide each year, and 1,023 cases of malaria were reported in the United States in 1988, most acquired outside the country. In Africa the mortality is concentrated mainly in younger age groups, with as many as a million infants and children dying per year of malaria [10]. Malaria transmission occurs in Central and South America, sub-Saharan Africa, India, Southeast Asia, the Middle East, and Oceania (Fig. 19-1). Historically the prevalence of malaria in the United States has paralleled U.S. military involvement abroad; however, the number of cases in the civilian population has been increasing steadily since the early 1980s. Most cases acquired in the United States result from transfusion,

but there is the possibility of transmission in some places where anopheles mosquitoes breed [11].

Life Cycle of the Parasite and Pathophysiology. Malaria is caused by four protozoan species of the genus *Plasmodium*: *P. falciparum*, *P. vivax*, *P. ovale*, and *P. malariae*. Female *Anopheles* mosquitoes transmit the disease by biting a mammalian host and inoculating sporozoites. The complete life cycle is illustrated in Fig. 19-2.

Clinical Manifestations. Initially malaria has a clinical presentation as an undifferentiated febrile illness, most commonly misdiagnosed as a flu-like or viral syndrome. Fever, malaise, headache, and nausea follow a usual incubation period of 10–16 days, which may last up to a month with *P. malariae* infection. Drug prophylaxis may suppress the initial attack for weeks to months for *P. falciparum* infection, and for months to years for *P. ovale* and *P. vivax* infections [12]. Periodic fevers occur with malaria caused by *P. falciparum*, *P. vivax*, *P. ovale* (48 hours), and *P. malariae* (72 hours), which have mature schizonts that can rupture synchronously;

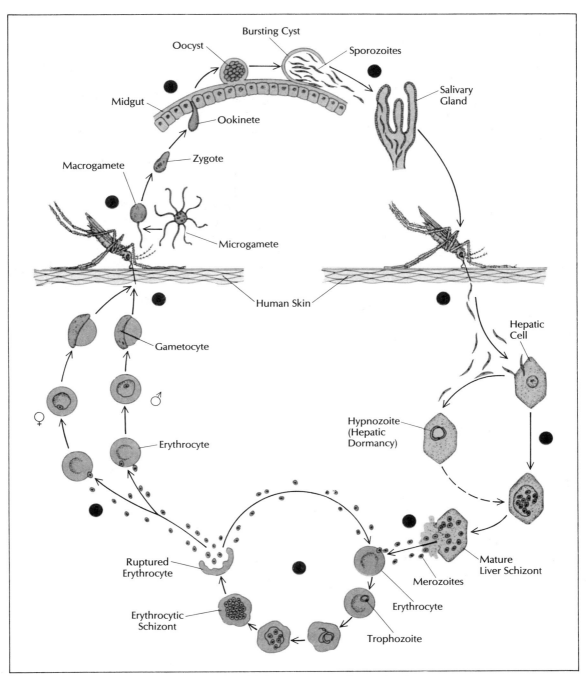

Fig. 19-2. Life cycle of the malaria parasite is divided between two hosts, the *Anopheles* mosquito (top) and a mammal, such as a human. In the mammal, *Plasmodium* sporozoites injected by mosquito bite (1) rapidly enter liver cells. There they proliferate (2) into merozoites. (*P. vivax* may, however, become dormant.) Rupture of the infected cells releases them into the blood (3), where they enter erythrocytes to begin a phase of asexual reproduction (4). Erythrocytic rupture is followed by reinfection of red cells and differentiation into sexual forms, or gametocytes (5). The latter, within their erythrocytes, can be ingested by a mosquito (6); lysis of the red cells frees them to develop into gametes. The male produces eight sperm-like microgametes, which fertilize the female macrogametes (7). The resulting zygotes become ookinetes, which penetrate the mosquito's midgut wall (8), develop into oocysts, and ultimately release sporozoites (9) that populate the insect's salivary glands. Nussenzweig V, Nussenzweig R. Progress toward a malaria vaccine. *Hosp Practice* 25: Fig. 1, 1990. Reprinted with permission.

fever is not periodic in severe *P. falciparum* infection and the first attack of infection with *P. vivax*.

Typical malarial paroxysms begin with a cold stage characterized by rigors and chills, followed by a hot stage lasting 3–4 hours with temperatures of 39°–40°C, and end with a sweating stage of several hours, in which the patient defervesces. Symptoms in the early stages of infection with *P. falciparum* may be relatively less severe than infection with *P. vivax*, which contributes to the chance of misdiagnosis in nonendemic areas. Patients may feel well intermittently between paroxysms, especially with forms of malaria other than that caused by *P. falciparum*. Mild jaundice, hepatosplenomegaly, and hemolytic anemia often develop in all types of malaria. Lymphadenopathy does not occur. *P. malariae* can produce chronic progressive nephritis. *P. falciparum* causes the most severe disease, with most of its mortality due to its high parasitemia and ability to obstruct microcirculation. Severe hemolysis may lead to hemoglobinuria and renal failure (blackwater fever). Multiorgan failure with pneumonia and respiratory distress syndrome may ensue.

Patient history should include a detailed travel itinerary in malaria-endemic areas. Even brief airport stopovers can provide sufficient exposure. In addition histories of blood transfusions and IV drug use in endemic regions should be queried. (Induced malaria acquired by intravenous routes may be particularly virulent.) A complete review of prior medication usage is mandatory, especially the use of any antimicrobial agents. A history of antimalarial chemoprophylaxis does not exclude the diagnosis of malaria. Moreover, the frequent use by international travelers of common antimicrobial agents with antimalarial activity (e.g., the tetracyclines and trimethoprim-sulfamethoxazole) can complicate the clinical picture.

Factors that increase the likelihood of malaria in patients recently returned from malarious areas include failure to maintain appropriate chemoprophylaxis; travel to rural areas of endemic countries, especially during evening hours; history of multiple mosquito bites; and the proximity of return date to the United States from endemic areas to onset of illness. Approximately 90% of cases of malaria caused by *P. falciparum* in the United States present within one month of date of entry, but onset of illness may be delayed as long as a year by factors such as chemosuppression.

Cerebral malaria, the most common complication of severe *P. falciparum* malaria, is a true emergency, with a 20%–50% mortality [13]. In endemic areas the disease typically presents in children less than 5 years old as malaise, headache, and vomiting, which rapidly progresses to somnolence, seizures, delirium, and coma [14]. Hypoglycemia is a frequent problem in children with cerebral malaria [15]. These patients require a lumbar puncture (LP) to rule out other pathogens. There may be a low-grade spinal fluid pleocytosis in cerebral malaria.

Diagnosis. The variety of clinical manifestations make consideration of malaria mandatory in anyone who has traveled to an endemic area. In the acute setting diagnosis is made by identifying parasites on Giemsa-stained blood smears (Fig. 19-3). Because

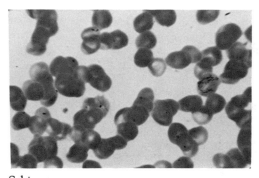

Schizont

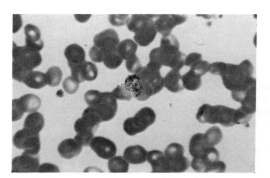

Trophozoite

Fig. 19-3. *Plasmodium malariae* identified on blood smear.

parasitemia can fluctuate, smears should be repeated every 12 hours for several days. Mixed infections can occur, so identifying one parasite does not exclude another. The density of parasitemia can identify those patients requiring emergent treatment. Parasitemia greater than 5% (250,000 parasites per milliliter of blood) or the presence of *P. falciparum* schizonts in peripheral blood smears are indicators of severe infection. Parasite counts above 500,000 per milliliter are associated with a greater than 50% mortality.

An indirect fluorescent antibody test, available through the CDC, is useful mainly for identifying transfusion malaria and corroborating the response to therapeutic trials. Therapeutic trials can be used diagnostically when the blood films are negative, but the suspicion is high.

Chemoprophylaxis. A malaria vaccine is a future possibility, but chemoprophylaxis currently is the most effective way to prevent malaria [16]. Before considering chemoprophylaxis, the traveler and the physician should look at a map that indicates countries at risk (see Fig. 19-1), and the traveler should investigate areas of risk within a given county, which usually are rural areas. The CDC publishes information yearly on malaria risk in each country.

Resistance of *P. falciparum* to chloroquine is widespread (see Fig. 19-1). For areas where chloroquine resistance has not been reported, chloroquine should be taken. For travel to areas with chloroquine-resistant *P. falciparum*, mefloquine should be taken (Table 19-7) [17]. Prophylactic efficacy is greater with mefloquine (92%) than with any other drug [18].

Doxycycline 100 mg daily is an alternative chemoprophylactic for those intolerant of mefloquine or in whom it is contraindicated.* Chloroquine should be used during pregnancy, in children less than 15 kg, and by those who cannot take doxycycline or mefloquine. Travelers on chloroquine who develop a febrile illness should take three tab-

---

* Mefloquine is contraindicated in those with a history of hypersensitivity, epilepsy, or psychiatric disorders, those taking betablockers, pregnant women, children less than 15 kg and those performing tasks requiring fine motor coordination and spatial discrimination, such as an airline pilot.

lets of pyrimethamine-sulfadoxine and immediately seek medical attention. The use of high-dose mefloquine for the treatment of presumptive malaria is controversial. Persons who have prolonged exposure in a malarious area where exposure to a species of relapsing malaria (caused by *P. vivax* and *P. ovale*) is probable should take primaquine for two weeks on leaving the endemic area (see Table 19-7). *P. ovale* is found in Africa, while *P. vivax* is found in Southeast Asia, South America, and Oceania. For children tablets may need to be pulverized and mixed with food to disguise chloroquine's bitter taste. Chloroquine is the only drug that can be used in pregnancy. Detailed recommendations are available through the CDC Malaria Hotline, 404-332-4555.

Treatment of Acute Illness. Oral chloroquine is used for all species except chloroquine-resistant *P. falciparum*. Primaquine should be added for *P. vivax* and *P. ovale* to kill parasites sequestered in the liver. Oral quinine, pyrimethamine, and a sulfonamide should be given for *P. falciparum* acquired in drug-resistant areas (see Table 19-7). Patients intolerant of pyrimethamine-sulfadoxine can be given tetracycline 250 mg qid for 7 days or clindamycin 900 mg tid for 3 days [19]. Single doses of mefloquine, another alternative to quinine, have cured 90%–100% of patients with resistant *P. falciparum* malaria, but rapidly emerging resistance and CNS toxicity are serious problems [20].

Patients who have *P. falciparum* malaria or who are severely ill, immunocompromised, or pregnant should be admitted to the hospital. In the United States patients often are admitted with lesser severity because malaria is uncommon and the workup can be expedited in a hospital.

Intravenous quinine was formerly recommended for severely ill patients in the same doses as oral quinine and infused over 2–4 hours [19]. It is no longer available in the United States. Quinidine gluconate is now recommended by the CDC in the United States, and it is well tolerated if given with cardiac monitoring [21]. A loading dose of 10 mg/kg (maximum 600 mg) in normal saline is infused over 1 hour, followed by a continuous infusion of 0.02 mg/kg/min for 3 days. Exchange transfusion may also need to be considered in severe malaria [22]. Other drugs, such as Qinghaosu, have

Table 19-7. Recommended chemotherapy and prophylaxis for malaria

Indication	Drug and route	Dosages	
		Adult	Pediatric
Uncomplicated infection with all species except chloroquine-resistant *Plasmodium falciparum*	Chloroquine phosphate PO	600 mg base (1 g) followed by 300 mg base (500 mg) in 6 hr, then 300 mg base (500 mg/day for 2 days)	10 mg/kg (base) to maximum of 600 mg followed by half this dose in 6 hr, then daily for 2 days
Patient unable to take oral medications	Chloroquine hydrochloride IM[a]	200 mg base (250 mg) q6h for maximum of 3 days	5 mg/kg (base) q12 h for maximum of 3 days
Severe (complicated) *P. falciparum* infection	Quinidine dihydrochloride IV[b]	600 mg q8h to maximum of 1.8 g/day or 10 mg/kg loading dose over 1- to 2-hour infusion followed by .02 mg/kg/min. infusion for 3 days	Same as for adults
Uncomplicated infection due to chloroquine-resistant *P. falciparum*[c]	Mefloquine PO	1250 mg in one dose	Not approved
	Combination of quinine sulfate PO	650 mg q8h for 7–10 days	25 mg/kg/day in 3 doses for 10 days
	plus		
	pyrimethamine PO	25 mg bid for 3 days	<10 kg: 6.25 mg/day 10–20 kg: 12.5 mg/day 20–40 kg: 25 mg/day
	plus		
	sulfadiazine or sulfisoxazole PO	500 mg qid for 5 days	100–200 mg/kg/day in 4 doses (maximum 2 g/day) for 5 days

Uncomplicated infection due to sulfonamide-pyrimethamine–resistant P. falciparum	Combination of quinine sulfate PO plus	650 mg q8h for 7–10 days	25 mg/kg/day in 3 doses for 10 days
	tetracycline PO	250 mg tid PO for 7–10 days	6 mg/kg tid PO for 7–10 days
Prevention of relapses due to Plasmodium vivax and Plasmodium ovale	Primaquine phosphate PO	15 mg base (26.3 mg) day for 14 days	0.3 mg base kg/day for 14 days
Chemoprophylaxis of all species except chloroquine-resistant P. falciparum[d]	Chloroquine phosphate PO	300 mg base (500 mg) once per week, begun 2 weeks before and continued for 6 weeks after leaving area	<1 year: 37.5 mg base[e] 1–3 years: 75 mg base 4–6 years: 100 mg base 7–10 years: 150 mg base 11–16 years: 225 mg base
Chemoprophylaxis of chloroquine-resistant P. falciparum	Mefloquine PO	250 mg once per week, begun 1 week before and continued for 4 weeks after leaving area	15–19 kg: 1/4 tab/wk 20–30 kg: 1/2 tab/wk 31–45 kg: 3/4 tab/wk >45 kg: 1 tab/wk
	Doxycycline PO	100 mg daily	> 8 years of age: 2 mg/kg day up to adult dose of 100 mg/day

Source: Adapted with permission from Mandell GL, Douglas RG, Bennett JE (eds.). *Principles and Practice of Infectious Diseases* (3rd ed.). New York: Churchill-Livingstone, 1990. P. 2064.

[a] May cause potentially fatal side effects. See text.

[b] Quinine dihydrochloride can be obtained in the United States from the Centers for Disease Control (Drug Service). Monitor vital signs and electrocardiogram. Should be replaced by oral medication as soon as possible. Quinidine can be used as an alternative. See text.

[c] Infection in patients with sulfonamide-pyrimethamine-resistant strains (such as those acquired in Southeast Asia) may recrudesce after this treatment. See text.

[d] In addition, patients returning from areas with high transmission rates of *P. ovale* should take primaquine phosphate in the doses indicated in the table.

[e] Since children may refuse to take chloroquine tablets because of their bitter taste, it may be necessary to disguise the taste by mixing ground tablets in food. Palatable liquid preparations for pediatric use are readily available in several countries in which malaria transmission occurs.

proved to be very effective in China but are not available elsewhere.

SCHISTOSOMIASIS

Schistosomiasis is a trematode infection that causes considerable morbidity and mortality in the developing world, especially in childhood and adolescence [23]. It is estimated that 200 million people worldwide are infected with schistosomes, although most do not have symptoms [24]. It is also a possible cause of undifferentiated fever in the returning traveler.

Pathogenesis and Risk. Exposure to schistosomiasis is a health hazard for those who travel to the Caribbean, South America, Africa, and Asia. Puerto Rico, St. Lucia, Egypt, most of sub-Saharan Africa, southern China, the Philippines, and Southeast Asia are the areas of greatest risk.

Schistosomiasis is acquired by wading or swimming in fresh water in rural areas where poor sanitation and the appropriate snail hosts are present. All types of schistosomiasis are acquired when free-swimming cercariae penetrate the intact skin of a person who comes in contact with infected fresh water. The life cycle of schistosomes is shown in Fig. 19-4. The intensity of infection does not appear to correlate with frequency and degree of water contact [25]. Potable water may also pose a risk, but the infection is not acquired in oceans or seas.

There are three major human parasites of the genus *Schistosoma*: *haematobium, mansoni,* and *japonicum. Schistosoma haematobium* is prevalent mostly in sub-Saharan Africa and Egypt. *Schistosoma mansoni* has the greatest worldwide distribution and is found in South America, the Caribbean, and sub-Saharan Africa. *Schistosoma japonicum* is found in China, Southeast Asia, and the Philippines. Less epidemiologically prevalent species, *Schistosoma intercalatum* and *Schistosoma mekongi,* can also cause disease, and certain species of avian and mammalian schistosomes can cause dermatitis. *S. mekongi* is found on the mainland of Indochina and Southeast Asia.

Clinical Manifestation. The traveler is most likely to suffer from symptoms of acute exposure. All types of schistosomiasis can produce a swimmer's itch from the cercarial dermatitis. However, the symptoms and signs of acute schistosomiasis

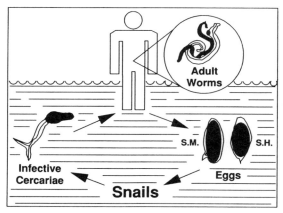

Fig. 19-4. Life cycle of human schistosomes represented by S. mansoni (S.M.) and S. haematobium (S.H.). Free-swimming cercariae penetrate intact skin in contact with infected fresh water. Adults developing within the human host mate and begin depositing eggs in the vasculature surrounding the intestine and the bladder. Eggs released into the stool or urine develop into forms infective for intermediate snail hosts when deposited into fresh water. Infected snails release cercariae to reinitiate the cycle. Reprinted with permission from Acute Schistosomiasis in U.S. Travelers Returning from Africa. *MMWR* 39:147, 1990.

occur more frequently than the dermatitis, especially in individuals heavily infected with *S. japonicum* and *S. mansoni*. There have been reports of at least five outbreaks among U.S. and European tourists since 1975 in travelers returning from Africa. In these five outbreaks the symptoms of acute schistosomiasis occurred in 40%–93% of those infected. Acute schistosomiasis, or Katayama fever, occurs as early as 2–3 weeks after water exposure. The most common symptoms are fever, lack of appetite, weight loss, abdominal pain, weakness, headaches, joint and muscle pain, diarrhea, nausea, and cough. Symptoms are thought to result from an immunological response to the maturation of adult worms and subsequent egg deposits in the vasculature surrounding the intestines or the bladder [26].

Diagnosis. The clinical manifestations of acute schistosomiasis often are very nonspecific. The disease needs to be sought to be diagnosed and should be suspected in anyone who has lived in or visited an endemic area. The diagnosis should be considered when eosinophilia is associated with fever, fatigue, headache, or GI distress in persons who have been exposed to fresh water in areas where schistosomiasis is endemic. One of the problems with diagnosis is that the number of eggs excreted during the acute stage may be small, and symptoms of acute infection may occur before detectable egg excretion. Definitive diagnosis is made by detecting ova in stool or urine. Sensitive and specific serologic tests such as the enzyme-linked immunoabsorbent assay (ELISA) can help establish the diagnosis before substantial egg deposition or excretion. Serologic techniques do not distinguish among the different species but should encourage intensive diagnostic attempts to verify the diagnosis. Sensitive filtration techniques detect ova in the urine, but egg detection in the stool is more difficult, even with thick-smear techniques. If the diagnosis is strongly suspected or the risk is high, a rectal biopsy should be performed [24].

Prevention. Fresh-water swimming in rural areas in endemic countries should be avoided because there is no way for a traveler to distinguish between infested and noninfested water. Chlorinated swimming pools are virtually always safe in endemic

countries and heating bathing water to 50°C for 5 minutes or treating it with iodine or chlorine in a manner similar to the precautions recommended for preparing drinking water will destroy cercariae. If accidental exposure to suspected water occurs, vigorous towel drying or rapid application of rubbing alcohol to the exposed areas may reduce the risk of infection. There are no chemoprophylactic agents [25].

Treatment. Single-day therapy with praziquantel 40–60 mg/kg is effective against all species of schistosomes. The treatment is divided into two or three doses over one day [19].

YELLOW FEVER

Yellow fever is the prototypical viral hemorrhagic fever. It is relatively common but underreported, with 100–300 annual cases in South America and 1,000 annual cases in Africa [27].

Distribution. Yellow fever occurs in tropical Africa and South America (Fig. 19-5). Two different mechanisms of spread are known. Urban yellow

Fig. 19-5. Yellow fever endemic zones in the Americas and Africa and the number of yellow fever cases reported to World Health Organization, 1980–1987. Reprinted with permission from Yellow Fever Vaccine: Recommendations of the Immunization Practices Advisory Committee (ACIP). MMWR 39:2, 1990.

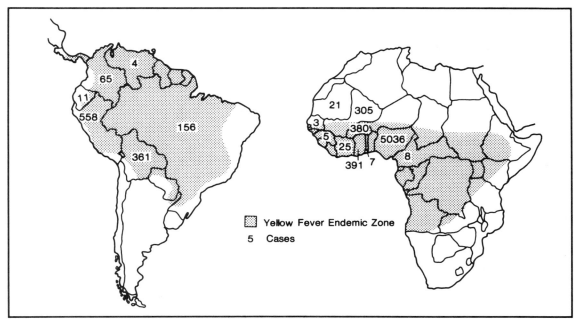

fever is an epidemic human disease spread by *Aedes aegypti* mosquitoes. Jungle yellow fever is an endemic disease spread by several species of *Aedes haemagogus* mosquitoes from primate hosts [28].

Symptoms and Signs. After an incubation period of 3–6 days most patients have only 48 hours of fever, headache, conjunctival injection, and myalgia, which vary in intensity. Half of cases are asymptomatic.

Hemorrhagic illness occurs in 10%–20% of symptomatic cases. The preceding symptoms are more severe with hemorrhagic fever. During the 3-day viremic phase nausea, vomiting, and minor bleeding may occur. Symptoms then improve, and the patient fever defervesces for a brief period (hours), then returns accompanied by a bleeding disorder due to disseminated intravascular coagulation (DIC). Multiorgan failure, including oliguric renal failure, with marked albuminuria, heart failure, and agitated delirium or coma may ensue; one-quarter to one-half of severe cases die.

Treatment. Treatment is supportive and may require short-term dialysis. A patient's blood is infective during the 3 days of early illness and occasionally throughout a severe case. The diagnosis can be confirmed by viral culture or antibody rise.

Prevention. Vaccine with a live attenuated strain provides long-term immunity (10–40 years) in 95% of recipients within 10 days. The vaccine causes a mild febrile reaction in 2%–5% of recipients. Vaccination of infants under 4 months is contraindicated because of the risk of vaccine-induced encephalitis. For infants between the ages of 4 and 6 months direct consultation with the CDC is recommended. Infants between 6 and 9 months can be vaccinated if their risk of contracting yellow fever is high, and children over 9 months can be vaccinated safely. The vaccine is contraindicated in immunosuppressed patients and those who are hypersensitive to eggs. Some countries require an international certificate of vaccination of all travelers, including those in transit, from countries where yellow fever is endemic. This requires vaccination within 10 years certified by a WHO-approved center. Consult the CDC's *Health Information for International Travel.* All state health

departments are approved to issue certificates, and one should be contacted for details. Mosquito repellent and netting can greatly decrease the risk.

OTHER VIRAL HEMORRHAGIC FEVERS

Dengue. Dengue is a recurrent epidemic disease spread by A. *aegypti* mosquitoes. The disease is common throughout the tropics of America, Africa, and Asia, with millions of cases reported yearly. The vector is the common urban mosquito, A. *aegypti*, in most of the tropics. A. *aegypti* mosquitoes are found in the southern United States, and dengue may spread to this region in the future.

Symptoms and signs of classic "breakbone" dengue are nonspecific, with sudden onset of fever, headache, conjunctival suffusion, eye pain, arthralgias, lymphadenopathy, and nausea, often followed in 3–5 days by an erythematous macular rash. There are four immunotypes with minimal cross-protection between types. Hemorrhagic fever is relatively rare in dengue occurring most commonly in children during a second attack. Dengue hemorrhagic fever is clinically similar to other viral hemorrhagic fevers but due to the requirement for a second attack, it is not a major problem among travelers [29, 30].

Other viral hemorrhagic fevers include Lassa fever, Junin (Argentine) fever, Bolivian hemorrhagic fever, Marburg virus disease, Ebola virus disease, Congo-Crimean hemorrhagic fever, Rift Valley fever, and Hanta virus disease (Table 19-8). The viral hemorrhagic fever syndrome is discussed in more detail in Chap. 12.

Fever and Multisystem Involvement

PLAGUE

Yersinia (formerly *Pasteurella*) *pestis*, which causes enzootic plague, is widespread among rodents in many parts of the world and is a possibility on every continent except Australia. Human disease is endemic in parts of Asia, Africa, and South America. Sporadic human cases still occur in the United States, primarily in the Southwest. The bacillus is carried by rodents and spread by fleas. Symptoms are rapid in onset, with fever, chills, tachycardia, headache, vomiting, delirium, and prostration. A bubo is pathognomonic. Plague, particularly the bubonic and pneumonic forms, is easy to confirm

Table 19-8. Other viral hemorrhagic fevers

	Lassa Fever	Junin Fever	Bolivian Hemorrhagic Fever	Marburg Virus	Ebola Virus	Congo-Crimean Hemorrhagic Fever	Rift Valley Fever	Hanta Virus and Korean and related hemorrhagic fevers
Geographic area	Central and West Africa	Maize-growing areas of Argentina	Grasslands of Bolivia	West and southern Africa	Sudan, Kenya, Zaire	Russia, Baltic States, Central and South Africa, Mideast and Pakistan	Egypt, sub-Saharan Africa	North Asia, Scandinavia, Central Europe to Greece
Transmission	Food borne	Unknown	Unknown	Blood borne	Blood borne	Tick borne	Mosquito borne, blood borne	Direct contact, fleas
Animal carrier	Rats	Rats	Rats	Monkeys	Humans, guinea pigs	Domestic animals	Domestic herbivores	Rodents
Common symptoms*	Cough, deafness, pharyngitis	Rash, petechiae, lymphadenopathy, facial edema	Similar to Junin fever	Severe headache, diarrhea, vomiting, conjunctivitis, rash, liver failure, bleeding	Similar to Marburg Virus	Liver failure and bleeding	Similar to but milder than yellow fever	Variable incubation up to 40 days; thrombocytopenia, renal failure
Isolation	Strict	Strict	Strict	Strict	Strict	Strict	Blood	Blood
Death rate	25%–50%	10%–20%	Not documented	25%	Varies, can involve several related viruses	50%	Low	Varies; Asian cases more severe
Treatment	Ribavivin	None	None	None	None	None	None	None
References in this chapter	31, 32, 33		34	35	35, 36	37		38, 39

* All symptoms may occur with any virus. This table lists the most common symptoms associated with each virus.

once suspected (see Chaps. 10 and 12). Septic plague is less common and harder to diagnose. The bacillus is resistant to penicillins and cephalosporins but sensitive to aminoglycosides, tetracyclines, and chloramphenicol.

AFRICAN TRYPANOSOMIASIS (SLEEPING SICKNESS)

Sleeping sickness is an acute or chronic disease limited to central Africa. Sleeping sickness is spread by tsetse flies and caused by two variants of *Trypanosoma brucei*: *T. brucei gambiense* and *T. brucei rhodesiense*. Trypanosomes are flagellated, blood-borne organisms that initially cause septic symptoms and eventually invade the CNS or the myocardium. Both forms of the disease are complicated by the parasites' ability to change surface antigenic components. This results in waves of blood-borne infection and recurrent symptoms as the host produces new antibodies to the currently active antigenic form. This also makes laboratory diagnosis more difficult. Aspirates from the chancre (see the discussion of Gambian sleeping sickness, next) and the lymph nodes and blood smears may be diagnostic, but repeat smears may be necessary. All patients suspected of having sleeping sickness should have a spinal tap. Diagnostic cerebrospinal fluid (CSF) findings require special stains, and CNS involvement must be determined before treatment is started.

Treatment is complex because the agents used are toxic, and the least toxic agents fail to penetrate the blood-brain barrier. Suramin and pentamidine are commonly used for early-stage disease. Melarsoprol, an extremely toxic arsenic-containing compound, remains the drug of choice for CNS disease. Mortality rate of both forms of the disease approaches 100% if not treated. Pentamidine is an effective prophylactic agent for the Gambian form of the disease. A single injection provides immunity for several months. However, it is not recommended for the Rhodesian form of the disease, since it is less effective and tends to mask the symptoms of the initial blood-borne infection, making diagnosis of the CNS stage far more difficult. The most important part of control is avoidance of highly endemic areas and the use of insect repellents (DEET), mosquito nets, and heavy, full-length clothing.

Gambian Sleeping Sickness. This form of sleeping sickness is limited to West Africa. There is no known animal host. Gambian sleeping sickness classically has three stages of infection. Within 1–2 weeks of a tsetse fly bite a painful circumscribed indurated chancre forms in approximately one-third of patients. This chancre resolves over a period of 2–3 weeks. There may be local lymph node enlargement. Within a few days of the appearance of the chancre, or within 1–3 weeks of the bite, a septic phase occurs, with high fever, malaise, headache, dizziness, diffuse joint pain, and tachycardia. These symptoms may remit, and several bouts of sepsis are common. Personality change, including irritability and insomnia, are common, particularly in non-Africans, as is an erythematous rash similar to erythema marginatum. The disease progresses to lymph node involvement with the posterior cervical nodes most frequently enlarged. The later stages of CNS invasion are usually of insidious onset over a period of months to years. Initial changes are subtle and involve personality change and difficulty with memory. With progression the patient loses initiative, speech may become more and more difficult, and cerebral atrophy occurs. Seizures and progressive mental deterioration occur late in the course and are followed by coma and death. Myocarditis occurs but only rarely with *T. brucei gambiense*. *T. brucei gambiense* is rare in travelers but common in immigrants due to the prolonged course of infection.

Rhodesian Sleeping Sickness. Rhodesian sleeping sickness is limited to the savannah areas of eastern Africa. Wild antelopes are the most common animal carrier, and this form of the disease is likely to be seen in visitors to animal parks. The Rhodesian form is similar to the Gambian form but is more fulminant, with only a half year from initial infection to death. Myocarditis is very common during the first month and is a more common cause of death than the CNS disease. Myocarditis is typified by conduction abnormalities and a dilated cardiomyopathy resulting in congestive heart failure.

AMERICAN TRYPANOSOMIASIS (CHAGAS' DISEASE)

Most acute cases of Chagas' disease are asymptomatic, but there may be mild fever, lymphadenopathy, hepatosplenomegaly, myocarditis, and meningitis. The bite of a reduviid bug may produce an erythematous nodule. Travelers with longer stays in rural areas may be at risk. Chagas' disease is discussed in more detail later in this chapter.

VISCERAL LEISHMANIASIS

Visceral leishmaniasis is a less likely disease in recreational travelers, but for those with longer stays in rural areas where there are sandflies it is a real possibility. Because of its long incubation period it can be a particularly difficult diagnosis for the American physician. Visceral leishmaniasis may occasionally acutely present with a minute papule or a sore; however, the incubation period for serious symptoms is 4–10 months. It often presents as a high fever, which may be intermittent or remittent with a periodicity resembling *P. falciparum* malaria. Splenomegaly develops in cases with gradual onset of symptoms. Leishmaniasis is discussed in more detail later in this chapter.

Traveler's Diarrhea

Traveler's diarrhea is by far the most common infection encountered among travelers to tropical countries. One-quarter to one-half of all international travelers develop diarrhea [31]. Traveler's diarrhea is ubiquitous, although it is most common among travelers going from developed countries to developing tropical countries. High-risk countries are found in Central and South America, India, Africa, and Asia. Intermediate risk is found in southern Europe, the former Soviet Union, some Caribbean islands, and China.

Most traveler's diarrhea is of sudden onset and only a few days' duration. The illness is rarely serious in terms of being a threat to life except, perhaps, in the very young, the very old, and the immunosuppressed. It can, however, be exceedingly inconvenient.

The onset of diarrhea is often 2–3 days after travel has begun. Untreated the symptoms last for 2–7 days. Stools are loose and watery, or if an invasive organism is present, they may have blood or mucus. Diarrhea may be explosive. Anorexia, nausea, and a low-grade fever are present. The unlucky traveler may experience recurrent episodes.

Several organisms are responsible for causing the disease, and polymicrobial infections are common [32]. Most of the organisms causing the disease are bacterial [33]. This makes antibiotic prophylaxis and treatment feasible. The most common organism is enterotoxigenic *Escherichia coli*, which is responsible for approximately 50% of cases. Other organisms include *Campylobacter jejuni*, *Salmonella* species, *Shigella* species, *Yersinia enterocolitica*, and several viruses (Table 19-9). Diagnosis depends on the classic clinical presentation, culture results, and the presence of leukocytes on a methylene blue or Gram's stain. Unfortunately enterotoxigenic *E. coli* is impossible to identify in most laboratories, and the stool leukocyte smear is negative. Fortunately antibiotic treatment is possible for most cases with or without a known causative agent.

Three antibiotic agents have been most popular for prophylaxis: trimethoprim-sulfamethoxazole (TMP-SMZ) one tablet daily, doxycycline 100 mg qd, and ciprofloxacin 250 mg qd. These agents are effective if given prophylactically, although most experts feel that unless the exposure is brief and the inconvenience to the traveler from the disease great, it is better to reserve the drugs for presumptive treatment once diarrhea starts. All three agents have significant side effects, and all are contraindicated in pregnancy. Doxycycline and ciprofloxacin are contraindicated in children. The photosensitivity induced by doxycycline and occasionally TMP-SMZ can be incapacitating in a tropical climate. For prophylaxis a single dose given in the morning beginning on the first day of travel and continuing for 2 days after returning home is probably adequate. Bismuth subsalicylate (Pepto-Bismol) in a dose of eight tablets daily is also effective. Unfortunately this is a relatively large dose and inconvenient to take. Serious side effects of this drug are unusual, but it does stain the tongue and stool black.

For most patients empiric therapy is perhaps more logical than prophylaxis. Patients with incapacitating diarrhea, particularly associated with fever, systemic effects, and bloody stool, can be treated with any of the above-mentioned antibiotics in a fully therapeutic dose. Loperamide in an initial dose of two capsules (4 ml) followed by one after each stool, up to eight capsules per day, is also effective in decreasing the number of stools.

Table 19-9. Traveler's diarrhea

Organism	Blood in stool	White blood cells in stool	Fever	Treatment	Method of diagnosis
Toxogenic Escherichia coli	No	No	No	Trimethoprim-sulfamethoxazole, doxycycline, ciprofloxacin, bismuth	Exclusion
Shigella species	Yes	Yes	Yes	Trimethoprim-sulfamethoxazole	Culture
Salmonella species	Yes	Yes	Sometimes	Rarely warranted	Culture
Campylobacter jejuni	Yes	Yes	Yes	Erythromycin, ciprofloxacin	Wet-prep, culture
Yersinia enterocolitica	Yes	Yes	Yes	Doxycycline, ciprofloxacin	Culture (cold-enriched)
Virus	No	No	Sometimes	None	Exclusion
Giardia lamblia	No	No	No	Quinacrine, metronidazole	Wet prep, O&P stain
Entamoeba histolytica	Yes	Yes	Yes	Metronidazole	Wet prep, O&P stain

Environmental precautions are probably helpful in decreasing the incidence of traveler's diarrhea. Unfortunately the pathogens all require only a small inoculum to cause disease, and extreme care must be taken to avoid exposure. Travelers should be warned that tap water, noncarbonated bottled water, ice, and fresh fruits and vegetables (except those that are peeled prior to eating) are all likely sources for the disease. Food that has been left out and potentially inoculated by flies should be avoided. Water purification must be meticulous. Iodine is by far the most effective chemical agent. When used properly, iodine kills all pathogens. Water filtration through a micropore filter designed for this purpose eliminates all pathogens except viral organisms. Brief boiling is also effective. Table 19-10 gives water-purification directions. Cooked food, peeled fruit and vegetables, carbonated and alcoholic drinks, and filtered or iodized water are probably the only safe products. The combination of meticulous environmental care and antimicrobial therapy plus loperamide if diarrhea starts is most reasonable for adults [34].

Infants under the age of 2 months are difficult to treat, although breastfeeding infants are extremely unlikely to get traveler's diarrhea. For children over the age of 2 months, TMP-SMZ is recommended for treatment of traveler's diarrhea. Although traveler's diarrhea is rarely serious in adults, it can be fatal in young children. Parents traveling with young children should carry powdered oral rehydration fluid with them or be prepared to make it. The following version is recommended by the CDC:

Glass number 1—8 oz. apple, orange, or other fruit juice (rich in potassium), 1/2 tsp. honey or corn syrup (contains glucose), and 1 pinch table salt

Glass number 2—8 oz. purified water, 1/4 tsp. baking soda

The patient should drink alternately from each glass until thirst is quenched. It is important that free water is supplied as desired to a person receiving salt solution [35].

Chronic diarrhea in returning travelers and immigrants is likely to be due to either the same organisms that cause acute traveler's diarrhea or parasitic infections, particularly Giardia or amebae.

Table 19-10. Water purification

Method	Agents	Directions
Disinfection	Iodine tablets or drops; iodine-crystal water-purification devices; tetraglycine hydroperiodide tablets (portable-agua)	Mix 30 minutes prior to drinking; double time and dose if water is turbid or cold.
Heat	—	Boil water 10 minutes; add 1 minute per 1000 feet elevation.

Most patients with amebiasis are asymptomatic. Others may occasionally have a few loose stools. Serious illness causes fever and bloody dysentery. The patient with Giardiasis may have intermittent symptoms consisting of bloating, gas, and constipation alternating with diarrhea. Diagnosis in these cases may be difficult. The patient should have a fresh stool specimen Gram-stained and tested for blood and fecal leukocytes (usually negative in Giardia). The specimen should be sent for ova and parasite examination. Cyst shedding may be intermittent, so multiple (three) specimens may be necessary.

The incidence of enteric parasite infection can be quite high, particularly among immigrants. However, few parasites cause diarrhea, and the diagnosis is usually made as an incidental finding on concentrated ova and parasite tests (Table 19-11).

Infection in Immigrants

There are at least 1 million immigrants to the United States yearly, mostly from Asia and Latin America [36]. Immigrants usually move from developing to developed countries. Developing-world peoples are a majority of immigrants to developed nations; for example, 84% of 643,000 immigrants to the United States in 1988 were of Latin-American or Asian origin [37]. While many of the diseases of immigrants and travelers are the same, the pres-

Table 19-11. Intestinal parasites

Disease and comments	Distribution	Medication	Comments
Amebiasis (trophozoites best seen in wet prep)	Widespread in tropics	Metronidazole (750 mg tid for 5 days); if symptomatic follow by iodoquinol	Metronidazole carcinogenic in rodents and mutagenic in bacteria; best avoided in pregnancy, especially first trimester; can cause antabuse reaction and GI and CNS symptoms.
Ascariasis (roundworm) (usually asymptomatic although massive infections cause pain and GI obstruction; migrates through lungs and can cause pulmonary symptoms)	Worldwide	Mebendazole (100 mg bid for 3 days, all ages), pyrantel pamoate (11 mg/kg once, max. 1 g)	All family members should be treated; mebendazole can cause diarrhea or abdominal pain, rarely agranulocytosis; pyrantel pamoate can cause GI disturbance, headache, rash, fever.
Clonorchiasis (adults reside in the biliary tree and cause hepatic symptoms)	Far East	Praziquantel (25 mg/kg tid × 2d)	Can cause GI disturbance or abdominal pain, rarely agranulocytosis.
Diphyllobothrium (fish) (caused by eating raw fresh water or anadromous fish)	Worldwide	Praziquantel (10–20 mg/kg once) or niclosamide (2 g chewed and swallowed, once; 11–34 kg, 1 g; 35–50 kg, 1.5 g)	Often causes malaise, headache, dizziness; can cause abdominal pain, fever, eosinophilia, rash.
Enterobiasis (pinworm) (causes perianal itching)	Worldwide, especially tropics	Mebendazole (100 mg once, all ages), pyrantel pamoate (11 mg/kg once, max. 1 g); repeat in 2 weeks	All family members should be treated; mebendazole can cause diarrhea or abdominal pain, rarely agranulocytosis; pyrantel pamoate may cause GI disturbance, headache, rash, fever.
Giardiasis (trophozoites best seen in wet prep)	Worldwide	Metronidazole (250 mg tid for 5 days), quinacrine Hcl (100 mg tid before meals for 5 days; 2 mg/kg tid for children)	Metronidazole carcinogenic in rodents and mutagenic in bacteria; best avoided in pregnancy, especially first trimester; can cause antabuse reaction, GI and CNS symptoms.
Hookworm infection (two species enter through bare feet [ground itch]; migrate through lungs and can cause pulmonary symptoms)	Worldwide, especially tropics	Mebendazole (100 mg bid for 3 days, all ages), pyrantel pamoate (11 mg/kg × 3d, max. 1 g/d)	All family members should be treated; mebendazole can cause diarrhea or abdominal pain, rarely agranulocytosis; pyrantel pamoate can cause GI disturbance, headache, rash, fever.

Infection	Distribution	Treatment	Comments
Paragonimiasis (pulmonary findings much more common than intestinal symptoms; migrates through lungs and may cause pulmonary symptoms)	Widespread in tropics	Praziquantel (25 mg/kg tid × 2d)	Can cause GI disturbance, headache, rash, fever.
Schistosoma japonicum infection	Japan, China, Philippines	Praziquantel (20 mg/kg/d divided tid for 1 day)	Often causes malaise, headache, dizziness; can cause abdominal pain, fever, eosinophilia, rash.
Schistosoma mansoni infection	Widespread in tropics, including Caribbean, Brazil, Near and Far East	Praziquantel (20 mg/kg/d divided tid for 1 day)	Often causes malaise, headache, dizziness; can cause abdominal pain, fever, eosinophilia, rash.
Schistosoma mekongi infection	Thailand, Cambodia, Laos	Praziquantel (20 mg/kg/d divided tid for 1 day)	Often causes malaise, headache, dizziness; can cause abdominal pain, fever, eosinophilia, rash.
Schistosomiasis (S. haematobium ova rarely passed in stools)			
Strongyloidiasis (larva, not ova, passed in stools; migrate through lungs and can cause pulmonary symptoms)	Southern U.S. and tropics	Thiabendazole (50 mg/kg/d divided bid for 2 days) (max. 3 g/d)	In disseminated disease and immuno-compromised patients treatment should be continued for at least 5 days. Often causes nausea, vomiting, vertigo; can cause leukopenia, CNS disturbances, erythema multiforme, convulsions, shock.
Taenia solium (pork) (larvae cause cysticercosis)	Worldwide, especially tropics and Eastern Europe	Praziquantel (10–20 mg/kg once) or niclosamide (2 g chewed and swallowed, once; 11–34 kg, 1 g; 35–50 kg, 1.5 g)	Often causes malaise, headache, dizziness; can cause abdominal pain, fever, eosinophilia, rash.
Tapeworm infection* Taenia saginata (beef) (usually asymptomatic)	Worldwide	Praziquantel (10–20 mg/kg once)	Often causes malaise, headache, dizziness; can cause abdominal pain, fever, eosinophilia, rash.
Trichuriasis (whipworm) (heavy infections can cause diffuse GI symptoms or even dysentery)	Worldwide	Mebendazole (100 mg bid for 3 days, all ages)	Can cause diarrhea or abdominal pain, rarely agranulocytosis.

*Echinococcosis is purely a tissue infection and is not covered here.

entation of these diseases differs enough that infection in immigrants is discussed separately.

Many immigrants are refugees and displaced persons from war and civil strife. Especially in refugees malnutrition is an important factor in the high mortality from measles, diarrheal disease, and acute respiratory infections [38]. Immigrants and travelers will of course get many of the same diseases. Immigrants often have chronic forms of diseases, such as schistosomiasis and amebiasis, or may be asymptomatic until an acute complication makes them seek medical attention. Some diseases, such as Brill-Zinsser disease (recurrence of epidemic typhus) and rabies, can appear years after the initial attack [39, 40].

There are often language barriers to obtaining a history that can be only partially overcome with an interpreter—details and nuance often are lost. Fear of a foreign medical system may cause an immigrant to delay in seeking appropriate medical attention, and cultural differences can mean that immigrants seek traditional healers before practitioners of "Western medicine" [36].

Large cities often have changing populations, but border areas and coastal cities usually have immigration patterns that are more predictable. Physicians should become knowledgable about disease prevalence and diagnosis in their communities, for example, amebic liver abscess as a cause of right upper quadrant pain in immigrants from Mexico and Clonorchis sinensis as a cause of cholangitis in immigrants from Asia [41, 42].

The physician should not assume that immigrants have had a screening examination. There are two major categories of visas to the United States: temporary visas for tourists and students and immigrant visas for persons planning to become U.S. citizens. Persons applying for a temporary visa need only complete a general two-page questionnaire and are asked to respond yes or no to whether they have contagious diseases or have suffered serious mental illness. Persons who are asymptomatic or who have an overwhelming desire to enter the United States obviously will answer no. The focus of the consular officer's inquiry is only to establish that the temporary immigrant will return to the country of origin and not overstay the visa [43]. All permanent immigrants get a standard screening examination on arrival in the United States by a physician contracted by the U.S. Immigration and Naturalization Service. The reasons for refusal are mental retardation, insanity, narcotic drug addiction or chronic alcoholism, and dangerous contagious diseases defined as active tuberculosis, Hansen's disease (leprosy), chancroid, gonorrhea, granuloma inguinale, lymphogranuloma venereum, and active syphilis. The main focus is to prevent aliens from becoming public charges. It is clear that a great many infectious diseases will not be screened and others will be asymptomatic [44]. See Table 19-6 for a summary of major clinical features of some of the important diseases discussed in this chapter.

Common Illnesses

Intestinal parasites are common in immigrants. Thirty-two percent of Southeast Asian refugees were found to have at least one intestinal parasite [45]. The most common intestinal parasites in Southeast Asian immigrants are hookworm, Giardia, strongyloides, and Hymenolepis nana; the most common parasites in Central American immigrants are trichuris, Giardia, and ascaris [45, 46]. Table 19-11 lists the diseases caused by intestinal parasites, their distribution, and treatment.

Tuberculosis remains an important world health problem, with 3 million deaths each year [47]. Twenty-four percent of the tuberculosis cases reported to the CDC in 1987 were in people born outside the United States. Schistosomiasis is especially common in immigrants from Puerto Rico and Yemen [48]. Other communicable diseases long since under control in the United States, including measles, rickettsial disease, hepatitis B, diphtheria, and typhoid fever, need to be considered in immigrants even though they may have been screened at the port of entry.

Eosinophilia is a common laboratory finding of people in developing countries and may offer a helpful clue to diagnostic possibilities (Table 19-12). In many cases it is caused by tissue-invading helminths and is often accompanied by vague abdominal pain. In some immigrants with eosinophilia a definitive diagnosis may not be possible; however, if combined with other clinical signs and symptoms it can be helpful.

Table 19-12. Conditions associated with peripheral eosinophilia

Parasites		Other diseases
Organism	Diseases	
Ancylostoma duodenale	Hookworm	Drug reactions
Anisakis species	Anisakiasis	Eosinophilic gastroenteritis
Ascaris lumbricoides	Ascariasis	Eosinophilia-myalgia syndrome
Brugia malayi	Filariasis	Hypereosinophilic syndromes
Clonorchis sinensis	Clonorchiasis	Inflammatory bowel disease
Dracunculus medinensis	Dracunculiasis	Malignancy
Echinococcus granulosus	Echinococcosis	Polyarteritis nodosa
Fasciola hepatica	Fascioliasis	Seasonal and environmental allergies
Loa loa	Loiasis	Tropical pulmonary eosinophilia
Necator americanus	Hookworm	
Onchocerca volvulus	Onchocerciasis	
Opisthorchis species	Opisthorchiasis	
Paragonimus westermani	Paragonimiasis	
Schistosoma species	Schistosomiasis	
Strongyloides stercoralis	Strongyloidiasis	
Toxocara species	Visceral larva migrans	
Wuchereria bancrofti	Filariasis	

Source: Manson-Bahr PEC, Apted FIC (eds.), *Manson's Tropical Diseases* (18th ed.). London: Bailliere Tindall, 1982. Pp. 38–71, 94–104. Used with permission.

Selected Syndromes in Immigrants

CNS SYMPTOMS

Cysticercosis. Cysticercosis is caused by infection with the larval form of the pig tapeworm *Taenia solium*. It is a major cause of morbidity in areas of Central and South America, Africa, India, and China. The adult parasite is rare in residents of North America, mainly because hogs in North America do not have access to human feces. Humans act as both definitive hosts and intermediate hosts, while pigs act only as intermediate hosts. Humans acquire the adult tapeworm by eating undercooked pork containing mature larvae. These cysticerci develop into adult tapeworms that reside in the human intestine and seldom cause symptoms (intermediate host). The clinical syndrome of cysticercosis develops when food or water contaminated by human feces containing tapeworm eggs is ingested. When ingested by human beings or swine, the eggs hatch in the small intestine, burrow into venules, and are carried to distant sites, usually the muscles and the brain. The eggs develop into

mature larvae, or cysticerci, that cause clinical symptoms. The incubation period for human cysticercosis ranges from 1–30 years [49]. Autoinfection can occur when persons infected with adult tapeworms contaminate their hands and ingest eggs. Patients who present with CNS manifestations may not have adult tapeworms in the GI tract; therefore, the stool ova and parasite (O & P) examination will be negative [50].

Cysticercosis can cause a variety of signs and symptoms, but the majority are CNS manifestations. The most common presentation is focal or generalized seizures, which occur in 30%–92% of patients. Headache, nausea, vomiting, and cranial nerve abnormalities may occur, depending on the location of the cysticerci. Cysts may also occur in clusters in the pia-arachnoid, or the larvae may migrate within ventricles, causing obstructive hydrocephalus and chronic granulomatous meningitis.

The diagnosis of cysticercosis should be suspected in any immigrant from an endemic country who presents with seizures or focal neurologic signs. Diagnosis has been greatly enhanced by the use of

CT scanning. Single or multiple cysticercial cysts usually appear as hypodense cystic lesions, but they may appear isodense or hyperdense. Administration of contrast material demonstrates ring enhancement [51]. Occasionally the presence of subcutaneous cysts that are available for biopsy provides the definitive diagnosis in combination with CT scanning. Currently an enzyme-linked immunoelectrotransfer blot (EITB) assay has been developed that is 98% sensitive and 100% specific [52]. Patients from endemic areas with neurologic symptoms should be screened by EITB.

Praziquantel, 50 mg/kg/day in three divided doses for 14 days, produces clinical improvement or cure in the majority of patients and with few side effects. Albendazole is a less expensive alternative. Corticosteroids often are used to suppress exacerbations of symptoms associated with treatment, most likely due to death of the cysts [19].

African Trypanosomiasis and Schistosomiasis.
West African immigrants may have chronic nonspecific neurologic symptoms from trypanosomiasis (see the section on trypanosomiasis earlier in this chapter).

Chronic *S. japonicum* is a major cause of focal epilepsy in Southeast Asia (see the sections on chronic schistosomiasis elsewhere in this chapter).

CARDIAC INVOLVEMENT
American Trypanosomiasis (Chagas' Disease).
Chagas' disease is a relatively common disease of tropical South America, particularly Brazil, Venezuela, and northern Argentina. The causative organism, *Trypanosoma cruzi*, is spread by reduviid bugs, also known as "kissing bugs." The infectious organism is common in many species of wild and domestic animals. Acute Chagas' disease is primarily a disease of children. A contaminated bite may produce an erythematous nodule. Most acute cases are asymptomatic or have only mild symptoms, but fever, lymphadenopathy, hepatosplenomegaly, myocarditis, and meningitis can occur. Trypanosomes are present in the peripheral blood and can be diagnosed with a blood smear. The acute phase passes over a few weeks, and the patient enters an asymptomatic phase that may last for life. Late Chagas' disease is typified by dilated cardiomyopathy, abnormal conduction with varying degrees of heart

block, and sudden death. The GI tract often is involved, with esophageal and colonic megacolon presenting as vomiting and constipation. Diagnosis is based on a typical clinical pattern, a positive serologic test, and in endemic areas xenodiagnosis using uninfected bugs. Chemotherapy is problematic. The available agents, nifurtimox and benzonidazole, are usually effective during acute Chagas' disease; however, no agents have much effect on the chronic symptoms, and symptomatic treatment is all that can be offered most patients. Prevention consists of the use of insecticides and avoidance of poorly thatched rural structures as sleeping quarters [53].

CUTANEOUS LESIONS
Leishmaniasis. Leishmaniasis is a widespread protozoan disease caused by an obligate intracellular parasite and with a spectrum of manifestations ranging from a cutaneous sore to visceral involvement. Wild rodents or domestic dogs, depending on the locale, are the animal reservoirs. Cutaneous leishmaniasis has an Old World form caused by *Leishmania tropica* and *Leishmania major*, with a distribution in southern Europe, Russia, Asia, and parts of Africa. The New World cutaneous form, caused by *Leishmania brasiliensis*, *Leishmania mexicana*, and other subtypes, is found throughout tropical South America, Central America, and the Yucatan area of Mexico. The disease-causing flagellated promastigotes are transmitted by the bite of the gnat-sized phlebotomine sandfly. Cutaneous disease usually begins as an erythematous macule at the site of the bite. The organisms change into amastigotes and multiply within macrophages, producing cutaneous ulcers on the face or limbs. The ulcers often persist for as long as a year, and particularly with *L. brasiliensis* mucocutaneous disease can cause extensive disfiguring lesions of the face.

The diagnosis should be suspected in anyone with a nonhealing ulcer who has been to an area of risk. The differential diagnosis of the cutaneous ulcer includes *Mycobacterium marinium*, yaws, and fungal ulcers such as sporotrichosis. The diagnosis is made by biopsy or aspiration of ulcer margins.

Sodium stibogluconate, a 10% pentavalent antimony compound, is the most effective drug, although toxic. It may be ineffective in patients with severe disease [54]. Amphotericin B has been effective in refractory cases [19]. Ketoconazole has been used with good results in cutaneous leishmaniasis and may also have potential in the treatment of visceral leishmaniasis [55]. Old World cutaneous ulcers usually heal spontaneously and may not require treatment. Only disfiguring New World ulcers and kala-azar usually require treatment.

Avoiding the sandfly bite by using netting, protective clothing, and insect repellent is the best way to avoid the disease, although the tiny size of the sandfly makes avoidance difficult.

Leprosy (Hansen's Disease). Leprosy is a chronic disease caused by Mycobacterium leprae. Leprosy is most common in Southeast Asia, sub-Saharan Africa, and India. It has, however, been reported from all parts of the world, and low-grade indigenous foci exist in the southwestern United States. Leprosy is an extremely indolent, slowly evolving infection with an incubation period as long as 20 years. Infection usually starts as a hypopigmented or mildly erythematous macule with subjective changes in sensation (indeterminate leprosy). Fully developed leprosy tends toward one of two forms, although most patients have some stigmata of both. Tuberculoid leprosy typically causes sharply demarcated macules with decreased sensation and hair loss within the macules. Peripheral nerve trunks commonly are damaged, and nerves may become palpable as they are infiltrated by bacteria. The loss of digits and damaged feet is secondary to loss of protective sensation and recurrent injury. Lepromatous leprosy is typified by slowly growing nodules within plaques, particularly in the cooler areas of skin, such as the arms and the face. These nodules are caused by direct infiltration by M. leprae, and the concentration of bacteria becomes enormous in the lesions. Diagnosis may be confirmed by biopsy of the lesions. Treatment requires long-term, multiple drug regimes, including dapsone, rifampin, and clofazimine. Despite its reputation leprosy is one of the least contagious of all contagious diseases, and no isolation is warranted [56].

HEPATITIS/JAUNDICE

The risk of all types of viral hepatitis is increased in travelers and immigrants, due to large reservoirs of infection and poor sanitary conditions. Vaccination and prophylaxis with immunoglobulin and meticulous purification of water greatly reduce the risk to the traveler.

Viral Hepatitis. Hepatitis B, by causing cirrhosis and hepatocellular cancer, is a major source of morbidity in the developing world. Non-A, non-B hepatitis and hepatitis C, which are major causes of transfusion-associated hepatitis, have also been associated with epidemic outbreaks [57].

Amebic Liver Abscess. A particular risk in immigrants is amebic liver abscess. The constellation of fever, leukocytosis, and right upper quadrant pain or tenderness, particularly in a male from a developing country, should remind the physician of this relatively common complication of chronic amebic infection. Ultrasound is diagnostic in nearly 100% of cases, and treatment with metronidazole is curative. This diagnosis must be made as quickly as possible; otherwise, the patient is likely to be subjected to needless surgery [41].

Clonorchis Sinensis. The Chinese, or oriental, liver fluke infects millions of people in China and southeast Asia. People become infected after consuming raw fish grown in ponds contaminated by animal or human feces. Most people are asymptomatic, but immigrants with a heavy fluke burden may present years after immigration with pyogenic cholangitis, in which bile ducts are occluded by the parasites. There is also a strong association between clonorchiasis and cholangiocarcinoma [58].

HEPATOSPLENOMEGALY

Schistosomiasis. In the United States an estimated 200,000 persons are infected with schistosomes, mostly immigrants from Puerto Rico, Brazil, the Middle East, and Southeast Asia [59]. Immigrants are most likely to suffer from chronic exposure to schistosomes. Chronic symptoms of schistosomiasis affect mostly children and adolescents who live in areas endemic for schistosomiasis [23]. With chronic S. mansoni infection, eggs deposited in the liver result in granuloma formation and fibrosis, which ultimately lead to hepatosplenomegaly and portal hypertension. The first manifestation of schistosomiasis may be hematoma and melena, and the usual cause of death is exsanguination. Egg deposits can occur in other organs, such as the vasculature of the lungs, with resulting pulmonary hypertension. The clinical manifestations of chronic infection with S. japonicum are similar to S. mansoni infection with two exceptions: S. japonicum has a much greater egg burden and is a major cause of focal epilepsy in Asia due to the deposits of egg aggregates in the venous system of the brain. Infection with S. mekongi is similar to S. japonicum infection, and treatment is the same [60]. S. haematobium causes urinary tract symptoms: dysuria, hematuria, and frequency. Eggs deposited in the urinary bladder and ureters cause granuloma formation, which obstructs urine flow, causing hydronephrosis and hydroureter. Carcinoma of the bladder has been associated with chronic S. haematobium infection.

Definitive diagnosis is made by detecting ova in the stool or urine. Ova may not be detected, especially in the immigrant. ELISA is a sensitive test but does not identify the species. Rectal biopsy may need to be performed if the suspicion is high and other tests are negative [24].

Single-day therapy with praziquantel 40–60 mg/kg is effective against all species of schistosomes. The treatment is divided into two or three doses over 1 day [19].

Visceral Leishmaniasis (Kala-azar). Some species of Leishmania disseminate hematogenously to the liver, spleen, bone marrow, and lymph nodes to cause visceral leishmaniasis, or kala-azar. Subtypes that cause visceral disease occur in India, Central and South America, Asia, southern Europe, and Africa. This form may present after an incubation period of 3–6 months with periodic fever. Immigrants may present with intermittent or relapsing fever that mimics malaria. The skin becomes dry and scaly. Petechiae and edema occur as massive splenomegaly develops. Jaundice is uncommon, but there is usually hepatomegaly. The typical patient with chronic kala-azar is emaciated with massive hepatosplenomegaly, petechiae, and edema. The disease is more common in children, and the petechiae with splenomegaly may cause it to be confused with leukemia. Many people in endemic areas develop immunity or have subclinical infection. During a 1975 epidemic in a valley in Italy clinical infection developed in 3% of the population while

there was an attack rate of 44% [61–67]. The disease has remarkably similar clinical features in all parts of the world.

Visceral disease should be considered in an immigrant or a traveler with fever; splenomegaly should add to the suspicion. Bone marrow aspiration with identification of Leishman-Donovan bodies and culture is the highest yield method to diagnose kala-azar. Demonstration of Leishman-Donovan bodies in a splenic aspirate may also yield the diagnosis. Skin tests and serology provide indirect evidence that should prompt a search for a definitive diagnosis.

Malaria. Immigrants usually do not present with P. falciparum malaria because of the short incubation period. However, drug prophylaxis may suppress the initial attack for weeks, and partial immunity can modify later attacks of P. falciparum, so that the immigrant may present with a tertian periodic fever like that of P. vivax. Immigrants with malaria will more likely present with hepatosplenomegaly or a relapsing fever characteristic of P. vivax, P. ovale, and P. malariae. They may lose their partial suppressive immunity on emigrating and develop relapsing fever.

Hepatosplenomegaly is often diagnosed as malaria empirically without laboratory confirmation in an endemic area. Splenomegaly with few other symptoms may be especially common in children, so much so that malaria prevalence is often estimated by the spleen rate or the proportion of children aged 2–10 who have enlarged spleens [62]. Immigrants from malaria-endemic areas may have a tropical splenomegaly syndrome manifested by hepatosplenomegaly, weight loss, anemia, and neutropenia.

The cause of this syndrome is not known. Patients have high antibody titers to plasmodia without circulating parasites and respond to antimalaria drugs, although the disease has a high mortality. This syndrome may represent a variant immune response to chronic malaria infection [13].

INTESTINAL PARASITES
Intestinal parasites are usually found as an incidental finding on O and P tests or in asymptomatic immigrants. (See Table 19-11 for a summary of their clinical importance and treatment.)

References

1. Bruce-Chwatt LJ. Global problems of imported disease. *Adv Parasitol* 11:75–114, 1973.
2. NIH Consensus Development Conference. Travelers' diarrhea. *JAMA* 253:2700–04, 1985.
3. Cossar JH, Reid D. Health hazards of international travel. *World Health Stat Q* 42:61–69, 1989.
4. Warren KS. Tropical diseases of travelers and migrants. In KS Warren, AAF Mahmoud (eds.), *Tropical and Geographical Medicine*. New York: McGraw-Hill, 1984. Pp. 1122–28.
5. Recommendations for the prevention of malaria among travelers. *MMWR* 39RR-3:1–16, 1990.
6. McKinney WP. Travelers' immunizations [letter]. *JAMA* 264:1812, 1990.
7. Cossar JH, Reid D. Health hazards of international travel. *World Health Stat Q* 42:61–69, 1989.
8. Insect repellents. *Med Lett Drugs Ther* 31:45–47, 1989.
9. Wyler DJ. Malaria-resurgence, resistance, and research (part I). *N Engl J Med* 308:875–78, 1983.
10. Division of Control of Tropical Diseases. World malaria situation, 1988. *World Health Stat Q* 43:68–78, 1990.
11. Greenburg AE, Lobel HO. Mortality from *Plasmodium falciparum* malaria in travelers from the United States, 1959 to 1987. *Ann Intern Med* 113:326–27, 1990.
12. Miller LH. Malaria. In KS Warren, AAF Mahmoud (eds.), *Tropical and Geographical Medicine*. New York: McGraw-Hill, 1984. Pp. 223–39.
13. Wyler DJ. Malaria. In GL Mandell, RG Douglas, JE Bennett (eds.), *Principles and Practice of Infectious Diseases*. New York: Churchill-Livingstone, 1990. Pp. 2056–66.
14. Brewster DR, Kwiatkowski D, White NJ. Neurological sequelae of cerebral malaria in children. *Lancet* 336:1039–43, 1990.
15. Phillips RE, Solomon T. Cerebral malaria in children. *Lancet* 336:1355–60, 1990.
16. Nussenzweig RS, Nussenzweig V. Antisporozoite vaccine for malaria: experimental basis and current status. *Rev Infect Dis* 11(suppl. 3):S579–85, 1989.
17. Change in mefloquine prophylaxis for malaria. *Med Lett Drugs Ther* 32:98, 1990.
18. Kozarsky PE, Lobel HO, Steppen R. Travel medicine 1991: new frontiers. ed. *Ann Intern Med* 115:574–75, 1991.
19. Drugs for parasitic infections. *Med Lett Drugs Ther* 32:23–30, 1990.
20. Mefloquine for malaria. *Med Lett Drugs Ther* 31:13–14, 1990.
21. CDC Drug Service. Treatment with quinidine gluconate of persons with severe *Plasmodium falciparum* infection: discontinuation of parenteral quinine. *MMWR* 40:21–23, 1991.
22. Miller KD, Greenburg AE, Campbell CC. Treatment of severe malaria in the United States with a continuous infusion of quinidine gluconate and exchange transfusion. *N Engl J Med* 321:65–70, 1989.
23. Doehring E. Schistosomiasis in childhood. *Eur J Pediatr* 147:2–9, 1988.
24. Mahmoud AAF. Schistosomiasis. In KS Warren, AAF Mahmoud (eds.), *Tropical and Geographical Medicine*. New York: McGraw-Hill, 1984. Pp. 443–460.
25. Centers for Disease Control. *Health Information for International Travel*. Atlanta: CDC, 1990. Pp. 116–17.
26. Centers for Disease Control. Acute schistosomiasis in US travelers returning from Africa. *MMWR* 39:141–48, 1990.
27. Centers for Disease Control. Yellow fever vaccine. *MMWR* 39, RR-6:1–6, 1990.
28. Monath TP. Yellow fever: a medically neglected disease. Report on a seminar. *Rev Infect Dis* 9:165–75, 1987.
29. Dengue and dengue hemorrhagic fever in the Americas, 1986. *MMWR* 37:129–31, 1988.
30. Caribbean: dengue epidemic. *Lancet* 336:236–37, 1990.
31. Dembert ML et al. Medical advice for foreign travel. *Milit Med* 151:211, 1986.
32. Taylor DN et al. Polymicrobial aetiology of travelers' diarrhoea. *Lancet* 1:381–83, 1985.
33. Dupont HL et al. Chemotherapy and chemoprophylaxis of travelers' diarrhea [editorial]. *Ann Intern Med* 102:260–61, 1985.
34. Blaser MJ. Environmental interventions for the prevention of travelers' diarrhea. *Rev Infect Dis* 8 (suppl. 2):S142–50, 1986.
35. Nahlen BL et al. International travel and the child younger than two years: II. Recommendations for prevention of travelers' diarrhea and malaria chemoprophylaxis. *Pediatr Infect Dis J* 8:735–39, 1989.
36. Kraut AM. Healers and strangers. Immigrant attitudes toward the physician in America: a relationship in historical perspective. *JAMA* 263:1807–11, 1990.
37. U.S. Department of Justice. *Statistical Yearbook of the Immigration and Naturalization Service*. Washington, DC: Immigration and Naturalization Service, U.S. Department of Justice, 1988.
38. Toole MF, Waldman RJ. Prevention of excess mortality in refugee and displaced populations in developing countries. *JAMA* 263:3296–302, 1990.

39. Green CR, Fishbein D, Gleiberman I. Brill-Zinsser: still with us [letter]. JAMA 264:1811–12, 1990.

40. Smith JS et al. Unexplained rabies in three immigrants in the United States. A virologic investigation. N Engl J Med 324:205–11, 1991.

41. Dozema D, Hauswald M. Amebic liver abscess: emergency department diagnosis. Am J Emerg Med 6:628–30, 1988.

42. Scully RE et al. Case records of the Massachusetts General Hospital. N Engl J Med 323:467–75, 1990.

43. Meyer B. Immigrants, international travelers, and HIV [letter]. N Engl J Med 323:1491–92, 1990.

44. U.S. Public Health Service. Guidelines for the Medical Examination of Aliens. U.S. Department of Health and Human Services. Atlanta: Centers for Disease Control, Division of Quarantine, 1985.

45. Molina CD, Molina MM, Molina JM. Intestinal parasites in Southeast Asian refugees two years after immigration. West J Med 149:422–25, 1988.

44. Salas SD, Heifetz R, Barrett-Connor E. Intestinal parasites in Central American immigrants in the United States. Arch Intern Med 150:1514–16, 1990.

47. Bloch AB et al. The epidemiology of tuberculosis in the United States. Implications for diagnosis and treatment. Clin Chest Med 10:297–313, 1989.

48. Warren KS. Helminthic diseases endemic in the United States. Am J Trop Med Hyg 23:723–28, 1974.

49. Pawlowski Z. Cestode infections. In KS Warren, AAF Mahmoud (eds.), Tropical and Geographical Medicine. New York: McGraw-Hill, 1984. Pp. 474–75.

50. Nash TE, Neva FA. Recent advances in the diagnosis and treatment of cerebral cysticercosis. N Engl J Med 311:1492–96, 1984.

51. Case Records of the Massachusetts General Hospital. Weekly clinicopathological exercises. Case 20-1990. A 16 year old boy with a lesion of the frontal lobe. N Engl J Med 322:1446–58, 1990.

52. Tsang VC, Brand JA, Boyer AE. An enzyme-linked immunoelectrotransfer blot assay and glycoprotein antigens for diagnosing human cysticercosis (taenia solium). J Infect Dis 159:50–59, 1989.

53. Kirchhoff LV, Gam AA, Gilliam FC. American trypanosomiasis (Chagas' disease) in Central American immigrants. Am J Med 82:915–20, 1987.

54. Franke ED et al. Efficacy and toxicity of sodium stibogluconate for mucosal leishmaniasis. Ann Intern Med 113:934–40, 1990.

55. Wali JP et al. Ketoconazole in treatment of visceral leishmaniasis. Lancet 336:810–11, 1990.

56. Pust RE, Campos-Outcalt D. Leprosy in the United States. Postgrad Med 77:151–59, 1985.

57. Velazquez O et al. Epidemic transmission of enterically transmitted non-A, non-B hepatitis in Mexico, 1986–1987. JAMA 263:3281–85, 1990.

58. Case Records of the Massachusetts General Hospital. Case 33-1990. N Engl J Med 323:467–75, 1990.

59. Warren KS. Helminthic diseases in the United States. Am J Trop Med Hyg 23:723–29, 1974.

60. Mahmoud AAF. Schistosomiasis: current concepts. N Engl J Med 297:4–6, 1977.

61. Kala-azar. In PEC Manson-Bahr, FIC Apted (eds.), Manson's Tropical Diseases (18th ed.). London: Bailliere Tindall, 1982. Pp. 94–104.

62. Malaria and babesiosis. In PEC Manson-Bahr, FIC Apted (eds.), Manson's Tropical Diseases (18th ed.). London: Bailliere Tindall, 1982. Pp. 38–71.

63. Centers for Disease Control. Health Information for International Travel. Updated yearly and available from the Superintendent of Documents, U.S. Government Printing Office, Washington, DC 20402, 202-783-3238.

64. Drugs for parasitic infections. Med Lett Drugs Ther 32:23–30, 1990.

65. Strickland GT (ed.). Hunter's Tropical Medicare (6th ed.). Philadelphia: Saunders, 1984.

66. PEC Manson-Bahr, FIC Apted (eds.). Manson's Tropical Diseases (18th ed.). London: Bailliere Tindall, 1982.

67. KS Warren, AAF Mahmoud (eds.). Tropical and Geographical Medicine. New York: McGraw-Hill, 1984.

20

Infection in the Patient with Alternative Living Circumstances

KNOX H. TODD
DAVID A. TALAN

The emergency department is often the sole source of medical care for those without access to traditional providers of primary care. This chapter addresses infectious diseases encountered in four groups of patients: the homeless, the incarcerated, the institutionalized, and the bed-bound. Infectious diseases common in these populations and factors that may influence the physician's ability to evaluate and treat them effectively will be covered. The chapter concludes with a discussion of compliance issues pertinent to these populations and to emergency department patients in general. Many infections discussed in this chapter have broad impacts on public health, and the benefits of appropriate evaluation and treatment of these high-risk patients are magnified in the community as a whole. The reader should refer to other sections of the text for a more detailed description of specific disease entities. Infection in the nursing home patient is discussed in Chap. 15.

The Homeless

It is estimated that there are at least 735,000 homeless persons in the United States and that in 1988 1.3–2.0 million persons were homeless at some time [1]. In addition to the stereotypical urban male alcoholic, the homeless population includes significant numbers of women, adolescents, and families with children [2]. Although medical disorders of the homeless are common, barriers to traditional sources of health care for this population are many, and the emergency department often serves as a primary provider of routine medical and social services. Researchers in San Francisco interviewed 170 homeless persons; 75% reported receiving medical care within the previous year, and 76% of these contacts were in an emergency department [3].

Physical and mental health problems can primarily cause, result from, or complicate homelessness. Psychiatric and substance use disorders are common causes of homelessness. A recent study of Baltimore homeless persons found a history of major mental disorder in 42% of men and 49% of women and a history of alcoholism or substance use disorder in 75% of men and 38% of women [4]. Homelessness increases the risk of many health problems, including trauma [5], respiratory diseases (particularly tuberculosis) [6], diseases of the extremities, including varicose veins, skin ulcers, and cellulitis [7], parasitic infestations, and periodontal disease [8]. Homelessness complicates any general health problem that requires adequate nutrition, bed rest, hygiene, medication, or frequent clinic visits.

Barriers to adequate health care for those who are homeless are numerous. Lack of medical insurance or money, problems with transportation, long waiting times at public hospitals or clinics, and negative attitudes of health care providers may discourage the homeless from seeking care.

Many homeless women have a history of past sexual abuse, which may lead to an avoidance of pelvic examinations. After medical evaluation the homeless patient may be unable to comply with treatment recommendations for various reasons. Illiteracy often renders written instruction useless [9]. The patient may misunderstand, and family members are unavailable to reinforce instructions. The cost of medication or supplies may be prohibitive. Routine discharge instructions such as "bed rest and elevation of extremity" may be impossible to follow. For those reasons health problems that might have been treated easily at an earlier stage often present to the emergency department in advanced stages and require inpatient treatment. Because homeless persons often present to the emergency department in the later stages of illness and because there is a shortage of community services to provide for outpatient care, they frequently require hospital admission. An experienced social work department should be available to the emergency department to optimize the utilization of community resources. In many private hospitals if a patient is to be treated as an outpatient, follow-up often includes a referral to a private subspecialist. This is unrealistic for most homeless patients, and more appropriate resources need to be identified.

The emergency department may be an important site for preventive care in the homeless. This population is more likely to be underimmunized against a variety of preventable infections. One recent study supported the administration of pneumococcal and influenza vaccines as part of routine emergency department care [10]. Immunization against tetanus and diphtheria is also appropriate. Other immunizations, such as against pneumococcus, influenza, and hepatitis B, should be considered. Information about alcohol and drug treatment programs as well as referrals to mental health centers, shelters, and other social services may be appropriate.

Soft-Tissue Infection

Cellulitis is the most common diagnosis of homeless inpatients, accounting for 12%–24% of discharge diagnoses [3, 11]. Predisposing factors for the development of cellulitis include prolonged standing with resultant dependent edema, pressure necrosis, venous insufficiency, and skin ulcers; minor trauma; alcoholism; intravenous drug use; and parasitic and fungal infections.

Whereas *Staphylococcus aureus* and *Streptococcus pyogenes* are the most common etiologies of uncomplicated soft-tissue infections in this population, these patients also are at risk for complicated infection involving other pathogens. The tendency for chronic and lower-extremity infection increases the likelihood of mixed infections with gram-negative bacilli and anaerobes in addition to S. *aureus* and S. *pyogenes*. This is also true for extremity infections related to IV drug use or "skin popping" [12]. In the setting of puncture wounds to the foot, especially those through the shoe, *Pseudomonas aeruginosa* should be considered [13] (see Chap. 33).

Unusual infections also are found in this population. Between 1972 and 1982 947 cases of cutaneous diphtheria were diagnosed among alcoholics living in Seattle's Skid Row [14]. These lesions were nondescript, chronic, nonhealing ulcers that were rarely associated with the typical dirty-gray pharyngeal membrane and toxin-related disease.

Dental Infections

Not surprisingly the homeless population has a higher prevalence of dental and periodontal disease than the general public. A community-based survey in Los Angeles found that although 27% of the homeless surveyed reported a toothache in the past month, only 10% of those sought dental care [8]. This prevalence of dental disease increases the risk of other local infections, including dental abscess, facial cellulitis, Ludwig's angina (see Chap. 36), and actinomycosis, as well as associated disorders such as aspiration pneumonia, empyema (see Chap. 22), and infective endocarditis (see Chap. 24).

Dental infection initially manifests as localized tooth pain, but it may progress to produce gingival swelling, exudate, and surrounding facial cellulitis. Dental infections may track along deep fascial planes of the head and neck and produce characteristic symptoms, including trismus and mandible pain (masticator space), cheek swelling (buccal space), upper lid, canine fossa and periorbital swelling (canine space), or swelling at the angle of the jaw (parotid space). Ludwig"s angina denotes infection of the sublingual, submaxillary, and submandibular spaces that presents as sublingual and submandibular swelling. This infection can progress rapidly and lead to upper airway obstruction. Other local complications of dental infection include involvement of deep spaces of the neck, jugular vein thrombosis, carotid artery erosion, cavernous sinus thrombosis, and mandibular osteomyelitis.

Poor dental hygiene also predisposes to actinomycosis ("lumpy-jaw syndrome"). This infection may present as an acute suppurative infection of the fascial tissue planes, or it may be a chronic, slowly progressive infection characterized by tissue induration and draining cutaneous fistulas.

Dental disease also increases the risk of infective endocarditis. In this setting the infection is usually subacute and due to viridans streptococci or members of the HACEK group of bacteria (i.e., *Haemophilus aphrophilus, Actinobacillus actinomycetemcomitans, Cardiobacter hominis, Eikenella corrodens* and *Kingella kingii*). Low-grade fever, nonspecific constitutional symptoms, a cardiac murmur, splenomegaly, and peripheral manifestations of endocarditis should suggest the diagnosis. Laboratory evaluation characteristically demonstrates normochromic normocytic anemia, microscopic hematuria, and an elevated sedimentation rate.

Dental extraction is beyond the scope of most emergency departments but may be appropriate if trained personnel are available. Information on local public dental clinics should be available in the department for patient referral. The presence of facial cellulitis or suspicion of endocarditis warrants admission in this difficult-to-follow population.

Pneumonia

Although routine lower respiratory infections such as mycoplasmal and streptococcal pneumonia are common among the homeless, pneumonia resulting from aspiration is particularly common due to concomitant alcoholism. The course of typical aspiration pneumonia is insidious and tends to involve the superior segment of the lower lobe or the posterior segment of the upper lobe. These infections frequently cause necrotizing pneumonia, lung abscess, and empyema. Putrid sputum is noted in approximately 50% of cases. Usually these infections involve oral anaerobes such as *Bacteroides* and *Fusobacterium*, but in chronically ill individuals they are more likely to be due to *S. aureus* and gram-negative bacilli. Aspiration pneumonia generally requires admission for IV antibiotics, but the patient with routine community acquired pneumonia who is not toxic can be treated with oral erythromycin and reevaluated in 2 days.

Tuberculosis

Although the prevalence of tuberculosis has decreased in the general U.S. population, groups at high risk continue to exist among homeless, jail, and nursing home populations. The prevalence of latent tuberculosis among the homeless ranges from 18%–51% in different surveys [15–18], while clinically active tuberculosis exists in 1.6%–6.8% of the homeless screened at selected clinics and shelters [17, 19, 20]. Homeless persons have multiple risk factors for reactivation of tuberculosis, including poor nutrition, alcoholism, and psychological stress. In addition crowded shelters are ideal locations for primary infection or exogenous reinfection with tuberculosis [21].

Any respiratory symptoms among the homeless should raise the index of suspicion for tuberculosis. Although nonmycobacterial respiratory infections are common among the homeless, all homeless patients with a productive cough should be evaluated with at least a chest x-ray. Depending on local health care organization, the emergency department may be an appropriate location for screening asymptomatic high-risk persons, including the homeless.

Optimally the homeless with newly diagnosed tuberculosis should be hospitalized to ensure initiation of therapy and prevention of spread [22]. Public health officials should be notified early in the patient's hospital stay. Although long-term beds for the completion of antituberculous therapy are scarce [23], they may be necessary, particularly for the mentally ill. For the patient who refuses treatment, court-ordered confinement may be necessary [24, 25]. In certain special circumstances continued long-term outpatient treatment has been successful in this population; however, selection of antimicrobial agents may be a problem. If the patient has been partially treated in the past, organisms may be resistant to the standard medications.

Parasitic Infestations

Scabies and pediculosis are common diagnoses among the homeless, as in any population in which crowding and inadequate sanitation are present. *Pediculosis humanis corporis*, the body louse, can serve as the vector for *Rickettsia prowazekii*, the cause of louse-borne epidemic typhus, and *Borrelia recurrentis*, the cause of louse-borne relapsing fever [26]. Epidemic typhus is a rare disease in the United States, but it occurs frequently in other parts of the world where crowding and poor hygiene exist. As with other rickettsial diseases the onset of illness is abrupt, with fever, chills, myalgias, and an intense headache. There is no eschar, and a maculopapular or petechial rash begins after several days on the trunk and in the axillary folds.

Louse-borne *B. recurrentis* is a spirochetal disease that causes relapsing fever. It is also rare in the United States but endemic in many parts of the world. Following several days of rigors, headache, myalgias, arthralgias, photophobia, and cough, the patient improves. This improvement is followed by the recurrence of a milder febrile illness in 7–10 days (see Chap. 12). Additional recurrences are uncommon in the louse form of disease. The diagnosis of pubic lice should prompt a screen for other sexually transmitted diseases which will be found in one-half to one-third of those infested [26]. Treatment with gamma benzine hexachloride (Kwell) is generally successful, but reinfestation is frequent.

Sexually Transmitted Disease

Although precise statistics of the prevalence of sexually transmitted disease (STD) among homeless persons are not available, workers in health care clinics for the homeless note that complaints related to STD are common. Appropriate cultures should be obtained, along with a rapid plasma re-

agin (RPR) test, an HIV antibody test, and a pap test. A method for follow-up should be addressed. Because of the difficulties in following this population, presumptive treatment is mandatory (see Chap. 30). Dispensing medications at the time of diagnosis is important to ensure compliance. In many cities care is available at free or reduced cost from public STD clinics.

AIDS

The prevalence of human immunodeficiency virus (HIV) seropositivity and AIDS among the homeless is unknown. Because homelessness is associated with IV drug use and STDs, the prevalence of HIV-related disease should be higher than that in the general population. A recent retrospective survey of hospitalized AIDS patients in New York City found that 13% of patients were homeless on admission. Homeless AIDS patients were more likely to be black, Hispanic, or IV drug users than were nonhomeless AIDS patients. Homeless AIDS patients also were more likely to present with tuberculosis and were more likely to be noncompliant, with 50% signing out of the hospital against medical advice and 81% lost to medical follow-up [27].

In some settings the emergency department can play an important role in identifying patients who may have early HIV infection. Testing of HIV serology in appropriate risk groups can be important to identify asymptomatic HIV-infected patients and to allow for continued medical care and patient education regarding means to prevent the spread of their infection. If HIV-antibody testing is done, appropriate counseling and follow-up must be made available.

The evaluation of patients suspected of symptomatic HIV-related disease is covered in detail in Chap. 17. In the homeless population with AIDS there are unique concerns. Pneumonia may be due to causes other than *Pneumocystis carinii*, such as tuberculosis, aspiration, influenza, or pyogenic bacteria such as *Streptococcus pneumoniae*, *Haemophilus influenzae*, or *Klebsiella pneumoniae*. For CNS-related symptoms, besides the frequent infections of *Toxoplasma gondii* and *Cryptococcus neoformans*, etiologies that include meningovascular syphilis, tuberculosis, pyogenic brain abscess, and, among immigrants, cysticercosis should be considered.

The Incarcerated

The emergency physician frequently evaluates prisoners, either at the time of arrest or after a period of incarceration. These consultations generally occur at night and on weekends, when most arrests occur and when jail medical resources are unavailable. Many features can confound these evaluations, including problems with security, communication between the referring institution and the emergency physician, and poor prisoner cooperation [28]. Although the American Correctional Association has set standards for medical facilities in jails, medical care varies at each institution. In some prisons, screening tests—such as skin tests for tuberculosis, tetanus immunizations, and chest x-rays, are performed routinely. Physicians who treat patients from a specific correctional institution with any regularity should become familiar with the institution's standards and capabilities. Those physicians also should not assume that compliance is ensured. A patient may be only temporarily in police custody and released in a short time. Some institutions may change antibiotic prescriptions to cheaper drugs or to drugs that require administration less frequently (e.g., to qd or bid drugs).

The incarcerated population is generally young and generally male. Of 1,420 new admissions to New York City jails in 1977 91% were male, and almost 75% were less than 30 years of age [29]. Common general health problems of prisoners include alcohol and substance abuse, seizure disorders, psychiatric illness, and trauma-related conditions [29–31]. Infectious diseases such as STDs, tuberculosis, and AIDS are more prevalent than in the general population.

STDs

Prison surveys report histories of gonorrhea in 10%–15% of inmates and histories of syphilis in 1.2%–4.0% [29, 32]. Gonorrhea-screening cultures were positive in 5.0%–7.5% of inmates [31, 32]. One survey of female inmates found a 12% prevalence rate of gonorrhea [33]. Because most prisoners serve short sentences and reenter the community rapidly, screening for and treating STDs are a public health priority. (Gonorrhea and other STDs are discussed in detail in Chap. 30.)

Tuberculosis

The prevalence of active and latent tuberculosis in the incarcerated population is similar to that of inner city communities and much higher than that of the general U.S. population. In a survey of 29 state health departments the incidence of tuberculosis in 1984 and 1985 among prisoners was three times higher than that of the general population. Since 1985 the Centers for Disease Control (CDC) has reported 11 prison outbreaks of tuberculosis in 8 states. The incidence of tuberculosis among California inmates in 1987 was 80.3 per 100,000, six times the national rate [34]. Clinical manifestations of active and potentially communicable tuberculosis are often subtle and can easily escape diagnosis in the prison setting. Thus, incarcerated individuals have a great potential to infect both their highly exposed co-inmates and the public at large upon their release [35]. Due to the increased risk of tuberculosis in HIV-seropositive patients, all newly diagnosed prisoners with tuberculosis should be screened for the HIV antibody [36, 37].

AIDS

Seroprevalence rates for HIV infection among prisoners reflect the high incidence of IV drug use. The rate of HIV seropositivity among incoming prisoners is 7% and 15% in Maryland and New York, respectively [38]. Unless segregated, HIV-seropositive prisoners can spread the virus through ongoing IV drug use and homosexual activity while incarcerated.

Hepatitis B

Hepatitis B is prevalent, consistent with the incidence of STDs and IV drug abuse in this population.

Wounds

The emergency physician will come into contact with incarcerated patients frequently because of wounds. These wounds may have been incurred in circumstances such as fights within the institution. A significant percentage of wounds may be human bites, which should be considered high-risk exposure for hepatitis B and HIV. Appropriate prophylactic steps should be taken (see Chap. 5).

The Institutionalized

The emergency physician often treats patients residing in institutional settings, particularly at night and on weekends. The institutionalized mentally retarded are particularly problematic because adequate histories often are unobtainable. This population is at risk for the usual communicable diseases affecting closed populations and at much higher risk for infections transmitted by the fecal-oral route, particularly GI infections and hepatitis.

Diarrheal Diseases

Enteric infections are common in any setting involving crowding and close person-to-person contact, including day care centers, military settings, and institutions for the mentally retarded. The combination of fecal incontinence and crowding particularly increases the risk of diarrheal illness in mental institutions. Many of the institutionalized are unable to practice standard hygiene procedures such as hand washing. While self-limited diarrheal illness in the general population rarely requires a specific etiologic diagnosis, institutionalized patients require routine stool culture and examination for ova and parasites in order to control the spread of enteric pathogens within the institution (see Chap. 25).

VIRAL GASTROENTERITIS
Viral gastroenteritis is frequent in this population. Norwalk-like viruses and rotavirus cause most cases, although the diagnosis is made by recognition of the typical syndrome (watery diarrhea, usually with vomiting) and exclusion of bacterial pathogens. A rapid enzyme immunoassay antigen test is available for rotavirus. Identification and isolation of the affected individual can help control spread of this illness.

BACTERIAL DIARRHEA
Common causes of acute bacterial diarrhea include Shigella, Salmonella, Campylobacter, and Yersinia organisms and enterotoxigenic Escherichia coli. Shigella species require a low inoculum (<200 organ-

isms) for infectivity and are particularly common in residential institutions for the mentally retarded. The incidence of shigellosis among the institutionalized mentally retarded is 80 times higher than the nationwide incidence [39]. Institutional outbreaks of hemolytic uremic syndrome, consisting of gastroenteritis with bloody diarrhea followed by hemolytic anemia, thrombocytopenia, and renal failure, can result from infections with Shigella or E. coli 0157:H7 [40].

PARASITIC INFECTIONS
Infection with Entamoeba histolytica and Giardia lamblia causes significant morbidity among the institutionalized mentally retarded, and prevalence rates are 20%–40% [41]. Recurrence after therapy is common due to person-to-person spread [42]. The nematode parasite Strongyloides stercoralis is frequently asymptomatic but can be associated with nonspecific abdominal symptoms and eosinophilia. In immunodeficient patients a disseminated and often fatal hyperinfection syndrome has been described [43].

Hepatitis

Hepatitis B is endemic among the institutionalized mentally retarded, with 10%–25% prevalence of hepatitis B surface antigen seropositivity [44]. Hepatitis rates increase with increased institutional crowding, less patient supervision, and more aggressive patient behavior [45]. Antigen seropositivity is markedly higher among patients with Down syndrome, perhaps due to impaired humoral immunity or higher rates of interpersonal contact [46]. Hepatitis B vaccine is warranted for all susceptible patients and staff of institutions for the mentally retarded.

Wounds

Institutionalized mentally ill persons are at risk for wounds, including human bites arising from aggressive behavior. Initial wound care may need to be more aggressive because the ability of this population to keep wounds clean may be decreased. Human bites and mucous membrane exposure to another's saliva should be considered significant exposures for hepatitis B and appropriate prophylaxis initiated (see Chap. 5).

The Bed-Bound

This section considers infections commonly affecting the bed-bound patient. Causes of immobility in this population are diverse and include spinal cord injury, hip fracture, stroke, and dementia. These patients share a defect in host defense mechanisms characterized by loss of mechanical barriers to infection. Loss of the normal cough reflex in stroke patients leads to aspiration pneumonia. Catheters required for feeding or urinary drainage bypass normal mucosal defenses, predisposing patients to urinary and respiratory tract infection. Loss of skin integrity due to pressure-induced ischemia leads to decubitus ulcers with resultant bacterial colonization and invasion.

Decubitus Ulcers

Important factors in the pathogenesis of pressure ulcers in the bed-bound patient include pressure, shearing forces, and friction [47]. These are potentiated by skin maceration caused by fecal and urinary incontinence. Ulcers occur under bony prominences, including the sacral, ischial, and trochanteric areas, and the heels and lateral malleoli.

All open wounds are colonized by bacteria. Cultures are useful only when systemic antibiotics are indicated. Low-grade ulcers should be treated with a vapor-permeable dressing to hasten healing [48, 49]. They should not be used on deeper or necrotic ulcers. The goal of treatment of the necrotic ulcer is to decrease bacterial counts so that spontaneous healing can occur. This can be achieved with débridement of necrotic tissue followed by wet to dry saline dressings three times a day. Prophylaxis for endocarditis is indicated prior to débridement for patients with valvular lesions. Antiseptic solutions such as hydrogen peroxide and povidone-iodine solutions should be avoided because they may impair wound healing. Ulcers with a purulent, malodorous discharge can be treated with a short course of silver sulfadiazine to achieve a clean ulcer base [50]. Systemic antibiotics should be used only for the decubitus ulcer with cellulitis, or when osteomyelitis or sepsis is suspected. These infections are polymicrobial, and pathogens include S. aureus, anaerobes, Enterobacteriaceae, Pseudomonas, and other gram-negative aerobic bacilli. Culture of purulent drainage from these ulcers can guide antibiotic therapy. Initial antimicrobial coverage should be broad spectrum with parenteral agents such as clindamycin and gentamicin, or single agents such as ampicillin-sulbactam, ticarcillin-clavulanate, cefoxitin, or cefotetan.

Catheter-Related Infections

SINUSITIS
Catheters placed through the nares induce mucosal edema that occludes the sinus ostia and predisposes to sinusitis. The diagnosis may be suggested by fever and purulent drainage around the tube, but the infection is often occult and discovered only after sinus radiographs or computed tomography scans. Treatment involves removing the tube, topical decongestants, and appropriate antibiotics. Common bacterial upper respiratory pathogens such as S. pneumoniae, H. influenzae, Moraxella catarrhalis, and group A streptococcus should be covered, however, since these nosocomial infections are often caused by S. aureus and gram-negative aerobic bacilli. Empiric therapy with an antistaphylococcal drug like nafcillin and a third-generation cephalosporin, or ampicillin-sulbactam alone, is indicated (see Chap. 34).

URINARY TRACT INFECTION
Bacteriuria is the rule in the chronically catheterized patient and is generally polymicrobial. Pyuria is common and does not correlate with the presence of symptoms or bacteriuria. Asymptomatic bacteriuria should not be routinely treated in these patients. In the patients with fever, flank pain, autonomic dysreflexia, or sepsis, antibiotic treatment should be started and urine cultures obtained after changing the catheter [51]. Minor infections can be treated with oral ampicillin, trimethoprim-sulfamethoxizole, or ciprofloxacin. Quinolones appear to be more efficacious than trimethoprim-sulfamethoxizole for treatment of complicated urinary tract disease and prostatitis. For serious infections an aminoglycoside is usually preferred and is often combined with a broad-spectrum

beta-lactam such as an antipseudomonal penicillin (e.g., mezlocillin) or a third-generation cephalosporin (e.g., ceftazidime) (see Chap. 29).

Aspiration Pneumonia

Loss of the cough reflex or presence of a nasogastric tube increases the risk of aspiration pneumonia in the bed-bound patient. These are generally mixed-anaerobic infections; however, in the nursing home setting, oral colonization with gram-negative rods leads to gram-negative pneumonia. Chest radiographs reveal infiltrates in gravity-dependent sections of the lung, usually in the superior segments of lower lobes, and posterior segments of upper lobes. The initial aspiration episode is rarely witnessed, and the patient's presenting symptoms may be subtle. High fever and rigors are rare. If untreated, aspiration pneumonia can progress to form a primary lung abscess or occasionally a necrotizing pneumonia or empyema (see Chap. 23).

There is little evidence to suggest that prophylactic antibiotic treatment of a witnessed aspiration is effective. This practice may select for resistant organisms. For patients with pulmonary infiltrates and clinical evidence of infection thought to be due to aspiration, one's prediction of the likely oropharyngeal flora of the patient guides the choice of antibiotic therapy. In healthy hosts with community acquired disease, penicillin or clindamycin alone will suffice to cover for oral anaerobes. More debilitated patients and those on H2-blockers that reduce gastric acidity or prior antibiotics are more likely to harbor S. aureus and gram-negative aerobic bacilli. Regimens such as clindamycin and gentamicin, the beta-lactamase inhibitor antibiotics, cefoxitin, or cefotetan have been employed with success.

Autonomic Dysreflexia

In paraplegic and quadriplegic patients infections such as urinary tract infections and decubitus ulcers are common. The patient is unable to localize pain or report detailed symptomatology. Autonomic dysreflexia may indicate infection or other noxious stimuli. The symptoms consist of a rise in blood pressure, bradycardia, sweating, and pilomotor reaction below the level of the neurologic lesion.

Compliance

Effective treatment of infectious diseases requires that the patient comply with the prescribed regimen. The populations discussed in this chapter are routinely noncompliant with physician directives. Unfortunately noncompliance is commonplace among the general emergency department population. A recent study of emergency department patients found that 21% failed to fill prescriptions for antibiotics [52]. The emergency physician has some advantages over the clinic physician in this regard. The emergency department patient usually is symptomatic—a patient seeking relief from symptoms is more likely to comply with the physician's directives than, say, the asymptomatic hypertensive patient. In addition prescriptions for antibiotics are usually for short periods of time, increasing the likelihood of compliance. Features of the emergency department setting that may adversely affect compliance include the often hectic nature of physician-patient interactions, allowing inadequate time for the establishment of physician-patient rapport or assessment of the patient's health beliefs and the presence of symptoms such as pain and fear that make the patient less attentive to directives. The hectic nature of the emergency department leads to the potential for misunderstood or not-understood directions. Problems less specific to the emergency department include the inability to pay for medications or arrange transportation for follow-up appointments, to arrange child care, or to get time off from work.

Before implementing measures to improve a patient's compliance it must be determined that the planned therapy is efficacious. In fact the physician's belief that a treatment is effective may enhance the patient's view of its effectiveness, thus improving compliance. The simplest way to ensure antibiotic compliance is to administer the antibiotic before the patient leaves the department. Intramuscular injection for gonorrhea, streptococcal pharyngitis, and primary syphilis or single-dose oral therapy for gonorrhea, trichomoniasis, and uncomplicated urinary tract infections guarantees total patient compliance. Simplifying the regimen with the use of single or twice-daily dosing will improve compliance rates [53], as will shortening the duration of therapy when possible (e.g., 3-day versus

7-day regimens for uncomplicated urinary tract infections or vulvovaginal candidiasis). Commonly prescribed medications can be dispensed in the emergency department, particularly when the patient's financial status is in question. The patient should be given both verbal and written instructions, preferably with family or friends present and if possible, in the patient's primary language. When possible, the emergency physician should learn what the patient understands about the disorder and attempt to educate where misinformation exists.

References

1. Alliance Housing Council. *Housing and Homelessness*. Washington, DC: National Alliance to End Homelessness.
2. Alperstein G, Arnstein E. Homeless children—a challenge for pediatricians. *Pediatr Clin North Am* 35(6):1413, 1988.
3. Surber RW et al. Medical and psychiatric needs of the homeless—a preliminary response. *Social Work* 33:116, 1988.
4. Breakey WR et al. Health and mental health problems of homeless men and women in Baltimore. *JAMA* 262(10):1352, 1989.
5. Gelberg L, Linn LS. Assessing the physical health of homeless adults. *JAMA* 262(14):1973, 1989.
6. Centers for Disease Control. Tuberculosis control among homeless populations. *MMWR* 36(17):257, 1987.
7. Brickner PW, Kaufman A. Case finding of heart disease in homeless men. *Bull NY Acad Med* 49:475, 1973.
8. Gelberg L. Dental health of homeless adults. *Spec Care in Dentistry* 8:167, 1988.
9. Powers RD. Emergency department patient literacy and the readability of patient-directed materials. *Ann Emerg Med* 17:124, 1988.
10. Polis MA et al. The emergency department as part of a successful strategy for increasing adult immunization. *Ann Emerg Med* 17:1016, 1984.
11. Morris W, Crystal J. Diagnostic patterns in hospital use by an urban homeless population. *West J Med* 151:472, 1989.
12. Webb D, Thadepalli H. Skin and soft tissue polymicrobial infection from abuse of drugs. *West J Med* 130:200, 1979.
13. Fitzgerald RH, Cowan JDE. Puncture wounds of the foot. *Orthop Clin North Am* 6:965, 1975.
14. Harnisch JP et al. Diphtheria among alcoholic urban adults: a decade of experience in Seattle. *Ann Intern Med* 111:71, 1989.
15. Sherman MN et al. Tuberculosis in single-room-occupancy hotel residents: a persisting focus of disease. *NY Med Q* 2:39, 1980.
16. Centers for Disease Control. Drug resistant tuberculosis among the homeless—Boston. *MMWR* 34(28):429, 1985.
17. Barry MA et al. Tuberculosis screening in Boston's homeless shelters. *Public Health Rep* 101:487, 1986.
18. Slutkin G. Management of tuberculosis in urban homeless indigents. *Pub Health Reports* 101:481, 1986.
19. Brickner PW et al. A clinic for male derelicts: a welfare hotel project. *Ann Intern Med* 77:565, 1972.
20. Brickner PW et al. Homeless persons and health care. *Ann Intern Med* 104:405, 1986.
21. Nardell E et al. Exogenous reinfection with tuberculosis in a shelter for the homeless. *N Engl J Med* 315:1570, 1986.
22. Schieffelbein CW, Snider DE. Tuberculosis control among homeless populations. *Arch Intern Med* 148:1843, 1988.
23. Yeager H, Medinger AE. Tuberculosis long-term care beds—have we thrown out the baby with the bath water? *Chest* 90:752, 1986.
24. *Balderas v Pitchess*. Civil no. CA000617, Superior Court, Los Angeles County, CA, 1980.
25. Mills M. Legal aspects of infectious disease practice. *Med Times* 111(8):83, 1983.
26. Gurevitch AW. Scabies and lice. *Pediatr Clin North Am* 32(4):987, 1985.
27. Torres RA et al. Homelessness among hospitalized patients with the acquired immunodeficiency syndrome in New York City [letter]. *JAMA* 258:779, 1987.
28. Lessenger JE, Bader T. Medical consultation for correctional institutions. *J Prison Jail Health* 4:96, 1984.
29. Novick LF et al. Health status of the New York City prison population. *Med Care* 15(3):205, 1977.
30. Derro RA. Admission health evaluation of inmates of a city-county workhouse. *Minn Med* 61:333, 1978.
31. Raba JM, Obic CB. The health status of incarcerated urban males: results of admission screening. *J Prison Jail Health* 3(1):6, 1983.
32. Felman YM. Sexually transmitted disease control services in a jail population: analysis and recommendations. *Bull NY Acad Med* 58(6):559, 1982.
33. Lucas JB. The national venereal disease problem. *Med Clin North Am* 56(5):1073, 1972.
34. Centers for Disease Control. Prevention and control

of tuberculosis in correctional institutions: recommendations of the advisory committee for the elimination of tuberculosis. *MMWR* 38(18):313, 1989.

35. Stead WW. Undetected tuberculosis in prison. *JAMA* 240(23):2544, 1978.

36. Braun MM et al. Increasing incidence of tuberculosis in a prison inmate population. *JAMA* 261(3):393, 1989.

37. Theur CP et al. Human immunodeficiency virus infection in tuberculosis patients. *J Infect Dis* 162:8, 1990.

38. Centers for Disease Control. AIDS and human immunodeficiency virus infection in the United States: 1988 update. *MMWR* 38(suppl. 4):1, 1989.

39. Rosenberg ML et al. Shigellosis in the United States: ten-year review of nationwide surveillance, 1964–1973. *Am J Epidemiol* 104:543, 1976.

40. Pavia AT et al. Hemolytic-uremic syndrome during an outbreak of *Escherichia coli* O157:H7 infection in institutions for mentally retarded persons: clinical and epidemiologic observations. *J Pediatr* 116:544, 1990.

41. Thacker SB et al. Parasitic disease control in a residential facility for the mentally retarded. *Am J Public Health* 69:1279, 1979.

42. Thacker SB et al. Parasitic disease control in a residential facility for the mentally retarded: failure of selected isolation procedures. *Am J Public Health* 71:303, 1981.

43. Igra-Siegman Y et al. Syndrome of hyperinfection with *Strongyloides stercoralis*. *Rev Infect Dis* 3:397, 1981.

44. Recommendation of the Immunization Practices Advisory Committee (ACIP). Recommendations for protection against viral hepatitis. *MMWR* 34(22): 313, 1985.

45. Perrillo RP, Strang S, Lowry OH. Different operating conditions affect risk of hepatitis B virus infection at two residential institutions for the mentally disabled. *Am J Epidemiol* 123:690, 1986.

46. Lohiya S, Lohiya G, Caires S. Epidemiology of hepatitis B infection in institutionalized mentally retarded clients. *Am J Public Health* 76:799, 1986.

47. Allman RM. Pressure ulcers among the elderly. *N Engl J Med* 320:850, 1989.

48. Oleske DM et al. A randomized clinical trial of two dressing methods for the treatment of low-grade pressure ulcers. *J Enterostomal Ther* 13:90, 1986.

49. Sebern MD. Pressure ulcer management in home health care: efficacy and cost effectiveness of moisture vapor permeable dressing. *Arch Phys Med Rehabil* 67:726, 1986.

50. Kucan JO et al. Comparison of silver sulfadiazine, povidone-iodine and physiologic saline in the treatment of chronic pressure ulcers. *J Am Geriatr Soc* 29:232, 1981.

51. Grahn D et al. Validity of urinary catheter specimen for diagnosis of urinary tract infection in the elderly. *Arch Intern Med* 145:1858, 1985.

52. Saunders CE. Patient compliance in filling prescriptions after discharge from the emergency department. *Am J Emerg Med* 5:283, 1987.

53. Greenberg RN. Overview of patient compliance with medication dosing: a literature review. *Clin Ther* 6:592, 1984.

III

Infections by Organ System

THE RESPIRATORY SYSTEM

21

Upper Respiratory Tract Infections

ROBERT D. HERR
STEVEN M. JOYCE

This chapter covers the emergency presentation and management of the common cold, acute pharyngitis (including tonsillitis), and infection of the parapharyngeal potential spaces.

Colds, influenza, and other acute upper respiratory infections (URIs) together accounted for 140 million visits to physicians in 1980 [1], caused 48% of all acute illnesses in the United States, and constitute the most frequent acute illness in the industrialized world [2]. Viruses and nonbacterial agents cause more than 90% of URIs [3].

The Common Cold

"Go to bed. Hang your hat on a bedpost. Drink whiskey until you see two hats."

—*Sir William Osler's "hat-trick" remedy for the common cold*

The average adult has two to four colds per year; the average preschool child, six to 10 [1]. The common cold is a major public health problem in the United States. In 1982 it caused 190 million days of restricted activity and 40% of the sick time lost in the work place [2]. Colds occur in several waves each year. Each wave is likely caused by a different virus or virus serotype, although one virus, rhinovirus,

accounts for 10%–25% of all colds [3]. The common cold is a self-limited, local disease, but—uncommonly—it can result in sinusitis or descend to cause lower respiratory tract infections.

Epidemiology and Population at Risk

TRANSMISSION

Person-to-person contact is implicated to explain why clusters of persons in the home [4], classroom [5], and military barracks [6] are shown to be infected with the immunotypically identical virus. In contrast office workers with colds have immunotypically different viruses [4]. These data also suggest that transmission requires prolonged, intimate contact. Transmission is known to occur during the first 3 days of symptoms, when viral shedding peaks. Research supports transmission by both self-inoculation and aerosol spread. Eleven of 15 volunteers caught colds after intentionally rubbing their hands in nasal secretions of people with colds, then touching their conjunctiva or nasal mucosa [7, 8]. Aerosol droplet spread is supported by students who contracted colds after playing poker with rhinovirus-infected students even when they wore arm restraints preventing self-inoculation of nose or eyes [9]. Spread by "fomites" was in vogue when rhinovirus could be cultured on skin after 2 hours and on a laboratory surface after 4 days [10]. Latest data show that although rhinovirus may survive, its transmissibility does not survive in dried nasal secretions on objects [11]. While debate rages, "fomite" transmission appears unlikely.

Although culture of nasal secretions yields rhinovirus in 10%–25% of adults and 5%–10% of children with colds [3], there is no evidence that other viruses implicated in colds are spread in the same way. For example, while experimental rhinovirus colds were contracted by only 1 of 16 students by "French" kissing, adenoviruses are known to be highly transmissible by oral contact [12].

SEASONALITY

Colds increase in the fall and the winter [13] in temperate climates and during the rainy season in the tropics [14], probably due to the aggregation of individuals indoors at school and home. Contrary to popular belief individual susceptibility is not seasonal. Human volunteers who received direct nasal inoculation of rhinovirus got colds with equal frequency in summer and winter months [1]. Nor does cold temperature per se increase susceptibility; volunteers induced to stand wet and naked in a draft had similar attack rates as warm, dry controls [15].

RESERVOIR AND CARRIER STATE

The noses of children are the main reservoir for rhinoviruses, yielding positive cultures in up to 6% of asymptomatic children and 2%–3% of adults [7, 10, 13]. Because subclinical infection occurs in 12%–37% of infected individuals, there is controversy over whether there is a true carrier state [3, 16].

POPULATION AT RISK

Children at school are most likely to get a cold and are most likely to bring it home with them [16, 17] (Table 21-1). Household contacts have a secondary attack rate of 20%–70%, depending on the serotype of rhinovirus [18]. Mothers of families have the highest and earliest chance of catching a cold after it has been introduced into the home [19].

GENETIC AND INDIVIDUAL SUSCEPTIBILITY

The following ethnic groups are said to be at a higher risk for colds than others [18]: Native American, including Eskimos, and those with the alpha antitrypsin genotype [20].

High-risk contacts include any individual who has high titers of virus in secretions or who has pronounced symptoms [18]. Why some people catch colds while others do not is the subject of research and speculation, with both implicating various factors of age, sex, exercise, psychosocial stress, living arrangements, and hormonal factors [2, 18, 21]. Susceptibility depends in part on levels of antibody derived from previous exposure [18]. After exposure serum-neutralizing antibody titers rise in 80% of infected individuals, and type-specific secretory antibody appears in nasal secretions [21]. Immunity is probably lifelong but confers poor protection against the next or future colds. This is due to the multiplicity of viral serotypes circulating, the lack of common antigens that confer protection, and evidence for antigenic drifts over time for rhinovirus [18, 21].

Patient Presentation

Sir William Osler described the common cold most notably in *The Principles and Practice of Medicine*:

> . . . the patient feels indisposed, perhaps chilly, has slight headache, and sneezes frequently. There is usually a slight fever. . . . At first the mucus membrane of the nose is swollen, "stuffed up," and the patient has to breathe through the mouth. A thin, clear irritating secretion flows, and makes the edges of the nostrils sore. . . . Usually, within thirty-six hours the nasal secretion becomes turbid and more profuse, the swelling of mucosa subsides . . . and gradually, within four or five days the symptoms disappear [18, 22].

A cold generally begins slowly with a scratchy, sore throat for 24–48 hours, then development of a nasal discharge or obstruction, usually with sneezing or coughing. There usually is no fever, but if one is present it is under 38.3°C. Malaise is frequent but not profound [23].

ROLE OF VIRUS IDENTIFICATION

Over 90% of causative organisms are nonbacterial; most are viruses [3]. Most viruses are of six respiratory virus families that cause clinically indistinguishable illnesses: rhinovirus, corona virus, in-

Table 21-1. Reference chart for the common cold

Population at risk	Likely organisms	Symptoms and signs	Appropriate treatment	Disposition
Adults and children in winter months	Picornaviruses (PV) Rhinoviruses (10%–25%) (RSV) Coxsackieviruses A & B Echoviruses Adenoviruses Coronaviruses Myxoviruses Influenza types A & B	For all but influenza type: Slow onset of sore throat, nasal congestion, sneezing, coughing, fever under 38.3°C For PV: also croup in children	(Symptomatic) Cough: Dextromethorphan/codeine, oral hydration, mist/steam Nasal blockage: topical/oral decongestants	Discharge from emergency department. Children: no day care or school. Croup: see Chap. 14 Bronchiolitis: see Chap. 14
Children	Parainfluenza virus	For RSV: also bronchiolitis in children For influenza A: fever over 38.3°C, myalgia, prostration	Treat croup if present (see Chap. 14)	Discharge if hydrated and taking PO; isolate to prevent spread; amantadine prophylaxis to household contacts
Children	Respiratory syncytial virus		Treat bronchiolitis if present (see Chap. 14)	
Adults and children with influenza A infection	Influenza type A		Amantadine 200 mg qd PO for the first 5 days of symptoms (if >65 years, given 100 mg qd)	

fluenza virus, adenovirus, parainfluenza virus, and respiratory syncytial virus (RSV) [3, 18]. An enzyme-linked immunosorbent assay (ELISA) for rhinovirus is being tested, but its accuracy can be measured only in subjects experimentally inoculated with rhinovirus of known serotypes [24]. Since therapy is symptomatic, and since the only specifically treatable cause (influenza A) can usually be recognized clinically, exact virus identification is unnecessary. Couch [25], however, has published some generalizations that may be of interest:

1. Adults are most likely to have rhinovirus.
2. Children who also have lower respiratory tract disease have parainfluenza or RSV causing the URI.
3. During influenza epidemics URI is most often caused by influenza virus.
4. Adults who also have conjunctivitis have URI due to adenovirus.

Differential Diagnosis

Definitive diagnosis requires identifying the patient with influenza and lower respiratory infection, differentiating symptoms from allergic rhinitis, and identifying acute bacterial infection, which is amenable to antibiotic therapy. Colds due to influenza cause systemic symptoms, which predominate over cold symptoms. Influenza should be diagnosed if a sore throat, stuffy nose and cough are accompanied by a fever over 38.3°C with headache, myalgia, fatigue, and weakness. Typically influenza is endemic in the community [23] (Table 21-2).

Allergic rhinitis is perennial, usually worse in summer, and includes watery, itchy eyes and rhinorrhea, which is thin and watery. There is a family or personal history of atopy, including nasal polyps or eczema. A nasal discharge that shows eosinophils is diagnostic of allergic rhinitis; the nasal discharge of the common cold shows polymorphonuclear neutrophils (PMNs), lymphocytes, and phagocytes [18].

In children the diagnoses of both bronchiolitis and laryngotracheobronchitis (croup) must be considered. Both present with dyspnea. Wheezing and expectoration alone in either child or adult may be the result of URI-induced bronchial hyperreactivity or of postnasal drip [26]. However, a peak expiratory flow meter showing a low rate may identify patients who will benefit from bronchodilating agents.

Pneumonia typically presents with fever over 38.3°C, pleuritic chest pain, and productive cough. Etiologies of the atypical pneumonia syndrome should be considered if a dry cough is accompanied by intermittent fevers or periodic (especially nocturnal) diaphoresis.

Table 21-2. Symptoms and signs in adult rhinoviral colds and influenza

Symptom or sign	Rhinoviral cold		Influenza	
	Percentage of patients	Severity	Percentage of patients	Severity
Nasal discharge or obstruction	80–100	Severe	20–30	Mild
Sneezing	50–70	Mild–moderate	30	Mild
Sore throat	50	Mild	50–60	Moderate–severe
Malaise	20–25	Mild	80	Severe
Headache	25	Mild	85	Severe
Hoarseness	30	Mild–moderate	10	Mild
Cough	40	Mild–moderate	90	Severe
Chills	10	Mild	90	Severe
Fever >38°C	0–1	Mild	95 +	—
Myalgia	10	Mild	60–75	Moderate–severe

Source: Adapted with permission from Lowenstein SR, Parrino TA. Management of the common cold. Adv Intern Med 32:207, 1987, and Douglas NG. Influenza in man. In ED Kilbourne (ed.), The Influenza Viruses and Influenza. New York: Academic, 1975. Pp. 395–488.

Bacterial upper respiratory infections with group A streptococcus typically have more prominent pharyngitis symptoms, including pharyngeal exudate, tonsillar enlargement, cervical adenopathy, and absence of cough and other upper respiratory symptoms [18].

Treatment

Except for influenza A–associated colds, treatment remains symptomatic. The search for the cure to rhinovirus through specific antiviral therapy is limited by lack of potent inhibitors, drug toxicity, and the inability to deliver the drug to the nasal mucosa, where viral replication occurs [27].

Colds get better regardless of treatment prescribed, leading to a proliferation of folk remedies. These range from "starve a fever, feed a cold" to insufflation of the nostrils with soap to therapy with zinc, aspirin, electric shock, special fans, and exposure to tear gas [18].

Only 5%–15% of colds are brought to medical attention. Why visit the doctor when promised relief is as close as the nearest supermarket? There are over 800 nonprescription cold tablets, capsules, elixirs, "tiny time pills," cough drops and syrups, nasal decongestants, sore throat lozenges, and medicating rubs, which together in 1988 exceeded $1.6 billion in retail sales [28]. This figure is due partly to the shift of prescription drugs into the over-the-counter (OTC) category, usually by lowering their potency. Enormous profits promise that this trend will continue. For example, Actifed, Sudafed, Dimetapp, and Drixoral, once available by prescription only, are now each among the top ten in sales. Some products contain up to six ingredients that may have antagonistic effects (e.g., caffeine and antihistamine).

The emergency physician must separate fact from fiction and provide a rationale (and at least one good suggestion) to the patient for treatment [18]. The physician should recommend drinking fluids to maintain hydration and cessation of smoking. Volunteers with common colds show impairment in their ability to perform tasks demanding manual dexterity and hand-eye coordination [29]. This impairment and the need to sneeze mandate that the patient avoid using dangerous equipment or engaging in other activities with the potential for injury.

Table 21-3. Classes of decongestants available as cold remedies

Pseudoephedrine
Release of norepinephrine from postsynaptic neuronal storage granules, resulting in stimulation of alpha and beta adrenergic receptors.

Phenylpropanolamine and Ephedrine 1% Spray
Amphetamine analogues release norepinephrine and stimulate alpha adrenergic receptors directly. Phenylpropanolamine is associated with serious hypertensive toxicity.

Phenylephrine
Direct alpha receptor stimulation.

For the same reason it is prudent to avoid all sedating medications.

Either oral or topical, all decongestants increase nasal patency, lower nasal resistance, and provide subjective relief [30, 31]. Most are alpha-adrenergic receptor agonists of the phenylephrine class (Table 21-3), which act in the nasal mucosa to prevent blood vessels from congesting, decreasing blood pooling, exudation of fluid, and mucosal edema [32]. Because systemic absorption of sympathomimetic amines causes generalized vasoconstriction and tachycardia, they should not be given to patients with hypertension or hyperthyroidism or those taking beta-blockers [31, 33, 34]. Absorption of tetrahydrozoline and naphazoline congeners have led to CNS depression and coma in infants [34]. Repeated use of topical decongestants causes tachyphylaxis and rebound hyperemia [30, 31]. This "after-congestion" can be minimized (though not eliminated) by not using a decongestant beyond 3 days [35]. Use beyond 3 weeks causes rhinitis medicamentosa, a condition of chronic nasal mucosal edema, which responds to stopping the decongestant [34]. Although decongestants improve eustachian tube function, there is no evidence that they relieve rhinorrhea, cough, or otalgia [18], or prevent sinusitis or otitis media [30, 32, 36].

Coughing is usually caused either by the irritation of cough receptors by postnasal drip or from bronchospasm by irritation of tracheobronchial receptors [18]. Lowenstein and Parrino [18] point out that cough is a protective reflex, and cough suppressants should be considered only if the cough is nonproductive, disrupts sleep or work, or is associated with nausea, vomiting, subconjunctival hemorrhage, or other complication.

Other cough medications are antitussives and expectorants. Antitussives reduce cough frequency and contain narcotics that are centrally acting suppressants of the medullary cough center. Codeine is most effective [18, 37], but dextromethorphan is nearly as effective as codeine with fewer side effects [37]. Keeping the mouth and throat moist may prevent drying and irritation. This rationale has appeal for those who prescribe cough drops, menthol lozenges, syrups, and alcohol, but it has never been proved to help [38]. If coughing results from bronchospasm, sympathomimetics should be considered effective antitussants [18].

Expectorants make sputum less viscous and promote its mobilization from the airways. The physician should suggest to the patient humidification of the airways by inhaling steam or simply prescribe oral liquids to promote hydration. Guaifenesin is commonly prescribed but it was shown by one study to be no more effective than a placebo [39]. No expectorant, including terpin hydrate and ipecac syrup, has been shown to increase mucociliary clearance or improve cold symptoms [40]. Prescribed expectorants hold no advantage over OTC ones. Most liquids are ethanol based and may be unsuitable for patients with a prior drinking history. Tussi-Organidin 1–2 tsp. q4 h (Wallace Labs) is an exception, being glycerol-based.

Acetaminophen is preferred to aspirin for analgesia and antipyresis. Both can relieve fever and mitigate malaise, but aspirin causes a decrease in mucociliary clearance and enhances viral shedding [41].

Controversial or Ineffective Therapies

Antibiotics are indicated only for treatment of associated streptococcal pharyngitis, sinusitis, or otitis media or if *Mycoplasma pneumoniae* is present. Its early use in the common cold does not prevent superinfection and leads to selection of resistant bacterial strains [3]. Oral amantadine 200 mg qd (100 mg qd for persons over 65) is indicated only for the first 5 days of influenza-associated colds. It will decrease symptoms only in those patients with influenza A strains [42].

Whereas everyone agrees that antihistamines

help in patients with allergic rhinitis, there is no convincing data that they are of benefit in colds. Histamine is not released in nasal mucosa during colds [43]. Therefore, relief through the use of H_1 antihistamines derives from atropinergic effects, which cause drying of nasal secretions. Their sedative effects may also blunt the unpleasantness of having a cold. High-dose chlorpheniramine (4 mg q4h on days 2 through 7 of experimental rhinovirus infection) has been shown to significantly reduce rhinorrhea and sneezing, but it does not decrease eustachian-tube obstruction [44]. Other studies show that nasal blockage and sinus congestion actually worsen with chlorpheniramine [18]. Side effects include urinary retention and sedation and retention of respiratory secretions in patients with a cough. Antihistamines should not be considered placebos. Antihistamines should be given only if the patient has responded to them in the past, or if the patient has allergic rhinitis and a common cold during hay fever season [36].

A 1986 review shows randomized double-blind trials of either megadose or maintenance doses of vitamin C during colds had negative results in 13 (including all 5 megadose studies), slight nonsignificant amelioration of symptoms in 5, and significant reduction in the duration of colds in 5 trials [45]. There may be a small therapeutic effect of vitamin C. Because megadosages are associated with diarrhea, they should be avoided. Prescription of low dosages does little physical harm, but calling it a cure tends to cast one's lot with paraprofessionals who use vitamins, macrobiotic diets, and homeopathic medicines without scientific support. A physician is wise to eschew even low dosages of vitamin C as a cure until the results of a clinical trial become incontrovertible.

Although it can decrease viral shedding, studies fail to show the efficacy of alpha, beta, and gamma interferon for prophylaxis [46–48]. Some studies show that treatment with nasal interferon prolongs experimental colds even when given on day 1 [49].

Studies have failed to show benefit in treatment or prophylaxis with zinc chloride [49].

One double-blind study of 62 patients who inhaled steam at 42°–44°C showed alleviation of cold symptoms and increased nasal patency [50]. Commercial heated nebulizer-sprayer devices have been marketed under Rhinotherm, Virotherm, and Viralizer, the third one being available without prescription for about $40. Studies financed by marketers have shown trends toward improved nasal symptoms and pharyngitis and decreased viral titers [29, 51], but an independent 1990 study [52] at Cleveland Clinic showed that the placebo-treated group (air at 20°–24°C) had improved symptoms over the treated (air at 40°–42°C). There is no evidence for beneficial effects of heated steam inhalation, and the use of such devices should be condemned pending further study, including comparison with decongestants. There is no evidence that the cold is shortened or cured [53].

Subsequent Therapy

Subsequent therapy is directed at complications of a URI. Bronchial hyperreactivity causes a reduction in pulmonary flow rates and should be treated with a sympathomimetic. Impetigo from group A streptococcal infection is found in children under age 4 following bloody rhinorrhea or nostrils that scale and crust. Acute otitis media follows in 2% of cases [18]; acute sinusitis in 0.5% of colds [18]. Both result from bacterial superinfection either after obstruction of the sinuses or eustachian tube or after viral-induced slowing of mucociliary transport of secretions from the middle ear and sinuses to the pharynx [18].

Prevention

No vaccine is available, but public health measures can decrease the spread of colds. Prevention is most effective by limiting the kinds of intimate contact implicated in cold transmission. Patients with colds should be segregated from living arrangements with someone who has an underlying pulmonary problem (e.g., chronic bronchitis). Children should be excused from day care, camp, or school. Because office work is not associated with the spread of rhinovirus colds, a return to the office is safe and reasonable provided a decrease in efficiency is anticipated. Hand washing and careful personal hygiene are helpful. A 4-year randomized study of mothers whose hands were treated with a virudicide had only 7% illness rate due to colds compared with 20% of mothers who did not [16]. Prevention of sneezing can decrease aerosolization of virus and in

theory could decrease spread. Patients should cover their noses during sneezing and deposit tissue in closed containers.

Chemotherapeutic prevention has been tried with alpha, beta, and gamma interferon without clear success. Alfa-2 interferon has been tested. Intranasal use daily prevented 39%–42% of colds, but only in rhinovirus infections and only at a high enough dose (5 MU/day) that causes a 10% risk of minor nasal bleeding [49]. There is no current retailer of this medication, and its cost would be prohibitive.

Vitamin C has no worthwhile effect in prevention. Of 22 studies reviewed, there was no significant effect over placebo in 15 studies, and prevention was inconclusive in the other 7 [45].

Acute Pharyngitis and Tonsillitis

Acute pharyngitis, or sore throat, is one of the most common illnesses encountered in the emergency department. Pharyngitis is defined as the inflammation of any structures of the pharynx, especially the pharyngeal mucosa and palatine tonsils. Tonsillitis refers to the inflammation of the palatine, pharyngeal (adenoid), or lingual tonsils, although common usage denotes the palatine tonsils. Acute tonsillitis is a subset of acute pharyngitis, and its inclusion is implied in the following discussion unless mentioned specifically.

Almost all pharyngitides are of infectious etiology [54] (Table 21-4). Most of the causative organisms are transmitted by aerosolized respiratory secretions. Other modes of infection exist, such as oral-genital contact (gonorrheal pharyngitis), or overgrowth of endogenous organisms (thrush, Vincent's angina). Infection may be limited to the mucosa, although hematogenous spread of the organism or its toxins usually causes some systemic symptoms. Most infectious pharyngitides are limited in duration without treatment, although local and systemic complications are not uncommon. The recent resurgence of acute rheumatic fever, as well as the possibility of other life- and health-threatening complications of pharyngitis, demands a serious approach to this common problem.

Noninfectious etiologies also can cause inflammation of the pharyngeal mucosa. Mechanical in-

Table 21-4. Reference chart for pharyngitis/tonsillitis

Organism	Population at risk	Relative frequency of occurrence, percentage of affected population	Season and syndrome	Specific signs and symptoms
Viruses				
Respiratory and enteroviruses	Children to adults, with decreasing frequency	27–30	Winter to spring, common cold; summer, herpangina	Coryza, pharyngeal vesicles, ulcers
Epstein-Barr virus and cytomegaloviruses	Adolescents and young adults	1–2	Spring and early fall, mononucleosis	Tonsillar edema, posterior cervical adenopathy, splenomegaly
Adenovirus	Children to adults, military recruits	5	Fall to spring, acute respiratory disease (ARD) and pharyngoconjunctival fever	Conjunctivitis, hoarseness, cervical adenopathy
Herpes simplex virus	Young children	4	Year-round	Vesicular gingivostomatitis, ulcerations
Bacteria and Other Organisms				
Streptococcus pyogenes, (GABHS)	All ages, but most common in 5–15-year-old group	15–35	Winter, strep throat	Fever, anterior cervical nodes, exudate, no cough

Chlamydia species and *Mycoplasma pneumoniae*	Children	Uncertain, 5–25	Nonseasonal	Nonspecific, may have lower respiratory signs
Neisseria gonorrhoeae	All those at risk for STDs	<1	Nonseasonal	Nonspecific, may have STD
Corynebacterium diphtheriae	Unimmunized children, poorly immunized adults	<1	Nonseasonal, diphtheria	Membrane, neck edema, dysphagia
Corynebacterium haemolyticum	Teenagers	<1	Nonseasonal	Scarlatiniform rash
Mixed anaerobes, oral flora	Poor oral hygiene	<1	Nonseasonal, Vincent's angina	Foul breath, ulcerative gingivitis
Legionella pneumophila	Adults	<1	Nonseasonal	Nonspecific, may have lower respiratory symptoms
Francisella tularensis	Animal-fur handlers	<1	Nonseasonal, tularemia	Pharyngeal ulcers, adenopathy
Other streptococci, not group A	Young adults	Uncertain, may be >10	Fall to spring	Nonspecific
Treponema pallidum	Adults at risk for STDs	<1	Nonseasonal, syphilis	Pharyngeal chancre, gumma
Candida albicans	Infants, immunocompromised	<1	Nonseasonal, thrush	White plaque over shallow ulcer

jury by trauma, drying, or chemical irritants is common. Neoplastic infiltration or autoimmune diseases can also cause pharyngitis.

There is much disagreement in the medical community regarding the proper approach to the patient with sore throat, varying from symptomatic treatment to dogmatic empiric antibiotic therapy. A simple, reliable scientific approach does not yet exist. However, consideration of the clinical presentation, combined with knowledge of various diagnostic schemes and laboratory tests, can lead the clinician to a cost-effective and rational approach.

Epidemiology and Population at Risk

EPIDEMIOLOGY OF PHARYNGITIS

Some studies estimate that sore throat accounts for over 15 million ambulatory-patient visits a year, with an annual cost of over $300 million in the United States [55]. Most pharyngitides are infectious in etiology, although a specific organism can be isolated in fewer than 50% of cases [56]. Table 21-4 lists the etiologic agents and their relative incidence as causes of acute pharyngitis.

Various respiratory viruses and enteroviruses are the most common viral causes, responsible for about 40% of cases with known etiology [57]. They cause sore throats in the winter and late summer/fall, respectively, usually in association with cold or flu syndromes. These common viral pharyngitides affect all age groups, with the highest incidence in children and tapering rapidly after age 60. Other viruses cause pharyngitis as part of specific syndromes. Adenovirus causes pharyngoconjunctival fever in children and adults, especially military recruits. Herpes simplex is associated with gingivostomatitis in young children and immunosuppressed patients. Either cytomegalovirus (CMV) or more commonly Epstein-Barr virus (EBV) cause mononucleosis syndrome, a prolonged illness in adolescents and young adults that begins with pharyngitis.

Bacteria and other single-celled organisms account for most of the remainder of infectious etiologies of pharyngitis. Group A, beta-hemolytic *Streptococcus pyogenes* (GABHS) is by far the most clinically important of these, due to its potential complications. GABHS is responsible for 15%–35% of infectious pharyngitides and is most

common in the 5-to-15-year age group [57]. Most infections occur during the winter months, and outbreaks are more common in institutional settings. GABHS assumes importance because it is the cause of acute rheumatic fever (ARF), a complication with an overall incidence of about 1–18 per 100,000 in the susceptible age group [58]. This inflammatory illness can result in severe carditis with lifelong morbidity, but it is completely preventable by timely treatment of GABHS infection. Other potential complications of GABHS include peritonsillar abscess (discussed elsewhere in this chapter), poststreptococcal glomerulonephritis (a nonpreventable complication with low incidence and low morbidity), and postanginal sepsis (a rare septic thrombophlebitis of the internal jugular vein, discussed later in this chapter [59]. GABHS may also be found in the throats of patients, usually children, with few or no symptoms. This so-called carrier state usually is not accompanied by a rise in streptococcal antibody titers, although some have questioned the reliability of this finding in excluding true infection [60]. The significance of all these factors in forming treatment decisions is discussed later.

Both M. pneumoniae and *Chlamydia pneumoniae* have been shown to cause pure pharyngitides, possibly in as many as 20% of cases [57]. Non–group A streptococci also have been implicated, particularly in endemic outbreaks of pharyngitis in young adults [61]. *Corynebacterium haemolyticum* causes a syndrome of pharyngitis and rash in teenagers.

Less common but nonetheless important as a cause of pharyngitis is *Corynebacterium diphtheriae*. Diphtheria occurs mostly in unimmunized children, although adults can get the disease if their immunization boosters are not up to date. Thanks to effective immunization the incidence in the United States has decreased to five or fewer cases each year throughout the 1980s [62]. Public mistrust of the safety of immunizations and an increase in the population without access to routine health care may cause a resurgence of this disease in the future. Morbidity and mortality are high in diphtheria, and due to either airway obstruction by the pharyngeal membrane or toxin-induced myocarditis or peripheral neuritis.

Other organisms have been implicated in the etiology of infectious pharyngitis in fewer than 1%

of cases [57]. Mixed anaerobic oral flora can cause Vincent's angina, an ulcerative gingivostomatitis/pharyngitis in young adults with poor dental hygiene. *Francisella tularensis* is a rare tick-borne disease causing pharyngeal ulceration and adenopathy. Syphilis may present as pharyngeal chancre, ulceration, or gumma. *Legionella pneumophila* can cause pure pharyngitis. *Candida albicans* can colonize the upper GI tract of neonates or immunocompromised adults, causing oropharyngeal thrush.

Only after treatable infectious etiologies have been considered should noninfectious causes of pharyngitis be entertained. These causes are usually suggested by the history. Trauma from foreign bodies or chemical or thermal burns is sudden in onset, and is usually apparent on exam. Pharyngitis due to mucosal involvement by inflammatory or neoplastic disorders is insidious in onset and more common in the older population. Various autoimmune diseases, such as systemic lupus erythematosus, erythema multiforme, and Stevens-Johnson syndrome, may first manifest themselves as pharyngitides in adults. Mucosal involvement by tumors or leukemic infiltration should be sought in patients over age 60 when an obvious cause of pharyngitis is not apparent. Smokers often have chronic pharyngeal inflammation, and those who mouth-breathe at night may experience mucosal drying. Psychogenic pharyngitis is infrequently the cause of an emergency department visit.

Epidemiology of Tonsillitis

The incidence of tonsillitis is unknown, but it occurs in many of the 11% of school-age children who seek medical care each year for acute pharyngitis [63]. Most of the 500,000 to 1 million tonsillectomies done each year in the United States are done to treat recurrent or chronic tonsillitis. While high this figure is one-half the annual number done throughout the 1960s and 1970s [64, 65].

The pathogenesis is multifactorial and related to tonsillar anatomy, immunology, and microbiology [66]. Since the decrease in tonsillitis after tonsillectomy is associated with an alteration in oropharyngeal flora, some attribute the occurrence of tonsillitis to an unfavorable alteration in the ecology of the microflora [67]. Infecting organisms are identical in type and incidence to those discussed under pharyngitis (see Table 21-4), with the addition of staphylococci, pneumococci, and *Haemophilus* species [65].

At higher risk are children, adolescents, and young adults, with this risk declining with age as the tonsillar tissue atrophies. Previous tonsillitis and previous GABHS infection increase the risk. Protective factors include tonsillectomy [68], but regrowth and reinfection of tonsillar tissue is common.

Patient Presentation

Pharyngitis

Symptoms. Most patients with sore throat present within several days of the onset of their symptoms seeking relief of throat pain and dysphagia, which interfere with the daily activities of eating, drinking, and sleeping. Most will have tried nonprescription remedies without success, and many will be under the impression that antibiotics will cure them.

Patients who complain of difficulty breathing or swallowing secretions are at risk for airway obstruction by one of several complications of pharyngitis and should be examined expeditiously.

Respiratory viruses and enteroviruses cause the recognizable cold and flu syndromes characterized by cough, coryza, malaise, myalgia, mild fever, and sometimes gastroenteritis. Patients with mononucleosis usually complain of sore throat with marked dysphagia followed by persistence of fatigue and fever for over 1 week and may report exposure to the illness. Adenovirus causes pharyngitis with marked rhinorrhea and conjunctivitis but without cough.

Bacterial pharyngitides usually are characterized by the absence of cold or flu symptoms. Streptococcal pharyngitis is characterized by sudden onset, fever, headache, and sometimes abdominal pain. Both GABHS and *C. haemolyticum* can cause a scarlatiniform rash along with sore throat. Pharyngitides caused by *Mycoplasma*, *Chlamydia*, and *Legionella* species may be accompanied by lower respiratory symptoms such as nonproductive cough, dyspnea, and pleuritic pain. In patients with sexually transmitted diseases and sore throat, gonorrhea should be suspected. Diphtheria may present as pharyngitis with severe dysphagia, nausea, vomiting, headache, and chills and should be suspected in unimmunized children and adults with uncertain immunization histories. Vincent's angina produces foul breath and no systemic symptoms. Patients whose immune systems are compromised by illness or corticosteroids or who are taking broad-spectrum antibiotics are more likely to have thrush.

The etiology of noninfectious pharyngitides often is suggested by the history. In cases of thermal or chemical burns or trauma, the causative agent can be tied to the sudden onset of symptoms. Mouth breathers with chronic drying are usually worse after sleep. In cases of neoplasm the onset is usually more insidious, and a history of smoking or alcohol abuse often obtained. Systemic symptoms of arthralgias, rash, and lassitude of varying duration often precede the sore throat in inflammatory disorders. Psychogenic pharyngitis usually has been longstanding and has failed to respond to multiple treatments.

Physical Examination. Patients who present with stridor, trismus, drooling, or voice changes should be examined quickly and carefully for the presence of peritonsillar or retropharyngeal abscess, epiglottitis, diphtheric pseudomembrane, or other causes of imminent airway obstruction. These conditions are discussed elsewhere in this chapter. Specific precautions are indicated in the examination of children with suspected epiglottitis.

The appearance of the throat is notoriously unreliable in determining the etiology of pharyngitis [55]. Attention also must be paid to the eyes, nose, lymph nodes, skin, and spleen.

The common viral pharyngitides are usually associated with mild pharyngeal mucosal edema and erythema, low-grade fever, coryza, and cough. Cervical adenopathy is usually absent. Various exanthems may be present, especially in children. Enteroviruses and herpesvirus can produce painful mucosal ulcerations. Adenovirus infection can cause marked tonsillar edema with variable exudate, conjunctivitis, high fever, and cervical adenopathy. The pharyngitis of mononucleosis can be severe, with marked tonsillar edema, exudate, palatine petechiae, high fever, generalized adenopathy, and perhaps splenomegaly.

Bacterial pharyngitides are likewise associated with a broad spectrum of physical findings. The "classic" strep throat is characterized by swollen, beefy-red pharyngeal and tonsillar mucosa, exudate in the tonsillar crypts, palatine petechiae, fever, anterior cervical adenopathy, and absence of coryza. However, GABHS also is likely to be present in the pharynx of a patient with mild sore throat and unimpressive mucosal erythema in a fair number of cases [60].

Lower respiratory findings may suggest *Mycoplasma, Chlamydia,* or *Legionella* infections in patients with a nonspecific appearance of the pharynx. A scarlatiniform rash may be seen in GABHS or *C. haemolyticum* infections. Pharyngeal ulcerations may be seen with Vincent's angina, tularemia, and syphilis.

Diphtheria classically presents as a white-to-gray exudate forming a pseudomembrane that becomes firmly adherent and extends beyond the tonsil as the disease progresses. Painful edema (not adenopathy) of the neck is characteristic early in the illness [69]. A low-grade fever is present, and the exam may reveal findings of carditis or peripheral neuropathies.

The oropharyngeal lesions of thrush are white patches on the mucosa covering shallow ulcerations that bleed easily.

Neoplasm may sometimes be evident as discrete tumor or demarcated mucosal infiltrate. Coagulation or liquefaction from burns usually affects both mouth and pharynx. A traumatic puncture site or scratch is discrete and often covered with white exudate. Inflammatory diseases can cause mucosal erythema; more often the diagnosis is suspected by the findings of rashes, joint effusions, and other characteristic lesions. A normal examination is the case in psychogenic pharyngitis.

PATIENT PRESENTATION OF TONSILLITIS

Acute Tonsillitis. Infection of the palatine tonsils, or palatine tonsillitis, is by far the most common form of tonsillitis. It is of highest incidence in adolescents and young adults, becoming much less frequent as these organs atrophy. The location of the palatine tonsils is shown in Fig. 21-1. Infecting organisms are identical in type and incidence to those discussed under pharyngitis (see Table 21-4), with the addition of staphylococci, pneumococci, and *Haemophilus* species [70]. The patient presents with a history of sore throat, sometimes preceded by

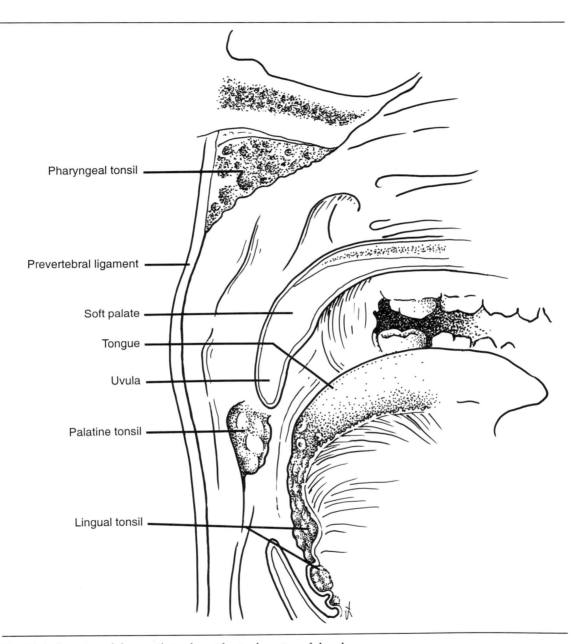

Fig. 21-1. Location of the tonsils in the midsagittal section of the pharynx.

cold symptoms. The patient complains of dysphagia, chills, malaise, and myalgia. Tender anterior cervical adenopathy and fever are usually present. Examination of the throat shows palatine tonsils that are erythematous with varying amounts of exudate, usually starting in the crypts. Gagging should be avoided because it causes medial movement of

the tonsils, giving the false impression of tonsillar enlargement. Occasionally, tonsillar swelling is so marked as to compromise the airway, most often in infectious mononucleosis. It must be remembered that inferior extension of tonsils can cause obstruction of the hypopharynx; therefore, the inferior pole should be visualized. If this is impossible, a soft-tissue lateral neck radiograph may identify the inferior extension of the tonsil, but it cannot be used to determine the size of the tonsils in relation to the airway.

Like most pharyngitides, palatine tonsillitis is a self-limited disease, lasting about a week. Peritonsillar cellulitis and abscess are specific complications discussed elsewhere in this chapter. Neoplasms can also affect the palatine tonsil, either by allowing bacterial overgrowth or by infiltration of the lymphoid tissues (e.g., leukemia, squamous cell carcinoma). Indications for laboratory testing and treatment are the same for acute tonsillitis as they are for other pharyngitides.

Acute inflammation of the lingual tonsil is, like other pharyngitides, usually infectious. The organisms responsible are probably similar in incidence and importance as those listed in Table 21-4. Acute lingual tonsillitis is probably often misdiagnosed, because of the nonspecific history and the lack of visible findings on pharyngeal exam. Clues to the diagnosis include a feeling of fullness in the throat, constant desire to swallow or clear the throat, and a tender mass palpable (but not always visible) at the base of the tongue [71]. The diagnosis may be confirmed by indirect laryngoscopy. Swabs for rapid strep test or culture should be obtained from the affected area. Treatment concerns are the same as those outlined below for all acute pharyngitides. The lingual tonsil may also be the site of an embedded foreign body, and abscess may result from this as well as from purulent infection. Neoplasms may also originate in the lingual tonsil.

Recurrent tonsillitis is defined in Table 21-5 [68].

Chronic tonsillitis is tonsillitis lasting longer than 1 week but also describes a syndrome of chronic sore throat with malodorous breath, tender cervical adenopathy, and often tonsilloliths [66]. When symptoms or signs persist after treatment for acute lingual tonsillitis, the condition is referred to as chronic lingual tonsillitis and can be treated by cryosurgery or laser surgery when chronic infection is the cause.

Laboratory Tests

INFECTIOUS PHARYNGITIS AND TONSILLITIS
The laboratory diagnosis and treatment of pharyngitis, including tonsillitis, are outlined in Table 21-6.

Table 21-5. Tonsillectomy: indications and contraindications

Indications
Infection:
  Recurrent tonsillitis despite medical therapy*
  Recurrent tonsillitis with:
    Airway obstruction
    Peritonsillar abscess (if under 40 or recurrent abscess)
    Abscessed cervical nodes
    Febrile seizure
    Cardiac valvular disease (with recurrent streptococcal tonsillitis)
  Persistent streptococcus carrier state despite medical treatment
  Chronic tonsillitis with:
    Persistent sore throat
    Halitosis
    Tender cervical adenitis
Obstruction:
  Tonsillar hyperplasia with obstruction
  Obstructive sleep apnea
  Cardiac or pulmonary disease exacerbated by upper airway obstruction
  Speech abnormalities

Contraindications
Anatomic:
  Cleft palate or submucous clefts (bifed uvula, midline furrow along the length of the soft palate, and notching of the posterior margin of the hard palate)
Hematologic:
  Coagulopathy
Medical condition:
  Presence of upper respiratory infection said to increase operative bleeding [86]

* Criteria for recurrent tonsillitis vary. The minimal acceptable criteria presented by the American Academy of Pediatrics and the AMA are four or more episodes within the preceding year, seven or more episodes in one year, five or more in each of two preceding years, or three or more episodes in each of three preceding years [86]. Tonsillectomy should be considered when recurrent tonsillitis causes sufficient morbidity to seriously jeopardize functioning at school or work [68].
Sources: Brodsky L. Modern assessment of tonsils and adenoids. *Pediatr Clin North Am* 36:1551–68, 1989; Fry TL, Pillsbury HC. The implication of "controlled" studies of tonsillectomy and adenoidectomy. *Otolaryngol Clin North Am* 20:409–13, 1986.

Viruses. Except for influenza type A, the common cold, flu, and other illnesses caused by respiratory viruses, adenovirus, and enteroviruses are self-limited, and no specific treatment is available. Hence, no attempt to identify the specific pathogen is routinely indicated in a clinical setting.

Table 21-6. Laboratory diagnosis and treatment of pharyngitis

Organism	Laboratory diagnosis	Treatment regimens
Viruses		
Respiratory and enteroviruses	Not practical	Symptomatic (see text)
Epstein-Barr virus and cytomegalovirus	>50% lymphocytosis, >10% atypical lymphocytes, monospot	Corticosteroids if airway compromised, hygiene and activity precautions
Adenovirus	Not practical	Symptomatic
Herpes simplex	Viral culture of vesicle base, but diagnosis usually clinical	Acyclovir, 200 mg PO 5 times/day for 10 days (not FDA approved, not for children)
Bacteria and Other Organisms		
Streptococcus pyogenes, GABHS	Clinical scoring, rapid strep screen, strep culture	Penicillin benzathine 1.2 million U IM >27 kg, 600,000 U <27 kg *or* Penicillin V K 250–500 mg PO qid (15 mg/kg/day in children) for 10 days *or* erythromycin 20–40 mg/kg/day bid–qid (max. 1 g) for 10 days, *or* cefadroxil 30 mg/kg/day 1–2 times/day for 10 days
Chlamydia species and *Mycoplasma pneumoniae*	Not practical, cold agglutinins not specific or sensitive	Need for treatment questionable; erythromycin as for GABHS *or* doxycycline 100 mg PO bid for 10 days
Neisseria gonorrhoeae	Culture on Thayer-Martin medium	Ceftriaxone 250 mg IM, *or* ampicillin 3.5 g PO with 1 g probenecid qd for 2 days, *or* tetracycline 0.5 g PO qid for 5 days, *or* doxycycline 100 mg PO bid for 10 days
Corynebacterium diphtheriae	Clinical to start treatment; membrane for immunofluorescence, Loeffler's or tellurate cultures	Diphtheria antitoxin 20,000–40,000 U IM (mild); 40,000–80,000 U, one-half IM, one-half IV (moderate–severe) *and* erythromycin 40 mg/kg/day *or* procaine penicillin G 600,000 U IM q12h; treat for 14 days
Corynebacterium haemolyticum	Not practical	Need for treatment questionable; erythromycin or penicillin as for GABHS
Mixed anaerobes	Not practical	Penicillin or erythromycin as for GABHS
Legionella pneumophila	Serology, culture, sputum fluorescent antibody	Erythromycin *or* doxycycline as for *Chlamydia*, for 14 days
Francisella tularensis	Tissue fluorescence, serology	Streptomycin 0.5–1 g IM bid for 10 days
Other streptococci, not group A	Not practical	Need for treatment questionable; penicillin *or* erythromycin as for GABHS
Treponema pallidum	Serology, dark-field exam of lesion swab	Penicillin *or* erythromycin, various doses depending on stage
Candida albicans	KOH wet mount of scraping (pseudohyphae) Gram's stain (budding yeast)	Clotrimazole troches *or* nystatin suspension until plaque gone, up to 14 days

Confirmation of mononucleosis has implications for the patient regarding hygiene and physical activity precautions. Early in the course of the illness, the WBC differential may reveal a relative (>50%) lymphocytosis or greater than 10% atypical lymphocytes. The heterophil antibody agglutination (monospot) test is positive in only about 60% of cases during the first week of illness, increasing to over 80% by the fourth week. The use of these tests may be reserved until the pharyngitis has persisted for a week or more, resulting in a higher yield and avoiding unnecessary testing of patients with self-limited illnesses.

GABHS Pharyngitis and Strep Throat. The best method for accurate and cost-effective identification of GABHS infections remains a much debated topic. Several clinical and laboratory tools are available; none is completely reliable or practical.

Several studies have proposed clinical scoring systems whereby children and adults with a high probability of having GABHS infections can be identified (Table 21-7). The positive predictive values of any of these scoring systems are limited, but their use may obviate the need for further laboratory testing in those with high scores, who can be treated empirically [72–74]. Table 21-8 lists the positive predictive values of scoring system III at various prevalences of the disease.

Until recently a throat culture selective for GABHS was considered the "gold standard" for diagnosis of strep throat. However, improper technique in obtaining or processing the specimen can result in false-negative culture results of over 10%, while the carrier state may account for up to 20% of positive results [55]. In addition cultures are expensive, delay treatment by several days, and allow for patient attrition.

The development of the rapid streptococcal antigen agglutination assay (rapid strep test) has provided some help to clinicians seeking early identification of strep throat. Studies have shown the sensitivity of these tests to be 72%–96% and specificity 90%–100% [75]. They are inexpensive and fast (most less than 30 minutes), but like cultures they will identify GABHS carriers as well as those truly infected.

A Gram's stain of the pharyngeal exudate may

be confirmatory in high-risk patients, with 10% false-negative and 33% false-positive rates [76]. Gram-positive ovoid cocci in association with polymorphonuclear leukocytes constitute a positive result.

Various schemes for cost-effective utilization of the above tests in the pharyngitis population have been proposed and are discussed in the section on treatment.

Other Organisms. Of the other organisms that can cause pharyngitis, few require identification for specific antibiotic therapy. Only those organisms will be discussed here.

Diphtheria requires prompt diagnosis and treatment. Gram's or methylene blue stains are not specific. A sample of the pseudomembrane should be sent to the laboratory, where initial immunofluorescence can confirm C. diphtheriae and toxinogenic strains subsequently identified from cultures on Loeffler's or tellurate media. Treatment is instituted based on clinical diagnosis and can be stopped or altered if these tests are negative.

C. albicans appears as branching pseudohyphae on a potassium hydroxide wet mount of a scraping from the plaque, although many clinicians diagnose thrush based on its appearance.

F. tularensis is identified by tissue fluorescence or serology, while Treponema pallidum is found on dark-field examination of a swab of the lesion or by serology.

A Gram's stain is not specific for gonorrheal pharyngitis; swabs of the pharynx or the affected genitalia

While both Mycoplasma and Chlamydia species can be identified by various tests of secretions or serum, it is not cost effective to do so, since pharyngitis caused by either organism is self-limited. The oral flora that cause Vincent's angina can be treated empirically (see Chap. 36).

NONINFECTIOUS PHARYNGITIS AND TONSILLITIS

Most cases of noninfectious pharyngitis and tonsillitis can be diagnosed clinically. A complete blood count and white cell differential should be ordered when neoplasm is suspected. Biopsy of solid tumors is diagnostic. In trauma from foreign bodies a lateral cervical radiograph may show the object or

Table 21-7. Three clinical scoring systems for GABHS pharyngitis

I. Pediatric Streptococcal Score Card [a]

SCORE

Month

Feb, Mar, Apr	_____	(4 points)
Jan, May, Dec	_____	(3 points)
June, Oct, Nov	_____	(2 points)
July, Aug, Sept	_____	(1 point)

Age

5 through 10 yr	_____	(4 points)
4 or 11–14 yr	_____	(3 points)
3 or 15+	_____	(2 points)
2 or younger	_____	(1 point)

WBC

<8,500	_____	(1 point)
8,500–10,400	_____	(2 points)
10,500–13,400	_____	(3 points)
13,500–20,400	_____	(5 points)
>20,400	_____	(6 points)
Not done	_____	(3 points)

Clinical Findings	Yes	No	Unknown
Fever 38° C or more	_____ (4 points)	_____ (2 points)	_____ (2 points)
Sore throat	_____ (4 points)	_____ (2 points)	_____ (2 points)
Cough	_____ (2 points)	_____ (4 points)	_____ (4 points)
Headache	_____ (4 points)	_____ (2 points)	_____ (2 points)
Abnormal pharynx	_____ (4 points)	_____ (1 point)	_____ (3 points)
Adenopathy	_____ (4 points)	_____ (2 points)	_____ (3 points)

Adult Scoring System

II. High-risk groups
   Enlarged or tender cervical nodes and pharyngeal exudate
   Enlarged or tender cervical nodes and recent streptococcal exposure

Moderate-risk groups
   No recent cough
   Recent cough and T ≥38°C

III. Risk factors[b] (one point each)
   Pharyngeal exudate
   Anterior cervical adenopathy
   Fever
   Absence of cough

[a]Consider score positive for streptococcal pharyngitis when the total score is ≥ 30.
[b]Risk factors associated with streptococcal pharyngitis. The presence of two or more risk factors suggests empiric oral antibiotic therapy. The presence of three or more risk factors supports empiric parenteral penicillin therapy on a cost-effective basis.
Sources: Centro RM, Meier FA, Dalton HP. Throat cultures and rapid tests for diagnosis of group A streptococcal pharyngitis. *Ann Intern Med* 105:892–99, 1986. Used with permission. Also adapted from Breese BB. *Am J Dis Child* 131:514–517, 1977. Copyright 1977, American Medical Association.

Table 21-8. Effect of prevalence of group A streptococcal pharyngitis on probability estimates

Symptom score	Prevalence		
	5.00%	10.00%	20.00%
0	0.64	1.34	2.96
1	1.71	3.55	7.65
2	4.53	9.10	18.38
3	11.42	21.39	37.97
4	25.95	42.52	62.47

Reprinted courtesy of Centro RM, Meier FA, Dalton HP. Throat cultures and rapid tests for diagnosis of group A streptococcal pharyngitis. *Ann Intern Med* 105:892–99, 1986.

air in the soft tissue. Inflammatory diseases are confirmed by various serologic and hematologic tests.

Differential Diagnosis

Very few conditions cause pain in the pharynx that do not fall under the definition of pharyngitis.

Infection of laryngeal structures often presents as sore throat, but examination reveals minimal or no inflammation of the pharynx. Epiglottitis and croup in children and laryngotracheitis in all ages are examples. Marked voice changes, brassy cough, and stridor may suggest these laryngeal infections.

Pain can be referred to the throat in ischemic heart diseases, although this is seldom an isolated symptom. Glossopharyngeal neuralgia is a rare condition that causes episodic severe throat pain in the absence of apparent pathology. Subacute thyroiditis may present as sore throat, but examination reveals an enlarged and tender thyroid gland and a normal-appearing pharynx.

Therapy

SYMPTOMATIC THERAPY

Treatment of acute pharyngitis is aimed at alleviating the severity and the duration of the patient's symptoms (the reason the patient came to the emergency department) and when possible at limiting spread of the illness and preventing serious complications.

Immediate stabilization of the airway takes precedence but is seldom a problem in uncomplicated pharyngitis. Symptomatic treatment will usually help patients through their illnesses. This includes pain control, fever therapy, and adequate fluid intake. Patients with significant discomfort may benefit from topical anesthetic sprays, lozenges, or gargles, which are available over the counter. Use of topical viscous lidocaine is probably best reserved for those with severe dysphagia, since it obtunds the gag reflex and is absorbed when swallowed. Systemic oral analgesic/antipyretic liquids, such as acetaminophen liquid with or without codeine, are indicated. Salt water gargle may help to relieve discomfort from mucosal edema and loosen secretions. Emphasis on adequate fluid and caloric intake in patients with dysphagia, especially children, is important. Outpatient IV volume repletion is sometimes needed.

PHARMACOLOGIC THERAPY

Viruses. As with most other viral illnesses, including the common cold, specific antibiotic therapy is seldom available or indicated. Prevention and treatment of influenza were discussed earlier in this chapter. Herpetic gingivostomatitis may respond to acyclovir 200 mg PO 5 times a day for 10 days. Acyclovir is not recommended for use in children.

Occasionally patients with mononucleosis and severe tonsillar edema may require treatment with oral or parenteral corticosteroids to prevent airway compromise. Mononucleosis patients should be cautioned to avoid strenuous activity if splenomegaly is present, but otherwise they can pursue normal activities as tolerated. Mononucleosis is transmitted by oral contact, and patients may remain infectious for months after the acute pharyngitis. These patients should be instructed to avoid oral contact and the sharing of eating and drinking utensils.

GABHS Pharyngitis/Tonsillitis and Strep Throat. Cost-effective treatment of GABHS pharyngitis is tied to its clinical and laboratory diagnosis. There is simply no one correct approach to this problem. Treatment of every pharyngitis with antibiotics is expensive and theoretically would result in a certain number of antibiotic allergies and thus anaphylaxis [77]. Proponents of this approach argue that the incidence of allergy so produced would probably be lower than that of acute rheumatic fever. At the other end of the spectrum are those who believe that patients should be treated only on the basis of a positive culture, thus avoiding treatment of non-GABHS pharyngitis but not GABHS carriers. The latter approach is also expensive and will miss a certain number of the true GABHS infections due to attrition and false-negative cultures. In addition evidence suggests that early treatment of GABHS pharyngitis may ameliorate symptoms and reduce the incidence of purulent complications [78, 79]. Consideration also must be given to the argument that the so-called carrier state may warrant treatment, if only to reduce the spread of GABHS.

Several authors [55, 77] agree on a conservative approach for patients with pharyngitis as follows. First, the following patients should be treated empirically: those with other causes of pharyngitis requiring specific treatment (e.g., diphtheria); those with a history of acute rheumatic fever (since recurrence is likely with each untreated GABHS infection); those with close family or institutional contacts with laboratory-proved GABHS; those who have taken antibiotics on their own; and those who have a high probability of GABHS pharyngitis based on clinical scoring (see Table 21-7). Remaining patients should be screened for GABHS with a rapid strep test and treated if the test is positive. Those with negative rapid strep tests should have a strep culture taken and treated if positive. This approach allows for cost-effective treatment of most cases of GABHS pharyngitis.

Once the decision has been made to treat a patient for GABHS pharyngitis, several options are available (see Table 21-6). Regardless of the regimen chosen, treatment must be instituted within 9 days of the onset of symptoms to adequately prophylax against rheumatic fever [57]. Penicillin still is considered by most to be the antibiotic of choice for GABHS pharyngitis. A single intramuscular dose of 1.2 million units of benzathine penicillin G (600,000 units in patients under 27 kg) will eradicate the organism in 75%–94% of cases [76]. Parenteral therapy has the advantage of ensured compliance, but it is also statistically more likely to result in a serious drug reaction [77]. Oral penicillin has a slightly decreased rate of eradication of GABHS and less risk for causing a reaction, but compliance is a major concern since oral therapy must be continued for 10 days to adequately prophylax against ARF [80]. Doses of oral antibiotics 2 to 3 times a day

may improve compliance rates (see Table 21-7). Other oral antibiotics have been advocated for initial treatment of GABHS or for penicillin treatment failures or allergies. Erythromycin is effective in eradicating GABHS 85%–95% of the time and has theoretical advantages in treating Mycoplasma and Chlamydia species and other causes of non-GABHS pharyngitis when given empirically [76, 81]. GI side effects are common, and one study has reported development of resistance to erythromycin when used for initial treatment [82]. Several authors recommend oral cefadroxil in a once-daily dosing regimen, citing a higher rate of eradication [76]. Several other alternative antibiotics have been studied (see Table 21-6). Tetracyclines and sulfas are not adequate in prophylaxing against ARF and should not be used [80].

Repeat cultures should be reserved for patients who remain symptomatic after treatment and for families in which a member has had ARF [82]. Some studies suggest that penicillin treatment failure may be the result of beta-lactamase produced by copathogens such as Staphylococcus aureus and Haemophilus influenzae [79]. In such cases treatment with cephalosporins, erythromycin, rifampin, dicloxacillin, amoxicillin-clavulanate, or clindamycin has been recommended.

Other Organisms. For diphtheria immediate treatment with a specific antitoxin should be initiated as soon as the clinical diagnosis is made. Time is of the essence, since only extracellular toxin can be neutralized. Dose varies depending on the severity of the pharyngitis, with 20,000 to 40,000 units given IM for mild to moderate cases and 40,000 to 80,000 units (half or all given by IV infusion) in severe cases with laryngeal involvement [83]. Skin testing for horse-serum sensitivity and pretreatment of sensitive patients with diphenhydramine and corticosteroids should precede antitoxin administration. Once antitoxin administration has begun, antibiotic therapy is indicated to eradicate the source of toxin and prevent spread to others. Table 21-6 lists adequate dosages of penicillin G and erythromycin. Nasopharyngeal cultures should be obtained from all close contacts, and those with adequate immunization histories given a toxoid booster (adult Td). Unimmunized contacts should receive 3,000 units of antitoxin intramuscularly, or have active immunization begun (not antibiotics). Any contacts with positive cultures or those who show signs of the illness should be treated with one of the antibiotic regimens mentioned above [83].

Pharyngitis and tonsillitis due to *Mycoplasma* and *Chlamydia* species, non-group A streptococci, *C. haemolyticum*, pneumococci, and staphylococci will respond to treatment with erythromycin in the same dosages as for GABHS pharyngitis (see Table 21-6). However, while some studies have suggested a slight amelioration of symptoms, a definite indication for antibiotic treatment in these self-limited illnesses has not been demonstrated.

Gonorrheal pharyngitis can be difficult to eradicate and should be treated with parenteral ceftriaxone (250 mg IM) or oral multiple-dose regimens using ampicillin with probenecid, doxycycline, or tetracycline [84] (see Table 21-6).

The mixed anaerobes of Vincent's angina respond to oral penicillin or erythromycin in the same dosages as listed for GABHS pharyngitis.

F. tularensis requires in-patient treatment with parenteral streptomycin or gentamicin. Syphilis is treated with penicillin or erythromycin in regimens described elsewhere.

Thrush is treated by nystatin suspension or tablets or clotrimazole troches until the plaque is gone or up to 14 days. Evaluation for underlying immunodeficiency should be undertaken if indicated.

Noninfectious Pharyngitis and Tonsillitis. Treatment is aimed at the underlying cause. Perforation due to mechanical injury can lead to infection of the parapharyngeal spaces and mediastinum, an emergency the treatment of which is described later in this chapter. The various neoplastic and inflammatory diseases mentioned in this section are treated by various approaches that are beyond the scope of this text.

TREATMENT OF RECURRENT AND CHRONIC TONSILLITIS

Treatment is directed against GABHS, the most common bacteria that cause infection. However, there is an increasingly recognized role of beta-lactamase—producing bacteria and encapsulated anaerobes (*Bacteroides melaninogenicus*, *Bacteroides oralis*, *Bacteroides ruminocola*) in producing chronic or hyperplastic tonsillitis [85]. This suggests that a therapeutic trial of other antibiotics, such as clindamycin, may be helpful if penicillin therapy is

Tonsillectomy remains the leading treatment for recurrent or chronic tonsillitis [70]. The stringent criteria of recurrent tonsillitis (see Table 21-5) are met by only 9% of patients referred to otolaryngologists for tonsillectomy [86]. In practice the patient should be referred for tonsillectomy whenever recurrent tonsillitis causes sufficient morbidity to seriously jeopardize functioning at school or work. Studies have shown a significant decrease in the incidence of recurrent throat infections during the 2 years following tonsillectomy with a strong trend over subsequent years [87]. The indications and contraindications for tonsillectomy are listed in Table 21-5 [87, 88].

Pharyngeal Abscesses

Peritonsillar, parapharyngeal, and retropharyngeal abscesses occur in a potential space that is invaded by the organisms of the pharyngeal space. Each begins as a cellulitis but tends to localize by the time diagnosis is made [89]. The anatomic location and contiguity can explain the spread of infection among the spaces, as illustrated in Fig. 21-2 (see also Fig. 36-5) [90, 91]. Each requires surgical drainage and, except for peritonsillar abscess, IV antibiotics and hospital admission. Table 21-9 is a reference table for these conditions.

Peritonsillar Abscess

EPIDEMIOLOGY AND PREDISPOSING FACTORS

Peritonsillar abscess is mainly a disease of young adults, ages 15 to 30 years (average age 22 years), who as a rule have coexistent tonsillitis [92]. There is, however, one case report of peritonsillar abscess after an adequately performed tonsillectomy [91]. About 70% of cases occur during winter months (October through February) [92]. In one study nearly 20% of patients were already taking penicillin at the time of diagnosis [92]. Peritonsillar abscess results from an invasion of organisms that cause tonsillitis through tonsillar capsule into the loose areolar tissue surrounding the tonsil.

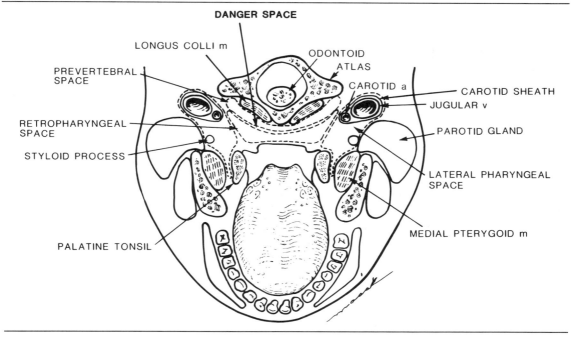

Fig. 21-2. Fascial spaces around the mouth and face. The anatomic location and contiguity can explain the spread of infection among the spaces. Reprinted from the Sept. 1991:44(3) issue of *American Family Physician*, published by the American Academy of Family Physicians, U.S. ed., with permission

PATIENT PRESENTATION

Most commonly young adults present with gradually increasing fever, dysphagia, and sore throat, symptoms similar to those of tonsillitis or pharyngitis. However, the patient also complains of ipsilateral ear fullness and otalgia and talks in a "hot potato" voice, due to swelling of soft palate and occlusion of the eustachian tube. Drooling is common. Physical examination shows tonsillar prolapse, a tender peritonsillar mass that displaces the uvula and soft palate (Fig. 21-3). While tender cervical adenopathy is present, trismus is less common and results from irritation of the internal pterygoid muscle [89, 93].

DIFFERENTIAL DIAGNOSIS

Peritonsillar cellulitis, in contrast to peritonsillar abscess, presents with no uvular deviation, no tonsillar prolapse, and a soft palate that is edematous. Every peritonsillar abscess is a potential lateral pharyngeal abscess (see Fig. 21-2 and Fig. 36-6) due to local invasion. A patient with lateral pharyngeal abscess will show not only tonsillar inflammation and swelling of the lateral pharyngeal wall but also have trismus, parotid swelling, and systemic toxicity [89, 94]. Also to be considered in the differential diagnosis are laryngitis, epiglottitis, foreign body, chemical or thermal burn, allergic edema, and aneurysms of the subclavian artery [89, 94].

THERAPY

Initial therapy in the emergency department includes antibiotics and surgical drainage. The antibiotic must cover GABHS and anaerobes, most commonly *Fusobacterium nucleatum* and *B. melaninogenicus*. First-line therapy is penicillin VK 250 mg qid PO for 10 days or penicillin G benzathine 1.2 million units IM. Penicillin-allergic individuals should be given erythromycin estolate 20 mg/kg PO or IV divided bid for 10 days. Surgical drainage has traditionally been by incision and drainage (I&D) by an otolaryngologist. In an I&D, the mucosa are incised sharply, then the abscess cavity is entered

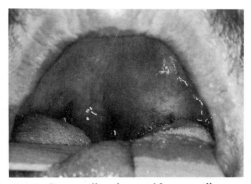

Fig. 21-3. Peritonsillar abscess. Note tonsillar prolapse and the tonsillar mass that displaces the uvula and soft palate contralaterally (one aspiration site is visible). Reprinted from the Sept. 1991:44(3) issue of *American Family Physician*, published by the American Academy of Family Physicians, U.S. ed., with permission

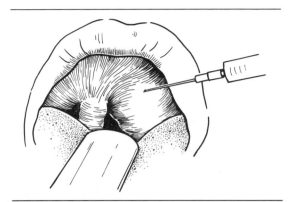

Fig. 21-4. Aspiration of peritonsillar abscess.

with a blunt hemostat to avoid damage to the carotid artery [95].

Immediate needle aspiration is becoming accepted for treating peritonsillar abscess [92, 96, 97]. It is technically easier and less painful than I&D in patients with trismus [92]. The proximity of the carotid artery should be considered. In one study the authors used an 18-gauge needle and aspirated at three points to get adequate drainage (superior pole, middle, and inferior pole) [92]. However, they found two immediate recurrences of peritonsillar abscess among 41 patients.

The classic technique consists of using a 1½-in., 18-gauge needle with a 10-cc syringe. After topical anesthesia has been given, the tonsil is aspirated midway between the base of the uvula and the posterior maxillary molar (Fig. 21-4). The needle is advanced approximately 1–2 cm while constant suction is applied. The abscess will usually be encountered and 1–10 cc of pus will be withdrawn. If the trismus is severe, an 18-gauge spinal needle will allow easy access to the tonsil. A single aspiration will resolve the problem in 90% of cases, with a second aspiration 24–48 hours later dealing with the 10% that fail initial therapy. Practitioners who are not head and neck specialists have been shown to be able to treat peritonsillar abscess competently in the emergency department setting [98].

Indications for admission are the following: (1) threatened airway embarrassment; (2) suspicion of spread to another fascial compartment; (3) inability to swallow fluids or antibiotics; (4) need for immediate tonsillectomy, or so-called "abscess tonsillectomy." Immediate tonsillectomy is appropriate for patients under 40 years with a history of recurrent tonsillitis or previous peritonsillar abscess. It has been shown to reduce the total period of hospitalization from an average of 7.2 to 3.9 days (compared with an I&D and interval tonsillectomy) [95]. Tonsillectomy is contraindicated in patients over age 40 and those with no previous history of tonsillitis. In this group recurrence of peritonsillar abscess is low [99, 100].

Discharge is indicated if drainage occurs, the patient is able to swallow, and there is no airway embarrassment. Follow-up should be in 24–48 hours to inspect for immediate recurrence.

Lateral Pharyngeal Abscess

The lateral pharyngeal space is also called the pharyngomaxillary space and the peripharyngeal space. Its exact location is crucial to appreciate how infection can spread [89, 90] (see Fig. 21-2 and Fig. 36-5). The lateral pharyngeal space is lateral to the superior pharyngeal constrictor muscle and its fascial covering and lateral to the oral cavity. It is closest to the peritonsillar space and is bounded laterally by the medial pterygoid muscle, the mandible, and the parotid gland. Posteriorly it extends to the prevertebral fascia and communicates with the retropharyngeal space. It is shaped like an inverted cone with its base on the sphenoid bone proximally and its apex at the hyoid bone distally.

The lateral pharyngeal space can be divided into

anterior and posterior compartments by the styloid process with its attached stylopharyngeous muscle and fascia (see Fig. 21-2). The anterior or muscular compartment contains fat, connective tissue, lymph nodes, and muscle. It is closest to the tonsillar fossa. The posterior or neurovascular compartment contains the carotid sheath (with carotid artery, internal jugular vein, and vagus nerve), the cervical sympathetic trunk, and cranial nerves IX through XII. Jugular lymph nodes cover the carotid sheath, and infection can cause the entire sheath to become indurated [90, 93].

EPIDEMIOLOGY AND PREDISPOSING FACTORS

Infection can arise from sources throughout the neck. Extension from peritonsillar infections can occur by direct penetration through the pharyngeal wall, by lymphatic spread, or via infection of perforating arteries and veins [90, 94]. Other sources are infection of the teeth, tonsils, adenoids, parotid gland, submandibular space, masticator space, or retropharyngeal space [90, 93].

PATIENT PRESENTATION

Anterior-compartment infection presents as dysphagia, trismus, or pain of the jaw, side of the head, or ear. Posterior-compartment infection may present as a history of pharyngitis 2 weeks previously, but history is usually unrevealing.

In anterior-compartment infection examination will show trismus, induration, and swelling at the angle of the mandible, medial bulging of the pharyngeal wall, and systemic toxicity [90, 94]. Posterior-compartment infection presents without lateral pharyngeal wall swelling, because it will be behind the palatopharyngeal arch and therefore missed [90, 94]. Swelling can be appreciated at three sites where the posterior compartment contacts mobile structures: the parotid space, the angle of the mandible, or the superior sternocleidomastoid muscle (here induration of the carotid sheath may be appreciated) [94]. Diagnosis is cryptic and often made only after a complication has occurred [90, 93, 94, 101].

Complications result from infection of all components of the carotid sheath and manifest as suppurative jugular thrombosis (termed postanginal sepsis) [90, 93, 94, 102, 103], carotid artery erosion and rupture [102, 104], laryngeal edema and obstruction [90, 94], retropharyngeal-space infection

[89, 94], and a poorly substantiated report of sudden death presumably caused by vagus nerve involvement [105], which is (unjustly) perpetuated through the literature [89, 90]. Suppurative jugular venous thrombosis is the most common vascular complication of lateral pharyngeal infection. Look for abrupt onset of chills, fever, and prostration with tenderness at the angle of the mandible or along the sternocleidomastoid muscle [89, 102, 106]. Dyspnea indicates that swelling has descended to involve the epiglottis and the larynx [93]. Head and neck CT scans are useful for identifying the abscess cavity; however, these studies will not show an isolated jugular venous thrombosis [89]. Occasionally gallium scanning can identify posterior compartment infection in a patient with sepsis of unknown cause, but it is plagued by false-negatives and delayed results [106].

DIFFERENTIAL DIAGNOSIS

In peritonsillar abscess patients will have fever, tonsillar prolapse, and less commonly trismus, but they will not have the parotid swelling or systemic toxicity associated with parapharyngeal-space infection. A masticator-space infection follows infection of the third molar and presents as trismus, pain, and swelling over the mandible, since this space contains all the muscles of mastication (see Chap. 36).

THERAPY

All patients require antibiotics, surgical drainage, and admission. Traditionally aqueous penicillin G 20 million units qd divided q4h. IV is used, but the latest data show an emergence of *Bacteroides* species that are penicillin resistant. Therefore, penicillin should be combined with metronidazole or clindamycin 600 mg q6h IV. Second-line treatment should be with amoxcillin-clavulonic acid (Augmentin) 500 mg q6h PO or ampicillin-sulbactam (Unasyn) 2 gs ampicillin/M/IV q6h. Chloramphenicol 1 g q6h IV is an alternate choice if there is penicillin allergy [101, 103, 106]. The surgical approach is always external to allow exposure to control potential carotid artery hemorrhage [107]. After admission the patient should be watched carefully for signs of infectious rupture of the internal carotid artery (56%), external carotid and its branches (25%), or common carotid artery (13%) [104]. Due to the protection afforded by the carotid sheath, vessel erosion is delayed for 1–2 weeks after onset of symptoms. It can erode even after surgical drainage, usually while the patient is still hospitalized. The following may herald carotid-artery rupture: small hemorrhages from nose, mouth, or ear (so-called herald bleeds), hematoma in the surrounding tissues, and onset of shock [102, 104]. Any suspicion of carotid-artery bleeding warrants investigation by angiography to localize the bleeding site and assess collateral flow with the immediate consultation of an ear, nose, and throat (ENT) surgeon or a vascular surgeon.

Retropharyngeal Abscess

The location of the retropharyngeal space reveals why infection can spread rapidly. It is bounded anteriorly by the pharyngeal constrictor and posteriorly by the alar fascia (see Figure 21-2) and is shaped like an inverted cone with its base against the skull and its apex terminating at C7 or T1, where the alar fascia fuses with the fascia of the pharyngeal constrictor [90, 94] (Fig. 21-5). The space contains loose areolar tissue and two chains of retropharyngeal lymph nodes located on either side of midline. If lymph nodes are the origin of the infection, this causes a pharyngeal mass to be seen to one side of the midline. These nodes drain the nose, nasopharynx, pharynx, middle ear, eustachian tube, and paranasal sinuses. If the source is a prevertebral space infection, swelling may be midline. The retropharyngeal space communicates with the "danger" space posteriorly (see Fig. 21-2 and shaded area in Fig. 21-5). Because the danger space extends nearly to the diaphragm, infection of this "highway to the mediastinum" should be considered concurrent with retropharyngeal infection [94]. Descending necrotizing mediastinitis is associated with a 40%–50% mortality, usually from sepsis and often within hours of diagnosis, even with IV antibiotics [89, 101].

EPIDEMIOLOGY AND RISK FACTORS
Children under 4 years are at greatest risk, because the retropharyngeal lymph nodes have not yet regressed [105, 108]. The infection may arise from suppuration of any of the sites of lymph node drainage [105]. In adults it most often results from extension from infection of the lateral pharyngeal space [89, 101, 102, 105] and can be concurrent with

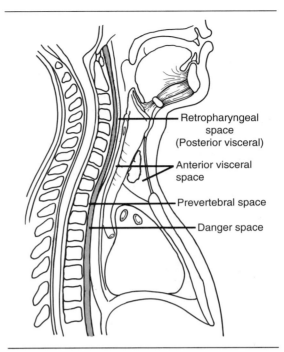

Fig. 21-5. Midline sagittal section showing deep spaces of neck and chest. Note how spread of infection from retropharyngeal space to the danger space (shaded) can spread to the mediastinum, thence to the lungs and pericardium

infection of other spaces. Other sources are trauma, including penetrating trauma and foreign bodies, and iatrogenic trauma, such as suctioning, endoscopy, and attempts at intubation [109].

Presentation of retropharyngeal abscess in children differs from that in adults. Children have vague symptoms of fever, irritability, dyspnea, dysphagia, and drooling [105]. Adult complaints are directly referable to the pharynx: fever, sore throat, noisy breathing, regurgitation, dyspnea, and stiff neck [105, 108]. Retropharyngeal abscess manifests after iatrogenic trauma as sore throat or neck pain 1–2 days after the procedure [109]. Severe respiratory distress, chest pain, or pleurisy suggests extension to the mediastinum or the pleura [89, 101]. Examination in children shows cervical adenopathy with the neck held rigid and tilting *away* from the infected side [105]. In contrast a lateral pharyngeal abscess involves head tilt *toward* the infected side. It is difficult to see or palpate any retropharyngeal mass in children. When present and seen early, swelling may be to the side of midline

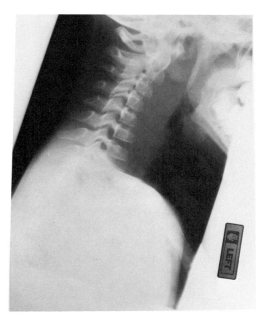

Fig. 21-6. Soft-tissue lateral neck radiograph in 7-year-old boy with retropharyngeal abscess. Note that prevertebral space is widened beyond the upper limit of 7 mm at C2 and 14 mm at C6. Reprinted from the Sept. 1991:44(3) issue of *American Family Physician*, published by the American Academy of Family Physicians, U.S. ed., with permission

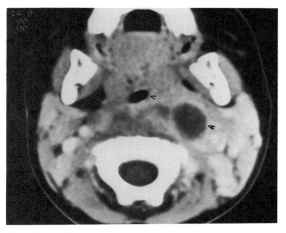

Fig. 21-7. CT scan with contrast showing retropharyngeal abscess in a child, with the abscess seen as a thick enhancing rim with central low-density zone. It typically lateralizes in children when one chain of bilateral retropharyngeal lymph nodes is suppurative. Reprinted from the Sept. 1991:44(3) issue of *American Family Physician*, published by the American Academy of Family Physicians, U.S. ed., with permission

when one but not both chains of retropharyngeal lymph nodes is suppurative [105]. In adults a midline pharyngeal mass is apparent. Care should be taken not to cause rupture of the abscess from digital pressure because death from aspiration can occur [105].

A soft-tissue lateral neck radiograph is imperative when a retropharyngeal abscess is a possibility. Diagnosis is supported by prevertebral soft-tissue widening, air or air-fluid levels, loss of cervical lordosis, or foreign bodies [89]. A proper radiograph has the neck in full extension and is taken during inspiration. In adults the upper limit of normal retropharyngeal soft-tissue width (measure from the posterior pharyngeal wall to the vertebral body) is 7 mm at C2 level, and normal retrotracheal width is 22 mm at C6. In children the numbers are 7 mm at C2 and 14 mm at C6 (Fig. 21-6). In infants it is 11 mm at C6. The radiologic diagnosis of retropharyngeal widening suggesting possible abscess formation in children is not uncommonly made and is rarely confirmed. A chest radiograph should be

obtained to evaluate for signs of mediastinal, pleural, and pulmonary spread. If mediastinal spread is suspected, however, a contrast-enhanced chest CT scan is more sensitive and can guide the surgical approach to drainage [89]. A contrast-enhanced CT scan can show the abscess as a thick enhancing rim with a central low-density zone, soft-tissue air, cystic appearance of fluid, and location consistent with a given fascial space (Fig. 21-7). Ultrasonography shows sensitivity of 95% in small studies but falsely reports hyperplastic lymph nodes for abscess 25% of the time [89].

DIFFERENTIAL DIAGNOSIS

The differential diagnosis includes infection of the cervical prevertebral space (Fig. 21-2 and Fig. 21-5), which also shows retropharyngeal swelling on lateral neck radiograph. The diagnosis must be entertained in any adult with fever and retropharyngeal swelling. A neck that is tender to palpation anteriorly or posteriorly (without swelling) suggests cervical prevertebral space infection. Another is history compatible with osteomyelitis of the cervical spine, which always predisposes to cervical prevertebral space infection [108]. Since the causative organism of cervical prevertebral abscess is S.

Table 21-9. Reference charts for parapharyngeal abscesses

Population at risk	Likely organisms	Appropriate treatment	Minimum data	Disposition
Peritonsillar Abscess				
Hx of tonsillitis, winter months	GABHS, α-hemolytic streptococcus Mixed anaerobes: *Fusobacterium nucleatum* *Bacteroides melaninogenicus* *Staphylococcus aureus*	Surgical drainage *and* penicillin VK 250 mg qid PO for 10 days *or* benzathine penicillin G 1.2 million U IM Erythromycin estolate 20 mg/kg PO or IV divided bid for 10 days (Confirm by culture) Dicloxacillin 500 mg qid PO for 10 days Erythromycin estolate 20 mg/kg PO or IV divided bid for 10 days	Hx: Fever, dysphagia, sore throat, muffled "hot potato" voice, otalgia, tender cervical adenopathy PE: Uvular deviation, tonsillar prolapse	Abscess drainage or immediate tonsillectomy for patients under 40 and with hx. of recurrent abscesses Discharge from emergency department if drainage occurs, patient can swallow and has no airway embarrassment; beware of airway obstruction with bilaterality, laryngeal edema, or retropharyngeal extension
Lateral Pharyngeal Abscess				
Hx of pharyngitis, sinusitis, otitis media	α-hemolytic streptococcus GABHS Pneumococcus *Eikenella corrodens* Anaerobic bacteroides sensitive to PCN Anaerobic bacteroides resistant to PCN *Staphylococcus aureus*	Surgical drainage with one of following: (1) penicillin 1.2 million U IV q4h *plus* metronidazole 750 mg tid PO *or* clindamycin 300–600 mg q6h IV (children: 20–40 mg/kg/day in 3 or 4 doses) IV or IM (2) amoxicillin-clavulanate 500 mg tid PO *or* ampicillin/sulbactam 2 g ampicillin q6h IV (3) For those with penicillin allergy: chloramphenicol 50 mg/kg/d divided q6h IV	Anterior compartment: 1. Trismus 2. Induration and swelling at angle of mandible 3. Medial bulging of pharyngeal wall 4. Systemic toxicity	Hospitalization, surgical drainage, IV antibiotics Evaluate head and neck CT
Recent (2 weeks previously) or no history of infection but presents with septic jugular thrombo-	α-hemolytic streptococcus GABHS Pneumococcus *Eikenella corrodens* Anaerobic bacteroids sensitive to PCN Anaerobic bacteroides resistant to PCN *Staphylococcus aureus*		Posterior compartment: Hx: dyspnea, hoarseness, neck pain PE: neck tilted away from abscess, systemic toxicity, swelling at angle of mandible or at superior sternocleidomastoid muscle	Hospitalization, surgical drainage, IV antibiotics Evaluate head and neck CT

phlebitis (post-anginal sepsis)			Lab/x-ray: Head and neck CT If septic jugular thrombophlebitis, may present with only fever, bacteremia (50%), and pulmonary emboli (50%)	

Retropharyngeal Abscess

Children with suppurative adenitis from infection of ear or respiratory structures	Mixed anaerobes/aerobes: *Bacteroides* species *Fusobacterium* species GABHS α-hemolytic strep β-lactamase producing *Bacteroides* species	(1) Penicillin G 12–20 million U/d (2) Cefoxitin 1–2 g q8h (3) Erythromycin and metronidazole	Children Hx: vague symptoms, fever, irritability, dyspnea, dysphagia, drooling PE: cervical adenopathy, nuchal rigidity, neck tilted toward abscess X-ray: ST lateral neck imperative	Hospitalization with surgical drainage
Adults with spread of adjacent infections, pharyngeal trauma	Mixed anaerobes/aerobes: *Bacteroides* species *Fusobacterium* species GABHS α-hemolytic streptococcus β-lactamase producing *Bacteroides* species	(1) Penicillin G 12–20 million U/d (2) Cefoxitin 1–2 g q8h (3) Erythromycin and metronidazole (For severe illness use penicillin G and metronidazole or clindamycin)	Adults Hx: fever, sore throat, dysphagia, noisy breathing, regurgitation, dyspnea, nuchal rigidity PE: pharyngeal mass X-ray: ST lateral neck imperative, chest x-ray	Hospitalization with surgical drainage
Institutionalized patients, diabetics, chronic alcoholics	Mixed anaerobes/aerobes: *Bacteroids* species *Fusobacterium* species GABHS α-hemolytic streptococcus β-lactamase producing *Bacteroides* species Gram-negative rods: *Escherichia coli* *Klebsiella pneumoniae* *Haemophilus influenzae*	(1) Penicillin G 12–20 million U/d (2) Cefoxitin 1–2 g q8h (3) Erythromycin and metronidazole (For severe illness use penicillin G and metronidazole or clindamycin)	Adults Hx: fever, sore throat, dysphagia, noisy breathing, regurgitation, dyspnea, nuchal rigidity PE: pharyngeal mass X-ray: ST lateral neck imperative, chest x-ray	Hospitalization with surgical drainage
Cervical osteomyelitis, external penetrating trauma	*Staphylococcus aureus* *Mycobacterium tuberculosis*	Nafcillin 1 g q4h IV *or* vancomycin		

aureus, prompt recognition is essential to select an antistaphylococcal antibiotic.

Severe croup and epiglottitis may present with fever and stridor. These can be evaluated by soft-tissue neck radiographs that show stippling or "pencil" sign on posteroanterior film in croup or by a lateral neck radiograph that shows swelling of the epiglottis or epiarytenoid folds in epiglottitis. Nuchal rigidity may result from meningitis as well as from retropharyngeal abscess. Meningitis can be diagnosed by positive lumbar puncture, negative pharyngeal exam, and normal soft-tissue lateral neck radiograph.

Peritonsillar abscess, especially if bilateral, can be mistaken for retropharyngeal abscess. In general patients with peritonsillar abscess do not present with the systemic toxicity and nuchal rigidity that patients with retropharyngeal abscess do. Often a contrast-enhanced CT scan is necessary to distinguish the two.

THERAPY

Antibiotics are begun and a surgical or an ENT consultation obtained emergently. Penicillin is the first-line antibiotic and can be used alone (Table 21-9). Localized abscesses can be drained transorally with local anesthesia. Spread to parapharyngeal spaces will require an anterior cervical approach. Subsequent therapy requires a high index of suspicion for complications, including meningitis, mediastinitis, epiglottitis, pneumonia, empyema, bronchial erosion, pyopneumothorax, purulent pericarditis, and spontaneous rupture with aspiration and asphyxiation. Worst among these is descending necrotizing mediastinitis, characterized clinically by symptoms of severe dyspnea, pleuritic chest pain, or retrosternal discomfort, as well as those complaints related to neck infection [93].

References

1. National Center for Health Statistics. *Physician Visits, Volume and Interval Since Last Visit, United States, 1980* (series 10, no. 144). Washington, DC: Public Health Service, 1983. U.S. Dept. of Health and Human Services publication PHS 83-1572.
2. National Center for Health Statistics. *Current Estimates from the National Health Interview Survey, United States, 1982* Washington, DC: Public Health Service, 1985. U.S. Dept. of Health and Human Services publication PHS 85-1578.
3. Liu C. The common cold. In PD Hoeprich, MC Jordan (eds.), *Infectious Diseases: A Modern Treatise of Infectious Processes* (4th ed.). Philadelphia: Lippincott, 1989. Pp. 231–56.
4. Dick Ed, Blumer CR, Evans AS. Epidemiology of infections with rhinovirus types 43 and 55 in a group of University of Wisconsin student families. *Am J Epidemiol* 86:386–400, 1967.
5. Beem MO. Acute respiratory illness in nursery school children: a longitudinal study of the occurrence of illness and respiratory viruses. *Am J Epidemiol* 90:30–44, 1969.
6. Mufson MA et al. Relationship of rhinovirus infection to mild upper respiratory disease. III. Further epidemiologic observations in military personnel. *Am J Epidemiol* 83:379–88, 1966.
7. Gwaltney JM Jr et al. Rhinovirus infections in an industrial population. I. The occurrence of illness. *N Engl J Med* 275:1261–68, 1966.
8. Gwaltney JM Jr, Moskalski PB, Hendley JO. Hand-to-hand transmission of rhinovirus colds. *Ann Intern Med* 88:463–67, 1978.
9. Dick EC et al. Aerosol transmission of rhinovirus colds. *J Infect Dis* 156:442–48, 1987.
10. Hendley JO, Wenzel RP, Gwaltney JM Jr. Transmission of rhinovirus colds by self inoculation. *N Engl J Med* 288:1361–64, 1973.
11. Jennings LC et al. Near disappearance of rhinovirus along a fomite transmission chain. *J Infect Dis* 158:888–92, 1988.
12. Gwaltney JM Jr. Epidemiology of the common cold. *Ann NY Acad Sci* 353:54–60, 1980.
13. Fox JP, Cooney MK, Hall CE. The Seattle virus watch. V. Epidemiologic observations of rhinovirus infections in families with young children (1965–1968). *Am J Epidemiol* 10:122–43, 1975.
14. Hatch MT et al. Stability of airborne rhinovirus type 2 under atmospheric and physiological conditions [abstract]. *Proc Am Soc Microbiol* 18:193–95, 1976.
15. Douglas RG, Lindgren KM, Cough RB. Exposure to cold environment and rhinovirus common cold. *N Engl J Med* 279:742–47, 1968.
16. Hendley JO, Gwaltney JM Jr. Mechanisms of transmission of rhinovirus infections. *Epidemiol Rev* 10:242–58, 1988.
17. Hamre D, Connelly AP Jr, Procknow JJ. Virologic studies of acute respiratory disease in young adults. IV. Virus isolation during four years of surveillance. *Am J Epidemiol* 83:238–49, 1966.
18. Lowenstein SR, Parrino TA. Management of the common cold. *Adv Intern Med* 32:207–33, 1987.

19. Fox JP et al. Rhinovirus in Seattle families, 1975–1979. *Am J Epidemiol* 122:830–46, 1985.

20. Martin NG et al. Association between alpha-1-antitrypsin types and the common cold. *Human Hered* 33:265–69, 1983.

21. Gwaltney JM. Rhinoviruses. *Yale J Biol Med* 48:17–45, 1975.

22. Osler W, McCrae T. *The Principles and Practice of Medicine* (9th ed). New York: D. Appleton, 1924. Pp. 371–72.

23. Douglas NG. Influenza in man. In ED Kilbourne (ed.), *The Influenza Viruses and Influenza*. New York: Academic, 1975. Pp. 395–488.

24. Nakib W, Dearden CJ, Tyrrell DA. Evaluation of a new enzyme-linked immunosorbent assay (ELISA) in the diagnosis of rhinovirus infection. *J Med Virol* 29(4):268–72, 1989.

25. Couch RB. Viral and mycoplasmal infections. In JP Sanford, JP Luby (eds.), *Infectious Diseases*. New York: Grune & Stratton, 1981. Pp. 4–70.

26. Hall WJ, Douglas RG Jr. Pulmonary function during and after common respiratory infections. *Ann Rev Med* 31:233–38, 1980.

27. Sperber ST, Hayden FG. Chemotherapy of rhinovirus colds. *Antimicrob Agents Chemother* 32:409–19, 1988.

28. Consumers Union. Cough remedies: Which ones work best? *Consumer Reports* Feb.:58–61, 1983.

29. Tyrrell DA. Hot news on the common cold. *Ann Rev Microbiol* 42:35–47, 1988.

30. Lampert RP, Robinson DS, Soyka LF. A critical look at oral decongestants. *Pediatrics* 55:550–52, 1974.

31. Gilman AG et al. (eds.). *The Pharmacological Basis of Therapeutics* (7th ed.). New York: Macmillan, 1985. Pp. 168–69.

32. Bluestone CD et al. Common cold: general discussion. *Ped Infect Dis J* 7(3):239, 1988.

33. White WB, Riotte K. Drugs for cough and cold symptoms in hypertensive patients. *Am Fam Physician* 31(3):183–87, 1985.

34. Physician's Desk Reference for Nonprescription Drugs. Oradell, NJ: Medical Economics, 1988. Pp. 735–36.

35. Berkow R (ed.). *The Merck Manual* (14th ed.). Rahway, NJ: Merck, 1982. Pp. 2415–16.

36. Bluestone CB et al. Common cold: consensus. *Ped Infect Dis J* 7:241, 1988. 7(3):241–42.

37. Matthys M, Bleicher B, Bleicher U. Dextromethorphan and codeine: objective assessment of antitussive activity in patients with chronic cough. *J Int Med Res* 11:92–100, 1983.

38. Irwin RS, Rosen MJ, Braman SS. Cough: a comprehensive review. *Arch Intern Med* 137:1186–91, 1977.

39. Kuhn JJ et al. Antitussive effect of guaifenesin in young adults with natural colds. *Chest* 82:713–18, 1982.

40. Ferguson JA. Progress in the treatment of coughs. *Am Pharm* 23:48–52, 1983.

41. Stanley ED et al. Increased shedding with aspirin treatment of rhinovirus infection. *JAMA* 231:1248–51, 1985.

42. M. Abramowicz (ed.). Viralizer for the common cold. *Med Lett Drugs Ther* 31(784):8, Jan. 27, 1989.

43. Naclerio RM et al. Is histamine responsible for the symptoms of rhinovirus colds? A look at the inflammatory mediators following infection. *Pediatr Infect Dis J* 7:215–22, 1988.

44. Doyle WJ et al. A double-blind, placebo-controlled clinical trial of the effect of chlorpheniramine on the response of the nasal airway, middle ear and eustachian tube to provocative rhinovirus challenge. *Pediatr Infect Dis J* 7:229–38, 1988.

45. Truswell AS. Ascorbic acid. *N Engl J Med* 315:708–9, 1986.

46. Monto AS, Schwartz SA, Albrecht JK. Ineffectiveness of postexposure prophylaxis of rhinovirus infection with low-dose intranasal alpha 2b interferon in families. *Antimicrob Agents Chemother* 33:387–90, 1989.

47. Sperber SJ et al. Ineffectiveness of recombinant interferon-beta serine nasal drops for prophylaxis of natural colds. *J Infect Dis* 160:700–5, 1989.

48. Higgins PG et al. Recombinant human interferon-gamma as prophylaxis against rhinovirus colds in volunteers. *J Interferon Res* 8:591–96, 1988.

49. Sperber SJ, Hayden FG. Chemotherapy of rhinovirus colds. *Antimicrob Agents Chemother* 32:409–19, 1988.

50. Ophir D, Elad Y. Effects of steam inhalation on nasal patency and nasal symptoms in patients with the common cold. *Am J Otolaryngol* 8:149–53, 1987.

51. Tyrrell D, Barrow I, Arthur J. Local hyperthermia benefits natural and experimental common colds. *Br. Med. J.* 298:1280–83, 1989.

52. Macknin ML, Mathew S, Medendorp SV. Effect of inhaling heated vapor on symptoms of the common cold. *JAMA* 264:989–91, 1990.

53. M. Abramowicz (ed.). *Med Lett Drugs Ther* 31:8, 1989.

54. Hedges JR, Lowe RA. Approach to acute pharyngitis. *Emerg Med Clin North Am* 5:335–51, 1987.

55. Joyce SM. Acute sore throat. In GC Hamilton (ed.), *Emergency Medicine: An Approach to Clinical*

Problem Solving. Philadelphia: Saunders, 1991. Pp. 547–60.

56. Todd JK. The sore throat: pharyngitis and epiglottitis. *Infect Dis Clin North Am* 2:149–62, 1988.

57. Lowe RA, Hedges JR. Pharyngitis. In ML Callaham (ed.), *Current Therapy in Emergency Medicine*. Toronto: Decker, 1987. Pp. 205–09.

58. Veasy LG et al. Resurgence of acute rheumatic fever in the intermountain area of the United States. *N Engl J Med* 316:421–27, 1978.

59. Shapiro J, Fried MP, Strome M. Postanginal sepsis. *Head Neck* 11:164–69, 1989.

60. Gerber MA, Randolph MF, Mayo DR. The group A streptococcal carrier state: a reexamination. *AJDC* 142:562–65, 1988.

61. Turner JC et al. Association of group C beta-hemolytic streptococci with endemic pharyngitis among college students. *JAMA* 264:2644–47, 1990.

62. Incidences of reportable diseases in the United States. *MMWR* 38:53–56, 1989.

63. Palumbo FM. Pediatric considerations of infections and inflammations of Waldeyer's Ring. *Otolaryngol Clin North Am* 20:311–16, 1987.

64. Bluestone CD. Effect of adenoids, tonsils and adenoidectomy (with or without tonsillectomy) on eustachian tube function. *Ann Otol Rhinol Laryngol* 194(S120):42, 1985.

65. Kornblut AD. A traditional approach to surgery of the tonsils and adenoids. *Otolaryngol Clin North Am* 20:349–63, 1987.

66. Brodsky L. Modern assessment of tonsils and adenoids. *Pediatr Clin North Am* 36:1551–68, 1989.

67. Sprinkle PM, Veltri RW. Quantitative alterations in the ecology of the oropharyngeal microflora subsequent to tonsillectomy and adenoidectomy. *Trans Am Acad Ophthalmol Otolaryngol* 78:ORL60–63, 1974.

68. Paradise JL et al. Efficacy of tonsillectomy for recurrent throat infections in severely affected children. Results of parallel randomized and nonrandomized clinical trials. *N Engl J Med* 310:674–83, 1984.

69. McCloskey RV et al. The 1970 epidemic of diphtheria in San Antonio. *Ann Intern Med* 75:495–503, 1971.

70. Kornblut AB, Bottone ME. Tonsillitis and peritonsillar abscess. In ML Callaham (ed.), *Current Therapy in Emergency Medicine*. Toronto: Decker, 1987. Pp. 209–12.

71. Puar RK, Puar HS. Lingual tonsillitis. *South Med J* 79:1126–28, 1986.

72. Breese BB. A simple scorecard for the tentative diagnosis of streptococcal pharyngitis. *AJDC* 131:514–17, 1977.

73. Wigton RS, Connor JL, Centor RM. Transportability of a decision rule for the diagnosis of streptococcal pharyngitis. *Arch Intern Med* 146:81–83, 1986.

74. Walsh BT et al. Recognition of streptococcal pharyngitis in adults. *Arch Intern Med* 135:1493–97, 1975.

75. Gerber MA. Comparison of throat cultures and rapid strep tests for diagnosis of streptococcal pharyngitis. *Pediatr Infect Dis J* 8:820–24, 1989.

76. Gerber MA, Markowitz M. Management of streptococcal pharyngitis revisited. *Pediatr Infect Dis* 4:518–26, 1985.

77. Hedges JR, Lowe RA. Streptococcal pharyngitis in the emergency department: analysis of therapeutic strategies. *Am J Emerg Med* 4:107–15, 1986.

78. Lowe RA, Hedges JR. Early treatment of streptococcal pharyngitis. *Ann Emerg Med* 13:440–48, 1984.

79. Pichichero ME. Controversies in the treatment of streptococcal pharyngitis. *Am Fam Physician* 4:1567–76, 1990.

80. Danjani AS et al. Prevention of rheumatic fever. *Circulation* 78:1082–86, 1988.

81. Marlow RA, Torrez AJ Jr, Haxby D. The treatment of nonstreptococcal pharyngitis with erythromycin: a preliminary study. *Fam Med* 21:425–27, 1989.

82. Maruyama S et al. Sensitivity of group A streptococci to antibiotics. *AJDC* 133:1143–45, 1979.

83. Hoeprich PD. Diphtheria. In PD Hoeprich, MC Jordan (eds.), *Infectious Diseases* (4th ed). Philadelphia: Lippincott, 1989. Pp. 318–26.

84. Hutt DM, Judson FN. Epidemiology and treatment of oropharyngeal gonorrhea. *Ann Intern Med* 104:655–58, 1986.

85. Brook I. The role of beta-lactamase-producing bacteria in the persistence of streptococcal tonsillar infection. *Rev Infect Dis* 6:601–7, 1984.

86. Witt RL. The tonsil and adenoid controversy. *Del Med J* 61:289–94, 1989.

87. Fry TL, Pillsbury HC. The implication of "controlled" studies of tonsillectomy and adenoidectomy. *Otolaryngol Clin North Am* 20:409–13, 1986.

88. Gates GA, Folbre TW. Indications for adenotonsillectomy. *Arch Otolaryngol Head Neck Surg* 112:501–2, 1986.

89. Blomquist IK, Bayer AS. Life-threatening deep fascial space infections of the head and neck. *Infect Dis Clin North Am* 2:237–63, 1988.

90. Hall C. The parapharyngeal space: an anatomical and clinical study. *Ann Otol Rhinol Laryngol* 43:793, 1934.

91. Roos K, Lind L. Peritonsillar abscess in spite of adequately performed tonsillectomy. *Arch Otolaryngol Head Neck Surg* 116:205, 1990.

92. Spires JR et al. Treatment of peritonsillar abscess: a prospective study of aspiration vs. incision and drainage. *Arch Otolaryngol Head Neck Surg* 113:984–86, 1987.

93. Scully RF, Galdabini JJ, McNeely BU. Case records of the Massachusetts General Hospital: weekly clinicopathological exercises. *N Engl J Med* 298:894, 1978.

94. Levitt GW. Cervical fascia and deep neck infections. *Laryngoscope.* 80:409–35, 1970.

95. McCurdy JA. Peritonsillar abscess: a comparison of treatment by immediate tonsillectomy and interval tonsillectomy. *Arch Otolaryngol* 103:414–15, 1977.

96. Herzon FS, Aldridge JH. Peritonsillar abscess: needle aspiration. *Otolaryngol Head Neck Surg* 89:910–11, 1981.

97. Schechter GL et al. Changing face of treatment of peritonsillar abscess. *Laryngoscope* 92:657–59, 1982.

98. Ophir D, Bawnik J, Poria Y. Peritonsillar abscess. *Arch Otolaryngol Head Neck Surg* 114:661–63, 1988.

99. Kronenberg J, Wolf M, Leventon G. Peritonsillar abscess: recurrence rate and the indication for tonsillectomy. *Am J Otolaryngol* 8:82–84, 1987.

100. Herbild O, Bonding P. Peritonsillar abscess. *Arch Otolaryngol* 107:540–42, 1981.

101. Wills PI, Vernon RP. Complications of space infections of the head and neck. *Laryngoscope* 91:1129–36, 1981.

102. Alexander DW, Leonard JR, Trai ML. Vascular complications of deep neck abscesses: a report of four cases. *Laryngoscope* 78:361–70, 1968.

103. Celikel TH, Muthuswamy PP. Case reports: septic pulmonary emboli secondary to internal jugular vein phlebitis (postanginal sepsis) caused by *Eikenella corrodens. Am Rev Resp Dis* 130:510, 1984.

104. Salinger S, Pearlman SJ. Hemorrhage from pharyngeal and peritonsillar abscesses. *Arch Otolaryngol* 18:464, 1933.

105. Shapiro SL. Deep cervical infection following tonsillectomy. *Arch Otolaryngol* 11:701–11, 1930.

106. Hadlock FP, Wallace RJ Jr, Rivera M. Pulmonary septic emboli secondary to parapharyngeal abscess: postanginal sepsis. *Radiology* 130:29–33, 1979.

107. Ramsey PG, Weymuller EA. Complications of bacterial infections of the ears, paranasal sinuses, and oropharynx in adults. *Emerg Med Clin North Am* 3:143–60, 1985.

108. Bryan CS, King BG, Bryant RE. Retropharyngeal infection in adults. *Arch Intern Med* 134:126–30, 1974.

109. Heath LK, Pierce TH. Retropharyngeal abscess following endotracheal intubation. *Chest* 72:776–77, 1977.

22

Respiratory Airway Infections

Chien Liu
Christopher M. Lowther

Respiratory infections are the most common illnesses that bring patients to a physician's office. Although these illnesses usually are not life threatening, many patients with upper or lower respiratory infections seek medical care in the emergency department. The emergency physician needs to assess the situation in sorting out those with potential serious consequences for hospitalization or emergency intervention.

The upper respiratory tract infections and the pneumonias are dealt with in Chap. 21 and Chap. 23, respectively). This chapter discusses the airway infections that occur between the epiglottis and the bronchioles.

Pathophysiology of Airway Infections

The respiratory tract is covered by a layer of ciliated epithelium from the naso-oropharynx to the bronchioles. The beating action of the ciliated cells is a powerful mechanism to rid the respiratory tract of foreign particles as well as infectious agents. Although natural specific defects of the microtubular structures of the respiratory cilia cells that interfere with the ciliary action have been reported, infection and cigarette smoking are probably the most important factors in damaging the ciliary action of these epithelial cells. Influenza viruses notably infect and destroy the ciliated epithelial cells [1], resulting in desquamation and denudation of the respiratory tract without functional ciliated cells. Influenza A virus infection has also been shown to cause airway hyperactivity and airway dysfunction [2]. In *Mycoplasma pneumoniae* infection the organisms are found to attach onto the ciliated epithelium. Possibly they liberate hydrogen peroxide or other toxic products, which may produce a ciliolytic effect to damage the bronchial epithelium.

Secretory IgA is the principal immunoglobulin in the respiratory secretions to exert a protective effect by preventing adherence of foreign substances, including microorganisms, onto the respiratory epithelium. Certain bacterial isolates such as *Streptococcus pneumoniae* and *Haemophilus influenzae* are known to produce IgA proteases that destroy the secretory IgA. This may explain why pneumococcus and *H. influenzae* are the most common bacterial colonizers in patients with chronic bronchitis and chronic obstructive pulmonary disease (COPD).

Supraglottitic Infections

Children with stridor and fever present a common and difficult diagnostic dilemma for the emergency department physician. The doctor is confronted

Table 22-1. Causes of supraglottic airway obstruction

Infectious Causes
Acute epiglottitis
Peritonsillar abscess
Retropharyngeal abscess
Diphtheric laryngitis

Noninfectious Causes
Acute spasmodic laryngitis*
Acute angioneurotic edema
Foreign body aspiration

*Cause unknown.

with differentiating infection of the supraglottic area (epiglottitis) from the syndrome of subglottic infection (croup). The croup syndrome describes diverse infectious and noninfectious entities, which include laryngitis and laryngotracheobronchitis. Other causes of upper airway obstruction include laryngeal diphtheria, retropharyngeal abscess, peritonsillar abscess, acute angioneurotic edema, spasmodic laryngitis, and foreign body aspiration (Table 22-1).

Childhood Epiglottitis

Acute epiglottitis is a life-threatening pediatric emergency (see Chap. 14). Between 5% and 10% of children with symptoms of acute upper airway obstruction have epiglottitis. In children who undergo aggressive airway support (intubation or tracheotomy) the mortality rate has decreased from 6.0% in closely monitored children to 0.9% in patients with airway support [3]. This fact argues for the immediate establishment of an artificial airway once the diagnosis has been established.

Surprisingly similar statistics exist for adults with epiglottitis. However, a consensus has not been reached in regard to the immediate establishment of an artificial airway in the adult [4].

Epiglottitis is caused by bacterial invasion of the epiglottis, the aryepiglottic folds, cartilage, and contiguous structures. The infection results in massive inflammation and edema. As swelling of the epiglottis increases, the pliable airway becomes compromised as the epiglottis dips into the laryngeal opening in inspiration, then relaxes with expiration, the so-called "ball-valve mechanism" [5]. Obstruction can be rapid and with little warning.

ETIOLOGY

H. influenzae type B (HiB) is the predominant organism in childhood epiglottitis, isolated in over 90% of patients in some series. Other organisms have been reported rarely in childhood epiglottitis, including *Staphylococcus aureus*, *S. pneumoniae*, and *H. parainfluenzae* (Table 22-2).

PATIENT PRESENTATION

Invasive diseases caused by *H. influenzae* type B are seen most commonly in the age group of 3 months to 3 years. The peak occurrence for epiglottitis is in children 2–4 years old, with one report that over 88% of children with epiglottitis are older than 2 years [5] and usually younger than 6. The onset is usually abrupt, with rapid progression of symptoms within the first 24 hours. The child attempts to sit upright with his head forward and will resist efforts to force him to lie supine. High fever, sore throat, drooling, dysphagia, hoarseness, and a barking cough are typical signs of epiglottitis. Retraction of the suprasternal notch and stridor are prominent with every breath [6]. Stridor is present on inspiration and absent on expiration.

The agitated child should be left sitting up. Excessive efforts at physical examination that would tend to agitate the patient further should be avoided. Direct visualization of the epiglottis and the posterior pharynx without preparation for immediate airway intubation if needed should be avoided, since this maneuver can precipitate abrupt obstruction.

DIAGNOSIS

If a child arrives in the emergency department with clinical symptomatology suggesting the possibility of acute epiglottitis, a timely diagnosis and early intervention are paramount. Efforts to coordinate immediate direct visualization of the epiglottis in the operating room by the most experienced personnel available, including a team of the emergency physician, a pediatrician, an anesthesiologist, and an otolaryngologist should be started as soon as clinical suspicion is aroused. If a staffed operating room is not available, visualization can be performed in an emergency department that is fully supplied with pediatric airway equipment.

The lateral neck x-ray may reveal an enlarged thumb-shaped epiglottis. Lateral neck x-rays are

Table 22-2. Airway infections and causative agents

Disease	Etiologic agents
Childhood epiglottitis	*Haemophilus influenzae* type B,* *Staphylococcus aureus*, *Streptococcus pneumoniae*, *Haemophilus parainfluenzae*
Adult epiglottitis	*H. influenzae* type B, *Streptococcus pyogenes*, *S. pneumoniae*, *S. aureus*, *Klebsiella* species, *Pasteurella multocida*, *Candida* species
Laryngitis	Influenza viruses, adenoviruses, rhinoviruses, RSV, *Moraxella catarrhalis*, *Corynebacterium diphtheriae*
Laryngotracheobronchitis	Parainfluenza viruses,* influenza viruses, RSV, adenoviruses, enteroviruses, coxsackieviruses, *Mycoplasma pneumoniae* (coinfections: *S. pneumoniae*, *S. pyogenes*, *S. aureus*, *H. influenzae*)
Bronchitis	Rhinoviruses, RSV, influenza viruses, parainfluenza viruses, adenoviruses, *M. pneumoniae*, *Chlamydia pneumoniae*, *Bordetella pertussis*, *Bordetella parapertussis*, (coinfections: *S. pneumoniae*, *H. influenzae*, *M. catarrhalis*)
Bronchiolitis (WARI)	RSV (infants),* *M. pneumoniae* (children),* parainfluenza viruses, influenza viruses, adenoviruses, rhinoviruses, (coinfections: *S. pneumoniae*, *H. influenzae*)

*Most common agent.

frequently misinterpreted, and normal-appearing x-rays do not exclude the diagnosis [7]. A CT scan will show the enlarged epiglottis, but this procedure can waste valuable time and is not recommended. If children are sent to x-ray for examinations, it is crucial to keep them under close observation.

Laboratory examinations are helpful in establishing an etiologic diagnosis ensuring appropriate antimicrobial therapy. Blood cultures are usually positive, and many series have reported greater than 90% positive growth of HiB. Pharyngeal cultures are often misleading, but a direct culture of the epiglottis taken after intubation often reveals the causative organism in typical and atypical cases. Latex agglutination of the urine or the blood for HiB may be positive.

DIFFERENTIAL DIAGNOSIS

The main differential diagnostic consideration is with acute laryngotracheobronchitis (croup), a subglottic airway infection process (Table 22-3). Laryngotracheobronchitis is more common than epiglottitis. The child with acute laryngotracheobronchitis typically has coryza for 2–3 days preceding a harsh, barking cough, hoarseness, and inspiratory stridor. Upper airway obstruction, although rare, may occur.

Acute spasmodic laryngitis usually occurs in children 2–4 years old who are emotionally labile. The attacks usually start at night and last for several hours. There is no fever, and the attacks respond to moist mist therapy.

Retropharyngeal abscess may present with laryngeal obstruction. Usually there is no hoarseness. Digital palpation of the intrapharyngeal mass may reveal the fluctuation of the abscess. Lateral neck x-rays and a CT scan of the neck can be helpful in differentiating cellulitis from true abscess. Retropharyngeal abscess is most common in young children less than 1 year of age.

Peritonsillar abscess is rare in young children and is usually seen in adolescents and young adults. Aspiration or incision and drainage of the mass ensures the diagnosis.

Foreign body aspiration is common in children of crawling age and toddlers. Direct laryngoscopy and bronchoscopy are indicated for diagnosis and removal of the foreign body.

Diphtheric laryngitis usually has a gradual onset with low-grade fever and a less abrasive cough. The patient grows progressively worse. Stridor may occur. A thick gray exudate and downward extending membrane may be visualized in the pharynx. A swab from the throat should be planted on a Loeffler's slant, a tellurite plate, and a blood agar plate. Peripheral neuritis and a myocardiopathy may develop [6].

Acute angioneurotic edema can occur at any age and is rapid in onset. The patient may have a history of allergy. Stridor, a swollen epiglottis on

Table 22-3. Diagnostic considerations in childhood epiglottitis and laryngotracheobronchitis (croup)

	Epiglottitis	Croup
Epidemiology		
Ages	6 months to 3 years	3–6 years
Sex	M > F	M > F
Season	Spring and fall	Nonseasonal
Clinical Features		
Toxicity	Moderate	Mild
Cough	Mild	Severe
Stridor	Severe	Mild
Drooling	Mild	None
Course	Rapid	Slow

lateral neck x-ray, and urticaria may be present. Death may occur without appropriate therapy.

THERAPY

The two basic principles in the treatment of acute epiglottitis are establishment of an adequate airway and control of the infection. Nasotracheal intubation usually is preferred to tracheostomy and results in shorter hospital stays. Intubation should be done in the operating room. Cricothyroidotomy can be performed in emergencies to establish a temporary airway. In emergency situations children with complete obstruction have responded to ventilation with a mask and bag.

Since 1974 strains of ampicillin-resistant HiB have been isolated from cereospinal fluid (CSF) and blood in children with meningitis, bacteremia, and epiglottitis. This resistance is mediated by plasmid-transferred beta-lactamase activity that is particularly active against the penicillin. Depending on the geographic locality, 12–40% of *H. influenzae* (type B and nontypable strains) are beta-lactamase positive and are therefore resistant to ampicillin. Strains of *H. influenzae* resistant to chloramphenicol have been reported but rare. In the United States HiB strains resistant to both ampicillin and chloramphenicol are very rare.

Due to the good experiences with ampicillin and chloramphenicol in treatment of invasive HiB illnesses, many physicians prefer conventional therapy of a combination of ampicillin 200–300 mg/kg/day and chloramphenicol 75–100 mg/kg/day in four divided doses given IV. However, since the *H. influenzae* isolates are exquisitely sensitive to the new cephalosporins, the current trend is to treat epiglottitis and other invasive HiB infections, such as meningitis, with IV ceftriaxone 50–75 mg/kg/day in two divided doses or cefuroxime 75–100 mg/kg/day in three divided doses. The duration of therapy in general is 7–10 days. The monobactam antibiotic aztreonam also has excellent antimicrobial activity against HiB. However, aztreonam lacks activity against gram-positive organisms and anaerobes; many physicians may not be comfortable to use it alone in treatment of patients with clinical symptomatology of sore throat.

CONTROL AND PREVENTION

Household and day-care contacts are considered to have increased risk for HiB infections. Prompt medical attention should be given to any exposed child who develops a febrile illness. Antimicrobial agents effective for invasive HiB infections should be administered when indicated, particularly for children under 4 years of age.

Rifampin is recommended as prophylaxis for all household contacts, both adults and children, in those households with at least one contact younger than 4 years of age and regardless of the immunization status of the contacts [8]. For adults the dosage of rifampin is 600 mg/day for 4 days. For children the recommended dosage is 20 mg/kg/day (not to exceed 600 mg/day) for 4 days. Rifampin prophylaxis should be started as soon as possible when an index case of HiB disease is diagnosed, because 54% of secondary cases occur in the first week after hospitalization of the index patient. Rifampin prophylaxis is not recommended if all contacts in a household are 4 years or older.

For day-care and nursery school contacts the risk

is probably less than household contacts, and prophylactic measures should be individualized. However, parents and supervisory personnel should be educated to have exposed children seek immediate medical attention if any febrile episodes develop in attendees of the facilities. Proposed guidelines for prophylaxis [8, 9] are (1) those exposed children less than 2 years old with 25 hours of contact per week should receive rifampin prophylaxis as recommended for household contacts; and (2) when a second or more index cases are diagnosed in a day-care center, all children attending the center as well as supervisory personnel should be put on rifampin prophylaxis. The effect of rifampin on the developing fetus is unclear; therefore, prophylaxis is not recommended for pregnant women. Rifampin is also recommended for the index case to eliminate the nasopharyngeal carriage. This is usually given concurrently during the last 4 days of hospitalization prior to discharging the patient home.

VACCINATION

A purified H. influenzae type B polysaccharide vaccine (PRP) licensed in 1985 is recommended for administration to children 24 months of age or older. This polysaccharide vaccine preparation does not elicit adequate antibody response when given to children under 18 months old. A conjugate HiB vaccine by covalently linking the HiB polysaccharide to diphtheria toxoid (PRP-D) has now been licensed and is antigenic when given to children 15–18 months of age [10]. The dose is 0.5 ml for both PRP and PRP-D. The former can be given SC or IM, while the latter is recommended for IM administration only. PRP-D is recommended for all children at 18 months of age, particularly those children at risk for contracting invasive HiB disease, for example, in day care centers.

Epiglottitis in Adults

Despite the potential severity of epiglottitis in adults, this diagnosis is often missed by physicians, including those staffing emergency departments. Although the clinical symptoms are somewhat different, the most common presenting symptoms of epiglottitis in adults are sore throat (90%), dysphagia (80%), fever (78%), and stridor (19%) [4]. Epiglottitis in adults is seen much less than in children. The rapidity of onset is usually slower, with sore throat present for 2–3 days prior to admission. However, the appearance of mild respiratory difficulty can be deceptive and may proceed to a rapid catastrophic decompensation. The disease is to be expected in the patient complaining of a severe sore throat but with a normal-appearing pharynx. As in children H. influenzae is the most common pathogen isolated from adult epiglottitis, although the frequency of positive blood culture is much lower (23%–26%) [11]. Other organisms, including group A streptococcus, pneumococcus, Klebsiella species, Pasteurella multocida [12], S. aureus, and Candida species [13], have been reported in the literature (see Table 22-2). Diagnosis and management of adult epiglottitis are similar to those described for children. A high index of suspicion in adults with sore throat, fever, and dysphagia should lead to direct visualization of the epiglottis as an emergency procedure. Laryngoscopy has rarely precipitated laryngeal obstruction in the adult, but the need remains for the ability to perform rapid intubation or tracheostomy when this procedure is undertaken. Sudden catastrophic obstruction has been reported in adults, often with little warning. The question whether all adults need establishment of an artificial airway still is controversial [14]. All patients should be admitted to the intensive care unit for maximal care.

Subglottic Infections

Subglottic infections usually are caused by viral and bacterial infections and historically have been referred to as croup. The term croup is derived from the Scottish term roup, which meant "to cry out in a shrill voice." Confusion continues to surround the term, since modern authors have used it freely when describing conditions of diverse etiology (Table 22-4).

Table 22-4. Subglottic airway infection

Laryngitis
Laryngotracheobronchitis (croup)
Bronchitis
Bronchiolitis

Laryngitis

Laryngitis is most commonly a viral infection of older children and adults [15]. Subglottic obstruction can occur but is rare. More severe cases need laryngoscopic evaluation.

ETIOLOGY

The predominant agents are influenza virus, adenovirus, rhinovirus, and respiratory syncytial virus (RSV). *Moraxella (Branhamella) catarrhalis* has been cultured from the nasopharynx in up to 55% of adults with acute laryngitis [16]. *Corynebacterium diphtheriae*, although rare in the United States, should be kept in mind, particularly for the following patients: those who have a history of foreign travel, recent immigrants from endemic areas, those who refuse vaccinations on religious backgrounds, and the elderly, in whom immunization may have lapsed (see Table 22-2).

PATIENT PRESENTATION

The typical clinical features of laryngitis are hoarseness and barking cough, which often is worse at night. Symptoms of the common cold (nasal stuffiness) may proceed the laryngeal involvement. Low-grade fever, myalgia, and headache may be present, or the patient may complain of little else but hoarseness. Infants with obstruction can become hypotonic from hypoxia.

DIAGNOSIS AND MANAGEMENT

Clinical diagnosis of laryngitis is not difficult. On the other hand, acute spasmodic laryngitis can be difficult to differentiate from infectious laryngitis in pediatric patients. However, spasmodic laryngitis usually occurs in children 2–4 years old who are emotionally labile. Its condition is generally less severe, and an attack lasts only a few hours. Congenital laryngeal stridor traditionally occurs early in neonatal life without signs of respiratory infection. Newborn infants with tetany can present with laryngeal spasm, which can be differentiated by the presence of hypocalcemia and increased muscular excitability (Chvostek's sign).

Laryngitis is usually a self-limited ailment of nonbacterial etiology and requires no specific treatment. In infants and small children if suggestive signs of obstruction and hypoxia are present, a laryngoscopic evaluation should be performed to rule out foreign body or supraglottic obstruction (epiglottitis). In an adult if hoarseness persists, laryngoscopy is indicated to rule out tumor growth as well as other noninfectious conditions.

Laryngotracheobronchitis

Laryngotracheobronchitis is almost exclusively a disease of children [17]. This severe infection extends downward from the larynx to include the trachea and the bronchial tree. Most children with laryngotracheobronchitis are 3 months to 3 years of age and more commonly are boys (see Chap. 14).

ETIOLOGY

Laryngotracheobronchitis usually is of nonbacterial etiology. Parainfluenza viruses type 1 and type 2 are considered the most common causative agents, accounting for approximately 50% of cases. Influenza viruses A and B, RSV, adenoviruses types 1, 2, 3, 5, and 7, enteroviruses, coxsackieviruses A and B, *M. pneumoniae*, and *Chlamydia pneumoniae* also have been implicated. Laryngotracheobronchitis in children older than 5 years often is secondary to influenza viruses or *M. pneumoniae* (see Table 22-2).

PATIENT PRESENTATION

The onset can be gradual over a period of several days and commonly occurs at night. Virus replication starts in the nasopharynx, with symptoms of upper respiratory involvement. When infection extends into the subglottic region, croup begins. The patient may soon develop a harsh barking cough (like the bark of a seal). As the process continues down the tracheobronchial tree, the symptoms increase in severity. Fever is higher, the child becomes more restless, and air hunger is apparent. In addition to suprasternal and supraclavicular retractions, substernal and intercostal retractions are prominent. In some cases nonsynchronous movements of the chest and abdomen during inspiration and expiration can be seen.

On auscultation fine inspiratory bronchitic rales and expiratory wheezes are present. The breath sounds vary, depending on the degree of obstruction and the quantity of bronchial exudates in affected areas. Fine to medium moist rales or rhonchi along with bronchophony, bronchial breathing sounds, and absent breath sounds from obstruction and atelectasis may be present. However, the child does not appear as toxic as in epiglottitis due to *H. influenzae* type B infection.

DIAGNOSIS

An experienced pediatrician can usually make a diagnosis of laryngotracheobronchitis (croup) on clinical grounds. Laboratory examinations generally are not very informative, with normal or slightly elevated WBC counts. Blood cultures usually are negative. Chest x-ray may sometimes demonstrate a narrow subglottic area or a widened hypopharynx, which is not thought to be very reliable and can be misinterpreted.

Definitive etiologic diagnosis depends on a virology laboratory with tissue-culture and serologic facilities. For isolation of parainfluenza viruses, primary monkey-kidney tissue culture is the best choice. Susceptible continuous culture cell lines, such as HeLa or Hep-2 cells, are useful for cultivation of respiratory syncytial virus and adenoviruses. Chick embryos or primary tissue-culture cells are used for isolation of influenza viruses. Serologic tests such as hemagglutination-inhibition, complement-fixation neutralization, or enzyme-linked immunosorbent assay (ELISA) tests are employed. Laboratory procedures for virologic studies are expensive and time consuming and usually are not available in most community hospitals. These procedures usually are not helpful in decision making for clinicians, particularly emergency department physicians, to manage their patients. They are useful as epidemiologic tools to follow community outbreaks of acute respiratory illnesses rather than for establishing etiologic diagnosis of sporadic cases.

TREATMENT

Because croup is caused mainly by viral agents, no consistent effective specific antimicrobial therapy is available [18, 19]. Considerable controversy has existed over the decades even as to the effectiveness in administration of steroids and humidification as supportive treatment. The following general guidelines are preferred by the authors.

Relief of anxiety and apprehension is paramount in handling sick children and their parents. It is important not to separate the child from the parents. Physical examination should be done swiftly by only one physician, and nonessential procedures should be avoided or be kept to a minimum.

Sedation should be used judiciously when the child is restless. This can help to relieve apprehension and anxiety. However, oversedation to the point of interfering with respiratory function should be avoided.

Early institution of mist therapy by nebulization is helpful [20, 21]. This can prevent inspissation of secretions and exudate in the small airways as well as minimize the desiccation of the inflamed respiratory epithelial cells, allowing easier removal of the bronchial secretions and debris by coughing. (Steam inhalation generally was used prior to the advent of the mist tent.) It is a convenient way of supplying moisture when caring for the patient at home. Most mist tents for hospital use deliver nebulization of cold air. The temperature of the nebulized air should not be unduly cold, which may be distressing to the sick child. It is advisable to have a parent be at the bedside when initiating the mist therapy, since the first encounter with a mist tent may be a frightening experience to the child. Oxygen administration should be used when needed but not routinely. Oxygen tends to dry up the bronchial exudate, rendering its removal more difficult by coughing.

Over the decades there have been a number of reports in the medical literature describing the use of corticosteroids for the treatment of croup, but it still remains controversial [22]. It is fair to say that the overall experience with steroids in treatment of laryngotracheobronchitis offers neither significant benefit nor excess risk if administered for only a short period of time. Since croup syndrome usually is not of bacterial etiology, antibiotic therapy would not be expected to be beneficial and should not be used routinely. However, in severe cases in which bacterial sepsis cannot safely be ruled out, judicious use of antimicrobials aiming at pathogens including *S. pneumoniae*, *S. aureus*, *S. pyogenes*, and *H. influenzae* is prudent.

In 1966 Jordan and associates introduced the use of racemic epinephrine by nebulization with intermittent positive pressure breathing (IPPB) to treat acute laryngotracheobronchitis [23, 24]. This method was soon adopted by many groups in the United States and other countries. Although impressive outcomes have been reported by the original inventors as well as by others, Gardner et al. [25] performed a double-blind controlled study using racemic epinephrine nebulized by compression without IPPB delivery. They found no significant benefit in racemic epinephrine recipients when compared to saline-treated controlled patients. Even in studies showing beneficial effect of racemic epinephrine administration, the effect is short lived, usually less than 2 hours. If racemic epinephrine treatment is to be given, observation over several hours in the emergency department or admission is required after its use, because rebound phenomenon can occur when the epinephrine effect wears off.

Bronchitis

Acute bronchitis is a common infectious process in both adults and children [26–28] characterized by inflammation of the upper respiratory tract and cough. The term tracheobronchitis is probably more accurate.

Because this disease process usually is self-limited in healthy individuals, knowledge of histopathology is scant. It is thought, however, that infection of the trachea leads to local inflammatory changes and increased bronchial secretions, with subsequent damage and inactivation to the ciliary escalator throughout the bronchial tree.

Chronic bronchitis, as defined by the American Thoracic Society, is characterized by excessive sputum production with cough, present on most days for at least 3 months in the year and not less than 2 successive years [29]. Cigarette smoking is directly associated with the development of chronic bronchitis.

Heredity, cold, damp climates, and air pollution may also play a role in the development and manifestation of chronic bronchitis. No consistent association has been made with mycoplasma, bacteria, or viral pathogens, although M. catarrhalis has garnered recent attention as a pathogen in recurrent exacerbations.

ETIOLOGY

The majority of bronchitis cases are thought to be of viral etiology. All the common viruses that affect the upper respiratory tract have been implicated as a cause of acute bronchitis in children. These include rhinoviruses, RSV, influenza viruses, and parainfluenza viruses. Adenoviruses (especially type 7) have been associated with acute bronchitis in children and in populations of military recruits. M. pneumoniae also has been shown to cause direct irritation to the bronchial tree, with subsequent damage and desquamation of the bronchial epithelium. Adults can serve as a reservoir for Bordetella pertussis with only an afebrile cough syndrome but place infants at risk for whooping cough. Bordetella parapertussis causes a protracted cough illness very similar to whooping cough but without the systemic toxicity. The prevalence of this organism in acute bronchitis has not been established, in part because B. parapertussis appears on agar as Haemophilus species and is often assumed to be "normal flora" and is reported as such by the microbiology laboratory. Adults with persistent cough without specific etiologic diagnosis should have cultures obtained for B. pertussis and B. parapertussis.

The TWAR agent (C. pneumoniae) may prove to be a significant newly characterized cause of acute bronchitis [28]. Acute bronchitis also can be a part of other specific infectious diseases such as measles, scarlet fever, and typhoid fever (see Table 22-2).

The significance of sputum cultures for S. pneumoniae, H. influenzae, and M. catarrhalis in the etiology of acute bronchitis remains unclear.

PATIENT PRESENTATION

The onset of acute bronchitis usually is preceded by a prodromal period of at least 24 hours with coryza and pharyngitis of varying severity. A dry cough heralds the early inflammation of the upper airway. The magnitude of constitutional symptoms of fever, headache, and myalgia depends on the etiologic agent involved and the age of the patient affected, with younger children often showing more marked temperature elevations.

On physical examination patients rarely appear toxic. As the illness progresses, the dry cough often progresses to a loose cough with mucopurulent sputum. Healthy patients rarely have dyspnea or appear cyanotic, but patients with underlying chronic pulmonary disease often show respiratory distress. Auscultation of the lungs may reveal clear breath sounds, rhonchi, or moist rales.

DIAGNOSIS

Diagnosis of bronchitis usually is a clinical process and a diagnosis of exclusion if the chest radiograph is without infiltrate. The white blood count, sputum, and blood cultures are not indicated in usual circumstances of acute or chronic bronchitis. The cell count is usually within normal limits; the sputum culture may show no predominant pathogen; and blood cultures will reveal no growth. In chronic bronchitis with exacerbation pneumococci, *H. influenzae* or *M. catarrhalis* is commonly recovered. Sputum cultures to direct anti-infective therapy are indicated in patients with persistent or relapsing illness who previously have received antibiotics. A chest radiograph often is needed to exclude pneumonia.

THERAPY

Acute bronchitis in immunocompetent individuals is a self-limited illness requiring no specific therapy. Bed rest and inhalation of warm, moist air are helpful. Aspirin or acetaminophen (650 mg for an adult, 10 mg/kg for a child) may be given every 4 hours for relief of fever and malaise. Aspirin should be avoided for children during the influenza season, because an association between aspirin and Reye's syndrome in children has been quite clearly linked. In young children, the elderly, COPD patients, and immunocompromised patients, the threshold for antibiotics is low. Parenteral therapy is rarely needed. Amoxicillin, ampicillin-clavulanate, trimethoprim-sulfamethoxazole, erythromycin (including the newer azithromycin and clarithromycin), and cefuroxime are all appropriate choices at usual dosages for 7–10 days.

In chronic bronchitic patients with purulent sputum production, administration of antimicrobials may shorten the course of acute exacerbation. However, most of the destructive changes in the respiratory tract from chronic bronchitis or emphysema are irreversible. In symptomatic patients with purulent sputum the following oral preparations can be prescribed: trimethoprim-sulfamethoxazole 800/160 mg bid, doxycycline 100 mg bid, amoxicillin 500 mg tid, erythromycin base 500 mg qid, cefaclor 500 mg qid, or cefoxime 400 mg qd. Such antimicrobials should be continued for 2–3 weeks. The fluoroquinolones are a rapidly expanding group of new antimicrobials. Currently norfloxacin, cip-

rofloxacin, and ofloxacin are licensed in the United States, but many others are under investigation and soon will be licensed. Norfloxacin does not achieve a significant serum level and is used mainly for treatment of urinary tract infections. Ciprofloxacin has a broad spectrum of antimicrobial activity against many gram-positive and gram-negative organisms. However, ciprofloxacin has rather poor antimicrobial activity against beta-hemolytic streptococci, pneumococci, *M. pneumoniae*, and anaerobes. Some staphylococci and *Pseudomonas aeruginosa* are relatively insensitive or resistant to ciprofloxacin. Frieden and Magi [30] cautioned practicing physicians on the inappropriate use of oral ciprofloxacin and stressed the fact that ciprofloxacin is not the drug of choice as initial therapy for respiratory infections, including otitis media, sinusitis, pharyngitis, and pneumonia.

In a study comparing ofloxacin with amoxicillin and erythromycin in treatment of community acquired lower respiratory infection, ofloxacin was found to be as effective clinically as amoxicillin and erythromycin and with the advantage of less frequent administration. The authors cautioned, however, that additional information is needed for S. *pneumoniae* due to the relatively high minimum inhibitory concentrations for this species [31].

Azithromycin and clarithromycin actually may be the agents of choice because of their spectrum of activity against respiratory pathogens (see Chap. 4 and Chap. 23). Higher costs may restrict their use to the more severely ill and the less immunocompetent.

Bronchodilators are helpful in those patients with airway obstruction. Theophylline 2–4 mg/kg q6h PO or terbutaline sulfate 2.5–5.0 mg/kg q8h PO can be given. Inhalation of aerosolized isoproterenol hydrochloride 0.5% solution, 0.65 mg/metered dose of metaproterenol sulfate, or 90 mcg/metered dose of albuterol is effective. Use of sedatives or narcotics is not recommended, and routine use of corticosteroids should be avoided.

Bronchiolitis

Bronchiolitis is an acute viral infection of infancy characterized by a prolonged expiratory phase and expiratory wheezing [32]. RSV is the predominant pathogen implicated in bronchiolitis in infancy.

During epidemics RSV is associated with over 80% of the cases. Some authors have used the term *wheezing-associated respiratory infection* (WARI) to include infection-induced wheezing for patients of all ages.

Henderson et al. [33] found the incidence of WARI highest in the first year of life, with 11.4 cases per 100 children per year (see Chap. 14).

ETIOLOGY
RSV is the predominant pathogen associated with bronchiolitis in infancy. In children 5–15 years of age M. *pneumoniae* may be the most common pathogen of WARI. In addition parainfluenza viruses, adenoviruses, influenza type A and B, and rhinoviruses have been associated with WARI. Even the role of RSV in infants may be underestimated, since infants aged 1–3 months may show RSV antigen in nasopharyngeal secretions without demonstrable serum antibody response. WARI peaks between December and March for children less than 2 years of age and in October and November for school-age children, which correlates with seasonal peaks of RSV and M. *pneumoniae* infections.

Viral infection in the respiratory tree causes necrosis of cilia and respiratory epithelium, marked edema, and obstruction of the small airways from mucus and cellular debris. The production of IgE increases with the severity of the illness, and virus-induced wheezing in early life may be mediated by virus-specific IgE [34].

Bacterial coinfection with RSV may be more common than previously thought [35]. In one recent study 35 of 90 children with RSV infection demonstrated serologic evidence of coinfection with S. *pneumoniae* and nontypable H. *influenzae* (see Table 22-2).

PATIENT PRESENTATION
Onset of bronchiolitis can be insidious, with 3–5 days of progressive illness characterized by coryza and cough. Fever may be low grade, and a high index of suspicion must be kept for hypoxia, since it may precede more dramatic clinical symptoms. As inflammatory changes in the airways progress, dyspnea, suprasternal and intercostal retractions, and cyanosis may become more apparent. Physical ex-amination generally reveals high-pitched wheezing that may vary from hour to hour. If bronchiolar obstruction is severe, breath sounds may become inaudible and herald respiratory failure. Dehydration with abnormal electrolytes is common.

DIAGNOSIS
In an infant with obstructive airway illness the clinical diagnosis of bronchiolitis is not difficult. Although acute bronchiolitis can be difficult to differentiate from bronchial asthma, the latter rarely is seen in infants under 18 months of age. A therapeutic trial of albuterol, epinephrine, or aminophylline may be helpful. Chest x-ray is of little help beyond the picture of hyperinflated lungs with a depressed and flattened diaphragm. If pneumonitis is present, patchy consolidations may be seen. The WBC count often is normal. Routine nasopharyngeal cultures usually do not yield bacterial pathogens. With dehydration and hypoxemia abnormal electrolytes and blood gases are common.

Etiologic diagnosis rests on viral isolation and serologic tests, which are of little value to an emergency department physician in the decision making for management. However, nasopharyngeal secretions from infected patients should be collected for viral culture and study. RSV is labile, and the specimens should be inoculated directly onto susceptible cell cultures without freezing. Rapid demonstration of RSV antigen with an immunofluorescence or ELISA test is available. For M. *pneumoniae* infections cold agglutinins and complement-fixation tests can be used for confirmatory diagnosis.

TREATMENT
The traditional and most valued therapy for bronchiolitis is oxygen and mist therapy. Physiotherapy, bronchodilators, and corticosteroids have not demonstrated therapeutic effects. Antibiotics have not been shown to be of proved benefit. However, if coinfection is seriously suspect, the clinician should keep in mind that S. *pneumoniae* and H. *influenzae* are the most commonly associated organisms. Because of increased mortality of RSV infection in patients with congenital heart disease, bronchopulmonary dysplasia, prematurity, and immunodeficiency, the American Academy of Pediatrics recommends the use of ribavirin in these patients, as well as in those children who are seriously ill with

PaO$_2$ less than 65 mm Hg, increasing PaCO$_2$, other congenital and neurologic anomalies or who are less than 6 weeks of age [36]. Ribavarin aerosol generally is administered 12–18 hours per day for 3–7 days, with improvement noted on the third to fifth day of treatment [37].

Management of Patients in the Emergency Department

Most cases of respiratory airway infection without involvement of the lungs are relatively benign and self-limited. Symptomatic treatment with or without oral antimicrobial agents usually suffices. Patients should be counseled that if symptoms worsen or persist longer than 3–4 days, a follow-up examination by their own physicians should be sought.

Acute epiglottitis is a medical emergency and should be handled with utmost expediency. These patients are at high risk for developing sudden unexpected airway obstruction. It is advisable to have a written protocol in each emergency department delineating procedures for transport, diagnostic studies, and management of a patient suspected to have acute epiglottitis. The roles and the cooperation of all care providers—pediatricians, otolaryngologists, anesthesiologists, and radiologists—are paramount and should be clearly defined to minimize confusion and serious complications. Although laboratory studies, including blood cultures, and parenteral antibiotics can be started in the emergency room, once the diagnosis of epiglottitis has been made or is suspected, the patient should be admitted to the floor for further treatment. With early recognition of the illness and skillful management, including elective intubation, the prognosis of acute epiglottitis is excellent.

Although laryngotracheobronchitis and bronchiolitis are less urgent medically than acute epiglottitis, patients who show signs of air hunger with chest wall retractions should not be treated as outpatients or sent home. It is prudent to admit such patients to the ward for treatment with mist tent and other therapeutic modalities. Patients with bronchitis in general can be dealt with as outpatients either symptomatically or by adding antimicrobials at the discretion of the attending physician.

References

1. Liu C. Studies of influenza infection in ferrets by means of fluorescein-labeled antibody. I. The pathogenesis and diagnosis of the disease. *J Exper Med* 101:665–76, 1955.
2. Little JW et al. Airway hyperactivity and peripheral airway dysfunction in influenza A infection. *Am Rev Respir Dis* 118:295–98, 1978.
3. Cantrell RW, Bell RA, Morioka WT. Acute epiglottitis: intubation versus tracheostomy. *Laryngoscope* 88:994–1005, 1978.
4. Mayosmith MF et al. Acute epiglottitis in adults: an eight-year experience in the state of Rhode Island. *N Engl J Med* 314:1133–39, 1986.
5. Daum RS, Smith AL. Epiglottitis (supraglottitis). In RD Feigin, JD Cherry (eds.), *Textbook of Pediatric Infectious Diseases.* Philadelphia: Saunders, 1987. Pp. 224–37.
6. Liu C. Epiglottitis, laryngitis, and laryngotracheobronchitis. In PD Hoeprich, MC Jordon (eds.), *Infectious Diseases.* Philadelphia: Lippincott, 1989. Pp. 328–32.
7. Stankiewicz JA, Bowes AK. Croup and epiglottitis: a radiologic study. *Laryngoscope* 95:1159–60, 1985.
8. In: Report of the Committee of Infectious Diseases—American Academy of Pediatrics Red Book: *Haemophilus influenzae* infections. Evanston IL: 1988. Pp. 204–10.
9. Jana H, Stutman HR, Marks MI. Invasive *Haemophilus influenzae* type B infections: a continuing challenge. *Am J Infect Control* 18(3):160–66, 1990.
10. Shapiro ED. New vaccine against *Haemophilus influenzae* type B. *Pediatr Clin North Am* 37:567–83, 1990.
11. Mustoe T, Strome M. Adult epiglottitis. *Am J Otolaryngol* 4:393–99, 1983.
12. Johnson RH, Rumans LW. Unusual infections caused by *Pasteurella multocida.* JAMA 237:146–47, 1977.
13. Haberman RS, Becker ME, Ford CN. *Candida* epiglottis. *Arch Otolaryngol* 109:770–71, 1983.
14. Baker AS, Eavey RD. Adult supraglottitis [editorial]. *N Engl J Med* 314:1185–86, 1986.
15. Gwaltney JM. Acute laryngitis. In GL Mandell, RG Douglas, JE Bennett (eds.), *Principles and Practice of Infectious Diseases.* New York: Churchill-Livingstone, 1990. P. 499.
16. Schalen L et al. High isolation rate of *Branhamella catarrhalis* from the nasopharynx in adults with acute laryngitis. *Scand J Infect Dis* 12:277–80, 1980.
17. Hall CB. Acute laryngotracheobronchitis. In GL Mandell, RG Douglas, JE Bennett (eds.), *Principles*

and Practice of Infectious Diseases. New York: Church-ill-Livingstone, 1990. Pp. 499–504.

18. Cherry JD. Croupi. In Feigin RD, Cherry JD (eds.), *Textbook of Pediatric Infectious Diseases*, Philadelphia: Saunders, 1987. Pp. 237–50.

19. Skolnik NS. Treatment of croup. *AJDC* 143: 1045–49, 1989.

20. Parks CR. Mist therapy: rationale and practice. *J Pediatr* 76:305–13, 1970.

21. Dulfano JM, Adler K, Wooten O. Physical properties of sputum. IV. Effects of 100 per cent humidity and water mist. *Am Rev Resp Dis* 107:130–32, 1972.

22. Kairys SW, Olmstead EM, O'Connor GT. Steroid treatment of laryngotracheitis: a meta-analysis of the evidence from randomized trials. *Pediatrics* 83 (5):683–93, 1989.

23. Jordan WS. Laryngotracheobronchitis—evaluation of new therapeutic approaches. *Rocky Mt Med J* 63:69–72, 1966.

24. Adair JC et al. Ten year experience with IPPB in treatment in acute laryngotracheobronchitis. *Anesth Analg* 50:649–55, 1971.

25. Gardner HG et al. The evaluation of racemic epinephrine in the treatment of infectious croup. *Pediatrics* 52:68–71, 1973.

26. Liu C. Bronchitis and bronchiolitis. In PD Hoeprich, MC Jordon (eds.), *Infectious Diseases*. Philadelphia: Lippincott, 1989. Pp. 333–39.

27. Brown RB. Acute and chronic bronchitis. *Postgrad Med* 85(8):249–54, 1989.

28. Grayston JT, Campbell LA, Kuo CC. A new respiratory pathogen: *Chlamydia pneumoniae* strain TWAR. *J Infect Dis* 161:618–25, 1990.

29. American Thoracic Society. Chronic bronchitis, asthma, and pulmonary emphysema. *Thorax* 15: 762–68, 1980.

30. Frieden TR, Mangi RJ. Inappropriate use of oral ciprofloxacin. *JAMA* 264:1438–40, 1990.

31. Stocks JM et al. Ofloxacin in community-acquired lower respiratory infections. *Am J Med* 87(suppl. 6C):6C–525–65, 1989.

32. Welliver R, Cherry JD. Bronchiolitis and infectious asthma. In Feigin RD, Cherry JD (eds.), *Textbook of Pediatric Infectious Diseases*. Philadelphia: Saunders, 1987. Pp. 278–88.

33. Henderson F, Clyde WA Jr, Collier AM. The etiologic and epidemiologic spectrum of bronchiolitis in pediatric practice. *J Pediatr* 95(2):183–90, 1979.

34. Welliver RC, Wong DT, Sun M. The development of respiratory syncytial virus-specific IgE and the release of histamine in nasopharyngeal secretions after infection. *N Engl J Med* 305:841–46, 1981.

35. Korppi M, Leinonen M, Koskela M. Bacterial coinfection in children hospitalized with respiratory syncytial virus infections. *Pediatr Infect Dis J* 8:687–92, 1989.

36. In: Report of the Committee of Infectious Diseases—American Academy of Pediatrics Red Book: *Haemophilus influenza* infections. Evanston, IL, 1988. Pp. 526–30.

37. Hall CB et al. Aerosolized ribavirin treatment of infants with respiratory syncytial viral infection. *N Engl J Med* 308:1443–47, 1983.

23

Pleuropulmonary Infections

PETER P. McKELLAR

The frequency of community acquired pneumonia in the United States is not known; it is not a reportable infectious disease, and the specific etiologic cause is often elusive. An estimated 4.5 million cases of pneumonia are treated in the outpatient setting yearly, and more than 500,000 patients are hospitalized each year [1]. The etiology of pneumonia requiring hospitalization may differ from that of pneumonia not requiring hospitalization. Most are treated empirically, and often little effort is made to document the etiology. The economic impact of pneumonia is enormous [2].

The pathogens that classically cause community acquired pneumonia are changing; the change is in part due to the identification of pathogens not previously recognized, such as Legionella species, *Coxiella burnetii* (Q fever), and *Chlamydia pneumoniae* [3]. Some of the change is due to new underlying diseases like AIDS, in which *Pneumocystis carinii* pneumonia has become a relatively common community acquired infection. There are regional differences in pneumonia etiologies: Pittsburgh finds a lot more Legionnaires' disease than does Phoenix, where a common cause of community acquired pneumonia is coccidioidomycosis. In rural Nova Scotia, Q fever pneumonia accounts for 20%

of community acquired pneumonias requiring hospitalization [4]. Many other factors may affect these regional differences, for example, socioeconomics, per-capita age, and access to health care.

The emergency department physician needs to determine expeditiously if the patient has pneumonia, what type, and how best to treat it. An understanding of the specific causes of pneumonia, the clinical presentations, and antibiotic resistance patterns combined with a sense of the type of host simplifies the patient's management.

A presumptive etiology often is ascribed and empiric therapy begun, because the mortality of community acquired pneumonia can be high [4–6]. The decision to hospitalize is a major one. Cost-containment issues have been highlighted by the large number of antibiotic strategies available. Many pneumonias can be treated on an outpatient basis, provided some common sense is used by both the physician and the patient. "Common things happen commonly" is a worthwhile adage to recall when considering an etiologic cause of pneumonia. Atypical manifestations of common pneumonias are more likely than uncommon causes of pneumonia. The clues to the type of pneumonia are often in the patient's history.

Pathogenesis of Pneumonia

Aspiration

There are three primary mechanisms for the development of bacterial pneumonia: aspiration, aerosolization, and hematogenous. Aspiration of oropharyngeal secretions is the most common mechanism. Aspiration of gastric contents occurs less frequently. Preceding aspiration is a change in the colonization immunity of the oropharynx, allowing colonization with the organisms that ultimately cause the patient's pneumonia. Often there is a viral respiratory infection preceding the onset of bacterial pneumonia. Most healthy people are relatively immune to colonizing their oropharynx with gram-negative bacteria. Illness changes this colonization immunity. Antibiotics also change the colonization immunity and allow the replacement of normal flora with more resistant bacteria. Occult aspiration is common and usually is cleared with ease by the mucociliary escalator defenses of the tracheobronchial tree. Atelectatic areas of the lung become the nidus for infection after occult aspiration.

Pneumonia caused by aspiration of gastric contents often is considered to be caused by anaerobic organisms, but it is more likely a polymicrobial (anaerobic and facultative) infection. Pure anaerobic pneumonia more commonly is seen in patients who chronically aspirate and have poor oral hygiene.

Aerosolization

Aerosolization as a mechanism for the development of bacterial pneumonia is particularly important in patients with home respiratory equipment that is not adequately cleansed. Bacteremia may be more common when pneumonia is due to aerosolization from contaminated respiratory equipment. *Mycobacteria tuberculosis*, *Legionella* species, *Coccidioides immitis* and other fungi, *Nocardia* species, *Mycoplasma pneumoniae*, *Chlamydia* species, and *Coxiella burnetii* are examples of pathogens acquired via aerosolization.

Hematogenous

The least common pathogenesis for pneumonia is the hematogenous route. IV drug abusers and hemodialysis patients are more prone to develop pneumonia hematogenously. Pulmonary infiltrates are seen in the lower lobes bilaterally in this setting because blood flow is predominantly to those areas.

Approach to the Diagnosis of Pneumonia

History

Undoubtedly the most important clinical skill in evaluating a patient is taking a history. In the emergency department, however, a comprehensive history may not be feasible, even though it is often the single most important clue to the diagnosis. A history is never complete, because there are always questions that were unasked, unanswered, or misinterpreted by all parties. A brief explanation of the importance of a careful history to both the patient and the family will help to allay some of their natural apprehension. The garnering of a history is an evolving process that often continues after the patient has left the emergency department. Telephone calls to family members may immediately open whole new vistas in the differential diagnosis. Initial questions to family members should be posed away from the patient to promote a freer exchange of information. Family history should not be neglected (e.g., tuberculosis tends to run in families).

Too frequently history is slighted in favor of technology. No laboratory test or radiographic exam can immediately compare to the value derived from the history. Some examples of this diagnostic value follow.

The diagnosis of *Pneumocystis carinii* pneumonia (PCP) is strongly aided by the history of risk factors for human immunodeficiency virus (HIV). PCP should be considered in infants with fever, failure to thrive, or adenopathy, with or without respiratory distress, particularly when risk factors for HIV exist in the family. Unfortunately there have been numerous examples of healthy adults with unsuspected HIV infection diagnosed only after PCP was demonstrated in their offspring.

Recurrent sinopulmonary infections suggest the need to rule out acquired hypogammaglobulinemia, immotile cilia syndrome, and even cystic fibrosis [7]. Recurrent pneumonia in the same lung area suggests a structural abnormality, such as focal bronchiectasis or bronchopulmonary sequestration.

Tobacco use in the family exposes children to the adverse effects of passive smoking, including more respiratory diseases [8].

Steroid use broadens the differential diagnosis to include many organisms not commonly found in healthy hosts, such as Nocardia species and aspergilli. There are many other medications that can directly affect the lungs; thus, a complete medication list on the patient with pneumonia is essential.

Aspiration of foreign bodies into the tracheobronchial tree can be occult and overlooked even in the adult [9]. Foreign-body aspiration is more commonly a problem in children, where a high index of suspicion is needed [10]. The new onset of wheezing and coughing in a young child should prompt a chest x-ray. Most aspirated objects are not radiopaque, but air trapping, atelectasis, and consolidation are major clues. Parents should be queried regarding any recent choking spells that may have seemed inconsequential. The diagnosis of a foreign body aspiration is often overlooked for more than 24 hours.

Pneumonia occurring in a female of childbearing age should spur a query regarding any recent pregnancy. Pulmonary infiltrates from gestational trophoblastic disease (hydatidiform mole) can present as an acute dyspnea with cough and hemoptysis. The history of pregnancy in the past year is of diagnostic import. Likewise, a very rare cause of pneumonia, the genital mycoplasma (*Mycoplasma hominis*) [11], can be associated with pregnancy and is resistant to many antibiotics, including beta-lactams and erythromycin.

Many other examples of the value derived from a careful patient history are emphasized throughout this chapter.

Clinical Setting of Pneumonia

The onset and the course of the pneumonia over time is important. The clinician must know the answer to the question, "On what day of this patient's illness am I seeing him?" The acute onset of pneumonia usually is obvious. A chronic pneumonia syndrome may be more subtle and requires a more thorough understanding of its evolution.

Pneumonia acquired in the community can be conveniently characterized as bacterial-like or atypical. Bacterial pneumonia typically has a sudden onset of fever, malaise, productive cough, and chest discomfort and is more often present in elderly persons with underlying disease. Atypical pneumonias are more likely to have increased constitutional symptoms, such as headache, myalgias, arthralgias, nonproductive cough, and less fever and suggest a nonbacterial origin (e.g., mycoplasmal, chlamydial, or viral). These nonbacterial-like pneumonias are more commonly present in younger, healthier people. The atypical presentation of pneumonia, like the compromised host, should encourage a much broader differential diagnosis. Unfortunately mixed or subtle presentations are sufficiently common to make any distinct categorization of limited value. The clinical manifestations of community acquired pneumonia are rarely specific for a particular microbe [12].

Knowledge of underlying disease is useful in determining if the pneumonia is a primary process or secondary to another disease. The elderly and patients with multiple myeloma, sickle cell disease, recent influenza, and so on, are prime candidates to develop pneumococcal pneumonia. Nursing home residents live in what amount to offshoots of hospitals. They are at risk for pneumonia due to antibiotic-resistant organisms. Patients with alcoholism, malnutrition, emphysema, chronic bronchitis, seizures, and pyorrhea similarly are at risk for pneumonia.

Most pneumonias are due to an infective process, but some are related to noninfections, such as collagen vascular disease, drug reactions, allergens, and neoplasia. A history of asthma with recurrent pneumonias suggests silent nocturnal, gastroesophageal reflux. Reflux symptoms need not be present [13]. Asthmatic symptoms in the presence of recurring pulmonary infiltrates should bring to mind bronchopulmonary aspergillosis, particularly in the presence of eosinophilia. Recurring pulmonary emboli, silent mitral stenosis, and other causes of pulmonary hypertension must be considered in the atypical asthmatic with pulmonary infiltrates on chest x-ray.

Physical Examination

The physical examination helps to distinguish noninfectious diseases from infectious ones, for example, congestive heart failure, signs of cancer peripherally, signs of thromboembolic phenomena, and hypertension with edema suggestive of renal dis-

Table 23-1. Diagnostic syndromes in pneumonia

Pneumonia + Relative Bradycardia
(Intracellular organisms)
  Viral pneumonia
  Mycoplasma infection
  Chlamydia infection
  Legionnaires' disease
  Salmonella typhi infection

Pneumonia with Rash (or Skin Lesions)
Atypical measles
Varicella
Fungal pneumonia
Nocardiosis
Staphylococcal pneumonia/bacteremia

Pneumonia with CNS Alterations
Tuberculosis
Coccidioidomycosis
Cryptococcosis
Legionnaires' disease
Infective endocarditis
Elderly patients with community acquired pneumonia

Pneumonia with Splenomegaly
Psittacosis
Typhoid fever
Brucellosis
Infective endocarditis

ease. Poor oral hygiene suggests aspiration pneumonia with mixed oral flora. Edentulous patients are less likely to develop aspiration pneumonia. Sinusitis with pulmonary infiltrates evokes the thought of Wegener's granulomatosis.

Fever is a nonspecific finding that is often present with pneumonia. Pulse-temperature dissociation (relative bradycardia for the level of fever) is seen in viral infections and other intracellular infections, for example, mycoplasma, chlamydia, legionella, and *Salmonella typhi* infections (Table 23-1). Antipyretics will obfuscate the presentation. The extremes of age may not have a febrile response; indeed, the elderly may demonstrate only confusion and tachypnea. Some compromised hosts, for example, alcoholics, may present with hypothermia and leukopenia when septic [14].

Tachypnea, nasal flaring, intercostal muscle use, pulsus paradoxus, and cyanosis are all signs of significant respiratory compromise. Splinting or decreased motion unilaterally suggests bronchial obstruction on that side.

Signs of consolidation on chest exam include dullness to percussion, increased tactile fremitus, increased clarity of whispered or spoken voice sounds, and bronchial (tubular) breath sounds with a shortened inspiratory phase and a prolonged expiratory phase. Inspiratory crackles usually are heard.

The absence of breath sounds and the presence of a tympanitic chest wall on percussion in a dyspneic patient indicates a pneumothorax. Sudden increase in dyspnea with cyanosis and shock implies a tension pneumothorax and the need for immediate aspiration of free air through the chest wall using a large needle. Spontaneous pneumothorax is a relatively common event. Occasionally there are subtleties involved that alter the management. Recurring pneumothorax associated with menstruation is one example [15].

Subcutaneous crepitance over the trachea or a precordial crunching sound during systole are clues to the presence of a pneumomediastinum. The lateral chest x-ray best demonstrates mediastinal air. Vomiting is often the initiating factor. The clinical differential diagnosis of pneumomediastinum includes spontaneous alveolar rupture and esophageal rupture. The distinction may be problematic since both conditions can present with severe substernal chest pain, fever, and leukocytosis [16].

Achalasia of the esophagus has been reported to cause acute upper airway obstruction by compressing the trachea at the thoracic inlet [17]. Soft, boggy supraclavicular neck fullness, along with cervical venous distension, is found on physical exam. The chest x-ray usually reveals a widened mediastinum. The acute postprandial onset of respiratory distress is a clue to this disorder. A prior history of achalasia is common.

Skin lesions can be diagnostic for atypical measles, varicella, and hypersensitivity reactions as well as offer rapid biopsy access to a specific diagnosis of disseminated pulmonary infection (e.g., coccidioidomycosis, cryptococcosis, blastomycosis, and nocardiosis (see Table 23-1). Palpable purpura associated with pulmonary infiltrates, severe asthma, eosinophilia, and a systemic process may represent allergic angiitis and granulomatosis of Churg-Strauss disease. The first clinical clues to meningococcal disease or Rocky Mountain spotted fever may be found on the skin exam. Jaundice ("toxic hepatitis") may develop in some patients with pneumonia, although it seems more probable that the mildly jaundiced patient will turn out to have Gilbert syndrome, a benign, chronic unconjugated hyperbilirubinemia.

Furuncles or a thumb paronychia in the context of multilobe pneumonia may be the source for bacteremic staphylococcal infection in young children. Needle track marks in the adult suggest a similar etiology.

Facial herpes simplex virus lesions are common with pneumococcal pneumonia but are not of diagnostic value. Herpes simplex virus pneumonia is very uncommon and usually manifests as a severe tracheobronchitis in an elderly or compromised host [18]. Isolating herpes simplex virus from respiratory secretions is of no value unless the clinical setting supports such a diagnosis. Neonates in contact with herpes simplex virus at birth are at significant risk of disseminated herpes simplex. A primary herpes simplex pneumonia can present in neonates without dissemination [19]. The rapid progression of pneumonia in the first 10 days of life suggests this diagnosis. Mucocutaneous lesions need not be present. Delayed prenatal care can be a risk factor for infection with herpes simplex virus.

A testicular mass suggests cancer with pulmonary metastases. Spermatic cord lesions are seen in tuberculosis and vasculitis syndromes.

Chronic arthritis implies a more complicated host. Acute arthritis in the context of pneumonia conjures the thought of a drug reaction. Symmetrical polyarthritis is very unlikely due to bacterial processes unless endocarditis is present. Collagen vascular disorders could cause both the pneumonia and the arthritis.

Clubbing and weight loss suggest a more chronic process (e.g., lung abscess, cancer). The presence of lymphadenopathy suggests a more complicated host and a site for biopsy if needed. Splenomegaly is seen with psittacosis, subacute infective endocarditis, typhoid fever, brucellosis, and a multitude of other illnesses (see Table 23-1).

Asplenic patients, whether surgically or functionally asplenic (as in sickle-cell anemia), are at increased risk of overwhelming bacteremia with infections due to *Streptococcus pneumoniae* and *Haemophilus influenzae*. The absence of a spleen is

important clinical information [20, 21]. Lethargy, confusion, and disorientation are seen more commonly in elderly patients and can be part of community acquired pneumonia, but they may also indicate underlying CNS infection. Infections like tuberculosis, coccidioidomycosis, and cryptococcosis may present with both pulmonary and CNS changes. Legionnaires' disease may be associated with mental status changes [22] (see Table 23-1). Hyponatremia and hypoxemia must be ruled out. Bacterial endovascular infection may present with meningitis and pneumonia concomitantly. The patient at risk for endocarditis may present with bilateral pulmonary infiltrates due to adult respiratory distress syndrome (ARDS). A heart murmur need not be present. The specific importance of blood cultures prior to antibiotics cannot be overstressed.

Radiographic Data

The radiographic findings are usually the definitive evidence for the presence of pneumonia, but they are rarely pathognomonic for a specific cause of pneumonia (Table 23-2). The chest x-ray helps to classify a pneumonia anatomically. Multilobar involvement is a bad prognostic sign and should prompt early hospitalization. Embolic pneumonia presents as bilateral lower lobe involvement because blood flow is greatest to those areas. Aspiration may present with multiple patchy areas of infiltrate as well as lobar and/or segmental infil-

Table 23-2. Radiographic differential diagnosis of pulmonary infiltrates

Infectious
Collagen vascular disease (CVD)
Cardiogenic pulmonary edema
Noncardiogenic pulmonary edema (ARDS)
Pulmonary hemorrhage
Radiation pneumonitis
Hypersensitivity pneumonitis
Lung cancer
Atelectasis
Sarcoidosis
Pulmonary alveolar proteinosis
Occupational lung diseases (e.g., silicosis, berylliosis)
Pulmonary emboli, infarction

trates; the specific location depends on the patient's position during aspiration.

Lack of infiltrates in the presence of fever, cough, and sputum production suggests tracheobronchitis, but small infiltrates hidden behind the diaphragm or the heart may be missed. This author has seen bacteremic pneumococcal disease present as an acute abdomen with profuse watery diarrhea, normal findings at laparotomy, and a minute retrocardiac infiltrate on chest x-ray. Similar presentations have been described [23].

Clinical information is important to the radiologist [24]. For example, wheezing in a young female with low-grade fevers and relatively clear lung fields but a straight left heart border may call to mind mitral stenosis. Collagen vascular diseases may present with pulmonary infiltrates in the absence of opportunistic infection [25]. Cardiogenic pulmonary edema usually presents as a bilateral butterfly distribution with relative sparing of the peripheral lung. Unilateral pulmonary edema is uncommon but well described [26]. Pulmonary hemorrhage from contusion and coughing can mimic a variety of lung infections. Radiation therapy to the lung can produce a pneumonitis that mimics infection with fever, cough, and dyspnea [27]. Onset is within 12 months of radiation exposure.

Underlying lung cancer is an important inciting reason for pneumonia. Cancer risk factors should be sought in the history. Volume loss on the initial x-ray early in pneumonia may be due to atelectasis; volume loss that persists is due to bronchial obstruction, and cancer must be considered. Severe bronchorrhea is a diagnostic clue to bronchioloalveolar carcinoma.

Alveolar proteinosis and sarcoidosis may produce chest x-ray findings that are worse looking than the clinical findings. Pulmonary alveolar proteinosis is a diffuse air-space disease that may present asymptomatically or with minimal symptoms of cough, dyspnea, and weight loss [28]. It is more common in men, predominantly in those 20–50 years old, and is occasionally associated with pulmonary nocardiosis.

A miliary pattern on the chest x-ray suggests tuberculosis, coccidioidomycosis, or histoplasmosis, but it can be due to bacterial sepsis. Cancer, sarcoidosis, silicosis, and berylliosis are in the differential diagnosis of pulmonary infiltrates but of-

ten have hilar or mediastinal lymphadenopathy. Mycoplasma pneumonia may present with mediastinal lymphadenopathy.

PCP can present in bizarre fashions [29]. The chest x-ray may be normal, although the patient is febrile and dyspneic. Cavitary upper-lobe infiltrates that mimic tuberculosis may even appear in patients who are not taking aerosolized pentamidine treatments [30]. Pleural effusions are very uncommon. The clinical history would be most useful in suggesting an atypical presentation.

Cavitary lung lesions may represent infiltrate around a lung bleb, or they may indicate a necrotizing pneumonia due to gram-negative or anaerobic organisms. Neoplasia, chemicals, and even pulmonary emboli can produce a similar picture. Pneumococcal pneumonia may mimic necrotizing gram-negative pneumonia in a patient with underlying emphysema. Pneumococcal pneumonia alone rarely causes cavitation [31]. *Legionella micdadei* can produce cavitation. Cavitation without much toxicity would bias the diagnosis toward noninfective causes (e.g., cavitary cancer). An old chest x-ray for comparison is extremely useful.

Abscess formation (consolidation with an air-fluid level) is common with anaerobes and gram-negative bacillary organisms but uncommon with pneumococcal infection. Tuberculous disease can necrose lung parenchyma and produce abscess. The rapid onset of multiple cavitary infiltrates in a toxic patient is seen with bacteremic *Staphylococcus aureus* pneumonia.

A pleural effusion may be suspected on physical examination and demonstrated on chest x-ray as a homogeneous density without air bronchograms. Subpulmonic pleural effusions are best seen on lateral decubital films. A pleural effusion associated with vomiting, severe chest pain, and dyspnea may be due to esophageal perforation [16]. The diagnosis can be confirmed by the presence of an exudative pleural fluid with an elevated amylase and low pH. Surgical exploration of the mediastinum, with repair of the perforation and drainage, becomes an emergency in this illness [32].

Pancreatic disease, subphrenic abscesses, and intrahepatic abscess are GI diseases that can produce exudative pleural effusions and mimic primary pleural disease [33, 34].

Adhesions are common between parietal and visceral pleura. Fluid in these areas can mimic tumors or dense consolidations (pseudotumors). Ultrasound is helpful in localizing pleural effusions, particularly loculated fluid. Hilar enlargement may be due to vascular engorgement from pulmonary hypertension (emphysema, pulmonary emboli, etc.) or may be lymphadenopathy. A CT scan of the chest is a sensitive but expensive means of defining hilar structures. Hilar nodes are not seen with the usual bacterial pneumonias; tuberculosis, pertussis, and pneumonic plague, or tularemia, are the exceptions. Cancer should be suspected when adenopathy is present. Occasionally a well-circumscribed mass may be seen in early pulmonary consolidation. This round pneumonia is more common in children [35].

Laboratory Data

The specific etiology of pneumonia is difficult to establish without a positive culture from blood, pleural fluid, or a direct lung puncture. Therefore, blood cultures are important.

A sputum Gram's stain and culture is a coarse mode of diagnosis that can be spurious, especially if acquired haphazardly [36]. The quellung test using antipneumococcal antisera may complement the Gram's stain in the rapid identification of pneumococcus [37]. The sputum culture is rarely diagnostic, since the distinction between colonization and infection by organisms in the sputum is difficult to make. The most common bacterial cause of pneumonia is S. pneumoniae, yet this organism may colonize the oropharynx of 20%–50% of asymptomatic people. Transtracheal aspiration to acquire a noncontaminated specimen of sputum has fallen out of favor because of the attendant risks of the procedure and because specimens from patients with chronic obstructive pulmonary disease (COPD) and patients on antibiotics are not reliable. Some organisms are always pathogenic in sputum, (e.g., M. tuberculosis, Legionella species).

The technique of sputum procurement is important but often slighted. The patient must first understand what is being requested. Written as well as verbal instructions are needed. The difference between saliva and sputum must be made clear. Full cooperation from the patient is essential. After instructions the patient ideally cleans the oral cav-

ity first by brushing the teeth and tongue areas followed by extensive gargling and rinsing of the mouth. A deep cough is requested and a produced sputum expeditiously sent to microbiology for Gram's stain and culture. The laboratory should routinely examine the Gram's stain for evidence of (1) adequacy of collection, that is, more than 25 WBCs and fewer than 10 squamous epithelial cells per high-power field and (2) a predominant organism and evidence of organisms within the WBCs. Few WBCs or many squamous epithelial cells are indicative of an inadequate sputum collection, since inflammatory cells are seen in pneumonia and squamous cells come from the oral cavity, not from the lower airway structures. Inadequate sputum collections should not be cultured. Instead the laboratory immediately should request a better sputum. The cooperative patient who is unable to produce sputum on coughing should have an aerosol of 3% saline nebulized over 10 minutes while sitting erect and breathing slowly through the mouth. A coughed specimen of sputum should be elicited at the end of this procedure after first rinsing the oral cavity again. This procedure can be repeated two more times before more invasive techniques are considered.

Inadequate patient instruction and lack of supervision in the induction of sputum are often reasons for failing to acquire a suitable specimen of lower respiratory secretions. In the emergency department the sputum Gram's stain is much more important than a culture, which will not be available for 48 hours (Table 23-3). A poorly collected sputum that is cultured provides no useful information and may be misleading.

Foul-smelling sputum suggests an anaerobic infection. Antibiotic use prior to sputum collection will make the interpretation of a Gram's stain and a culture more difficult since they change the normal oral flora quickly.

Sputum Gram's stains that demonstrate many WBCs but no organisms suggest a "stealth organism" such as a virus, a mycoplasma, Chlamydia pneumoniae, a Legionella species, P. carinii, Coxiella burnetii (Q fever), M. tuberculosis, and some fungi. These organisms need to be considered in the atypical pneumonia setting, where special smears, cultures, and possibly serologies are indicated. Occasionally aspergilli found in the sputum of an

Table 23-3. Sputum Gram's Stain analysis to guide empiric antibiotic therapy

Gram-positive Cocci
S. pneumoniae
S. aureus

Gram-negative Coccobacilli
H. influenzae
M. catarrhalis

Gram-negative Bacilli
Enteric bacilli (i.e. *Klebsiella* and *Enterobacter*
  species, etc.)
Pseudomonas species

Mixed Flora
Oral contamination
Mixed aerobes/anaerobes

Organism Absent
Viruses
Mycobacteria
Fungi
Mycoplasma
Chlamydia
Coxiella burnetii
Legionella
Pneumocystis carinii

Table 23-4. Parapneumonic effusions

Infectious Causes
S. pneumoniae
M. tuberculosis
Other bacteria

Noninfectious Causes
Malignancy
Pulmonary infarction
Rheumatoid lung disease
Pancreatitis
Allergic pneumonitis
Congestive heart failure

immunocompetent host with pneumonia are significant [38].

A parapneumonic effusion may be demonstrated on lateral chest x-ray by blunting the posterior costophrenic angles (Table 23-4). When the pleural-fluid thickness on a lateral decubitus x-ray is more than 10 mm, a diagnostic thoracentesis is done for Gram's stain and culture of the fluid using a heparinized syringe. If sufficient fluid is obtained, a cell count with differential, pH, protein and lactic acid dehydrogenase (LDH) levels, Gram's stain, and cultures are requested. The distinction between transudate, which usually is not related to pleural disease (e.g., congestive heart failure [CHF] or hypoproteinemia), and exudate, which indicates pleural disease (e.g., infection, malignancy, or pulmonary embolus), is arbitrary but easily made. Exudative pleural fluids have protein levels greater than one-half the serum protein level, an LDH that is greater than 60% of the serum LDH level, and/or an LDH that is more than two-thirds the upper normal serum limits [39].

The initial thoracentesis helps to distinguish between a complicated and an uncomplicated parapneumonic effusion. Most parapneumonic effusions are uncomplicated and resolve on antibiotic therapy alone. About 10% of parapneumonic effusions are complicated and will not resolve without tube drainage [39]. A grossly purulent pleural effusion is an empyema and demands drainage by either repeated pleurocentesis or insertion of a chest tube. Thinner effusions may be seen in a variety of pleural processes. S. pneumoniae causes most community pneumonias and has a parapneumonic effusion in about 50% of cases (more if the patient waits longer for therapy), yet rarely is associated with a positive pleural fluid culture [40]. Tuberculosis can have a high protein and is frequently associated with a positive skin test. Partially treated bacterial pneumonias are often associated with thin exudative effusions. Mycoplasma pneumonia usually has minimal exudative effusion similar to most viral pneumonias [41].

Noninfective processes such as malignancy, pulmonary infarction, rheumatoid disease, and pancreatitis can produce exudative effusions. Allergic pneumonitis has been reported to cause effusions. Chest trauma has produced eosinophilic pleural effusions [42]. Thoracoscopy may offer a safe and convenient technique for diagnosing pleural disease when thoracentesis and needle biopsy fail [43].

White blood count, electrolytes, renal and liver function tests, and arterial blood gases do not provide significant clues to the specific etiology of pneumonia [12]. There can be considerable spontaneous variability in the arterial blood gas determinations even in stable patients [44]. An elevated

WBC count above 15,000 cells per centimeter is very suggestive of a bacterial infection. A depressed WBC count is associated with a poor outcome and is seen most commonly in alcoholic patients [45]. Pancytopenia is more suggestive of miliary tuberculosis, histoplasmosis, or a metastatic neoplasm. Anemia suggests a more chronic process. Urinalysis for protein, hematuria, RBC casts, and so on, is important. Glomerulonephritis may present with nonproductive cough, edema, pulmonary infiltrates, and low-grade fever. Wegener's granulomatosis can mimic bacterial pneumonia with sinusitis, but usually it will have evidence of glomerulonephritis. Tuberculosis may have sterile pyuria present.

Acute and convalescent serologies can be helpful but rarely in the acute setting. Cold agglutinins are not specific for mycoplasma pneumonia and are positive in only about 50% of cases. Very high titers seem to correlate with severity of disease.

The future availability of very specific and sensitive DNA probes may revolutionize the way certain pneumonias are rapidly diagnosed [46].

Differential Diagnosis Considerations in Pneumonia

Clinical acumen is essential because blood and pleural fluid cultures are uncommonly positive, sputum Gram's stain and culture are difficult to interpret, and the clinical manifestations of pneumonia are rarely specific for a single microbial organism (Table 23-5). The clinician can often focus on the most likely etiology using the clinical history and a well-collected and examined Gram's smear of sputum. Compromised hosts, nursing home residents, and patients already receiving antibiotic therapy will require broader antibiotic coverage and a more accelerated, invasive diagnostic workup. Reactivation of latent disease, such as tuberculosis, coccidioidomycosis, histoplasmosis, cytomegalovirus infection, pneumocystosis, toxoplasmosis, and strongyloidiasis must all be recalled in the compromised host at risk.

Positive blood cultures can take 24 hours; the sputum Gram's stain takes minutes. If the sputum is a good collection, that is, there are many WBCs and few epithelial cells, the predominant organism should be treated (see Table 23-3). A repeat sputum

Table 23-5. Clinical clues often overlooked in LRI

Clue	Possible Causes
Clubbing	Lung abscess or cancer
Chronic paroxysmal cough	*Bordetella pertussis,* *B. parapertussis*
Pneumonia recurring in the same segment	Foreign body, bronchopulmonary sequestration, bronchiectasis
Purulent sputum with no organisms on Gram's stain	Stealth bugs (e.g., M. tuberculosis, Legionella species, Coxiella burnetii, Pneumocystis carinii, mycoplasma, chlamydia, fungi), viruses
Pneumonia not responding to a beta-lactam antibiotic	Stealth bugs (e.g., M. tuberculosis, Legionella species, Coxiella burnetii, Pneumocystis carinii, mycoplasma, chlamydia, fungi), viruses, postobstructive pneumonia, noninfectious causes

for Gram's stain only will reduce the sampling error of the first smear. *S. pneumoniae* is most common; *H. influenzae* is second. *M. pneumoniae, Legionella* species, *C. pneumoniae, Moraxella (Branhamella) catarrhalis,* gram-negative bacillary organisms, and *S. aureus* then must be considered. There are regional differences in pneumonia (e.g., coccidioidomycosis in the southwestern deserts) just as there are host differences (e.g., prior antibiotic usage, underlying illness, age of patient).

Staphylococcal pneumonia is relatively uncommon and presents as a toxic patient with high fevers, pleuritic chest pain, and tachypnea. Sheets of gram-positive cocci in clusters should be apparent on sputum smear. It may be a superinfection following influenza, but more commonly it is secondary to septic pulmonary emboli in IV drug abusers.

Gram-negative bacillary pneumonia likewise is uncommon in the community setting, although prior antibiotic therapy, nursing home residence, alcoholism, and poorly cleaned home respiratory equipment are definite risk factors. The presence of gram-negative bacteria on sputum culture is common and leads to a major error in diagnosis if a concomitant sputum Gram's smear is not inspected. The smear should show many gram-negative rods.

Anaerobes predominate in the oral cavity but rarely cause pulmonary infection on their own, unless repeated aspiration is a problem and periodontal disease is in evidence. Most aspiration pneumonia is polymicrobial in origin, with anaerobes predominating.

General Therapeutic Considerations in the Emergency Department

The emergency department physician's responsibilities include initiating the diagnostic workup with blood cultures and sputum examination as well as other laboratory parameters. The patient's disposition is often decided by the emergency department physician. Unlike the setting of meningitis, empiric antibiotic therapy for pneumonia may not need to start in the emergency department. However, in the critically ill patient cultures should be promptly acquired and antibiotic therapy started without delay. Critically ill patients require a broader antibiotic regimen on day 1. Subsequent daily evaluations may call for modification of the initial therapy or may indicate the need for a more rapidly aggressive diagnostic effort. When there is no sputum produced, the clinical history and the clinical condition of the patient dictate how aggressively the patient should be evaluated and treated. Invasive tests are indicated early if failure of empiric therapy would lead to rapid clinical deterioration. Invasive tests include fiberoptic bronchoscopy, needle aspiration of lung, and open lung biopsy.

Which patients with community acquired pneumonia need hospitalization? The answer, of course, depends a lot on clinical severity, but there are other considerations. Community resources and family or caretaker reliability must be assessed. Are follow-up evaluation and compliance unlikely? For some patients a short stay in the hospital and IV antibiotic therapy is optimal. For other patients daily outpatient intramuscular injections of long-acting antibiotics (e.g., ceftriaxone or cefonocid) until improvement is seen may help to balance the high costs of hospitalization with compliance and oral absorption concerns. The clinician's "diagnos-

tic and therapeutic tenesmus" is stimulated by many forces, but the ultimate decision calls for clinical acumen.

In an effort to standardize the hospitalization decision in community acquired pneumonia, a model has been developed that identifies risk factors for a complicated course [47]. This model identifies five predisposing risk factors: (1) high-risk etiology of the pneumonia (staphylococcal, gram-negative bacillary, aspiration, or postobstructive), (2) immunosuppression in the host, (3) comorbid illness (diabetes, congestive heart failure, renal failure, hospitalization within 1 year), (4) age greater than 65, and (5) temperature greater than 38.3°C. The model is derived from a prospective cohort study and needs to be confirmed by others. Unfortunately the study has a very narrow definition of comorbid disease, which excludes HIV disease, chronic lung disease, cancer, splenectomy, and dementia, among others. Since the high-risk pneumonia etiology often is unknown in the emergency department, the emergency department physician may not be able to assess this predisposing risk factor. The cost-containment aspects of this type of study are admirable, but they fail to reconcile the litigious environs of the emergency department. Published studies such as this one are useful as guidelines, but they must never be substitutes for clinical decision making. Criteria for admitting pneumonia patients to the hospital are varied and often confounded by many tenuous factors that do not fit into clinical algorithms [48]. Hospitalization is advised for patients who (1) have multilobe infiltrates, (2) are over 65 years of age, (3) have had a splenectomy or are immunodeficient in other ways, (4) have chronic lung disease, (5) have hypoxemia, or (6) are septic (Table 23-6).

Table 23-6. Indications for hospitalization

Multilobe infiltrates
Age > 65 years
Splenectomy
Immunodeficient status
Chronic lung disease
Hypoxemia
Sepsis
Poorly responding pneumonias

Adjunctive pneumonia therapies like hydration, chest physical therapy, oxygen, and bronchodilators need to be individualized. Cough suppressants probably should be avoided in the patient with copious sputum production, since cough is a valuable defense mechanism. Chest physical therapy and intermittent positive pressure breathing have not been shown to be of therapeutic value in uncomplicated pneumonias [49].

Table 23-8. Causes of viral pneumonia in healthy patients

Adults	Children
Influenza A and B	Herpes simplex virus
Measles	Respiratory syncytial virus
Atypical measles	Rhinovirus
Varicella	Influenza A and B
	Parainfluenza
	Adenovirus

Specific Clinical Syndromes in Pneumonia

Viral Pneumonias

Viral pneumonias are seen much more often in children. In fact, symptomatic viral respiratory infections are more common than any other type of infection in childhood (Table 23-7).

Viral illness in the adult remains primarily confined to the upper respiratory structures (Table 23-8). Adults rarely develop flagrant viral pneumonia in the absence of influenza virus. Adenoviral bronchitis or pneumonia in closed populations such as military barracks or prisons occurs, but severe disease is uncommon and primarily a risk for the immunocompromised patient [50]. Cytomegalovirus (CMV) pneumonia is seen only in the severely compromised host.

In the past the diagnosis of viral pneumonia has

been a clinical call relying on clues such as seasonal prevalence, community and family outbreaks, and patient age and contacts. The diagnosis should be suspected when the clinical presentation and the epidemiologic factors fit. Viral-like symptoms of rhinorrhea, conjunctivitis, sore throat, and raspy cough are emphasized. In the 1990s viral isolation and seroconversion are needed for definitive diagnosis. We can anticipate that the DNA probe era will greatly facilitate the identification of viruses [46].

INFLUENZA

There are more than 45 million cases of influenza in the United States each year, with the brunt of the cases falling on the elderly and the very young. More than 3 million people in the United States are hospitalized yearly due to influenza, and the mortality of the disease is astounding (over 20,000 each year) [51]. People with underlying cardiac or pulmonary problems are at particularly high risk of dying, but healthy young adults also die from influenza [52].

Influenza is typically abrupt in onset with high fever, headache, chills, cough, myalgias, and intense prostration. Photophobia and conjunctivitis are seen. The elderly and the very young may have a more insidious onset with a prodromal period of several days. Rhinorrhea, sore throat, and a dry irritative cough can last for weeks. The time to resolution of fever is variable, and full recovery may take several weeks. In the recovery phase a protracted cough may be indicative of hyperreactive airways and may respond well to bronchodilator therapy.

The diagnosis of influenza is often clinical. Viral isolation and serology are confirmatory but require

Table 23-7. Causes of pneumonia in young children

Age	Possible pathogens
Newborn	Group B streptococcus
	Herpes simplex virus
2–6 weeks	Chlamydia trachomatis
< 2 years	Respiratory syncytial virus
	Rhinovirus
	H. influenzae
	S. pneumoniae
2–5 years	Parainfluenza types 1 and 3
	Influenza A and B
> 5 years	Mycoplasma pneumoniae
	S. pneumoniae
	B. pertussis
All ages	Influenza A and B
	Adenovirus

days to weeks. Rapid diagnostic tests for influenza are available and being improved [53]. These tests offer the hope of early treatment intervention, especially since amantadine has value in the first 48 hours of influenza A illness.

Therapy for most patients with influenza entails rest, oral fluids, and a "tincture of time." Aspirin in children should be avoided because of the possibility of Reye's syndrome. Patients in need of hospitalization often require supplemental oxygen.

The value of yearly influenza vaccination in the population at highest risk should not be forgotten. Emergency department personnel should receive and dispense the vaccine each fall. The target groups for influenza vaccine include high-risk persons and their close contacts. The recommendations are published yearly by the Centers for Disease Control (CDC) [54] (see Chap. 5).

Amantadine as a prophylactic agent during an outbreak of influenza A is useful, but only while the patient is awaiting the vaccine's protective benefit, which may take two weeks. Amantadine is dosed at 100 mg bid PO (less in renal impairment and the elderly) and has no value in influenza B disease. Prophylactic antibiotic therapy is inappropriate. Secondary bacterial infections do occur, but antibiotics serve only to select a more resistant superinfecting organism. The patient is better served by a careful explanation of why antibiotics are not helpful initially and what signs to look for in the event of a superinfection. As is commonly the case in the emergency department setting, written as well as verbal explanations are advised.

MEASLES

The rashes of measles and varicella quickly suggest the diagnosis. More than 27,000 cases of measles were reported to the CDC for 1990. The classic measles rash commences centrally and spreads peripherally. Measles pneumonia in a young military population has been described as clinically very severe but with a relatively benign outcome [55]. Fatal measles pneumonia has been well characterized [56]. Bacterial superinfection with *S. aureus, S. pneumoniae, Streptococcus pyogenes,* or *H. influenzae* is a major risk (see Chap. 9).

A modified form of measles is being noticed [57]. These patients have had well-documented vaccinations, but they develop typical measles with all the complications. Rash and the three Cs (coryza, cough, conjunctivitis) are common. Koplik's spots may be found on the oral mucosa.

Atypical measles occurs in young adults who had their childhood vaccinations in 1964–1968 [58]. These patients may have received killed vaccine, which sets the stage for a hypersensitivity reaction when they are exposed to the wild virus. A peripherally distributed rash that can be mistaken for varicella, Rocky Mountain spotted fever, Henoch-Schonlein purpura, drug reactions, and even toxic shock syndrome has been the key presentation. Atypical measles tends to be quite severe, with toxic fevers, peripheral edema, interstitial pulmonary infiltrates with pulmonary edema, and hepatitis. These patients are not contagious since measles virus is not isolated. The diagnosis is made by the clinical picture and the presence of very high measles-antibody titers. Treatment is supportive.

VARICELLA

Varicella, like most childhood diseases, can be particularly severe in adults. Varicella pneumonia in the nonimmune adult is relatively common (approximately 20% of varicella cases). About 15% of adults have no immunity to varicella. An approach to adults who develop varicella skin lesions is to place them on high-dosage acyclovir (4 g/day, divided every 8 hours). Varicella-zoster virus is a lot more resistant to acyclovir than is herpes simplex virus, thus the large dose. The duration of this therapy is unclear. Mild cases may not need therapy; severe cases may need 10 days [59]. The usual length of treatment is 7 days.

VIRAL PNEUMONIA IN CHILDREN

The actual incidence of viral pneumonia is unknown, but it probably is more common than suspected because so few patients are sufficiently ill to warrant hospitalization. In the first 3 years of life more than 90% of acute respiratory disease is viral.

The clinical presentations are often diagnostic in children with croup (stridor) or bronchiolitis (wheezing). Other epidemiologic data, such as age, season of the year, and contact in the community to illness, are important in assessing the nature of a respiratory syndrome. Fever, rhinorrhea, pharyngitis, headache, nonproductive cough, and chest discomfort are common. Physical examination may demonstrate cervical lymphadenopathy, pharyngeal erythema, or myringitis. Localized or diffuse crackles, wheezes, and diminished breath sounds may be heard. The presence of cyanosis or crackles on physical exam has been shown to correlate better than tachypnea in assessing severity of acute bronchiolitis in children [60]. Occasionally a friction rub or the presence of a pleural effusion is noted. Unfortunately the clinical distinction between viral and bacterial pneumonia is difficult to make [61].

The chest x-ray in viral pneumonia may reveal bilateral patchy infiltrates prominent in the lower lobes but involving multiple lobes, unlike the single-lobe, dense infiltrate of bacterial pneumonia. Hilar adenopathy may be seen. Small pleural effusions can be expected. Unfortunately the value of the pediatric chest x-ray in determining bacterial versus viral pneumonia is poor [62]. The major respiratory viruses can produce areas of atelectasis or consolidation similar to bacterial pathogens. The need for a chest x-ray in children with clinically diagnosed pneumonia has been questioned [63]. A chest x-ray is advised in the following instances: when toxicity or physical findings suggest the need for therapeutic intervention (e.g., pleural fluid); when the source of a fever is not clear but could be occult pneumonia; and in older children, where the likelihood of viral pneumonia is much less. Arterial oxygen saturation by oximetry gives a more useful assessment of lung function in the child with pneumonia.

Sputum production in viral pneumonia is minimal with clear secretions usual, although purulence may be noted, particularly in the child with chronic lung disease. A slight leukocytosis with lymphopenia is common. Clinical findings of cyanosis, tachycardia, nasal flaring, and the use of accessory respiratory musculature mandate immediate oxygen therapy and prompt admission. Less ill children can be followed as outpatients. The emergency department evaluation of suspected childhood viral pneumonia depends on the underlying health of the host and the severity of the pneumonia. Compromised children with suspected viral pneumonia need a more aggressive diagnostic approach than do those who are basically healthy.

Respiratory Syncytial Virus

Respiratory syncytial virus (RSV) and parainfluenza types 1 and 3 are common causes of pneumonia and bronchiolitis in children during the winter and the early spring. RSV is the single most important respiratory pathogen of infancy and early childhood worldwide [64]. Typically RSV is more common in children under the age of 2, parainfluenza is more common between the ages of 2 and 5, and the nonviral agent, mycoplasma, is common after the age of 5. Influenza A and B and adenovirus can produce severe pneumonia in any age. The clinical disease patterns produced by RSV and rhinoviruses are identical [65]; both are major causes of bronchiolitis and pneumonia in normal children less than 3 years old.

Each year RSV is associated with prominent winter outbreaks in children under 2 years of age; 95,000 children in the United States are hospitalized because of RSV infection and more than 4,500 die [66]. RSV is also a major nosocomial pathogen and requires strict isolation at the time of admission. Very rapid antigen detection tests for RSV permit isolation procedures to start within 1 hour of admission. Oxygen saturation by pulse oximetry in the emergency department will identify the hypoxemic patient who needs admission [60, 67]. Most of these infants have been ill for several days and are congested and not feeding. Nasal suction, oxygen, and bronchodilators will improve many of them promptly. Antibiotics should not be used in RSV infections unless secondary bacterial infection is clearly documented by clinical deterioration and appropriate cultures [68]. RSV also has been found to cause pneumonia in elderly and compromised adults [69, 70].

Diagnosis

The diagnosis of viral pneumonia can be made by a nasopharyngeal or throat swab transmitted in viral transport media to an appropriate microbiology laboratory. Viruses isolated from the upper respiratory tract in the setting of pneumonia usually are assumed to be the cause of the pneumonia. In some compromised hosts the finding of CMV [71] or herpes simplex virus [72] in respiratory secretions is not synonymous with infection. Since viral therapy is limited and nonviral causes of pneumonia are common, diagnostic diligence is important.

Rapid viral diagnosis has been facilitated by sensitive viral antigen detection techniques using immunofluorescence and enzyme immunoassay [73].

Treatment

Treatment for viral pneumonia at the present is limited (Table 23-9). Costs, safety, and efficacy

Table 23-9. Definitive treatment of community acquired pneumonia

Etiology	Therapy of choice (adult dosages)	Alternate choices
Viruses		
RSV	Ribavirin (aerosolized)	
Influenza A	Amantadine 100 mg bid PO	
Influenza B	± Ribavirin (aerosolized)	
Varicella zoster	Acyclovir 800 mg 5 times/day for 7–10 days	
Bacteria		
Streptococcus pneumoniae	Penicillin G 30 mg/kg/day	Erythromycin, first-generation cephalosporin, TMP-SMX[a]
S. pneumoniae (PR)[b]	Vancomycin 1 g q12h	Cefotaxime
Haemophilus influenzae	Ampicillin 2 g q4–6h	TMP-SMX, second- or third-generation cephalosporins, fluoroquinolones, ampicillin-sulbactam
H. influenzae (+ ase)[c]	Cefotaxime 2 g q8h	TMP-SMX, second- or third-generation cephalosporins, fluoroquinolones, ampicillin-sulbactam
Klebsiella pneumoniae	Cefotaxime 2 g q8h	Other third-generation cephalosporins, cefazolin + aminoglycoside, fluoroquinolone, TMP-SMX
Moraxella catarrhalis	Cefotaxime 2 g q8h	TMP-SMX, second- or third-generation cephalosporins, fluoroquinolones, ampicillin-sulbactam
Staphylococcus aureus	Nafcillin 2 g q4–6h	Cefazolin, vancomycin
S. aureus (MRSA)[d]	Vancomycin 1 g q12h	—
Situations		
Atypical pneumonia syndrome (otherwise healthy)	Erythromycin 2 g/day	(see Table 23-11)
COPD + pneumonia	Second- or third-generation cephalosporin ± erythromycin 2 g/day	Tetracycline, ampicillin/sulbactam, fluoroquinolones, TMP-SMX
Critically ill	Erythromycin 2 g/day + third-generation cephalosporin	Imipenem, tetracycline, ampicillin-sulbactam, ticarcillin-clavulanate, fluoroquinolones, TMP-SMX, aminoglycosides
Aspiration	Clindamycin 900 mg q8h	Penicillin G, ampicillin-sulbactam
Recent hospitalization	Ceftazidime 2 g q8h ± aminoglycosides	Imipenem, other third-generation cephalosporins
Postinfluenza	Cefazolin 2 g q8h	Nafcillin, vancomycin, erythromycin

[a] TMP-SMX = trimethoprim-sulfamethoxazole
[b] PR = penicillin resistant
[c] + ase = Beta lactamase positive
[d] MRSA = methicillin resistant S. aureus

concerns have strictly limited the use of aerosolized ribavirin to RSV-infected patients with specific clinical criteria [74]. Adenovirus, influenza virus B, and parainfluenza viruses have no specific therapy. Amantadine is of some value only in the first 48 hours of influenza A (not influenza B). Aerosolized ribavirin may be effective in severe influenza B illness [75].

POSTVIRAL BACTERIAL COLONIZATION
Viral respiratory infections readily set the stage for bacterial colonization with gram-negative bacteria,

S. aureus, and S. pneumoniae [76]. There is no evidence that "expectant" antibacterial therapy does any more than change the respiratory flora to a more resistant flora. Patients diagnosed as having a "viral-like" respiratory syndrome should be advised both verbally and in writing of the need for immediate follow-up if fever, sputum production, and cough worsen or reoccur after an initial period of clinical improvement. An explanation as to why antibiotic therapy is not presently indicated would be important. Mindless antibiotic prescribing adversely affects the colonization immunity of the host as well as his or her finances [77].

Bacterial Pneumonias

BACTERIAL PNEUMONIA IN CHILDREN

The specific etiology of bacterial pneumonia in a child is difficult to identify (see Table 23-7). Invasive procedures are rarely indicated, sputum often is not available, and blood cultures are frequently negative. S. pneumoniae and H. influenzae type B are most commonly isolated when blood culture or lung aspiration is used to define the etiology of the pneumonia. Even the clinical, laboratory, or chest x-ray distinction between bacterial and viral pneumonia is difficult to discern [61]. The management of the child with presumed bacterial pneumonia depends on the child's age and clinical presentation. In a toddler with the acute onset of fever and cough combined with a leukocytosis, left shift, and a lobar infiltrate the likelihood of bacterial pneumonia is high. The absence of viral signs such as runny nose and pharyngitis adds further support to a bacterial etiology. The child who is not in respiratory distress, not toxic appearing, and is able to take food and fluids does not need admission. A blood culture should be drawn even though the yield will be low. Antigen detection tests on the urine and blood have an even lower yield at present. A sputum specimen is unlikely to be produced by a 3-year-old; children tend to swallow their sputum. A skin test for tuberculosis should be done in the patient at risk (family history or immigrant from high-risk area). Vaccination status with conjugate H. influenzae B vaccine must be known. The most likely bacterial organism in this setting is S. pneumoniae or H. influenzae, so amoxicillin is an appropriate antibiotic to start provided no allergy exists.

In many communities beta-lactamase–resistant

H. influenzae makes up as much as 40% of the isolates. Because of ampicillin resistance concerns, one can make a strong case against using amoxicillin as a primary therapy even though the nontoxic child can be observed for therapeutic effect. Beta-lactamase–resistant antibiotics (e.g., amoxicillin-clavulanate [Augmentin], cefaclor [Ceclor], and cefuroxime-axetil [Ceftin]) are more expensive, but they are appropriate alternatives. Erythromycin-sulfisoxazole (Pediazole), or trimethoprim-sulfamethoxazole (Bactrim or Septra) could be substituted as well, and they are relatively inexpensive. The combination of erythromycin-sulfisoxazole has an additional attraction because M. pneumoniae, Bordetella pertussis, and Chlamydia organisms are covered. Cefuroxime-axetil (Ceftin) does not yet come in a liquid form and is difficult to give to young children.

Much less likely causes of pneumonia in the toddler are S. aureus, group A streptococcus, M. pneumoniae, and Neisseria meningitides. Tuberculosis and fungal infections are even lower in the differential diagnosis.

The child should be reevaluated within 48 hours and, if improved, oral therapy should continue for 7–10 days. Lack of improvement suggests the following: (1) antibiotic resistance, (2) poor oral absorption, (3) incorrect antibiotic administration by the parents, (4) a complication such as empyema, or (5) a nonbacterial infection. Oral absorption may be diminished in the presence of diarrhea. Ceftriaxone [78] 50 mg/kg IM or IV once daily avoids the malabsorption concerns. If the child is worse after 48 hours of therapy, a repeat chest x-ray to look for pleural fluid is indicated. If the child still does not require hospitalization, a switch to a beta-lactam–resistant antibiotic like cefaclor or erythromycin-sulfisoxazole can be tried. Written and verbal instructions regarding what to do and what to look for in the child must be given to the family. Follow-up plans need to be carefully explained. Continued lack of improvement is an indication for hospitalization.

Some parents can provide their office-based physicians with reliable clinical observation by phone. With very few exceptions the emergency department physician should request a reexamination by a physician within 48 hours and not rely on telephone follow-up. Written instructions are important to avoid confusion.

School-aged children presenting to the emergency department with 24 hours of fever and cough combined with leukocytosis, a left shift, and a lobar infiltrate can be treated with erythromycin, since mycoplasmal infection is as likely as pneumococcal infection.

Tetracycline has excellent activity against mycoplasma, but it is not a good substitute because of increasing pneumococcal resistance. Tetracycline is contraindicated in pregnancy and in children under the age of 8 years.

The same 8-year-old would be handled more cautiously if sickle cell disease were a risk factor. Sickle cell disease would make the child functionally asplenic and at risk for a more severe pneumonia [79]. Pneumococcal and *H. influenzae* pneumonia are high in the differential diagnosis. Mycoplasmal pneumonia is more severe in these hosts. *C. pneumoniae* has been noted to be prevalent in children with sickle cell disease and the acute chest syndrome, consisting of fever and new pulmonary findings [80]. Pneumonia in the sickle-cell patient requires hospitalization for adequate hydration and IV antibiotic.

Table 23-10. Adult-patient predispositions to specific pneumonias

Patient condition	Pathogen
Healthy	*Streptococcus pneumoniae*
	Mycoplasma (< 40 years of age)
Alcoholic	*S. pneumoniae*
	Gram-negative bacilli
	Mixed anaerobes
	Tuberculosis
IV drug abuser	*Staphylococcus aureus*
	Pneumocystis carinii
COPD	*S. pneumoniae*
	Haemophilus influenzae
	Moraxella catarrhalis
	Legionella species
Following influenza	*S. pneumoniae*
	S. aureus
	H. influenzae
Nursing home or recent hospitalization	Gram-negative enteric bacilli
	S. aureus
	Pseudomonas aeruginosa
Asplenic	*S. pneumoniae*
	H. influenzae

BACTERIAL PNEUMONIA IN ADULTS

Pneumonia occurring in the adult should be categorized, if possible, into bacterial and atypical depending on the history and the physical exam along with sputum examination. Typical bacterial pneumonia begins abruptly with chills, fever, pleuritic pain, cough, and a purulent sputum production. An antecedent upper respiratory illness is often mentioned. Consolidation changes are noted on physical examination. Atypical pneumonias are more subtle in presentation. The patient is less likely to be toxic appearing. Chills, pleuritic pain, and sputum production are uncommon. The chest examination is rather banal in comparison to the chest x-ray. Unfortunately there are sufficient variations in hosts, organisms, and presentations to make a dogmatic division of pneumonia types impossible.

The initial question of bacterial versus atypical pneumonia helps to generate a differential diagnosis. Even more important is the assessment of the host (Table 23-10). Compromised hosts will always need more careful scrutiny. Compromising conditions are legion; they include age, underlying health, medications, and all the concerns that are paramount to a careful patient history. Pending isolation of a pathogen from a normally sterile site (blood, pleural fluid), the specific etiologic diagnosis of pneumonia is tentative. Empiric therapy is guided by the Gram's stain of sputum and the historical information.

Healthy Host. Community acquired bacterial pneumonia in a healthy host is most often pneumococcal. The classic presentation includes a single shaking chill, fever, pleuritic chest pain, and rusty colored sputum production. Penicillin V (30 mg/kg/day in four equal doses PO) is still the drug of choice. The penicillin-allergic patient who does not develop anaphylaxis from penicillin can be treated with cephalexin (Keflex) or cephradine (Velosef). Trimethoprim-sulfamethoxazole (Bactrim, Septra) and erythromycin are alternatives, particularly in the patient with hypersensitivity to penicillin (see Table 23-9). Penicillin-resistant pneumococcal strains are increasing throughout the world but are uncommon in the United States [81, 82]. Prior beta-lactam antibiotic use is a risk factor for penicillin-resistant pneumoccal pneumonia. Alternatives to penicillin when resistance exists include vancomycin and cefotaxime. The more common use of the pneumococcal vaccine should be encouraged, although data regarding its effectiveness in the United States are meager.

There are many preparations of erythromycin, not all with the same gastrointestinal side effects. Often these GI side effects are dose dependent and can be ameliorated by smaller doses given more frequently. Erythromycin has a GI stimulating effect, which is responsible for this toxicity [83].

New long-acting erythromycin congeners are being developed that have high levels of activity and fewer side effects. Clarithromycin [84] has much better GI tolerance and can be given less often, but like erythromycin it has limited activity against *H. influenzae*. Azithromycin [85] is a new 15-membered macrolide that is considerably more active than erythromycin against many organisms, including all the common causes of community acquired pneumonia. Azithromycin has unique pharmacokinetic properties, achieving high intracellular-tissue concentrations which are sustained for days. Controlled, comparative studies of azithromycin with other commonly used antibiotics are needed to establish its role in the treatment of community acquired pneumonia.

A 3-day supply of medication with instructions to purchase more if no side effects occur is cost effective. Implicit in this strategy is the clear understanding that some antibiotic is indicated for a defined period of time. An informed patient is more likely to be a compliant patient; thus, a careful explanation of the therapy and the consequences of noncompliance should be given to the patient and family.

The duration of antibiotic therapy for most infections is empiric. Host-defense considerations must be weighed with organism-virulence factors. Rarely is more than 10 days necessary in the therapy of uncomplicated community acquired pneumonia. Pneumococcal pneumonia probably needs no more than 3 days of antibiotic once the patient becomes afebrile.

The response to therapy must be cautiously assessed. Therapy does not substitute for a diagnosis,

so the prudent clinician should keep an open mind. A temporary improvement or a partial response calls for further evaluation. An obstructing neoplasia, an underlying subtle immune defect, an adverse medication effect, or the wrong initial diagnosis could be the problem. Furthermore, the empiric antibiotic therapy may obfuscate the clinical picture and delay appropriate therapy, for example, in the patient with concurrent endocarditis or meningitis.

A repeat chest x-ray in an uncomplicated pneumonia that responds well to therapy is needed in 6–8 weeks. Lack of complete clearing of the infiltrate at that time would heighten the concern for an underlying malignancy. Delayed resolution of chest x-ray changes is common, particularly in the elderly and patients with chronic lung disease [86]. Where there is no reason to suspect any underlying pathology (e.g., a healthy young person with a first episode of pneumonia and quick response to therapy), there is no reason to obtain a follow-up film.

Pneumonia occurring in a patient less than 40 years of age and with less convincing evidence of bacterial origin can be treated with erythromycin (500mg qid PO) from the outset (see Table 23-9). In that way pneumococci and mycoplasma are adequately covered. Legionnaires' disease may not respond to oral erythromycin, so the lack of response does not rule out legionella pneumonia.

Unhealthy Host. The adult with chronic lung disease who develops increasing cough, purulent sputum, fever, shortness of breath, and chest discomfort with a lung infiltrate is more problematic. That patient may have pneumococcal pneumonia but is prone to other pathogens such as *H. influenzae* [87, 88]. Unencapsulated and nontypable *H. influenzae* have become common causes of pneumonia in the elderly, the chronic bronchitic patient, and the alcoholic. Unlike the encapsulated *H. influenzae* type B, these *H. influenzae* rarely cause bacteremia. *M. (Branhamella) catarrhalis* and other gram-negative organisms are also more common. Prior antibiotic therapy broadens the differential diagnosis to include resistant organisms. Steroid use, alcohol abuse, and other underlying conditions further confuse the picture. Gram's stains can be misleading in these hosts because a multitude of organisms may be seen, and their sputa are always full of WBCs. Legionnaires' disease should be considered, especially when there is poor response to beta-lactam antibiotics. Many of these patients warrant hospitalization until they are stable (see Table 23-9).

Some community acquired pneumonia patients are extremely ill and require intensive care. When no specific pathogen is immediately apparent by Gram's stain, the critically ill patient can be started on a third-generation cephalosporin and IV erythromycin (4 g/day). If there is a history of hospitalization in the past two months or the patient uses a small volume nebulizer at home, ceftazidime should be used initially to cover *Pseudomonas aeruginosa*. Home respiratory equipment that is not being adequately cleansed is a risk factor for bacteremic community acquired gram-negative pneumonia. In-hospital therapy can then be modified when the diagnosis becomes more apparent (see Table 23-9).

Chronic aspiration-prone patients (alcoholics, epileptics, stroke patients, etc.) with severe periodontal disease are at high risk for anaerobic pneumonia and empyema formation. Poor oral hygiene adds to the enormous number of anaerobes in the oral cavity. Bacterial aspiration pneumonia is usually insidious in onset with weight loss, fatigue, and anemia that may mimic tuberculosis or lung cancer [89]. The diagnosis of an anaerobic lung infection usually is made by the clinical clues of chronic cough, putrid sputum, weight loss, fever, night sweats, and evidence of necrotizing pneumonia on chest x-ray with lung abscess or empyema. A setting conducive to chronic aspiration is supportive evidence. Only 50% of anaerobic pleuropulmonary infections are associated with a foul-smelling sputum. Gram's smears usually show mixed flora. Cultures are not useful unless obtained through transtracheal aspiration or protected brushing via the fiberoptic bronchoscope. Therapy needs to be initiated in the hospital. Clindamycin has been shown to be superior to penicillin in this setting [90, 91] (see Table 23-9). The correction of any underlying pyorrhea will help reduce the risk of recurrent anaerobic lung infection.

The less common acute aspiration pneumonia may mimic pneumococcal pneumonia [92]. In comparison to the patient with pneumococcal pneumonia the acute anaerobic aspiration pneumonia

patient is more likely to be aspiration prone, more likely to have poor oral hygiene, and less likely to be bacteremic. Outpatient therapy in this setting is probably best with clindamycin (300 mg q6h PO) or amoxicillin-clavulanate (Augmentin) (500 mg/125 mg q8h PO). The specific etiologic diagnosis is often unknown, however, and there are no controlled, comparative studies (see Table 23-9).

Daily outpatient ceftriaxone (1–2 g IM) may be an effective option in the stable chronic lung patient with pneumonia who has reliable home caretakers. Outpatient IV and IM antibiotic therapy commonly has been used with a variety of infectious diseases. Pneumonia therapy may be more challenging, but it is feasible if the patient and family are willing and backup support is readily available in the form of home-visiting nurse services. Since the chronic lung patient with pneumonia has less pulmonary reserve, the decision to start with a parenteral antibiotic seems prudent. Some patients, however, will do very well on oral antibiotics alone, and most can readily be switched to oral therapy once clinical improvement becomes apparent.

Oral antibiotic choices in the chronic obstructive lung disease patient include trimethoprim-sulfamethoxazole (Bactrim, Septra) 160/800 mg double strength bid, cefuroxime-axetil (Ceftin) 250–500 mg bid, or amoxicillin-clavulanate (Augmentin) 500/125-mg or 250/125-mg tablets tid. Ampicillin or amoxicillin alone has the risk of beta-lactamase inactivation by some *H. influenzae* and many *M. catarrhalis* organisms. Erythromycin is active against moraxella but much less active against *H. influenzae*. Azithromycin (discussed previously) may eventually become a very useful antibiotic in the COPD patient, but controlled comparative studies are needed first. Tetracycline, including doxycycline, is not reliably active against *S. pneumoniae*. Ciprofloxacin is therapeutic against *H. influenzae* and moraxella organisms, but it is not recommended for initial outpatient therapy of community acquired pneumonia, since *S. pneumoniae*, *M. pneumoniae*, and oral anaerobic flora are common. None of the latter three types of organism is appropriately treated with ciprofloxacin. The frequently inappropriate use of ciprofloxacin has been noted [93]. Chloramphenicol is very active against most of the above bacterial pathogens and is well absorbed, but it is rarely used today because of potential bone marrow toxicity and the availability of less toxic antibiotics.

The time to resolution of bacterial pneumonia is variable and depends on the host and the type of pneumonia. When signs of fever and respiratory compromise persist, the clinician should not automatically assume that the antibiotic regimen is failing. Sequestered infection, such as an abscess or an empyema, may preclude clinical improvement. Endovascular infection, particularly on the tricuspid valve, may be a source of delayed resolution. Drug fever may be present. A reexamination of the sputum and a repeat chest x-ray are needed before any change in antibiotics is made. Bacterial superinfection is uncommon and presents late in therapy as a recurrence of fever, dyspnea, and productive cough. Clinical improvement comes long before any improvement is noted on the chest x-ray. Similarly clinical cure invariably exists long before bacteriologic cure comes to the sputum.

Some objective criteria for nonresolving pneumonia have been published recently [94]. These authors found that bronchoscopy in nonresolving pneumonia yielded a significant alternative diagnosis most commonly in patients less than 55 years old, with no preexisting pulmonary disease, and with multilobar infiltrates of at least 4 weeks' duration. Opportunistic infections (often in the context of AIDS), alveolar neoplasms, and idiopathic inflammatory disorders like Wegener's granulomatosis, eosinophilic pneumonia, and bronchiolitis obliterans predominated. The causes of community acquired pneumonia are changing, and both diagnostic diligence and vigilance are needed

[95]. The patient with a poorly responding pneumonia often requires hospitalization.

Atypical Pneumonias (Stealth Bugs)

The presentations of atypical pneumonia have some of the clinical features of both viral and bacterial pneumonias. They are "atypical" because they present with constitutional symptoms and extrapulmonary findings that often overshadow the pulmonary findings. A nonproductive cough, headache, and myalgias predominate. Symptoms may overlap with bacterial processes, but there is a distinct lack of benefit from beta-lactam antibiotics. Unfortunately the signs and symptoms of community-acquired pneumonia are of limited value in predicting the specific origin of the pneumonia [12]. The differential diagnosis of atypical pneumonia includes *Pneumocystis carinii* pneumonia, mycoplasma pneumonia, Legionnaires' disease, *C. pneumoniae* (TWAR) pneumonia, psittacosis, Q fever, tuberculosis, and fungal pneumonias (Table 23-11).

PNEUMOCYSTIS CARINII PNEUMONIA

Pneumocystis carinii pneumonia (PCP) has become a common cause of atypical pneumonia (see Chap. 17). The manifestations of PCP depend on the host. Oncology patients undergoing chemotherapy are likely to have a rapid progression of fever and dyspnea leading to severe hypoxia within 1 week. The HIV-infected patient, however, commonly has an insidious onset of fever, fatigue, weight loss, cough, and exertional dyspnea, which may last weeks to months before pulmonary symptoms pre-

Table 23-11. Atypical pneumonia syndrome

Disease	Etiology	Treatment choices
Mycoplasma infection	*Mycoplasma pneumoniae*	Erythromycin, tetracycline
Chlamydia infection	*Chlamydia pneumoniae*	Tetracycline, erythromycin
Psittacosis infection	*Chlamydia psittaci*	Tetracycline, erythromycin
Q fever	*Coxiella burnetii*	Erythromycin ± rifampin
Legionnaires' disease	*Legionella pneumophila* (and other species)	Erythromycin ± rifampin, doxycycline
Pneumocystis pneumonia	*Pneumocystis carinii*	TMP/SMX, pentamidine
Acute tuberculosis	Mycobacteria	See Table 23-12
Acute fungal pneumonia	*Histoplasma capsulatum, Coccidioides immitis*	See Table 23-12

dominate. Even with pulmonary symptoms present, the chest x-ray may appear normal.

Early diagnosis and therapy clearly improve the prognosis of PCP. Unfortunately the diagnosis may be suspected but elusive. Definitive diagnosis requires microscopic identification of the *P. carinii* organism. Bronchoscopy with bronchoalveolar lavage and transbronchial biopsy has replaced the open lung biopsy as the "gold standard" for PCP diagnosis [96]. There is a reluctance to bronchoscope the patient who has only mild symptoms because of inconvenience, cost, and the occasional morbidity of bronchoscopy. The induced sputum to diagnose PCP is a sensitive test in the right setting. Emergency departments that often see patients at high risk for PCP should arrange with respiratory therapy and microbiology to have a well-coordinated approach to obtaining and promptly processing sputum for *P. carinii*. Since appropriate management often includes the early use of corticosteroids [97] along with specific antipneumocystis drugs, a definitive diagnosis is optimal. Gallium radioisotope scanning and pulmonary function testing are sensitive but lack specificity. Unfortunately the number of projected AIDS cases in the United States will make the empiric rather than the specific diagnosis of PCP necessary. History (HIV risk factors), physical findings (oral lesions of thrush or hairy leukoplakia), laboratory data (LDH greater than 220 IU/l, sedimentation rate greater than 50 mm/hr), combined with an abnormal chest x-ray, may assist in the empiric diagnosis of PCP [98]. The recent description of PCP in five elderly patients without AIDS or identifiable risk factors reminds us that we have a lot to learn about *P. carinii* and its epidemiology [99].

When considering the diagnosis of PCP, the clinician should not forget that bacterial pneumonia is common in the AIDS patient [100, 101]. Antibiotic resistance likewise is common, particularly to trimethoprim-sulfamethoxazole.

Mycoplasma Pneumoniae Pneumonia

Mycoplasma pneumoniae is the most common cause of atypical pneumonia. Mycoplasma pneumonia is age dependent, being much more common in children and young adults [102]. Transmission is by respiratory secretions and aided by close, prolonged contact in families, schools, or the work force. The incubation time is 3 weeks, which allows for a slow progression through households. Unlike viral pneumonias, which tend to peak in the fall and winter, mycoplasma pneumonia occurs throughout the year. Children often are not sufficiently ill to warrant therapy. As is typical of many childhood infections, older adults who contract mycoplasma pneumonia may be more severely afflicted. The few adults who become very ill with mycoplasma pneumonia have a hypersensitivity reaction, which contributes to the severity of their illness. Mycoplasma pneumonia becomes much less common in patients past the age of 40 [103]. Most mycoplasma pneumonia is self-limited. The majority of mycoplasmal illness involves respiratory infection without pneumonia, but there is a wide range of clinical presentations in the adult [104]. The usual clinical presentation includes a predominance of headache, malaise, and fever combined with a nonproductive cough and substernal chest pain. The chest x-ray appears worse than would be anticipated from the physical findings. Occasionally normal hosts have very severe disease [105].

The initial diagnosis of mycoplasma pneumonia is made clinically. A severe headache, nonproductive cough, and absence of the usual toxicity associated with bacterial infections are common. Nasopharyngeal and constitutional symptoms predominate. A clue to the presence of mycoplasma is a history of contact with children, young adults, or family members with recent respiratory illness.

Laboratory diagnosis is delayed because of the current dependence on serologies. Cold agglutinins in high titer are suggestive of mycoplasmal infection, but they are seen only in severe disease and are not very sensitive or specific. Complement-fixation serologies require a convalescent titer at 2 weeks and may not be confirmatory. An indirect immunofluorescence test for *M. pneumoniae* is both sensitive and specific. This test allows separate measurement of antibodies of IgG and IgM classes and, thus, can distinguish between current (IgM antibody) and past (IgG antibody) infections. Culture of the organism is difficult and requires days to weeks to become positive. Cultures often stay positive despite therapy. Most promising for the rapid diagnosis of mycoplasma pneumonia are the DNA probes, which are now beginning to be marketed [46].

Tetracycline (only in patients who are older than 8 years and who are not pregnant) or erythromycin for at least 2 weeks is the therapy for mycoplasma pneumonia. Relapses may occur with less protracted therapy. In uncommonly severe cases steroids have been used to reduce the hypersensitivity reaction that accounts for much of the lung tissue inflammation.

CHLAMYDIAL PNEUMONIAS

Chlamydial pneumonia (TWAR) due to C. pneumoniae is a newly described chlamydial respiratory infection with person-to-person transmission, unlike psittacosis, which is caused by C. psittaci [106]. C. pneumoniae infection often starts as a pharyngitis, sometimes with hoarseness, and gradually over days to weeks becomes pneumonia. The onset is slower than mycoplasma or viral infections. Fever may be minimal. The white blood count often is normal. Chest x-ray may show a single infiltrate or multiple infiltrates, depending on the severity. The spectrum of disease ranges from subclinical to severe pneumonia. Clinical illness is uncommon in children less than 5 years old. University students are more likely to present with 10 days of sore throat or hoarseness, minimal fever or leukocytosis, with abnormal breath sounds and a pneumonia by chest x-ray [107]. Older adults have a more severe clinical presentation. Diagnosis is by epidemiologic evidence and confirmed with convalescent serologies. Specific serologies (microimmunofluorescence test) generally are not available. The chlamydia complement-fixation test commonly is used for the presumptive diagnosis, although it does not distinguish among antibodies to C. pneumoniae, Chlamydia psittaci, and Chlamydia trachomatis. Therapy is best with tetracycline 500 mg qid PO for at least 14 days. Doxycycline 100 mg bid or erythromycin 500 mg qid for 14 days can be used. Persistent cough and malaise after therapy may necessitate a repeat course of therapy. Adult-onset asthma recently has been associated with chlamydial pneumonia [108].

The diagnosis of psittacosis (C. psittaci) is considered when there is contact with infected poultry and pet birds, usually illegally imported. There are 200–300 cases reported each year in the United States. The clinical presentation is variable. Severe headache, malaise, myalgias, arthralgias, and a dry cough are common. Splenomegaly and a pulse-temperature disparity may be noted. The differential diagnosis includes most of the causes of atypical pneumonia. Like Legionnaires' disease, psittacosis does not respond to beta-lactam antibiotics. Tetracycline is the preferred therapy; erythromycin will work.

C. trachomatis presents in infants 2–12 weeks old as a chronic interstitial pneumonia that gradually worsens [109]. A mucoid conjunctivitis and a peripheral eosinophilia may be evident. The child is afebrile with a persistent, dry hacking cough, tachypnea, diffuse crackles and wheezes, and hyperinflated lungs. Diagnosis is made clinically and confirmed with direct fluorescent antibody staining of conjunctival or respiratory secretions. Culture of tracheal secretions is most specific but requires cell-culture capability in the laboratory. Chlamydial colonization rather than infection of the respiratory tract may occur, so other potential pathogens need to be sought. Some infants improve without therapy, but erythromycin or sulfisoxazole shortens the clinical illness time. Newborn infants are also at risk for group B streptococcal pneumonia, presumably from maternal vaginal flora (see Chap. 14).

PERTUSSIS

Cases of pertussis in children less than 4 years old are increasing in the United States [110]. More than 10,000 cases were reported to the CDC in 1986–1988 [111]. The vaccination status of all children in the emergency department should be assessed. Severe cough is common. Paroxysmal cough lasting more than 14 days is a clinical clue to pertussis. Minimal fever and interstitial infiltrates may be present. Complications include pneumonia, seizures, and encephalopathy. The complications of chronic paroxysmal cough include all the physical sequelae of increased intra-abdominal and intrathoracic pressures. A marked lymphocytosis is common. Culture by calcium alginate nasopharyngeal swab for B. pertussis is negative late in the course of the illness. Cultures need to be plated in the emergency department because B. pertussis does not survive well in transport media. Rapid diagnosis is made by direct immunofluorescent antibody staining of nasopharyngeal secretions. Therapy with erythromycin (40 mg/kg/day for 2 weeks) is effective even when started late and reduces the spread of the disease.

Adults are at greater risk for pertussis than realized because of waning immunity. Adults with the illness may present with chronic cough, or they may be asymptomatic transmitters of the organism [112]. Adults may represent the major reservoir of pertussis in the United States [113]. Because immunity wanes, fully immunized adults are not protected and thus need to be given erythromycin prophylaxis when exposed to pertussis.

Q Fever

Q fever (C. burnetii) is a rickettsial pathogen associated with cattle, sheep, goats, and most recently parturient cats in a closed-space environment [114]. The incubation period is 2–4 weeks. Symptoms vary from benign, self-limited disease to overwhelming pneumonia. Headache, myalgias, chills, fever, sweats, and cough are common. Physical examination may be relatively normal, similar to other causes of atypical pneumonia. The white blood count may be slightly elevated and the liver transaminases increased two to three times normal. Diagnosis is made by a fourfold rise between acute and convalescent serologies. The complement-fixation test is the most convenient serology. The therapy of Q fever is with tetracycline or erythromycin. Although erythromycin is the drug of choice for the "unknown" atypical pneumonia, therapeutic failures have been noted in severe cases of Q fever, and the addition of rifampin (600 mg bid PO) may be useful [115].

Legionnaires' Disease

Legionella pneumonia usually is sporadic in occurrence, but it can be epidemic. The legionella organism is a gram-negative bacterium that does not stain well. Pneumonias caused by this pathogen share clinical features of both acute bacterial pneumonia and atypical pneumonia [116]. A water source for the organism is common; even misting sprays in the vegetable displays of grocery stores have been incriminated. All age groups can be involved, but elderly persons, chronic lung disease patients, and compromised hosts are most likely to demonstrate rapid and severe infection. The spectrum of clinical illness ranges from fever with headache, malaise, and no pneumonia to severe pneumonia. An initially nonproductive cough may become productive. The acute onset of high fever and chills is common. A pulse-temperature dissociation is seen occasionally. Diarrhea and encephalopathic changes are prominent [117]. These changes are suggestive but are not unique to Legionnaires' disease [12]. A major clue to Legionnaires' disease is the lack of response to beta-lactam antibiotics. Direct fluorescent antibody (DFA) staining for legionella antigen in sputum may be rapidly diagnostic, but it requires an experienced microbiologist [118]. A negative stain does not rule out Legionnaires' disease; the sensitivity of the DFA stain is less than that of culture. Urinary legionella-antigen detection for Legionella pneumophila serogroup 1 antigen has been shown to have high specificity and sensitivity [119]. Unfortunately other legionellae that are less common but still important are not detected. Sputum should be cultured on special media for the legionella organism.

Legionnaires' disease should be treated in the hospital. Erythromycin (4 g IV initially) is usually given for 3 weeks. Severe cases may benefit from the addition of rifampin (600 mg bid PO or IV). Alternative therapies in the erythromycin-intolerant patient include doxycycline or trimethoprim-sulfamethoxazole plus rifampin. There is much more clinical experience with erythromycin.

Fungal Pneumonias

Histoplasma capsulatum is an uncommon cause of acute pneumonia (histoplasmosis). This fungus is found throughout the United States, Central America, and South America; the endemic areas in the United States are in the Mississippi River valley and the Ohio River valley. Infection occurs following inhalation of soil contaminated by bird or bat feces. Pneumonia is most likely after heavy exposure to contaminated soil in such settings as a chicken coop or a construction site that formerly was a bird roost or after using a chainsaw to cut decayed wood. A flu-like syndrome consisting of dyspnea, nonproductive cough, arthralgias, chills, and low-grade fever are the typical symptoms. Most infections are asymptomatic. Solitary or multiple small, calcified granulomas are produced in the lung. Hilar nodes often calcify with histoplasmosis. Hematogenous dissemination in primary disease is common, judging by the frequency of calcified granulomas containing the organism being found on incidental autopsy studies. Therapy rarely is needed in the normal host.

C. immitis is an endemic fungus in the arid southwestern Sonoran deserts and causes coccidioidomycosis. Subclinical illness is common. Clinical disease presents with pleuritic chest pain, dry cough, malaise, and fever. Most pneumonia is self-limited. In some cases primary progressive coccidioidomycosis occurs. High initial inocula also produce more severe clinical illness. A travel history is important. Sputum fungal smears and culture are the primary diagnostic aids. Serologies are available to help in the diagnosis. Therapy usually is not indicated except in progressive disease or compromised hosts.

Other fungal infections of limited importance in the normal host include blastomycosis and cryptococcosis. Blastomyces dermatitidis is a dimorphic fungus that is endemic to the central and southeastern United States. It can produce primary pneumonia or reactivation disease. The organism has an affinity for skin, bones, and the prostate. Pulmonary disease mimics tuberculosis and cancer [120]. Definitive diagnosis requires culture of the fungus. Presumptive diagnosis can be made by special stains, which demonstrate the distinctive morphology of the yeast phase.

Candida species are rare causes of pneumonia, even in compromised hosts. Sputum may frequently become colonized with Candida species, but treatment is not required. Neutropenic patients are the exception, since they invariably require empiric amphotericin B when febrile.

TUBERCULOUS PNEUMONIAS
Tuberculosis in adults may present in the lower lobes as a primary infection [121, 122]. Most tuberculous pneumonias represent reactivation of latent apical disease and present as subacute clinical illnesses. Rarely tuberculosis presents as acute disease with multilobar involvement. The insidious onset of low-grade fever, night sweats, and a nonproductive cough is much more common. As with most entities in clinical medicine the diagnosis of tuberculosis is relatively easy, once one thinks of it. The clue to the diagnosis is to remember that tuberculosis tends to run in families; is most often found in the elderly, American Indians, Asian immigrants, and crowded intercity populations; is increasing in the United States; and looks like a "stealth bug" on a Gram's stain because it does not pick up the stain. Therapy for tuberculosis is becoming more complicated because of increased drug resistance. Confirmatory cultures are necessary to distinguish the pathogen from atypical mycobacteria and to assess drug susceptibility. There are three basic tenets of therapy: (1) never use only one drug; (2) never add a single agent to a failing regimen; (3) when resistance is likely, use four drugs until susceptibility data are available. The public health ramifications of tuberculosis mandate careful, long-term follow-up.

MELIOIDOSIS
Melioidosis is caused by Pseudomonas pseudomallei, a gram-negative bacterium that can mimic tuberculosis in chronicity and upper-lobe cavitation. Because this pathogen is predominantly acquired in Southeast Asia, Vietnam veterans may still harbor the organism [123]; thus the importance of the medical history in evaluating the patient with infection.

Chronic and Recurrent Pneumonias

Chronic pneumonias are by definition pneumonias that last longer than 3 or 4 weeks. Often they are due to tuberculosis or chronic fungal infection. Occasionally the culprit is an unrecognized foreign-body aspiration or an underlying malignancy. An indolent aspiration pneumonitis with abscess formation may present with fatigue, weight loss, chronic cough, and pulmonary infiltrate. Noninfective causes need to be considered: Wegener's granulomatosis, hypersensitivity lung disease, sarcoidosis, and others. Definitive diagnosis of a chronic pneumonia often requires culture or histology. Table 23-12 lists the etiologies and treatment choices of chronic pneumonias.

Recurrent pneumonia, as distinct from relapsing pneumonia, represents multiple, separate episodes of pneumonia. The list of potential causes is long. The history often provides the major clues to the presence and the etiology of recurrent pneumonia [124].

Table 23-12. Chronic pneumonias

Disease	Etiology	Treatment choices
Tuberculosis	Mycobacteria species	INH, + rifampin, ± pyrazinamide, ± ethambutol, ± streptomycin, ± others*
Fungal Pneumonias		
Coccidioidomycosis	*Coccidioides immitis*	Amphotericin B, ke-
Histoplasmosis	*Histoplasma capsulatum*	toconazole, flu-
Cryptococcosis	*Cryptococcus neoformans*	conazole,
Blastomycosis	*Blastomyces dermatitidis*	itraconazole
Aspergillosis	*Aspergillus* species	
Melioidosis	*Pseudomonas pseudomallei*	Ceftazidime, trimethoprim-sufamethoxazole, imipenem
Nocardiosis	*Nocardia asteroides*	Trimethoprim-sufamethoxazole, sulfonamide, minocycline
Actinomycosis	*Actinomyces* species	Penicillin, tetracycline
Aspiration pneumonia	Anaerobes	Clindamycin, am-picillin-sulbactam, penicillin

*Ethionamide, cycloserine, capreomycin, ciprofloxacin, clofazimine, amikacin.

Mimics of Infective Pneumonia

Mimics of infective pneumonia are listed in Table 23-13.

PULMONARY EMBOLI

The distinction between pulmonary embolus and atypical pneumonia can be difficult to make, especially when there is coexistent pulmonary disease [125]. Fever, cough, dyspnea, leukocytosis, and a pulmonary infiltrate on chest x-ray may be due to an embolus and pulmonary infarction. A clue to the diagnosis is the sudden onset of dyspnea and chest pain in a patient with risk factors for emboli. These risk factors include birth control or other estrogen use in women who also smoke, recent trauma, and protracted immobilization, particularly in older patients. A family history of hypercoagulability should be sought. The lower extremity should be carefully examined, even though the sensitivity and the specificity of physical findings in deep-vein thrombosis are low.

HYPERSENSITIVITY PNEUMONIAS

The list of drugs that cause pulmonary disease [126] is extensive and includes some common medications like aspirin, nitrofurantoin, dilantin, and gold salts, as well the less commonly used cytotoxic drugs. Even ophthalmic preparations can produce significant pulmonary complications [127]. Onset of dyspnea, cough, and fever can be abrupt or gradual. The mechanisms of pulmonary toxicity and the clinical features vary. The role of underlying illness may be important in many of these drug reactions. The clinician evaluating a patient with a pulmonary process must recall that more than 20 noncytotoxic agents have been associated with pulmonary injury. Since the end result of many types of lung injury is pulmonary fibrosis, early intervention is important.

Recurrent pneumonias due to a hypersensitivity reaction to thermophilic actinomycetes in building air vents have been well documented [128]. The onset may be rapid with chills, fever, cough, and

Table 23-13. Mimics of infective pneumonia

Foreign body aspiration
Pulmonary emboli
Mitral stenosis
Eosinophilic pneumonias
Hypersensitivity pneumonias
Collagen vascular disease
Molar pregnancy (choriocarcinoma)
Pulmonary hemorrhage
Congestive heart failure
Pulmonary alveolar proteinosis
Allergic bronchopulmonary aspergillosis

dyspnea beginning within hours of exposure to antigen. The chest x-ray may show patchy alveolar infiltrates in the lower lobes. Alternatively there may be a more indolent onset with cough, dyspnea, weight loss, and fibronodular infiltrates. The clue to this diagnosis is in the seasonality of the disease and its relation to air conditioning, humidification, or heating system contact. An occupational and home exposure history is vital in any patient with recurrent pneumonia or unexplained interstitial lung disease. Hot tubs, indoor pools, and vaporizers are all potential reservoirs for organic substances that can produce hypersensitivity pneumonitis [129].

EOSINOPHILIC PNEUMONIAS

Acute eosinophilic pneumonias are uncommon [130]. Their etiologies often are unknown. They present as acute febrile illness, severe hypoxemia, and diffuse pulmonary infiltrates in the absence of infection or history of an atopic illness. Unlike chronic eosinophilic pneumonia [131] acute eosinophilic pneumonias may have a normal peripheral eosinophil count. They can be clinically indistinguishable from an acute infective pneumonia or adult respiratory distress syndrome. Diagnosis is made by bronchoalveolar lavage (BAL) and finding more than 5% eosinophils in the lavage fluid without evidence of infection. A myriad of interstitial lung diseases, including sarcoidosis and lupus, and drugs also can cause increased BAL eosinophils. Likewise, coccidioidomycosis, aspergillosis, AIDS-related pneumonias, and helminthic diseases can demonstrate increased eosinophils in the BAL. Di-

agnosis is made in the hospital after careful consideration of these other potential causes. Prompt resolution of the pneumonia comes in response to a brief course of corticosteroids. Relapse does not occur.

Chronic eosinophilic pneumonia more typically presents as a patient who has had repeated courses of antibiotics for suspected recurrent bacterial pneumonia. Cough, fever, dyspnea, night sweats, and weight loss are apparent. An atopic history may be present, but asthma is not a problem. Most patients have an eosinophilia, anemia, and an elevated sedimentation rate. The chest x-ray shows bilateral, peripherally distributed infiltrates, the "photographic negative" of pulmonary edema. This chronic illness mimics tuberculosis, coccidioidomycosis, lymphoma, bronchopulmonary aspergillosis, Churg-Strauss vasculitis, and bronchiolitis obliterans with organizing pneumonia (BOOP). Rather than receive another course of antibiotics, the patient with "poorly responding bronchitis, recurrent pneumonia" should be hospitalized for definitive diagnosis, which often requires a lung biopsy.

Miscellaneous Causes of Bacterial Pneumonias

Nocardia asteroides is a bacterial respiratory pathogen that is particularly common in steroid-dependent hosts [132]. It is occasionally seen as a pathogen in patients with COPD or alveolar proteinosis. Nonspecific cough, fever, and weight loss are common. The chest x-ray infiltrates are more nodular initially but can become cavitary like tuberculosis. Dissemination to brain, skin, and adrenals occurs. Gram-positive filamentous rods on Gram's stain are often diagnostic. Culture of this aerobic bacterium may take 2 weeks. Therapy is with sulfonamides in high doses and for months. Controlled, comparative antibiotic trials in nocardia infection have never been done.

Actinomyces species (actinomycosis) are anaerobic organisms indigenous to the oral cavity. Pleuropulmonary disease is chronic and initially quite subtle. An early pneumonic focus may progress with minimal symptoms to involve the pleura and adjacent structures. Typically there is no pleural effusion or empyema, and tissue planes and anatomical barriers like bone are ignored. The result is an indolent, destructive infection with bony erosion and cutaneous fistulas. The infection mimics tuberculosis or cancer. A chest-wall mass that extends through the pleura is a major clue. Poor dentition commonly is present. Diagnosis is by anaerobic culture, but a Gram's smear demonstrating filamentous gram-positive rods is suggestive. The drainage of sulfur granules (partially calcified masses of actinomyces) is characteristic. Therapy is with high-dose penicillin (20 million U/day) for 4–6 weeks followed by oral penicillin for months. The tetracyclines are effective substitutes in the penicillin-allergic patient.

Group B streptococcus (*Streptococcus agalactiae*) [133], group Y *meningococcus* [134], and group A streptococcus are uncommon causes of pneumonia.

References

1. Garibaldi RA. Epidemiology of community-acquired respiratory tract infections in adults. *Am J Med* 78 (suppl 6B):32–37, 1985.
2. Dixon RE. Economic costs of respiratory tract infections in the United States. *Am J Med* 78 (suppl. 6B):45–51, 1985.
3. Fick RB, Reynolds HY. Changing spectrum of pneumonia—news media creation or clinical reality? *Am J Med* 74:1–8, 1983.
4. Marrie TJ, Durant H, Yates L. Community-acquired pneumonia requiring hospitalization: 5-year prospective study. *Rev Infect Dis* 11:586–99, 1989.
5. Pachon J et al. Severe community-acquired pneumonia. *Am Rev Respir Dis* 142:369–73, 1990.
6. Fine MJ et al. Prognosis of patients hospitalized with community-acquired pneumonia. *Am J Med* 88 (5N):1–8, 1990.
7. Davis PB. Clinical characteristics of the adult patient with cystic fibrosis. *Intern Med* 6(3):79–84, 1985.
8. Tager IB. Health effects of "passive smoking" in children. *Chest* 96:1161–64, 1989.
9. Limper AH, Prakash UBS. Tracheobronchial foreign bodies in adults. *Ann Intern Med* 112:604–9, 1990.
10. Muth D, Schafermeyer RW. All that wheezes. *Ped Emerg Care* 6:110–13, 1990.
11. Word BM, Baldridge A. *Mycoplasma hominis* pneumonia and pleural effuson in a postpartum adolescent. *Pediatr Infect Dis J* 9:295–96, 1990.
12. Fang GD et al. New and emerging etiologies for community-acquired pneumonia with implications for therapy: a prospective multi-center study of 359 cases. *Medicine* 69:307–16, 1990.
13. Irwin RS et al. Chronic cough as the sole presenting manifestation of gastroesophageal reflux. *Am Rev Respir Dis* 140:1294–1300, 1989.
14. Lewin S, Brettman LR, Holzman RS. Infections in hypothermic patients. *Arch Intern Med* 141:920–25, 1981.
15. Carter EJ, Ettensohn DB. Catamenial pneumothorax. *Chest* 98:713–16, 1990.
16. Maunder RJ, Pierson DJ, Hudson LD. Subcutaneous and mediastinal emphysema; pathophysiology, diagnosis, and management. *Arch Intern Med* 144:1447–58, 1984.
17. Dominguez F et al. Acute upper airway obstruction in achalasia of the esophagus. *Am J Gastroenterol* 82:362–64, 1987.
18. Sherry MK et al. Herpetic tracheobronchitis. *Ann Intern Med* 109:229–33, 1988.
19. Barker JA et al. Primary neonatal herpes simplex virus pneumonia. *Pediatr Infect Dis J* 9:285–89, 1990.
20. Doll DC, List AF, Yarbro JW. Functional hyposplenism. *South Med J* 80:999–1006, 1987.
21. Styrt B. Infection associated with asplenia: risks, mechanisms, and prevention. *Am J Med* 88 (5N):33–42, 1990.
22. Johnson JD, Raff MJ, Van Arsdall JA. Neurological manifestations of Legionnaires' disease. *Medicine* 63:303–10, 1984.
23. Guerin JM, Meyer P, Habib Y. Severe diarrhea in pneumococcal bacteremia [letter]. *JAMA* 257:1897–98, 1987.
24. Tew J, Calenoff L, Berlin BS. Bacterial or nonbacterial pneumonia: accuracy of radiographic diagnosis. *Radiology* 124:607–12, 1977.
25. Hunninghake GW, Fauci AS. Pulmonary involvement in the collagen vascular diseases. *Am Rev Resp Dis* 119:471–503, 1979.
26. Calenoff L, Kruglik GD, Woodruff A. Unilateral pulmonary edema. *Radiology* 126:19–24, 1978.
27. Gross NJ. Pulmonary effects of radiation therapy. *Ann Intern Med* 86:81–92, 1977.
28. Claypool WD, Rogers RM, Matuschak GM. Update on the clinical diagnosis, management, and pathogenesis of pulmonary alveolar proteinosis (phospholipidosis). *Chest* 85:550–58, 1984.
29. Edelstein H, McCabe RE. Atypical presentations of *Pneumocystis carinii* pneumonia in patients receiving inhaled pentamidine prophylaxis. *Chest* 98:1366–69, 1990.

30. Milligan SA et al. *Pneumocystis carinii* pneumonia radiographically simulating tuberculosis. *Am Rev Respir Dis* 132:1124–26, 1985.

31. Leatherman JW, Iber C, Davies SF. Cavitation in bacteremic pneumococcal pneumonia. *Am Rev Respir Dis* 129:317–21, 1984.

32. Finley RJ et al. The management of nonmalignant intrathoracic esophageal perforations. *Ann Thorac Surg* 30:575–81, 1980.

33. Light RW. Exudative pleural effusions secondary to gastrointestinal diseases. *Clin Chest Med* 6:103–11, 1985.

34. Lorch DG, Sahn SA. Pleural effusions due to diseases below the diaphragm. *Semin Respir Med* 9:75–85, 1987.

35. Charles OH, Panaro V. Round pneumonia in adults. *Arch Intern Med* 148:1155–57, 1988.

36. Rein MF et al. Accuracy of Gram's stain in identifying pneumococci in sputum. *JAMA* 239:2671–73, 1978.

37. Merrill CW et al. Rapid identification of pneumococci; gram stain vs. the quellung reaction. *N Engl J Med* 288:510–12, 1973.

38. Karam GH, Griffin FM. Invasive pulmonary aspergillosis in non-immunocompromised, non-neutropenic hosts. *Rev Infect Dis* 8:357–63, 1986.

39. Light RW. *Pleural Diseases.* Philadelphia: Lea & Febiger, 1990. Chap. 5.

40. Light RW et al. Parapneumonic effusions. *Am J Med* 69:507–11, 1980.

41. Fine NL, Smith LR, Sheedy PF. Frequency of pleural effusions in mycoplasma and viral pneumonias. *N Engl J Med* 283:790–93, 1970.

42. Beekman JF, Bosniak S, Canter HG. Eosinophilia and elevated IgE concentration in a serous pleural effusion following trauma. *Am Rev Respir Dis* 110:484–89, 1974.

43. Menzies R, Charbonneau M. Thoracoscopy for the diagnosis of pleural disease. *Ann Intern Med* 114:271–76, 1991.

44. Thorson SH et al. Variability of arterial blood gas values in stable patients in the ICU. *Chest* 84:14–18, 1983.

45. Perlino CA, Rimland D. Alcoholism, leukopenia, and pneumococcal sepsis. *Am Rev Respir Dis* 132:757–60, 1985.

46. Tenover FC. Diagnostic deoxyribonucleic acid probes for infectious diseases. *Clin Micro Rev* 1:82–101, 1988.

47. Fine MJ, Smith DN, Singer DE. Hospitalization decision in patients with community-acquired pneumonia: a prospective cohort study. *Am J Med* 89:713–21, 1990.

48. Fine MJ. Pneumonia in the elderly: the hospital admission and discharge decisions. *Sem Resp Infect* 5:303–13, 1990.

49. Graham WGB, Bradley DA. Efficacy of chest physiotherapy and intermittent positive pressure breathing in the resolution of pneumonia. *N Engl J Med* 299:624–27, 1978.

50. Zahradnik JM, Spencer MJ, Porter DD. Adenovirus infection in the immunocompromised patient. *Am J Med* 68:725–32, 1980.

51. Glezen WP. Serious morbidity and mortality associated with influenza epidemics. *Epidemiol Rev* 4:25–44, 1982.

52. Langmuir AD, Schoenbaum SC. The epidemiology of influenza. *Hosp Pract* 11 (Oct):49–56, 1976.

53. Sullivan CJ, Jordan MC. Diagnosis of viral pneumonia. *Sem Resp Infect* 3:148–61, 1988.

54. Centers for Disease Control. Prevention and control of influenza: recommendations of the Immunization Practices Advisory Committee. *MMWR* 40 (no. RR-6):1–15, 1991.

55. Gremillion DH, Crawford GE. Measles pneumonia in young adults. *Am J Med* 71:539–42, 1981.

56. Sobonya RE et al. Fatal measles (rubeola) pneumonia in adults. *Arch Pathol Lab Med* 102:366–71, 1978.

57. Edmonson MB et al. Mild measles and secondary vaccine failure during a sustained outbreak in a highly vaccinated population. *JAMA* 263:2467–71, 1990.

58. Frey HM, Krugman S. Atypical measles syndrome: unusual hepatic, pulmonary, and immunologic aspects. *Am J Med Sci* 281:51–55, 1981.

59. Feder HM Jr. Treatment of adult chickenpox with oral acyclovir. *Arch Intern Med* 150:2061–65, 1990.

60. Mulholland EK, Olinsky A, Shann FA. Clinical findings and severity of acute bronchiolitis. *Lancet* 335:1259–61, 1990.

61. Turner RB et al. Pneumonia in pediatric outpatients: cause and clinical manifestations. *J Pediatr* 111:194–200, 1987.

62. McCarthy PL et al. Radiographic findings and etiologic diagnosis in ambulatory childhood pneumonias. *Clin Pediatr* 20:686–91, 1981.

63. Hall CB, Disney FA, Marcy SM. Chest roentgenograms in children with clinically diagnosed pneumonia. *Pediatr Infect Dis J* 8:895–96, 1989.

64. Publication of Centers for Disease Control. Respiratory syncytial virus and parainfluenza virus surveillance–United States, 1989–90. *MMWR* 39(46):832–34, 1990.

65. Kellner G et al. Clinical manifestations of respira-

tory tract infections due to respiratory syncytial virus and rhinoviruses in hospitalized children. *Acta Pediatr Scand* 78:390–94, 1989.

66. Hall CB, McBride JT. Respiratory syncytial virus— from chimps with colds to conundrums and cures [editorial]. *N Engl J Med* 325:57–58, 1991.

67. Shaw KN, Bell LM, Sherman NH. Outpatient assessment of infants with bronchiolitis. *AJDC* 145:151–55, 1991.

68. Hall CB et al. Risk of secondary bacterial infection in infants hospitalized with respiratory syncytial viral infection. *J Pediatr* 113:266–71, 1988.

69. Englund JA et al. Respiratory syncytial virus infection in immunocompromised adults. *Ann Intern Med* 109:203–08, 1988.

70. Takimoto CH, Cram DL, Root RK. Respiratory syncytial virus infections on an adult medical ward. *Arch Intern Med* 151:706–08, 1991.

71. Millar AB et al. Cytomegalovirus in the lungs of patients with AIDS: respiratory pathogen or passenger? *Am Rev Resp Dis* 141:1474–77, 1990.

72. Ramsey PG et al. Herpes simplex virus pneumonia: clinical, virologic, and pathologic features in 20 patients. *Ann Intern Med* 97:813–20, 1982.

73. Sullivan CJ, Jordan MC. Diagnosis of viral pneumonia. *Sem Resp Infect* 3:148–61, 1988.

74. Marks MI, Wald E. Ribavirin therapy for respiratory syncytial virus infections. *Pediatr Infect Dis J* 9:S84, 1990.

75. Knight V, Gilbert BE. Ribavirin aerosol treatment of influenza. *Infect Dis Clin North Am* 1:441–57, 1987.

76. Ramirez-Ronda CH, Fuxench-Lopez Z, Nevarez M. Increased pharyngeal bacterial colonization during viral illness. *Arch Intern Med* 141:1599–1603, 1981.

77. DiNubile MJ. Antibiotics: the antipyretics of choice? *Am J Med* 89:787–88, 1990.

78. Leibovitz E et al. Once daily intramuscular ceftriaxone in the outpatient treatment of severe community-acquired pneumonia in children. *Clin Pediatr* 11:634–39, 1990.

79. Zarkowsky HA et al. Bacteremia in sickle cell hemoglobinopathies. *J Pediatr* 109:579–85, 1986.

80. Miller ST et al. Role of *Chlamydia pneumoniae* in acute chest syndrome of sickle cell disease. *J Pediatr* 118:30–33, 1991.

81. Feldman C et al. Community-acquired pneumonia due to penicillin-resistant pneumococci. *N Engl J Med* 313:615–17, 1985.

82. Rauch AM et al. Invasive disease due to multiple resistant *Streptococcus pneumoniae* in a Houston, Texas day care center. *Am J Dis Child* 144:923–27, 1990.

83. Janssens J et al. Improvement of gastric emptying in diabetic gastroparesis by erythromycin. *N Engl J Med* 322:1028–31, 1990.

84. Neu HC. The development of macrolides: clarithromycin in perspective. *J Antimicrob Chemother* 27 (suppl. A):1–9, 1991.

85. Girard AE et al. Pharmacokinetic and in vivo studies with azithromycin (CP-62, 993), a new macrolide with an extended half life and excellent tissue distribution. *Antimicrob Agents Chemother* 31:1948, 1987.

86. Jay SJ, Johanson WG, Pierce AK. The radiographic resolution of *Streptococcus pneumoniae* pneumonia. *N Engl J Med* 293:798–801, 1975.

87. Levin DC et al. Bacteremic *Haemophilus influenzae* pneumonia in adults: a report of 24 cases and a review of the literature. *Am J Med* 62:219–24, 1977.

88. Musher DM et al. Pneumonia and acute febrile tracheobronchitis due to *Haemophilus influenzae*. *Ann Intern Med* 99:444–50, 1983.

89. Bartlett JG. Anaerobic bacterial infections of the lung. *Chest* 91:901–9, 1987.

90. Levison ME et al. Clindamycin compared with penicillin for the treatment of anaerobic lung abscess. *Ann Intern Med* 98:466–71, 1983.

91. Gudiol F et al. Clindamycin vs. penicillin for anaerobic lung infections. *Arch Intern Med* 150:2525–29, 1990.

92. Bartlett JG. Anaerobic bacterial pneumonitis. *Am Rev Respir Dis* 119:19–23, 1979.

93. Frieden TR, Mangi RJ. Inappropriate use of oral ciprofloxacin. *JAMA* 264:1438–40, 1990.

94. Feinsilver SH et al. Utility of fiberoptic bronchoscopy in non-resolving pneumonia. *Chest* 98:1322–26, 1990.

95. Sen RP. Making bronchoscopy count. *Chest* 98:1314–15, 1990.

96. Davey RT, Masur H. Minireview: recent advances in the diagnosis, treatment, and prevention pf *Pneumocystis carinii* pneumonia. *Antimicrob Agents Chemother* 34:499–504, 1990.

97. Bozzette SA. The use of corticosteroids in *Pneumocystis carinii* pneumonia. *J Infect Dis* 162:1365–69, 1990.

98. Katz MH, Baron RB, Grady D. Risk stratification of ambulatory patients suspected of *Pneumocystis* pneumonia. *Arch Intern Med* 151:105–10, 1991.

99. Jacobs JL et al. A cluster of *Pneumocystis carinii* pneumonia in adults without predisposing illnesses. *N Engl J Med* 324:246–50, 1991.

100. Schlamm HT, Yancovitz SR. *Haemophilus influenzae* pneumonia in young adults with AIDS, ARC, or risk of AIDS. *Am J Med* 86:11–14, 1989.

101. Polsky B et al. Bacterial pneumonia in patients with the acquired immunodeficiency syndrome. *Ann Intern Med* 104:38–41, 1986.

102. Cotton EM, Strampfer MJ, Cunha BA. *Legionella* and *Mycoplasma pneumoniae*—a community hospital experience with atypical pneumonias. *Clin Chest Med* 8:441–53, 1987.

103. Foy HM et al. Long-term epidemiology of infections with *Mycoplasma pneumoniae*. *J Infect Dis* 139:681–87, 1979.

104. Murray HW et al. The protean manifestations of *Mycoplasma pneumoniae* infection in adults. *Am J Med* 58:229–42, 1975.

105. Koletsky RJ, Weinstein AJ. Fulminant *Mycoplasma pneumoniae* infection. *Am Rev Respir Dis* 122:491–96, 1980.

106. Grayston JT. *Chlamydia pneumoniae*, strain TWAR. *Chest* 95:664–69, 1989.

107. Thom DH et al. *Chlamydia pneumoniae* strain TWAR, *Mycoplasma pneumoniae*, and viral infections in acute respiratory disease in a university student health clinic population. *Am J Epidemiol* 132:248–56, 1990.

108. Hahn DL, Dodge RW, Golubjatnikov R. Association of *Chlamydia pneumoniae* (strain TWAR) infection with wheezing, asthmatic bronchitis, and adult-onset asthma. JAMA 266:225–30, 1991.

109. Wilfert CM, Gutman LT. *Chlamydia trachomatis* infections of infants and children. *Adv Pediatr* 33:49–76, 1986.

110. Bass JW, Stephenson SR. The return of pertussis. *Pediatr Infect Dis* 6:141–44, 1987.

111. Publication of Centers for Disease Control. U.S. Department of Health and Human Services/ Public Health Service. Pertussis surveillance– United States, 1986–88.

112. Mortimer EA. Pertussis and its prevention: a family affair. *J Infect Dis* 161:473–79, 1990.

113. Herwaldt LA. Pertussis in adults. *Arch Intern Med* 151:1510–12, 1991.

114. Langley JM et al. Poker players' pneumonia: an urban outbreak of Q fever following exposure to a parturient cat. *N Engl J Med* 319:354–56, 1988.

115. Marrie TJ. *Coxiella burnetii* (Q fever). In GL Mandell, RG Douglas, JE Bennett (eds.), *Principles and Practice of Infectious Diseases* (3rd ed.). New York: Churchill-Livingstone, 1990. P. 1474.

116. Helms CM et al. Comparative features of pneumococcal, mycoplasmal, and Legionnaires' disease pneumonias. *Ann Intern Med* 90:543–47, 1979.

117. Johnson JD, Raff MJ, Van Arsdall JA. Neurological manifestations of Legionnaires' disease. *Medicine* 63:303–10, 1984.

118. Edelstein PH. The laboratory diagnosis of Legionnaires' disease. *Sem Resp Inf* 2:235–41, 1987.

119. Ruf B et al. Prevalence and diagnosis of *Legionella* pneumonia: a 3-year prospective study with emphasis on application of urinary antigen detection. *J Infect Dis* 162:1341–48, 1990.

120. Brown LR et al. Roentgenologic features of pulmonary blastomycosis. *Mayo Clin Proc* 66:29–38, 1991.

121. Khan MA et al. Clinical and roentgenographic spectrum of pulmonary tuberculosis in the adult. *Am J Med* 62:31–38, 1977.

122. Berger HW, Granada MG. Lower lung field tuberculosis. *Chest* 65:522–26, 1974.

123. Dance DAB. Melioidosis: the tip of the iceberg? *Clin Micro Rev* 4:52–60, 1991.

124. Geppert EF. Recurrent pneumonia. *Chest* 98:739–45, 1990.

125. Kelley MA et al. Diagnosing pulmonary embolism: new facts and strategies. *Ann Intern Med* 114:300–06, 1991.

126. Cooper JA, White DA, Matthay RA. Drug-induced pulmonary disease. *Am Rev Resp Dis* 133:488–505, 1986.

127. Prakash UBS, Rosenow EC. Pulmonary complications from ophthalmic preparations. *Mayo Clin Proc* 65:521–29, 1990.

128. Hodgson MJ et al. An outbreak of recurrent acute and chronic hypersensitivity pneumonitis in office workers. *Am J Epidemiol* 125:631–38, 1987.

129. Sharma OP. Hypersensitivity pneumonitis. *Dis Mon* 37:409–71, 1991.

130. Allen JN et al. Acute eosinophilic pneumonia as a reversible cause of noninfectious respiratory failure. *N Engl J Med* 321:569–74, 1989.

131. Jederlinic PJ, Sicilian L, Gaensler EA. Chronic eosinophilic pneumonia: a report of 19 cases and a review of the literature. *Medicine* 67:154–62, 1988.

132. Wilson JP et al. Nocardial infections in renal transplant recipients. *Medicine (Baltimore)* 68:38–57, 1989.

133. Verghese A et al. Group B streptococcal pneumonia in the elderly. *Arch Intern Med* 142:1642–45, 1982.

134. Irwin RS, Woelk WK, Coudon WL. Primary meningococcal pneumonia. *Ann Intern Med* 82:493–98, 1975.

THE CARDIAC SYSTEM

24

Cardiovascular Infections and Mediastinitis

GEORGE L. STERNBACH
MICHAEL JAY BRESLER

Infections involving the cardiovascular system are relatively uncommon. However, they are important from the standpoint of potential morbidity and mortality. Moreover, the subtle and nonspecific modes of presentation of some of these infections render their recognition difficult.

Infective Endocarditis

Endocarditis is an infection of the endothelial surface of the heart, typically occurring on the surface of the cardiac valves. Nonvalvular endocarditis can occur on the endothelium of such structures as ventricular septal defects. The frequency of infective endocarditis ranges from 0.03%–0.3% of hospital admissions [1]. The term *infective endocarditis* has supplanted the previously used *bacterial endocarditis* in recognition of the fact that rickettsiae, chlamydiae, and fungi can serve as infecting organisms.

Nomenclature formulated in the preantibiotic era subclassified endocarditis into acute, subacute, and chronic forms, depending on the rate of progression of the disease to a fatal outcome. Acute endocarditis was a fulminant disease that presented with high fever and systemic toxicity and pro-

gressed along a natural course to a fatal outcome in days to weeks. Subacute and chronic forms followed slower and more indolent courses (6 weeks to 3 months for subacute, more than 3 months for chronic) and were likely to present with more nonspecific findings. The distinction between acute and subacute endocarditis is of less clinical significance than previously believed, however, because there is considerable overlap of manifestations between the acute and subacute forms. Moreover, advances in medical and surgical therapy have dramatically changed the clinical course of endocarditis. Consequently this classification is now utilized to a lesser extent. However, there is some utility to the distinction, in that a more fulminant presentation is likely to represent infection with specific organisms, such as *Staphylococcus aureus*, *Streptococcus pyogenes*, or *Streptococcus pneumoniae*.

Pathogenesis

The development of endocardial infection depends on a number of factors in addition to bacteremia. Loss of cellular or tissue integrity, turbulent blood flow, and possibly humoral immunologic impairment are required for the process to develop [2]. Experimental endocarditis has proved difficult to

571

initiate solely through the intravascular injection of bacteria in the absence of any alteration of cardiac valve structure [3].

Damage to the endothelial surface of a valve leads to exposure of underlying collagen. This process in turn causes the aggregation of platelets. The platelet thrombus may then stimulate the deposition of fibrin to form a sterile vegetation. Microbial colonization of the vegetative mass may follow, especially in the wake of bacteremia. Although such bacteremia often is caused by a recognizable infection or inoculation via IV drug use, relatively innocuous activities such as dental extraction or even tooth brushing can lead to microbial colonization. Incision and drainage of infected tissue and genitourinary or gastrointestinal procedures also can instigate the bacteremia that leads to endocarditis.

The resulting septic lesion leads to additional fibrin deposition and enlargement of the valvular vegetation. The classic vegetation is located on the atrial surface of the atrioventricular valves or the ventricular surface of the semilunar valves. Vegetations can be single or multiple and vary in size from a few millimeters to several centimeters. A lack of vascularization of the vegetation and the consequent minimal inflammatory response account for the resistance of infective endocarditis to normal host defenses, as well as the necessity for intensive and prolonged antibiotic treatment.

Almost any type of structural heart disease may predispose to the development of endocarditis, especially when the deficit results in turbulence of blood flow. The mitral and aortic valves are most commonly involved [4]. Infection involving the tricuspid valve is less frequent and often appears in the setting of IV drug abuse [5]. Pulmonic valve endocarditis is extremely uncommon.

Although rheumatic heart disease is still the most common underlying cause of endocarditis, the proportion of cases with other structural cardiac pathology has been increasing over the past several decades [6]. The mitral valve is involved in the majority of cases of rheumatic heart disease–based endocarditis.

Congenital and degenerative heart disease and idiopathic hypertrophic subaortic stenosis also predispose to the development of endocarditis. The congenital lesions that can be the focus of infective endocarditis are those that result in high-pressure

Table 24-1. Risk factors for development of endocarditis

Congenital heart disease
Acquired valvular disease
Mitral valve prolapse
Idiopathic hypertrophic subaortic stenosis
IV drug abuse
Recent urinary or gastrointestinal tract surgery or instrumentation
Presence of intravascular device (intravenous catheter, cardiac pacemaker)
Source of infection (e.g., dental caries, cutaneous abscess, decubitus ulcer)
Previous endocarditis
Prosthetic heart valve
Atrioventricular shunt

Sources: Reference 11 and Friedland G et al. Nosocomial endocarditis. *Infect Control* 5:284, 1984; Terpenning MS, Buggy BP, Kauffman CA. Hospital-acquired infective endocarditis. *Arch Intern Med* 148:1601, 1988. Used with permission.

gradients (e.g., patent ductus arteriosus, ventricular septal defect, tetralogy of Fallot, pulmonary stenosis, and coarctation of the aorta). Endocarditis is relatively rare in atrial septal defect [1]. Mitral valve prolapse also has been implicated as a risk factor for the development of endocarditis. At increased risk for endocarditis are those patients with mitral valve prolapse accompanied by a systolic murmur, particularly males and those above the age of 45 years [7].

Patients at risk for the development of endocarditis are listed in Table 24-1. The majority of patients with IV drug abuse who develop endocarditis have no history of prior valvular disease. It is postulated that endocarditis occurs in these patients because IV injection of particulate matter damages the valvular endothelium or because intravenous injection of drugs causes antigenic damage to cardiac valves.

Microbiology

Although any microorganism is capable of producing infective endocarditis, the majority of cases are caused by streptococci and staphylococci (Table 24-2) [8]. The most frequent streptococcal pathogens are the viridans streptococci, with enterococci and other streptococci being less common causes.

Table 24-2. Common causative organisms of infective endocarditis

Type of endocarditis and causes	Approximate incidence, %
Native-Valve	
Streptococci	60–80
Viridans species	30–40
Enterococci	10
Others	20–30
Staphylococci	10–30
S. aureus	9–27
S. epidermidis	1–3
Gram-negative bacilli	3–10
Haemophilus aphrophilius	
Haemophilus parainfluenzae	
Eikenella corrodens	
Others	
Fungi	2–4
Prosthetic-Valve	
Staphylococci	
Coagulase-negative staphylococci	20–35
S. aureus	10–20
Gram-negative bacilli	10–20
Streptococci	10–20
Fungi	5–15
IV Drug Use–Related	
S. aureus	40–60
Pseudomonas aeruginosa	5–10
Candida	5–15
S. viridans	5–10
Enterococci	5–10

Sources: References 2, 13, and Kaye D. Infecting microorganisms. In D Kaye (ed.), *Infective Endocarditis.* Baltimore: University Park, 1976. Pp. 43–54. Used with permission.

S. aureus is the most frequent variety responsible for staphylococcal-induced illness, with *staphylococcus epidermidis* occurring in only a small proportion of cases of endocarditis affecting native valves [2]. A smaller number of cases are produced by gram-negative bacilli, though the proportion of these has increased over the past several decades [8].

Fungi account for less than 5% of endocarditis [1]. Fungal endocarditis is most frequently caused by *Candida* and *Aspergillus* species. Infection with these agents is particularly likely to occur in patients with intravascular catheters who receive corticosteroids, antibiotics, or cytotoxic agents.

The organisms involved in prosthetic-valve endocarditis are different from those infecting native

valves. *S. epidermidis* is the most common infecting pathogen, occurring with particular frequency during the first several months following valve replacement [2].

Endocarditis associated with illicit IV drug use also has a distinctive microbial spectrum. The most common organism isolated from IV drug users with endocarditis is *S. aureus* [9]. Gram-negative bacilli and fungi also account for a substantial proportion of infecting organisms. The relative frequency of infection with various gram-negative pathogens varies from one geographic region to another [2].

Clinical Findings

GENERAL FINDINGS

Any organ system can be affected by endocarditis. Manifestations can, furthermore, be multisystemic. The clinical presentation particularly may be atypical in the elderly, in whom many of the classic findings tend to be absent [10]. Table 24-3 lists common signs of infective endocarditis. The frequency with which these signs are encountered varies. In one long-term study a heart murmur was present in 89% of patients, and fever of greater than 38°C was present in 77%. Clinically recognized embolic episodes to the brain, lung, coronary arteries, extremities, spleen, eyes, and intestines were present in 50%. Half of the patients displayed skin manifestations of infective endocarditis, and splenomegaly was present in 28%. Septic complications (such as pneumonia and meningitis) occurred in 19% of cases [11]. Clinical manifestations may be the result of the infectious process itself, embolic phenomena, immunologic consequences of infection, or the cardiovascular sequelae of valvular damage. Fever, the cardinal sign of infection, is usually present but is typically low grade, rarely exceeding 39.4°C. It may, however, be absent in the elderly, in persons with renal insufficiency, and in very debilitated patients. Because fever may be only intermittently present, it may be absent during the time the patient is in the emergency department.

Constitutional symptoms of malaise, anorexia, weight loss, fatigue, weakness, and nausea frequently are present but are nonspecific. Musculoskeletal manifestations (arthralgia, myalgia, back pain) are common but likewise lack specificity.

Table 24-3. Common symptoms and signs of infective endocarditis

Symptom	Present in percentage of cases	Physical finding	Present in percentage of cases
Fever	80	Fever	90
Chills	40	Heart murmur	85
Weakness	40	Changing murmur	5–10
Dyspnea	40	New murmur	3–5
Sweats	25	Embolic phenomenon	>50
Anorexia	25	Skin manifestations	18–50
Weight loss	25	Osler's nodes	10–23
Malaise	25	Splinter hemorrhages	15
Cough	25	Petechiae	20–40
Skin lesions	20	Janeway's lesion	<10
Stroke	20	Splenomegaly	20–57
Nausea/vomiting	20	Septic complications	20
Headache	15	(pneumonia, meningitis, etc.)	
Myalgia/arthralgia	15	Mycotic aneurysms	20
Edema	15	Clubbing	12–52
Chest pain	15	Retinal lesion	2–10
Abdominal pain	10–15	Signs of renal failure	10–15
Delirium/coma	10		
Hemoptysis	10		
Back pain	10		

Source: Reprinted with permission from Scheld WM, Bande MA, Endocarditis and intravascular infections, in Mandell GL, Douglas RG, Bennett JE (ed.). Principles and Practice of Infectious Disease 3rd ed. New York: Churchill Livingstone, 1990. P. 677.

Confusion also arises in patients whose nonspecific symptoms have been treated with antibiotics.

Cardiovascular Findings. A heart murmur is found in the majority of cases, but the presence of a new or changing murmur, though classic, is rare. Murmurs may be particularly difficult to hear or may be absent with right-sided valvular involvement. Furthermore, the character and the intensity of a murmur may be influenced by fever or anemia even in the absence of endocarditis.

Congestive heart failure may be the end result of longstanding illness or the consequence of acute hemodynamically significant valvular insufficiency. It is a common cause of death in endocarditis.

The Abdomen and Kidneys. Splenomegaly in endocarditis represents an immunologic consequence of infection. It may be present in as many as half of patients, being most commonly seen in cases of endocarditis of long duration [2]. It is a far more frequent finding in left- than right-sided endocarditis. Immune complex deposition also is a cause of renal damage, probably a more frequent one in endocarditis than is embolization. This may lead to abnormalities of the urinalysis and an increase in serum creatinine.

The Skin. A number of classic cutaneous findings of endocarditis have been thought to be the consequence of emboli (though some of these may, in fact, have an immunologic pathogenesis). Cutaneous findings include subungual splinter hemorrhages, conjunctival petechiae, Osler's nodes (small, tender nodular lesions on the fingers and toes) (see Color Plate 7), Janeway's lesions (macular, erythematous nontender lesions of the extremities) (see Color Plate 8), and Gannet lesions (painless, macular, sometimes hemorrhagic lesions usually involving the palms and the soles).

Petechiae are found in 20%–40% of patients

with endocarditis [6], being seen most often in patients with prolonged illness. The most common sites of appearance are the palate, the buccal mucosa, the conjunctiva, and the extremities. Splinter hemorrhages appear as dark linear streaks beneath the fingernails or toenails. Both splinter hemorrhages and petechiae must be differentiated from traumatic lesions. It may be helpful to count splinter hemorrhages initially, since an increase in the number of hemorrhages while the patient is at bed rest is suspicious for bacterial endocarditis. Clubbing of the nails occasionally is seen, particularly in longstanding cases.

The Eyes. The best-known ocular findings of endocarditis are Roth's spots, which arise from embolization. These spots are bright-red, oval retinal lesions with pale centers. They are not pathognomonic for endocarditis, however, occasionally being seen in severe anemia or collagen-vascular disease. If the fundus cannot be adequately visualized, the pupils can be dilated with a short-acting mydriatic to aid examination.

The CNS. Approximately a third of cases of endocarditis are complicated by CNS involvement [12]. Cerebral embolism is the most common form of neurologic compromise in endocarditis. A variety of clinical deficits may be produced, including hemiplegia, sensory loss, visual field cut, aphasia, ataxia, and alteration of mental status. Major cerebral emboli are more common in older patients with endocarditis [10]. However, endocarditis should particularly be considered if neurologic impairment develops abruptly in a young individual. Neurologic deficit can also be produced by enlargement or rupture of a cerebral mycotic aneurysm. This entity is discussed later in the chapter.

SPECIFIC TYPES OF INFECTIVE ENDOCARDITIS
Native-Valve Endocarditis. Most classic descriptions of endocarditis refer to subacute native-valve involvement. The left-sided cardiac valves typically are involved. Clinical findings include audible murmurs of mitral or (less frequently) aortic insufficiency. Fever and splenomegaly may be present, and congestive heart failure may be produced. Petechiae and splinter hemorrhages are frequent cutaneous manifestations, whereas Osler's nodes and Roth's spots are less common.

Endocarditis Related to IV Drug Use. Endocarditis is an important infection in drug users (see Chap. 18), but the incidence is difficult to calculate in this population. It has been estimated to occur in 1 to 20 IV drug abusers per 10,000 per year [13]. Endocarditis is found in 10%–20% of IV drug abusers who present with fever and lack a cutaneous source of infection [14]. Although suspicion of endocarditis is a common reason for hospital admission in drug abusers, clinical judgment has been shown not to be sensitive in predicting which patients who present with fever ultimately turn out to have infective endocarditis [15].

The tricuspid valve is affected predominantly. Aortic-valve involvement occurs in 20%–30% of cases, mitral-valve involvement in 15%–20%, and multiple-valve involvement in 10%–20% [13]. Intravenous drug abusers may be at risk for development of recurrent infection within 12 months of an initial episode of infectious endocarditis. S. aureus is the most common infecting organism.

The presentation is typically one of an acute febrile illness, with the duration of symptoms usually being a week or less. Almost all patients give a history of fever, and an elevated temperature is documented in 95% of patients upon admission [16]. Cutaneous manifestations are encountered in a minority of patients [17]. Cardiac murmurs frequently are absent. Presenting symptoms may be those of pneumonia with cough, chest pain, dyspnea, and hemoptysis being prominent complaints. Abnormalities on the chest roentgenogram, including pulmonary infiltrates, cavitary nodules, and pleural effusion are common [9].

Prosthetic-Valve Endocarditis. Prosthetic-valve endocarditis is an infrequent complication of cardiac valvular replacement, occurring with an incidence of 1%–4% [18]. However, it constitutes 12%–33% of reported endocarditis [1]. Both mechanical and porcine valves are susceptible to infection. Prosthetic-valve endocarditis is customarily divided into that with early (less than 60 days after surgery) and late onset. Infection occurring within 60 days of surgery often reflects surgical contamination.

Patients are usually febrile, and new or changing murmurs are present in about one-half of cases [1]. Cutaneous manifestations, splenomegaly, and

Roth's spots usually are absent. *S. epidermidis* is a major cause of both early and late prosthetic-valve endocarditis.

Diagnosis

PITFALLS

The diagnosis of endocarditis is often a difficult one to establish on clinical grounds. This difficulty is exemplified in one series from a university hospital in which in 32% of cases of endocarditis the diagnosis was not even considered in the differential at the time of hospital admission [4]. Repeated examination over time may be required for microvascular signs (e.g., splinter hemorrhages, Roth's spots, Osler's nodes) and other findings of endocarditis to evolve.

Errors in diagnosis are significantly more common in elderly patients with endocarditis [10]. Such patients tend to present more frequently with nonspecific complaints, such as weakness, anorexia, and fatigue. New and changing murmurs are less common findings in elderly patients with endocarditis. Confusion is a frequent presenting sign in the elderly, and this also serves to limit the historical information that can be obtained from these patients [10].

LABORATORY EVALUATION

Laboratory evaluation is of little specificity. Anemia is frequently present, usually exhibiting normocytic normochromic indices. A mean hematocrit of 35% was found in one series, with the lowest hematocrits present in gram-negative and culture-negative cases [11]. The anemia tends to worsen with the duration of the illness. Leukocytosis may be present, especially with an acute fulminant presentation. The erythrocyte sedimentation rate nearly always is elevated, with a mean of 57 reported in one large series [11]. Abnormalities are often evident on urinalysis. Proteinuria, pyuria, microscopic or gross hematuria, or bacteriuria may be present. Red or white blood cell casts may be observed in the urinary sediment. Proteinuria is seen in 50%–65% of cases, microscopic hematuria in 30%–50% [19].

Because bacteremia tends to be continuous in endocarditis, positive blood cultures are the rule. Furthermore, organisms frequently are isolated from early blood cultures. In patients with infective endocarditis who have not received antibiotics, the causative organism can be isolated from one of the first two blood culture sets in 95% of cases [8].

Blood cultures should be performed on any patient suspected of having infective endocarditis. This includes the febrile patient at risk for the development of endocarditis (see Table 24-1). Of particular importance is obtaining cultures in patients with prosthetic cardiac valves or other intravenous devices or a history of valvular disorder or IV drug abuse and patients who display findings of peripheral embolization, unexplained neurologic changes, or ongoing constitutional symptoms. In an acute presentation a series of three cultures should be drawn over 15–45 minutes [5]. With a more subacute onset, three cultures drawn over 24 hours are sufficient. In the patient with a subacute course, initial blood cultures can be obtained in the emergency department, and subsequent cultures drawn and treatment initiated by the inpatient service. Blood cultures are negative in a small number of cases, often due to prior administration of antibiotics. In some cases negative cultures are the result of infection with slow-growing, nutritionally fastidious, or nonbacterial organisms (fungi, rickettsia, or chlamydia).

RADIOLOGIC EVALUATION

The chest radiograph may reveal signs of congestive heart failure, pleural effusion, or evidence of septic embolization (especially present in right-sided drug abuse–related staphylococcal endocarditis as single or multiple peripheral circular, wedge-shaped, or irregular infiltrates). The electrocardiogram may show nonspecific changes or be normal. Electrocardiographic evidence of ischemia should raise consideration of coronary artery embolization.

Echocardiography often is employed in evaluating the patient with endocarditis. The sensitivity of two-dimensional echocardiography in detecting vegetations is approximately 80% [20]. A negative echocardiogram, however, does not rule out the presence of infectious endocarditis, and a positive one in a patient with a history of endocarditis does not necessarily indicate acute infection. Although the procedure can be performed in the emergency department, it more commonly is done as part of the inpatient assessment. It can, however, be considered part of the emergency evaluation of the patient with an acute disease course.

DIFFERENTIAL DIAGNOSIS

The differential diagnosis is broad, including all entities causing fever of unknown origin. Difficulties in diagnosis may be related to the clinical variability of endocarditis. Infectious involvement of various organ systems may present in a fashion similar to endocarditis. Consequently the differential diagnosis includes upper respiratory infection, viral syndrome, pneumonia, urinary tract infection, gastroenteritis, hepatitis, and meningitis. Collagen vascular diseases, such as systemic lupus erythematosus, have a number of features in common with endocarditis, including fever, arthralgia, and renal abnormalities. When the presentation is with a neurologic deficit, endocarditis must be distinguished from entities such as cerebrovascular accident, subarachnoid hemorrhage, meningoencephalitis, and cerebral tumor. A presentation with congestive heart failure requires differentiation from failure produced by other cardiac and noncardiac causes.

Treatment

Parenteral antibiotic therapy is required for the treatment of endocarditis. The course of this therapy is necessarily prolonged, on the order of 4–6 weeks in duration so valvular vegetations can be sterilized and relapse prevented. Use of bactericidal rather than bacteriostatic agents is required, because the relatively avascular nature of valves and hence the vegetation may protect the infecting organisms from host defenses.

When the presentation of endocardial infection is indolent or subacute, institution of antibiotics can await identification of the infecting organism through blood culture. In the patient who is acutely ill or hemodynamically unstable, however, empiric antibiotic therapy should be instituted immediately after the collection of the initial three blood cultures.

Table 24-4 contains recommended initial antibiotic regimens for infective endocarditis [21]. Treatment subsequently can be adjusted as culture and sensitivity results become available. Patients with a

Table 24-4. Recommended empiric antibiotic therapy for endocarditis

Native-Valve Endocarditis
Aqueous crystalline penicillin G 20 million U/d (children: 200,000–300,000 U/kg) in 6 divided doses IV
plus
Nafcillin 2 q4h (children: 150–200 mg/kg/d, maximum 12 g) IV if staphylococcal infection is suspected
plus
Gentamicin 1.5–2 mg/kg (children 2 mg/kg, maximum 80 mg) q8h IV *or* streptomycin 7.5 mg/kg (children 15 mg/kg, maximum 500 mg) q12h IM
For patients with penicillin allergy:
Cephalothin 2 g (children 100–150 mg/kg/d, maximum 12 g/d) q4h IV *or* Cefazolin 1–2 g (children: 80–100 mg/kg/d, maximum 3 g/d) q8h IV or IM *or* vancomycin 30 mg/kg/d (children: 40 mg/kg/d, maximum 2 g/d) in 2 or 4 divided doses IV

Prosthetic-Valve Endocarditis
Vancomycin 30 mg/kg/d (children: 40 mg/kg/d, maximum 2g/d) in 2 or 4 divided doses IV
plus
Gentamicin 1.5–2 mg/kg (children: 2 mg/kg, maximum 80 mg) q8h IV
plus
Rifampin 300 mg (children 20 mg/kg, maximum 600 mg/d) q12h PO

IV Drug Use–Related
Nafcillin 2g q4h (children: 150–200 mg/kg/d, maximum 12 g/d) IV
plus
Gentamicin 1.5–2 mg/kg (children: 2mg/kg, maximum 80 mg) q8h IV
For patients with penicillin allergy:
Replace nafcillin with cephalothin, cefazolin, or vancomycin

Source: Reference 21. Reprinted with permission.

history of IV drug abuse should be considered to have infection with *S. aureus*. Such patients should have treatment initiated with nafcillin and gentamicin. Those with suspected endocarditis in the presence of a prosthetic valve or other prosthetic material should be treated with a combination of vancomycin, gentamicin, and rifampin. This regimen is utilized to take advantage of the synergy of these agents in the treatment of coagulase-negative staphylococcus.

Patients with acute native-valve endocarditis should be treated initially with a combination of penicillin G, nafcillin, and either gentamicin or streptomycin. Evaluation of the patient should identify historical factors or physical findings that implicate a particular group of organisms. Likely portals of entry of microorganisms into the circulation (e.g., oral mucosa, GI or genitourinary tract) should be sought. For example, an elderly man, particularly one with a recent history of urinary tract instrumentation or infection, has a higher likelihood of infection with enterococcus. Such a patient initially should be treated with a combination of penicillin or ampicillin and gentamicin [2]. In the penicillin-allergic patient, vancomycin should be substituted.

The patient should be observed closely for signs of hemodynamic deterioration. The majority of patients with infective endocarditis can be managed with antibiotics and supportive care. Some patients, however, will require consultation with a cardiac surgeon for consideration of valvular replacement. These patients include those with severe heart failure that does not respond to therapy, early prosthetic-valve endocarditis, and findings suggestive of myocardial abscess (e.g., development of heart block in a patient with aortic-valve endocarditis) or one or more major embolic events [2].

Antibiotic Prophylaxis

Patients who have underlying abnormalities that make them susceptible to endocarditis (Table 24-5) should be given antibiotic prophylaxis prior to undergoing procedures that may produce bacteremia (such as dental treatment and surgical procedures or instrumentation involving mucosal surfaces or contaminated tissue) [22]. Prophylaxis also should be considered in patients with indwelling transvenous cardiac pacemakers, arteriovenous shunts for hemodialysis, and ventriculoatrial hydrocephalus shunts. Table 24-6 lists procedures for which endocarditis prophylaxis is indicated. Prophylaxis is not recommended for patients on the basis of having undergone coronary artery bypass grafting.

Dental procedures prior to which prophylaxis should be administered include routine cleaning and tooth extraction. Although prophylaxis is recommended prior to rigid bronchoscopy, endo-

Table 24-5. Conditions for which endocarditis antibiotic prophylaxis is indicated

Prosthetic heart valves
Rheumatic and other acquired valvular dysfunction
Most congenital cardiac malformations
Idiopathic hypertrophic subaortic stenosis
Mitral valve insufficiency
History of bacterial endocarditis

Table 24-6. Procedures for which antibiotic prophylaxis is indicated

All dental procedures likely to induce gingival bleeding
Surgical procedures involving the respiratory mucosa
Bronchoscopy
Incision and drainage of infected tissue
Various genitourinary and gastrointestinal procedures and instrumentation

tracheal intubation is not an indication for prophylaxis. Bacteremia often accompanies surgery and instrumentation of the genitourinary and GI tracts. Consequently prophylaxis is recommended prior to a variety of procedures involving these systems, including urethral catheterization. Prophylaxis is not required prior to performance of a barium enema or a proctosigmoidoscopy (unless accompanied by biopsy). Likewise, unless concurrent infection is suspected, dilatation and curettage and removal of an intrauterine contraceptive device do not require prophylaxis. Table 24-7 lists the prophylactic antibiotic regimens recommended by the American Heart Association [23]. These recommendations are based on a number of studies and experimental models, but it should be emphasized that no definitive controlled clinical trials of antibiotic regimens for the prevention of endocarditis have been conducted.

Although weight-based dosages are recommended for children, such dosages should not exceed the maximum adult dose. It is important that antibiotics be administered within the time frame recommended, which involves one-half to one hour rather than days prior to the procedure. Note that different regimens are suggested for dental and respiratory tract procedures compared to GI and genitourinary procedures. Endocarditis following genitourinary and GI surgery or instrumentation

Table 24-7. Prophylactic antibiotic regimens against infective endocarditis

Dental and Respiratory Tract Procedures
Standard regimen:
 Amoxicillin 3.0 g (children: 50 mg/kg) orally 1 hour before procedure, then 1.5 g 6 hours after initial dose
For patients unable to take oral medications:
Ampicillin 2 g (children: 50 mg/kg) IV or IM 30 minutes before procedure, then 1.0 g 6 hours after initial dose
For patients allergic to penicillin, ampicillin, or amoxicillin:
 Erythromycin ethylsuccinate 800 mg or erythromycin stearate 1 g (children: 20 mg/kg) PO 2 hours before the procedure, then half the dose 6 hours later
or
Clindamycin 300 mg (children: 10 mg/kg) IV 30 minutes or PO 1 hour before procedure and 150 mg PO or IV 6 hours after initial dose
For high-risk patients (those with prosthetic heart valves, history of endocarditis, or surgically constructed systemic-pulmonary shunts)
 Ampicillin 2 g IM or IV and gentamicin 1.5 mg/kg IM or IV (children: 2 mg/kg) 30 minutes prior to procedure, followed by amoxicillin 1.5 g PO 6 hours later
For high-risk patients allergic to penicillin, ampicillin, or amoxicillin:
 Vancomycin 1 g (children 20 mg/kg) IV over 1 hour starting 1 hour prior to procedure

Gastrointestinal and Genitourinary Procedures
Standard regimen:
Ampicillin 2 g IM or IV and gentamicin 1.5 mg/kg IM or IV 30 minutes prior to procedure, followed by amoxicillin 1.5 g PO 6 hours after initial dose
For patients allergic to penicillin, ampicillin, or amoxicillin:
Vancomycin 1 g IV over 1 hour and gentamicin 1.5 mg/kg IM or IV 1 hour before procedure; repeat dose in 8 hours

Minor Procedures (e.g., Urinary Catheterization):
Amoxicillin 3 g (children 50 mg/kg) PO 1 hour before procedure; 1.5 g 6 hours later

Source: Dajani AS et al. Prevention of bacterial endocarditis. Recommendations by the American Heart Association. JAMA 264:2919, 1990. Reprinted with permission.

most often is caused by enterococci [23]. Consequently prophylaxis in this setting is aimed primarily against these organisms. Alpha-hemolytic (viridans) streptococci are the most common cause of endocarditis following dental procedures.

Pericarditis

Pericarditis, an inflammation of the fibrous cardiac envelope, can result from a variety of etiologies, which may be either infectious or noninfectious. It is a common but often subclinical entity. Its true incidence is uncertain because the disease frequently is self-limited and consequently goes undiagnosed and because pericardial inflammation may constitute an unrecognized aspect of a systemic infection [24].

Etiology

Although the relative incidence of specific types of pericarditis varies from institution to institution, the most common type overall is probably idiopathic pericarditis [25]. This form likely is due to viral infection in most instances. A number of viruses are known to be highly cardiotropic, with the coxsackie B group being especially likely to cause pericarditis and myocarditis [26]. Other viruses known to produce pericarditis are listed in Table 24-8 [27].

Bacterial pericarditis has been a recognized entity for many centuries, but its incidence has declined in the antibiotic era [22]. *S. aureus*, once by far the foremost causative pyogenic organism, remains the single most frequent bacterial etiologic microbe but no longer causes the overwhelming preponderance of cases [28]. The proportion of cases caused by *S. pneumoniae* also has diminished. There has, furthermore, been a progressive expansion of the bacterial spectrum over the past three decades (Table 24-9). Gram-negative aerobic bacilli have accounted for an increasingly greater proportion of purulent pericarditis during this period [24, 25].

The pericardium is rarely the site of primary

Table 24-8. Common viral causes of pericarditis

Coxsackie virus B
Echovirus 8
Adenovirus
Mumps
Influenza A and B
Epstein-Barr virus
Varicella-zoster virus

Table 24-9. Common bacterial causes of pericarditis

Staphylococcus aureus
Streptococcus pneumoniae
Haemophilus influenzae
Neisseria meningitidis
Klebsiella pneumoniae
Mycobacteria tuberculosis

bacterial infection, purulent pericarditis almost always occurring as a complication of another illness. Patients particularly predisposed to the development of purulent pericarditis are those who (1) are debilitated; (2) have undergone extensive thoracic or cardiac surgery; (3) have uncontrolled myocardial or endocardial infection; or (4) have preexisting nonpyogenic pericarditis [28].

Spread of infection to the pericardium from a primary site occurs via one of the following mechanisms: (1) direct extension from a pulmonary focus; (2) hematogenous spread; (3) septic embolization due to endocarditis or rupture of a myocardial abscess (the risk of development of purulent pericarditis is especially high in patients with S. aureus endocarditis); (4) perforation of the chest wall (either surgical or traumatic); or (5) extension of a subdiaphragmatic suppurative focus [29]. Transdiaphragmatic spread is the least common of these mechanisms.

Tuberculosis was once the most common cause of pericarditis. It is now rare, occurring in only 1%–2% of patients with pulmonary tuberculosis [30]. Although fungal and parasitic infections of the pericardium may occur, these are uncommon in the United States [31].

Clinical Findings

UNCOMPLICATED PERICARDITIS

In most instances, acute pericarditis results in an inflammatory process that produces no significant increase in the volume of pericardial fluid [32]. The presentation of pericarditis varies depending on the etiology. The clinical manifestations of viral pericarditis may follow an upper respiratory infection. Fever, dyspnea, and chest pain are typical complaints. Purulent pericarditis usually presents as a fulminant febrile illness. By contrast tuberculous pericarditis has a more insidious onset, presenting with the gradual development of fever, malaise, anorexia, and weakness.

Pain is the most important feature of pericarditis. It is a particularly prominent feature of viral pericarditis, where its absence is unusual. The pain is characteristically sharp and pleuritic, becoming dramatically worse with cough or inspiration. The pleuritic nature of the pain may be the result of inflammation of pleura adjacent to the involved pericardium. Pain may be of sudden onset and is usually retrosternal or precordial. There may be a wide area of radiation, with pain felt in the neck, back, left shoulder, and occasionally the left arm or epigastrium. Radiation often extends to one or both trapezius ridges, a feature particularly characteristic of pericarditis [33]. Pain is usually aggravated by recumbency and eased by sitting upright and leaning forward. Occasionally it is felt at the cardiac apex synchronous with each heart beat.

Dyspnea is frequently present, though its pathogenesis is incompletely understood. In some instances the patient may experience difficulty breathing because of pain produced by deep inspiration. Dyspnea, however, is not invariably related to chest pain. Other signs and symptoms that occur with variable frequency include cough, fever, hiccups, nausea, vomiting, dizziness, malaise, anorexia, and palpitations. Odynophagia (pain on swallowing) occurs occasionally. When pericarditis is due to coxsackievirus infection, there also may be considerable skeletal muscle pain.

The pericardial friction rub is the physical finding that is pathognomonic of pericarditis. It is not always present, however. Furthermore, it can vary in intensity, be audible intermittently, or change in quality from one examination to the next. It is a scratching, grating, high-pitched sound. It is classically described as having three components that correspond to cardiac motion during atrial systole, ventricular systole, and early diastole. The ventricular systolic component is the one most consistently heard. The rub is heard more easily with the stethoscope diaphragm than with the bell and with the patient leaning forward and maintaining full expiration.

PERICARDIAL EFFUSION

Pericardial effusion can be clinically silent or produce chest pain by distending the pericardium. A variety of other symptoms (cough, dysphagia, hiccups, and hoarseness) may be produced by compression of mediastinal structures adjacent to the pericardium. The development of increased intrapericardial pressure depends largely on the absolute volume of an effusion, as well as the rate of fluid accumulation. Slowly developing effusions are accommodated much more readily than is rapid fluid accumulation.

Infectious pericarditis is not a common cause of cardiac tamponade because the volume of pericardial fluid generally is small and the rate of accumulation relatively slow. Although cardiac tamponade can result from pericarditis of any cause, this is most often a complication of malignant disease [34]. Idiopathic pericarditis does, however, lead to cardiac tamponade in a small number of cases.

Diagnosis

The electrocardiogram is an important diagnostic tool in pericarditis. Stages of electrocardiographic changes through the course of the illness are listed in Table 24-10 and are illustrated in Fig. 24-1. The changes of stage I are virtually diagnostic. These changes are generally present at the time of onset of

Table 24-10. Electrocardiographic changes in pericarditis

Stage I: ST segment elevation (concave upward)

Stage II: Return of ST segments to baseline
  T wave flattening
  PR segment depression

Stage III: T wave inversion
Stage IV: ECG normalization

pain and may last for several days. They consist of ST segment elevations that are concave upward and are usually present in all leads except aVR and V_1. The electrocardiogram may be atypical when there are preexisting ECG changes due to other illness.

The echocardiogram is the primary diagnostic modality in detecting pericardial effusion. It is extremely sensitive, being capable of identifying effusions as small as 15 ml [35]. The cardiac silhouette as seen on the chest radiograph also may be altered by an effusion. However, because this does not occur until at least 250 ml of fluid has accumulated, a normal radiograph of the chest does not exclude the presence of a clinically significant pericardial effusion.

Differential diagnosis of infectious pericarditis

Fig. 24-1. EKG suggestive of pericarditis. Note the depressed PR segment and diffuse ST elevation, which is changed from a prior EKG.

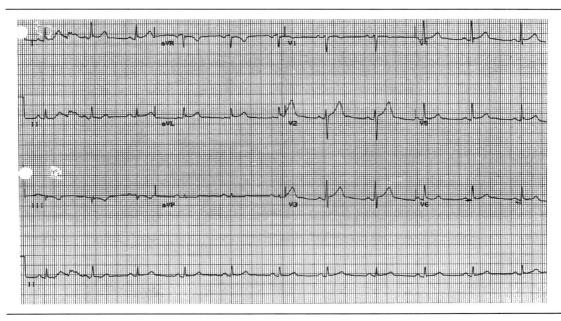

includes pericarditis due to systemic illness, such as collagen vascular disease (rheumatoid arthritis, systemic lupus erythematosus, scleroderma), rheumatic fever, sarcoidosis, and renal failure. The distinction between pericarditis and acute myocardial infarction is occasionally challenging. The pattern of pain may be similar, as may be the electrocardiographic changes. Dressler's syndrome, a syndrome of fever and pleural and pericardial inflammation classically appearing weeks to months after myocardial infarction, may also be similar in presentation to infectious pericarditis. When pleuritic pain is present, pericarditis must be distinguished from pneumonia, pulmonary embolism, and pleurisy.

Treatment

The organism responsible for a particular case of infectious pericarditis seldom will be known at the time of the patient's presentation to the emergency department. The patient with suspected purulent pericarditis should be hospitalized. Blood cultures should be obtained, as should cultures of any areas of suspected primary infection. Empiric antibiotic therapy can be initiated following the obtaining of such cultures, with coverage for staphylococci and gram-negative organisms being of primary importance. The patient with purulent pericarditis may also require pericardial drainage as part of definitive therapy, this being accomplished either via pericardiectomy or pericardiocentesis [36].

Treatment of the patient with suspected viral pericarditis is aimed primarily at relieving pain. The patient can be managed as an outpatient if stable but should be hospitalized if severely symptomatic, if a significant pericardial effusion is suspected, or if the diagnosis is in doubt. Nonsteroidal anti-inflammatory agents are effective for alleviating pain and reducing fever. Ibuprofen should be administered at a dose of 400–800 mg q8h PO [32]. Aspirin 650–900 mg q6h PO can be used if there is an inadequate response to ibuprofen. Alternatively indomethacin 25–50 mg q6h PO can be administered.

Myocarditis

Myocarditis, the inflammation of the myocardium, can be of infectious etiology. It also, however, can be the consequence of a variety of noninfectious conditions, such as systemic illness or toxic or hypersensitive drug effects. Myocarditis is characterized histologically by the presence of lymphocytic infiltrates and myocardial cell necrosis [37]. These changes may be the result of injury by infectious organisms or their toxins or be caused by an autoimmune response triggered by infection.

Etiology

Every major type of infectious agent—bacteria, viruses, protozoa, rickettsia, helminths, and fungi—has been implicated as a causative agent in myocarditis [38]. In the United States the majority of cases are related to viral infection. Coxsackie B and echovirus infections in particular are known to produce myocarditis as a sequel to systemic infection [39]. The human immunodeficiency virus also has been associated with myocarditis [40]. Other viruses known to cause myocarditis include cytomegalovirus, influenza A and B viruses, and Epstein-Barr virus.

In this country the most common bacterial causative agents are staphylococcus, streptococcus, pneumococcus, meningococcus, gonococcus, clostridia, and brucella [41]. Bacteria-induced myocarditis is less common. Although myocarditis is a recognized complication of infection with *Corynebacterium diphtheriae*, diphtheria is rare in the United States. Myocardial inflammation is produced by bacterially released toxins in the cases of diphtheria, clostridial infection, and some streptococci. In the remainder myocarditis is produced by direct bacterial invasion.

Worldwide the causes of myocarditis are more diverse. In South America, for example, the greatest proportion of myocarditis results from infection with *Trypanosoma cruzi* (Chagas' disease; see Chap. 19). Myocardial infestation with *Toxoplasma gondii* and *Trichinella spiralis* also can produce myocarditis.

Clinical Findings

The essential physiologic derangement of myocarditis is depressed myocardial contractility. Consequently clinical manifestations reflect congestive heart failure and inadequate perfusion. Symptoms are often those of pulmonary congestion: dyspnea, orthopnea, decreased exercise tolerance, and nocturnal cough. In patients (especially children) with the acute onset of myocarditis, the presenting findings may reflect acute hepatic congestion. Abdominal distention, right upper quadrant pain, and nausea may predominate.

A history of a recent systemic viral illness, especially one producing prominent myalgia or symptoms of pericarditis, should raise the suspicion of infection with a cardiotropic virus. However, historical identification of such a viral prodrome is the exception rather than the rule [38]. Consequently the presentation of myocarditis usually is removed temporally from the episode of inciting infection.

Physical findings vary from extremely subtle and nonspecific ones to those that reflect overtly depressed cardiac output. Pallor or cyanosis may be present, as may tachycardia (out of proportion to fever, when fever is present). Jugular venous distention may be found, and an audible S_3 gallop is extremely common. Hypotension may reflect significantly depressed left ventricular systolic function. Pulsus alternans is common in such patients, indicating beat-to-beat changes in ventricular volume [42].

Diagnosis

Diagnosis on clinical grounds may be difficult, especially given the subtle presentation that is characteristic of subacute cases. The diagnosis most generally is considered when a young patient presents with unexplained congestive heart failure or cardiac dysrhythmias. The electrocardiogram is typically nonspecific and may reveal low-voltage or ST-T wave abnormalities. Occasionally patterns resembling Q-wave myocardial infarction can be seen and are believed to reflect myonecrosis. [38]

The chest radiograph may display cardiomegaly and various degrees of pulmonary venous congestion. Findings of interstitial edema, particularly peribronchial cuffing and Kerley B lines, are frequently present prior to alveolar rales being audible [43]

Although echocardiography may be useful in identifying the physiologic and morphologic aspects of myocarditis, its employment is rarely required in the emergency department. Differential diagnosis includes congestive heart failure of other cause. A clinical presentation with predominantly respiratory symptoms and findings may be erroneously diagnosed as being due to bronchial infection or asthma. A picture produced by acute hepatic congestion may lead to the mistaken diagnosis of hepatitis or biliary disease.

Treatment

The patient with the initial presentation of myocarditis should be hospitalized for further diagnostic evaluation and treatment. Management of congestive heart failure can be initiated if the patient is significantly symptomatic. Diuretics are the traditional therapeutic modalities for congestive heart failure due to cardiomyopathy, with vasodilators representing the next level of pharmacologic management. However, such therapy must be balanced against the effects on cardiac output. In unstable patients optimum medication regimens may be derived only through invasive cardiac hemodynamic monitoring.

Vascular Infection

Septic Thrombophlebitis

The two major predisposing factors to the development of septic thrombophlebitis are the presence in situ of polyethylene IV catheters and IV drug abuse. The introduction of a bacterial inoculum at the time of IV injection or cannulation is an obvious instigating event. In addition other factors can predispose to thrombosis and perivenous inflammation, including intimal injury produced by the needle or catheter and the injection of noxious or hyperosmolar solutions. Thrombophlebitis related to IV catheters develops more commonly when the catheter is left in place for 48 hours or longer. Patients with burn injuries appear particularly susceptible to infection at catheter sites. A high mortality accompanies this complication in burn patients [44].

Pain is the typical presenting complaint, with fever, swelling, and purulent drainage also being frequently encountered. Physical examination usually reveals local erythema and edema. The presence of abscess, a palpable venous cord, and lymphadenopathy are less common findings [45]. When the involved vessels are deep (e.g., the femoral, jugular, or subclavian vessels), local physical findings may be minimal, the presentation being that of systemic infection.

Complications of septic thrombophlebitis include septic embolization, proximal thrombosis, and bacteremia. Septic embolization is the most frequent complication, the lung being the most common site of embolism. This event is particularly likely to occur in IV drug users.

Bacteremia is a potentially life-threatening complication of intravascular devices and has been reported in 2%–8% of patients with central venous catheters [46]. Bacteremia must begin with a localized infection of the dermal cannula entrance wound. The infection rate is lower per catheter day with prolonged IV access devices (such as Hickman and Broviak catheters) that are tunneled beneath the skin than for simple percutaneous central venous lines [47].

Staphylococci, streptococci, and gram-negative bacilli (especially *Klebsiella* and *Enterobacter*) are the most common infecting organisms [45, 48]. Positive blood cultures usually can be obtained in most cases [45]. Initial treatment includes: (1) removal of the needle or catheter, (2) elevation of the involved extremity, (3) application of topical heat, and (4) the institution of parenteral antibiotics. Catheters suspected of being infected should be cultured. Coverage for staphylococci and gram-negative organisms should be initiated pending the results of blood cultures. Nafcillin plus an aminoglycoside or a third-generation cephalosporin is recommended. Patients who do not respond to such management may require surgical excision of the involved venous segment. Such therapy may be required because vascular seeding from an infected focus can persist even in the setting of appropriate antibiotic treatment.

Central Venous Catheter Infection

DEFINITION

Central venous catheter infections are identifiable as three clinical syndromes: (1) exit site infections characterized by cellulitis and/or purulent drainage from the catheter exit site (see Color Plate 9); (2) tunnel infection characterized by erythema and tenderness along the catheter tunnel without drainage at the exit site; and (3) sepsis from infection of the intravascular portion of the catheter. Half of these infections are at the exit site, 20% are tunnel infections, and a third result in sepsis [49].

Table 24-11. Organisms commonly implicated in central venous catheter infections

Staphylococcus, coagulase-negative
Staphylococcus aureus
Candida albicans and other species
Streptococcus viridans
Groups A, B, and D streptococci
Escherichia coli
Klebsiella species
Enterobacter species
Pseudomonas species
Bacillus species
Corynebacterium

Source: Reference 49. Reprinted with permission.

PATHOGENESIS

Infection of central venous catheters results in three ways: (1) movement of organisms along the catheter tunnel, (2) hematogenous seeding, and (3) contamination of infusate. Table 24-11 lists the organisms imnplicated in central venous catheter infections. *Candida* species are frequently implicated when parenteral nutrition is being given through a central venous catheter.

DIAGNOSIS

The reported incidence of central venous catheter infection ranges from 0.10–0.28 infections per 100 catheter days [49]. While clinical signs of exit site and tunnel infections will be found if sought, line sepsis is more subtle and must be considered in all febrile patients without a source and with an indwelling catheter. Since only 25% of the catheters suspected of being infected are infected, diagnostic maneuvers that do not require removal of the IV line are recommended. One method is to compare colony counts of blood cultures drawn through the line and a separate IV site. Another relies on the culture of the exit site. A positive exit site culture has a positive predictive value of 60%, and a negative culture has a negative predictive value of 96.7% [50]. Definitive diagnosis however, usually mandates removal of the catheter tip.

MANAGEMENT

Exit site infections can be treated with oral antibiotics in the patient who is not neutropenic or otherwise severely immunosuppressed. Patients who fail to improve within 48 hours should then be treated with IV antibiotics. A Gram's stain and a culture should always be obtained from purulence from the exit site to guide the treatment.

In neutropenic patients, the severely immunosuppressed, and those with tunnel site infections or sepsis, admission and IV antibiotics are required. If no clinical improvement or positive blood cultures are noted after 48–72 hours, the catheter should be removed. Sometimes the tunnel will need to be surgically opened and drained. Empiric antibiotic therapy consists of vancomycin and gentamicin.

In nonneutropenic patients line sepsis can be treated with IV antibiotics with or without thrombolytic agent without removal of the catheter. The patient requires hospitalization and the risks and benefits of such an approach must be considered. This is not a decision for the emergency department physician.

Neutropenic patients will not develop the usual local signs of indwelling catheter infection (i.e., erythema, edema, purulent discharge) and may have only very minor tenderness over the tunnel. The diagnosis of catheter-associated infection in the patient is difficult but should be suspect, particularly if no other source is evident. Inpatient workup and management are indicated.

Mycotic Aneurysm

Mycotic aneurysm is an acquired aneurysm produced by infection on the vessel wall. Such aneurysms can develop consequent to a number of mechanisms: (1) septic embolization of the arterial lumen with occlusion of the vasa vasorum; (2) direct spread of infection and invasion of the arterial wall from a contiguous site of infection; (3) contamination from penetrating arterial injury or surgery; (4) infection of a previously formed atherosclerotic aneurysm; and (5) arterial-wall injury resulting from immune complex deposition. Although mycotic aneurysm is well known in its relation to infective endocarditis, other causes have been increasingly implicated in recent reports [51, 52]. For example, mycotic aneurysms have been observed with increasing frequency secondary to IV drug use [52].

When mycotic aneurysm is related to endocarditis, lesions usually develop during active disease, although they may not become clinically evident until much later. Their most common site is the cerebral circulation. They are recognized clinically in 2% of cases of endocarditis and in 5%–10% of autopsy cases [12]. However, they can occur at other sites in the arterial circulation.

Cerebral mycotic aneurysms most typically involve distal branches of the middle cerebral artery. Although they usually are single, multiple aneurysms may be present. The aneurysm is generally asymptomatic until it ruptures, although an enlarging aneurysm may produce headache, nuchal rigidity, or cranial nerve palsies. Aneurysmal rupture is an abrupt life-threatening event, producing the typical clinical picture of subarachnoid, intraventricular, or intracerebral hemorrhage. A CT scan may be helpful, but arteriography is the only means of diagnosing intracranial mycotic aneurysm.

Mycotic aneurysms can involve the aorta. Such lesions have a grave prognosis and had been considered to be invariably fatal until relatively recently. Although a successful outcome is uncommon, the combination of early diagnosis, antibiotic therapy, and surgical intervention can lead to survival [49]. Bacterial endocarditis remains a risk factor for the development of an aortic mycotic aneurysm, but other predisposing factors have become increasingly recognized, including arterial trauma (self-induced, accidental, or iatrogenic), immunocompromise (due to diabetes, alcoholism, collagen vascular disease, use of corticosteroids or cytotoxic agents, and malignant neoplasms), and sepsis [51].

Mycotic aneurysms of the peripheral arterial circulation nearly always present with fever and a painful pulsatile mass (Fig. 24-2). A bruit, a thrill, or a diminished peripheral pulse may be evident. The popliteal artery is the site of about 70% of peripheral aneurysms [53]. Many of these are atherosclerotic aneurysms that become infected in the course of bacteremia. Ultrasonography or dynamic CT scanning usually will confirm the diagnosis. Initial management should include the administration of broad-spectrum antibiotics, as in bacterial endocarditis (such as cefazolin and gentamicin), and surgical consultation.

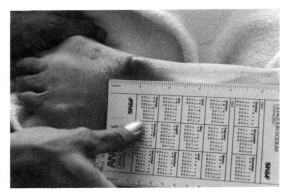

Fig. 24-2. Mycotic aneurysm of dorsal pedalis artery secondary to arterial line

Mediastinitis

The extrapleural portion of the thoracic cavity between the two pleural spaces is a potential space known as the mediastinum. Infection in this area is rarely primary, most commonly representing secondary involvement due to injury or infection of some other structure. Acute mediastinitis usually arises from esophageal perforation, occasionally from extension of infection in surrounding regions (head, neck, lungs, pleura, vertebrae, or retroperitoneal space), and as a complication of cardiac surgery.

Although the mediastinum is subdivided into a number of fascial planes, mediastinal fascia do not necessarily constitute adequate barriers to the containment of infection. Mediastinal infection is rendered more likely by proximity to the pharynx, there being no tissue barrier between the pharynx and the mediastinum. Negative intrathoracic pressure generated during inspiration is another aid to the spread of infection, acting to draw the contents of a perforated esophagus from the neck or retroperitoneum into the mediastinum.

Most cases of mediastinitis are the consequence of esophageal perforation. This can occur as a result of instrumentation (e.g., endoscopy or dilatation), trauma, or foreign-body or caustic ingestion or be subsequent to vomiting (Boerhaave's syndrome). Trauma is the least common of these causes, instrumentation the most frequent.

Spread of infection to the mediastinum from adjacent sites (upper respiratory tract, lung, pleura, vertebrae, and abdomen) or hematogenous seeding from remote foci have become progressively less common in recent years. However, mediastinitis that complicates infection of the oropharynx (known as descending necrotizing mediastinitis) remains one of the most lethal forms of the disease [54]. The origin of descending necrotizing mediastinitis can be odontogenic infection (especially that originating from the second or third mandibular molars), peritonsillar or retropharyngeal abscess, or Ludwig's angina. Mediastinal infection also complicates cardiac surgery in 0.5%–5.0% of patients [55].

A more indolent form of mediastinitis is the consequence of granulomatous infection, such as histoplasmosis or tuberculosis. This is termed fibrosing mediastinitis. Pathogenesis may relate to the rupture of caseated mediastinal lymph nodes.

Etiology

Most forms of mediastinitis, including descending necrotizing mediastinitis, are polymicrobial processes. Anaerobic organisms are predominant, with anaerobic streptococci being the most commonly isolated anaerobic organisms. Among aerobic bacteria group A beta-hemolytic streptococci are the most frequent. Gram-negative bacilli also are commonly isolated [54].

The most common organism causing mediastinal infection following cardiac surgery is staphylococcus. *S. epidermidis* has, in particular, emerged as a primary pathogen in this setting, possibly due to the routine use of prophylactic antistaphylococcal antibiotic treatment. Such treatment likely selects out resistant staphylococcal strains, since pathogens are frequently resistant to the antibiotic used in perioperative prophylaxis [56]. Infection with gram-negative organisms is less common [55]. There is a small but increasing occurrence of mediastinal infection caused by *Candida* species [57]. Fibrosing mediastinitis is most often caused by *Histoplasma capsulatum* [58].

Clinical Findings

The clinical findings in mediastinitis vary widely, depending on the extent and the nature of the infection. The patient frequently appears acutely ill. Esophageal perforation generally has a painful presentation. Pain following esophageal perforation is typically severe, and varies in location from the neck to the substernal region to the epigastrium. Radiation may be to the neck, left chest, shoulder, or back. The nature of the pain may be pleuritic.

Respiratory distress often represents pleural involvement, which produces rapid, shallow respirations. When pneumothorax or pleural effusion is present, physical findings of either entity may be observed. Pneumomediastinum can be heralded by subcutaneous emphysema (best palpable in the region of the suprasternal notch) or an audible mediastinal crunch. Abdominal findings, including tenderness, guarding, rebound tenderness, and diminished bowel sounds, may be present. Fever is often low grade initially but may become sustained with the passage of time. Dysphagia is characteristic of acute mediastinitis due to esophageal perforation.

Mediastinitis following cardiac surgery usually is seen within 2 weeks of the operation. Drainage from the incision is the pathognomonic finding, especially when it is noted to bubble through an unstable sternotomy wound. However, postoperative mediastinitis can present as sepsis without any demonstrable sternal or wound abnormalities [55]. Fibrosing mediastinitis may present as superior vena caval syndrome.

Diagnosis

The diagnosis of mediastinitis is frequently difficult on clinical grounds, and delay in diagnosis is common. Laboratory data are usually of little diagnostic value. Although leukocytosis or a leftward shift of the WBC differential may be present, these are nonspecific. Suggestive findings may, however, be present on the chest or lateral neck roentgenogram. These include pneumomediastinum, pleural effusion, mediastinal widening, pneumothorax, and gas in the soft tissues. Plain roentgenograms may, however, be nonspecific, and a CT scan of the thorax can be extremely valuable in the diagnosis of mediastinitis. [59]

Contrast esophagography is considered the definitive diagnostic study in cases of suspected esophageal rupture. Extravasation of swallowed radiographic contrast material is seen in about 75% of cases. There is some debate regarding whether bar-

ium or water-soluble contrast is the agent of choice [60, 61].

Treatment

Initial treatment includes the assurance of a patent airway and ventilation, as well as the management of septic or hypovolemic shock. Monitoring of vital signs, urinary output, and arterial blood gases is essential in severely ill patients. Chest-tube drainage may be required for pleural effusion or pneumothorax. Broad-spectrum antibiotic coverage should be administered initially, with intravenous penicillin G and metronidazole recommended for suspected descending necrotizing mediastinitis. An aminoglycoside or third-generation cephalosporin should be added for suspected gram-negative infection. Antistaphylococcal coverage is imperative in postsurgical mediastinitis. Imipenem 500 mg q6h is a good option in the treatment of mediastinitis. This antibiotic is active against nearly all common bacteria, including those resistant to aminoglycosides and the newer cephalosporins. Its spectrum includes anaerobic and aerobic bacteria and both gram-positive and gram-negative organisms [62].

In addition to supportive care and antibiotic administration, early surgical consultation is needed. The form of surgical intervention required depends on the type of mediastinitis involved. Mediastinal drainage and repair of injured mediastinal structures frequently are essential to patient survival. Aggressive approaches to surgical intervention have been advocated recently [59].

References

1. Oikawa JH, Kay D. Endocarditis: epidemiology, pathophysiology, management and prophylaxis. *Cardiovasc Clin* 16(2):335, 1986.
2. Smilack JD, Horn VPH. Acute infective endocarditis. *Cardiol Clin* 2:201, 1984.
3. Freedman LR. *Infective Endocarditis and Other Intravascular Infections.* New York: Plenum, 1982.
4. Von Reyn CF et al. Infective endocarditis: an analysis based on strict case definitions. *Ann Intern Med* 94:505, 1981.
5. Pankey GA. Infective endocarditis: changing concepts. *Hosp Pract* 21(3):103, 1986.

6. Cherubin CE, Neu HC. Bacterial endocarditis at the Presbyterian Hospital in New York City from 1938 to 1967. *Am J Med* 51:83, 1971.

7. MacMahon SW et al. Mitral valve prolapse and infective endocarditis. *Am Heart J* 113:1291, 1987.

8. Wilson WR et al. General considerations in the diagnosis and treatment of infective endocarditis. *Mayo Clin Proc* 57:81, 1982.

9. Chambers HF, Korzeniowski OM, Sande MA. *Staphylococcus aureus* endocarditis: clinical manifestations in addicts and nonaddicts. *Medicine* 62:170, 1983.

10. Terpenning MS, Buggy BP, Kauffman CA. Infective endocarditis: clinical features in young and elderly patients. *Am J Med* 83:626, 1987.

11. Pelletier LL, Petersdorf RG. Infective endocarditis: a review of 125 cases from the University of Washington Hospitals, 1963–72. *Medicine* 56:287, 1977.

12. Lerner PI. Neurologic complications of infective endocarditis. *Med Clin North Am* 69(2):385, 1985.

13. Roberts R, Slovis CM. Endocarditis in intravenous drug abusers. *Emerg Med Clin North Am* 8(3):665, 1990.

14. Chambers HF. Infection in the parenteral drug user. In M Callaham (ed.), *Current Therapy in Emergency Medicine*. Toronto: Decker, 1987. Pp. 788–92.

15. Marantz PR et al. Inability to predict diagnosis in febrile intravenous drug abusers. *Ann Intern Med* 106:823, 1987.

16. Reisberg BE. Infective endocarditis in the narcotic addict. *Prog Cardiovasc Dis* 22:193, 1979.

17. Tuazon CU, Cardellis TA, Sheagren JN. Staphylococcal endocarditis in drug users. Clinical and microbiological aspects. *Arch Intern Med* 135:1555, 1975.

18. Calderwood SB et al. Risk factors for the development of prosthetic valve endocarditis. *Circulation* 72:31, 1985.

19. Mandell GL. The laboratory in diagnosis and management. In D Kaye (ed.), *Infective Endocarditis*. Baltimore: University Park, 1976. Pp. 155–66.

20. Melvin ET et al. Noninvasive methods for detection of valve vegetations in infective endocarditis. *Am J Cardiol* 47:271, 1981.

21. Bisno AL et al. Antimicrobial treatment of infective endocarditis due to viridans streptococci, enterococci, and staphylococci. *JAMA* 261:1471, 1989.

22. Shulman ST et al. Prevention of bacterial endocarditis. *Circulation* 70:1123A, 1984.

23. Dajani AS et al. Prevention of bacterial endocarditis. Recommendations by the American Heart Association. *JAMA* 264:2919, 1990.

24. Roberts WC, Ferrans VJ. A survey of the causes and consequences of pericardial heart disease. In PS Reddy et al. (eds.), *Pericardial Disease*. New York: Raven, 1982. Pp. 49–75.

25. Hancock EW. Pericardial disease—differential diagnosis and management. *Hosp Pract* 18(4):101, 1983.

26. Burch GE. Acute viral pericarditis. *Cardiovasc Clin* 7(3):149, 1976.

27. Fulton DR, Grodin M. Pediatric cardiac emergencies. *Emerg Med Clin North Am* 1(1):45, 1983.

28. Rubin RH, Moellering RC Jr. Clinical, microbiologic and therapeutic aspects of purulent pericarditis. *Am J Med* 59:68, 1975.

29. Klacsmann PB, Bulkey BH, and Hutchins GM. The changed spectrum of purulent pericarditis. An 86 year autopsy experience in 200 patients. *Am J Med* 63:666, 1977.

30. Larrieu AJ et al. Recent experience with tuberculous pericarditis. *Ann Thorac Surg* 29:464, 1980.

31. Poland GA, Jorgensen CR, Sarosi GA. *Nocardia asteroides* pericarditis: report of a case and review of the literature. *Mayo Clin Proc* 65:819, 1990.

32. Spodick DH. Pericarditis, pericardial effusion, cardiac tamponade and constriction. *Crit Care Clin* 5(3):455, 1989.

33. Spodick DH. Acute pericardial disease: pericarditis, effusion and tamponade. *J. Continuing Educ Cardiol* 14:9, 1979.

34. Guberman BA et al. Cardiac tamponade in medical patients. *Circulation* 64:633, 1981.

35. Horowitz MS et al. Sensitivity and specificity of echocardiographic diagnosis of pericardial effusion. *Circulation* 50:239, 1974.

36. Magobunje OA et al. Surgical management of pericarditis in Zaire, Nigeria. *Thorax* 36:590, 1981.

37. Aretz HT et al. Myocarditis: a histopathologic definition and classification. *Am J Cardiovasc Pathol* 1:3, 1986.

38. Stevenson LW, Perloff JK. The dilated cardiomyopathies. *Cardiol Clin* 6(2):187, 1988.

39. Reyes MP, Lerner AM. Coxsackievirus myocarditis—with special reference to acute and chronic effects. *Prog Cardiovasc Dis* 27:373, 1985.

40. Cohen IS et al. Congestive cardiomyopathy in association with the acquired immunodeficiency syndrome. *N Engl J Med* 315:628, 1986.

41. Kopecky SL, Gersh BJ. Dilated cardiomyopathy and myocarditis: natural history, etiology, clinical manifestations and management. *Curr Prob Cardiol* 12:569, 1987.

42. Harris LC et al. Severe pulsus alternans associated with primary myocardial disease in children. *Circulation* 34:948, 1966.

43. Meszaros WT. Lung changes in left heart failure. *Circulation* 47:859, 1973.

44. O'Neill JA et al. Suppurative thrombophlebitis: a

lethal complication of intravenous therapy. *J Trauma* 8:256, 1968.

45. Baker CC, Peterson SR, Sheldon GF. Septic phlebitis: a neglected disease. *Am J Surg* 138:97, 1979.

46. Sugarman B, Young EJ. Infections associated with prosthetic devices: magnitude of the problem. *Infect Dis Clin North Am* 3(2):187, 1989.

47. Reed WP et al. Prolonged venous access for chemotherapy by means of the Hickman catheter. *Cancer* 52:185, 1983.

48. Garrison RN, Richardson JD, Fry DE. Catheter-associated septic thrombophlebitis. *South Med J* 75:917, 1892.

49. Toltzis P, Goldmann DA. Central venous catheter infections. *Immunocomp Host* 4:2, 1986.

50. Cercenado E et al. A conservative procedure for the diagnosis of catheter related infections. *Arch Intern Med* 150:1417, 1990.

51. Johansen K, Devin J. Mycotic aortic aneurysms. *Arch Surg* 118:583, 1983.

52. Patel YD, Norowitz DB. Ruptured mycotic aneurysms. *Cardiovasc Intervent Radiol* 11:86, 1988.

53. Gaylis H. Popliteal arterial aneurysms: a review of 55 cases. *S Afr Med J* 48:75, 1974.

54. Estrera AS et al. Descending necrotizing mediastinitis. *Surg Gynecol Obstet* 157:545, 1983.

55. Sarr MG, Gott VL, Townsend TR. Mediastinal infection after cardiac surgery. *Ann Thorac Surg* 38:415, 1984.

56. Bor DH et al. Mediastinitis after cardiovascular surgery. *Rev Infect Dis* 5:885, 1983.

57. Glower DD et al. Candida mediastinitis after a cardiac operation. *Ann Thorac Surg* 49:157, 1990.

58. Wieder S, Rabinowitz JG. Fibrous mediastinitis: a late manifestation of mediastinal histoplasmosis. *Radiology* 125:305, 1977.

59. Wheatley MJ et al. Descending necrotizing mediastinitis: transcervical drainage is not enough. *Ann Thorac Surg* 49:780, 1990.

60. Curci JJ, Horman MJ. Boerhaave's syndrome: the importance of early diagnosis and treatment. *Ann Surg* 183:401, 1976.

61. del Castillo J et al. Atraumatic panmural rupture of the esophagus: Boerhaave syndrome. *Ann Emerg Med* 12:385, 1985.

62. Sobel JD. Imipenem and aztreonam. *Infect Dis Clin North Am* 3(3):613, 1989.

THE GASTROINTESTINAL SYSTEM AND ABDOMEN

25

Diarrheal Disease and Gastroenteritis

LARRY J. GOODMAN

JOHN SEGRETI

Worldwide, diarrheal disease is among the most common infectious syndromes in all age groups. In developing nations diarrheal illness is the leading cause of death in children, with an estimated 5 million deaths annually in children less than 5 years old [1]. Estimates from the Centers for Disease Control (CDC) suggest that in the United States 25 million cases of enteric infections occur annually, with over 10,000 deaths [2]. Persons at greatest risk to die from an acute diarrheal illness include those already dehydrated, malnourished, or debilitated and persons at the extremes of age. In some diarrheal conditions, however, fluid loss can be so rapid that otherwise healthy adults will not survive without adequate volume replacement. Bacteremia, intestinal emergencies (e.g., perforation, toxic megacolon), and malabsorption of vital oral medications are additional complications that can limit survival.

Diarrheal disease is most common in children under 1 year of age. Diarrhea can also be a false localizing sign. An infant with otitis media, meningitis, torsion of a testicle, or Kawasaki's disease may also present with diarrhea and thus represent a difficult diagnostic challenge. In adults pneumonia, intra-abdominal abscess, ischemic colitis, inflammatory bowel disease, toxic shock syndrome, Rocky Mountain spotted fever, and intestinal ob-struction may all present with diarrhea. While there are some data indicating the annual rate of diarrhea in children in various settings, few similar data exist on adults [3]. There appears to be a second peak in the incidence of some bacterial diarrheas, particularly *Campylobacter jejuni*, in young adults attending college [4]. For compromised hosts nausea, vomiting, or diarrhea can complicate treatment of the underlying condition (e.g., chemotherapy for certain cancers) or apparently be specifically associated with the underlying process (e.g., human immunodeficiency virus [HIV] infection).

No widely accepted definition of diarrhea exists. Most patients have at least three or four stools per 24-hour period, with the stool loose enough to take the shape of the container in which it is placed. In most studies of diarrheal illness a large percentage of patients, often the majority, have no pathogen identified. Despite the large number of pathogens that are known to cause diarrhea, most microbiology laboratories evaluate specimens for only a small fraction of these. Furthermore, even for commonly identified pathogens, isolating an organism from stool, the most heavily contaminated specimen received by the laboratory, is a formidable task. Methods commonly employed, such as plating stool on selective media containing antibiotics, may inhibit the growth of the pathogen sought [5]. Other pathogens may not survive transportation to the laboratory [6].

Diarrhea has a broad differential diagnosis, including both infectious and noninfectious processes. The age of the patient, travel and exposure history, underlying condition, medications, physical examination, and stool examination for cells all provide important information that assists in the development of a rational approach, and all are available to the emergency department physician. Most patients should also have stool sent for culture for the presence of common bacterial pathogens. Studies for viruses, parasites, and other pathogens should be obtained on an individualized basis. Table 25-1 lists the clinical and laboratory clues that can assist in the diagnosis of GI infections and intoxications.

Development of Diarrheal Disease and Gastroenteritis

With rare exceptions enteric infections are acquired from eating contaminated food or beverages or through the ingestion of contaminated material via fecal-oral spread with hands or fomites as intermediaries. The GI system, therefore, represents the first point of contact of the pathogen with the host. Interactions of invader and host at this level are critical in determining which patients will become symptomatic and which will transiently excrete the organism without symptoms.

There are four major host defenses against enteric infections in the GI system: (1) gastric acidity, (2) small-bowel motility, (3) the colonic flora, and (4) local antibody production. The most important of these is gastric acidity. Fasting gastric pH, which is normally less than 4, is toxic to most enteropathogens, although spores are minimally affected. Colony counts can be reduced by greater than 90% by this exposure. Conversely patients who are achlorhydric or who have their stomach pH raised by other means are at greater risk to develop an enteric infection [7, 8]. This also helps to explain why 10 people can eat the same contaminated meal and only 3 become ill. Those who eat the contaminated portion of the meal first have maximal stomach acidity and are less likely to become ill than those who eat the contaminated portion of the meal

after their stomach acidity has been buffered by other foods.

After leaving the stomach, surviving organisms enter the small bowel. Moving down the small bowel, the normal flora become more dense, with approximately 10^6 colony-forming units per milliliter of fluid, and more similar to colonic flora with a predominance of anaerobes and gram-negative organisms. Normally the small bowel is constantly in motion. This peristaltic activity decreases the contact time for pathogens that act by attachment and invasion. Factors that decrease this peristaltic activity, such as an ileus or antimotility medications may, therefore, increase the severity of illness for invasive pathogens [9, 10].

In the colon there are approximately 10^9 to 10^{11} colony-forming units per gram of feces, with anaerobes outnumbering aerobes 10,000 to 1 and a predominance of gram-negatives. This large number of resident flora provides an important defense in several ways. Nonpathogens take up attachment sites, compete for nutrients, and produce chemicals toxic to some pathogens [11, 12]. Finally local antibody production in the small bowel and the colon may also be important in the defense against some pathogens [13, 14].

An illustration of how important these host factors are can be found in studies in which enteric pathogens are administered orally to volunteers in an attempt to cause disease. Pretreatment with antacids to buffer stomach acidity or antibiotics with activity against the colonic flora each significantly decreased the amount of organism necessary to cause disease [15, 16].

A number of organism factors also play important roles in permitting the pathogen to survive outside the host, avoid host defenses, and resist attempts at eradication through the use of antimicrobial agents. Organisms with a spore phase, such as *Bacillus cereus* and *Clostridium difficile*, are particularly well suited to survive for prolonged periods on surfaces. *B. cereus* has caused outbreaks of diarrhea with fried rice as the vehicle [17]. It is postulated that in these cases the organism exsporulates on the cooked stored rice and is not killed by the reheating process. *C. difficile*, among the most common of nosocomial infections, has been cultured from hospital carpeting, beds, and walls [18]. These spores are particularly difficult to eradicate and may play a

Table 25-1. Gastroenteritis, diarrheal disease, food-borne/water-borne intoxications: clinical and laboratory clues that may assist in diagnosis

Clue	Possible cause
Symptoms (History)	
Incubation period <1 hour	Heavy metal intoxication, scromboid, puffer fish poisoning
Incubation period >1 week	*Giardia lamblia, Entamoeba histolytica*
Symptoms present >3 weeks	*G. lamblia, E. histolytica, Yersinia enterocolitica*, postinfectious malabsorption, *C. difficile* colitis, inflammatory bowel disease
Neurological symptoms	Ciguatera, paralytic shellfish poisoning, neurotoxic shellfish poisoning, amnesiac shellfish poisoning, puffer fish poisoning, botulism
Suspected Vehicle	
Milk	*Campylobacter jejuni, Y. enterocolitica, Salmonella* species
Untreated water	*G. lamblia*, Norwalk virus, enterotoxigenic *Escherichia coli*
Poultry, eggs	*Salmonella* species, *C. jejuni*
Raw fish, shellfish	*Vibrio* species, anasikiasis, paralytic shellfish poisoning, neurotoxic shellfish poisoning, amnesic shellfish poisoning, Norwalk virus
Physical Examination	
Mimics appendicitis	*Y. enterocolitica, Salmonella* species, *C. jejuni, C. difficile, E. histolytica, Angiostrongylus costaricensis*
Toxic megacolon	*Y. enterocolitica, Salmonella* species, *C. jejuni, E. histolytica, Angiostrongylus costaricensis*; also consider ischemic colitis and inflammatory bowel disease
Perianal vesicles	Herpes simplex virus
Anal ulcer	*Treponema pallidum* (syphilis), *E. histolytica*, inflammatory bowel disease, trauma
Laboratory Findings	
Diarrhea and eosinophilia	*Strongyloides stercoralis, Ascaris lumbricoides, Trichinella spiralis, Schistosoma* species (Katayama fever), *Isospora belli, Dientamoeba fragilis*, eosinophilic gastroenteritis
Findings on Stool Smear	
Curved gram-negative rods	*Campylobacter* species, *Vibrio* species
Acid-fast stain positive	*Cryptosporidium* species, *Mycobacterium* species, Cyanobacteri, *I. belli*
Many RBCs (gross blood) but rare WBCs	Verotoxin-producing *E. coli*, ischemic colitis, CMV colitis in compromised host, GI bleed
Many RBCs and mononuclear WBCs	*E. histolytica*

role in the acquisition of disease. Organisms with pili, fimbriae, and other attachment or adhesion factors are better able to attach to host cells. Plasmids, bits of extrachromosomal DNA, may code for toxins, other virulence factors, or enzymes that inactivate antimicrobial agents. Just as host factors are, to some extent, predictive of outcome, these organism factors help explain why some members of a genus are pathogenic for humans and others are mere commensals.

Approach to the Patient with Diarrhea

Commonly identified diarrheal pathogens typically cause disease by (1) elaboration of an enterotoxin, producing an afebrile watery diarrhea syndrome; (2) partially invading the mucosa, producing a syndrome characterized by fever and cells in the stool and occasionally frank dysentery; or (3) completely invading the mucosa, producing fever and cells in the stool. Dysentery in this third group is rare, but some patients will develop mesenteric adenitis. The incidence of bacteremia is highest in this group. A fourth distinct syndrome consisting of an acute diarrhea with GI bleeding recently has been described. Organisms producing this syndrome produce a cytotoxin that lyses mucosal cells. Patients are afebrile. It should be noted that these syndromes may overlap and that some organisms produce an enterotoxin and have invasive potential. Nevertheless, this approach does help to orient the physician toward the most likely etiologies and to identify patients who might benefit from antibiotic treatment or develop specific complications.

The major clinical clues in distinguishing among these syndromes are (1) the incubation period, (2) the presence or absence of fever, and (3) cells in the stool. Each of these factors provides important information for patients with diarrhea. Of these factors the incubation period is the most difficult of which to be confident, except during an outbreak in which multiple people are ill and only shared one common meal or when the vehicle is already known at the time of the examination. Although patients may blame their illness on a food that smelled, tasted, or looked "bad" or a food that was unusual for them, in most cases contaminated foods are indistinguishable from other foods.

Enterotoxin-Mediated Diarrhea

Organisms in this group cause disease by producing an enterotoxin that stimulates fluid movement from the intravascular spaces to the small-bowel lumen, usually via stimulation of cyclic adenosine monophosphate (AMP) or guanosine monophosphate (GMP). The enterotoxin may be elaborated inside the host or already be present on the food. In the latter case further preparation (cooking) of the food may kill the organism, leaving only the preformed toxin. Since the site of activity is the small bowel and the toxin already may have been present on the ingested food, the incubation period is short, often 6–18 hours. There is little or no local inflammatory reaction to the toxin, so WBCs or RBCs are rarely seen in the stool and fever is uncommon. Bacteremia and metastatic infection almost never are seen, and antimicrobial therapy is necessary only occasionally.

In summary an enterotoxin-associated diarrheal illness is characterized by a short incubation period, voluminous watery diarrhea often associated with nausea and vomiting, an absence of fever or cells in the stool, and a very low risk of bacteremia or metastatic infection with the offending organism. The illness usually lasts hours to a few days, with the major risk to the patient being dehydration.

ENTEROTOXIGENIC ESCHERICHIA COLI
Enterotoxigenic *Escherichia coli* is the most commonly identified cause of traveler's diarrhea [19]. An *E. coli* may contain a plasmid that codes for a heat-stable toxin, a heat-labile toxin, both, or neither (20). Morphologically enterotoxigenic organisms are identical to other *E. coli* found in the stool. Most microbiology laboratories do not currently identify this organism. Prophylactic antibiotics (trimethoprim-sulfamethoxazole, ampicillin, ciprofloxacin, norfloxacin, and others) or prophylactic bismuth subsalicylate have been effective in preventing disease [21–23]. Also, antibiotic treatment if administered early may shorten the duration and the severity of illness [24]. The incubation period is usually 24 hours or less, and the untreated illness typically lasts less than 5 days.

STAPHYLOCOCCUS AUREUS
Approximately 10% of all bacterial food-borne outbreaks of diarrhea in the United States are due to enterotoxin (enterotoxin B)–producing *Staphylococcus aureus* [25]. In most cases food handlers carrying the organism on their skin contaminated food that was then only partially cooked (26). Symptoms usually last only about 8 hours or less, and antibiotic treatment is unnecessary.

CLOSTRIDIUM PERFRINGENS
Most outbreaks of diarrhea due to *Clostridium perfringens* occur 8–24 hours after ingestion. The toxin is rarely present on the food in sufficient quantity to cause disease but is produced in the host. The most common presenting symptoms are diarrhea and abdominal pain. Meats and poultry that were cooked and then reheated frequently are identified as vehicles [17]. Symptoms typically last less than 2 days, and antibiotics have not been shown to be of benefit in shortening the duration of the disease or lessening the symptoms.

BACILLUS CEREUS

Bacillus cereus is present in many raw foods, particularly cereals and spices (17). This organism may cause a vomiting (emetic) syndrome, usually within 5 hours of ingesting a contaminated meal. The most commonly identified vehicle in these cases is fried rice. The organism exsporulates on the cooked rice at room temperature and the heat-stable toxin survives reheating. Symptoms usually last less than 24 hours, and antibiotics have not been demonstrated to be of benefit. *B. cereus* also may cause a diarrheal syndrome with a slightly longer incubation period (8–16 hours). Again, symptoms usually resolve within 24 hours.

VIBRIO CHOLERA

Vibrio cholera is found primarily in coastal areas near salt water, with raw shellfish a common vehicle. While the organism may be identified using routine enteric media, selective media (e.g., thiosulfate-citrate-bile salts-sucrose agar [TCBS]) are recommended for optimal recovery [27]. Patients with diarrhea due to toxigenic *V. cholera* may lose up to 1 liter of fluid per hour by rectum. In addition to rehydration therapy, antibiotics (doxycycline, furazolidone) may decrease the duration of shedding of the organism and shorten the illness [28, 29]. *V. cholera* and other *Vibrio* species also can be found inland, particularly on fresh fish transported to suppliers and restaurants.

Patients with severe liver disease (cirrhosis, hemachromatosis) are at particular risk for bacteremia with *Vibrio* species. A syndrome of fever, shock, and hemorrhagic bullae has been reported with bacteremia due to *Vibrio vulnifercus* and other *Vibrios*. (See Chap. 16.)

GIARDIA LAMBLIA

Infections with *Giardia lamblia* are among the most common parasitic infections in the United States and are distributed worldwide. The organism typically is acquired from ingesting fecally contaminated water or from person-to-person spread. After ingestion of the infective particle, the cyst, there is excystation, multiplication, and attachment to the GI surface. After a 1- to 2-week incubation period, patients may become asymptomatic cyst passers, develop an acute diarrheal illness, or develop a chronic diarrhea. The chronic diarrhea may persist for months and be associated with weight loss, mal-

aise, "gas" symptoms, and abdominal pain. Diagnosis is via identification of the organism on stool sample or samples of small-bowel aspirate or biopsy. Patients are typically afebrile, and there are no WBCs or RBCs in the stool. *Isospora belli, Balantidium coli, Dientamoeba fragilis*, and *Cryptosporidium* species may produce a similar clinical syndrome. Of these, *B. coli* is unique in its ability to progress to a severe colitis, with bloody diarrhea and possible intestinal rupture.

Mucosal Invasion (Incomplete)— The Dysentery Syndrome

Dysentery is defined as diarrhea that contains gross blood and mucus. Organisms in this group generally act by attaching to mucosal cells in the distal small bowel and colon and are locally invasive. This stimulates a local inflammatory response with WBCs (usually polymorphonuclear leukocytes) moving to the area of damage and spilling into the lumen. The inflamed tissue often is friable and bleeding. In most cases red cells and white cells are seen on microscopic examination of the stool. In severe cases gross blood and pus or mucus are present, producing a dysentery syndrome. There is often a systemic inflammatory response manifest by fever and an elevated WBC count. Microbial invasion is rarely through the full thickness of the bowel wall. Intestinal perforation and bacteremia are uncommon complications. Since the organism must reach the distal bowel, attach, and invade before the patient develops symptoms, the incubation period is longer than for the enterotoxin-mediated diarrheas, usually 1–3 days.

Antimicrobial therapy is often effective in eradicating these organisms from the stool, but it has not been consistently demonstrated to shorten the clinical syndrome.

In summary diarrhea due to organisms that invade primarily the superficial mucosal layers of the bowel are characterized by an incubation period of 1–3 days, the presence of white and red cells in the stool, and fever. Some patients have a dysentery syndrome, with gross blood and pus in the stool. Untreated patients typically are ill less than 7 days. Complications such as bacteremia or intestinal rupture are rare. Antimicrobial therapy may decrease the duration of shedding of the pathogen and, in some cases, may shorten the clinical illness by about 1 day [30].

CAMPYLOBACTER JEJUNI

Campylobacter jejuni has been identified as the most common bacterial cause of diarrhea in nearly every country and age group in which it was studied [31–33]. It is found in many animals, particularly poultry and cows. Chicken and unpasteurized milk have been identified sources from several outbreaks [34, 35]. Campylobacter organisms are curved gram-negative rods. Seeing this morphology on a Gram's stain of stool from a patient with diarrhea is a strong clue for Campylobacter and was found in about 50% of cases in one study [36]. Vibrio species are also curved gram-negative rods that cause diarrhea. C. jejuni grows best at 42°C in a microaerobic atmosphere [37]. Selective media are usually required to inhibit the growth of other stool organisms. Treatment with erythromycin 500 mg qid PO usually will clear the organism from the stool and may shorten the duration of diarrhea if begun early in the course of the illness [38]. Resistance to erythromycin is rare. Fluoroquinolones, such as ciprofloxacin 500 mg bid PO and norfloxacin 400 mg bid PO, also are effective [30, 39].

SHIGELLA

Infection with the Shigella organism is one of the most communicable of diarrheal diseases. The ingestion of as few as several hundred organisms can cause clinical illness [40]. Person-to-person spread is, therefore, of particular concern, especially among family members or in confined populations. Most patients initially have a watery diarrhea that over the subsequent 1 or 2 days evolves into a more typical invasive syndrome. Patients with Shigella dysenteriae 1 (the shiga bacillus) usually have a more severe illness than those infected with other serotypes (Shigella boydii, Shigella flexneri, and Shigella sonnei). This organism, like the verotoxin-producing E. coli (VTEC), has been associated with disseminated intravascular coagulation (DIC) and the hemolytic uremic syndrome. In the United States the most common serotype is S. sonnei. Treatment is indicated for patients with moderate to severe illness or to eradicate the organism from the stool

when the risk of transmission to others is high. Trimethoprim-sulfamethoxazole or a fluoroquinolone for a total of 3–5 days is usually effective [41, 42].

CLOSTRIDIUM DIFFICILE

Clostridium difficile is the most common identified cause of antibiotic-associated diarrhea and is the primary cause of pseudomembranous colitis [43]. The majority of patients with diarrhea due to this pathogen have recently been on antibiotics or cancer chemotherapy, although as many as 5% of community onset diarrheas may be due to C. difficile. Unlike other organisms in this group C. difficile is not directly invasive. It produces diarrhea and occasionally a true dysentery picture by producing several toxins, including an enterotoxin and a cytotoxin. Diagnosis can be made by culture, latex agglutination, or cytotoxin assay. It should be noted that a high percentage of infants may be cytotoxin positive with no symptoms and therefore need not be treated [44]. Similarly a significant percentage of hospitalized persons may be culture positive without clinical symptoms [44]. Proctosigmoidoscopy or colonoscopy usually is necessary to determine the extent of pseudomembranous colitis. Many patients will improve if the antibiotic therapy they are receiving is discontinued. For those needing specific treatment, vancomycin and metronidazole are both effective and should be administered orally unless contraindicated [45–48]. Metronidazole is less expensive, so many consider it the drug of choice. However, for the most severe cases, vancomycin is often recommended. Approximately 20% of patients will relapse after stopping either treatment [45, 49, 50]. Most of these patients will respond to a second course of treatment, even with the same drug.

ENTAMOEBA HISTOLYTICA

Amebiasis is among the most common of parasitic infections. In developing countries many persons are colonized with this organism without apparent ill effects. Recent studies have demonstrated that there are pathogenic and nonpathogenic strains, separated by isoenzyme (zymodeme) typing [51, 52]. Entamoeba histolytica invades mucosal cells and causes cell lysis. A wide range of mucosal changes has been described, including the classic flask-shaped mucosal ulcers. Nearly every patient with amoebic colitis has red cells in the stool [53, 54]. White cells (often mononuclear cells) and Charcot-Leydin crystals also may be seen in stool smears. Trophozoites with ingested RBCs is a diagnostic finding.

There are several important differences in the clinical illness seen due to E. histolytica compared to the other organisms in this group. The incubation period is longer (1–2 weeks), and the onset of the disease may be gradual over several weeks. Also, patients may have a more prolonged or even chronic illness, suggesting inflammatory bowel disease rather than an infectious process. Local complications, such as toxic megacolon, ameboma, fulminant colitis with colon necrosis, and metastatic disease, such as amoebic liver abscess, may occur in up to 1% of cases.

Amoebic colitis is diagnosed by finding cysts or trophozoites in the stool. Barium, antacids, and some antibiotics obscure these findings. Fresh stool should be examined. A single stool specimen will detect approximately one-third of cases. Endoscopy with mucosal scrapings may detect cases missed on stool examination. Scrapings of the ulcer edge or pipetted liquid stool from the proctoscope should be examined by a direct mount in saline for the presence of motile trophozoites (linear motility) or trophozoites with ingested erythrocytes. Serological studies may also assist in the diagnosis of invasive disease.

Invasive amoebic rectocolitis can be treated with metronidazole followed by diiodohydroxyquin. For proven or suspected perforation, IV metronidazole and parenteral dehydroemetine are recommended. When perforation is suspected, coverage for bowel flora also is indicated.

Complete Mucosal Invasion

A third group of organisms also attach to and penetrate the mucosa, but they rarely cause dysentery. Stool examination usually reveals red and white cells but fewer than seen in Shigella infection or amoebic disease. Many patients have fever. Organisms in this group may penetrate through the full thickness of the bowel and reach regional lymph nodes. Mesenteric adenitis, mimicking acute appendicitis, may precede the first diarrheal stool. Bacteremia and subsequent metastatic infection is most common with these organisms.

Diarrhea due to organisms that more completely invade the colon is characterized by an incubation period of 1–3 days, fever, and white and red cells in the stool. Dysentery is rare. Mesenteric adenitis and bacteremia with metastatic infection are seen occasionally and are more common for these organisms than for any other diarrheal pathogens.

SALMONELLA

Over 2000 serotypes of Salmonella have been described. These have been found throughout the world in domestic and wild animals, birds, reptiles, and insects [55]. Many of these serotypes are pathogenic for humans. Approximately 2 million cases of salmonellosis occur in the United States yearly, with 30,000–60,000 of these reported annually to the CDC [56]. Common serotypes include Salmonella typhimurium, Salmonella enteriditis, Salmonella heidelberg, Salmonella newport, and Salmonella infantis. Outbreaks frequently are traced to contaminated eggs, milk, or poultry. Infected pets, platelets, and pharmaceutical products have also been sources [57, 58]. Salmonella typhi, the most common cause of typhoid fever, is confined to humans as its only host. Salmonella species, particularly Salmonella cholerae-suis, have a propensity to infect vascular surfaces, such as vascular grafts and aneurysms [59, 60].

In most cases, diarrhea due to Salmonella species is self-limited. Earlier studies demonstrated that antimicrobial therapy did not shorten the duration of illness but in fact prolonged the excretion of the organism [61]. Therefore, fluid replacement and supportive care are usually the main therapies. Recently quinolones have been shown to eradicate Salmonella organisms from the stool in most cases [62]. Therefore, for severe illness or for patients prevented from returning to work because of a positive stool culture, treatment with ciprofloxacin or norfloxacin should be considered. A chronic Salmonella carrier is an individual who excretes the organism in the stool or urine for more than one year. Nearly all chronic carriers are without symptoms. If treatment is indicated, ciprofloxacin and norfloxacin have been effective in several small studies [63–65].

YERSINIA ENTEROCOLITICA

Yersinia enterocolitica is an infrequent cause of diarrhea in the United States but a common pathogen in northern Europe. Unlike most of the other pathogens discussed here, its incidence increases in the winter months. It grows at 4°C, which explains why contaminated refrigerated meat products and milk are important sources of infection. It causes a syndrome similar to that caused by *Salmonella* species; however, there is an increased incidence of metastatic infection with abscess formation in the spleen, liver, and lungs, particularly in compromised hosts. Patients on steroids or cirrhotics or those receiving desferrioxamine for iron overload are particularly prone to this complication [66]. A second *Yersinia* species, *Yersinia pseudotuberculosis* is an important cause of mesenteric adenitis. *Y. enterocolitica* is usually susceptible to the fluoroquinolones, trimethoprim-sulfamethoxazole, and aminoglycosides. Up to 8% of patients with *Y. enterocolitica* may have an accompanying exudative pharyngitis. Erythema nodosum has been reported in up to 30% of cases.

Hemorrhagic Colitis

After an incubation period of about 4 days, patients with hemorrhagic colitis develop crampy abdominal pain and watery diarrhea that becomes bloody, usually within 1 day. Most patients are afebrile and have no white cells in the stool. Bacteremia, local complications, and metastatic infection are rare. The differential diagnosis includes other causes of GI bleeding, particularly ischemic colitis. The illness typically lasts 2–9 days. This syndrome is caused by VTEC. Serotypes associated with verotoxin production include 0157:H7, 04, 05, 026, 0111, 0125, and 0145. Hemolytic uremic syndrome and thrombotic thrombocytopenic purpura may complicate diarrhea due to VTEC [67].

Viral Gastroenteritis

Adenovirus types 40 and 41, calcivirus, astrovirus, Norwalk virus, Norwalk-like agents (Snow Mountain, Ditchling, Hawaii), and rotavirus have all been identified as etiological agents in patients with diarrhea. They most commonly present as watery diarrhea (similar to enterotoxin-mediated bacterial process) with vomiting a prominent part of the symptom complex. Of these agents rotavirus and Norwalk virus are the best studied.

Rotavirus

After an incubation period of 1–3 days patients develop a severe watery diarrhea. Infants and children up to 2 years old are most affected, with adults typically being asymptomatic or only mildly symptomatic [68]. Disease occurs primarily in the winter as sporadic cases. In the United States rotavirus accounts for nearly half of pediatric diarrhea cases that require hospitalization [69]. Fever is occasionally present in severe cases. White cells usually are not seen in the stool. The diagnosis is made by enzyme-linked immunosorbent assay (ELISA) testing. Treatment is supportive.

Norwalk Virus

Infection with Norwalk virus typically affects older children and adults, with infants often being spared [69]. It occurs year round, often in epidemics. The incubation period is usually about 24 hours, with symptoms including watery diarrhea, nausea, and vomiting. Fever and cells in the stool are not seen. Contaminated shellfish, water, and raw vegetables have been among identified vehicles [70]. Diagnosis is limited by the lack of widely available commercial detection kits. Treatment is supportive with symptoms usually abating in 1–3 days.

Sexually Transmitted Diseases

Several common sexually transmitted diseases (STDs) may present as rectal pain, discharge, bleeding, or diarrhea. These diseases are particularly important considerations in patients who are recipients of anal intercourse. Physical examination of the perianal area for the presence of vesicles, warts, fissures, or chancres may be diagnostic. Similarly a rectal Gram's stain showing gram-negative diplococci and WBCs is highly suggestive of *Neisseria gonorrhoeae*. Sigmoidoscopy assists in identifying the extent of disease, which limits the differential diagnosis [71]. For patients with proctitis (disease limited to distal 15 cm), the most common pathogens are *N. gonorrhoeae*, herpes simplex virus, *Chlamydia trachomatis*, and *Treponema pallidum*. A Tzanck smear and culture (for herpes virus) of perirectal vesicles or dark-field examination of any ulcers (syphilis) assist in making the diagnosis. Patients with sigmoidoscopic abnormalities extending beyond 15 cm (proctocolitis) may have *Lymphogranuloma venereum* or a common enteric pathogen (*Shigella*, *Campylobacter* species, or *Entamoeba histolytica*). As in other settings the diagnosis of one sexually transmitted infection should prompt a consideration of others, including HIV.

Diarrhea in the Patient with HIV Infection

The differential diagnosis of diarrheal disease in patients infected with HIV is very broad and includes common bacterial and viral causes, opportunists, malignancies, and primary infection (see Chap. 17). Abnormal D-xylose absorption, steattorhea, and jejunal and rectal biopsy abnormalities have all been attributed to infection with HIV [72]. Giant aphthous ulcerations, Kaposi's sarcoma, and lymphoma are important noninfective processes that may present with GI symptoms or findings [73].

Cryptosporidium species, *I. belli*, cytomegalovirus (CMV), *Mycobacterium* species, and *Histoplasma capsulatum* are opportunistic processes that can produce diarrhea or other abdominal symptoms in patients with HIV infection. An acid-fast stain of the stool or sugar flotation smear assists in the diagnosis of *Cryptosporidium* organisms. *Mycobacterium avium* complex also can be detected by an acid-fast stain of the stool. Biopsy may be necessary to diagnose histoplasmosis or CMV. In patients with no pathogen identified, antimotility medications may decrease symptoms.

Recurrent bacteremia with *Salmonella* species has been reported in patients with HIV infection and may occur in the absence of GI symptoms [74, 75]. Breakthrough bacteremia has occurred on several different regimens. In one small study a 4-week course of ciprofloxacin prevented breakthrough bacteremia and recurrence, although follow-up was limited [76].

Diagnosis

A history of nausea and vomiting associated with a diarrheal syndrome is suggestive of a viral or an enterotoxin-mediated process. Patients should be questioned concerning the foods they have ingested during the several days prior to illness. For patients presenting with vomiting and watery diarrhea, foods ingested during the previous 12 hours are most suspect. An ingestion history of raw clams or oysters with a watery diarrhea syndrome makes *Vibrio* species and Norwalk virus important considerations. Well water may be a vehicle for *G. lamblia* and unpasteurized milk for *Salmonella*, *Campylobacter*, or *Yersinia* species. A history of exposure to other ill persons may assist in identifying the vehicle (a single common meal) or the pathogen if the contact has already been diagnosed.

Travel history is also important. In addition to enterotoxigenic *E. coli*, an important cause of traveler's diarrhea characterized by a watery diarrhea syndrome, travelers to developing nations are at higher risk to acquire parasitic infections. *Pleisiomonas shigelloides* and *Salmonella* species have been seen more commonly in travelers from Mexico and *G. lamblia* in travelers from Russia and western U.S. ski resorts [77, 78]. Malaria may present with fever and GI symptoms. This should be considered in travelers from malarious areas, particularly if there are no cells in the stool and the patient is anemic. Patients should also be asked about medicines they are taking, preexisting illnesses, and associated symptoms.

The presence of fever on physical examination is suggestive of an invasive pathogen. The patient's state of hydration should be carefully assessed. Orthostatic blood pressure and pulse measurements, assessment of skin turgor, mucous membranes, and mental status assist in this determination.

Most patients with diarrhea have normoactive or hyperactive bowel sounds. Patients with hypoactive or absent bowel sounds should be evaluated carefully for the presence of toxic megacolon or some other process that may require surgery. An abdominal mass or focal abdominal pain is also a clue to something other than an uncomplicated diarrheal syndrome.

The rest of the examination can also yield important information. The presence of a skin rash with desquamation beginning at the distal extremities and a swollen red tongue should suggest the possibility of toxic shock syndrome. Diarrhea and hypotension frequently are part of this process. Other illnesses associated with characteristic rashes—Rocky Mountain spotted fever, measles, Kawasaki's disease, and the hemorrhagic fevers (e.g., dengue)—often present with abdominal symptoms, including diarrhea.

The presence of focal neurologic abnormalities with diarrhea may be due to botulism (usually descending cranial nerve palsies), neurotoxic or paralytic shellfish poisoning, puffer fish intoxication, or ciguatera poisoning.

Of the laboratory information available in the emergency department the microscopic examination of the stool is particularly useful. The presence of WBCs is usually indicative of an invasive pathogen. If red cells are absent, invasive amebiasis is unlikely. The presence of red cells without white cells supports a diagnosis of VTEC. If curved gram-negative rods are seen, *Campylobacter* or *Vibrio* organisms are the most likely pathogens. Stains for ova and parasites also are often available while the patient is still in the emergency department. Stool cultures should be obtained in most cases if cells are noted in the stool and, for febrile or toxic-appearing patients, blood cultures are advised. Other blood studies may provide important information, but they are rarely diagnostic.

The Decision to Admit or Manage as an Outpatient

The most common reason a patient may require hospital admission is an inability to maintain a hydrated state. While rehydration usually can be achieved in the emergency department, the physician should consider whether it is likely the patient will remain hydrated after discharge. For example, a patient having five to seven stools per hour with frequent vomiting is likely to become dehydrated again quickly. Other patients who may require hospitalization include patients with neurologic abnormalities, abdominal examinations suggestive of a complication that may require surgery, serious underlying illnesses, and high fever and toxicity.

If patients are sent home, they should be instructed on methods of remaining hydrated and signs of dehydration (e.g., dizziness when standing). Several oral rehydration therapies have been demonstrated to effectively rehydrate and maintain hydration [79]. Dairy products should be avoided initially. Diet can be advanced from clear liquids as tolerated.

Patients with diarrhea should not prepare food for others, particularly food that is handled after cooking or food served uncooked (salads, fruits). They should be instructed to wash their hands thoroughly after using the bathroom. Separate bathroom facilities or other forms of isolation at home usually are not required. Siblings of infants and children with diarrhea are at high risk to acquire the illness due to cross-contamination while playing. Most efforts to control this situation are not practical.

Patients should be instructed to return to a physician if the illness worsens significantly or persists longer than 3–5 days. There should also be some method of contacting the patient for culture results.

Empiric antibiotic treatment should be considered in patients with an invasive syndrome who are moderately to severely ill, immunocompromised patients, and patients with a local or systemic complication (toxic megacolon, intestinal rupture, bacteremia). A fluoroquinolone (e.g., ciprofloxacin 500 mg bid PO) or the combination of erythromycin (500 mg qid PO) and trimethoprim-sulfamethoxazole (one double-strength bid) or a third-generation cephalosporin (e.g., cefotaxime 2 g q6h IV) will cover most common bacterial enteric pathogens. Antimicrobials can be given parenterally when there is a question of ulcer or intestinal rupture or when the patient cannot retain the regimen due to vomiting. It should be noted that quinolones are not approved for use in children or pregnant women. Additional coverage for amebiasis and the GI flora should be considered on an individual basis.

Postinfectious Complications

Most infectious diarrheal syndromes in immunocompetent patients are self-limited, with diarrhea rarely lasting longer than 7 days. Parasitic infections (e.g., amebiasis or giardiasis) and *Y. enterocolitica* are important exceptions, with diarrhea in these syndromes occasionally lasting weeks to months. Persistent diarrhea following an acute diarrheal syndrome may be due to one of these pathogens, or it may have a noninfectious etiology. After a bout with acute infectious diarrhea, some patients will slough a portion of their small bowel mucosal surface, resulting in a postinfectious malabsorption syndrome. Like other patients with malabsorption, diarrhea is worse after eating or drinking and minimal when intake is limited. Stool cultures are negative. The diagnosis is confirmed by small-bowel biopsy. Treatment is dietary, with the use of foods that are easily absorbed without intestinal enzyme degradation. Unlike patients with sprue, who have a similar biopsy picture, the mucosal surface regenerates over time. G. *lamblia* may produce a similar clinical picture. Stool examination for ova and parasites may be negative in giardiasis. In those cases small-bowel aspirate or biopsy is required for diagnosis.

A second postinfectious syndrome seen after some diarrheal illnesses is Reiter's syndrome. Reiter's syndrome includes an asymmetric arthritis, often involving large joints and the axial skeleton, keratoderma blennorrhagica (a thickening of the skin of the palms and soles, seen primarily in postvenereal Reiter's), conjunctivitis/uveitis, and urethritis. Not all these components are necessary to make a diagnosis. The presenting symptom in most patients is urethritis, with other symptoms following over the next 1–6 weeks. Reiter's syndrome may follow a diarrheal infection (infection with *Campylobacter*, *Salmonella*, *Shigella*, or *Yersinia* species and antibiotic-associated diarrhea) or an STD (gonorrhea, mycoplasma, and chlamydia). The majority of patients are positive for the HLA-B27 histocompatibility antigen, and most are male. Reiter's syndrome is treated with anti-inflammatory agents, particularly nonsteroidals.

The hemolytic uremic syndrome has complicated diarrheal illnesses, particularly those due to certain *E. coli* serotypes (primarily verotoxin-producing organisms), *S. dysenteriae*, and some enteroviruses (coxsackieviruses A4, B2, and B4 and echovirus 22). No specific therapy has been demonstrated to be consistently effective in the treatment of this syndrome.

Food-Borne Illnesses

A food-borne outbreak is defined as two or more persons having GI and/or neurologic symptoms within 72 hours of a common meal. The specific symptoms, food-specific attack rates, geographic location, and other factors assist in identifying the pathogen and the vehicle. In addition to reporting to public health officials numbers of patients and culture results, emergency departments can collect important epidemiologic information during outbreaks. Information that includes incubation periods, the specific foods each ill person ate from a common meal, and characteristics of the illness can greatly assist public health officials in their evaluation of the outbreak.

Scromboid

Also called histamine fish poisoning, scromboid usually occurs within 1 hour of ingesting a contaminated fish [80]. This syndrome consists of flushing, headache, dizziness, cramps, and sometimes diarrhea. Rarely urticaria and bronchospasm occur. Symptoms last only several hours and may respond to antihistamines. It is due to histamine and enzyme inhibitors present in the flesh of some fish, including tuna, mackerel, yellowjack, bluefish, and dolphin (mahimahi). The coastal areas of California and Hawaii are the most common geographic locations in the United States for scromboid syndrome. The Chinese restaurant syndrome, shellfish poisoning, and niacin poisoning are in this differential diagnosis.

Ciguatera

Ciguatera is the most common food-borne chemical intoxication. Ciguatoxin is found in a number of marine fish (including sea bass, grouper, and snapper), particularly near the Caribbean and Indo-Pacific islands. The toxin is produced in a dinoflagellate and passed up the food chain, eventually to humans. The toxin produces no noticeable change in the taste or other characteristics of the fish and is not inactivated by cooking, smoking, or other methods of preparation. No routine test is available to identify tainted fish. Symptoms usually occur within hours of eating the fish and consist of abdominal pain, paresthesias, temperature dysesthesias, weakness, and headache. Hypotension and bradycardia may occur and, rarely, respiratory failure. Symptoms may persist for months. Treatment is supportive, although mannitol provided relief of symptoms in one study [81]. Opiates, barbiturates, and alcohol can worsen symptoms.

Paralytic Shellfish Poisoning

Paralytic shellfish poisoning is another syndrome caused by ingesting a contaminated shellfish (mussel, clam, or scallop) that harbors a toxin produced by a dinoflagellate. It is most common during the summer months, with most cases in the United States reported from the Northeast and Pacific coastal states. There is a greater risk of poisoning during times of dinoflagellate blooms (red tides). The toxin is unaffected by steaming or routine cooking methods. Symptoms begin 30–45 minutes after ingestion and are primarily neurologic, consisting of paresthesias, ataxia, vertigo, paralysis, and cranial nerve dysfunction. Gastric lavage may remove some toxin, otherwise treatment is supportive. Airway management is particularly important. The mortality rate from this intoxication is nearly 10%, with most deaths occurring in the first 12 hours from respiratory failure. When suspected, patients should be observed for at least 24 hours or until neurologic symptoms are improving.

Neurotoxic Shellfish Poisoning

Neurotoxic shellfish poisoning is caused by a different toxin, which can contaminate mollusks. Symptoms usually occur within 3 hours of ingestion and are less severe than those seen in paralytic shellfish poisoning. Recovery usually occurs in 24–72 hours, with no fatalities reported. In the United States the toxin is found mainly in mollusks along the coast of Florida. The aerosolized toxin also can cause reversible rhinorrhea, conjunctivitis, and cough during red tides.

Amnesiac Shellfish Poisoning

In 1987 there was an outbreak in Canada of a syndrome consisting of diarrhea, abdominal pain, severe headache, and loss of short-term memory occurring within 48 hours of eating mussels [82]. Seizures, coma, and blood pressure instability complicated some cases. Severely affected patients had persistent memory deficits and motor neuropathies. Epidemiologic investigation traced this outbreak to contamination of mussels with domoic acid produced by a form of marine vegetation. Autopsy studies showed the hippocampus and amygdala to be particularly involved [83]. While no new cases have been reported, routine screening of mussels for this toxin does not occur.

Puffer Fish Poisoning

The puffer fish, or fugu, contains a potent neurotoxin (tetrodotoxin) concentrated in its skin and viscerae. Individuals who prepare this fish are required to undergo special training and to be licensed. The toxin is related to the toxin that causes paralytic shellfish poisoning and is associated with a mortality rate of nearly 60% [79]. Symptoms include lethargy, vomiting, paresthesias, hypotension, bradycardia, and paralysis. Gastric lavage may decrease further toxin absorption. Treatment is mainly supportive with careful attention to airway management and respiratory support. Most deaths occur within the first 24 hours.

Botulism

Botulism is caused by the elaboration of one of the botulinus toxins from Clostridium botulinum. Of the eight toxins that have been identified, three account for most disease in humans (types A, B, and E). The first symptoms usually begin about 12–36 hours after ingestion and consist of dizziness and malaise, progressing to a descending symmetrical paralysis. Nausea, vomiting, diarrhea, ulcer, and urinary retention are seen occasionally. Most patients complain of dry mouth. Patients are alert and afebrile. Postural hypotension and ocular findings (dilated pupils, palsies, ptosis) often are present.

Infant botulism occurs in infants under 1 year of age. Apparently due to a lack of inhibitory products found in adult GI flora, C. botulinum spores may generate in the infant's GI tract and produce toxin. In the United States infant botulism is now the most common form of botulism seen. Wound botulism can occur when a wound becomes contaminated with *C. botulinum* and anaerobic conditions exist, allowing toxin elaboration.

The diagnosis is confirmed by identifying the toxin in blood, stool, or food or identification of *C. botulinum* in stool or food. Treatment is primarily supportive, including early respiratory support. Antitoxin administration and penicillin treatment to eradicate stool carriage are recommended, although data to support penicillin therapy are lacking.

Heavy-Metal Intoxication

Ingestion of heavy metals, usually via contaminated beverages, produces a syndrome of nausea and vomiting. The incubation period is among the shortest for any illness, typically 15 minutes or less. Cadmium, zinc, tin, and copper have all produced this syndrome, with symptoms attributed to direct irritation of gastric mucosa. Symptoms usually resolve with emesis.

Anisakiasis

Anisakis larvae, which live in the gut of several different types of fish, may migrate to the muscle of the fish if it is not refrigerated. If the fish is then served without being fully cooked, the larvae penetrate the gastric mucosa, producing abdominal pain, nausea, and occasionally hematemesis several hours after ingestion. The larvae may produce eosinophilic granulomas in the small bowel or migrate to the oropharynx and stimulate coughing. Treatment is removal of the larvae via gastroscopy.

Mass Psychogenic Illness

Occasionally nausea and vomiting in one or two persons will precipitate similar symptoms in large numbers of observers. Ill persons often do not have a shared exposure. This most commonly occurs in persons aged 9–14 with symptoms of dizziness, itching, and rash, in addition to nausea and vomiting.

References

1. Snyder JD, Merson MH. The magnitude of the global problem of acute diarrheal disease: a review of active surveillance data. *Bull WHO* 60:605, 1987.

2. Bennett JV et al. Infectious and parasitic diseases. *Am J Prev Med* 3 (suppl.):102, 1987.

3. Koopman JS et al. Patterns and etiology of diarrhea in three clinical settings. *Am J Epidemiol* 119:114, 1984.

4. Tauxe RV, Deming MS, Blake PA. *Campylobacter jejuni* infections on college campuses: a national survey. *Am J Public Health* 77:659, 1985.

5. Rahaman MM, Huq I, Dey CR. Superiority of MacConkey's agar over *Salmonella-Shigella* agar for isolation of *Shigella dysenteriae* type 1. *J Infect Dis* 131:700, 1975.

6. Rahaman MM et al. An outbreak of dysentery caused by *Shigella dysenteriae* type I on a coral island in the Bay of Bengal. *J Infect Dis* 132:15, 1975.

7. Giannella RA, Broitman SA, Zamcheck N. Influence of gastric acidity on bacterial and parasitic enteric infections: a perspective. *Ann Intern Med* 78:271, 1973.

8. Gitelson S. Gastrectomy, achlorhydria and cholera. *Isr J Med Sci* 7:663, 1971.

9. Sprinz H. Pathogenesis of intestinal infections. *Arch Pathol* 87:556, 1969.

10. DuPont HL, Hornick RB. Adverse effect of Lomotil therapy in shigellosis. *JAMA* 226:1525, 1973.

11. Price DJE, Sleigh JD. Control of infection due to *Klebsiella aerogenes* in a neurosurgical unit by withdrawal of all antibiotics. *Lancet* 2:1213, 1970.

12. Mentzing LO, Ringertz O. *Salmonella* infection in tourists. 2. Prophylaxis against salmonellosis. *Acta Pathol Microbiol Scand* 74:405, 1968.

13. Bodey GP et al. Quantitative relationships between circulating leukocytes and infection in patients with acute leukemia. *Ann Intern Med* 64:328, 1966.

14. Yolken RH et al. Infectious gastroenteritis in bone-marrow transplant recipients. *N Engl J Med* 306:1009, 1982.

15. Hornick RB et al. The Broad Street pump revisited: response to volunteers to ingested cholera vibrios. *Bull NY Acad Med* 47:1181, 1971.

16. Ryan CA et al. Massive outbreak of antimicrobial-resistant salmonellosis traced to pasteurized milk. *JAMA* 258:3269–74, 1987.

17. Lund BM. Foodborne disease due to *Bacillus* and *Clostridium* species. *Lancet* 336:982–86, 1990.

18. Fekety R et al: Epidemiology of antibiotic-associated colitis. Isolation of *Clostridium difficile* from the hospital environment. *Am J Med* 70:906, 1981.

19. Gorbach SL, Edelman R. Introduction. *Rev Infect Dis* 8:S109, 1986.

20. Doyle MP. Pathogenic *Escherichia coli, Yersinia enterocolitica,* and *Vibrio parahaemolyticus*. *Lancet* 336:1111–15, 1990.

21. Sack DA et al. Prophylactic doxycycline for traveler's diarrhea. N Engl J Med 298:758–63, 1978.

22. DuPont HL et al. Antimicrobial agents in the prevention of travelers' diarrhea. Rev Infect Dis 8:S167, 1986.

23. Steffen R, Heusser R, DuPont HL. Prevention of travelers' diarrhea. Rev Infect Dis 8:151–59, 1986.

24. Ericsson CD et al. Ciprofloxacin or trimethoprim-sulfamethoxazole as initial therapy for travelers' diarrhea. Ann Intern Med 106:216–20, 1987.

25. Tranter HS. Foodborne staphylococcal illness. Lancet 336:1044–46, 1990.

26. Bean NH et al. Foodborne disease outbreaks, 5-year summary, 1983–1987. MMWR 39:15–57, 1990.

27. Thorne GM. (Moellering RC, Gorbach SL (eds.)). Diagnosis of infectious diarrheal diseases. Infect Dis Clin North Am 2:747–74, 1988.

28. De S et al. Doxycycline in the treatment of cholera. Bull WHO 54:177, 1976.

29. Rahaman MM et al. Effects of doxycycline in actively purging cholera patients: a double-blind clinical trial. Antimicrob Agents Chemother 10:610, 1976.

30. Goodman LJ et al. Empiric antimicrobial therapy of domestically acquired acute diarrhea in urban adults. Arch Intern Med 150:541–46, 1990.

31. Blaser MJ et al. Campylobacter enteritis in the United States. Ann Intern Med 98:360–65, 1983.

32. Bokkenheuser VD et al. Detection of enteric campylobacteriosis in children. J Clin Microbiol 9:227–32, 1979.

33. Blaser MJ et al. Isolation of Campylobacter fetus subsp. jejuni from Bangladeshi children. J Clin Microbiol 12:744–47, 1980.

34. Harris NV, Weiss NS, Nolan CM. The role of poultry and meats in the etiology of Campylobacter jejuni/ coli enteritis. Am J Public Health 76:407–11, 1986.

35. Harris NV et al. A survey of Campylobacter and other bacterial contaminants of pre-market chicken and retail poultry and meats, King County, Washington. Am J Public Health 76:401–6, 1986.

36. Sazie ESM, Titus AE. Rapid diagnosis of Campylobacter enteritis. Ann Intern Med 96:62, 1982.

37. Penner JL. The genus Campylobacter: a decade of progress. Clin Microbiol Rev 1:157–72, 1988.

38. Salazar-Lindo E et al. Early treatment with erythromycin of Campylobacter jejuni–associated dysentery in children. J Pediatr 109:355, 1986.

39. Goodman LJ et al. Comparative in vitro activity of ciprofloxacin against Campylobacter spp. and other bacterial enteric pathogens. Antimicrob Agents Chemother 25:504–6, 1984.

40. DuPont HL et al. Protection induced by oral live vaccine or primary infection. J Infect Dis 125:12, 1972.

41. Nelson JD et al. Trimethoprim-sulfamethoxazole therapy for shigellosis. JAMA 235:1239, 1976.

42. DuPont HL et al. Treatment of travelers' diarrhea with trimethoprim/sulfamethoxazole and with trimethoprim alone. N Engl J Med 307:841, 1982.

43. Larson HE et al. Clostridium difficile and the etiology of pseudomembranous colitis. Lancet 1:1063, 1978.

44. Batts DH et al. Treatment of antibiotic-associated Clostridium difficile diarrhea with oral vancomycin. J Pediatr 97:151, 1980.

45. Silva J, Batts DH, Fekety R. Treatment of Clostridium difficile colitis and diarrhea with vancomycin. Am J Med 71:815, 1981.

46. Tedesco F et al. Oral vancomycin for antibiotic-associated pseudomembranous colitis. Lancet 2:226, 1982.

47. Pashby NL, Bolton RP, Sherriff RJ. Oral metronidazole in Clostridium difficile colitis. Br Med J 1:1605, 1979.

48. Cherry RD et al. Metronidazole: an alternate therapy for antibiotic-associated colitis. Gastroenterology 82:849, 1982.

49. Bartlett JG et al. Symptomatic relapse after oral vancomycin therapy of antibiotic-associated pseudomembranous colitis. Gastroenterology 78:431, 1980.

50. Walters BAJ et al. Relapse of antibiotic-associated colitis: endogenous persistence of Clostridium difficile during vancomycin therapy. Gut 24:206, 1983.

51. Sargeaunt PG, Williams JE, Grene JD. The differentiation of invasive and noninvasive Entamoeba histolytica by isoenzyme electrophoresis. Trans R Soc Trop Med Hyg 72:519, 1978.

52. Sargeaunt PG et al. The epidemiology of Entamoeba histolytica in Mexico City. A pilot survey I. Trans R Soc Trop Med Hyg 74:653, 1980.

53. Adams EB, MacLeod IN. Invasive amebiasis. II. Amoebic liver abscess and its complications. Medicine (Baltimore) 56:325–34, 1977.

54. Juniper K. Parasitic diseases of the intestinal tract. In M Paulson (ed.), Gastroenterologic Medicine. Philadelphia: Lea & Febiger, 1969. Pp. 172.

55. Bennett IL Jr, Hook EW. Infectious diseases (some aspects of salmonellosis). Annu Rev Med 10:1, 1959.

56. U.S. Department of Health and Human Services. Centers for Disease Control Salmonella surveillance. Annual Summary. Washington, DC: U.S. Department of Health and Human Services, 1985.

57. Cohen ML et al. Turtle-associated salmonellosis in the United States. JAMA 243:1247, 1980.

58. Baine WB et al. Institutional salmonellosis. J Infect Dis 128:357, 1973.

59. Kanwar YS et al. Salmonellosis associated with abdominal aortic aneurysm. Arch Intern Med 134:1095, 1974.

60. Cohen PS et al. The risk of endothelial infection in adults with salmonella bacteremia. *Ann Intern Med* 89:931, 1978.

61. Aserkoff B, Bennett JV. Effect of antibiotic therapy in acute salmonellosis on the fecal excretion of salmonellae. *N Engl J Med* 281:636, 1969.

62. Pichler HET et al. Clinical efficacy of ciprofloxacin compared with placebo in bacterial diarrhea. *Am J Med* 82:329–32, 1987.

63. Diridl G, Pichler H, Wolf D. Treatment of chronic salmonella carriers with ciprofloxacin. *Eur J Clin Microbiol* 5:260–61, 1986.

64. Gotuzzo E et al. Use of norfloxacin to treat chronic typhoid carriers. *J Infect Dis* 157:1235–39, 1988.

65. Ferreccio C et al. Efficacy of ciprofloxacin in the treatment of chronic typhoid carriers. *J Infect Dis* 157:1235–39, 1988.

66. Chiu HY et al. Infection with *Yersinia enterocolitica* in patients with iron overload. *Br Med J* 292:97, 1986.

67. Harris AA. Hemorrhagic colitis and *Escherichia coli* 0157:H7—identifying a messenger while pursuing the message. *Mayo Clin Proc* 65:884–88, 1990.

68. Wenman WM et al. Rotavirus infection in adults: results of a prospective family study. *N Engl J Med* 301:303, 1979.

69. Fairchild PG, Blacklow NR. (Moellering RC, Gorbach SL (eds.)). Viral diarrhea. *Infect Dis Clin North Am* 2:677–84, 1988.

70. Morse DL et al. Widespread outbreaks of clam and oyster associated gastroenteritis: role of Norwalk virus. *N Engl J Med* 314:678–81, 1986.

71. Quinn TC et al. The polymicrobial origin of intestinal infections in homosexual men. *N Engl J Med* 309:576–82, 1983.

72. Gillin JS et al. Malabsorption and mucosal abnormalities of the small intestine in the acquired immunodeficiency syndrome. *Ann Intern Med* 102:619–22, 1985.

73. Bach MC et al. Aphthous ulceration of the gastrointestinal tract in patients with the acquired immunodeficiency syndrome (AIDS). *Ann Intern Med* 112:465–67, 1990.

74. Fischl MA et al. *Salmonella* bacteremia as manifestation of acquired immunodeficiency syndrome. *Arch Intern Med* 146:113–15, 1986.

75. Glaser JB et al. Recurrent *Salmonella typhimurium* bacteremia associated with the acquired immunodeficiency syndrome. *Ann Intern Med* 102:189–93, 1985.

76. Jacobson MA et al. Ciprofloxacin for *Salmonella* bacteremia in the acquired immunodeficiency syndrome (AIDS). *Ann Intern Med* 110:1027–29, 1989.

77. Holmberg SD et al. *Plesiomonas* enteric infections in the United States. *Ann Intern Med* 105:690–94, 1986.

78. Ryan CA, Hartgrett-Ben NT, Blake PA. *Salmonella typhi* infections in the United States, 1975–1984: increasing role of foreign travel. *Rev Infect Dis* 11:1–8, 1989.

79. Balistreri WF. Oral rehydration in acute infantile diarrhea. *Am J Med* 88:30S–33S, 1990.

80. Eastaugh, J, Shepherd S. Infectious and toxic syndromes from fish and shellfish consumption: a review. *Arch Intern Med* 149:1735–40, 1989.

81. Palafox NA et al. Successful treatment of ciguatera fish poisoning with intravenous mannitol. *JAMA* 259:2740–42, 1988.

82. Perl TM et al. An outbreak of toxic encephalopathy caused by eating mussels contaminated with domoic acid. *N Engl J Med* 322:1775–80, 1990.

83. Teitelbaum JS et al. Neurologic sequelae of domoic acid intoxication due to the ingestion of contaminated mussels. *N Engl J Med* 322:1781–86, 1990.

26

Hepatitis and Hepatic Abscess

HAROLD A. KESSLER
JOHN C. POTTAGE, JR.

Acute hepatitis is most commonly caused by the hepatotropic viruses hepatitis A virus (HAV), hepatitis B virus (HBV), the viruses that cause non-A, non-B hepatitis (NANB), hepatitis C virus (HCV), hepatitis D virus (HDV), and hepatitis E virus (HEV). Other viruses also have been implicated as a cause of hepatitis. These include Epstein-Barr virus (EBV), cytomegalovirus (CMV), herpes simplex virus, measles virus, enteroviruses, and adenoviruses. In persons traveling to certain parts of the world, hepatitis caused by viruses such as the yellow fever virus can develop. The viral causes of hepatitis are listed in Table 26-1. Acute hepatitis is also associated with bacterial sepsis, autoimmune illnesses, and drug or toxin exposure.

Viral hepatitis typically causes an asymptomatic to mildly symptomatic infection. However, a severe to fulminant course leading to death can sometimes occur. The major roles for the emergency department physician in the evaluation of viral hepatitis are threefold: (1) initiation of diagnostic testing, (2) determination of the severity of the illness and the need for hospitalization, and (3) prophylaxis for and counseling of patients exposed to various forms of viral hepatitis.

Signs and Symptoms of Viral Hepatitis

Symptomatic acute viral hepatitis progresses through three stages: incubation, clinical illness, and convalescence. During the incubation stage

the patient is asymptomatic. The period of clinical illness has two phases [1]. The preicteric phase, which lasts 2–10 days, is characterized by non-specific symptoms without jaundice—fatigue, malaise, anorexia, distaste for cigarettes, nausea, vomiting, and abdominal pain. In addition a low-grade fever and headache may be present. Some patients with hepatitis B or, rarely, with hepatitis A or NANB hepatitis may develop a serum sickness syndrome, with urticarial rash, migratory arthralgias, and a low-grade fever.

The onset of jaundice signals the transition to the icteric phase. Initially the patient notices darkening of the urine or lightening of the feces. Pruritus often occurs. Toward the conclusion of the icteric phase, which generally lasts 2–4 weeks, the non-specific symptoms begin to recede.

As jaundice disappears, the patient enters the convalescent stage. This stage varies in length and is characterized by fatigue and malaise. With the exception of hepatitis B and its associated serum sickness syndrome, it is impossible to distinguish among the various causes of viral hepatitis on the basis of symptoms [1].

The most frequent physical examination findings relate to the skin and the abdomen. Jaundice is most common; urticaria, excoriations resulting from pruritus, and spider angiomas also may be present [1]. Signs of chronic liver disease, such as ascites, dependent edema, and prominent abdominal veins, are usually absent. Tenderness is often elicited in the right upper quadrant of the abdo-

607

Table 26-1. Viral causes of acute hepatitis

Hepatotropic Viruses
Hepatitis A virus
Hepatitis B virus
Hepatitis C virus
Hepatitis D virus
Hepatitis E virus

Herpes Viruses
Epstein-Barr virus
Cytomegalovirus
Herpes simplex virus
Varicella-zoster virus

Other
Measles virus
Paramyxovirus
Rubella virus
Enteroviruses (coxsackie-virus A and B, echovirus)
Adenoviruses
Yellow fever virus
Lassa virus
Ebola virus
Marburg virus

men. Fifty to 70% of patients with viral hepatitis have hepatomegaly; 25% have splenomegaly [1].

Routine biochemical testing reveals at least a tenfold increase in the serum transaminases, alanine aminotransferase (ALT), and aspartate aminotransferase (AST). The transaminases become abnormal during the late incubation and early pre-icteric periods. Hepatocellular enzymes peak during the icteric period and return to normal during the convalescent period. The levels of alkaline phosphatase (ALP) and other enzymes indicative of cholestasis, such as serum leucine aminopeptidase and 5'-nucleotidase, are only minimally elevated, as is lactic dehydrogenase. On rare occasions a cholestatic picture can predominate and may persist well into the convalescent phase.

The prothrombin time (PT), a measure of hepatic synthetic function, serves as a rough guide to the severity of acute hepatitis. Individuals with markedly prolonged PTs usually require hospitalization for closer observation and treatment of severe hepatic dysfunction. Patients with severe hepatic dysfunction and encephalopathy may also have elevated ammonia levels.

The CBC count tends to be normal, as does the WBC differential, but lymphocytosis may occur. A large number of atypical lymphocytes (> 10%) suggests the possibility of an EBV or CMV infection.

The constellation of previously described signs and symptoms, in the presence of marked elevations of transaminases and bilirubin but without other organ-system involvement, makes the diagnosis of viral hepatitis clinically secure. Serologic assays are required to identify the cause; unfortunately they are not always conclusive. Patients with hepatitis B have a less favorable prognosis than those with hepatitis A; hepatitis B and hepatitis C can cause chronic disease. Chronic disease (> 6 months) is never seen with hepatitis A virus.

Specific Etiologies of Viral Hepatitis

Hepatitis A

VIROLOGY
HAV is a single-stranded RNA enterovirus 27 nm in diameter that is a member of the *Picornavirus* family. The virus has an icosahedral shape and is surrounded by a nucleocapsid containing the antigenic determinants. It has no lipid envelope [2, 3].

EPIDEMIOLOGY
HAV has a worldwide distribution and is transmitted primarily via the fecal-oral route. Close personal contact with an infected person accounts for most cases of HAV infection. Ingestion of sewage-contaminated water and food is another important source for infection. The most common foods implicated in transmission of HAV are bivalve shellfish and mollusks, including clams, oysters, and mussels. Of note is the fact that there is no way to screen for contamination, and infected shellfish appear normal. Therefore, any history of ingestion of raw shellfish should raise suspicion to hepatitis A [2, 4, 5]. Outbreaks associated with infected food handlers in restaurants, cafeterias, and college dormitories have been well described. Additionally outbreaks associated with day care centers have been described [2, 6, 7]. Sexual transmission of HAV occurs particularly among homosexual men who engage in oral-anal contact [8].

Depending on the country and the regional sanitation, 25%–80% of the adult population have antibodies to HAV. After the virus is ingested, it initially replicates in the upper GI tract, and a brief viremia period follows. HAV then localizes in the liver, where it replicates. It is then secreted into the GI tract and the feces [2, 3].

CLINICAL PRESENTATION

Clinical illness follows an incubation period of 14–45 days. Maximal viral shedding into the feces occurs late in the incubation period, several days before clinical symptoms occur. As with all types of viral hepatitis, it is impossible to distinguish clinically the exact viral etiology [2, 3, 7]. Other clinical signs and symptoms associated with HAV infection include a mild erythematous maculopapular rash, arthralgias, and mild diarrhea [2, 9]. Diarrhea occurs more commonly in children, but it is also seen in approximately 18% of adult patients with hepatitis A [2]. The diarrhea typically is mild and noninflammatory with no WBCs seen on a Wright stain. A sore throat, cough, and upper respiratory tract symptoms are sometimes seen [10]. Rarer presentations include renal failure due to glomerulonephritis, vasculitis, and meningoencephalitis [2, 9].

DIAGNOSIS

Measurement of serum antibodies confirms the diagnosis. Anti-HAV-IgM antibodies appear in the serum just before the onset of clinical symptoms, peak shortly thereafter, and usually are detectable for 1–3 months. Detection of these antibodies using currently available immunoassays confirms the presence of acute HAV infection. Anti-HAV-IgG antibodies begin to rise during the period of clinical illness and generally persist for the life of the patient. These antibodies are neutralizing and afford lifelong protection against reinfection [1, 2, 7]. Chronic lifelong illness with HAV does not occur, although prolonged illness with evidence of viral replication over several months does occur rarely [9, 11].

Hepatitis A should be suspected clinically if there is no history of exposure to blood or other body fluids. The patient may have a close contact with similar symptoms. Emergency department management of hepatitis A is discussed later in this chapter.

Hepatitis B

VIROLOGY

HBV is a member of the *Hepadnaviridae* family. The infectious HBV virion is 42 nm in diameter and circular with a double-stranded DNA genome within a nucleocapsid core surrounded by a outer lipoprotein envelope. Determinants of the hepatitis B core antigen (HBcAg) are associated with the core protein, while the hepatitis B virus surface antigen (HBsAg) determinants are associated with the outer lipid envelope. Hepatitis B e antigen is a protein associated with the HBV core particle, which is antigenically distinct. A unique HBV DNA polymerase enzyme is also found associated with the HBcAg particle [12, 13].

EPIDEMIOLOGY

Hepatitis B is a worldwide health problem. It is predominantly a blood-borne viral infection that is transmitted via percutaneous inoculation or contamination of mucous membranes with infected blood or body fluids. Virtually all body fluids of acute or chronically ill infected patients have been shown to contain HBsAg, but transmission has been documented only by blood, blood products, saliva, and semen. The incubation period of clinical illness averages 75 days, although it may be as short as 40 days or as long as 180. Evidence of viral replication in the host can be detected as early as 7 days following exposure. HBV particles circulate in the blood of actively infected patients for weeks to months, as indicated by the presence of HBsAg, HBV-DNA, or HBV-DNA polymerase activity. Approximately 90% of HBV-infected patients will clear the virus from the bloodstream within 6 months and are considered to have recovered from the infection. Disappearance of HBsAg and appearance of antibodies to HBsAg (anti-HBs) is evidence of recovery. An additional 5% clear the infection in 12–18 months. In the United States the remaining 5% of patients remain chronically infected for life and constitute the reservoir for transmission of the virus [12, 13].

Although HBV infection is relatively uncommon among the general population in the United States, certain groups of people have a high prevalence rate. These groups include those who acquired the disease through perinatal transmission in parts of the world where the rates of HBV endemicity are high. Persons from Southeast Asia, China, Africa, the Pacific Islands, and the Amazon basin and Alaskan natives are included in this group [14–16]. Persons with high-intensity exposure to blood or blood products also have an increased rate of HBV infection. This group includes IV drug users; health care workers, particularly laboratory technologists; nurses, especially those working in the emergency department, hematology/ oncology units, operating rooms, and dialysis units; and physicians, surgeons, gynecologists, and pathologists. Other groups include persons from institutions for the developmentally disabled, male prisoners, sexually active homosexual men, and sexually promiscuous heterosexuals who do not practice safe sex. The incidence of cases of acute hepatitis B has decreased significantly in homosexuals and health care workers over the past several years. There has been a disturbing increase however, in IV drug users and heterosexually active individuals [14–16].

CLINICAL PRESENTATION
Hepatitis B can present with a serum-sickness-type syndrome, characterized by an urticarial rash, migratory arthralgias, and a low-grade fever [17]. Although this occurs most commonly with hepatitis B, it has been described with hepatitis A and hepatitis C. After this prodrome signs and symptoms of hepatitis B occur, indistinguishable from the signs and symptoms of other types of viral hepatitis. These include fatigue, malaise, anorexia, nausea, vomiting, and abdominal pain. Rare accompanying symptoms that can occur include glomerulonephritis; skin lesions, including acrodermatitis and erythema nodosum; hematologic manifestations, including aplastic anemia, agranulocytosis, and thrombocytopenia; and neurologic manifestations, including aseptic meningitis, meningoencephalitis, and Guillian-Barré syndrome [12, 13, 17].

DIAGNOSIS
Immunologic methods to detect HBV antigens and antibodies are used to confirm the diagnosis. The earliest identifiable marker of HBV infection is HBsAg, which is present as early as 7–14 days following infection. It is detected in 96% of patients and tends to decrease in titer as the patient's clinical condition improves. Antibodies to HBsAg appear weeks to months after the onset of acute infec-

tion. The appearance of anti-HBs antibodies indicates that the patient's blood is no longer infectious and the patient has successfully recovered from the infection [12, 13].

HBcAg particles are found only in infected hepatocytes and are never detectable in the serum. Antibodies to HBcAg, however, appear shortly after HBsAg is detectable. These antibodies are present for the life of the patient and are the best single serologic marker for current, recent, or past HBV infection. The presence of anti-HBc IgM denotes active or recent infection and it is generally present in the serum for 1–3 months following the acute infection [12, 13].

HBVe antigen (HBeAg) is present in the serum at the onset of clinical symptoms. HBeAg appears to be a protein constituent of the HBV core particle that is antigenically distinct from HBsAg and HBcAg. Detection of HBeAg in the serum of infected patients is correlated with active replication of HBV in the liver. Typically as the infection progresses, HBeAg disappears from the serum and antibodies to HBeAg (anti-HBe) appear. The disappearance of HBeAg indicates that HBV replication has decreased or ended and that the infectivity of the patient's serum is markedly diminished. Of note, however, is that all blood and body fluids positive for HBsAg must be considered potentially infectious, whether or not HBeAg is present. The disappearance of HBeAg and the appearance of anti-HBe is always a good prognostic finding and is generally followed by a decrease in transaminase levels [12, 13]. Emergency department management of hepatitis B is discussed later in this chapter.

Hepatitis D
VIROLOGY
First referred to as the delta agent, HDV is a replicative defective RNA virus that uses the outer lipid envelope of HBV, that is, HBsAg, to complete its replication, resulting in a 35-nm to 37-nm particle resembling hepatitis B. HBsAg determinants are found on its surface, and the internal component is the delta agent, which has hepatitis D antigen determinants [18–20].

EPIDEMIOLOGY
HDV infection is dependent on a coincident or concurrent HBV infection and, therefore, is always associated with hepatitis B virus infections. In the

United States HDV is found almost entirely among hemophiliacs and IV drug abusers [18–20].

CLINICAL PRESENTATION

Simultaneous infection with HBV and HDV may cause the typical acute viral hepatitis syndrome or subclinical disease. The acute illness may sometimes be biphasic with two peaks of transaminase elevation. HDV is also important to consider when a patient who is a chronic carrier of HBsAg develops a new episode of icteric hepatitis. When HBV infection is associated with a simultaneous or sequential HDV infection, it is thought to be more severe, have a higher mortality, and to be associated with a greater incidence of chronic active hepatitis [18–20].

DIAGNOSIS

Serologic tests for IgM and IgG antibodies to HDV performed in a sequential fashion will establish the diagnosis.

Non-A and Non-B Hepatitis

Until recently the causes of NANB hepatitis have remained unidentified. The diagnosis was made in patients who had clinical or biochemical evidence of hepatitis and serologies that excluded infections by HAV, HBV, HDV, EBV, and CMV. In 1989, however, a serologic assay was developed through recombinant DNA technology that identified the most common cause of the parenteral transmitted type of NANB hepatitis in the United States. This virus is HCV [21, 22]. Additionally a second virus, HEV, has been associated with an enterically spread epidemic variety of NANB hepatitis [23, 24].

HEPATITIS C

Virology. HCV is a lipid-enveloped RNA virus measuring 30–60 nm in diameter. The virus has tentatively been classified as a flavivirus [21, 22].

Epidemiology. HCV infections are common, with approximately 1% of the U.S. population being infected [25]. Hepatitis C virus is spread via parenteral contact and is the most common cause of posttransfusion hepatitis in the United States. Now that blood can be screened for hepatitis C prior to transfusion, the incidence should decrease. The

risk factors for acquiring HCV mimic those of acquiring HBV [26]. Of note, however, is that spread via close personal contact does not seem to occur as commonly as it does for hepatitis B [27]. The incubation period is between that of HAV and HBV, ranging from 14–120 days, with a peak at 42–56 days.

Clinical Course. The clinical course of the disease is similar to that of hepatitis B, with the majority of patients being asymptomatic. As with all causes of viral hepatitis, the signs and symptoms of hepatitis C are indistinguishable from other types of the disease. Associated symptoms that rarely occur with acute HCV include a serum sickness syndrome with arthralgia and rash. Pancreatitis also has been described in association with HCV disease [26, 28].

Diagnosis. Although measurement of antibodies to HCV will confirm the diagnosis of this infection, the antibody response usually is delayed. Therefore, most patients with acute HCV infections will not demonstrate a positive antibody response when seen in the emergency department. The antibody response occurs approximately 3 months after initial infection. The diagnosis of acute HCV infection continues to be a diagnosis of exclusion [29]. Fulminant hepatitis due to HCV is rare and is less common than that associated with hepatitis B. The mortality rate for HCV infection is between those of HAV and HBV, at approximately 0.5%–1.0% of patients with icteric hepatitis. Fulminant hepatitis due to HCV may occur more frequently in those with underlying liver disease, such as alcoholic liver disease [26, 30, 31]. Of special note is that there is a high incidence (50%) of chronic liver disease following acute HCV infection. For the most part chronic disease due to HCV is mild and continues for many years. Development of cirrhosis, hepatic failure, or hepatocellular carcinoma can occur. HCV infection is probably the most common cause of cryptogenic liver disease in the United States [26, 32].

HEPATITIS E

HEV has been associated with several water-borne outbreaks in India, central Asia, Africa, Mexico, and Central America. The specific virologic classification is unknown at present but may be related to the calciviruses, which are GI pathogens in lower animals. Viral particles measuring 27–32 nm that are unrelated to HAV or other enteroviruses have been isolated in stool suspension of infected patients [23, 24, 33].

The disease caused by HEV is transmitted via the fecal-oral route, and outbreaks have been associated with water contaminated by sewage. Cases have occurred worldwide; however, virtually all cases in the United States have been imported [24].

The signs and symptoms of HEV infection are similar to those of other types of hepatitis. The incubation period is approximately 40 days. Transaminases are usually only moderately elevated, although the disease seems to be more severe in pregnant women. Chronic disease has not been associated with HEV infection [24, 33, 34].

The diagnosis of disease due to HEV is one of exclusion. The disease should be considered likely in patients with acute hepatitis who have recently traveled to areas of the world where HEV infection has been described. Serologic testing is not available at present.

Other Causes of Viral Hepatitis

Acute hepatitis can occur in association with a mononucleosis syndrome characterized by fever, sore throat, and lymphadenopathy. On the peripheral blood smear atypical lymphocytes are present. Viruses associated with this syndrome include EBV, CMV, and the human immunodeficiency virus (HIV). The vast majority of these patients have EBV.

Approximately 90% of patients with EBV mononucleosis have elevated transaminases. Only a small percentage, however, develop icteric hepatitis. Although atypical lymphocytes can be seen with primary viral hepatitis, a large percentage (> 10%) of atypical lymphocytes is seen almost exclusively with EBV. Patients suspected of having EBV infection but presenting in atypical fashion should have specific EBV serologic testing, because the nonspecific heterophile antibody (i.e., Monospot type tests) may be falsely positive in acute HBV infections. The presence of IgM antibodies to the viral capsid antigen of the EBV will confirm the diagnosis.

Acute CMV infection also is frequently associated with elevated transaminases. Mononucleosis associated with CMV tends to have less intense symptomatology, with a milder or even absent pharyngitis and less prominent lymphadenopathy, than that seen in EBV infection (see Chap. 10). Atypical lymphocytes may not be as prominent as in EBV infection. A CMV-induced "post-pump" syndrome characterized by prolonged low-grade fever, lymphocytosis, and mild elevation of transaminases has been reported in patients following open heart surgery. In addition to a pattern of elevated transaminases, CMV can also cause a cholestatic hepatitis, with elevation of alkaline phosphatase and bilirubin and minimal transaminase elevation. Diagnosis rests with obtaining acute and convalescent IgM and IgG serology. Additionally, urine and blood can be sent for culture or cytopathology.

An acute HIV infection can sometimes present as a mononucleosis syndrome characterized by skin rash, fever, sore throat, and lymphadenopathy. Transaminases may be elevated but are generally less than five times normal values. Confirmation of diagnosis consists of demonstration of positive serology [35].

A fulminant progressive hepatitis has been described in association with herpes simplex virus [36]. Although the majority of these patients are immunocompromised (usually transplant patients), pregnancy also seems to be a risk factor. A marked elevation in transaminase levels and disseminated intravascular coagulation characterize this infection. Serologic testing is not useful, and diagnosis depends chiefly on review of pathologic specimens and viral culture of liver tissue [36]. Varicella-zoster virus also can be associated with a severe hepatitis in the immunocompromised host.

Childhood exanthematous illnesses, particularly measles and rubella, have been associated with hepatitis [37–39]. The majority of patients with measles hepatitis have the characteristic rash of measles, although measles hepatitis has been described in patients without the rash. Recent outbreaks of measles in the United States have made measles hepatitis more common, and measles should be considered in the differential diagnosis of hepatitis, particularly if there is an outbreak in the community. Associated symptoms of cough, coryza, and conjunctivitis should alert the emergency department physician to the diagnosis of measles. For the most part measles hepatitis follows a benign course [37, 38]. Rubella hepatitis also is benign [39].

Recently a form of hepatitis presenting as a severe form of NANB hepatitis and characterized by large syncytial giant hepatocytes has been described. Particles resembling paramyxoviruses can be seen with an electron microscope, but staining with antimeasles antibody is negative, indicating that this virus is distinct from measles [40].

Other viruses associated with transient elevations of transaminases include enteroviruses (particularly coxsackievirus B) and adenoviruses. Hepatitis usually is found incidentally and follows a benign course. The diagnosis usually is made with acute and convalescent serology [41].

Several types of viral hepatitis need to be considered in persons returning from Africa, Central America, or South America, including infections caused by yellow fever virus, Lassa virus, Marburg virus, and Ebola virus. The incubation period for yellow fever is short (4–7 days), and the disease is characterized by a biphasic course with a 1- or 2-day period of nonspecific symptoms (fever, malaise, headache, nausea, and vomiting) followed by improvement and then worsening symptoms characterized by progressive hepatic and renal failure and GI bleeding. Diagnosis rests on serology or viral culture of the blood [42]. Hepatitis associated with Lassa, Marburg, and Ebola viruses is usually part of a hemorrhagic fever syndrome [43].

Bacterial Causes of Hepatitis

Bacterial infections can occasionally present as an acute hepatitis syndrome mimicking viral hepatitis. Infections in this group include syphilis, leptospirosis, and granulomatous hepatitis. Although secondary syphilis can present as an acute hepatitis syndrome with elevated transaminases, jaundice, and right upper quadrant pain, other signs and symptoms pointing to the diagnosis of syphilis usually are present. These signs include diffuse lymphadenopathy and the characteristic maculopapular rash. In congenital syphilis an infant may present with hepatosplenomegaly, jaundice, rash, and the "snuffles." Diagnosis rests with obtaining specific syphilis serology, either the fluorescent treponemal antibody (FTA) or the microhemagglutination assay–*Treponema pallidum* (MHA-TP). Nonspecific

syphilis serology such as the rapid plasma reagin (RPR) or VDRL may be falsely positive with autoimmune causes of hepatitis [44].

Severe forms of leptospirosis can present with hepatic dysfunction in association with fever, renal failure, thrombocytopenia, altered mental status, hypotension, and cardiac dysfunction. Of special note is that the hepatic dysfunction of leptospirosis is characterized by only slight transaminase elevation (two to five times the normal level) accompanying a marked elevation in the bilirubin (10–20 times the normal level). Liver biopsy shows minimal hepatic necrosis. The diagnosis usually is made with serology. Epidemiologic clues for the diagnosis of leptospirosis include a history of exposure to water contaminated with the urine of infected animals. Animals typically implicated in the United States are dogs, cattle, and pigs [45]. (See Chap. 12.)

Granulomatous hepatitis generally is characterized by nonspecific signs and symptoms. Prolonged fever and fatigue are common presenting symptoms. Less commonly patients will have abdominal pain. On physical examination hepatomegaly or splenomegaly is seen in more than 50% of patients. Signs of chronic liver disease occur in fewer than 10% of the patients [46, 47]. Typically in granulomatous hepatitis, the transaminases are only slightly elevated and the ALP is markedly elevated. Bilirubin usually is normal. A large number of bacteria, fungi, and viruses have been associated with granulomatous hepatitis. Since the diagnosis of granulomatous hepatitis requires a liver biopsy, the role of the emergency department physician is limited to recognizing the possibility of the diagnosis and assessing the severity of the illness. Most diagnostic testing is done after the patient has left the emergency department. A list of infectious causes of granulomatous hepatitis is presented in Table 26-2 [46, 47].

Finally nonspecific elevations in transaminases and bilirubin can be seen with a variety of bacterial syndromes. This has been well described with bacterial pneumonia as well as sepsis. Liver biopsy shows nonspecific changes and little necrosis, and the clinical course is benign [48]. Diseases of the biliary tract, such as cholecystitis and cholangitis, can result in an increase of transaminases and bilirubin (see Chap. 27.)

Table 26-2. Infectious causes of
granulomatous hepatitis

Bacteria
Mycobacterium tuberculosis
Atypical mycobacteria
Mycobacteria leprae
Tularemia
Brucellosis
Melioidosis
Granuloma inguinale
Listeria
Syphilis
Nocardia
Actinomycosis

Rickettsia
Coxiella burnetti (Q fever)

Fungi
Histoplasmosis
Coccidioidomycosis
Blastomycosis
Paracoccidiodomycosis
Candidiasis
Aspergillus
Cryptococcosis

Parasites
Schistosomiasis
Ascaris
Toxocara species
Amebiasis
Fascioliasis

Noninfectious Causes of Hepatitis

There is a variety of noninfectious causes of the acute hepatitis syndrome. Medication-, alcohol-, and toxin-induced hepatitis closely mimic infectious hepatitis; thus, all patients in the emergency department with hepatitis should be closely questioned about medication, alcohol, and toxin exposure. Medications most associated with hepatitis include acetaminophen, aspirin, phenytoin, phenothiazines, monoamine oxidase inhibitors, alpha methyldopa, and antibiotics, including sulfa drugs, isoniazid, rifampin, oxacillin, erythromycin, and ketoconazole (see Chap. 4). Typically the transaminase and bilirubin levels are markedly elevated. Erythromycin and the phenothiazines usually present as a cholestasis syndrome. Serologic testing for viral hepatitis may be required to differentiate toxin-induced hepatitis from viral hepatitis.

Alcoholic hepatitis is seen frequently in emergency department patients. Patients who are HBsAg carriers are more susceptible to developing alcoholic hepatitis even at low levels of alcohol intake. Transaminase levels may be several times normal but usually are not as elevated as in viral hepatitis. Furthermore, in alcoholic hepatitis AST levels usually are higher than ALT levels.

Ingestion of poisonous mushrooms can cause a fulminant hepatitis. *Amanita phalloides* is most associated with hepatic dysfunction. A history of collecting and ingesting mushrooms from the woods usually should be obtained.

Other conditions leading to abnormal liver function tests include right-sided heart failure, Wilson's disease, hepatic vein thrombosis, and space-occupying diseases of the liver.

Fulminant Hepatitis

Fulminant hepatitis is a rare complication of viral hepatitis that can lead to death. It is most commonly associated with hepatitis B but can occur with hepatitis A and the various forms of NANB hepatitis. It can occur at any time in the course of acute viral hepatitis and is characterized by massive hepatic necrosis leading to hepatic encephalopathy, coma, GI bleeding, and possibly death. Signs and symptoms associated with fulminant hepatitis include fetor hepaticus, progressive jaundice, shrinkage of the liver, GI bleeding, and changes in mental status. Mental status changes may be subtle at first and consist of only mild lethargy. In more advanced cases stupor and coma may be present. Laboratory studies usually show markedly elevated transaminases, bilirubin, and ammonia levels. The PT is markedly prolonged and usually does not respond to vitamin K therapy. Patients with fulminant hepatitis need immediate hospitalization. Therapy includes a low-protein diet, cleansing enemas, lactulose, and vigorous treatment of coagulation defects and electrolyte abnormalities. Corticosteroids often are used in this situation. Other considerations for therapy include emergency liver transplantation [49–51].

Table 26-3. Testing for viral hepatitis*

Serologic test results			
HAV IgM	HBsAg	Anti-HBc IgM	Interpretation
Negative	Negative	Negative	Possible NANB hepatitis; check EBV, CMV serology
Negative	Negative	Positive	Possible active or recent HBV: check anti-HBs, anti-HBe
Negative	Positive	Positive	New HBV infection
Positive	Positive	Negative	HAV infection in patient with chronic HBV
Positive	Negative	Negative	New HAV infection
Negative	Positive	Negative	Early HBV infection

*Delta hepatitis should always be considered when there is evidence of new or old active HBV infection.

Management in the Emergency Department

No specific treatment of viral hepatitis is available; therefore, treatment is supportive. A patient suspected of having viral hepatitis by history or physical examination should have blood taken for a complete blood count, platelet count, electrolytes, BUN, creatinine, glucose, and liver studies, including AST, ALT, ALP, and bilirubin. It is important that the PT also be determined. The initial blood for diagnostic testing also should be drawn in the emergency department. This should include a HAV/IgM, HBsAg, and anti-HBcIgM. If the white blood cell differential shows more than 10% atypical lymphocytes and the liver transaminases are minimally elevated, the mononucleosis syndrome, especially EBV mononucleosis and acute HIV infection, should be pursued with EBV-IgM and HIV serology. CMV mononucleosis also can be diagnosed by serologic testing, but in most situations of normal immunocompetent hosts it is not indicated. The interpretation of these studies is listed in Table 26-3. In cases of fulminant hepatitis anti-HDV also should be obtained.

Although most patients with acute viral hepatitis can be managed as outpatients, there are indications for those who need to be hospitalized (Table 26-4). The need for hospitalization roughly correlates with the severity of the illness. Patients showing signs of dehydration as a result of nausea and vomiting may need admission for IV fluids. Evidence of severe hepatic destruction as manifested by a prolonged PT (> 50%) is also indicative of the need for hospitalization. These patients are at risk for fulminant hepatic failure. Bleeding as a result of a prolonged PT also may occur. Stool should be checked for the presence of occult blood. A close examination of the patient for signs and symptoms of hepatic encephalopathy is extremely important. Testing for asterixis should be done. Minor alterations of mental status and restlessness may be early clues to the presence of hepatic encephalopathy. These patients clearly need to be hospitalized. Admission criteria need to be individualized for those patients who are debilitated, have underlying disease, or have poor social situations, as in the homeless or alcoholic patient.

For patients who are only mildly symptomatic and have a normal PT, hospitalization is not necessary. The patient should be advised to stay home and rest until symptoms have abated. Patients should be monitored on a weekly or biweekly basis by a physician. In a patient without signs of encephalopathy, no special diet needs to be followed, although all patients should be cautioned against the use of alcohol during the acute phase of the illness. Sedatives should be used cautiously. Instructions concerning the transmission of the various forms of hepatitis and personal hygiene should be given to the patient and family members. Hepatitis A,

Table 26-4. Indications for hospital admission

Dehydration
Prolonged prothromblin time (> 50% normal)
Bleeding
Hepatic encephalopathy

through fecal-oral transmission, is particularly infectious. The patient should be placed in relative isolation and should not work if employment involves food preparation or close contact with people (e.g., health care). Strict handwashing is required, and disposable dishware should be used.

For patients and family members with exposures to the various forms of hepatitis, prophylaxis and/or vaccination may be appropriate. The following section, as well as Chapter 5, outlines the various regimens that are recommended by the CDC [14].

Treatment of Patients with Hepatitis Exposure

Hepatitis A

Measures included in preventing hepatitis A consist of immune globulin (IG) injection. Currently no vaccine is commercially available, although an inactivated and an alternated live vaccine are under development.

PREEXPOSURE PROPHYLAXIS

Preexposure prophylaxis is recommended for persons traveling to areas of the world where poor sanitation exists. The recommended regimen consists of a single dose of IG (0.02 ml/kg). If travel is to be prolonged, IG should be given at a dose of 0.06 ml/kg every 3–5 months.

POSTEXPOSURE PROPHYLAXIS

Postexposure prophylaxis should be given as soon as possible after a potential exposure. IG needs to be given within 2 weeks after the exposure. The recommended dose is a single IM dose of IG (0.02 ml/kg). Postexposure prophylaxis should be given to the following individuals:

1. Household and sexual contacts of persons with HAV infection
2. Staff and attendees of day care centers that have children in diapers
3. Residents and staff of facilities for the developmentally disabled
4. Residents and staff of prisons
5. Persons exposed to a common source in which the food-borne or water-borne contamination has been discovered early.

IG is not recommended if symptoms and signs of HAV infection already have begun to occur.

Contacts at elementary and secondary schools, offices, and factories usually do not result in virus transmission, and routine postexposure prophylaxis is not recommended. Routine postexposure prophylaxis also is not recommended for hospital personnel caring for patients with hepatitis A. IG should be given to hospital personnel who have an unprotected exposure to the feces of a person or an infant who is fecally incontinent [14].

Hepatitis B

Measures used for protection from HBV infection include hepatitis B immune globulin (HBIG) and the HBV vaccine.

PREEXPOSURE PROPHYLAXIS

Hepatitis B vaccines available in the United States include two recombinant DNA–derived HBsAg particle vaccines for routine use. The original human plasma–derived HBsAg particle vaccine is no longer produced in the United States and is limited to hemodialysis patients, immunocompromised hosts, and patients with an allergy to yeast. The currently licensed recombinant hepatitis vaccines are produced in the yeast Saccharomyces cerevisiae.

The recommended series of injection consists of three IM injections in the deltoid at 0, 1, and 6 months or 1, 2, and 12 months. This induces an adequate antibody response in more than 90% of healthy adults and more than 95% of infants and children.

The most common adverse effect of the vaccine includes soreness at the injection site. Guillian-Barré syndrome is thought not to be related to the HBV vaccine. Additionally, there is no risk of transmission of other infectious agents, such as HIV.

Persons at risk for hepatitis B virus infection should receive vaccination. These groups include the following:

1. Persons with occupational risk, such as health care workers and public safety workers
2. Patients and staff of institutions for the developmentally impaired
3. Hemodialysis patients
4. Sexually active homosexual men
5. Prisoners and IV drug users

6. Patients with clotting disorders who receive a large amount of blood products
7. Household and sexual contacts of patients with HBV infections
8. Immigrants of countries with high HBV endemicity
9. International travelers, particularly if long-term visits to areas of the world with high levels of HBV endemicity.

The current vaccine policy in the United States has failed to decrease the incidence of acute HBV infection, particularly in IV drug abusers and heterosexually active individuals who do not practice safe sex. Therefore, use of the vaccine may be expanded to a routine childhood vaccination in the next several years [14, 16].

POSTEXPOSURE PROPHYLAXIS

Postexposure prophylaxis should be given to persons with the following exposures:

1. Accidental percutaneous or perimucosal exposure to HBsAg positive blood
2. Sexual exposure to an HBsAg positive person
3. Perinatal exposure of an infant born to an HBsAg positive mother
4. Household exposure of an infant less than 12 months of age to a primary care giver who has acute hepatitis B virus infection.

Persons exposed to blood that contains or might contain HBsAg and who have not been previously vaccinated or have not completed the vaccination schedule should be given a single dose of HBIG (0.06 ml/kg) IM. HBV vaccine should then be begun either simultaneously (at a separate site in the deltoid) or within 7 days. If the exposed person had begun the vaccination schedule prior to exposure, HBIG should be given and the vaccine completed as scheduled. HBIG should be given as early as possible, and for sexual exposures within 14 days. If a person has completed the HBV vaccine series and is known to have responded and is now exposed to HBsAg, anti-HBs levels should be tested. HBIG or a vaccine dose does not need to be given at this time. Once the anti-HBs level is known and is adequate, nothing further needs to be done. An adequate antibody level is defined as a level greater than or equal to 10 IU/ml or 10 sample ratio units by radioimmunoassay (RIA) [14]. If the level is inadequate, a booster vaccine dose should be given and a single dose of HBIG (0.06 ml/kg).

If a person has completed the HBV vaccine series and is known to have not responded to the vaccine and is now exposed to HBsAg-containing blood, HBIG (0.06 ml/kg) should be given immediately and repeated in 1 month. A dose of the HBV vaccine also may be given.

Infants born of HBsAg positive mothers should receive HBIG (0.5 ml) IM within 12 hours of birth, and HBV vaccine also should be given at this time at a separate site. Subsequent dosing should be done according to the recommendations of the specific vaccine [14].

Hepatitis D

Since HDV is dependent on hepatitis B virus for replication, prevention of HBV infection will effectively prevent HDV infection.

Hepatitis C

Although parenteral transmission is important for the spread of HCV, the role of person-to-person contact and the importance of sexual spread are not clear. Therefore, firm preexposure and postexposure prophylaxis recommendations cannot be made at this time. However, if a person is exposed percutaneously to a person with known HCV infection, IG (0.06 ml/kg) should be given, although several reports of failure of this regimen have been reported recently [14, 52].

Hepatitis E

No specific recommendations regarding prophylactic treatment of HEV exposure can be made at this time.

Hepatic Abscess

Pyogenic Abscess

The clinical presentation of hepatic abscess is similar to that of hepatitis: fever, right upper quadrant pain, nausea, and vomiting. On examination right upper quadrant tenderness is appreciated. The history may help distinguish viral hepatitis from hepatic abscess. Most patients will have an antecedent illness. Hepatic abscess most commonly follows cholangitis or other biliary infections. Other intra-abdominal infections, such as diverticulitis or appendicitis, may spread to the liver via portal vein. Less commonly bacterial seeding of the liver occurs during hematogenous spread from another focus of infection elsewhere in the body [54]. The incidence of hepatic abscess is increased in those with underlying conditions such as malignancy, diabetes, alcoholism [53], and history of transplant [54].

In contrast to viral hepatitis liver function tests in hepatic abscess are only mildly elevated, if at all. Mean AST and ALP levels are two to four times normal [53], while mean bilirubin is only slightly elevated. In one study of 37 patients, ALP was most likely to be abnormal (92%), while bilirubin was least likely to be abnormal (51%) [54]. Chest x-rays may demonstrate an elevated right hemidiaphragm, right basilar atelectases, or right pleural effusion. Although an abscess may be demonstrated by ultrasound or radionuclide scan, an abdominal CT scan is most accurate at identifying all abscesses.

Most liver abscesses are polymicrobial. The most common aerobic organism noted is *Escherichia coli*, although *Klebsiella* and *Proteus* species, enterococci, streptococci, and staphylococci are also found [53, 54]. *Bacteroides fragilis* is the most common anaerobe, followed by *Fusobacterium* species and other *Bacteroides* species [53, 54]. Identification of gas in an abscess points to anaerobic involvement. Because anaerobes are difficult to isolate from cultures of either blood or the abscess, their presence should be assumed, even with a culture negative for anaerobes.

Antibiotic therapy must be directed against gram-negative bacilli, gram-positive cocci, and anaerobes. Usual dosages of metronidazole, which is active against all anaerobic bacteria as well as *Entamoeba histolytica* (amebiasis), plus a third-generation cephalosporin (e.g., cefotaxime, ceftriaxone) or an aminoglycoside (e.g., gentamicin) for gram-negative aerobic coverage are appropriate antibiotic choices. Clindamycin can be substituted for metronidazole, although it is not active for amebic abscess. Broad-spectrum agents, such as imipenem, ticarcillin-clavulanate, and ampicillin-sulbactam, may be useful as single agents for pyogenic abscesses. Ultimately therapy is best guided by the culture results obtained by CT scan or ultrasound-guided needle aspiration. Percutaneous drainage of a single large abscess also will decrease mortality.

Amebic Liver Abscess

Patients presenting with fever and right upper quadrant pain and tenderness may have an amebic hepatic abscess. Epidemiologic factors will aid in distinguishing this from a pyogenic abscess. Patients with amebic liver abscess will have a history of living in or extensive travel in an area endemic for amebiasis. Patients in the United States most often contract amebiasis in Mexico [55, 56]. Unlike pyogenic abscess amebic abscess often occurs in young men [55, 56] without prior history of gallbladder or other underlying disease. A minority of patients will have a history of antecedent or active intestinal amebiasis (see Chap. 25).

Fever will be present in 75%–100% of patients [55, 57–59]. Right upper quadrant pain is found in 89% of patients on average [55]. Pooling of several studies indicates that ALP, AST, and bilirubin are elevated in 69%, 39%, and 22% of cases, respectively. Positive amebic serology is the rule. Diagnosis of abscess can be made on ultrasonographic examination, although it is slightly less sensitive than a CT scan (Fig. 26-1).

Fig. 26-1. CT scan showing a large amebic liver abscess

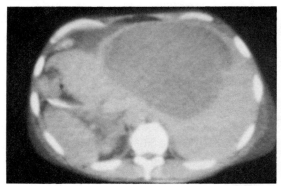

References

1. Hoofnagle JH. Type A and type B hepatitis. *Lab Med* 14:705, 1983.
2. Lemon SM. Type A viral hepatitis: new developments in an old disease. *N Engl J Med* 313:1059, 1985.
3. Gust ID et al. The biology of hepatitis A virus. In F Deinhardt and J Deinhardt (eds.), *Viral Hepatitis: Laboratory and Clinical Science.* New York: Dekker, 1983. P. 201.
4. Mackowiak PA, Caraway CT, Portnoy BL. Oyster associated hepatitis: lessons from the Louisiana experience. *Am J Epidemiol* 103:181, 1976.
5. Portnoy BL et al. Oyster associated hepatitis: failure of shellfish certification programs to prevent outbreaks. *JAMA* 233:1065, 1975.
6. Hadler SC et al. Hepatitis A in day care centers: a community-wide assessment. *N Engl J Med* 302:1222, 1980.
7. Hollinger FB, Melnick JL. Epidemiology. In FB Hollinger, JL Melnick, WS Robinson (eds.), *Viral Hepatitis. Biological and Clinical Features, Specific Diagnosis and Prophylaxis.* New York: Raven, 1985. P. 101.
8. Corey L, Holmes KK. Sexual transmission of hepatitis A in homosexual men: incidence and mechanism. *N Engl J Med* 302:435, 1980.
9. Inman RD et al. Arthritis, vasculitis, and cryoglobulinemia associated with relapsing hepatitis A virus infection. *Ann Intern Med* 105:700, 1986.
10. Routenberg JA et al. A food-borne outbreak of hepatitis A: clinical and laboratory features of acute and protracted illness. *Am J Med Sci* 778:123, 1979.
11. Jacobson IM, Nath BJ, Dienstag JL. Relapsing viral hepatitis type A. *J Med Virol* 16:163, 1985.
12. Hoofnagle JH. Type B hepatitis: virology, serology, and clinical course. *Sem Liver Dis* 1:7, 1981.
13. Robinson WS. Hepatitis B virus. In FB Hollinger, JL Melnick, WS Robinson (eds.), *Viral Hepatitis. Biologic and Clinical Features, Specific Diagnosis, and Prophylaxis.* New York: Raven, 1985. P 19.
14. Centers for Disease Control. Protection against viral hepatitis: recommendations of the Immunization Practices Advisory Committee (ACIP). *MMWR* 39:1, 1990.
15. Kane MA et al. Hepatitis B infection in the United States. Recent trends and future strategies for control. *Am J Med* 87(3A):115, 1989.
16. Alter MJ et al. The changing epidemiology of hepatitis B in the United States. Need for alternative vaccination strategies. *JAMA* 213:1216, 1990.
17. Gocke DJ. Extrahepatic manifestations of viral hepatitis. *Am J Med Sci* 270:49, 1975.
18. Rizzetto M, Canese MG, Arico S. Immunofluorescence detection of a new antigen system (delta/anti-delta) associated to the hepatitis B virus in the liver and the serum of HBsAg carriers. *Gut* 18:997, 1977.
19. Hadziyannis S, Hatzakis A, Karamanos B. Clinical features of chronic delta infection. In GN Vyas (ed.), *Viral Hepatitis.* Philadelphia: Franklin Institute, 1984. P. 701.
20. Hoofnagle JH. Type D hepatitis. *JAMA* 261:1321, 1989.
21. Choo QL et al. Isolation of a cDNA clone derived from a blood-borne non A, non B viral hepatitis genome. *Science* 244:359, 1989.
22. Kuo G et al. An assay for circulating antibodies to a major etiologic virus of human non A, non B hepatitis. *Science* 244:362, 1989.
23. Kraczynski K, Bradley DW, Kane MA. Virus associated antigen of epidemic non A, non B hepatitis and specific antibodies in outbreaks and in sporadic cases of non A, non B hepatitis. *Hepatology* 8:1223, 1988.
24. Gust ID, Purcell RH. Report of a workshop: waterborne non A, non B hepatitis. *J Infect Dis* 156:630, 1987.
25. Stevens CE et al. Epidemiology of hepatitis C virus: a preliminary study in volunteer blood donors. *JAMA* 263:49, 1990.
26. Dienstag JL. Non A, non B hepatitis. I. Recognition, epidemiology, and clinical features. *Gastroenterology* 85:439, 1983.
27. Melbye M et al. Sexual transmission of hepatitis C virus. Cohort study among European homosexual men. *Br Med J* 301:210, 1990.
28. Eugene C et al. Acute pancreatitis associated with non A, non B hepatitis. Report of a case. *J Clin Gastroenterol* 12:195, 1990.
29. Alter HJ et al. Detection of antibody to hepatitis C virus in prospectively followed transfusion recipients with acute and chronic non A, non B hepatitis. *N Engl J Med* 30:1494, 1989.
30. O'Grady JG et al. Early indicators of prognosis in fulminant hepatic failure. *Gastroenterology* 97:439, 1989.
31. Bodenheimer HC et al. Histological and clinical correlations in chronic hepatitis C. *Hepatology* 12:844, 1990.
32. Davis GL et al. Treatment of chronic hepatitis C with recombinant interferon alpha: a multicenter randomized controlled trial. *N Engl J Med* 321:1501, 1989.
33. Kane MA et al. Epidemic non A, non B hepatitis in Nepal. Recovery of a possible etiologic agent and transmission studies in marmosets. *JAMA* 252:3140, 1984.

34. Centers for Disease Control. Enterically transmitted non A, non B hepatitis—Mexico. *MMWR* 36:36, 1987.

35. Tindall B et al. Characteristics of the acute clinical illness associated with human immunodeficiency virus infection. *Arch Intern Med* 148:945, 1988.

36. Chase RA et al. Herpes simplex viral hepatitis in adults. Two case reports and review of the literature. *Rev Infect Dis* 9:329, 1987.

37. Shalev-Zimels H et al. Extent of measles hepatitis in various ages. *Hepatology* 8:1138, 1988.

38. Gavish D et al. Hepatitis and jaundice associated with measles in young adults. *Arch Intern Med* 143:674, 1983.

39. Zeldis JB, Miller JG, Dienstag JL. Hepatitis in an adult with rubella. *Am J Med* 79:515, 1985.

40. Phillips MJ et al. Syncytial giant cell hepatitis—sporadic hepatitis with distinctive pathological features, a severe clinical course, and paramyxoviral features. *N Engl J Med* 324:455, 1991.

41. Lansly LL, Krugman S, Juq G. Anicteric coxsackie B hepatitis. *J Pediatr* 94:64, 1979.

42. Monath TP. Flavivirus. In GL Mandell, RG Douglas, JE Bennett (eds.), *Principles and Practice of Infectious Diseases*. New York: Churchill-Livingstone, 1990. P. 1248.

43. Murphy FA, Kiley MP, Fisher-Hoch SP. Filoviridae, Marburg, and Ebola viruses. In BN Fields, DM Knipe (eds.), *Virology*. New York: Raven Press, 1990. P. 933.

44. Lee RV, Thornton GF, Conn HO. Liver disease associated with secondary syphilis. *N Engl J Med* 284:1423, 1971.

45. Heath CW, Alexander AD, Galton MM. Leptospirosis in the United States. Analysis of 483 cases in man 1949–1961. *N Engl J Med* 273:857, 1965.

46. Simon HB, Wolff SM. Granulomatous hepatitis and prolonged fever of unknown origin. A study of 13 patients. *Medicine* 52:1, 1973.

47. Guckiam JG, Perry JE. Granulomatous hepatitis: an analysis of 63 cases and review of the literature. *Ann Intern Med* 65:1081, 1966.

48. Zimmerman HG et al. Jaundice due to bacterial infection. *Gastroenterology* 77:362, 1977.

49. Dernan J, Rueff B, Benlamou JP. Fulminant and subfulminant liver failure: definition and causes. *Sem Liver Dis* 67:97, 1986.

50. Auslander MO, Gitnick GL. Vigorous medical management of acute fulminant hepatitis. *Arch Intern Med* 137:599, 1977.

51. Bismuth H et al. Emergency liver transplantation for fulminant hepatitis. *Ann Intern Med* 107:337, 1987.

52. Kiyosawa K et al. Hepatitis C in hospital employees with needle stick injuries. *Ann Intern Med* 115:367, 1991.

53. McDonald MI et al. Single and multiple pyogenic liver abscesses. *Medicine* 63:291, 1984.

54. Galvin G, Dayton MT. Factors contributing to improved survival in pyogenic hepatic abscess. *Contemp Surg* 37:11, 1990.

55. Doezema D, Hauswald M. Amebic liver abscess: emergency department diagnosis. *Am J Emerg Med* 6:628, 1988.

56. Abuabara SF et al. Amebic liver abscess. *Arch Surg* 117:239, 1982.

57. Adams EB, MacLeod IN. Invasive amebiasis. II. Amebic liver abscess and its complications. *Medicine* 56:325, 1984.

58. Thompson JE, Florenza S, Verma R. Amebic liver abscess: a therapeutic approach. *Rev Infect Dis* 7:171, 1985.

59. Merten DF, Kirks DR. Amebic liver abscesses in children: the role of diagnostic imaging. *AJR* 143:1325, 1984.

27

Intra-Abdominal Infections and Perirectal Abscess

Donald E. Fry

Despite the increased technology available to the contemporary clinician, the correct diagnosis of intra-abdominal infection remains largely a clinical judgment. The correct diagnosis will usually follow when an exacting history is obtained and a careful physical examination is performed. Optimum results in the management of these patients begin with the correct diagnosis. Avoidable morbidity and deaths will occur if the diagnosis is not made when the patients are initially evaluated. A thorough understanding of the natural history and pathophysiology of intra-abdominal infection will allow the emergency department clinician to establish the correct diagnosis and to direct the patient into definitive treatment.

Intra-abdominal infection encompasses a vast array of very different disease processes that may have very different clinical presentations. Because the processes are all within the anatomic confines of the abdominal cavity, these diseases are commonly considered together.

In one hospital abdominal pain was the chief complaint for 5% of patients [1]. Many patients with abdominal pain will not have an etiology of their pain determined at the time of emergency department visit. In one study a small number had appendicitis (4.3%) or acute cholecystitis (2.5%), which are considered in this chapter. Eight percent

had gastroenteritis or gastritis (see Chap. 25), while 6%–7% had pelvic inflammatory disease (see Chap. 30) and 7% had urinary tract infection (see Chap. 28). The remainder had noninfectious related diseases of the kidney, GI, and reproductive tracts [1].

Most infectious disease processes considered as intra-abdominal infection have common features that the emergency department physician must constantly bear in mind. First, these diseases usually, but not always, begin as peritonitis. While the diagnosis of peritonitis periodically may be proved definitively by the objective identification of air beneath the diaphragm when an upright chest roentgenogram is obtained, usually the diagnosis is a clinical one based on a careful history and a discriminating physical examination. Second, missed diagnoses of intra-abdominal infection, with the patient being sent home from the emergency department, commonly result in significant morbidity and even death. The emergency department physician must accumulate considerable experience in the evaluation of the abdomen and should get additional opinions when equivocal or unclear findings are present. Third, in the final analysis most cases of intra-abdominal infection become surgical diseases for definitive management. It is important that the emergency physician and the surgical consultant have a good working relationship, so case management can proceed as soon as the diagnosis is reasonably assured.

Pathophysiology of Peritonitis

Peritonitis has a natural history that, if understood, makes the clinician more perceptive and better equipped to make the diagnosis clinically. If the perforation is associated with minimal bacteria in a clinically competent host, findings of rebound tenderness and abdominal rigidity may be striking, but systemic toxicity of the patient may be surprisingly mild. A correct diagnosis with subsequent repair of the source of contamination will result in a favorable outcome. If contamination is massive, diffuse peritoneal findings are accompanied by shock, mental confusion, spiking fevers, and a patient in extremis; not infrequently the patient's fate may have been sealed by prehospital events, with even prompt diagnosis and treatment offering little. The patient with an illness of several days' standing but with localized findings, with or without systemic toxemia, may well have a loculated perforation with pus.

Because the diagnosis of peritonitis is principally a clinical one, an understanding of the pathophysiology of the process is critical to an understanding of the clinical findings. A generic consideration of the peritonitis process follows to illustrate the issues.

Contamination

The contamination event usually follows after a perforation of the biliary-enteric tract occurs. Intraabdominal contents extravasate into the free peritoneal cavity. The clinical magnitude of the infectious process is dictated by the inoculum of bacteria that is released into the peritoneal space from the time of perforation until definitive closure or repair is achieved by surgical intervention. The bacterial inoculum may be small or insignificant, as is commonly seen in the acutely perforated peptic ulcer, where the greatest component of the acute peritoneal inflammation is chemical in nature from the acidic contents of the stomach. Bacterial densities may be much greater in perforated appendicitis,

because of the greater bacterial densities of the cecal region of the GI tract. Free perforation of the rectosigmoid colon into the peritoneal cavity has particularly grave consequences because of the $10^{10}-10^{11}$ organisms per gram of stool in this distal location of the gut. In the latter situation diagnostic delay with a consequent delay in operative intervention has grave prognostic implications for the patient. Because perforative events are acute events, patients commonly will identify the precise time when "something happened." Each patient may describe the event differently, but a seminal clinical event within the abdomen can be identified by the astute clinical historian.

Dissemination

The peritoneal cavity normally contains free fluid. This clear transudate probably represents extracellular water that extravasates from mesenteric tissues secondary to tissue hydrostatic pressures. Fluid accumulation likely increases during the day, while the body is in the upright position, and is likely cleared at night, when the body is in the recumbent position.

Peritoneal fluid has a defined circulation [2]. It moves as a function of our body position and as a consequence of pressure gradients that are created with each expiration from the normal human ventilatory cycle. With expiration the subdiaphragmatic space has a relatively negative potential space, and the normal movement of fluid is toward the diaphragm, particularly when the body is in a supine position. This diaphragmatic direction for movement of peritoneal fluid is to facilitate the clearance of fluid through the millions of lymphatic fenestrations that are present only on the diaphragmatic surface of the peritoneal cavity [3]. Peritoneal fluid enters the lymphatic system at the diaphragmatic fenestrations, and the fluid is then passed into the thoracic duct and ultimately into the left subclavian vein. In essence the peritoneal space is a large lymphocele with constant and active fluid movement.

When bacterial contamination of the peritoneal cavity occurs with biliary or enteric perforation, the potential pathogens are immediately disseminated throughout the peritoneal space by virtue of this natural peritoneal-fluid movement. The dissemination of organisms actually serves a nonspecific host defense purpose. The density of organisms at the primary site is effectively reduced, and the biologic interface between the host and the microorganisms is increased. The movement of the contaminant toward the diaphragm may actually result in the clearance of bacteria into the lymphatic system [4]. To the clinician, dissemination means that following a free intestinal perforation localized abdominal findings will rapidly, over a few hours, proceed to diffuse tenderness and rebound across the entire abdomen. Board-like rigidity on physical examination is the end result. In many cases no localized findings can be appreciated, and only the patient's history can provide even a clue as to the anatomic origin of the process.

Inflammation

Contamination and dissemination are accompanied virtually simultaneously by the onset of the inflammatory response [5, 6]. The inflammatory response dictates the severity of clinical findings that the physician will observe at the time of patient presentation. Bacteria and foreign material (e.g., fecal material) elicit the activation of mast cells with the immediate release of inflammatory proteins. Vascular permeability of the peritoneal lining immediately occurs, and plasma proteins render the contaminated soft tissues rapidly edematous. Complement proteins within the edema fluid are activated, and complement cleavage products serve as "sirens" to focus neutrophil mobilization into the area of bacterial transgression. The circulating neutrophils are activated, by complement cleavage products and other chemical signals, to marginate to the endothelial cell. Then via the process of *diapedesis* under the direction of *chemotactic* signals from the inflammatory area, they phagocytose bacteria. The process is completed by intracellular killing of the ingested pathogen. When the numbers of bacteria are excessive, or adjuvant factors (e.g., hemoglobin, dead tissue, foreign bodies) amplify bacterial virulence, the neutrophils may be killed in the attempt to ingest and kill the bacterial pathogens. Exudative tissue fluid with dead leukocytes, bacteria, and bacterial cell products becomes the essence of pus.

Within the peritoneal cavity, some resident mac-

rophages may be present, but most macrophages arrive following the neutrophils and invade the area 12–48 hours after inflammation has begun. These macrophages then release many soluble mediators (i.e., cytokines) that diffuse into the systemic circulation and become important activators of systemic responses. For example, pyrogens released by macrophages stimulate the hypothalamus and activate the febrile response [7]. Because of the delay between the onset of inflammation and actual cytokine release, early peritonitis may not be accompanied immediately by clinical fever.

Essentially three potential outcomes are identified with acute peritonitis. First, the inflammatory process with its attendant phagocytic response may completely eradicate the pathogens, with resolution of the process. Second, the magnitude and virulence of bacterial contamination may overrun the containment effects of host defense, with bacteremia, septic shock, and death of the patient being a common outcome. Third, a physiologic standoff may occur between the host defenses and the pathogen, with abscess being the product.

Loculation

When the peritoneal cavity encounters densities of bacteria-laden peritoneal fluid that cannot be eliminated either by the lymphatic fenestrations or by phagocytic cells, then loculation becomes the court of last resort to contain the infectious process. These pools of bacteria-rich fluid usually occur in the physiologic drainage basins of the peritoneal cavity, specifically in the subphrenic space, pericolic gutters, or the pelvis. Since the movement of peritoneal fluid normally is toward the diaphragm, when the lymphatic fenestrations become occluded from fibrin and inflammatory exudate, then the contaminated peritoneal fluid naturally will settle in the subphrenic space. Densities of bacteria anywhere within the peritoneal sac may elicit the loculation process much earlier in the process, as the peritoneal cavity attempts to contain the source of bacterial contamination. Thus, abscess may already be present about the perforated appendix or diverticulum at the time of clinical presentation. Localized peritoneal findings may reflect the end stages of an acute peritonitis event rather than the early events prior to dissemination. The value of an accurate history at the time of patient presentation to the emergency department will facilitate the correct diagnosis. Abscess can be a stable clinical infection, or it can be accompanied by severe septic symptoms. The diagnosis of abscess can be made clinically, but will usually require objective confirmation by inpatient imaging techniques.

Abdominal Pain and Intra-Abdominal Infection

Pain is the common clinical denominator of the patient with intra-abdominal infection. The location and the character of the pain must be carefully elicited from the patient, since subtle details may give the emergency physician the "big scoop" in diagnosis over the specialist consultants.

Referred Pain

Referred pain commonly is present as an early part of the fundamental disease responsible for the peritonitis or abscess infection that occurs in these patients. Appendicitis, acute cholecystitis, and diverticulitis are inflammatory processes within the organ so affected, but they are contained and have not yet led to peritonitis or abscess. In each of these clinical cases inflammation and distention in the wall of each anatomic structure elicits referred pain for the patient. Referred pain is usually poorly defined and is midline in location. Referred pain provides characteristics consistent with the embryonic origin of the anatomic structure that is inflamed and distended. Foregut derivatives refer pain to the epigastrium. Thus, GI structures from the foregut or those proximal to the ligament of Treitz refer pain to the epigastric area. The stomach, duodenum, gallbladder, and pancreas are the principal anatomic structures. Midgut derivatives refer pain to the periumbilical area and usually include the disease processes of appendicitis, regional enteritis (distal ileum), or Meckel's diverticulum. Hindgut derivatives refer pain to the suprapubic, hypogastric area of the abdomen. Referred pain to this area is commonly diverticular disease and occasionally colon cancers.

Somatic Pain

Somatic pain fibers are in the parietal peritoneum. When the inflammatory process becomes sufficiently severe that the parietal peritoneum is involved, findings of pain and tenderness are localized to the anatomic area of the disease. Somatic pain then becomes the localized right lower quadrant pain of appendicitis or the right upper quadrant pain of acute cholecystitis. Being able to historically trace the transition of a patient's pain complex from the referred stage to the somatic stage can improve accuracy in establishing the clinical diagnosis. The peculiar features of the referred-somatic relationship are further discussed with each specific disease process.

Appendicitis

Acute appendicitis continues to be the most common cause of emergency abdominal surgery and occurs in about 7% of the U.S. population. Perforated appendicitis remains the most common cause of secondary bacterial peritonitis. The significant morbidity and even occasional deaths from the process of acute appendicitis leading to perforation can be avoided by the astute diagnostician in the emergency department setting. Earlier diagnosis usually will be translated into quicker appendectomy, which means fewer perforations.

Pathophysiology

The process of acute appendicitis begins with mechanical obstruction of the narrow lumen of this anatomic structure [8, 9]. An appendolith usually obstructs the lumen of the appendix at or near its proximal orifice, which communicates with the lumen of the cecum. The appendolith is usually composed of a relatively desiccated concretion of fecal material. Impaction of the appendolith into the appendiceal opening results in a closed loop of bacterial stasis in the appendix. The obstructing appendolith elicits a reflex contraction of smooth muscle in the appendiceal wall to expel the obstruction. The combined effects of efforts to expel the obstruction and the proliferation of stagnant bacteria in the distal portion of the appendix result in a local inflammatory response.

Necrosis of the appendiceal wall with resultant perforation can occur by two separate mechanisms. First, transmural inflammation and edema result in lymphatic compromise, which may embarrass effective arterial perfusion at the microcirculatory level with resultant appendiceal necrosis. Second, the transluminal inflammation may result in thrombosis of adjacent arterial branches from the appendiceal artery with segmental or complete necrosis being the sequelae. At operation either mechanism can be seen, with some patients having a necrotic or perforated appendix with the appendiceal artery patent, and other circumstances where thrombosis of the arterial branches clearly is evident.

The end result of tissue ischemia combined with bacterial proliferation in the obstructed appendix is transmural necrosis and gangrenous appendicitis. The necrotic tissue then perforates with the release of the intraluminal contents of the appendix into the peritoneal cavity. Perforation commonly occurs at or immediately distal to the appendolith, with resultant decompression of luminal obstruction. This can result in free communication of the cecal lumen into the peritoneal cavity.

Dissemination and inflammation in the peritoneal cavity then are initiated. Because transmural inflammation may elicit an early response from the peritoneal cavity, the loculation process actually may be initiated prior to frank perforation and the attendant massive release of bacteria into the peritoneal cavity. Adherent omentum and loops of small intestine to the nonperforated but inflamed appendix may mean that a disseminated peritonitis phase may not be seen in some patients. When the appendix is located in a retrocecal position, this means that necrosis and perforation may occur with no intraperitoneal inflammation and, hence, only minimal or subtle physical findings on abdominal examination. When perforation occurs at the appendiceal base, particularly if the diagnosis is delayed, the inflammation and necrosis may extend onto the cecal wall itself, with necrosis and perforation of the cecum being an occasional complication. In every case earlier diagnosis affords the best opportunity for the patient to avoid the morbidity attendant to the next stage of the disease.

Clinical Presentation

Acute appendicitis begins with feelings of malaise and anorexia. It is unusual for patients to have acute appendicitis and not be nauseated or have frank vomiting. Patients being evaluated for appendicitis usually will not have eaten recently nor will they express the wish to have something to eat.

Abdominal pain commonly begins as the poorly defined referred pain of a midgut derivative, with the pain being dull in character and poorly localized about the umbilicus. As transmural inflammation of the appendix occurs, the parietal peritoneum becomes inflamed, and the pain shifts to the right lower quadrant.

A history of peritoneal irritation and inflammation can also be established by questioning the patient about the journey to the hospital. As the car went over the bumps or around turns, did the pain increase in the right lower quadrant? Was getting out of the car or walking to the examining room uncomfortable, and did the pain increase in the right lower quadrant? Does the pain increase when the patient coughs?

If the pain was severe in character, lasted for 24 hours or more, and is followed by an interlude of abrupt relief, the clinician should not take any solace that the crisis has passed. Acute relief followed within an hour or so by severe peritoneal signs is proof positive that perforation has occurred. The interlude of pain relief simply reflects the decompression of the distended appendix into the peritoneal cavity. In essence, a well-taken history may ensure the diagnosis, even without an examination, if the clinician is attuned to the correlation of the pathophysiology of the disease with the history that is relayed by the patient.

The physical examination of the abdomen should be viewed as an art form by emergency department physicians. The examiner should stand somewhat away from the patient while the history is being told. Leaning over the patient for a simultaneous examination while the history is being solicited will result in a tense patient giving a poor history and a compromised examination because of anxiety. The physician should try to get the patient to relax during the history. A little humor is even in order, since a short chuckle by a relaxed patient may result in the patient's clutching the right lower quadrant as affirmation of the diagnosis. During the history the physician should watch how the patient positions the right leg, since flexion of the iliopsoas muscle may well reflect the irritation on the anterior surface of that muscle from a "hot" appendix.

When approaching the examination of the abdomen, the physician should begin the palpation away from the right lower quadrant. A useful approach can be for the clinician to bump the bed or litter with his or her hip. Not infrequently the patient will respond to the bump by clutching the right lower quadrant or by flexing the right leg at the hip. Such response is evidence of acute appendicitis.

Flexion of the right leg at the hip joint can be useful when equivocal findings are present on the abdominal exam. The practitioner should gently flex the leg and observe the patient's response. In selected cases pressure on the heel of the extended right lower extremity may exacerbate symptoms. By and large if the physician has to ask the patient, "Did that hurt?" then the findings are inconclusive. A spontaneous response to the physical examination is always the real clue to the diagnosis of acute appendicitis.

A rectal examination may be helpful for the diagnosis of a retrocecal appendix or in the patient where perforation and abscess have already occurred. Exquisite and localized right rectal-wall tenderness is the important finding in the retrocecal appendix. A fluctuant mass may be identified if abscess has already occurred.

The pelvic examination is essential for the female patient with suspected appendicitis. The female patient has numerous alternative diagnoses that may present in a similar or identical fashion to acute appendicitis. Uterine size, adnexal masses, and bladder tenderness are important observations. Even culpotomy may be useful in evaluating other potential problems.

Interpretation of fever and leukocytosis patterns in the patient with appendicitis is difficult at best. Patients may be afebrile and have a normal white count but still have acute appendicitis. Conversely patients may have temperature elevations to 38.5°C or above with dramatically elevated white counts and not have appendicitis. It must be remembered that fever and white cell count elevations are the nonspecific consequences of the release of inter-leukin-1 from stimulated macrophage cells. Elevations in temperature and white cell count indicate that the patient has an inflammatory focus, which may or may not be appendicitis. Of course if the appendicitis is early in the natural history of the disease, the patient may not have mounted any inflammatory response, and hence no fever or leukocytosis is present.

In a study of 1,000 patients with appendicitis, the mean temperature of patients with nonperforated appendicitis was 37.8°C ($\pm 0.6°$). In patients with localized peritonitis mean temperature was 38.3°C ($\pm 0.8°$). The mean WBC count of patients without perforation was 15,570 μl ($\pm 5,370$), and in patients with localized peritonitis it was 15,240 μl ($\pm 5,000$) [10]. In other studies normal WBC counts have been noted in 10%–18% of adults [11, 12]. Normal WBC counts in children have ranged from 4%–20% [13–15]. In 100 patients 50 years and older with appendicitis, 30% had normal white blood counts compared with 14% of a younger group [16].

Abdominal roentgenograms commonly are performed when patients are suspected of having acute or perforated appendicitis. These studies often are unproductive. Rarely an appendolith may be identified. Because of the critical location of the appendix with respect to the ileocecal valve, appendiceal perforation may be associated with intestinal obstruction. Extraluminal air may be identified in such cases and significantly add to diagnostic accuracy (Fig. 27-1). An adynamic ileus or sentinel loop may be identified, but it is nonspecific.

Considerable recent interest has focused on the potential use of ultrasound in the diagnosis of appendicitis. Ultrasound remains of unproved value in the clinical evaluation of the most difficult cases. This technique is investigational at the present time and cannot solely be relied on for a decision to proceed with an operation [17]. The accuracy of the diagnosis is largely dependent on the skill and experience of the examiner. Ultrasound may be of value in identifying other diseases that may mimic appendicitis [18].

Differential Diagnosis

The number of alternative diagnoses that can mimic appendicitis are many. In pediatric patients

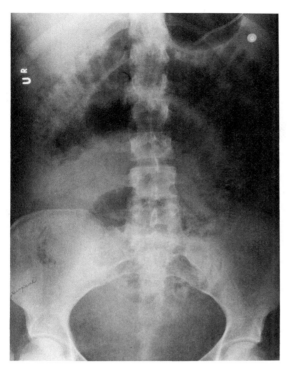

Fig. 27-1. Abdominal roentgenogram of a patient with a perforated appendix and associated intestinal obstruction. The multiple air-fluid levels are evident from the obstruction. There is no colon gas. Extra-luminal air in the right lower quadrant reflects gas within the abscess cavity, which subsequently was confirmed at operation

nonspecific mesenteric lymphadenitis from viral infection or other bacterial infection is the greatest mimic and probably represents the most common cause for removal of a normal appendix. While the tendency in a child with a recent upper respiratory tract infection may be to presume the clinical diagnosis of mesenteric lymphadenitis, the physical examination must be the final arbiter of the clinical decision.

In female patients numerous genital tract problems can mimic appendicitis. Ectopic pregnancy or a threatened spontaneous abortion require that the pregnancy test accompany each evaluation of women of reproductive age. Pelvic inflammatory disease, tubo-ovarian abscess, ovarian cysts, and ovarian torsion also can give localized findings. The presence of a right adnexal mass may represent one of these "pretenders," or it may be an appendiceal abscess. Urinary tract infection is commonly discussed as a potential alternative diagnosis, but it is really an infrequent competing diagnosis to the discriminating examiner. A urine sample of the patient with appendicitis may contain some white cells from the proximity of the inflamed appendix to the ureter or bladder, but generally it should not contain bacteria.

Other diagnoses in the adult should be considered regardless of the patient's gender. Cecal diverticular disease and regional enteritis are alternative considerations. Meckel's diverticulitis is commonly discussed as an alternative but is really seldom seen. Renal calculi in the right urinary collecting system may be seen, and occasionally a perforated peptic ulcer may mimic appendicitis as succus entericus from the perforation pools into the right lower quadrant and simulates localized inflammatory findings in that area of the abdomen.

Management

Once a presumed diagnosis of appendicitis has been made, the management of the patient is surgical [19]. The patient should be kept from any oral intake prior to the operative procedure. IV fluids should be started with either Ringer's lactate or 0.9% sodium chloride solution. If perforation already has occurred, then significant volume administration of isotonic resuscitation fluids may be required. Foley catheterization is required only in the most severe cases.

The patient with an inconclusive clinical presentation for appendicitis represents a difficult dilemma for the emergency department physician. Admission of the patient for continuous follow-up of changes in the physical examination has generally been the safest recourse. Observation in an emergency department observation ward for 6–12 hours is also a reasonable option. In selected patients follow-up the following morning or a scheduled return to the emergency department for a second visit in 12–24 hours may also be a reasonable approach for the dependable patient.

Antibiotics should not be initiated until a firm decision has been made for the patient to go to the operating room for appendectomy. The administration of antibiotics while the patient is under clinical evaluation may alter the natural progression of

Table 27-1. Antibiotic use in intra-abdominal infections

Disease	Antibiotic	Dosage
Appendicitis*	Cefoxitin	1–2 g q6h IV
Diverticulitis		
(outpatient)	Tetracycline or erythromycin	500 mg q6h PO
(inpatient)	Gentamicin plus	3–5 mg/kg/day IV
	clindamycin	600–900 mg q6–8h IV
	(or metronidazole)	750 mg q12h IV/PO
	or cefoxitin	2 gm q6h IV
Cholecystitis	Cefazolin	1–2 g q8h IV
Cholangitis	Imipenem or	500 mg q6h IV
	gentamicin plus	3–5 mg/kg/day IV
	metronidazole	750 mg q12h IV
Pancreatic abscess or infected pseudocyst	Cefoxitin or	2 g q6h IV
	imipenem	500 mg q6h IV
Perforated ulcer	Cefazolin or	1–2 g q8h IV
	ampicillin-sulbactam	3 g q6h IV
Intra-abdominal trauma	Cefoxitin	2 g q6h IV
Peritonitis, primary (SBP)	Cefotaxime (or like cephalosporin)	2 g q8h IV

* Only when diagnosis is secure and patient is scheduled for surgery.

physical findings. The altered presentation of clinical findings can result in the patient evolving from relatively mild signs of tenderness to frank perforation. Indeed, antibiotics may not be justified at all if the diagnosis is that of acute appendicitis without perforation. If clinical peritonitis is present, antibiotics are clearly warranted and should be initiated immediately. A single antibiotic with activity against both enteric aerobic and anaerobic bacteria (e.g., cefoxitin) will be adequate (Table 27-1).

Occasionally the emergency department physician will see patients who recently have been discharged from the hospital following appendectomy. The emergency department visit by the patient will usually relate to complaints of fever. It will be important to elicit from the patient or family whether the appendix was perforated at the time of appendectomy. The major sources of postoperative fever will be "where the hands of man have been." The wound should be carefully inspected for evidence of inflammation. Draining pus is proof positive of wound infection. Palpation of the abdomen will be compromised in these patients, who have residual incisional tenderness, and the physician cannot expect to palpate masses or define deep-seated localized tenderness. The rectal exam may define fluctuance from abscess. If abscess is truly suspected, then an abdominal CT scan will be required.

Diverticulitis

Diverticulitis of the human colon is very common in Western cultures where highly refined diets are enjoyed [20, 21]. As many as 50% of persons in the United States will have diverticula at age 65 years. Fortunately most cases do not become clinically significant. Acute attacks of diverticulitis or other more severe manifestations of diverticula-associated infection are fairly common among patients in the sixth decade of life and older. Of interest is that recent trends in diverticular disease suggest that younger patients are presenting more frequently than in the past with acute diverticulitis.

Pathophysiology

Diverticula are generally thought to be consequences of increased intra-abdominal colonic pressure generated by the straining and spasm of passing of low-bulk stool. The increased intra-abdominal pressure results in the herniation of colonic mucosa through weakened areas of the colonic seromuscular coat [22]. These weak areas typically are located at the site where nutrient blood vessels of the colonic blood supply penetrate the seromuscular layers and communicate into the submucosal anastomotic arcade of vessels. The herniation of mucosa alone creates saccular protrusions that are actually pseudodiverticula, since true diverticula (e.g., duodenal diverticula) actually have all layers of the intestinal wall represented in the pouch. In diverticula of the colon the opening into the native colonic lumen may really be quite small compared to the cross-sectional diameter of the saccular diverticular lesion. This disproportional relationship of the actual volume of the diverticular lesion compared to the opening into the lumen sets the stage for infectious complications.

The formed diverticulum then has the potential for infection in much the same way that infection occurs in appendicitis. A fecalith is found in the diverticular lumen. Since the nutrient vessel to the colon is immediately adjacent to the diverticulum opening, erosion of the fecalith concretion can provoke acute colonic bleeding. The obstruction of the diverticular opening sets the stage for stasis with bacterial proliferation and an inflammatory response (e.g., diverticulitis).

The natural history of the process in the absence of any clinical intervention can have one of several outcomes. The inflammatory process may generate considerable pressure within the lumen of the diverticulum with dislodgement of the impacted fecalith back into the colonic lumen and spontaneous resolution of the process. The edema and inflammation may become progressively circumferential, with colonic obstruction being the outcome. The acute inflammation may provoke acute perforation into the peritoneal cavity with acute peritonitis. Finally inflammation in acute diverticulitis may result in an adjacent omentum and small intestine adhering to the inflamed colonic segment. A perforation into a phlegmon provides containment and sets the stage for diverticular abscess. Those segments of the colon that are normally retroperitoneal will have functional containment of perforation, and abscess commonly will be identified in these areas rather than free intraperitoneal perforation.

Clinical Presentation

The typical case of acute diverticulitis begins with vague lower abdominal referred pain that commonly proceeds within a few hours to localized pain in the left lower quadrant. The localization occurs as the overlying parietal peritoneum becomes involved in the process. Among those patients with multiple previous episodes of diverticulitis, adhesions between the inflamed segment of colon to the abdominal wall will result in immediate left lower quadrant pain with subsequent episodes, because of the proximity of the abdominal wall to the colon.

As in appendicitis, fever and leukocytosis may or may not be present with acute diverticulitis. In a study of 216 patients with diverticulitis, mean temperature was 38.2°C (range 36.7°C–40.0°C) [23]. The clinical diagnosis really requires only localized left lower quadrant tenderness on palpation of the abdomen. Staging the severity of the diverticular infectious process can be tricky. Before a clinical diagnosis of diverticulitis can be accepted, the examining physician must be convinced that no element of colonic obstruction or significant peritonitis is present. Abdominal distention means obstruction, and that means admission to the hospital. A clinically toxic picture with high fever, major white count elevations, hyperglycemia, and so on, means that abscess already may be present. Since many patients will provide a history of previous diverticular events, there may be a temptation to send these patients home with oral antibiotic therapy. Each episode must be individually managed, and patients with localized tenderness and rebound should be hospitalized for intensive antibiotic therapy and more extensive assessment of the disease.

In the emergency department setting the laboratory and radiology services are of little help in the assessment of the diverticulitis patient. WBC counts invariably are done and seldom affect clinical decisions in the evaluation of the acute abdomen. In the study of 216 patients with diverticulitis, the mean white blood count was 9,200 per μl (3,000–22,000), and the mean erythrocyte sedimentation rate (ESR) was 40 mm/hr (range 3–148) [23]. Three-way abdominal films also are commonly performed and, except for the identification of free-air or air-fluid levels, seldom demon-

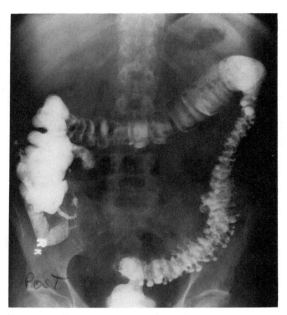

Fig. 27-2. Barium enema performed in a patient with suspected acute diverticulitis. The disease can be extensive, as is illustrated in this case, or it may involve only a relatively short segment of the sigmoid colon.

strate clinically significant problems. In difficult cases for diagnosis, an urgent barium enema may be necessary and will usually prove accurate (Fig. 27-2). When free perforation into the peritoneal cavity is suspected, a barium enema is contraindicated.

Differential Diagnosis

The differential diagnostic considerations for diverticulitis are generally less demanding than for appendicitis. Because the patient population with diverticulitis generally is older than appendicitis patients, ectopic pregnancy, pelvic inflammatory disease, and acute ovarian cysts are lesser concerns. The pelvic examination is nevertheless a necessary part of the evaluation.

Perforating or obstructing colon cancer can be clinically indistinguishable from diverticulitis. Renal calculi in the left collecting system also can be within the differential consideration, although the character of pain in these patients is usually quite different from that of diverticulitis. In the elderly patient severe constipation and fecal impaction may present with abdominal pain, diffuse abdominal tenderness, and perhaps even low-grade fever. In those cases it is the physician's responsibility to differentiate diverticulitis and diverticular abscess from these less significant but very vexing problems. Hospitalization is commonly necessary for these patients with confusing physical examinations.

Management

The overall management attitude toward patients with diverticulitis is variable. Initial episodes are managed with antibiotics. Mild cases in otherwise healthy patients may be treated on an ambulatory basis, while more severe cases will require inpatient management with intensive antibiotic management (enteric aerobic and anaerobic coverage). Those cases that have frequent recurrences of acute episodes and those cases not responding to antibiotic therapy will require resection. Those cases presenting with complications of diverticulitis (e.g., obstruction, perforation, abscess) will require resection of the diseased segment of colon.

Oral antibiotic regimens include tetracycline (500 mg qid) or erythromycin (500 mg qid), since both drugs will provide a measure of aerobic and anaerobic bacterial coverage. With significantly enhanced anaerobic activity azithromycin may be an ideal agent and can be administered once daily. Adding bulk to the diet also is desirable, and ambulatory diverticulitis patients should be taking psyllium seed (Metamucil) or some similar agent for this purpose. Follow-up and continuity of care for diverticulitis patients are vitally important, because many will be refractory to ambulatory medical management and will need in-patient or surgical management. Clinical toxicity and the presence of peritoneal signs (e.g., rebound) are reasons for admission.

When hospitalization occurs, antibiotic therapy for diverticulitis needs to be more aggressive but still with aerobic and anaerobic coverage. Combination therapy with gentamicin (4–5 mg/kg/day) and clindamycin (600–900 mg q6–8h) or a cephalosporin with reasonably good anaerobic activity (e.g., cefoxitin, cefotaxime, ceftizoxime) will usually be effective (see Table 27-1). Nonresponsive patients to systemic antibiotic therapy will commonly have a diverticular abscess and will require operation. Evidence of perforation or obstruction at the time of admission will ordinarily mean immediate abdominal exploration.

Biliary Tract Infection

Infection in the biliary tract is another intra-abdominal infection that commonly is seen in the emergency department. The prevalence of stone disease in the biliary tract is generally very high in the United States, but it is extraordinarily high in the Hispanic and Native American populations. Biliary calculi are the usual prerequisites for biliary infection, and those patients at greatest risk for stone disease define the population that will present with acute attacks.

Pathophysiology

There are essentially two requirements for an acute infectious event in the biliary tract: (1) stasis of bile flow and (2) bacteria in the bile. Stasis can occur at two anatomic sites: either at the cystic duct with the creation of acute cholecystitis or by common duct obstruction and evolution of ascending cholangitis.

Gallbladder stones nearly always are the cause of acute cholecystitis, although acute cholecystitis as a clinical event occurs in only 10%–15% of patients with cholelithiasis. The physiologic contraction of the gallbladder following food intake may propel stones within the gallbladder toward the cystic duct. Small stones may be forcibly expelled into the common duct, and large stones (> 1 cm in diameter) may be pushed into the internal opening of the cystic duct. In either scenario patients will have symptoms of biliary colic, which is relieved when either the stone is passed (only to result in other problems) or the gallbladder relaxes and the wedged stone falls back into the gallbladder lumen with relief of symptoms. When stones are of a particular size (0.5–1.0 cm), however, they cannot navigate the entire length of the cystic duct nor are they expelled from the cystic duct back into the gallbladder lumen. Acute cholecystitis is the result.

Acute cholecystitis then either becomes a me-

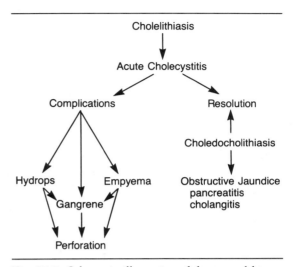

Fig. 27-3. Schematic illustration of the natural history of acute cholecystitis. The exact percentages involved in each possible outcome really are not known. Unrecognized diagnosis or delays in the treatment of acute cholecystitis can have enormously serious consequences.

chanical obstruction with associated inflammation of the gallbladder wall secondary to pressure and distention, or if bacteria are trapped in the retained distention or the retained bile, bacterial infection occurs. The natural history of acute cholecystitis has several potential outcomes (Fig. 27-3). The obstructing stone may pass or retract into the gallbladder with spontaneous resolution of the acute event. Bacterial infection actually may proceed to empyema of the gallbladder [24]. Severe hydrops of the gallbladder may develop from nonbacterial progressive distention secondary to the refractory cystic-duct obstruction. When the pressure in the gallbladder due to either infection or pure mechanical obstruction exceeds the perfusion pressure of the gallbladder wall, then gangrenous cholecystitis occurs, with free perforation into the peritoneal cavity becoming the next and commonly fatal event [25].

Occasionally acalculous cholecystitis can be seen in ambulatory patients. While more commonly an illness of very ill, hospitalized patients, acalculous cholecystitis can occur from tumor obstruction of the cystic duct, sclerosis and narrowing of the cystic-duct passage for any number of reasons: dyskinesia of biliary flow, or ischemia related to mesenteric vascular disease. Acalculous disease can be clinically occult in onset because the patients usually do not have the crampy pain of biliary colic as a prodrome. When intense acute acalculous cholecystitis is present, the right upper quadrant constellation of symptoms is similar to that seen in calculous disease.

A scenario similar to acute cholecystitis can be constructed to describe ascending, or suppurative, cholangitis. Obstruction of the common duct results in progressively increasing pressure in the ductal system. If no bacteria are present in the common duct, then simple mechanical obstruction with progressively increasing jaundice occurs. If bacteria are present, the static but contaminated bile results in the proliferation of bacteria and cholangitis. Because there is access of the evolving infection into the ductal system within the liver parenchyma itself, the proximal ascent of the infection results in a fulminant septic process that will take otherwise healthy patients to the brink of a septic demise within hours.

In the setting of both acute cholecystitis and ascending cholangitis, bacteria probably gain access to the bile via lymphatics from the GI tract. The potential for bacterial contamination may exist via retrograde movement from the duodenum through the ampulla of Vater. However, since *Escherichia coli*, *Klebsiella* species, and the enterococcus are the most commonly encountered bacteria in bile [26], and these bacteria are of distal ileum and colonic (not duodenal) origin, it is more likely that lymphatic spread to the bile is the mechanism. Factors that govern why one patient has bactobilia and another does not are unclear. Clinical factors that favor bactobilia include age ($\geq$ 50 years) and stone disease. Bactobilia is probably a random and transient event among all humans, but it becomes a more persistent finding with aging or when stones are present in the bile. The critical variable of calculi in part addresses why ascending cholangitis occurs much more frequently when stone disease is responsible for common duct obstruction rather than neoplasm.

Clinical Presentation

Table 27-2 lists the clinical characteristics of biliary tract disease to assist the physician in differentiating cholelithiasis, cholecystitis, and cholangitis. Right upper quadrant abdominal pain is the critical complaint of the patient with acute inflammation

Table 27-2. Clinical characteristics of biliary tract disease

Characteristic	Cholelithiasis	Cholecystitis	Cholangitis
Pathophysiolgy	Mechanical obstruction	inflammation of gallbladder (stone associated 90%)	Ascending bacterial infection of biliary ducts, usually from complete ductal obstruction
Pain	Acute onset lasts 1–4 hrs. Epigastrium and RUQ	Constant, severe; lasts for days	Constant, severe acute onset; rapidly progressive
Other symptoms	Focal RUQ pain, no rebound	Nausea, vomiting; history of biliary colic	Chills, rigors
Physical exam	Well appearing, focal RUQ tenderness, no rebound	Ill appearing, RUQ tenderness, rebound, palpable gallbladder $\pm$; jaundice $\pm$	Toxic appearing, RUQ tenderness, rebound; gallbladder not palpable, rapidly evolving jaundice
Temperature	Normal	Mild elevation	Marked elevation (> 39°C)
Leukocytosis	No	Mild	Marked (> 20,000 μl)
Liver function tests	↑ bilirubin; ↑ alkaline phosphotase	$\pm$ ↑ bilirubin, $\pm$ ↑ alkaline phosphotase; $\pm$ ↑ amylase, $\pm$ ↑ transaminases	↑ bilirubin; ↑ alkaline phosphotase; ↑ transaminases
Radiologic testing	Gallstones on ultrasound; $\pm$ abnormal radionuclide scan	Gallstones on ultrasound; abnormal radionuclide scan	Ductal gallstones on ultrasound

in the biliary tract. Gallbladder stones occur three to six times more frequently in women. The most common age range is the fourth to eighth decade. The pain is ordinarily accompanied by nausea and vomiting. Initial pain symptoms arise from gallbladder distention in acute cholangitis, which will be clinically manifest as vague, epigastric midline pain. Extension of the inflammation to the parietal peritoneum then localizes the pain into the right upper quadrant.

A careful history is important to differentiate biliary colic from acute cholecystitis. Colic pain usually is transient as either the stone passes or regresses back into the gallbladder. With acute cholecystitis the pain is constant and severe. Patients will literally writhe from the severe and incapacitating nature of the pain.

The palpation examination of the abdomen must be approached carefully. Again, the examination should be begun away from the area of complaint, and the right upper quadrant examined last. Localized tenderness usually will be found in the midclavicular line in the subcostal area of the right upper quadrant. If the physician can get the patients to relax at all, the gallbladder dome actually may be palpable. Rebound tenderness that is generally evident in the entire right upper quadrant or that extends to other areas may reflect that perforation already has occurred. Such patients customarily are quite toxic. A toxic patient with complaints referable to the right upper quadrant but without palpable tenderness may well have ascending cholangitis. This is particularly true when rapidly emerging jaundice is present. These patients are surgical emergencies and must be treated in that fashion.

Fever and leukocytosis are nonspecific signs in patients with acute cholecystitis. Fever greater than 38°C and white counts greater than 18,000–20,000 cells/μl will suggest a bacterial component to the patient's illness rather than inflammation from mechanical obstruction. Because inflammation is a nonspecific response, the magnitude of fever and leukocytosis must be used cautiously since the duration of the patient's acute cholecystitis may be a more important determinant in these responses than the presence or absence of bacteria in the process.

Clinical jaundice may be observed. Low-grade hyperbilirubinemia or faintly detectable jaundice noted in the sclera of the eyes may be seen with acute cholecystitis without common duct obstruction [27, 28]. If the history from the family or the patient is that of rapidly evolving jaundice, then ascending cholangitis or gallbladder empyema is present, and urgent surgical intervention is essential. In acute cholecystitis the process must have been present for days before elevation of liver enzyme profiles can be seen. The acute septic response from any source within the abdomen may be responsible for liver enzyme abnormalities, particularly if the patient has been ill for several days.

In general routine roentgenographic studies that are ordered in the emergency department do not add to diagnostic accuracy. Only about 10% of biliary calculi are radiopaque (Fig. 27-4). The occasional patient may even have air evident within the biliary tract, "milk of calcium" gallbladder shadow (Fig. 27-5), or even an air-fluid level within the gallbladder. Usually the history and the carefully performed physical examination make laboratory and radiographic studies of relatively little value.

In patients with equivocal findings and in elderly patients, an ultrasound study may be useful in the identification of biliary calculi. Because inflammation in the wall of the gallbladder in not reliably

Fig. 27-4. The occasional abdominal roentgenogram that identifies radiopaque stones in the gallbladder

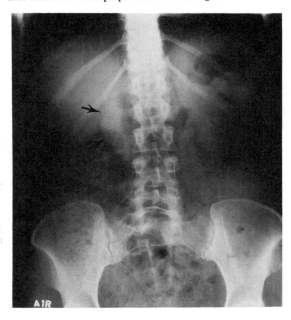

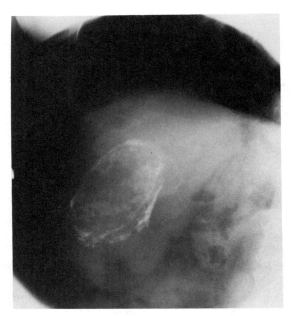

Fig. 27-5. "Milk of calcium" bile in a patient who presented with symptoms of acute cholecystitis

identified on ultrasound studies, the presence of gallstones on the ultrasound scan does not always mean that they are responsible for the symptoms that have precipitated the patient's illness. A radionuclide scan with HIDA, PIPIDA, or DESIDA may confirm the diagnosis of acute cholecystitis [29]. These technetium-tagged analogues of bilirubin are removed by the hepatocyte from the patient's blood and are excreted into the bile. When the right upper quadrant is scanned after administration, acute cholecystitis is confirmed by the absence of identification of the gallbladder. The radionuclide studies probably are best ordered and followed by the admitting physician.

It is important to emphasize that the clinical presentation of acute cholecystitis and ascending cholangitis can be quite similar. In general patients with ascending cholangitis are much more toxic and have had a more rapid development of the disease. They commonly will have percussable tenderness over the liver and more commonly will be clinically jaundiced. The jaundice of ascending cholangitis develops in a very rapid fashion. Chills, rigors, marked temperature elevation (> 39°C), and very marked leukocytosis (> 20,000 μl) all favor ascending cholangitis (or gallbladder perforation). Usually emergency operative intervention is necessary to establish the specific diagnosis.

Differential Diagnosis

Right upper quadrant pain may be a component of the disease complex of all anatomic structures that arise from foregut derivatives. Thus, in addition to biliary tract disease, peptic ulcer disease and acute pancreatitis are important components of the differential diagnosis. Patients with fulminant acute hepatitis, particularly secondary to alcoholism, can present with findings very similar to biliary tract infection. A liver enzyme profile will usually provide useful information in eliminating hepatocellular disease. Occasionally proximal urinary tract calculi on the right side may mimic symptoms of acute cholecystitis. Rarely the adhesive bands from the tubo-ovarian complex may extend to the right upper quadrant and give a right upper quadrant component of pain to pelvic inflammatory disease or tubo-ovarian abscess.

Management

Patients with acute cholecystitis are best managed by urgent cholecystectomy [24, 25]. A nasogastric tube is placed and IV volume is administered with Ringer's lactate or 0.9% sodium chloride. If vomiting has been present, hypokalemia may need to be corrected. Antibiotics appropriate for E. coli and Klebsiella species are started. This author prefers cefazolin 1 g q8h IV until operation for the straightforward acute cholecystitis patient (see Table 27-2). Demerol analgesia with a antiemetic remains preferred. The operation is performed within 24 hours of admission.

Some surgeons prefer nonoperative management during acute cholecystitis [30]. Patients are treated with nasogastric suction and antibiotics, and it is hoped that the acute cholecystitis will resolve by spontaneous movement of the obstructing stone from the cystic duct. This form of therapy should be reserved only for very-poor-risk patients (e.g., recent myocardial infarction). The benefits of immediate surgical removal of the acute gallbladder, in terms of both economics and patient suffering, are far superior to the nonoperative approach.

In those patients with suspected ascending cholangitis, operative intervention on an emergency basis is essential. Procrastination in making the diagnosis in the emergency department area or delays in operative decompression of the obstructed common duct in these patients may prove fatal.

Pancreatitis

Pancreatitis is a complex illness that remains poorly understood in terms of its causative factors. Clinical associations with acute pancreatitis generally have been grouped into those that are alcohol related, those that are biliary stone related, and a broad group of idiopathic syndromes. The idiopathic syndromes have association with chlorthiazide diuretics, hyperlipidemia, mumps, and so on. Even congenital abnormalities (pancreatic divisium) have been associated with pancreatitis [31]. Most surgeons have cared for acute pancreatitis patients where a specific association could never be identified. The wide range of different clinical associations makes a unifying hypothesis to explain the pathophysiology of the disease for all patients essentially impossible.

Pathophysiology

Pancreatitis is initially a disease of inflammation and not an infectious disease. The pathogenesis of pancreatitis can be viewed as generally having its origin in the obstruction to the normal flow from the pancreatic exocrine duct. In acute alcoholism spasm of the ampulla of Vater may be responsible for impaired exocrine flow [32]. With alcohol causing increased secretin production from the duodenum, a working hypothesis could be that the volumes of pancreatic secretion would be stimulated against a functional resistance or spasm at the ampullary region. The increased ductal pressure would then provoke inflammation with self-digestion of pancreatic parenchyma by pancreatic enzymes.

With biliary obstruction from calculi in the common duct, the stone becomes wedged at the ampulla and results in anatomic obstruction of both the biliary and the pancreatic ductal systems [33]. An important issue in biliary pancreatitis is

thought to be the reflux of bile acids into the pancreatic duct. The bile acids are felt to augment significantly the inflammatory response in the pancreas.

While the above-defined "obstructive" etiologies of pancreatitis are attractive, there remain unanswered questions about the real origin of pancreatitis. For example, why does alcohol cause ampullary spasm in only certain patients and not others? There certainly appears to be a genetic predisposition to the development of alcoholic pancreatitis. A single drinking episode commonly will provoke an acute episode in certain individuals, while others may drink heavily for life with no adverse sequelae. It is interesting that the overwhelming majority of alcoholic cirrhotic patients who undergo operations of the abdomen usually have a very normal pancreas. There is no apparent dose-effect relationship in the onset of pancreatitis and the number of years of alcoholism. Indeed, alcoholic pancreatitis can be seen in the very young patient.

Likewise, biliary obstruction is not always associated with pancreatitis even though simultaneous obstruction of the pancreatic duct also may be present. Proximal malignancy in the pancreas invariably is associated with pancreatic duct obstruction but is infrequently associated with clinically significant pancreatitis. Certain drug-induced pancreatitis and infectious pancreatitis (e.g., mumps) are probably direct injury of the pancreatic parenchymal cell or the pancreatic ductal system.

Acute pancreatitis is initially a sterile inflammation. It is characterized by severe edema of the pancreatic parenchyma. Adjacent retroperitoneal structures become edematous, and significant interstitial edema is identified in and about the acutely inflamed pancreas. The natural history of the disease is summarized in Fig. 27-6 and can be quite unpredictable. In selected cases the acute inflammation spontaneously resolves without any residual ductal damage in the gland. The patients become asymptomatic until a subsequent encounter with a physiologic provocateur. Damage to the ductal system may leave the individual with stenotic and obstructed ducts within the pancreas. This sets the stage for recurrent, relapsing, and chronic pancreatitis, even though no additional stimuli (e.g., alcohol consumption) are encountered. Chronic pancreatitis results in progressive disin-

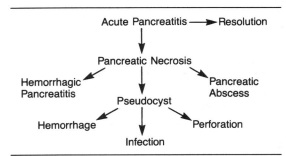

Fig. 27-6. Schematic illustration of the natural history of acute pancreatitis. Fortunately with prompt treatment and elimination of the offending focus, most of these patients do not have the severe adverse sequelae that can attend this disease

tegration of the entire gland, with both pancreatic endocrine and exocrine insufficiency being the end result. Pain from this chronic smoldering process and the adjacent perineuritis of celiac and other retroperitoneal sensory nerve structures commonly becomes unrelenting and incapacitating.

Severe acute pancreatitis can result in additional acutely morbid complications. Severe inflammation can result in disruption of a major pancreatic duct with extravasation of enzymes into the lesser sac area. This results in an acute pancreatic pseudocyst. The pseudocyst may become acutely infected or may rupture into the peritoneal cavity and cause acute chemical peritonitis. Hemorrhage into the pseudocyst can cause a life-threatening emergency. The severity of the acute pancreatitis may actually compromise the microcirculation to the gland, which results in necrosis. Necrosis leads to the sloughing of the gland. This focus of the necrotic gland then becomes secondarily infected with GI bacteria, and pancreatic abscess is the result.

Clinical Presentation

The clinical features of acute pancreatitis are pain, nausea, and vomiting. The referred pain is in the epigastrium. Because the overlying parietal peritoneum of the anterior abdominal wall becomes involved in the inflammatory process only very late, vague and poorly localized anterior pain is the characteristic complaint of the acute pancreatitis patient. The retroperitoneal location of the pancreas results in retroperitoneal somatic pain fibers being

stimulated. This results in the classic "burrowing" back pain that is commonly localized by the patient as between the scapulae on the back. With a careful history of the evolution and nature of the pain, combined with an evaluation of potential clinical associations (e.g., alcohol ingestion, biliary calculi), the diagnosis of acute pancreatitis can be made without fancy diagnostic methods.

The physical examination in the acute pancreatitis patient can be highly variable. In acute, early pancreatitis there will be no peritoneal signs, and tenderness can be elicited only with deep abdominal palpation, if at all. In severe cases board-like rigidity of the abdomen will suggest that catastrophic pancreatitis with fulminant peritonitis is present. In actuality the peritonitis is only a severe chemical peritonitis. If the patient has been ill for a number of days prior to presentation, pancreatic abscess may already be in evolution. The patient may have full-blown septic shock and all associated sequelae.

Patients with infected pancreatic pseudocysts or pancreatic abscess will present in a common fashion. Both will commonly have palpable and tender masses. The patients are clinically quite toxic appearing. Ultrasound and CT scan evaluation may prove to differentiate the two processes. One can be too academic with the septic patient and a palpable epigastric mass. Both need drainage and need it quickly.

Pancreatitis commonly is complicated by respiratory distress [34]. With severe cases adult respiratory distress syndrome may emerge rapidly and be apparent at presentation or may rapidly evolve during emergency department evaluation. Endotracheal intubation may be necessary. Patients with tachypnea should have arterial blood gases done immediately both to evaluate current oxygenation and to serve as a baseline for monitoring of future developments.

Fever and WBC counts may be normal or distinctly abnormal and are of little help in the diagnostic process. Elevated serum amylase and lipase will establish the diagnosis for most patients. Patients who have had multiple and severe previous bouts with pancreatitis essentially may have "burned out" their pancreas. Acute exacerbations in these patients may be associated with minimal or no amylase elevation, because insufficient pancreatic parenchyma remains. Patients with severe end-stage pancreatitis may actually present as hyper-osmolar nonketotic coma.

Differential Diagnosis

Clinical presentations of pancreatitis may be confused with other disease processes arising from the embryonic foregut. Acute cholecystitis is most notable because of both referred epigastric pain and the back pain that is seen in gallbladder patients. Biliary disease and pancreatitis go hand in hand, and both may be seen together in a large number of patients.

Penetrating peptic ulcers commonly involve the pancreatic head. A diagnosis of acute pancreatitis may be correct in these patients, but in reality they have peptic ulcer disease and should be managed accordingly.

The CT scan has significantly improved the diagnostic accuracy of evaluating the patient with pancreatitis. Acute edematous pancreatitis, pseudocysts, and pancreatic abscesses can be accurately determined with this methodology. The utility of the CT scan has made the ultrasound of little value in these patients.

Traumatic pancreatitis from blunt abdominal injury is common. An amylase determination is appropriate in the evaluation of patients with blunt abdominal trauma. The emergency department physician must beware of the low-grade hyper-amylasemia of the trauma patient, because it may reflect severe pancreatic injury. In multiple-trauma patients, craniofacial trauma may elevate amylase concentration because of salivary gland trauma also. The low-grade amylase elevation must be treated with respect. Not infrequently CT scans or even laparotomy may be required to discern whether a pancreatic injury has occurred. Because pancreatic enzyme concentrations are elevated within the proximal small intestine, duodenal or proximal jejunal disruption may give an increased serum amylase with or without any associated pancreatic injury.

Management

Several aspects of the management of acute pancreatitis can be initiated in the emergency department. Expansion of extracellular volume is essential, since the retroperitoneal process results in the massive sequestration of volume in the inflammatory area. A Foley catheter usually will be necessary for purposes of monitoring urine output as soon as volume resuscitation has been started. A nasogastric tube should be placed as soon as the diagnosis has been made. For acute edematous pancreatitis antibiotic therapy should not be started either in the emergency department or after admission. Antibiotics should be started only when an infected pseudocyst or a pancreatic abscess is strongly suspected (see Table 27-1).

Total management goals for these patients need to be individualized. Nasogastric suction and IV fluid support are the essentials of the management of acute pancreatitis. Acute pseudocysts commonly are managed nonoperatively, and many will resolve. Large pseudocysts will develop a mature rind and at that point, the cystic mass is internally drained into the GI tract surgically. The timing of surgical intervention for pseudocysts is best predicted by the abdominal CT scan, which will identify the thickness of the cyst wall necessary for internal drainage. Infected pseudocysts need to be drained immediately with either open surgical drainage to the exterior or percutaneous CT-directed drainage by a radiologic interventionalist.

Is there a role for outpatient management of patients with acute pancreatitis? In the author's judgment, acute pancreatitis needs nasogastric suction, IV fluids, and hospitalization. When the destruction of the pancreatic gland from a single episode or multiple recurrent episodes of pancreatitis results in permanent destruction of the pancreatic ductal structure, chronic pancreatitis will be the consequence. Ambulatory management of acute episodes can be undertaken only with caution and when the physician is very familiar with the patient and has dealt with acute episodes previously.

Perforated Ulcer

Perforated ulcers remain a common cause of the acute abdomen that will bring patients to the emergency department for evaluation. While the overall incidence of peptic ulcer disease appears to be declining, acute perforation even when the individual has no antecedent history of peptic ulcer disease continues to be a problem. Perforated gastric ulcers and perforated gastric cancers will present in a similar clinical fashion, but gastric cancers usually present in patients in their fifth decade of life or older. Perforation from a primary gastric lesion is less common than is perforation from peptic ulcer disease.

Pathophysiology

Acute perforated peptic ulcer is the consequence of excessive gastric acid production, which results in peptic digestion of the vulnerable tissues of the bulb, or first portion, of the duodenum. Intestinal mucus and the alkaline effects of biliary and pancreatic secretions in the duodenum constantly provide protection against peptic digestion. When acid secretion exceeds a critical threshold, mucosal breakdown occurs. When the acute ulcer occurs on the anterior antimesenteric site of the duodenum, free perforation into the peritoneal cavity can occur. Ulcers on the posterior or mesenteric site of the duodenum will penetrate into the pancreas (and cause a local pancreatitis) or burrow into the retroperitoneal area and provoke major hemorrhage as the gastroduodenal arterial complex becomes involved in the inflammatory process.

Perforation customarily favors the patient with acute-onset peptic ulcer disease. When a patient has had ulcer disease for a period of time, the scar formation in and about the longer-standing lesion probably provides a measure of protection against perforation. However, the scarring and contraction process does predispose the patient to gastric-outlet obstruction.

The causes of perforation from benign gastric ulcer and gastric cancer are less well understood. Benign gastric ulcer is not associated with hyperacidity. Benign gastric lesions probably are a consequence of the loss of gastric-barrier function and hence probably represent some element of peptic digestion from normally innocuous concentrations of acid. Since gastric-carcinoma patients characteristically are achlorhydric, the occasional perforation in these cases is secondary to transmural growth of tumor cells.

Clinical Presentation

The precipitous and abrupt onset of upper abdominal pain characterizes the acute perforated ulcer. The patients will relate that they were feeling fine

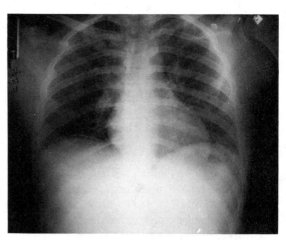

Fig. 27-7. Abdominal roentgenogram that illustrates free air underneath the diaphragm in a patient who subsequently proved to have a perforated peptic ulcer

but then were doubled over by acute pain, as though they had been struck in the abdomen. The patients commonly will relate the exact time of the perforation. When first seen in the emergency department, the patients usually will be clutching the epigastric area of the abdomen. A history of prior peptic ulcer pain may or may not be identified. In the author's experience about one-third of patients with perforated peptic ulcer have had no previous symptoms, about one-third will have had recent onset of peptic ulcer symptoms and may have currently started medical management, and about one-third are long-standing ulcer patients.

The abdominal examination will show acute peritoneal signs. Rebound tenderness almost always will be present. In large perforative lesions with massive peritoneal contamination or in those perforations where there was a considerable delay in getting to the emergency department, board-like rigidity from spasm of the abdominal wall muscles will be seen. The presence or absence of fever and leukocytosis usually will depend on the interval between perforation and clinical assessment. Upright chest roentgenogram will often show free air under the diaphragm (Fig. 27-7). Selected cases, particularly in older patients, may have an equivocal history or equivocal physical findings. Occasionally a Gastrografin swallow may be necessary to define extravasation of contents.

Differential Diagnosis

Any perforative event in the abdominal cavity can mimic a perforated ulcer, and similarly a perforated ulcer can mimic other events. Every experienced surgeon can relate a case in which a McBurney incision was made to remove an acute appendix only to find peas or carrots in the right pericolic gutter from a perforated ulcer. It is vitally important for the emergency department physician to understand that one can be too precise in trying to diagnose the cause of peritonitis. The most compelling question to be answered in the patient with an acute abdomen is, "Does this patient need an emergency operation or not?" Diffuse rebound tenderness of the abdomen may arise from any number of sources. The important issue is whether operative intervention is necessary, and management objectives need to be focused in that direction.

Diseases arising from foregut derivatives can be confusing. Equivocal tenderness may require a Gastrografin swallow to differentiate severe penetrating ulcer from perforation. Ultrasound may identify cholelithiasis. Amylase determination may define the acute pancreatitis. On many occasions the emergency department physician will be expected to be actively involved in efforts to define the source of a patient's acute abdomen. Decisions in the emergency department commonly will dictate whether patients are admitted to the ward or proceed to the operating room.

Management

The management of the perforated ulcer remains surgical. When the diagnosis is evident, IV isotonic sodium chloride or Ringer's lactate should be begun immediately. A nasogastric tube should be placed. Antibiotic therapy is started before the operation, even though a large number of acutely perforated peptic ulcers result in a sterile peritonitis. Antibiotic coverage should focus on aerobic gram-negative rods. Any of the cephalosporin antibiotics is adequate for this purpose. Cefazolin (1–2 g q8h) remains an inexpensive and effective antibiotic for these patients. Anaerobic microflora from upper GI tract perforation usually are derived from the mouth and are quite sensitive to most antibiotics employed for peritonitis (see Table 27-1).

The rapidity of proceeding with the operation is dictated by the severity of the patient's illness. Most patients will benefit from some volume resuscitation, nasogastric decompression, and antibiotic therapy. If the patient is severely toxic and has hemodynamic instability, then emergency operation is necessary. Ideally all patients should undergo laparotomy for a perforated ulcer within 8 hours of the primary event.

While it is beyond the scope of this presentation to provide a dissertation about the controversial issues in the surgical management of acute perforations, the patient's history commonly is an important variable in how the acute peptic perforation is managed. If the patient has no prior history of peptic ulcer disease, many surgeons would favor simple plication of the ulcer. If the patient has been having symptoms of peptic ulcer disease for weeks to months prior to the perforation, then vagotomy and a drainage procedure would be favored. If the duration of perforation has been less than 8–12 hours, that would favor the performance of an ulcer procedure (e.g., vagotomy and pyloroplasty), whereas a perforation that has been present for much longer periods of time might favor a plication of the ulcer. The documentation of these historic details from either patients or families may be uniquely available to the emergency department physician and may influence subsequent surgical management.

Intra-Abdominal Infection After Trauma

Intra-abdominal infection following traumatic injury of the abdomen is quite frequent. Infectious morbidity is most commonly identified after penetrating injuries rather than blunt injuries because of the marked increase in the frequency of GI disruption in the penetrating cases. Blunt disruption actually is rare, but it can be diagnostically treacherous when it occurs. The prevention and treatment of posttraumatic peritoneal infection begin in the emergency department. It is important that the emergency department physician and the trauma surgeon have a consensus opinion about antibiotic initiation for these patients.

Pathophysiology

Penetrating injuries can violate any structure in the peritoneal cavity. The infectious implications of a GI injury are obvious, but the potential morbidity depends on the anatomic site of injury, the magnitude of the contamination, the presence of adjuvant factors, and the velocity of the missile causing the injury. As noted in earlier discussions the average patient will have few bacteria in the stomach and relatively small numbers of bacteria in the proximal small intestine. Disruptions in the proximal portions of the abdominal GI tract have the least risks for infection. The mid-to-distal ileum has bacterial concentrations of 10^5–10^6 organisms per milliliter, and the bacterial species at this level demonstrate a mix of both aerobic and anaerobic species. This differs from the proximal gut, where the limited numbers of bacteria are primarily aerobic. The right colon will have bacterial counts of 10^7–10^8 organisms per gram of content, and the rectosigmoid lumen will contain 10^{10}–10^{11} organisms per gram. Major disruptions of the distal gut clearly portend a high risk for subsequent infectious morbidity.

In earlier discussions about the pathophysiology of peritonitis in general the role of adjuvant factors was discussed. In the abdomen that has sustained a penetrating injury, adjuvant factors are of major importance. Free hemoglobin, soft-tissue hematomas, and dead tissue are of particular importance in the injured abdomen. Foreign bodies from the injury and particulate matter released from the injured bowel all become adjuvants when present in the peritoneal cavity. Thus, the gastric injury that results in massive soilage of recently eaten food into the peritoneal cavity will have a relatively high likelihood of infection, even though the actual number of contaminating bacteria is relatively small.

Both blunt and penetrating injuries of the abdomen can disrupt solid viscus structures, which may have the consequences of accentuating potential infectious risks. Liver injuries even after repair for active bleeding will continue to have a weeping, bloody effluent from the injury. Bile leaks will establish an inflammatory response and will reduce the number of bacteria necessary to cause peritonitis or abscess. Repaired splenic injuries may have dead tissue retained in the patient or may have

parenchymal hematomas, which can be morbid variables if a GI injury is also present. Perhaps the most morbid injury for infectious complications is the pancreatic injury. The release of potent digestive enzymes into the peritoneal cavity commonly will result in infection, even though the intestine has not been disrupted. The severe inflammation generated by the pancreatic injury will result in bacterial translocation into the phlegmon with subsequent abscess. If GI injury accompanies a major pancreatic injury, then intra-abdominal infectious morbidity is virtually certain. A major pancreatic and colonic combination commonly is an ultimately fatal tandem.

In blunt injuries intestinal injuries are infrequent but have interesting features [35]. Intestinal injury can occur from direct compression and disruption from an external force. Compressive trauma of the abdomen may compress a closed loop of intestine thereby increasing intraluminal pressure and cause a burst injury. Finally sheering forces from deceleration may cause disruption at points of intestinal fixation. Thus, the ligament of Treitz and the ileum at the ileocecal valve are common areas of disruption.

Blunt disruption can be very subtle. The midportion of the duodenum may be disrupted immediately over the midline vertebral bodies of the spine. If disruption occurs without a rent or injury of the overlying peritoneum, the contamination will be totally confined within the retroperitoneum. There will be no peritonitis and no clinical findings of peritonitis. Thus, the infectious process can be extensive among the retroperitoneal structures before abdominal findings are present. Retroperitoneal injury without contamination in the peritoneal cavity also is possible with the ascending colon, the descending colon, and the rectum below the peritoneal reflection.

Clinical Presentation

Penetrating injuries usually are secondary to either firearms or sharp instruments. In general all gunshot wounds below the nipples and above the groin require abdominal exploration. The uncertainty of the course of the missile makes further diagnostic efforts useless. All should be assumed to have intestinal injury.

The clinical decisions in stab wounds remain

somewhat controversial. Routine exploration is advocated only if the patient is hemodynamically unstable or there is ready evidence of intra-abdominal injury (e.g., eviscerated omentum or bowel). Other wounds of less certain significance may be locally explored, may require peritoneal lavage, or may be observed for the development of peritoneal signs.

Blunt abdominal injuries can be evaluated by physical examination if the patient has not had an associated head injury or is not intoxicated. Acute peritoneal signs require surgical intervention, particularly if any hemodynamic instability is present. When the patient has an altered mental status or has equivocal physical findings, then either a CT scan or a diagnostic peritoneal lavage is necessary.

Because of the significance of a pancreatic injury a serum amylase should be done in these patients, since pancreatic and retroperitoneal injuries can be quite subtle in some patients. The presence of abdominal pain out of proportion to physical findings, early postinjury fever, or an elevation of the serum amylase should raise the suspicion of a pancreatic or retroperitoneal duodenal injury. Also early postoperative fever and disproportionate abdominal pain relative to physical findings may herald other retroperitoneal intestinal injury (e.g., right or left colon). Seat belt abrasions and other upper abdominal wall contusions should sensitize the examining physician to the potential of a pancreatico-duodenal injury.

Differential Diagnosis

In general, attempts to detail intra-abdominal injury in the trauma patient are not necessary. The decision that must be made in these patients is whether abdominal exploration is necessary. The specifics of intra-abdominal injury can be fully defined with a comprehensive abdominal exploration.

Management

The management of the abdominal-trauma patient requires establishment of an airway, adequate ventilation, and volume resuscitation, as would usually be the case for all trauma patients. Full restoration of tissue perfusion and oxygenation is of major significance in bolstering host defenses against major

contamination that may or may not have occurred from the injury.

Preventive antibiotics are important for the abdominal-trauma patient and should be administered as soon as the decision to pursue operation has been made [36]. The single most important issue in preventive antibiotics is timing of administration. The antibiotics must be administered preoperatively and as close to the time of the injury as possible. Antibiotics may reduce the number of viable organisms that have contaminated the soft tissues of the peritoneal cavity. Adequate antibiotic concentrations are vitally important for the surgical wound, since these drugs clearly have been shown to reduce surgical wound infections in the postoperative period.

The pathogens likely to be encountered in the injured abdomen are numerous. Both enteric facultative bacteria (e.g., *E. coli*) and obligate anaerobes (e.g., *Bacteroides fragilis*) are encountered if the distal ileum or the colon has been perforated. Penetrating injuries can carry staphylococci from the skin and external areas into the peritoneal cavity. Lapses in surgical technique associated with the urgent surgical procedure of the trauma patient make the risks of staphylococcal contamination from the procedure itself significant. Preventive antibiotics generally are felt to need coverage of the Enterobacteriaceae, obligate anaerobes, and staphylococci. Second- and third-generation cephalosporins that have this comprehensive profile generally are preferred by most trauma surgeons. Cefoxitin (2 g q6h IV) is probably the most popular choice for the trauma patient that is about to undergo laparotomy. For the emergency department physician an understanding should be reached with the trauma division about antibiotic use. When this agreement exists, the emergency department physician can initiate antibiotic therapy as soon as possible when the indications for abdominal exploration clearly are present (see Table 27-1).

Spontaneous Bacterial Peritonitis

Spontaneous bacterial peritonitis represents the classic misnomer in medicine. Spontaneous generation was soundly disproved by Louis Pasteur 150 years ago. Primary peritonitis is perhaps a better term. The disease occurs when there is the absence of an anatomic defect or intra-abdominal disease process that serves as the source of the bacterial contamination.

Pathophysiology

Since no disease process of the intra-abdominal compartment is present, primary peritonitis requires that bacteria gain access to the peritoneal cavity via the bloodstream or the lymphatic system. Remote infections can serve as a means of bacterial seeding of the peritoneal space. Thus, pneumococci may actually become pathogens of primary peritonitis. The recent resurgence of interest in bacterial translocation reflects the concern that bacteria may gain access to the peritoneal cavity via visceral lymphatics or by migration across the intestinal barrier. Of significance is that this translocation phenomenon appears to involve only aerobic bacterial species.

While bacteremia is a relatively common phenomenon in clinical medicine, spontaneous bacterial peritonitis is uncommon. Either the organism must have a particular affinity for seeding the peritoneal cavity (e.g., *Mycobacterium* species) or the peritoneal cavity must have biological conditions that favor lodging of the bacteremic organisms (e.g., ascites). The patient with hepatic cirrhosis and ascites represents the prototype patient of the current era that has both compromised defenses, and the fluid-filled compartment that is vulnerable to blood-borne or lymphatic-borne contamination [37].

Clinical Presentation

Primary peritonitis is suspected in the patient with ascites who develops an acute febrile illness and abdominal tenderness [37, 38]. Patients commonly will have diffuse rebound tenderness as a nonspecific sign of an acute abdomen. Because the patient with ascites commonly will have altered host defenses related to the fundamental underlying disease (e.g., cirrhosis), the physical examination of the abdomen may not always demonstrate dramatic signs of peritonitis. A fever, tachycardia, abdominal pain, or altered mental status may be the only indicators, and the clinician must maintain a high index of suspicion for the diagnosis.

Paracentesis of ascites for a Gram's stain, culture, and white cell count usually will establish the diagnosis. Polymorphonuclear WBC counts of more than 250/μl generally are associated with the diagnosis [39, 40]. Intracellular organisms within phagocytic cells on Gram's stain likewise are useful. See Chap. 18 for a more complete discussion of spontaneous bacterial peritonitis in the alcoholic patient.

Differential Diagnosis

The critical diagnostic consideration in these patients is whether the peritonitis is from a primary lymphatic or hematogenous seeding or whether the patient has secondary peritonitis due to a biliary or enteric source. Gram-positive diplococci on Gram's stain from the ascitic fluid would confirm primary peritonitis. Gram-negative rods may still indicate primary peritonitis, but this diagnosis must be approached cautiously since biliary or other sources in the abdomen may be responsible. The author would be cautious about a diagnosis of primary peritonitis in a patient with clearly a polymicrobial microflora on Gram's stain. A surgical consultation for the evaluation of secondary sources would seem prudent for the patient with suspected polymicrobial primary peritonitis. The differentiating characteristics of the ascitic fluid in spontaneous bacterial peritonitis, secondary bacterial peritonitis, and culture-negative neutrocytic ascites can be found in Table 18-5.

Management

The general management of these patients should be similar to the management of patients with peritonitis regardless of cause. Intravascular volume support should be appropriate to the patient's need, but caution should be exercised relative to excessive volume administration in the patient with ascites. Urine output becomes a difficult clinical monitor in the patient with ascites, and the Swan-Ganz catheter may be required for volume management.

Antibiotic management usually will be started prior to the availability of cultures and will require a certain dependence on the Gram's stain. Initial therapy with a third-generation cephalosporin (e.g., cefotaxime) is recommended to cover suspected *E. coli*, *Streptococcus* species, *Klebsiella* species, and other enteric gram-negative bacteria. Usually only a single pathogen is isolated from the ascitic fluid in spontaneous bacterial peritonitis. Because of concerns about nephrotoxicity, aminoglycosides are discouraged for many of these patients. For suspected polymicrobial infections, broad aerobic and anaerobic coverage is initiated. Drug therapy usually will be tailored to cultured pathogens in 48 hours (see Table 27-1).

Perirectal Abscess

Pathophysiology

Anorectal abscesses probably result from blockage of mucus-secreting anal glands, which ordinarily drain into anal crypts. The abscesses are usually mixed infections of aerobes and anaerobes. Organisms include *E. coli* and *Proteus, Bacteroides,* and *Streptococcus* species. Anal abscesses can involve several potential spaces, including perianal, submucosal, ischiorectal, and supralevator. Anal fissures from Crohn's disease and ulcerative colitis also can lead to abscess formation.

Clinical Presentation

PERIANAL ABSCESS
Perianal abscesses are the most common anal abscesses and the easiest to diagnose. Patients will report anal pain, which is increased with defecation or straining. Most patients are afebrile. A tender, erythematous fluctuant mass is evident in the perianal area with a normal rectal exam. Small abscesses can be drained in the emergency department, but care must be taken to determine that the abscess does not involve other anal potential spaces. Other contraindications to emergency department drainage include inability to achieve pain control, immunosuppression, advanced age or debilitation, morbid obesity, and evidence of systemic infection such as high fever, hypotension, or other evidence of sepsis.

SUBMUCOSAL ABSCESS
Patients with submucosal abscess will complain of rectal pressure, pain, and fullness. Fever is not usually noted. External examination will be normal,

while rectal examination will demonstrate a tender mass above the pectinate line. Drainage can be done in the emergency department if adequate visualization can be obtained.

ISCHIORECTAL AND SUPRALEVATOR ABSCESS
Patients with these abscesses will experience dull pain deep in the buttocks. Rectal, pelvic, or abdominal pain also may be present. Fever is common. With ischiorectal abscess buttock asymmetry or cellulitis may be evident on physical exam. The abscess can be best evaluated with one finger in the rectum and another on the buttock. The supralevator abscess is the deepest and hence the most difficult to diagnose. Tenderness or induration may be appreciated on rectal exam, or a fullness between the coccyx and rectum discerned. These abscesses are deep and may be extensive, so incision and drainage in the operating room is necessary.

Management

Incision and drainage in the emergency department is preceded by analgesia, which may include intradermal lidocaine or bupivacaine, systemic narcotic analgesia, or the administration of nitrous oxide. The excision is made, loculations broken up, the cavity cleaned out and loosely packed. The patient should be asked to return in 48 hours for packing removal and recheck. If symptoms persist, adequate drainage may not have been achieved, and a surgical consultation is recommended. All patients should have surgical referral because of fistula formation and abscess recurrence. Antibiotics are not necessary unless extensive cellulitis or underlying disease is present. In those cases consideration should be given to admission.

References

1. Brewer RJ et al. Abdominal pain: an analysis of 1,000 consecutive cases in a university hospital emergency room. *Am J Surg* 131:219, 1976.
2. Autio V. The spread of intraperitoneal infection. Studies with roentgen contrast medium. *Acta Chir Scand* 123(suppl. 321):5–31, 1964.
3. Tsilibary EC, Wissig SL. Absorption from the peri-

toneal cavity: SEM study of the mesothelium covering the peritoneal surface of the muscular portion of the diaphragm. *Am J Anat* 149:127, 1977.

4. Hau T, Simmons RL. Heparin in the treatment of experimental peritonitis. *Ann Surg* 187:294–98, 1978.

5. Hau T, Ahrenholz DH, Simmons RL. Secondary bacterial peritonitis: the biological basis of treatment. *Curr Probl Surg* 16(10):1, 1979.

6. Fry DE, Polk HC Jr. Host defense in the trauma patient. In JD Richardson, HC Polk Jr, LM Flint (eds.), *Trauma: Clinical Care and Pathophysiology*. Chicago: Year Book, 1987. Pp. 41–77.

7. Dinarello CA, Cannon JG, Wolff SM. New concepts on the pathogenesis of fever. *Rev Infect Dis* 10:168–89, 1988.

8. Wangensteen OH, Dennis C. Experimental proof of the obstructive origin of appendicitis in man. *Ann Surg* 110:629, 1939.

9. Burkitt DP. The aetiology of appendicitis. *Br J Surg* 58:695, 1971.

10. Lewis FR et al. Appendicitis: a critical review of diagnosis and treatment in 1000 cases. *Arch Surg* 110:677, 1975.

11. Hyman P, Westring DW. Leukocytosis in acute appendicitis. *JAMA* 229:1630, 1975.

12. Lee PWR. The leukocyte count in acute appendicitis. *Br J Surg* 60:618, 1973.

13. Doraiswamy NV. Leukocyte counts in the diagnosis and prognosis of acute appendicitis in children. *Br J Surg* 66:782, 1979.

14. Lansden FT. Acute appendicitis in children. *Am J Surg* 106:938, 1963.

15. Bower RJ, Bell MJ, Ternberg JL. Diagnostic value of the white blood cell count and neutrophil percentage in children. *Surg Gynecol Obstet* 152:424, 1981.

16. Hubbell DS, Barton WK, Solomon OD. Leukocytosis in appendicitis in older person. *JAMA* 175(2):163, 1961.

17. Schwartz SI. Tempering the technological diagnosis of appendicitis. *N Engl J Med* 317:703, 1987.

18. Puylaert JBCM et al. A prospective study of ultrasonography in the diagnosis of appendicitis. *N Engl J Med* 317:666, 1987.

19. Lewis FR et al. Appendicitis: a critical review of diagnosis and treatment in 1000 cases. *Arch Surg* 110:677, 1975.

20. Painter NS, Burkitt DP. Diverticular disease of the colon: a deficiency disease of Western civilization. *Br Med J* 2:450, 1971.

21. Almy TP, Howell DA. Diverticular disease of the colon. *N Engl J Med* 302:324, 1980.

22. Slack WW. The anatomy, pathology, and some clinical features of diverticulitis of the colon. *Br J Surg* 50:185, 1962.

23. Wahlby L, Knutsen OH. Leukocyte counts, ESR and fever in the diagnosis of diverticulitis. *Acta Chir Scand* 148:623, 1982.

24. Fry DE, Cox RA, Harbrecht PJ. Empyema of the gallbladder: a complication in the natural history of acute cholecystitis. *Am J Surg* 141:366–68, 1981.

25. Fry DE, Cox RA, Harbrecht PJ. Gangrene of the gallbladder: a complication of acute cholecystitis. *South Med J* 74:666–68. 1981.

26. Chetlin SH, Elliott DW. Biliary bacteremia. *Arch Surg* 102:303–7, 1971.

27. Cheung LY, Maxwell JG. Jaundice in patients with acute cholecystitis. *Am J Surg* 130:746–48, 1975.

28. Dumont AE. Significance of hyperbilirubinemia in acute cholecystitis. *Surg Gynecol Obstet* 142:855–57, 1976.

29. Suarez CA et al. The role of HIDA/PIPIDA scanning in diagnosing cystic duct obstruction. *Ann Surg* 191:391, 1980.

30. Matolo NM, LaMorte WW, Wolfe BM. Acute and chronic cholecystitis. *Surg Clin North Am* 61(4):875, 1981.

31. Delhaye M, Engelholm L, Cremer M. Pancreas divisium: congenital variant or anomaly? Contribution of endoscopic retrograde dorsal pancreatography. *Gastroenterology* 89:951, 1985.

32. Schapiro H, Wruble LD, Britt LG. The possible mechanism of alcohol in the production of acute pancreatitis. *Surgery* 60:1108–11, 1966.

33. Acosta JM, Pelligrini CA, Skinner DB. Etiology and pathogenesis of acute biliary pancreatitis. *Surgery* 88:118, 1980.

34. Ranson JHC et al. Respiratory complications in acute pancreatitis. *Ann Surg* 179:557, 1974.

35. Hunt KE, Garrison RN, Fry DE. Perforating injuries of the gastrointestinal tract secondary to blunt abdominal trauma. *Am Surg* 46:100–104, 1980.

36. Fullen WD, Hunt J, Altemeier WA. Prophylactic antibiotics in penetrating wounds of the abdomen. *J Trauma* 12:282, 1972.

37. Conn HO. Spontaneous bacterial peritonitis in cirrhosis: variations on a theme. *Medicine* 50:161–97, 1971.

38. Hoefs JC et al. Spontaneous bacterial peritonitis. *Hepatology* 2:399–407, 1982.

39. Garcia-Tsao G, Conn HO, Lerner E. The diagnosis of bacterial peritonitis: comparison of pH, lactate concentration and leukocyte count. *Hepatology* 5:91–96, 1985.

40. Yang C-Y et al. White count, pH, and lactate in ascites in the diagnosis of spontaneous bacterial peritonitis. *Hepatology* 5:85–90, 1985.

THE GENITOURINARY TRACT

28

Infections of the Urinary Tract and Male Genitalia

CHARLES STEWART
RAQUEL L. GIBLY
JUDITH C. BRILLMAN

Urinary Tract Infection in Women

Urinary tract infection (UTI) is one of the most common entities encountered by the physician. Approximately 25%–30% of otherwise healthy women 20–40 years of age will suffer from at least one episode of UTI [1], and 10%–20% of all women will suffer from UTI at some point during their lifetime [2]. Because of the acute nature of this problem the emergency physician will be the initial source of care for many of these patients. Accurate diagnosis and treatment in the emergency department will allow the most cost-effective patient management with the lowest rate of complications.

Lower Tract Infection

Lower urinary tract infection results from superficial bacterial infection of the urethra and the bladder [2]. These infections develop when uropathogens, usually from colonization of the anus, vaginal introitus, or periurethral area, enter the urethra [1], resulting in a urethritis. If the pathogens ascend farther, the infection presents as a cystitis or may ultimately result in an upper tract infection and pyelonephritis.

EPIDEMIOLOGY AND RISK FACTORS

Any factor that results in the movement of bacteria from the rectum anteriorly is a predisposing factor for a UTI. Sexual intercourse, probably through mechanical effect, has been shown to be one of the most important risk factors in the development of an uncomplicated UTI in the sexually active female. Other sexual behaviors, such as masturbation and oral sex, have not been implicated. The use of a diaphragm has been associated with increased incidence of UTI, as has anything that changes the vaginal pH, such as spermicides. The pH of the urine may also play a role in the development of UTIs [1].

Other predisposing factors include anatomical variations that facilitate movement of bacteria from the periurethral tissues into the urethra, as occurs with a short urethra, or close proximity between the urethra and the introitus; pregnancy, which causes anatomical changes that lead to an increased potential for partial urinary obstruction; increased bladder pressure, which causes vesicoureteral reflux; and acute obstruction secondary to cancer in the bladder or the pelvis, stricture of the urethra, or stones anywhere from renal pelvis to urethra [3, 4].

Table 28-1. Risk factors for development of UTIs

Anatomical
  Short urethra
  Proximity of urethra to periurethral tissues
Sexual intercourse
Diaphragm use
Change in pH
  Spermicide use
Pregnancy
Obstruction
  Stone
    Upper tract (renal pelvis, ureter)
    Lower tract (bladder, urethra)
  Tumor
    Pelvic or abdominal cancer with impingement
      on urinary tract
    Primary urinary tract cancer
  Stricture
Manipulation
  Postcatheter
  Postsurgical
Vesicoureteral reflux
  Increased bladder pressure
  Anatomic abnormality
Underlying medical factors

Sources: References 1–5. Used with permission.

Table 28-1 lists the various risk factors for the development of UTI.

COMPLICATING FACTORS

When complicating factors are present, pathogenesis is different and antimicrobial resistance may be more common. Approximately one-third of these patients will have occult upper tract infections, as diagnosed by antibody-coated bacteria testing (ACBT), bladder washout techniques, and ureteral catheterization [2, 5]. These patients may need to be monitored more closely because systemic complications may be more frequent. Risk factors for complicated UTIs are listed in (Table 28-2) [2, 6].

BACTERIOLOGY

The most common urinary pathogen, *Escherichia coli*, is responsible for 80%–95% of all uncomplicated UTIs [1, 2]. This organism is a fastidious gram-negative uropathogen and will often show greater than 10^5 colony-forming units (CFUs) on bacterial culture. *Staphylococcus saprophyticus*, a

Table 28-2. Risk factors for complicated UTIs

Demographic factors
  Presentation to an urban ED
  Lower socioeconomic status
Pregnancy
Recent hospitalization (within 2 weeks)
Recent manipulation or instrumentation
  Indwelling catheter
  Kidney tubes
  Cystoscopy
Obstruction
  Stricture
  Stone
  Cancer
Recent infection or relapse
Recent antibiotic therapy (within 3 weeks)
Previous UTIs
  Before age 12
  More than three in the past year
  Recent pyelonephritis
Symptoms for more than 7 days
Other medical conditions
  Diabetes
  Immunocompromise
  Cancer
  Neurologic conditions
    Spinal cord dysfunction
    Cerebral palsy
    Muscular dystrophies

Sources: References 1–5. Used with permission.

gram-positive uropathogen, is responsible for 5%–15% of all UTIs, is a much slower growing organism than *E. coli*, and will often grow only 10^2–10^4 CFUs on a routine culture. This organism, although a true urinary pathogen, often is reported as *Staphylococcus epidermidis* or as a contaminant. *S. saprophyticus* can easily be distinguished in the laboratory from *S. epidermidis* by Novobiocin antibiotic resistance [7]. Other common uropathogens include *Proteus mirabilis* (3%–6%) [8, 9], *Klebsiella* species (3%–5%) [9, 10], *Citrobacter freundii* (< 2%) [8], and enterococci (< 3%) [9]. In patients with complicating factors *Serratia*, *Enterobacter*, and *Pseudomonas* species also are noted [7]. *Lactobacillus* species, *Gardenerella vaginalis*, and *Mycoplasma* species have also been implicated as causative organisms in UTI [1].

In women with acute urethral syndrome (pyuria and dysuria without bacterial growth on culture) or with vaginal discharge, sexually transmitted diseases (STDs) such as *Chlamydia trachomatis*, *Neisseria gonorrhoeae*, *Trichomonas vaginalis*, and herpes simplex also must be considered. None of these will grow on routine cultures.

PRESENTATION

The most common presenting symptom of lower UTI is dysuria, which can be described as internal or external. External dysuria is a sensation of burning or pain caused by the passage of urine over inflamed periurethral or introital tissues [3, 4]. The patient presents with a sharp, burning sensation while or after she urinates. The sensation often is relieved by sitting in warm water. External dysuria occasionally occurs with a urethritis, but the causes usually are nonurinary. Infectious causes include herpes simplex, condyloma accuminatum, candida, or a periurethral abscess [3, 4]. Vaginitis often presents this way, and a pelvic exam with appropriate cultures must be considered in patients with multiple sexual partners, new sexual partners, vaginal discharge, or symptoms of pelvic inflammatory disease (PID) [7]. Chalmydia can cause a concurrent vaginitis and urethritis and must be considered in women with a mucopurulent endocervical discharge and dysuria with sterile pyuria [11, 12]. Noninfectious causes include sexual trauma, manipulation, foreign body, allergies, irritants, atrophic vaginitis (seen in women with estrogen deficiencies), and cancer or dysplasia [13]. When any of these is suspected, a thorough genital exam is warranted.

Internal dysuria is a dull visceral pain that may be constant or may occur only with urination. It may be sensed as an urgency or fullness by the patient and reflects inflammation of the urethra or the bladder. If pyuria and bacturia are present, a urethritis or cystitis can be diagnosed, with the most common pathogens being *E. coli* or *S. saprophyticus*. In the woman with pyuria without bacturia (sterile pyuria), infection with *Chlamydia* species, *N. gonorrhoeae*, *T. vaginalis*, or gram-positive cocci also must be considered [11]. Renal tuberculosis can also present as sterile pyuria and must be suspected in the patient with appropriate clinical history. Sterile pyuria may also result from noninfectious inflammatory conditions of the kidney and structures adjacent to the genitourinary tract (e.g. appendicitis), endocarditis, drugs (steroids, cyclo-phasphamide), recent antibiotic therapy for UTI, and trauma.

The terms *acute urethral syndrome* (AUS) and *pyuria-dysuria syndrome* (PDS) are most often used to describe a patient with pyuria without bacteruria. Chlamydial urethritis or a low-grade bacterial urine infection (10^2–10^4 CFUs) usually are suspected [3, 4, 11, 12]. The terminology can be confusing. Both AUS and PDS present with internal dysuria and can be thought of as urethritis (Table 28-3).

If a woman with internal dysuria also complains of vaginal discharge, coexisting urinary tract and vaginal infections must be considered, and a pelvic exam with appropriate cultures should be performed [11].

When urethral infection goes untreated, bladder mucosa becomes involved. Cystitis, which is the inflammation of bladder mucosa, often presents with more symptoms than just dysuria. Urinary frequency, urgency, incontinence, and nocturia are frequent complaints [3, 4]. Patients may have a sensation of fullness or soreness in the suprapubic area; although found in only 10% of patients, subprapubic tenderness on exam is very specific for cystitis [2]. Patients may also complain of foul-smelling, cloudy, or discolored urine [2, 13].

If back or flank pain is present and if the patient has any systemic symptoms or signs such as malaise, fever, nausea, or vomiting, the patient probably has an upper tract infection.

LABORATORY FINDINGS

Urinalysis. Urinalysis can detect pyuria, hematuria, and bacturia and is invaluable in the diagnosis of a UTI. Microscopic and dipstick methods can be used and are described next.

Pyuria is defined as more than 5–10 WBCs per high-power field of centrifuged, clean-catch-midstream specimen (CCMS), of urine [11]. Pyuria can be detected by direct microscopic exam or via dipstick, which detects the leukocyte esterase (LCE) contained in the WBCs [13]. Demonstration of more than 5 WBCs per high-power field is 90%–95% sensitive for urine cultures growing more than 10^5 colony counts and is 70% sensitive for urine cultures growing 10^2–10^5 colony counts [11]. LCE is highly specific for pyuria (94%–98%), but sensitivity is highly variable (74%–96%) [11]. This

Table 28-3. Differential diagnosis of dysuria

| | Nonurinary | | Urinary | | | |
| | Infectious | Noninfectious | Urethritis | | Cystitis | Pyelonephritis |
			Classic	AUS/PDS		
Dysuria	External	External	Internal	Internal	Internal	Internal
Other symptoms	Lesions, vaginal discharge, itching	Trauma, manipulation, foreign body, irritation, lesions		± Vaginal discharge	Frequency, urgency, suprapubic pain, fullness, hematuria	Back/flank pain, abdominal pain, fever, myalgias, malaise, nausea/vomiting
Pyuria	No	No	Yes	Yes	Yes	Yes
Bacteria/Cx	No/Neg	No/Neg	Yes/$10^2 - 10^5$	No/$<10^2$	Yes/$\geq 10^5$	Yes/$\geq 10^5$
Common organism	N. gonorrhoeae; Chlamydia, Trichomonas, Candida, herpes, Condyloma	None	E. coli, S. saprophyticus, other gram-negative bacilli	N. gonorrhoeae, Chlamydia species, Herpes simplex virus	E. coli, S. saprophyticus, other gram-negative bacilli	E. coli, S. saprophyticus, other gram-negative bacilli

Sources: References 3, 4, 11–13. Used with permission.

is because the number of WBCs in the urine is dependent on many factors, including bladder dwell time and patient hydration, while the presence of LCE depends on a certain amount of WBC lysis [13]. Therefore, microscopic exam using a hemocytometer for cell count may be necessary in the patient who has a high clinical probability of UTI but a negative dipstick. Sensitivity of LCE is increased by ensuring that the pad is read after 2 full minutes of exposure.

Hematuria, either microscopic or gross, can be found in 40%–60% of patients with acute cystitis and is rarely found in patients with isolated urethritis [2]. Microscopic hematuria is defined as greater then 2–5 RBCs per high-power field in a centrifuged urine specimen, and gross hematuria is defined as enough RBCs present that the unspun urine appears grossly bloody. The urine dipstick, which measures hemoglobin released from lysed RBCs, is sensitive enough to measure the hemoglobin from 2–5 RBCs per high-power field of spun urine and therefore is very sensitive [13, 14]. Hypotonic urine allows for a greater sensitivity than hypertonic urine, because it promotes RBC lysis [15]. Dipstick urinalysis for hematuria is 91%–100% sensitive and 65%–99% specific [14].

The degree of hematuria is not related to the severity of the infection, and hemorrhagic cystitis (when gross hematuria is present) need not be treated differently from nonhemorrhagic cystitis [7]. Patients with symptoms typical of a UTI and concurrent bacteria or pyuria should be treated for UTI. If hematuria alone is present, other causes, such as stones, cancer, polyps, trauma, coagulopathies, glomerulonephritis, systemic lupus erythematosis, tuberculosis, schistosomiasis, a foreign body, endocarditis, and sickle cell disease, must be ruled out [13]. Drugs, such as anticoagulants, nonsteroidal anti-inflammatory agents, steroids, and some antibiotics, also have been known to cause hematuria [13, 15].

Bladder catheterization itself may cause up to 4 RBCs per high-power field and may rarely cause gross hematuria [16]. Catheter-induced hematuria can be caused by abrasions to the urethra or the bladder, or it can be secondary to disturbance of strictures, polyps, or cancerous growths.

Significant bacteriuria is the presence of one bacterium per oil-immersion field in CCMS, uncentrifuged, gram-stained urine. This correlates with 10^5 or more bacteria per milliliter of urine [13]. Stamm and colleagues found that in up to 33% of cases of women with dysuria and pyuria, low bacterial counts of 10^2–10^4 were found [12, 18, 19]; this lower threshold for positive culture should be used by the clinician [17]. The primary organisms were *E. coli*, *S. saprophyticus*, and *Proteus* species, both true uropathogens. These low-count infections may not be picked up by the dipstick, and direct microscopic exam may be necessary to ensure high sensitivity [13].

The dipstick nitrite test detects nitrite produced by bacteria in the urine (other than *Enterococcus* species) that reduce urinary nitrate to nitrite. It is highly specific (92%–100%), but its sensitivity is only 35%–85% [14]. This test depends on the dwell time and the concentration of bacteria in the bladder.

Protein also may be present in the urine of a patient with acute UTI [11]. Specificity and sensitivity of this dipstick test is 95%–99% [14]. Urinary pH is usually around 5, so a pH greater than 7 may be useful in suggesting the presence of urea-splitting organisms such as *Proteus* species, which also may be associated with struvite stones [11]. If any test for LCE, nitrite, protein, or blood is positive, sensitivity for diagnosing UTI is 95%, but specificity is only 66%–80%

False-Negative Results. Detection of WBCs, RBCs, and bacteria in the urine is dependent on many factors. A patient who has voided recently or who has frequency may have a short bladder dwell time (less than 6 hours). This may not allow the adequate migration of WBCs or enough time for the production of nitrite by bacteria. This may cause a falsely negative result on dipstick or microscopic urinalysis [6]. Consuming large amounts of liquid can cause a dilutional effect on all elements of the urine and may cause falsely low WBC, RBC, or bacterial counts [13].

False-negative dipsticks can be due to the use of expired or improperly stored dipsticks. Not reading the dipstick at the specified time can cause both false negatives and false positives. False-negative cultures also can be caused by incorrectly obtained CCMS or catheter urine specimens in which antiseptic solutions have been used for the pre-void

Table 28-4. Causes of false-negative results

All components
    Problems involving dipstick
        Outdated
        Improperly stored
        Improperly read
    Short bladder dwell time or recent voiding
    Dilutional effect
Culture
    Use of antiseptic agents in prevoid cleaning
    Improper plating
Hematuria
    Hypertonic solution
    Presence of reducing agents
    Urine pH < 5.1

Sources: References 6, 11, 12, 15. Used with permission.

Table 28-5. Causes of false-positive results

All components
    Contamination (vaginal, fecal, handling)
Hematuria
    Presence of oxidizing agents
    Induction of hematuria
        Catheterization
        Drugs (steroids, nonsteroidal anti-inflammatory
            agents, antibiotics, anticoagulants)
Pseudohematuria
    Drugs (Pyridium)
    Food products (vegetable dyes, beets)
    High concentration of urates
    Hemoglobin
    Myoglobin
Bacteria
    Improper sample handling or processing

Sources: References 6, 11, 12, 15, 16, 23. Used with permission.

cleaning. Antiseptic agents should not be used because they can enter the urine sample and inhibit bacterial growth [11]. False negatives can also result from improper plating of the specimen (wrong culture medium, use of too hot a loop), which can result in bacterial death.

Hematuria by dipstick may not be detected when urine is hypertonic, decreasing the amount of RBC lysis and free hemaglobin. It also may be falsely negative when the pH is less than 5.1 or reducing agents are present [15].

The various causes of false-negative urinalysis results are listed in Table 28-4.

False-Positive Results. False-positive results can occur when contamination from vaginal or fecal reservoirs brings WBCs, bacteria, or blood into the urine specimen. Contamination is suspected when the urine specimen contains a large number of squamous epithelial cells. Contamination can be avoided by obtaining a urine specimen by catheterization. False-positive results also can occur by improperly read dipsticks.

Hematuria can be invoked by catheterization [20] and certain drugs, while the dipstick may be falsely positive in the presence of oxidizing agents [21, 22].

Pseudohematuria, a red or pink color to the urine, can be caused by foods (beets, berries, food colorings), a high concentration of urates, Pyridium (often used in the UTI patient for symptomatic relief of dysuria), and porphyria. On microscopic exam no RBCs will be present because there

is no actual hematuria. Free hemiglobin or myoglobin will also discolor the urine, as well as cause a positive urine dipstick with a negative microscopic exam, and must be considered when urine is red or brown in color [13, 15, 23]. A microscopic exam is recommended when urine is discolored.

Bacteria counts may be falsely elevated if urine is improperly handled or allowed to sit at room temperature longer than 20 minutes after collection.

The various causes of false-positive urinalysis results are listed in Table 28-5.

Need for Culture. According to a study by Wigton and colleagues, there are five independent predictors of positive urine culture in patients suspected of UTI: history of UTI symptoms, back pain, pyuria, hematuria, and bacturia. This study showed that if two or more findings were present, there was a 73% chance of a positive urine culture [24]. In fact, pyuria is found in 90%–95% of patients with lower UTI and greater than 10^5 CFUs and in 70% of patients with 10^2–10^4 CFUs [11].

Carlson et al. found that routine use of pretherapy cultures in patients with suspected lower tract infection increased the cost of treatment by 40% but decreased the overall duration of symptoms only 10% (from 3.1 days to 2.7 days) [12]. Therefore, symptoms suggestive of UTI has hematuria, bacteriuria, pyuria, or a combination of these are sufficient to treat a woman for a lower UTI, and urine culture may be omitted. Empiric antibiotic therapy in uncomplicated lower urinary tract infections is highly effective and rarely altered by culture results. A urine culture should be obtained when an upper tract infection is suspected, in patients with complicating factors (see Table 28-2) [2, 12], or when unusual or resistant organisms may be identified.

Routine urine culture is of no value in diagnosing C. trachomatis, N. gonorrhoeae, Candida species, or viruses; if these are suspected, appropriate specimens and cultures should be obtained.

Tests of cure are of little value with lower tract infections. Virtually all relapses or reinfections will present symptomatically and the patient can be reevaluated and cultured at that time [11].

CATHETERIZATION

In most nonmenstruating women and older children, a CCMS urine sample is adequate to evaluate for a UTI. A study by Walter of 105 asymptomatic, nonmenstruating women found no statistically significant difference in nitrite, LCE, significant microscopic bacteriuria, or pyuria when catheter and CCMS urines were compared [23]. If the patient is instructed to clean with sterile water or saline and a nonbacteriostatic soap, a CCMS sample should be adequate in most older children and adults [13].

Catheterization may be necessary in patients who are menstruating, have severe vaginal discharge, or are otherwise not able to give a CCMS urine sample (patients who are bedridden, incontinent, or physically disabled). Bladder catheterization can cause bacteriuria in 1%–3% of healthy, young patients and in up to 20% of elderly debilitated patients [13]. It also can induce hematuria [16], which can cause false-positive test results. The use of suprapubic catheterization also has the risk of introducing bacteria, but it often is the only option in infants [11] and may occasionally be necessary in adults with urethral obstruction.

ASYMPTOMATIC PATIENTS

In asymptomatic pregnant women with bacteriuria 20%–40% will develop symptomatic UTI. Because they also are at higher risk for premature and low-birth-weight infants, treatment of this class of asymptomatic individuals is recommended [2, 14]. There is little evidence, however, to support the treatment of asymptomatic females under the age of 60 who are not pregnant and who have no compli-

cating factors (see Table 28-2) [11]. In these uncomplicated patients treatment should be started only if two or more consecutive urine specimens demonstrate significant bacteriuria [3, 4, 17].

At least 20% of women over the age of 65 have asymptomatic bacteriuria. In uncomplicated patients there is no convincing evidence that treatment leads to any increase in well-being or survival [25]. For those women who are institutionalized or who have complicating factors, the treatment of asymptomatic bacteriuria may reduce the incidence of symptomatic UTI and therefore should be considered [14].

TREATMENT REGIMENS

The traditional approach to infections of the lower tract has been 7–14 days of treatment with oral antibiotics. It has been shown, however, that since urethritis and cystitis are superficial infections, many can be treated with a single dose [2, 8–10] or a 3-day course of antibiotics [7, 26].

Single-dose therapy has been proved to be an effective and inexpensive way to treat urethritis and cystitis. It has been found to be equally as effective as 10-day therapy with any drug chosen (90% vs. 95%, respectively) but with fewer side effects (8% vs. 26%, respectively), making single-dose therapy a cost-effective choice [13, 27]. The advantages include decreased allergic reactions, decreased side effects, lower cost, and better patient compliance [2, 7]. Lack of response to a single-dose regimen also may be diagnostic in that patients who fail to respond to therapy may have an occult upper tract infection. On the other hand, 40%–70% of patients with occult upper tract infections diagnosed by ACBT have been found to respond to single-dose therapy [1, 2, 28–30], so an occult upper tract infection is a poor predictor of individual response to single-dose therapy [2].

Since no treatment failures or relapses have been reported to present with worse than the original presenting symptoms, the single-dose regimens are recommended [9, 27]. Patients with signs of upper tract infection, recurrence after single-dose therapy, or complicating factors are not candidates for short-course therapy. It has been suggested that patients with hemorrhagic cystitis or symptoms for more than 48 hours may also fare less well on single-dose therapy, and therapy for 3–7 days is recommended [12].

A study of 140 women with symptoms of lower UTI by Tolkoff-Rubin et al. showed single-dose trimethoprim-sulfamethoxizole (TMP-SMZ) to cure 93% of patients versus a 95% cure in patients on 10-day therapy with the same drug. The side effects were 4% for the one day group, and 24% for the 10 day group. This study also showed no difference in cure rates in patients with occult pyelonephritis as documented by positive ACBT [28]. A study by Fihn of 260 women that compared single-dose to 10-day treatment with TMP-SMZ in women with dysuria-pyuria syndrome concluded that single-dose treatment is as effective as 10-day treatment (86% vs. 91%, respectively) but causes significantly fewer side effects (7% vs. 22%) [27]. TMP-SMZ also has been shown to be effective in the treatment of the acute urethral syndrome secondary to C. trachomatis [31] and has been suggested to eradicate upper tract infections better than other regimens [2]. Therefore, TMP-SMZ is an ideal drug of choice for the primary treatment of lower UTIs [28].

Higher cure rates have been noted with TMP-SMZ than with ampicillin and the related beta-lactams or cephalosporins regardless of duration of treatment or site of infection [1, 32]. After single-dose treatment with TMP-SMZ the cure rate is 85%–95% versus 50%–85% with the beta-lactams [1, 29]. The differences probably are due to three reasons. One is the high resistance of E. coli to ampicillin (25%–35%) [1]. The second is the duration and concentration of the antibiotic in the renal tissues and in the urine. Amoxicillin is excreted quickly [33], while TMP-SMZ can be found in therapeutic concentrations in the urine and serum up to 24 hours after administration [10]. TMP also is concentrated in the renal tissue to a greater extent than ampicillin [2, 10]. The third reason may be that TMP-SMZ has been shown to better suppress periurethral, vaginal, and fecal flora, which are the primary sources of UTI [10]. Three- to 10-day therapy with the drug seems to be necessary to effectively eradicate flora in these areas [1, 2, 10]. Cephalexin has a 67%–87% cure rate with single-dose therapy, with better results obtained in ABCT-negative patients [34], and a single IM injection of aztreonam was found to be 84%–93% efficacious [35]. Single-dose ciprofloxacin shows a success rate of 90% [36], but norfloxacin has not been well studied as a single-dose agent [1].

Three-day treatment has been suggested as an alternative short-course therapy. There is high compliance secondary to symptoms of infection often lasting 2–3 days, and there may be greater patient satisfaction than with single-dose treatment, since the patient is taking an antibiotic for all the days she is symptomatic [26]. This regimen is also as efficacious as longer (10–14 days) therapy but with side effects comparable to single-dose treatment [1, 2, 26]. A 3-day regimen of norfloxacin and ciprofloxacin has been shown to be highly effective (greater than 90% cure rate) and well tolerated [36–38]. These drugs are considerably more expensive than previously described regimens and should be reserved for patients who cannot tolerate the less expensive antibiotics [1, 26].

Standard therapy for 7–14 days is recommended for women with complicating factors or in whom symptoms recur or do not resolve by the end of short-course therapy [20]. Cultures should be obtained, and therapy with an appropriate susceptible agent should be instituted [2]. There has been no proof that therapy longer than 14 days in this population increases cure rates or lowers rates of reinfection. In fact treatment regimens longer than 2 weeks may potentiate reinfection with resistant organisms that may be harder to eradicate [21]. The same antibiotics recommended for short-course therapy are adequate for regimens of 7–14 days. Table 28-6 compares common therapies for UTI.

Upper Tract Infection

Patients who have a lower tract infection that is not treated or that is inadequately treated may go on to develop infection of the upper urinary tract, known as pyelonephritis. Pyelonephritis is a tissue infection that affects the renal parenchyma and collecting system. Inadequately diagnosed and treated pyelonephritis can lead to systemic complications.

EPIDEMIOLOGY AND RISK FACTORS

Patients with complicating factors (see Table 28-2) are more likely to develop occult upper tract infections and subsequent symptomatic pyelonephritis. These patients must be followed closely so that the clinician can ensure eradication of the infecting organism.

Table 28-6. Common oral therapies for UTI

Antibiotic[a]	Single-dose therapy, number of tablets	Single-dose efficacy	3- or 14-day therapy[b]
TMP (160 mg)-SMZ (800 mg)[c]	2	85%–95% [1, 25]	1 bid
SMZ (500 mg)[d]	4	85%–95% [26]	1 qid
TMP (100 mg)[d]	4	85%–95% [1]	1 bid
Nitrofurantoin (100 mg)[d]	—		1 qid
Ampicillin (500 mg)	7	50%–85% [1, 25]	1 qid
Amoxicillin (500 mg)	6	50%–85% [1, 25]	1 tid
Cephalexin (500 mg)	4	67%–87% [30]	1 qid
Ciprofloxacin (250 mg)	1	81%–90% [1, 32]	1 bid
Ofloxacin (200 mg)	1	—	1 bid
Norfloxacin (400 mg)[d]	—	—	1 bid
Amoxicillin-clavulanate (500 mg)	1	50%–95% [1, 2]	1 tid

[a] Listed in approximate increasing cost.
[b] 3-day therapy is for uncomplicated lower UTI only.
[c] Preferred antimicrobial agent [2].
[d] Minimum suggested dosing is 3 days.
Sources: References 1, 2, 7, 22, 29, 34, 36, 37. Used with permission.

PRESENTATION

The patient with a lower UTI most often will present with dysuria, while the patient with acute pyelonephritis most often will complain of renal pain reflected as back or flank pain. In some women abdominal pain may be the major complaint, and physical examination should help the clinician distinguish if it is truly the kidneys that are tender (costovertebral angle, flank, or deep abdominal tenderness over the kidney areas). In any woman with abdominal complaints PID, appendicitis, and GI disease must be ruled out.

The complaints are usually unilateral, but severe infection can lead to bilateral pain. Constitutional symptoms such as total body aches, malaise, fevers, and chills often are present. Urinary symptoms such as dysuria, frequency, and hematuria may or may not be present. Nausea, vomiting, and diarrhea are not uncommon, and these patients may need IV antibiotic therapy as well as rehydration [3, 4].

OCCULT UPPER UTI

Occult upper tract infection refers to the patient who presents with symptoms of a lower urinary tract infection but who has bacterial invasion of the tissues of the upper urinary tract. Occult upper tract infection must be suspected in the patient who has been treated with short-course or standard therapy for lower tract infection, but who does not respond as expected (27).

Several direct and indirect methods are used to detect occult upper tract infection. The direct methods are considered the most reliable, but they are invasive and uncomfortable for the patient. They include ureteral catheterization, bladder washout, and water loading, which consists of forced diuresis to cause diuresis-induced bacteria. Indirect methods are easier to perform and much better tolerated by the patient, but they tend to be less specific than direct methods [5]. Indirect methods include urine enzyme assays, assessment of maximal urine concentrating ability, urinary leukocytes/casts, and serum or urine antibody assays [5].

A commonly used test is the antibody-coated bacteria test (ACBT), an inexpensive immunofluorescence study performed on urine that detects antibodies manufactured by the kidney and excreted in the urine against invading bacteria. When performed on patients with lower UTIs, a positive test assumes that the kidneys have been exposed to the bacteria, and therefore an occult upper tract infection is present. The sensitivity of this test is 72%–100%, while specificity is 50%–100% [5].

False negatives can be caused by reader variability, impaired immune response, extremes of age, acute infection with bacterial exposure time too short for antibody production, superimposed cystitis, bladder dysfunction, low-bacterial-count infections, recent antibiotics, and pseudomonal infections (due to their production of extracellular polysaccharide, which blocks antibody adherence to the organisms). False positives can occur secondary to contamination, cross-reactivity, ileal conduits, and bladder lesions [5].

Although ACBTs have been used to confirm the diagnosis of occult upper tract infection in women with symptomatic lower UTIs, the influence of a positive result on treatment regimens is not totally clear. Some studies have shown a decreased cure rate in women with positive ACBT results who are treated with short-course therapy [27, 30], while other studies have shown no significant difference in the cure rates of positive and negative ACBT patients in both short-course and standard-treatment regimens [10, 17, 27, 28].

Higher rates of positive ACBT results have been found in women with longer duration of symptoms and poorer access to medical care [8]. A positive test in itself is a poor prediction of individual response to therapy [9, 27] and does not reliably identify women at greater risk for treatment failure or with a higher recurrence rate [10, 17].

Some studies suggest that response to single-dose therapy may be a more accurate clinical predictor than a positive ACBT for localization of UTI. If a symptomatic patient with a lower UTI does not improve after single-dose therapy, an occult upper tract infection may be present, and conventional therapy should be instituted [8, 27].

Regardless of the controversies on this topic the clinician must be aware of the presence of occult upper tract infections in women presenting with symptoms of lower UTI. Many of these patients will be cured by single-dose or short-course therapy. It is these patient who remain symptomatic after a therapeutic trial who are of concern; with these patients repeat urinalysis, urine culture, and conventional therapy [27] with an appropriate antibiotic should be instituted. The patient should be closely followed so the progression of the infection can be stopped.

ADMISSION CRITERIA

Although some sources advocate hospital admission for all patients with pyelonephritis, adequate cost-effective management of the uncomplicated, nonpregnant, and nondiabetic female with mild pyelonephritis can be attempted on an outpatient basis [39]. For the patient who can tolerate oral intake, a 10–14-day course of oral antibiotics on an outpatient basis should be sufficient. These patients must be instructed to follow up with a physician and to return if their symptoms get any worse or do not improve in 3 days [2].

If the patient is vomiting, is not able to tolerate oral fluids, or shows signs of dehydration, IV antibiotics and fluid therapy are recommended until the patient is symptomatically improved and tolerating oral intake [2]. Since this improvement can occur within 24 hours, these patients may be candidates for an emergency department observation unit. If an observation unit is not available, admission must be considered.

For the severely ill patient with high fevers, severe pain, or marked disability, admission must be considered [13]. Patients with complicating factors (see Table 28-2), such as concurrent medical illness, diabetes, immunocompromise, renal stones, or an indwelling catheter or who recently have been discharged from the hospital (within 2 weeks) are also candidates for admission. In these patients infection with *Pseudomonas*, *Serratia*, and *Enterobacter* species and resistant organisms are not uncommon, and renal and systemic complications are more frequent [2, 6].

In the patient with an uncertain social situation or in whom noncompliance may be a problem, hospitalization is indicated [1]. In addition, all pregnant women with pyelonephritis should be treated aggressively with admission and IV antibiotics.

LABORATORY FINDINGS

Pyuria and bacturia invariably are present in upper tract infections. Bacterial counts are usually greater than 10^5, although 5%–10% of women may have lower counts [11]. Therefore, for the patient with symptoms of an upper tract infection but no growth on bacterial culture the clinician should reconsider the diagnosis. Hematuria and proteinuria are also seen in upper tract infections [11].

The hallmark of renal involvement in the infectious process is the presence of casts in the urine. Casts are formed when elements such as RBCs or WBCs gather in the renal tubules and are then washed into the urine. These can be seen on microscopic exam of spun or unspun urine [3, 4], although the centrifugal force applied to spun urine may break the casts apart. WBC casts often are seen with pyelonephritis, while RBC casts are rarely seen with that disease and suggest an underlying glomerular disease such as glomerulonephritis [40].

Concentrating defects (the inability to raise specific gravity greater than 1.023) and subsequent glucosuria are signs of renal disease and may be present in pyelonephritis [3, 4].

Leukocytosis is a finding with any systemic infection and so may be seen with pyelonephritis [3, 4]. A shift to the left (a high number of polymorphonuclear cells) is common.

All patients suspected of having an upper tract infection must have a urine culture sent. Follow-up urinalysis and culture are justified in this patient population, since this is a tissue infection and is harder to eradicate than the superficial infection of urethritis or cystitis. Follow-up cultures should be obtained 2–3 days after completion of therapy. Repeat cultures should be obtained sooner if a patient fails to respond to therapy [11].

TREATMENT REGIMENS

Oral Therapy. In the patient with acute, uncomplicated pyelonephritis, antibiotics are required for 10–14 days. Some sources state that the 14-day regimen is optimal [2, 20], because the upper tract infections are tissue infections. To effectively eradicate the organism, antibiotic levels must be maintained at adequate tissue levels for long periods of time. There is no justification for treatment longer than 14 days in this group of patients. In fact, patients treated with longer antibiotic regimens (2–6 weeks) have been shown to have more side effects and higher relapse rates [21]. All the antibiotics listed in Table 28-6 are appropriate for treatment of pyelonephritis if continued for 10–14 days.

In the patient in whom oral antibiotics are appropriate, TMP/SMZ is the drug of choice. It exhibits good oral absorption and tissue penetration, and its twice daily dosing adds to patient compliance.

Alternative first-line agents are fluoroquinolones—ciprofloxacin and ofloxacin. They exhibit good gram-negative and gram-positive coverage and have been proved to be equally or more effacious than TMP-SMZ with fewer side effects [1, 20, 37, 41]. These are dosed twice daily. Although norfloxacin is highly efficacious for lower UTI's [42], it should not be used in pyelonephritis due to low tissue levels. Ciprofloxacin and ofloxacin have been shown to have higher tissue levels and enhanced pseudomonal coverage and are therefore the drugs of choice in complicated infections [2]. Both of these agents are more expensive than TMP-SMZ and should be used as a first line agent only in the patient who is complicated or who cannot tolerate TMP-SMZ. The fluoroquinolones are contraindicated in pregnant women, children, and adolescents.

Common second-line oral agents include TMP, amoxicillin, amoxicillin-clavulanate, and the cephalosporins [1]. TMP alone has been shown to be efficacious in renal infection, although there is a concern that the synergistic action of SMZ may be needed to enhance its effect [2]. Amoxicillin also has been used, with cure rates of 65%–73% [21, 32], but it is not recommended due to the high resistance exhibited by E. coli. The physician can start with another agent and switch to ampicillin after the culture sensitivities are known [20].

Amoxicillin-clavulanate has been shown to be more efficacious than amoxicillin alone in the treatment of UTI [2]. Its spectrum is similar to that of ampicillin-sulbactam (IV) and should be considered in the patient who cannot tolerate TMP-SMZ, in a recurrent infection, or when ampicillin-resistant E. coli or Klebsiella species are suspected [2].

Cephalexin also has been used as a second-line agent, with an efficacy comparable to amoxicillin and a similar side-effect profile [32].

IV Therapy. In patients who are vomiting or who cannot tolerate oral antibiotics, IV antibiotics should be used until the patient can tolerate oral agents. They then should be switched to an additional 14-day course with a susceptible oral antibi-

Table 28-7. IV antibiotics in UTI with tissue invasion

Antibiotic[*]	Dose	Interval
Gentamycin[a]	2 mg/kg loading 1.5–2.0 mg/kg (adjust for renal function)	q12h
Ampicillin	1.0–1.5 g	q6h
Cefazolin	1.0–1.5 g	q8h
Ampicillin-sulbactam	1.5–3.0 g ampicillin	q6h
TMP-SMZ[a]	160 mg/800 mg	q12h
Aztreonam	1–2 g	q8h
Ticarcillin-clavulanate	3.1 g	q6h
Ceftriaxone	2 g	q24h
Ciprofloxacin	500 mg	q12h
Imipenem-cilastatin	0.5–1.0 g	q8h

[*] Arranged in approximately increasing order of cost.
Source: Reference 2. Used with permission.

otic. Recommended first-line agents include aminoglycosides, TMP-SMZ, and third-generation cephalosporins (Table 28-7) [1, 2].

Traditionally ampicillin and gentamicin have been the first-line agents for IV therapy. Since the aminoglycosides exhibit good gram-negative coverage, and approximately 25% of *E. coli* are resistant to ampicillin, this regimen is more costly but no more efficacious than gentamicin alone. It also has been shown to increase the number of side effects [1, 39]. Studies comparing tobramycin to gentamicin show no difference between the two agents in the treatment of uropathogens, and since the cost of tobramycin is three to four times greater, gentamicin is recommended as a first-line aminoglycoside [43]. In the complicated patient or the male patient suspect for group D enterococcal infection, adding ampicillin to gentamicin may provide a broader coverage needed by these patients and is therefore justified [1]. A Gram's stain of the centrifuged urine can determine the need for better gram-positive coverage. Nephrotoxicity is always a concern with long-term use (10 days) of aminoglycosides but should not cause a problem in the uncomplicated patient with normal renal function [39]. Monitoring BUN and creatinine in all patients receiving aminoglycosides is important.

Another first-line antibiotic available in IV form is TMP-SMZ. The IV preparation is expensive, but it is an excellent first-line antibiotic with broad-spectrum coverage and efficacy comparable to its oral use [1, 2].

The beta-lactamase-inhibiting antibiotics, such as ampicillin-sulbactam and ticarcillin-clavulanate, have been shown to be less efficacious than TMP-SMZ or the aminoglycosides, and are second-line agents. Ampicillin-sulbactam has been shown to be as efficacious as its oral equivalent, amoxicillin-clavulanate. Ticarcillin-clavulanate studies have been variable, with cure rates as low as 29% [2, 6, 44]. It therefore is not recommended in a primary treatment of this disease [2].

In the class of cephalosporins, cefazolin has exhibited a cure rate for UTI of 74%, comparable with that of ampicillin, and is recommended as a second-line agent [43, 45]. Third-generation cephalosporin agents are more reliable against gram-negative pathogens, making them first-line agents for nosocomial pyelonephritis [1, 2].

For extended-spectrum penicillin derivatives, such as piperacillin and mezlocillin, a high amount of resistance by both community and hospital acquired pathogens has been demonstrated. They are not recommended as monotherapy in this group of patients [2, 44].

Imipenem combined with cilastatin has been used successfully in serious, complicated UTIs and should be reserved to treat resistant infections [2].

Aztreonam, a monobactam, exhibits good penetration into the renal cortex [35]. It covers aerobic gram-negatives, including *Klebsiella* species and most *Pseudomonas* species, but it is not active against gram-positive organisms or anaerobes. In a study by Swabb et al. of 625 patients with UTI the cure rate using aztreonam 0.5–1.0 g 8–12h ranged from 89% in patients with primary UTIs to 82% in patients with recurrent UTIs. Microbiologic cure rates in these patients were 76% in patients with *Pseudomonas* species, 87% in patients with *E. coli*, and 90% in patients with *Klebsiella*, *Enterobacter*, or *Serratia* species [35]. Aztreonam should be considered when other treatment regimens have failed or are contraindicated [2].

IV ciprofloxacin is useful in those patients who cannot tolerant oral therapy. After 24–72 hours of hydration and resolution of nausea and vomiting, oral ciprofloxacin can be instituted. The effectiveness of therapy with ciprofloxacin for pyelonephritis is comparable to that with first-line agents. This agent is useful in treating infections caused by resistant organisms.

Urinary Tract Infection in Men

A male who presents to the emergency department with symptoms of urinary hesitancy, urgency, frequency, penile discharge, or dysuria may have disease ranging from the meatus to the kidney and extending to any of the adjacent structures, such as the prostate, vas deferens, seminal vesicles, epididymis, or testes. Organisms reach the genitourinary tract via retrograde flow from the urethra or, less commonly, through the bloodstream. Table 28-8 is a summary of the diagnoses and treatments of diseases of the male genitourinary tract.

When all parts of the male genitourinary tract are considered, male UTIs occur with the same incidence as female UTIs. However, UTIs in males are more complex than those in females. Infections in males may be difficult to treat (prostatitis), be difficult to distinguish from other serious processes (epididymitis from testicular torsion or testicular cancer), or indicate underlying urologic abnormality (cystitis). All males diagnosed with disease of the genitourinary tract deserve careful evaluation in the emergency department and urologic follow-up to ensure the best chances for cure.

The microbiology of genitourinary infections in the male fall into two major groups: those associated with STD and those infections arising from enteric organisms. Urethritis is almost exclusively related to STD and is discussed in detail in Chap.

30. Prostatitis and epididymitis may fall into either group. These entities are discussed in detail in this chapter, but treatment recommendations for those whose etiology is an STD are discussed in Chap. 30.

History

The hallmark of genitourinary infectious disease is dysuria in either sex. Other historic details may include increased frequency of urination with scant amounts of urine, cloudy or foul-smelling urine, hematuria, urgency, or suprapubic pain. Symptoms of difficulty with initiation of urinary stream (hesitancy), post-void dribbling, intermittent urination, and decreased force of urine stream are symptoms of bladder-outlet obstruction and implicate the prostate or other more distal processes, such as urethral stricture. Urethritis is more specifically suspected if penile discharge, underwear staining, or initial voiding dysuria is noted. Testicular pain, coupled with a recent urethritis, trauma, vasectomy, or urethral discharge may indicate epididymitis or orchitis. The possibility of testicular torsion should always be considered in these patients. The presence of fever, chills, or back pain may indicate an upper tract infection and tissue invasion.

A history of prior UTIs, previous diagnostic tests, and treatment should be elicited. The patient's sexual preference, recent sexual contacts, and history of STD is mandatory. The history of food and fluid intake in the last day or two may help assess the severity of illness and state of hydration. Medication, allergy, and past medical history are essential.

Pneumaturia is rare but may indicate infection with a gas-forming organism, but it usually results from formation of a vesicoenteric fistula. A history of recent colonic surgery or cancer may be obtained. In some cases unusual sexual practices can cause pneumaturia, particularly in younger patients or those with psychiatric histories. A history compatible with this problem may be deliberately concealed by the patient.

Physical Examination

During the physical examination general condition, vital signs, and toxicity should be assessed.

Table 28-8. Diagnosis and treatment of diseases of the male genitourinary tract

Disease	Symptoms and signs	Laboratory findings	Organisms	Antibiotics
Urethritis	Penile discharge, initial voiding dysuria, underwear staining, partner with STD	WBC count $\geq$ 5 on Gram's stain of penile discharge, organisms on Gram's stain, VB1 urine specimen abnormal	N. gonorrhea, chlamydia	Ceftriaxone, doxycycline (see Chap. 30)
Acute bacterial prostatitis	Dysuria, fever, chills, back pain, perineal pain, tender prostate	Gram-negative organisms on urine Gram's stain, EPS or VB3 urine specimen abnormal, urine culture $\geq 10^5$ CFUs	E. coli, P. aeruginosa, enterococci	Norfloxacin, ciprofloxacin TMP-SMX, ampicillin (treat 4 weeks)
Chronic bacterial prostatitis	Continued relapsing dysuria, fever, perineal pain, back pain, prostate $\pm$ tender	Gram-negative organisms on urine Gram's stain, EPS or VB3 urine specimen abnormal, urine culture $\geq 10^5$ CFUs	E. coli, P. aeruginosa, enterococci	Norfloxacin, ciprofloxacin *TMP-SMX, ampicillin (treat 4–12 weeks)
Epididymitis	Unilateral scrotal swelling, pain, dysuria $\leq$ 50%, fever, epididymis swollen and tender, underlying urologic abnormality	Pyuria in 24%, Gram's stain urethral discharge	Men < 35 years or multiple sexual partners: GC, chlamydia Men > 40 years: E. coli and other enteric bacteria, staphylococci	Ceftriaxone, doxycycline, norfloxacin ciprofloxacin TMP-SMX ampicillin ampicillin-gentamicin (see Chap. 30)
Cystitis and pyelonephritis	Dysuria, fever, back pain, history of urethral insult, trauma or urologic abnormality, suprapubic tenderness, costovertebral tenderness	VB2 urine specimen abnormal, urine culture > 10^5 CFUs	E. coli; Klebsiella, Enterobacter, Proteus, Citrobacter, Pseudomonas species	TMP-SMX, ampicillin, norfloxacin, ciprofloxacin, ampicillin-gentamicin

The abdomen and back should be examined for masses, abdominal tenderness or guarding, costovertebral angle tenderness, and bladder fullness and tenderness. The scrotum should be examined for tenderness and masses; the prepuce retracted and inspected for lesions or discharge, and the perineum inspected for lesions. A rectal exam should include inspection for perianal sores, tenderness, and fissures; examination of the stool for blood; and evaluation of the prostate for tenderness and texture. Inguinal lymph nodes should be evaluated for size, tenderness, and mobility. The physician must be gloved for the entire exam to prevent transmission of infectious diseases.

Laboratory Findings

Urine can be obtained by routine voiding as a CCMS does not improve diagnostic accuracy in the male [46]. Prior to voiding, the foreskin, if present, should be retracted and the prepuce cleaned. Urethral catheterization is necessary only if obstruction prevents spontaneous voiding. If catheterization is impossible, a suprapubic needle cystostomy will both relieve a distended bladder and provide an uncontaminated specimen.

If urethritis is suspected, specimens should be obtained for Gram's stain, culture for gonococcus, and for chlamydia testing. Penile discharge can be expressed directly onto a slide and two swabs inserted into the urethral meatus to obtain specimens for evaluation for gonococcus and chlamydia. The discharge is best obtained when the patient has not voided for several hours, since urination dilutes urethral organisms. If discharge is not present spontaneously, it often can be expressed by "milking" the penile shaft. The swab for a chlamydia specimen should be inserted several centimeters into the urethra and rotated to obtain cells, because chlamydia is an intracellular organism. A calcium alginate (Calgonate) swab should be used for urethral specimens, since cotton swabs can inhibit the growth of gonococcus. Calcium alginate swabs are small in diameter and therefore more comfortable. Urethritis is present if a Gram's stain reveals 15 or more leukocytes per high-power field.

If discharge is not present, UTIs can be localized by the four-glass urine technique (Table 28-9). Infection of the bladder, the kidney, or the prostate

Table 28-9. Four-glass technique for localization of genitourinary tract infection in males

1. Collect first 10 ml of voided urine (VB1) and culture.
2. Collect sample of midstream urine (VB2) and culture.
3. Instruct patient to stop voiding before bladder is empty.
4. Massage prostate, express fluid (EPS), and culture.
5. Collect remaining voided urine (VB3) and culture.

may result in some bacteria in all urine specimens. To localize infection, sequential urine samples should be obtained from the urethra, the bladder, and the prostate, and leukocyte and bacterial colony counts compared. The utility of this technique is limited by the fact that prostatic massage should not be done if initial urinalysis indicates prostatic infection, or if prostatitis is indicated by rectal exam.

The four-glass urine technique is carried out as follows: The first 10 ml of voided urine is the VB1 specimen. Then 100–200 ml are voided, and the next 10 ml (VB2) collected. The patient is then instructed to interrupt voiding. The prostate is massaged by the physician, and any expressed prostatic secretions (EPS) are collected. The remaining urine is voided (VB3) [47].

If the VB1 specimen has the most leukocytes or the most colonies of bacteria, the infection is presumed to be in the urethra. A one-log increase in bacterial count in the VB2 specimen indicates a bladder or renal infection. Similar abnormalities of the EPS or VB3 specimen indicate prostatitis. If urinalysis demonstrates infection of the VB1 or VB2 specimen, administration of antibiotics that are active in the urine but that do not diffuse well into the prostate, such as amoxicillin or nitrofurantoin, should be administered for 2–3 days prior to prostatic massage [48]. Antibiotics should be stopped 24 hours prior to prostatic massage to clear the urine of antibiotics.

If the EPS or VB3 specimen cannot be obtained, a semen specimen is useful. Seminal fluid, however, is likely to be contaminated with urethral organisms, since massage of the distal urethra occurs during masturbation [49].

Urethritis is considered in detail in Chap. 30.

Table 28-10. Clinical classification of prostatitis

	Acute bacterial prostatitis	Chronic prostatitis		Prostatodynia
		Bacterial	Nonbacterial	
Evidence of inflammation (EPS)	Yes	Yes	Yes	No
Culture positive (EPS)	Yes	Yes	No	No
Culture positive (bladder)	Yes	Yes	No	No
Etiology	E. coli*	E. coli*		None
Rectal examination	Abnormal	Normal	Normal	Normal

* Plus all Enterobacteriaceae.
Reprinted with permission from Stewart C. Genitourinary tract infections in men, in Schillinger D, Harwood-Nuss A, ed. Infections in Emergency Medicine Vol. 2. New York: Churchill Livingstone, 1990. P. 188.

Prostatitis

Prostatitis refers to a poorly defined but common syndrome of prostatic inflammation. It can be classified into three categories based on microscopic examination and culture of the EPS specimens. These categories are acute prostatis, chronic prostatis, and prostatodynia. In acute and chronic prostatitis urine, prostatic secretions, and semen will demonstrate leukocytosis, and frequently an organism can be cultured from these specimens. It is estimated that 50% of males will have some symptoms of prostatitis during their lifetime. Prostatitis may result in acute or recurrent UTIs. Prostatodynia is not associated with infection, and there is no inflammation of prostatic specimens. However, it shares many of the symptoms of acute or chronic prostatitis.

Chronic prostatitis can be divided into bacterial and nonbacterial categories. Chronic bacterial prostatitis represents 10% of cases. Chronic nonbacterial prostatitis accounts for up to 80% of diagnoses, and although evidence of inflammation is present, organisms cannot be cultured from urine or prostatic specimens. Table 28-10 summarizes these categories.

ACUTE PROSTATITIS

Epidemiology and Etiology. Prostatitis from Enterobacteriaceae becomes more frequent with advancing age. The most common pathogens are E. coli, Pseudomonas aeruginosa, and enterococci [49]. Less commonly Salmonella species, Clostridium species, N. gonorrhoeae, tuberculosis, and fungi also can cause acute prostatitis [50].

Presentation. The patient will present with the acute onset of fever, chills, dysuria, and urinary urgency, frequency, or retention [51, 55]. Pain, often in the lower back, rectum, or perineum is common. Initial signs of infection are nonspecific and include malaise, fever, arthralgias, and myalgias. Acute bacterial prostatitis may have a dramatic presentation, leading the clinician to suspect pyelonephritis or urosepsis. Once renal and rectal pathology are ruled out, the diagnosis may be obvious.

Prostatic examination in full-blown prostatitis can be difficult and limited, due to extreme tenderness of the inflamed prostate. The prostate will be swollen, markedly tender, warm, and indurated. The literature notes that rectal examination of the prostate may result in bacterial seeding and thus should be avoided. It is difficult to understand, however, how a clinical diagnosis of prostatitis can be made without prostatic examination. A reasonable compromise would be to ensure that only one gentle rectal examination is done. Urine obtained after rectal exam may show more pyuria than the preexamination specimen. Prostatic massage in the patient with acute prostatitis should never be performed.

Laboratory Tests. Because the urethra must pass through the prostate, urine will usually contain the organism that has infected the prostate [52]. Urine should be obtained for microscopic analysis and culture. Growth of 10^5 CFUs of bacteria on culture is good evidence of bacterial prostatitis. Lower colony counts will indicate infection in the male and should be considered to be significant. The four-glass technique is not necessary to make a diagnosis of acute prostatitis.

Differential Diagnosis. Prostatitis shares with cystitis and pyelonephritis symptoms such as dysuria, urgency, frequency, back pain, and fever. Cystitis and pyelonephritis are to be considered more likely if the patient is known to have pathology of the urinary tract. Patients with urethritis are likely to have a penile discharge and not likely to have prostatic tenderness. The specimen with maximal abnormality in urethritis is the VB1 specimen.

Treatment. Because of the inflammation present, acute bacterial prostatitis is quite responsive to antibiotics that do not normally enter the prostate well. Most patients should be admitted for IV antibiotics since they often appear toxic and have urinary retention, concurrent underlying disease, or altered immune response. Empiric therapy for men older than 35 years of age includes a combination of ampicillin and an aminoglycoside (see Table 28-7). Antibiotics can be changed if necessary after urine culture sensitivities and response to empiric therapy are known.

Outpatient therapy of prostatitis is reserved for the well-appearing, healthy man. TMP-SMX often is used initially because of its excellent prostatic penetration and low cost, although the fluoroquinolones are being used more frequently as first-line drugs because of their greater efficacy. The fluoroquinolones have good prostatic penetration plus an expanded spectrum of activity (see Table 28-6 for dosages). Antibiotic therapy should be continued in all patients for 4 weeks, despite clinical improvement. Many of these patients often actually have chronic bacterial prostatitis, and urologic referral and treatment for 3 months may be necessary.

Supportive care includes ensuring adequate fluid replacement, analgesics, antipyretics, and stool softeners. Spasmolytics and bed rest may also increase patient comfort. Nonsteroidal anti-inflammatory agents are a necessary part of treatment.

Instrumentation of the urinary tract usually should be avoided. Urinary retention from prostatitis should be treated with suprapubic bladder catheterization using the Seldinger technique.

Commercial kits are available that allow this procedure to be done easily. A urethral catheter may be painful and can provoke the hematogenous release of bacteria. Some practicing urologists, however, do gently pass a small urethral catheter to avoid use of a suprapubic catheter.

Despite adequate antibiotic treatment irritative voiding symptoms may be noted for several months. The prostate may be firm and hard during this period. The patient should be reexamined for relapse and must be examined serially until induration resolves. Otherwise, biopsy may be necessary to rule out prostatic cancer.

PROSTATIC ABSCESS

Once a common complication of bacterial prostatitis, prostatic abscess is now rare, except in the immunosuppressed, diabetic, or untreated patient. Urinary tract obstruction or a foreign body predispose to abscess formation. Continued elevated temperature, rectal symptoms, and leukocytosis despite therapy may indicate prostatic abscess. Symptoms of urosepsis may be present. Prostatic abscess is also a complication of urethritis, epididymitis, and cystitis. Patients will experience continued dysuria and urinary frequency. The patient may present with urinary obstruction due to the abscess. A fluctuant prostatic mass felt on rectal examination is diagnostic of this disease; however, only prostatic tenderness or enlargement may be appreciated. The cautions about vigorous rectal examination in acute prostatitis also apply to the patient suffering from prostatic abscess. Pyuria and positive urine cultures usually are present, but occasionally the urine may be normal. A transrectal ultrasound examination [53] or a CT scan [54] of the prostate may be necessary for diagnosis.

Treatment is surgical drainage, for which a urologist should be consulted. Drainage may be external through the perineum or internal via cystoscopy. Hospitalization and IV antibiotics are mandatory. Antibiotic selection is the same as for the hospitalized patient with acute prostatitis (see Table 28-7).

CHRONIC PROSTATITIS

Chronic prostatitis is difficult both to diagnose and to treat. Although symptoms are similar, it is divided into two classifications. In chronic bacterial whereas no such organism can be identified in chronic nonbacterial prostatitis.

Epidemiology and Etiology. Chronic bacterial prostatis compromises about 10% of all cases of prostatitis; however, it is probably the most common cause of recurrent UTI [56]. In most cases the pathogen is *E. coli*, but *Pseudomonas, Proteus, Enterobacter,* and *Klebsiella* species and enterococcus are found [57, 58]. *N. gonorrhoeae* and tuberculosis are uncommon in industrialized countries. Fewer than 10% of cases are the result of infection with more than one organism [59, 60].

Chronic nonbacterial prostatitis may be noninfectious, or it may be that the offending organism or organisms have not yet been identified. The roles of chlamydia, *U. urealyticum, Trichomonas vaginalis,* and *Mycoplasma hominis* as causative agents in prostatitis are unclear [61–65]. Some studies have implicated gram-positive commensals such as micrococci, streptococci, diphtheroids, and coagulase-positive staphylococci as contributing to this condition. Conversely all these organisms may be found in the anterior urethra of normal men and may represent contaminants [66]. The widespread ability to identify chlamydia easily and inexpensively has occurred only recently and may represent an opportunity to better delineate the role of this organism in chronic prostatis. Unfortunately it is still difficult to separate urethral organisms from prostatic organisms.

Presentation. Clinical manifestations of chronic prostatis include mild to moderate symptoms of urinary frequency, urgency, dysuria, suprapubic pain, testicular pain, low back pain, and perineal pain. Fever and chills are uncommon. The symptoms are relapsing and indolent, with occasional acute exacerbations. Patients may or may not have had a preceding episode of acute bacterial prostatitis. Physical examination often is noncontributory. The prostate may be normal or tender, boggy or firm.

Recurrent UTI is a common presentation of chronic bacterial prostatis. Antibiotic treatment will sterilize the urine temporarily and result in an abatement of symptoms. The pathogen may persist in the prostate and reinfect the urine when antibiotics are discontinued.

Laboratory Tests. The diagnosis is based on the finding of inflammatory cells in expressed prostatic secretions. Microscopic examination of EPS and VB3 will give a leukocyte count and may identify an infecting organism on Gram's stain. A normal EPS will have a leukocyte count of less than 10 leukocytes per high-power field. A diagnosis of chronic prostatitis is likely if there are more than 10 leukocytes per high-power field of EPS [55]. Recent sexual activity, including masturbation, can elevate the EPS leukocyte count and must be sought on the history. Lipid-laden macrophages also are more common in symptomatic men [52]. Identification of an organism on Gram's stain or culture allows the diagnosis of chronic bacterial prostatitis; failure to identify a pathogen leads to the diagnosis of nonbacterial chronic prostatitis. In chronic bacterial prostatitis infection is presumed to be a sequestered, rather than a diffuse, tissue infection. Therefore, colony counts of bacteria may be low. The colony counts of the EPS or VB3 specimen, however, should be 10 times the counts in the VB1 or VB2 specimen.

Differential Diagnosis. Chronic prostatitis can be distinguished from acute prostatitis by the course of onset. Whereas the patient with acute prostatitis will have acute onset of symptoms, the patient with chronic prostatitis will experience an insidious onset and a relapsing course of symptoms. The patient with chronic prostatitis may have been treated in the past for acute prostatitis. In contrast to the patient with prostatodynia, evidence of inflammation is present in the urine of the patient with chronic prostatitis. Prostatic symptoms also may be evidence of tumor and should not be ignored. The patient with continued symptoms must be evaluated by a urologist, and biopsy may be necessary to rule out cancer.

Treatment. Treatment of chronic prostatitis can be frustrating for both the patient and the practitioner. Antibiotic therapy does not eradicate the organism in a high percentage of patients with chronic bacterial prostatitis, and in chronic nonbacterial prostatitis, no organism is implicated.

Prostatic infections without a great deal of inflammation are difficult to treat because most antibiotics penetrate poorly into the prostate [67]. Organisms are thought to persist within the prostate despite therapy because most drugs do not reach adequate concentrations within prostatic tissue [68, 69]. Drugs that do diffuse into the prostate must be un-ionized, lipid soluble, and poorly protein bound. Drugs that best meet this profile include the fluoroquinolones, doxycycline, erythromycin, and TMP-SMX. The only penicillin found to be effective is carbenicillin, used for chronic pseudomomas infection, although this drug has not been well studied for use in prostatic infection. All antibiotics produce higher cure rates with prolonged therapy (4–12 weeks) than with 2-week treatment. Ciprofloxacin penetrates prostatic tissue readily and was found to be efficacious in small, short-term studies [70, 71]. The results of treatment of *Pseudomonas* and *Enterococcus* species have not been as good. Norfloxacin and ofloxacin also are good choices [48], although there is debate about whether tissue levels of norfloxacin are adequate for treatment.

Treatment of recurrent prostatitis with chronic suppressive therapy (TMP-SMX, one single-strength tablet daily) has given good results during treatment, but relapses are common when antibiotics are stopped. Recurrence may be due to infection of prostatic calculi, which are common and may be visible on pelvic radiographs [72] or on prostatic ultrasound. These stones can serve as a nidus of infection from bacteria inside the stone being protected from antibiotics [73]. Surgical removal may cure recurrent prostatitis. Other surgical intervention has not been found to be very effective in eradicating this condition.

Drug regimens have been used with mixed results in chronic nonbacterial prostatitis [74]. Current evidence supports the empiric use of antibiotics active against chlamydia and *Ureaplasma* infections. Nonsteroidal anti-inflammatory drugs often are effective in eliminating pelvic pain and dysuria.

PROSTATODYNIA
Prostatodynia is the term used to describe the existence of symptoms referable to the prostate, but there is no evidence of inflammation, and no organisms can be cultured. Prominent symptoms include pain and discomfort in the low back, perineal, suprapubic, penile, scrotal, or groin areas. Irritative and obstructive voiding symptoms also are present.

Prostatodynia has been considered a "wastebasket" diagnosis. Various etiologies have been postulated including bladder neck obstruction without prostatic hypertrophy, bladder neck dysfunction, abnormal pelvic floor tension, urethral spasm, and psychological factors.

Patients with this syndrome should be referred to a urologist for evaluation for bladder tumor, interstitial cystitis, or prostatic carcinoma. Chronic bacterial prostatitis must be ruled out by culture of EPS. Patients can be treated with nonsteroidal anti-inflammatory drugs.

SEMINAL VESICULITIS
Seminal vesiculitis is an acute inflammation of the seminal vesicles. The patient will usually present with ejaculatory pain and hematospermia. The workup is the same as for acute prostatitis. A semen specimen can be particularly helpful in identifying the causative organism, but it is not usually necessary. Seminal vesiculitis almost always is a benign disease with intense psychic overlay. The major problem is often reassurance of the patient of the benign course of this disease. The patient then should be started on either TMP-SMX or ciprofloxacin and referred on a routine basis to a urologist for follow-up.

Epididymitis

The patient with acute epididymitis presents with scrotal pain, swelling, and tenderness. Epididymitis generally is an infectious process.

EPIDEMIOLOGY AND ETIOLOGY
Epididymitis occurs most commonly between the ages of 19 and 35, although it may be seen in older adults and less commonly in children [75–78]. It occurs in up to 600,000 men per year and represents 19% of military urologic admissions [75]. Epididymitis at the extremes of age may be the first manifestation of an underlying urologic abnormality, or it may occur in the normal host.

Positive bacterial cultures are found in two-thirds of epididymitis cases [75]. *E. coli* and other enteric bacteria are found in 60% of cultures and *Staphylococcus* species are responsible for the remainder [79]. Among 19- to 35-year-old men, the etiology often is related to STDs, and there is no underlying urologic abnormality. The pathogenic organisms are *N. gonorrhoeae* (30%), *C. trachomatis* (50%–67%), or *U. urealyticum* [75, 80]. In men over 40 an underlying structural lesion, such as benign prostatic hypertrophy, often is noted. An underlying urologic abnormality is seen in 12% of patients under age 50 and in 45% of men over age 50 [81]. In men over 40 enteric bacteria predominate, particularly *E. coli*. Organisms that rarely cause epididymitis include *Brucella* species, *Blastomyces dermitis*, *Mycobacterium tuberculosis*, and *Coccidioides immitis* [82].

Organisms probably gain access to the epididymis by traveling from the prostate and up the vas deferens. Urine may also reflux into the ejaculatory duct and has been noted in patients with neurogenic bladder disorders [83]. Epididymitis also occurs more frequently in those who have had a vasectomy or a prostatectomy or who have an indwelling urinary catheter or other urinary tract instrumentation within weeks to months.

PRESENTATION

Patients most commonly present with complaints of unilateral scrotal swelling and pain. The pain is usually severe and develops rapidly over 24 hours. A history of "unfulfilled" arousal, a recent extended episode of intercourse, heavy lifting, or trauma may be given, but the relationship of these events to epididymitis is unclear and is probably unrelated. Dysuria occurs in about 50% of sexually active patients and may be a manifestation of a preceding urethritis [81]. Dysuria is less common in older men and children [55]. The patient may walk with a broad-based gait to avoid pressure on the scrotum.

The patient may be febrile or look toxic. In advanced cases, the scrotum is swollen, tender, and erythematous. Because of the degree of swelling, it may be difficult to identify the epididymis itself, although it should be in its normal posterolateral location. Maximal tenderness will be located over the epididymis. Scrotal elevation may relieve pain (Prehn's sign), although this can also occur in testicular torsion.

Often patients will present earlier in the course of disease and will not exhibit all the characteristic signs. In those cases inflammation of the epididymis is less pronounced. Early on epididymal inflammation will be readily localized, and the entire hemiscrotum will not be involved. Appropri-

ate therapy at this early stage may allow resolution of symptoms in several days in contrast to the protracted 2- to 3-week course of patients with more advanced disease.

LABORATORY TESTS

Urinalysis and urine culture should be obtained, but only 24% of patients will have pyuria [58]. Because of the association with sexually transmitted organisms, the patient must be checked for urethral discharge, and specimens obtained for testing for these organisms. Evaluation of sexual partners for sexually transmitted organisms will be helpful for identifying causative pathogens. Direct aspiration of the epididymis may be the best means of obtaining accurate cultures, but this is not necessary in the emergency department [81, 84].

It is impossible to distinguish clinically between epididymitis caused by enteric pathogens and that caused by sexually transmitted organisms. If coliforms or gonococci are seen on the Gram stain's, the differentiation is clear. If midstream urinalysis and Gram's stain both are negative, chlamydia is suspected, especially if the patient is less than 35 years of age or if an older man has more than one sexual partner, has a sexual partner who is symptomatic for or known to have an STD, or recently has had an STD.

The patient with an acutely swollen, tender scrotum deserves urologic consultation to prevent complications such as testicular ischemia.

DIFFERENTIAL DIAGNOSIS

Testicular torsion also presents with a unilateral swollen, painful, tender, red scrotum of acute onset. In torsion the epididymis may be high riding or rotated, whereas in epididymitis its location is normal. The exact location of the epididymis may be difficult to ascertain in the face of scrotal swelling. Pain relief with elevation of the involved scrotum may occur in both conditions. The onset of symptoms generally is more abrupt in testicular torsion, but onset may be gradual. Fever and pyuria are less common in testicular torsion. The peak age for testicular torsion is 12–14 years, with a range of 7–24 years. Differentiation of testicular torsion from epididymitis is not easy, and surgical exploration is the gold standard of diagnosis of the acutely inflamed scrotum. If there is any doubt, immediate urologic consultation is indicated in view of the consequences of unrecognized testicular torsion. Although Doppler ultrasound examination or technetium scanning can be used to demonstrate absence of blood flow, if torsion is suggested, surgical exploration should be undertaken without additional diagnostic testing to avoid delay in detection. Both Doppler ultrasound and nuclear scans have a significant error rate. Prepubescent and early adolescent males *must* be presumed to have torsion until proved otherwise. Epididymitis is relatively rare in these early age groups, but torsion is not. Urgent urologic consultation is indicated for *all* prepubescent males with scrotal swelling.

Torsion of the testicular or epididymal appendage must be considered in the differential of the swollen, tender scrotum. Initially the torsed appendage may be identifiable as a tender, pea-sized, cyanotic nodule in the upper scrotum (the "blue-dot" sign). If the swelling has advanced significantly, differentiation from testicular torsion or epididymitis may be difficult. Other entities to be considered include tuberculosis, testicular tumors, testicular trauma, and orchitis.

TREATMENT

Patients in whom a sexually transmitted etiology is suspected generally are treated with ceftriaxone and doxycycline, as in other sexually transmitted infections such as urethritis. (See Chap. 30 for complete treatment regimens.) Men over the age of 40 in whom an STD is not suspected are treated for 2 weeks with TMP-SMX, fluoroquinolones, or ampicillin (see Table 28-6 for dosages). Elevation of the scrotum with an athletic supporter, bed rest, and analgesics will improve patient comfort. Nonsteroidal anti-inflammatory agents will provide pain relief as well as shorten the clinical course of the disease.

If the patient appears toxic, has failed outpatient management, or has underlying genitourinary or immunosuppressive disease, he should be hospitalized for IV antibiotics and observation. Fluoroquinolones, ampicillin and an aminoglycoside, TMP-SMX, or a third-generation cephalosporin can be used (see Table 28-7). Nonsteroidal anti-inflammatory agents are again necessary.

COMPLICATIONS

Spermatic vessels can be compressed by epididymal swelling, which can lead to ischemia of the testicular vascular system. Such ischemia is suspected clinically when the scrotum is fixed over the testicle. In this circumstance surgical decompression may be indicated to salvage the testicle [85, 86].

Orchitis may result from the vasovasitis, which often accompanies epididymitis. As the epididymitis resolves, so will the orchitis. Other complications include chronic inflammation of the epididymis, obliteration of the vas deferens, and epididymal abscess formation. Infertility, oligospermia, and testicular atrophy are all seen after an episode of epididymitis that has been inadequately treated or untreated or occasionally following appropriate treatment [87]. Patients must receive urologic follow-up until induration resolves, since 15% of patients with testicular cancer will present with epididymitis.

Cystitis and Pyelonephritis

Differentiation of an upper from a lower tract urinary infection in men has less clinical significance than in women. On the basis of an ACBT even prostatitis and epididymitis involve tissue invasion and are therefore more analogous to upper tract infection than lower. Furthermore, the difficulty in differentiating an upper from a lower tract infection on clinical grounds alone is well known [88, 89]. Therefore, every UTI in a male must be treated as if it were an upper tract infection.

EPIDEMIOLOGY AND ETIOLOGY

In the adult male cystitis and pyelonephritis are rare without underlying abnormality or insult [90]. This is because in the normal male the long distance between the urinary meatus and the bladder discourages retrograde travel of organisms to the bladder. Retrograde spread of organisms is facilitated by congenital abnormalities such as hypospadias [91], trauma to the bladder or urethra, or instrumentation of the urethra. After 3 days of indwelling urinary catheterization, almost 100% of patients will have a UTI [92, 93]. Autoerogenous intraurethral insertion of foreign objects can precipitate an infection with unusual bacterial flora.

Abnormalities of the genitourinary tract are found in up to 80% of men with a UTI and no history of trauma or instrumentation. Anatomic abnormalities predisposing to infection include ureteral ectopia, bifid ureter, or renal scarring from prior renal infections. Other conditions that contribute to infection include abnormal bladder physiology from neurologic trauma, urinary retention, urinary obstruction, and foreign bodies such as stones or catheters. Urinary retention is common in patients with neurologic abnormalities, including the neurogenic bladder of diabetics. The most common cause of urinary obstruction is benign prostatic hypertrophy.

E. coli is the most common causative organism, followed by Klebsiella, Enterobacter, Proteus, Citrobacter, and Pseudomonas species [94, 95]. In one study 4% of cystitis was due to M. tuberculosis [90]. Staphylococcus aureus renal infections usually are associated with hematogenous spread, and a primary source should be sought. Grampositive organisms are unusual etiologic agents and may be associated with diabetes, immunocompromise, or tumors. Candida may be present in the urine of patients with diabetes or indwelling urinary catheters.

In the first year of life UTIs are more common in boys than in girls (1.5:1), due to the greater frequency of congenital urinary tract abnormalities in male infants. After the first year until the fifth decade cystitis is more common in females with a male-female ratio of 1:10 in the preschool years and 1:50 in the reproductive years. After the fifth decade the male-female ratio of cystitis and pyelonephritis rises to 1:1 [96].

PRESENTATION

The patient will present with the acute onset of dysuria. Urinary urgency, hesitancy, frequency, or change in the color or the smell of urine may be noted. The patient may have flank, back, or abdominal pain. The patient may relate a history of recent urinary tract instrumentation, trauma, or other urologic abnormality. Fever or evidence of sepsis, such a tachypnea, tachycardia or hypotension, may be evident. The patient may have costovertebral angle tenderness or suprapubic tenderness.

LABORATORY TESTS

Urinalysis and urine culture should be obtained. Coliform organisms may be identified on Gram stain's. According to the four-glass technique, maximal abnormality of the VB2 specimen will indicate bladder or kidney infection.

Studies such as a renal ultrasound or intravenous pyelography (IVP) should be considered to rule out underlying urologic abnormalities. IVP in the face of dehydration and infection can precipitate acute tubular necrosis due to the increased hyperosmolar load. Because of this risk IVP should not be done unless the serum creatinine is normal and the patient is well hydrated [97, 98]. Other diagnostic modalities such as ultrasound and noncontrasted CT scan can be used for diagnosis of obstruction [93].

DIFFERENTIAL DIAGNOSIS

In uncomplicated renal colic, flank pain and hematuria are present, but fever or pyuria should raise concerns about concomitant infection. Pyelonephritis in the presence of an obstruction is a medical emergency, because a renal abscess or pyonephrosis may ensue with subsequent loss of renal tissue and severe generalized sepsis. This patient requires immediate urologic consultation and a diagnostic upper tract study.

Other diseases of the male genitourinary tract, such as prostatitis and epididymitis, can cause systemic symptoms with abnormal urine sediment. Infection of the bladder or kidney also can be confused with urethritis. The four-glass technique for localizing UTIs in men is useful. In urethritis a penile discharge may be noted, and maximal urine abnormalities will be on the VB1 specimen. In prostatitis the EPS and VB3 specimens will be most abnormal. Acute prostatitis and pyelonephritis are pathophysiologically similar, since both conditions involve tissue invasion of the genitourinary tract. Contiguous spread from prostate to bladder with a resulting cystitis is quite common. Indeed, the most common cause of recurrent cystitis in the noncatheterized male is a chronic bacterial prostatitis.

TREATMENT

Empiric therapy to eradicate coliform bacteria using antibiotics such as TMP-SMZ, quinolones, or ampicillin should be initiated. Antibiotic treatment should be continued for 10–14 days. Short-course therapy has not been well studied, and in light of the high likelihood of urologic abnormalities and tissue invasion, it is not recommended. Fluoroquinolones are appropriate if less expensive antibiotic regimens have failed. (See Table 28-6 for dosages.)

The patient who appears toxic and has nausea, vomiting, or temperature greater than 39°C should be admitted. Appropriate IV antibiotics would include TMP-SMX or ampicillin plus gentamicin or other agents listed in Table 28-7. Patients suspected of having obstruction, urinary retention, or foreign bodies also should be admitted. A urologic consult should be obtained for all men with a first episode of

Orchitis

MUMPS ORCHITIS

Mumps orchitis is seen most frequently in postpubertal males. About one-third of postpubertal males with mumps develop orchitis. Men from 15 to 29 years of age are most likely to be affected, although orchitis has been found in boys as young as 3 years.

Orchitis begins near the end of the first week of illness. Fever is noted first, followed by severe scrotal pain, swelling, erythema, and tenderness. Orchitis is unilateral 60%–80% of the time and may occur before or in the absence of parotitis. A marked leukocytosis with left shift is common. Complications include atrophy, and bilateral atrophy can lead to sterility. Treatment is symptomatic and includes analgesics and scrotal support.

MISCELLANEOUS ORCHITIS

Orchitis also may be found in association with prostatitis, seminal vesiculitis, and gonorrhea. Testicular inflammation may be found as a manifestation of systemic diseases such as tuberculosis, leptospirosis, melanosis, tuberculosis, relapsing fever, chickenpox, brucellosis, and lymphocytic chorioretinitis. Inflammation of the epididymis can be confused with inflammation of the testes. Testicular torsion must be considered in the patient with unilateral swollen, tender testes. Tumor or trauma also can cause similar symptoms.

Complications of Bladder and Kidney Infections

When inadequate treatment of pyelonephritis occurs, many localized and systemic complications can occur. These complications occur more fre-

quently in patients with complicating factors, especially diabetes.

Recurrence versus Reinfection in Women

Recurrence, or relapse, means that the patient initially improves but subsequently presents with an infection with the same organism as the original infection. This indicates that the original organism was never adequately eradicated from the patient's urinary tract [1]. Repeat cultures should be sent and appropriate therapy instituted for 10–14 days. If the infection persists, urologic referral is necessary.

Reinfection occurs when the primary infection has been eradicated, and the patient presents with another infection. There is usually an asymptomatic period of more than 6 weeks between infections, and the organism is usually different from that in the primary infection. The clinician should treat a patient with reinfection the same as any other patient presenting with a UTI.

For women with more than two symptomatic UTIs over a 6-month period or more than three over a 1-year period, prophylactic antibiotics may be warranted. In these women postcoital, intermittent, or continuous prophylaxis has been demonstrated to be successful, depending on symptomology [1]. These patients should be followed regularly. If a woman on prophylaxis presents with symptomatic infection, prophylaxis should be stopped, urine cultures sent, and treatment started with an appropriate antibiotic.

In uncomplicated patients with recurrent lower tract infections, abnormal pathology almost never is found, and a full urologic workup is rarely necessary [1, 6]. Urologic workup, starting with an ultrasound to rule out abnormal pathology and obstruction, is recommended in the patient with more than two recurrences of upper tract infection [1].

Acute Focal Bacterial Nephritis

Acute focal bacterial nephritis is a severe form of pyelonephritis that localizes in a single lobule and that may be suspected in a patient with a persistent or indolent infection. It usually occurs in diabetic patients. Acute focal bacterial nephritis is hard to eradicate but usually resolves with 4–6 weeks of antibiotic therapy [99, 100]. If this infection is suspected, renal ultrasound and urologic consult should be obtained.

Chronic Pyelonephritis

Chronic pyelonephritis is a term used to describe a chronic inflammatory process that results in scarring and contraction of the renal tissue. It was originally thought to occur as a result of recurrent UTIs but has been shown to occur with other syndromes such as chronic obstruction and nephropathies. Because *chronic pyelonephritis* is a pathologic term used to describe the appearance of the kidneys, it should not be used to describe chronic or recurrent renal infections [99, 100].

Papillary Necrosis

Papillary necrosis occurs as a result of ischemic insult to the renal papilla and is most commonly associated with diabetes, pyelonephritis, obstruction, sickle cell disease, and analgesic abuse. Sixty-six percent of the patients who develop this disease have some sort of urinary tract infection. Symptomology is similar to pyelonephritis, with patients most commonly presenting with hematuria, flank pain, abdominal pain, chills, and fever. It may be accompanied by acute renal failure, oliguria, or anuria. It may be asymptomatic only rarely [3, 4]. Diagnosis can be made with renal contrast studies [99, 100].

Emphysematous Pyelonephritis

Emphyematous pyelonephritis is a rare, life-threatening complication of pyelonephritis that usually is seen in diabetics and that results in intraparenchymal gas formation. The most common causative organisms are *E. coli, Klebsiella* species, and *Proteus* species. Aggressive medical and surgical therapy is warranted. Diagnosis can be made by ultrasound or CT scan [99, 100].

Renal Abscesses

Renal abscesses can be categorized as cortical, corticomedullary, or perinephric. Cortical abscesses arise from hematogenous seeding of the kidney and are usually caused by *S. aureus* (90%). Skin lesions are the most common source of infection, followed by cardiac valvular infection. Patients predisposed to *S. aureus* bacteremia, such as the immunocompromised, diabetics, hemodialysis patients, and IV drug abusers, are more susceptible to this complication [99, 100].

Corticomedullary abscesses most commonly are caused by ascending infection with gram-negative bacilli [99, 100]. Patients generally have urinary tract abnormalities, such as obstruction from tubular scarring from recurrent infections, renal calculi, or vesicoureteral reflux, particularly children [46]. Underlying illness, such as diabetes mellitus, is a predisposing factor.

Perinephric abscesses are usually a result of direct spread of infection from an abscess in the renal parenchyma to the perinephric space. Occasionally hematogenous spread or direct extension from other nearby infected structures can cause this infection.

Clinically the physician should suspect abscess formation when patients with the symptoms of pyelonephritis present with an insidious onset of disease or do not respond to a standard course of antibiotics. Chills, flank pain and tenderness, diffuse abdominal pain, nausea, vomiting, and hematuria are frequent. Fewer than 40% of patients complain of typical urinary symptoms such as dysuria, frequency, and urgency. Occasionally a renal mass or an enlarged liver can be palpated. Urinalysis usually shows pyuria and bacturia, but it may be normal if the infection does not communicate with the collecting system (cortical and perinephric abscess) [99, 100]. Leukocytosis is often present.

If renal abscess is suspected, an ultrasound or CT scan should be obtained, to rule out other renal masses such as carcinoma and hematoma [100].

When abscess is present, the patient should be admitted for percutaneous aspiration, aggressive IV antibiotics, and surgical intervention as needed [99, 100]. Antibiotic therapy for cortical abscess is directed against *S. aureus* and may include nafcillin, a first-generation cephalosporin, or in penicillin allergy, vancomycin. Treatment of corticomedullary abscess involves the antibiotics usually used for pyelonephritis (see Table 28-7). The patient with cortical or corticomedullary abscess may respond to antibiotic therapy alone, whereas surgery is necessary in the treatment of perinephric abscess. Adjuvant antibiotic therapy for perinephric abscess is directed against gram-negative uropathogens as well as *S. aureus*.

Urosepsis

The urinary tract is frequently the site of origin for gram-negative bacteremia. This bacteremia may be transient and respond to the treatment for the UTI, or it may result in a symptomatic septic patient (urosepsis). Urosepsis is generally a complication of pyelonephritis or renal abscess. The incidence is increased in patients with urinary tract obstruction, an indwelling catheter, immunocompromise, debilitation, or any underlying medical illness. In these patients rapid diagnosis and treatment can prevent progression to hemodynamic instability, metabolic acidosis, coagulation abnormalities, renal failure, and death [100]. (See Chap. 6)

All patients suspected of having urosepsis should have a full septic workup, including standard blood work such as electrolytes, BUN, creatinine, and glucose. Urine and blood cultures should be sent, as well as culture of sputum and cerebrospinal fluid as warranted by physical exam. Confirmation of urosepsis occurs when the same organism is cultured from both the urine and the blood.

Catheter-Related Infections

The presence of a urinary catheter provides a portal of entry into the urinary tract for bacteria and provides a foreign surface to colonize. Bacteriuria occurs at a rate of 5%–10% per catheter day [99, 100, 101]. The most serious consequence of bacteriuria is bacteremia, which occurs in 2%–4% of catheterized patients with bacteriuria [102, 103].

Prevention of Bacteriuria

Utilizing an alternative to an indwelling urinary catheter will decrease the risks associated with its use. For incontinence diapers or condom catheters for males can be used. Intermittent catheterization has successfully replaced indwelling catheters for many patients with urinary retention.

A closed catheter-and-collecting-bag system is essential to limit bacteriuria. One study found that the insertion of a urinemeter between the catheter and the collecting bag decreased bacteriuria [104]. Continuous bladder irrigation or instillation of antimicrobial substances does not decrease bacteriuria. Antibiotics may decrease bacteriuria initially, but they are not effective for chronic use. Some urologists recommend administration of a single dose of antibiotics with every in-and-out catheterization.

Microbiology

Infections in patients with short-term catheterization (< 30 days) are generally with the same etiologic agents that cause urinary infections of noncatheterized patients and include *E. coli*, *Klebsiella pneumoniae*, *P. mirabilis*, *P. aureginosa*, *S. epidermidis*, and enterococci [105]. Infections in patients with long-term catheterization are polymicrobial, and etiologic agents include common pathogens as well as *Providencia stuartii* and *Morganella morganii*.

Management

The urine sediment of patients with long-term indwelling urinary catheters invariably will be abnormal. Antibiotic treatment in the asymptomatic patient is not effective because bacteriuria will reoccur when treatment is discontinued. The febrile patient with a urinary catheter may be a diagnostic dilemma. Extraurinary causes of infection must be diligently sought. Catheter obstruction and renal abscess must be ruled out. The well-appearing patient with a low-grade fever may be admitted and observed without antibiotics; most low-grade fevers in one study were short-lived and self-limited [106]. The patient with a temperature higher than 38.9°C or other evidence suggestive of bacteremia should be admitted for antibiotic therapy [106]. Appropriate antibiotics include a second- or third-generation cephalosporin or a combination of ampicillin or a first-generation cephalosporin plus an aminoglycoside.

References

1. Hooten TM, Stamm WE. Management of acute uncomplicated urinary tract infection in adults. *Med Clin North Am* 75:2:339–57, 1991.

2. Johnson JR, Stamm WE. Urinary tract infections in women: diagnosis and treatment. *Ann Intern Med* 111:906–17, 1989.

3. Holmes KK, Handsfield HH. Sexually transmitted diseases. In E Braunwald, K. Isselbacher, RG Petersdorf (eds.), *Harrison's Principles of Internal Medicine* (11th ed.). New York: McGraw-Hill, 1987. Pp. 508–12.

4. Stamm WE, Turck M. Urinary tract infection, pyelonephritis and related conditions. In E. Braunwald, K. Isselbacher, RG Petersdorf (eds.), *Harrison's Principles of Internal Medicine* (11th ed.). New York: McGraw-Hill, 1987. Pp. 1189–95.

5. Giamarellou H. Antibody-coated bacteria in urine: when, where and why? *J Antimicrob Chemother* 13:95–99, 1984.

6. Gebhart RJ et al. Timentin in the treatment of symptomatic complicated urinary tract infections in adult patient. *Am J Med* 79(suppl 5B):101–5, 1985.

7. McCue JD. Urinary tract infection and dysuria. *Postgrad Med* 80(5):133–42, 1986.

8. Rubin RH, et al. Single dose amoxicillin therapy for urinary tract infection: multicenter trial using antibody-coated bacteria localization technique. *JAMA* 244(6):561–64, 1980.

9. Tolkoff-Rubin NE et al. Single-dose amoxicillin therapy of acute uncomplicated urinary tract infections in women. *Antimicrob Agents Chemother* 25 (5):626–29, 1984.

10. Iravani A, Richard GA, Baer H. Trimethoprim once daily vs. nitrofurantoin in treatment of acute urinary tract infections in young women, with special reference to periurethral, vaginal and fecal flora. *Rev Infect Dis* 4(2):378–87, 1982.

11. Komaroff AL. Urinalysis and urine culture in women with dysuria. *Ann Intern Med* 104:212–18, 1986.

12. Carlson KJ, Mulley AG. Management of acute dysuria: a decision-analysis model of alternative strategies. *Ann Intern Med* 102:244–49, 1985.

13. Harwood-Nuss AL. Genitourinary disease. In P Rosen et al. (ed.). *Emergency Medicine: Concepts and Clinical Practice* (2nd ed.). St. Louis: Mosby, 1988. Pp. 1539–72.

14. U.S. Preventive Services Task Force. Screening for asymptomatic bacturia, hematuria and proteinuria. *Am J Fam Pract* 42(2):389–95, 1990.

15. JM Sutton. Evaluation of hematuria in adults. *JAMA* 263(18):2475–80, 1990.

16. Sklar DP, Diven B, Jones J. Incidence and magnitude of catheter-induced hematuria. *Am J Emerg Med* 4(1):14–16, 1986.

17. Fihn SD, Stamm WE. Interpretation and comparison of treatment studies for uncomplicated urinary tract infections in women. *Rev Infect Dis* 7(4):468–78, 1985.

18. Stamm WE et al. Treatment of the acute urethral syndrome. *N Engl J Med* 304(16):956–58, 1981.

19. Stamm WE et al. Diagnosis of coliform infection in acutely dysuric women. *N Engl J Med* 307:463–68, 1982.

20. Ronald AR. Optimal duration of treatment for kidney infection [editorial]. *Ann Intern Med* 106:467, 1987.

21. Stamm WE, McKevitt M, Counts GW. Acute renal infection in women: treatment with trimethoprim-sufamethoxazole or ampicillin for two to six weeks. *Ann Intern Med* 106:341–45, 1987.

22. Lohr JA et al. Three-day therapy of lower urinary tract infections with nitrofurantoin macrocrystals: a randomized clinical trial. *J Pediatr* 99(6):980–83, 1981.

23. Walter FG, Knopp RK. Urine sampling in ambulatory women: midstream clean-catch versus catheterization. *Ann Emerg Med* 18(2):166–72, 1989.

24. Wigton RS et al. Use of clinical findings in the diagnosis of urinary tract infection in women. *Arch Intern Med* 145:2222–27, 1985.

25. Baldassarre JS, Kaye D. Special problems of urinary tract infection in the elderly. *Med Clin North Am* 75(2):375–90, 1991.

26. Charlton CAC et al. Three-day and ten-day chemotherapy for urinary tract infections in general practice. *Br Med J* 1:124–26, 1976.

27. Savard-Fenton M et al. Single-dose amoxicillin therapy with follow-up urine culture. *Am J Med* 73:808–13, 1982.

28. Tolkoff-Rubin NE et al. Single dose trimethoprim-sulfamethoxazole for urinary tract infection in women. *Rev Infect Dis* 4(2):444–48, 1982.

29. Hooton TM, Running K, Stamm WE. Single-dose therapy for cystitis in women. *JAMA* 253(3):387–90, 1985.

30. Buckwold FJ et al. Therapy for acute cystitis in adult women. *JAMA* 247(13):1839–42, 1982.

31. Fihn SD et al. Single-dose trimethoprim/sulfamethoxazole for women with acute dysuria [abstract]. *Clin Research* 34:816A, 1986.

32. Brumfitt W, Pursell R. Double-blind trial to compare ampicillin, cephalexin, cotrimazole, and trimethoprim in treatment of urinary tract infection. *Br Med J* 2:673–76, 1972.

33. Bodey GP, Nance J. Amoxicillin: in vitro and pharmacological studies. *Antimicrob Agents Chemother* 1(4):358–62, 1972.

34. Cardenas J et al. Single-dose cephalexin therapy for

acute bacterial urinary tract infection and acute urethral syndrome with bladder bacteriuria. *Antimicrob Agents Chemother* 29(2):383–85, 1986.

35. Swabb EA, Jenkins SA, Muir JG. Summary of worldwide clinical trials of aztreonam in patients with urinary tract infections. *Rev Infect Dis* 7(suppl 4):772–77, 1985.

36. Garlando F et al. Single-dose ciprofloxacin at 100 versus 250 mg for treatment of uncomplicated urinary tract infections in women. *Antimicrob Agents Chemother* 31(2):354–56, 1987.

37. Sabbaj J, Hoagland VL, Shih WJ. Multiclinic comparative study of norfloxicin and trimethoprim-sulfomethoxazole for treatment of urinary tract infections. *Antimicrob Agents Chemother* 27(3):297–301, 1985.

38. Kirby CP. Treatment of simple urinary tract infections in general practice with a three day course of norfloxacin. *J Antimicrob Chemother* 13(suppl B):107–12, 1984.

39. Safrin S, Siegel D, Black D. Pyelonephritis in adult women: inpatient versus outpatient therapy. *Am J Med* 85:793–98, 1988.

40. Schiff SF, Dretier SP. Urologic emergencies. In EW Wilkins, Jr. (ed.). *Emergency Medicine: Scientific Foundations and Correct Practice* Baltimore: Williams & Wilkins, 1989. Pp. 674–700.

41. Goldstein EJC et al. Norfloxacin in the treatment of complicated and uncomplicated urinary tract infection: a comparative multicenter trial. *Am J Med* 82(suppl 6B):65–69, 1987.

42. Schaeffer AJ. Multiclinic study of norfloxacin for treatment of urinary tract infections. *Am J Med* 82(suppl 6B):53–58, 1987.

43. Preheim LC. Complicated urinary tract infection. *Am J Med* 79(suppl 2A):62–66, 1985.

44. Sanders CV et al. Safety and effectiveness of ticarcillin plus clavulanic-acid in the treatment of community-acquired acute pyelonephritis in adult women. *Am J Med* 79(suppl 5B):96–100, 1985.

45. Cox CE. Cefazolin therapy of urinary tract infection. *J Infect Dis* 129(suppl):397–98, 1973.

46. Lipsky BA et al. Is the clean catch midstream void procedure necessary for obtaining urine culture specimens from men? *Am J Med* 76:257, 1984.

47. Fairly KF. Determination of the site of urinary tract infection. *Proc 5th Internat Cong Nephrol, Mexico* 3:236, 1972.

48. Aagaar J, Madsen PO. Bacterial prostatitis: new methods of treatment. *J Urol* 37(suppl):4–8, 1991.

49. Stamey TA. Prostatitis. *J R Soc Med* 74:22, 1981.

50. Pfau A. Prostatitis: a continuing enigma. *Urol Clin North Am* 13(4):695, 1986.

51. Meares EM Jr. Urinary tract infection in men. In JH Harrison et al. (eds.), Campbell's *Urology* (4th ed.). Philadelphia: Saunders, 1978.

52. Ireton RC, Berger RE. Prostatitis and epididymitis. *Urol Clin North Am* 11:83, 1984.

53. Suago H, Takiuchi H, Sakurai T. Transrectal longitudinal ultrasonography of prostatic abscess. *J Urol* 136:1281, 1986.

54. Vaccaro JA et al. Prostatic abscesses: computed tomography scanning as an aid to diagnosis and treatment. *J Urol* 136:1318, 1986.

55. Meares EM Jr. Urinary tract infection in men. In JH Harrison et al. (eds.), Campbell's *Urology* (4th ed.). Philadelphia: Saunders, 1978. Pp. 509–37.

56. Hanus PM, Danzinger LH. Treatment of chronic bacterial prostatitis. *Clin Pharm* 3:49, 1984.

57. Meares EM. Bacterial prostatitis vs. prostatosis: a clinical and bacteriological study. *JAMA* 224:1372, 1973.

58. Meares EM, Stamey TA. Bacterial localization patterns in bacterial prostatitis and urethritis. *Invest Urol* 5(5):492, 1968.

59. Fair WR et al. A re-appraisal of treatment in chronic bacterial prostatitis. *J Urol* 121:437, 1979.

60. Ristuccia AM, Cunha BA. Current concepts in antimicrobial therapy of prostatitis. *Urology* 20:338, 1982.

61. Mardh PA et al. Role of *Chlamydia trachomatis* in non-acute prostatitis. *Br J Vener Dis* 54:330, 1982.

62. Brunner H, Weidner W, Schiefer HG. Studies on the role of *Ureaplasma urealyticum* and *Mycoplasma hominis* in prostatitis. *J Infect Dis* 147:807, 1983.

63. Peeters MF et al. Role of mycoplasmas in chronic prostatitis. *Yale J Biol Med* 56:551, 1983.

64. Brunner H, Weidner W, Schiefer HG. Quantitative studies on the role of *Ureaplasma urealyticum* in non-gonococcal urethritis and chronic prostatitis. *Yale J Biol Med* 56:545, 1983.

65. Vinje O et al. Laboratory findings in chronic prostatitis with special reference to immunological and microbiological aspects. *Scand J Urol Nephrol* 17:291, 1983.

66. Meares EM. Prostatitis and related diseases. *Dis Mon* 26(8):1, 1980.

67. Meares EM JR. Prostatitis: review of pharmacokinetics and therapy. *Rev Infect Dis* 4(2):475, 1982.

68. Winningham DG, Nemoy NJ, Stamey TA. Diffusion of antibiotics from plasma into prostatic fluid. *Nature* 219:139, 1968.

69. Stamey TA, Meares EM, Winningham DG. Chronic bacterial prostatitis and the diffusion of drugs into prostatic fluid. *J Urol* 103:187, 1970.

70. Dan M et al. Concentration of ciprofloxacin in human prostatic tissue after oral administration. *Antimicrob Agents Chemother* 30:88, 1986.

71. Weidner W, Schiefer HG, Dalhoff A. Treatment of chronic bacterial prostatitis with ciproloxacin: results of a one-year follow-up study. *Am J Med* 82 (suppl 4A):280, 1987.

72. Fox M. The natural history and significance of stone formation in the prostate gland. *J Urol* 89:716, 1963.

73. Meares EM Jr. Infection stones of the prostate gland. Laboratory diagnosis and clinical management. *Urology* 4:560, 1974.

74. Thin RN, Simmons PD. Review of results of four regimens for treatment of chronic non-bacteria prostatitis. *Br J Urol* 55:519, 1983.

75. Surfin G. Acute epididymitis. *Sex Tran Dis* 8:132, 1981.

76. Hermansen MC, Chusid MJ, Sty JR. Bacterial epididymo-orchitis in children and adolescents. *Clin Pediatr* 19:812, 1980.

77. Williams CB, Litvak AS, McRoberts JW. Epididymitis in infancy. *J Urol* 121:125, 1979.

78. Gislason T, Noronha RFX, Gregory JG. Acute epididymitis in boys: a 5-year retrospective study. *J Urol* 124:533, 1980.

79. Likinukul S et al. Epididymitis in children and adolescents. *AJDC* 141:41, 1987.

80. Harnisch JP et al. Aetiology of acute epididymitis. *Lancet* 1:819, 1977.

81. Tam MR et al. Culture independent diagnosis of *Chlamaydia trachomatis* using monoclonal antibodies. *N Engl J Med* 310:1146, 1984.

82. Chen KT. Coccidiomycosis of the epididymis. *J Urol* 130:978, 1983.

83. Holmes KK. Acute epididymitis. *Cur Ther Res* 26:738, 1979.

84. Berger RE et al. The clinical use of epididymal aspiration cultures in the management of selected patients with acute epididymitis. *J Urol* 124:60, 1980.

85. Witherington R, Harper IV, WM. The surgical management of acute bacterial epididymitis with emphasis on epididymotomy. *J Urol* 128:722, 1982.

86. Surfin G. Acute epididymitis. *Sex Tran Dis* 8:132, 1981.

87. Ireton RC, Berger RE. Prostatitis and epididymitis. *Urol Clin North Am* 11(1):83, 1984.

88. Abraham E, Brenner BE, Simon RR. Cystitis and pyelonephritis. *Ann Emerg Med* 12:228, 1983.

89. Busch R, Huland H. Correlation of symptoms and results of direct bacterial localization in patients with urinary tract infections. *J Urol* 132:282, 1984.

90. Booth CM et al. Unheralded urinary tract infection in the male: a clinical and urodynamic assessment. *Br J Urol* 53:270, 1981.

91. Mandell J et al. Ureteral ectopia in infants and children. *J Urol* 126:219, 1981.

92. Kaye D. Urinary tract infections in the elderly. *Bull NY Acad Med* 56:209, 1980.

93. Riff LJM. Evaluation and treatment of urinary tract infection. *Med Clin North Am* 62(6):1183, 1978.

94. Brumfitt W, Reeves DS. Recent developments in the treatment of urinary tract infection. *J Infect Dis* 120:61, 1969.

95. Roberts JA. Pathogenesis of pyelonephritis. *J Urol* 129:1102, 1983.

96. Sant GR. Urinary tract infection in the elderly. *Semin Urol* 5:126, 1987.

97. Finger MA, Ramsey A. Contrast nephropathy. *Am Fam Physician* 35(6):171, 1987.

98. Fontanarosa PB. Radiologic contrast-induced renal failure. *Emerg Med Clin North Am* 6(3):601, 1988.

99. Garibaldi RA et al. Factors predisposing to bacteriuria during indwelling urethral catheterization. *N Engl J Med* 291:215, 1974.

100. Kunin CM, McCormack RC. Prevention of catheter-induced urinary-tract infections by sterile closed drainage. *N Engl J Med* 274:1155, 1966.

101. Lapides J et al. Further observation on self-catheterization. *J Urol* 116:169, 1976.

102. Bryan C, Reynolds K. Hospital acquired bacteremic urinary tract infection: epidemiology and outcome. *J Urol* 132:494–98, 1984.

103. Gordon R et al. Diagnostic criteria and natural history of catheter-associated urinary tract infections after prostatectomy. *Lancet* 1:1269–71, 1983.

104. Blenkharn JJ. Prevention of bacteriuria during urinary catheterization of patients in an intensive care unit. Evaluation of the "Ureofix 500" closed drainage system. *J Hosp Infect* 6:187–93, 1985.

105. Warren JW. Catheter associated urinary tract infections, *Infect Dis Clin North Am* 1(4):823, 1987.

106. Warren JW et al. Fever, bactermia and death as complications of bacteriuria in women with with long-term urethral catheters. *J Infect Dis* 155:1151–58, 1987.

29

Gynecologic and Obstetric Infections

CATHY L. DRAKE

In this chapter are considered infections unique to women because of anatomic and physiologic factors. Infections of uniquely female anatomic areas including the vagina, bartholin's glands and breast are discussed first. Infectious disease concerns of pregnancy make up the remainder of the chapter, and include discussion of urinary tract infection in pregnancy, teratogenic infections, immunizations during pregnancy, and post-partum endometritis. Cervicitis and pelvic inflammatory disease is discussed in Chapter 30.

Vaginitis

The Normal Vaginal Environment

The vagina possesses a dynamic environment composed of secretions, exfoliated cells, and a variety of bacteria. Lubricating and cleansing glandular secretions, cervical mucous, endometrial fluid, and vaginal transudate contribute to the production of a normal vaginal discharge [1]. The discharge has a life of its own that is dependent on hormonal cycles of estrogen and progesterone, sexual activity, age, and a variety of other factors, such as tampon and contraceptive use, douching, and medications [1–3].

Normal vaginal secretions are described as clear or white, viscous, and homogenous. One author reports them to be odorless [1]. Extensive attempts have been made to describe odors; because of the many factors that influence vaginal secretions, even normal vaginal secretions seem to be perceived as having a variety of odors [2]. The amount of normal vaginal discharge also varies with the menstrual cycle, with the maximum amount occurring midcycle [4].

Estrogen, pH, and bacterial composition affect vaginal conditions. Estrogen produces glycogen deposition in vaginal epithelial cells. Breakdown of glycogen to lactic acid produces an acidic environment conducive for *Lactobacilli* growth [1]. Normal vaginal secretions in adult women are considered to have a pH value of less than 4.5, but in pregnancy they may be more acidic [5]. The normal genital tract contains a host of bacteria, with *Lactobacilli* species dominating. *Diphtheroid* species, *Staphylococci epidermidis*, beta-hemolytic group B streptococci, alpha-hemolytic group B streptococci, and nonhemolytic *Streptococcus* species, *Enterococcus*, *Escherichia coli*, *Peptococcus magnus*, *Peptococcus prevotii*, *Peptococcus asaccharolyticus*, *Peptostreptococcus anaerobius*, *Peptostreptococcus micros*, *Bacteroides fragilis*, *Bacteroides corrodens*, *Bacteroides melaninogenicus*, *Candida albicans*, and *Gardnerella vaginalis* are some of the organisms most often seen [6]. Individual vaginal sampling varies significantly, but increased colony counts are found premenstrually, with mainly anaerobes accounting for the increase. Although decreased colony counts are seen during menstruation, there is an increase in the varieties of organisms [6, 7]. Changes in pH from decreased estrogen or the introduction of more alkaline secretions from blood or semen can alter the bacterial complement present. These changes may produce a discharge that is abnormal due to changes in odor, consistency, volume, pruritus, and local irritation.

Etiology

Vaginitis is the clinical result of these changes in the vaginal environment, and three types are primarily identified: candidal, trichomonal, and bacterial. Bacterial vaginosis is the current nomenclature of this last controversial category, because it lacks the inflammation seen in the other two types. The bacterial etiology is multifactorial and results from a collective bacterial overgrowth of anaerobic organisms.

Vaginitis results from either (1) sexually transmitted organisms (trichomoniasis) or (2) overgrowth or disturbance of normal flora (candida, bacterial vaginosis) [8]. Single or concurrent infections are possible. Exclusion of chlamydial and gonorrheal cervicitis (see Chap. 30) as a cause of abnormal vaginal discharge is necessary. Tumor, malignancy, and other noninfectious agents must be considered. Retained foreign objects (tampons, diaphragms); allergic reactions to contraceptive creams, douches or semen; and atrophic vaginitis can all produce abnormal vaginal discharge and irritative symptoms of odor, pruritus, or burning [9]. Atrophic vaginitis should be suspected in postmenopausal women.

Epidemiology

The frequency of each type of vaginal discharge varies somewhat with the population studied, with sexual activity being a variable factor. Riordan and colleagues reported the evidence of bacterial vaginosis, candidiasis, and trichomoniasis having equal prevalence in women with symptoms who presented either for vaginal/gynecologic complaints or for contraceptive advice at four inner city family

planning clinics [10]. Only half of the women who visited because of vaginal symptoms had signs of infection. Women with lower genital symptoms in a French hospital clinic were found to have culture evidence of G. vaginalis in 37%, C. albicans in 30%, and T. vaginalis in 3% [11]. A community based population visiting their family practitioners had positive culture results for G. vaginalis in 33%, C. albicans in 25%, and Trichomonas vaginalis in 14% [12]. Over half of these women complained of vaginal or pelvic symptoms, with the rest were being seen for routine exams or contraception.

Presentation

Patients presenting to the emergency department with gynecological complaints often describe an abnormal vaginal discharge, itching, odor, or pain. The discharge may be described as fitting one of the following descriptions: (1) thick and cheesy with associated pruritus (candidiasis); (2) thin, foamy, yellowish-green or gray perhaps with spotting, intense irritation, and external dysuria (trichomoniasis); or (3) milky but often nondescript except for a fishy or musty odor (bacterial vaginosis). Table 29-1 summarizes these conditions. A history of contraceptive use, medications, other medical conditions (such as pregnancy, diabetes, sexually transmitted disease [STD] exposure), and prior vaginitis should be elicited. If vital signs are abnormal, then other more serious diagnoses should be explored. Abdominal pain is not usually a significant factor of the complaint, but other sexually transmitted infections can be associated with trichomoniasis or bacterial vaginosis. Further investigation for pelvic inflammatory disease (PID), urinary tract infection (UTI), ectopic pregnancy, endometriosis, or appendicitis should be pursued with the complaint of abdominal pain.

Physical Examination

The physical examination is focused on the abdomen and genitalia, and a tentative clinical diagnosis can be made based on symptoms, risk factors, and description of the discharge. The external genitalia should be examined for lesions, rash, and labial irritation, and the Bartholin's and Skene's glands should be inspected. Next a moistened speculum should be inserted gently, and the vagina inspected for discharge, odor, lesions, erythema, and foreign bodies. The cervix should be visualized for lesions or discharge.

Samples should be taken for Pap smear, gonococcal culture (GC), and chlamydia identification; cultures or other tests for trichomoniasis or candidiasis could be considered, especially in those patients in whom there have been treatment failures or recurrent complaints. The vaginal discharge should be assessed for color, consistency, odor, and quantity. If no blood is present, the discharge pH can be determined by placing nitrozene paper on the vaginal wall or in the secretions pooled on the speculum after its removal. Taking a large swab of the discharge and placing the Q-tip in a tube with 0.2–0.5 ml normal saline to suspend the discharge is an easy and fast way to make individual slides in the laboratory after the pelvic examination. The patient can hold the tube in her hand to maintain body temperature of the suspension, or the tube can be put in warm water to help keep any *Trichomonas* organisms alive and motile. A slide for Gram's stain of an endocervical sample can be made if the suspicion of GC cervicitis exists, but should be made from the cervical discharge only after swabbing the cervix first to remove vaginal secretions. Gram's stain or methylene blue stain of the vaginal secretions have been advocated to increase the ability to diagnose bacterial vaginosis or candidiasis.

Bacterial Vaginosis

DIAGNOSIS
Bacterial vaginosis is diagnosed by using the following criteria: (1) presence of > 20% clue cells (vaginal epithelial cells with adherent bacilli) with debris obscuring the cells or floating in clumps on wet prep; (2) pH greater than 4.5 (with no blood present); (3) positive "whiff test" (on addition of 10% potassium hydroxide to the discharge a fishy odor from liberation of amines is produced); (4) homogeneous or milky, nonspecific discharge [13–15]. The presence of three of these criteria is necessary for the diagnosis. On Gram's stain variable coccobacillary forms are seen. Gram's stain is the most reliable method for identifying bacterial vaginosis

but is dependent on an experienced examiner and is time consuming [1, 14, 15]. Interestingly the odor of the discharge is more significant than its change in color, consistency, or amount.

Proline aminopeptidase assay may prove to be another way to confirm the diagnosis of bacterial vaginosis [14, 21]. The bacteria associated with bacterial vaginosis produce aminopeptidase, and when vaginal fluid is incubated with a substrate an enzymatic reaction can be detected by a simple color change. If positive this test establishes the presence of aminopeptidase and the diagnosis of bacterial vaginosis with a sensitivity of 81% and a specificity of 90% [21]. More elaborate chromatography examination for fermentation products does not appear to be effective or cost or labor efficient [21, 22].

ETIOLOGY
Bacterial vaginosis is the most confusing type of vaginitis because of the variety of names used for it in the past, as an understanding of its etiology evolved. Originally called nonspecific vaginitis after the exclusion of other agents like trichomoniasis, yeast, and gonorrhea, it was first thought to be from bacterial overgrowth [15]. Dukes and Gardner next identified the persistent presence of a bacteria which was named *Haemophilus vaginalis*, then *Corynebacterium vaginale*, and later G. *vaginalis* in those patients who had met the criteria described above [13]. Currently the explanation is that the original idea of an aberrant bacterial state probably is correct, but whether *Gardnerella* produces the vaginitis is unclear, and *Gardnerella* is probably not the singular infecting agent [13–15]. Studies in which pure cultures of G. *vaginalis* were introduced into the vagina produced clinical infection in less than 10% of volunteers, but fluid from women diagnosed clinically with bacterial vaginitis produced an infection in 11 of 15 women [15]. Contributing to the development of bacterial vaginosis are the shift from a predominance of lactobacilli to the more anaerobic G. *vaginalis* and the newly identified presence of *Mobiluncus* species and *Bacteroides* species. *Bacteroides bivus, Bacteroides disiens*, black-pigmented bacteroides, *P. prevotti, P. asaccharolyticus, Mobiluncus curtisii, Mobiluncus mulieris*, and *Mycoplasma hominis* assume dominant

Table 29-1. Vaginitis diagnosis and treatment

Infection	Discharge	Odor	pH	Micro/wet prep/gram's stain	PAP/culture	Treatment
Bacterial vaginosis	Thin, adherent, homogenous	Musty or fishy	>4.5	1. + clue cells 2. No WBC 3. Gram's stain: gram-negative, gram-variable, pleomorphic bacteria, floating clumps 4. "Whiff" test	Not helpful	Metronidazole 300 mg bid for 7 days Metronidazole 2 g on day 1, repeat on day 3 Clindamycin 300 mg bid for 7 days Topical metronidazole or clindamycin per vagina when available Symptomatic treatment: vinegar water douche—2 T vinegar in 2 qt water; Povo-iodine douche—2 T in 2 qt water (contraindicated in pregnancy)
Trichomoniasis	Gray, yellow, or green, spotting	None	>4.5	1. + motile trichomonas 2. + WBC	Pap ± Diamond/ Feinberg Kupferberg	Metronidazole 2 g single dose, with concurrent treatment of sexual partners Metronidazole 500 mg bid for 7 days Symptomatic treatment: Clotrimazole cream/suppositories; vinegar-water douche

| Vaginal can-didiasis | White/cheesy | None | <4.5 | 1. KOH hyphae, yeast
2. + WBC
3. Methylene blue or Gram's stain helpful | Pap ± Nickerson's | Clotrimazole 2, 100 mg vaginal tablet qhs for 3 days (Gyne-Lotromin, Mycelex-G)
100 mg vaginal tablet qhs for 7 days
500 mg vaginal tablet qhs for 1 day
1% cream, 5 g qhs for 7–14 days
Miconazole 200 mg vaginal suppository qhs for 3 days (Monistat)
100 mg vaginal suppository qhs for 7 days
2% cream, 5 g qhs for 7 days
Nystatin 100,000-U vaginal tablet qhs for 14 days (My-costatin, Nilstat)
Butoconazole 2% cream, 5 g qhs for 3–6 days (Femstat)
Terconazole 80 mg vaginal suppository qhs for 3 days (Ter-azol); .4% cream, 5 g qhs for 7 days |

roles in bacterial vaginosis [3, 15]. There is an increased incidence of bacterial vaginosis in women with more sexual partners. Bacterial vaginosis is not considered an STD, but frequent intercourse alters the pH of the vagina, which can allow overgrowth. G. vaginalis is cultured in 30% of asymptomatic women and still can be cultured after treatment despite clinical resolution or failure to meet the criteria described previously on reexamination. Consequently test of cure is not considered worthwhile [3], and culture for G. vaginalis is not definitive.

THERAPY

Current therapy for bacterial vaginosis is metronidazole 500 mg bid for 7 days, which has a higher and longer curative percentage than single-dose therapy of 2 g [17, 18]. Despite the fact that G. vaginalis and Mobiluncus species are insensitive in vitro to metronidazole, other anaerobes are susceptible, and treatment probably alters the vaginal bacterial environment allowing regrowth of lactobacilli. A single dose of 2 g metronidazole on day 1 and repeated on day 3 has been found to have a 90% cure rate [1, 8]. Clindamycin 300 mg bid for 1 week also has been used as an effective alternative [19]. Amoxicillin and ampicillin have 50%–70% efficacy but at the same time eliminate lactobacilli, which allows for a continued altered vaginal balance and candida overgrowth [15, 19]. Local therapy with 150 mg chlorhexidine (Hibiclens) pessaries is as effective as single-dose metronidazole, with similar recurrence rates [20]. Sulfa drugs, tetracycline, and erythromycin are considered ineffective [1, 15]. Intravaginal metronidazole tablets and sponges, lactate-gel per vagina, along with topical intravaginal clindamycin recently has been found to be effective [16]. Vinegar-water, betadine, or hydrogen peroxide douches may be ameliorating measures but are not therapeutic or prophylactic [15, 16]. Pure cultures of human lactobacillus can repair the vaginal ecosystem, but yogurt-based products have not been useful [15]. Concurrent treatment of sexual partners is not warranted except if problems recur.

The concern over the treatment of bacterial vaginosis has special implications in pregnancy, since bacterial vaginosis has been linked to the development of premature labor, intra-amniotic, post-cesarean [23, 24], and episiotomy infections [8]. Metronidazole is contraindicated in the first trimester of pregnancy, but its use in later trimesters to treat bacterial vaginosis is advocated to prevent the complications described. The use of topical agents such as clindamycin as well as alternative oral therapy with clindamycin or amoxicillin may prove to be of value in pregnant patients.

Trichomoniasis

ETIOLOGY

Trichomoniasis is caused by a family of motile parasites, of which T. vaginalis infects only the lower genitourinary tract, including the urethra, vagina, prostate, and Skene's glands [26, 27]. It is predominantly a sexually transmitted organism, although there has been some evidence that T. vaginalis can live in urine and semen and on wet cloths and toilet seats, consequently providing familial infections [28] (thus the saying "catching it from toilet seat"). T. vaginalis is a strict anaerobe and lives in a wide range of pH, but its motility markedly decreases in an acidic environment [26, 27]. This provides for the synergistic development of bacterial vaginosis.

CLINICAL PRESENTATION AND DIAGNOSIS

Classic symptoms are a profuse, frothy gray, yellow, or green discharge with vulvar pruritus and dysuria. No specific odor is described. Erythema of the vagina and vulva, occasionally with punctate hemorrhages or "strawberry spots," can be seen. As many as 50% of women and 90% of men can harbor trichomonas asymptomatically [26]. 30% of women become symptomatic in 6 months if left untreated [26]. Five to twelve percent of infected women will complain of lower abdominal pain [27].

Diagnosis can be made with a wet prep slide by looking first under low power (100 ×) for motile organisms and confirming T. vaginalis on high power. Only motile trichmonads are easily identified, because their size is close to that of a leukocyte. Current studies have reported a 50%–80% sensitivity of wet preps for diagnosis of trichomoniasis [26–30]. Gram staining is not reliable, and Pap smears can result in false positives and false negatives [3, 26, 30]. Culture media are sensitive and specific (Diamond/Feinberg or Kupferberg) but require 5–7 days of incubation [1, 3, 26–30]. New monoclonal and immunofluorescent studies may prove helpful, and approach cultures in sensitivity and specificity [1, 29–30].

THERAPY

Treatment is with metronidazole is a single 2-gram dose, with concurrent treatment of any sex partners [1, 3, 16, 18, 26, 27]. For recurrent cases 500 mg bid of metronidazole for 7 days is suggested. Metronidazole is contraindicated in the first trimester of pregnancy due to concern over teratogenic effects. Clotrimazole vaginal suppositories or cream is effective in 50% of cases; vinegar-water or povidone-iodine douches may help alleviate discomfort, but they do not eliminate T. vaginalis [1, 16, 26–27].

An association of T. vaginalis as a vector for other diseases, such as PID and GC, and other viruses is not clear. Definite association with bacterial vaginosis and the subsequent risk of premature rupture of membranes and prematurity suggest that treatment in later trimesters of pregnancy is advisable [8, 27].

Candidal Vaginitis

ETIOLOGY AND CLINICAL SYMPTOMS

C. albicans and Candida (torulopsis) glabrata are considered to be the main agents of candidal vaginitis [1, 31]. Candida species often are found as members of normal vaginal flora. Opportunistic overgrowth resulting from a variety of factors can produce a spectrum of vulvar and vaginal inflammation [32]. In addition, candidal vaginitis can occur as an isolated episode, although some women have frequent and recurrent infections [8, 25, 33]. Candidal vulvovaginitis is a very common type of vaginitis, with 20% of all women experiencing an episode once in their lifetime [3]. Classic symptoms include a minimal or white, lumpy, "cottage-cheese" discharge without malodor and complaints of vulvar/vaginal burning, itching, and labial erythema. These symptoms obviously become blurred in the setting of a mixed infection.

PREDISPOSING FACTORS

Several factors are believed to contribute to the development of candidal or yeast vaginitis, but the literature is quite confusing in documentation [12]. Diabetes, obesity, oral contraceptives, pregnancy,

corticosteriods, tight-fitting or moisture-retaining clothing, antibiotic therapy, and immunosuppression have all been associated [1, 3, 12, 16, 34]. Some disruption of the mucous membranes from associated irritation with moisture retention from nylon undergarments may be a mechanism of infection [8]. This may be manifested predominantly as a vulvitis [16]. Antibiotic-induced vulvovaginitis is presumed to be the result of candidal overgrowth after the vaginal bacterial balance is altered. Pregnancy estrogen predominance, oral contraceptive medications, corticosteroids, and diabetes increase the glycogen in the vaginal epithelial cells, subsequently providing a substrate for candidal growth [32]. A reduced cell-mediated immunity in pregnancy [8] or Candida-specific suppressor lymphocytes in nonpregnant women [8, 32] may allow for decreased host resistance. A local hypersensitivity response also has been proposed to occur in men and women [3, 31]. Although yeast vaginitis is not considered an STD, colonization of a sex partner's urethra and foreskin can be a source of recurrent infection [33]. Lastly initial and recurrent contamination from the GI tract or an anal reservoir also has been proposed as a source.

DIAGNOSIS

To make a diagnosis of candidal vaginitis, the clinical symptoms and associated factors are of some help. The traditional method of diagnosis relies on examination by light microscopy of a sample of vaginal secretions warmed to bubbling with a few drops of 10% potassium hydroxide. The potassium hydroxide will dissolve cells and debris to reveal fungal forms. Gram's stain or methylene blue has been reported to be helpful in increasing identification of budding yeast and pseudohyphae [25]. Examination of several fields is necessary. Despite being considered an adequate method of diagnosis, light microscopy has been reported to fail in identification of yeast in 30%–50% of symptomatic women with positive yeast cultures [1]. Culture using Nickerson's medium or others is very sensitive but not specific for the clinical presence of candidal vaginitis [3]. Twenty-five percent of asymptomatic women are reported to have positive cultures [1]. Normal pH of less than 4.5 and a negative whiff test can contribute to making a diagnosis. Once again mixed infections can obscure these neat categories.

Pap smears have not been considered to be sensitive, but newer latex particle agglutination and culture slides may become useful in aiding diagnosis [12].

THERAPY

Treatment for vulvovaginal candidiasis is with local antifungal therapy. Polyene antifungal agent (Nystatin) has been the treatment of choice in the past, in the form of vaginal suppositories or cream intravaginally for 1–2 weeks. Currently imidazole antifungals (miconazole and clotrimazole) are effective treatment choices, with a dosing pattern of 100-mg suppositories or 2% vaginal cream nightly for 1 week or 200-mg suppositories nightly for 3 days [16]. An even shorter single-dose regimen of clotrimazole as a 500-mg suppository has equal efficacy [16, 31]. The higher dose has been found to maintain vaginal drug levels for 2–3 days, essentially providing the same effect as therapy for 3–7 days with the ease of patient compliance [35–38].

Shorter treatment intervals have been linked to recurrent infection. Treatment success has been based on negative follow-up cultures after treatment, and these rates have been similar. With any modality 20%–25% of patients are found to have positive vaginal cultures 30 days after treatment [31, 33]. Positive cultures do not mean an infection is present, but monthly self-treatment in some symptomatic women seems to be an effective approach [37].

The newer imidazoles (butoconazole and ketoconazole) also are available. Butoconazole used as a topical antifungal cream or as suppositories has not been found to be any more effective than clotrimazole or miconazole, but it requires only 3 days of treatment [16, 39]. Ketoconazole has been used systemically, especially in recurrent cases. While it is effective during treatment, a similar rate of recurrence is seen after therapy is stopped [16, 4]. Given the risk of hepatic toxicity, ketoconazole is best reserved for severe, recalcitrant cases.

Boric acid powder and gentian violet, both used intravaginally, have been used with success, but concerns of toxicity and local irritation limit their use [8, 16]. Yogurt douches and lactobacilli preparations have not been proved to be efficacious, but they may temporally provide relief, as may vinegar-water douches [31].

Clotrimazole and miconazole now are available as an over-the-counter medications, which may help women with simple recurrent infections. One problem for physicians will be that "ping-pong" vaginitis [32], resulting from partial treatment of a second overgrowth phenomena, may make diagnosis and treatment difficult. This is no different, however, than the current dilemma that douching and other home remedies can produce by obscuring microscopic identification.

Treatment during pregnancy can be difficult and prolonged. The imidazole antifungals have some systemic absorption [8]; nystatin clearly is safe, but it often is ineffective. Serum levels of clotrimazole and miconazole are low, without any reported known effects and theoretically should not be used in the first trimester of pregnancy [8, 31, 39]. One approach is to use lower-dose regimens for longer periods of time [39].

Finally recurrent vulvovaginal candidiasis requires consideration of treatment of an infected sex partner, systemic therapy, chronic intermittent dosing, and immunotherapy [31, 34, 40]. Immunotherapy involves injection of a *Candida* preparation, similar to other allergy desensitization techniques, to increase anti-*Candida* antibodies [34].

Bartholin's Gland Duct Infection

The Bartholin's glands are located deep in the perineum on both sides of the vagina, in the posterior third of the fourchette. Also called the major vestibular glands, they produce lubricating fluid for the vagina and vulva. Each Bartholin's gland empties through a duct about an inch long. The duct openings are just outside the hymenal ring of the vagina, one at 5 o'clock and one at 7 o'clock [41–43].

Clinical Presentation

Initially a blocked duct causes a cystic collection of mucus in the Bartholin's glands [41–47]. The patient will complain of a unilateral swelling in the labia around the vagina. If the mucus becomes infected, then an erythematous and exquisitely tender duct infection can occur. This abscess, if not drained, can extend, causing a cellulitis of the labia with significant edema and erythema. It is the duct,

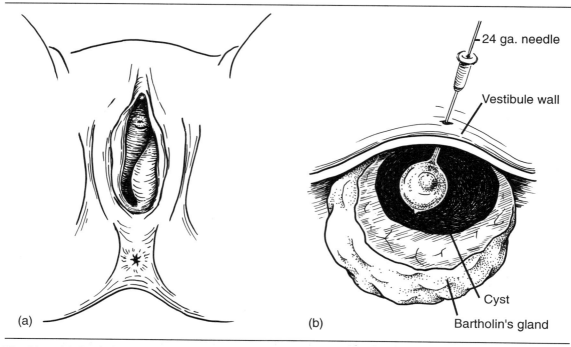

Fig. 29-1. (a) Bartholin's gland duct abscess (b) with insertion of Word catheter

not the gland, that becomes infected, although back pressure from the blocked duct stops the Bartholin's gland production of lubricating fluid [43].

Etiology

Colonizing flora such as *E. coli*, bacteroides, and anaerobes are the probable infecting agents in Bartholin's gland duct infections, but culture and treatment for *Neisseria gonorrhoeae* and *Chlamydia trachomatous* also must be considered [46, 47]. Although cystic collections and infections often recur, carcinoma of the Bartholin's glands should always be suspected, especially in perimenopausal and menopausal women [42–43, 47].

Therapy

Warm soaks and antibiotics (ampicillin, amoxicillin, penicillin, erythromycin, and cephalosporin) may be useful in resolving the acute cellulitis [44, 46, 47]. Therapy for *N. gonorrhoeae* with ceftriaxone may also provide coverage for a surrounding cellulitis. Simple incision and drainage of

the duct cyst or abscess will initially be successful, but fistulization of the duct is necessary to prevent recurrent problems [43]. Dr. B. Word has written eloquently on the treatment of Bartholin's gland duct cysts and abscesses while developing a single-lumen, bulb-tipped catheter that bears his name [43–44]. He recommends using a simple stab incision parallel and just outside the posterior hymenal opening of the duct on the mucosal surface. The incision should be just large enough (about 1 cm) to allow the insertion of the catheter; the bulb then is inflated with 2–4 ml saline. A small gauge needle like a tuberculin syringe, no larger than 25 gauge, helps keep the puncture small enough so the bulb won't deflate (Fig. 29-1). The end of the catheter can be tucked up into the vagina and reportedly is not cumbersome to the patient, even to the point of allowing intercourse. The catheter ideally should remain in place 4–8 weeks to allow the tract to epithelize [43, 44, 47].

The physician can improve the effectiveness of the Word catheter by (1) using saline or water, not air, to fill the catheter; (2) using a small stab incision to allow drainage but not expulsion of the catheter; and (3) using just enough fluid to inflate the bulb so it won't be expelled but not so much as to occlude drainage or cause pain.

Local infiltration of an anesthetic for drainage of a cyst is necessary, but if inflammation is present it may cause excessive pain during injection without producing adequate anesthesia. IV or IM pain medications, midazolam, and/or nitrous oxide are essential when the catheter is placed. Without adequate anesthesia, the labia are too tender to allow exposure for proper placement of the catheter near the hymen. A main advantage of the catheter is that excess manipulation is not necessary, because once the infected cyst has been entered it can be allowed to drain. Traditional incision and packing in a patient with significant inflammation probably should be done with general anesthesia or a pudendal block.

Marsupialization has been considered the definitive treatment for recurrent duct abscesses or cysts [46–48]. Downs and colleagues have successfully used emergency department marsupialization with pudendal anesthesia in patients with Bartholin's gland duct cysts or abscesses larger than 3 cm [45].

Infections of the Breast

Infections of the female breast are of two distinct kinds: puerperal (lactational) and nonpuerperal. puerperal mastitis is an infectious or inflammatory process of the breast that occurs in lactating women. Marshall et al. reported in 1975 a 2.5% incidence of mastitis in nursing women [49]. Due to the recent popularity of breast-feeding, mastitis is likely to be seen with greater frequency in the emergency department.

Anatomy

A review of breast anatomy and development may aid in an understanding of infections of the breast. The breast is a modified sweat gland that consists of a collection of gland lobules radiating out from a common collection site of ducts at the areola and nipple (Fig. 29-2) [50]. Fat, a rich lymphatic system, and fibrous divisions are found between the lobules. The breast lies dormant until puberty, when the glands proliferate under the influence of estrogens. Cellulitis of the nonlactating but mature

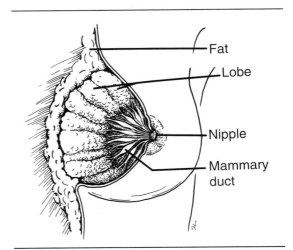

Fig. 29-2. Breast anatomy

breast is rare and occurs because the ducts and sinuses become plugged with keratin. Subareolar accumulation of abnormal ductal proliferation or glandular secretions may occur. In pregnancy placental hormones cause further glandular and alveolar proliferation until delivery. The withdrawal of these hormones, along with prolactin stimulation, causes secretion of the alveolar lining to produce milk. This process can produce a spectrum of physical changes that must be considered when evaluating for mastitis.

Puerperal (Lactational) Mastitis

Puerperal (lactational) mastitis is divided into endemic and epidemic types. Endemic (sporadic infectious) mastitis [49, 51–56] is a cellulitis of the tissue between the glands of the breast and is the most common type of mastitis seen. It is caused by breast-skin contamination or by the baby's oral bacteria, either of which can produce a local infection and lymphatic involvement.

ENDEMIC MASTITIS

Etiology. Staphylococcal bacteria (*Staphylococcus aureus*, *S. epidermis*), coagulase-negative streptococcus (*enterococcus*, nonhemolytic streptococcus, group A and group B hemolytic streptococci), diphtheroids, and *E. coli* are the most common organisms that cause endemic mastitis [49, 55, 57, 58].

Irritation or fissuring of the nipple has been presumed to be the portal of entry for the bacteria.

Milk stasis, from missed feedings or weaning, has been associated with endemic lactational mastitis. Marshall et al., however, reported only 8 of 65 women as having nipple fissuring, and just 9 as having any history of milk stasis [49].

Clinical Findings. Endemic puerperal mastitis causes a unilateral, V-shaped, erythematous, tender, warm, and indurated area of the breast radiating out from the areola [50, 53–56, 58–60]. A fever as high as 38.9°–40.6°C, malaise, and rigors can be seen. The nipple should be inspected for cracks, fissures, and other lesions. Since this kind of mastitis is a cellulitis, purulent discharge from the nipple is rare. Lactational mastitis can occur anytime during nursing, but it most often is seen during the first few weeks of breast-feeding [51, 52, 57].

Adapting from veterinary medicine a technique of using breast-milk leukocyte counts and cultures, Thomsen describes a spectrum of disease ranging from inflammatory to infectious mastitis. He reports that cell counts greater than 10^6 and cultures greater than 10^3 are found in lactational mastitis [57, 58] (Table 29-2).

Therapy. The treatment of endemic puerperal mastitis is to continue frequent and regular nursing or emptying of the breast, if possible or desired, and antibiotics. Warm soaks and massage of the affected area is also helpful. Traditionally nursing has been interrupted because of fears of infecting the baby or the baby's experiencing side effects from the antibiotics, as well as continued infection from baby's

Table 29-2. Comparison of puerperal and nonpuerperal mastitis

Puerperal (lactational) endemic mastitis	Nonpuerperal mastitis
Unilateral	Unilateral
V-shaped wedge for areola	Subareola abscess with cellulitis
Erythema	
Tenderness	Purulent discharge
Warmth	
Indurated	Recurrence
Fever, malaise	Rare systemic symptoms
Rare purulent discharge	

mouth to breast [58]. Although the literature on mastitis is limited, current reports indicate that continued nursing produces few problems for the baby and is almost essential in resolving mastitis [49, 51, 52, 55, 58, 61]. Thomsen's randomized treatment of infectious mastitis showed that continued nursing without antibiotics in the infectious mastitis group had a good outcome in only 51% of the cases. The addition of antibiotics provided for a good outcome in 96% and shortened the duration of symptoms to 2 days [58]. Abscess formation occurred only in the group that did not continue emptying of the breast, regardless of antibiotic use. Antibiotics are excreted in breast milk in limited amounts [62].

Antistaphylococcal antibiotics are recommended, so cephalosporins, dicloxacillin, and erythromycin are the drugs of choice [57–58]. Penicillin [49] and trimethoprim-sulfasoxazole [52] have been used with good results. Ten to fourteen days of antibiotics by mouth is usually adequate.

Administering an initial dose of a long-acting parenteral antibiotic in those patients with high fever, rigors, or significant cellulitis or in those in whom treatment has been delayed could be considered. IV or IM ceftriaxone, antibiotics by heplock, or short-term hospitalization should be considered in this group. Failure to defervesce in 24–48 hours also should be managed with IV antibiotics, and the patient evaluated for abscess formation, as discussed later in this chapter.

Treatment failure can be better managed if a breast-milk culture is obtained. There is one report of methicillin-resistant *Staphylococcus aureus* mastitis occurring in a contralateral breast that responded to vancomycin after successful treatment with cephalexin in the other breast [63]. A few cases of toxic shock syndrome related to lactational mastitis have been reported [64].

Differential Diagnosis. One to three days after delivery, milk fever [65] from glandular engorgement can occur. Low-grade fever may be seen, along with bilateral "rock-hard" breasts. Unlike mastitis, no cellulitis will be present. Resolution begins in less than 24 hours in most nursing women.

If a single gland becomes blocked and fails to empty, a firm, tender area of focal engorgement without erythema can result [51, 55]. A galactocele [50, 54, 55] is a tender mass of focal engorgement,

Table 29-3. Spectrum of endemic mastitis

	Milk stasis	Inflammatory mastitis	Infectious mastitis
Breast-milk cell counts	$<10^6$ WBC/ml milk	$>10^6$ WBC/ml milk	$>10^6$ WBC ml/milk
Breast-milk culture	$<10^3$ CFU bacteria/ml	$>10^3$ CFU bacteria/ml	$>10^3$ CFU bacteria/ml

Sources: References 57, 58. Used with permission.

usually centrally located, that occurs in women who have stopped nursing. Local inflammation with subsequent erythema can develop due to extravasation from this milk cyst. Diagnosis is possible by aspiration of milky fluid or expression of a milky discharge.

Milk stasis is engorgement caused by incomplete emptying of lactating breasts and can present with tender, swollen breasts, usually without fever or erythema [52, 55]. According to Thomsen et al, normal breast-milk WBC counts and cultures define patients with milk stasis (Table 29-3). To prevent the unnecessary use of antibiotics, continued nursing was used to shorten the duration of symptoms. A good outcome was produced in 96% of cases, compared to 21% in the group that stopped nursing [58].

Inflammatory carcinoma must be considered in any patient with breast inflammation or mass. This cancer has been found to result in a worse outcome in the peripregnant period.

Preventive Care. Prevention of mastitis and its recurrence by limiting drying and irritation of the nipples can be accomplished by some simple practices. The nipples can be toughened up during pregnancy by buffing them with a rough washcloth and limiting excess washing with drying soaps. Several breast and nipple creams are marketed to prevent drying. Limiting the initial duration of nursing and gradually increasing the time of suckling also is suggested. In addition, not skipping feedings and encouraging equal and effective nursing on both breasts helps prevent milk statis and any engorgement.

EPIDEMIC MASTITIS
Epidemic puerperal mastitis [49, 51–53, 55, 56] is caused by virulent staphylococcal outbreaks in hospital nurseries with colonization of the babies' mouth flora. This kind of mastitis is an adenitis that

involves the lactiferous glands, which produce purulent breast milk. Shortened postpartum hospital stays and improved nursery hygienic practices have reduced the incidence of epidemic mastitis.

LACTATIONAL BREAST ABSCESS
A complication of puerperal (lactational) mastitis is the development of a breast abscess. The incidence of lactational breast abscesses has been reported to be 5%–11% of patients with mastitis [49, 52]. While puerperal breast abscesses would seem to be the most common kind of breast abscess seen, in a report of patients hospitalized for breast abscesses, only 33% were related to lactation [59]. Early recognition and aggressive treatment with continued nursing and antibiotics may explain the low frequency of abscess formation. Delay in therapy of mastitis beyond 24 hours has been associated with abscess formation [52]. In a recent study it was noted that only 6 of 339 cases of lactational mastitis progressed to abscess formation, and in all of these cases breast emptying had not been continued [58].

Identification of an abscess can be clinically difficult and should be considered in those patients with mastitis who show little improvement, have persistent systemic symptoms, or develop fluctuance. Peripheral location of lactational abscess is most common [66]. If a suspicion of abscess exists, needle aspiration with a large-bore needle (18 or 19 gauge) could be attempted [49, 52, 67, 68]. Aggressive pain medication administration and local anesthesia should be used. Ultrasound examination with directed needle aspiration is more exact and less disconcerting for patient and physician.

The classic treatment for any breast abscess is incision and drainage by a surgeon and under general anesthesia, often with packing or a drain, which requires several days of care [50, 54]. Another approach is incision and drainage along with curettage of the abscess cavity and then closure of the deep space and skin with sutures [66]. This process prevents the recurrent dressing changes and secondary closure and granulation of such a sensitive area, along with the hope of a better cosmetic result. A curved incision is usually made along the skin lines [54], although some argue for a radial incision in the upper half of the breast, with a curved incision in the lower or inferior quadrants along the skin lines of tension [53]. Superficial collections pointing near the areola should be drained with periareolar incisions.

Antibiotics are recommended for rapid resolution of the associated cellulitis [54, 66]. Antistaphylococcal antibiotics such as the cephalosporins, dicloxacillin, and erythromycin are used, since S. aureus is the organism most often cultured from abscess fluid [54, 66].

Nonpuerperal Mastitis

Nonpuerperal mastitis most often is a localized abscess of the subareolar ducts with a surrounding cellulitis [54, 59, 60]. Two types of nonpuerperal mastitis are identified. In younger women a process of squamous metaplasia with plugging and dilation of the ducts is described [54, 59, 60]. This plugging produces collections that often point to the overlying skin or discharge from the nipple. In older women nonpuerperal mastitis is thought to develop from duct ectasia and nipple eversion [53, 59, 60, 69]. However, the nipple eversion could also be the sequelae of recurrent infections and scarring [53, 54, 59]. (See Table 29-2 for a comparison of the clinical features of nonpuerperal mastitis to those of puerperal mastitis.)

BACTERIOLOGY

S. aureus, S. epidermitis, Proteus mirabilis, and Streptococcus milleri are the most common organisms cultured in nonpuerperal mastitis [67, 70–72]. More recent studies have revealed an equal predominance of anaerobic organisms, including peptostreptococci and Propionibacterium and Bacteroides species [70, 72, 73]. Mixed infections are common, suggesting the synergism of the two groups. Some researchers speculate that oral stimulation or transient bacteremia during sexual intercourse may transfer anaerobic vaginal organisms to the breast, explaining the anaerobic etiology of nonpuerperal mastitis [74].

THERAPY

An antistaphylococcal/streptococcal antibiotic in addition to anaerobic coverage is recommended as treatment for nonpuerperal mastitis. A cephalosporin, dicloxacillin, or erythromycin in combination with metronidazole or clindamycin; single-dose therapy with ciprofloxacin; or amoxicillin-sulbactam should provide optimum coverage [70, 72, 73, 75]. Initial infections may respond to antibiotics alone and spontaneously drain. If an abscess is present, needle aspiration or incision and drainage should be used. Needle aspiration may require repeated aspirations for reaccumulations of pus [68, 71, 76]. Ultrasound-directed aspiration also is very helpful, because it identifies the extent of abscess formation. Mammography and CT scans also may be useful in evaluating for malignancy and localizing the abscess. Simple incision and drainage of a small localized abscess with a periareolar incision may be necessary. After resolution of the acute infection, a sinus tract may remain that requires excision. The definite treatment is excision of the involved ducts.

DIFFERENTIAL DIAGNOSIS

Inflammatory carcinoma [53, 69] is the most dangerous masquerader to consider when evaluating inflammatory and infectious processes in the breast. Inflammatory breast carcinoma presents with a red, tender area that becomes a large, hard mass. Pregnancy is not protective of any breast carcinoma, and changes in host defenses may allow for accelerated growth [66, 67]. Inspection and examination should not be ignored during pregnancy and lactation. In fact, pregnancy is associated with a worse outcome of breast cancer. Pregnancy itself may result in both a delay of diagnosis and treatment [66, 67]. Biopsy is to be considered in any case of breast mass to rule out carcinoma.

A localized, discrete rubbery, spherical lump that becomes red and tender, usually with a blocked punctum, can be an infected sebaceous cyst [60]. Infected sebaceous cysts are treated similarly to those of any other part of the body.

Fat necrosis after trauma can cause a tender, firm area of the breast that might be mistaken for an early cellulitis, abscess, or tumor [50, 53, 60]. Mammography can reveal the calcific stippling and stellate contraction seen in carcinoma. Large pendulous breasts may be more prone to this injury. Although involution of the mass generally occurs within 2 weeks, biopsy may be the best way to obtain a certain diagnosis, since trauma is reported in only 50% of cases. Warm soaks may speed recovery.

Mondor's disease, or thrombophlebitis of the superficial veins of the breast and chest, can present with a red, tender, hard cord usually near the lateral aspect of the breast [53, 60]. A "bowstring" or furrow may be produced when the patient lifts her arm. Trauma is the main etiology. Mondor's disease is not benefitted by anticoagulation and will improve with heat.

Tuberculosis of the breast is usually from nodal involvement and associated with pulmonary tuberculosis, usually in young women [53–54]. A "cold abscess," that is, a mass without tenderness or warmth, is described.

Urinary Tract Infections in Pregnancy

Urinary tract infections are common medical complications of pregnancy and require special consideration in the emergency department. Detection of asymptomatic bacteriuria in pregnant women who use the emergency department as their initial source of prenatal care allows for early treatment and prevention of pyelonephritis. UTIs are also discussed in Chap. 28.

Asymptomatic Bacteriuria (ASB)

Asymptomatic bacteruria (ASB) refers to the culture of more than 10^5 colony forming units (CFUs) of a single pathogen from two consecutive clean-catch midstream (CCMS) urine specimens in patients without complaints. The importance of ASB detection in pregnancy is that left untreated 20%–40% of these patients subsequently will develop pyelonephritis [80–82]. Pyelonephritis is 70%–80% preventable if bacteriuria is eradicated [82]. ASB is often detected on a first prenatal visit. The use of an emergency department as the location of that first visit requires ASB screening to help prevent pyelonephritis.

FREQUENCY AND PREDISPOSING FACTORS

ASB is reported in 2%–9% of pregnant patients [80–82], which is similar to the rate of ASB in nonpregnant but sexually active women [81, 83]. Women with sickle cell trait, lower socioeconomic status, and possibly increasing parity and age all have a higher incidence of ASB [80–84].

ASB may in fact be a preexisting condition in some women that happens to be detected on screening during pregnancy, or it may reflect asymptomatic or subclinical renal disease. Pregnancy may allow this smoldering condition to become apparent.

Hormonal and mechanical changes of the urinary tract during pregnancy do not increase the frequency of ASB, but they may predispose to the subsequent development of upper tract infection [84]. Decreased bladder tone, increased bladder capacity, incomplete emptying, and increased urinary pH may allow for bacterial growth [81].

BACTERIOLOGY

In all cases of UTIs in pregnancy the predominant organisms originate from GI tract contamination. Gram-negative bacilli are the main offenders, with 80% of infections due to E. Coli [80–84]. Proteus species, P. mirabilis, Klebsiella pneumoniae and other species, and Enterobacter species are other gram-negative organisms frequently cultured [80, 81, 83, 84]. Staphylococcus, saprophyticus, S. epidermidis, and group B beta-hemolytic streptococci also are found [80, 81, 83, 84].

DIAGNOSIS

As described earlier the classic definition of ASB requires two consecutive cultures from a CCMS sample with one organism of 10^5 or more CFUs per milliliter [1, 4] in an asymptomatic patient.

Patients who should be cultured include those who have an abnormal result on urine dipstick screening (blood, protein, nitrates, or leukocyte esterase) and high-risk patients [83]. Urine for culture can be collected with a CCMS or mini-catheterization technique. If a CCMS specimen is used, collection after cleaning the vulvar area with water and soap but not an antiseptic is recommended. The prevalence of ASB in a CCMS specimen is comparable to that in a catheterized collection [82].

The exclusion of vaginal or skin contamination is necessary, so a mini-cath technique may be needed. This technique is avoided as a standard procedure because of the 1%–5% risk of introducing infection with catheterization [81].

Other considerations in specimen collection include the timing of specimen collection. Ideally a first-voided morning sample is the standard; repeat dilute specimens may not meet the culture criteria. Some reports recommend 2–4 hours of bladder dwell time between specimens. In addition the specimen needs to be promptly plated, usually in less than 2 hours, to prevent bacterial overgrowth. In clinical practice a second specimen is not necessary unless contamination or specimen collection is suspect [84].

TREATMENT

Empiric therapy using sulfisoxazole, nitrofurantoin, ampicillin, or a first-generation cephalosporin for 10–14 days is reported to eradicate 65% of ASB [80]. Although the main risk of trimethoprim-sulfamethoxazole is near term, this drug is not recommended in pregnancy [84]. Culture sensitivity can be followed with continued surveillance for bacteriuria by urinalysis or culture, since these patients are asymptomatic. Monitoring every 4–6 weeks is recommended [80, 83].

Some recent studies have advocated single-dose therapy as a way to determine who will require more conventional therapy. Single-dose therapy has the advantages of increasing compliance and decreasing side effects, with a cure rate of 69%–77% [85, 86]. This approach is ideal for many emergency department patients because it is simple, effective, and inexpensive, and potential side effects are limited. However, follow-up is paramount, since a third of patients will fail this therapy and remain asymptomatic until a possible presentation with pyelonephritis. Because pregnancy may simply reveal subclinical pyelonephritis, some percentage of recurrence is expected [82]. Although controversial, it could be that single-dose therapy does not fail but identifies those patients who will require continued surveillance and therapy. Localization studies have not helped in defining what duration of therapy is necessary [84]. Conventional therapy is warranted for those patients who fail single-dose therapy or who suffer reinfection or relapse [80,

Table 29-4. Oral therapy for asymptomatic bacteriuria and cystitis in pregnancy

Antibiotic	Dosage
Amoxicillin*	3 g single dose
Ampicillin*	3.5 g single dose
Sulfisoxazole	2 g single dose
Sulfisoxazole	500 mg q6h for 10–14 days
Nitrofurantoin	50–100 mg q6h for 10–14 days
Ampicillin	500 mg q6h for 10–14 days
Amoxicillin	500 mg q8h for 10–14 days
First-generation cephalosporin (cephalexin, cephradine, velosef)	250 mg q6h for 10–14 days

* Can substitute probenecid 1 single dose.

84–86]. Antibiotic regimens are listed in Table 29-4.

Cystitis

Cystitis is identified by a variety of symptoms that suggest bladder inflammation. In addition cystitis is defined by the absence of any systemic symptoms or signs of upper tract involvement. Urinary frequency, urgency, dysuria, suprapubic pain, bacteriuria, occasionally hematuria without fever, nausea and vomiting, costovertebral angle (CVA) tenderness, or other systemic symptoms characterize cystitis [80, 83, 84, 87, 88] (see Chap. 28.) Urethritis and vaginitis must be excluded. A positive urine culture confirms the clinical diagnosis. Fluorescent antibody testing has been used as a technique to determine the location of infection in the urinary tract. WBCs not labeled with fluorescent antibodies suggest lower tract infection. (See Chap. 28.)

INCIDENCE AND PREDISPOSING FACTORS

Cystitis occurs with an incidence of 1.3%, most commonly in the second trimester [81, 84, 87, 88]. Unlike ASB most patients who subsequently develop cystitis have negative urine cultures on initial visits [87, 88]. The bladder changes described during pregnancy probably allow for the growth of pathogens introduced after sexual intercourse.

In one study of second-trimester patients with a UTI, 94% had cystitis by fluorescent antibody studies [88].

BACTERIOLOGY

E. coli is again the most common urine isolate, found in 71% of cases with cystitis [88]. P. mirabilis, K. pneumoniae, and group B beta-hemolytic streptococci were isolated in 8% of the remaining cases.

DIAGNOSIS

A CCMS specimen yielding a single pathogen of 10^5 or more CFUs per milliliter in a patient with symptoms of bladder involvement and no fever or CVA tenderness confirms the diagnosis of cystitis. A dilute or forced urine specimen or a catheterized specimen may have single pathogens on culture with 10^2 or more CFUs per milliliter. In a symptomatic patient this count should be considered positive [80, 81, 89].

The differential diagnosis of dysuria includes urethritis and vaginitis. Chlamydial and herpes urethritis and vaginal infections can cause external dysuria. Performing a speculum exam for a Pap smear and cervical cultures is important in identifying concurrent infections. A catheterized urine specimen is considered the most exact method to eliminate contamination.

THERAPY

The recommended treatment of cystitis is similar to that of ASB (see Table 29-4). Single-dose therapy can be considered [80] if follow-up for clinical improvement is possible, but studies are limited. Single-dose therapy is more likely to be successful in patients with a brief duration of symptoms, which suggests that upper tract involvement is minimal. After 10-day therapy, recurrence is reported in only 17% of cases [88], which is half the frequency of recurrence with ASB. Follow-up cultures throughout pregnancy are recommended [84, 88]. If a clinical response is noted despite lack of sensitivity on culture, repeat cultures are recommended with a change in antibiotics only if continued infection is documented [87]. Pyridium is safe in pregnancy and may help symptoms, but vitamin C is to be avoided [83].

Pyelonephritis

Pyelonephritis is an infection of the renal parenchyma. Symptoms and findings include fever, flank pain, and CVA tenderness by fist percussion, along with pyuria, bacteriuria, and a positive urine culture [80, 81, 83, 84, 87] (see Chap. 28). Chills, nausea or vomiting, and occasionally a history of urinary frequency, urgency, and dysuria are reported. A decreased urine-concentrating ability may be a marker for renal involvement [82, 90]. Fluorescent antibody testing can be used for study purposes but has not been used clinically. Symptoms develop rapidly [80]. A spectrum of illness can be seen, with progression to sepsis, end-organ instability, and shock, mandating vigilance in diagnosis and treatment [80, 84, 87].

The focus of aggressive therapy has been based on an association of premature labor, low birth weight, and some degree of subsequent chronic maternal renal disturbance. The association between these complications and pyelonephritis has recently come into question [91].

INCIDENCE

The incidence of pyelonephritis increases in the second and third trimesters [81, 84, 87, 92–95]. Pyelonephritis develops in 20%–40% of women with ASB if left untreated [80–81], and some authors believe that two-thirds of pyelonephritis can be prevented by screening and treatment for ASB [80–82, 87]. In addition pyelonephritis may recur in at least 10% of pregnant women after a successful initial treatment [80, 83, 84, 94, 96], with some reports of recurrence as high as 60% [95]. Recurrent or prolonged symptoms also suggest coexisting renal anomalies or calculi.

PATHOGENESIS

Significant hormonal, anatomic, and physiologic changes beginning in the first trimester of pregnancy produce the dilated renal collecting system, which contributes to the development of renal infection [81, 84, 87, 96]. Progesterone-induced smooth-muscle relaxation decreases ureteral tone, and uterine enlargement causes ureteral compression, creating physiologic hydroureter. This mechanism is more pronounced on the right side [81, 84,

96]. Similar delayed emptying of the bladder and subsequent ureterovesicular reflux allows for bacterial ascension from GI contamination of the perineum. Hematogenous and lymphatic spread also can occur.

BACTERIOLOGY

The organisms cultured from patients with pyelonephritis are the same as those cultured in ASB and cystitis. *E. coli* is the most common infecting organism, cultured in 75%–90% of cases [80, 83, 84, 87, 90]. *K. pneumoniae* is the second most common, followed by *P. mirabilus*, *Pseudomonas aeruginosa*, *Enterobacter* species, and *Staphylococci* species. Group B beta-hemolytic streptococcus is considered a pathogen during pregnancy, and confirmation by catheterization is suggested [87].

DIAGNOSIS

The diagnosis of pyelonephritis in pregnancy includes the clinical parameters of fever or flank pain along with a positive urine culture. The seriousness of pyelonephritis probably warrants a catheterized urine specimen. Pyuria and bacteriuria are essential in supporting the diagnosis on initial presentation. However, if the urine is dilute, it may not meet the criterion of 1 or 2 bacteria per high-power field on an unspun specimen or more than 10 bacteria on a spun specimen, which corresponds with a 10^5 culture result [80, 93]. Likewise, whereas standard urine cultures are considered 95% accurate when 10^5 CFUs per milliliter are seen, cultures of more than 10^3 CFUs may be considered positive in the setting of a symptomatic patient. In addition 6% of women are found to have negative cultures, probably from prior antibiotic use [80]. Subclinical pyelonephritis from prolonged lower tract infection also must be considered. Approximately 10% of women with pyelonephritis have positive blood cultures [84].

Creatinine clearance and serum creatinine alterations will be found in 20%–30% of pregnant patients with pyelonephritis [80]. A creatinine clearance of less than 80 milliliters per minute and a serum creatinine of greater than 0.8 mg/dl point to renal dysfunction. These levels can rapidly return to normal 3–8 weeks after successful therapy.

The complications of pyelonephritis in preg-

nancy include sepsis and shock, renal deterioration, and respiratory insufficiency [80, 81]. Endotoxemia is implicated in both pulmonary complications and thermoregulatory instability [80, 81, 98, 99]. Acute renal failure in pregnancy from pyelonephritis is possible but usually preventable with appropriate therapy [100].

THERAPY

The current practice is to hospitalize pregnant patients with pyelonephritis [80, 81, 83, 84, 87, 92]. Current recommendations include IV ampicillin or a first-generation cephalosporin with the consideration of adding an aminoglycoside (Table 29-5) [80, 81, 84, 87, 92]. More recent literature has pointed out that many uropathogens on culture results are resistant to ampicillin, so the use of a first-generation cephalosporin has been encouraged as the initial single drug [81, 97]. The in vitro sensitivities may not correlate with the in vivo clinical response [97], but knowledge of bacterial sensitivities in the physician's practice area is helpful. The potential renal toxicity of aminoglycosides in patients with renal compromise is worrisome, and its use is best reserved for those patients who do not respond clinically to initial therapy. The choice of antibiotics also must take into consideration fetal safety, and aminoglycosides, especially tobramycin, are categorized as less safe than ampicillin and cephalosporins. Second- and third-generation cephalosporins are reserved for poorly responding infections (table 29-5).

IV fluid is necessary since dehydration is often present, but replacement should not be excessive because of possible renal dysfunction. Urine output can be monitored to maintain 30–60 ml/hour, and another approach is to infuse 1 liter over 4 hours.

One approach is to continue IV antibiotics until the patient is afebrile for 24 hours, then switch to antibiotics by mouth, with discharge if the patient remains afebrile for another 24 hours. Urine-culture sensitivities should be reviewed prior to discharge. Outpatient therapy includes a 21-day course of antibiotics [87, 92]. Another approach calls for 5 days of parenteral antibiotics, followed by oral medications for a total of 10–14 days [84]. The clinical response may not produce sterile urine cultures, so repeating urine cultures on treatment day

Table 29-5. Therapy for pyelonephritis

Antibiotic	Dosage
Ampicillin	1–2 g q6h PO
First-generation ceph- alosporin (cephalexin, cephalothin, cefazolin)	1–2 g q6–8h PO/IV
Carbenicillin	1 g q4h IV
Penicillin/beta-lactamase[b] (Amoxicillin-clavulo- nate)	500 mg q8h PO
Ampicillin-sulbactam	1.5 gm q6h PO

Consider Addition of One of the Following Aminoglycosides:[a]

Gentamicin	1.5 mg/kg loading dose, then dose for renal function IV
Cefoxitin	1–2 g q8h IV
Ceftriaxone	1–2 g q24h IM/IV
Cefamandole	1 g q6h

For Penicillin-Allergic Patients:
Consider cephalosporin or gentamicin

Trimethoprim-sulfa- methoxazole[c]	5 mg SMX/kg q12h

[a] Avoid use of tobramycin.
[b] Unstudied but presumed safe.
[c] During pregnancy use only in second trimester.

2 for confirmation of response is suggested [80, 81, 83, 84, 87]. If bacteria continue to be found, then a change in antibiotics is warranted.

The outpatient treatment of nonpregnant patients with pyelonephritis has prompted consideration of oral antibiotic therapy in pregnant patients with pyelonephritis. Excluding any patient with the possibility of sepsis (i.e., hypotension, lethargy, tachypnea), preterm labor, inability to drink, or other medical problems, outpatient treatment was found in one study to be safe and effective [93]. A compromise that warrants consideration would be 24 hours of initial IV therapy on an inpatient basis or in an observation unit. It appears that a significant cost savings without fetal risk could be made if such flexibility existed, and this warrants further study.

Suppressive therapy or close surveillance and monitoring for recurrent disease are essential. Some authors recommend chronic suppressive therapy, especially if underlying renal disease, urinary cal-

culi, or a history of recurrent infections exists [80, 81, 83, 87, 95]. Others suggest a monthly surveillance culture, with suppressive therapy if a second infection develops.

Antibiotic Use in Pregnancy

Antibiotic use in pregnancy occasionally is unavoidable and should not be withheld if it is necessary. The choice of antibiotics needs to be guided by a risk-benefit analysis with consideration of both patients: fetus and mother. The dilemma of developing a scientific database regarding the adverse effects of any drug is the difficulty in controlling all the factors during a pregnancy that can affect fetal development. The impact of embryonic sharing of any medication is crucially important during the first 12 weeks of pregnancy, when organogenesis occurs. The fetal participation in any drug use continues during fetal maturation. Equally important is the risk to fetal well-being from a maternal illness or a severe drug reaction.

Animal studies have not always correlated with human studies on the actual outcome of medications during pregnancy [101]. Controlled human studies in pregnant women are limited. Thalidomide serves as an example of a drug that was not found to have an adverse outcome in pregnant rats or mice [101]. Conversely sulfonamides have an association with cleft palate in mice but no reports of documented complications in many years of human use [102].

Maternal, placental, and fetal involvement influence the pharmacokinetics of drugs during pregnancy [101–103]. Increased renal function and expanded blood volume in pregnancy can lower the serum levels of some medications. The placenta allows only unbound portions of medications to cross to the fetus. This significantly reduces fetal exposure but subsequently can lower the maternal drug level and the drug's effectiveness. Fetal circulation allows a higher distribution of drugs to the fetal brain and kidneys. Although the level of most medications may be lower in the fetus, poorly developed fetal drug metabolism can lead to potentially toxic levels.

Last, the specific interval of pregnancy and fetal development influence drug selection [101–103].

Table 29-6. FDA classification of drugs

Category	Description
A	No fetal risk from controlled studies in first trimester; proved safe during pregnancy.
	Controlled studies in women have failed to demonstrate a risk to the fetus in the first trimester (and there is no evidence of a risk in later trimesters), and the possibility of fetal harm appears remote.
B	Fetal risk not demonstrated in animal or human studies.
	Either animal-reproduction studies have not demonstrated a fetal risk but there are no controlled studies in pregnant women, or animal-reproduction studies have shown an adverse effect (other than a decrease in fertility) that was not confirmed in controlled studies in women in the first trimester (and there is no evidence of risk in later trimesters).
C	Fetal risk unknown; no adequate human studies and some adverse effects in animal studies.
	Either studies in animals have revealed adverse effects on the fetus (teratogenic, embryocidal, or other) and there are no controlled studies in women or studies in women and animals are not available. Drugs should be given only if the potential benefit justifies the potential risk to the fetus.
D	Some evidence of fetal risk. Acceptable in some cases if necessary to use drug.
	There is positive evidence of human fetal risk, but the benefits from use in pregnant women may be acceptable despite the risk (e.g., if the drug is needed in a life-threatening situation or for a serious disease for which safer drugs cannot be used or are ineffective).
X	Proved fetal risk. Contraindicated for use during pregnancy.
	Studies in animals or human beings have demonstrated fetal abnormalities or there is evidence of fetal risk based on human experience or both, and the risk of the use of the drug in pregnant women clearly outweighs any possible benefit. The drug is contraindicated in women who are or may become pregnant.

Sources: References 103–105. Used with permission.

From conception to implantation, toxicity is considered an all or nothing phenomenon, resulting in spontaneous abortion or an unaffected pregnancy. Days 15 to 55 after conception is the period most crucial to organogenesis, when teratogenicity can occur. Drug exposure occurring during that time is reported to account for 2%–3% of birth defects [102]. After the first trimester growth and maturation of the CNS system, teeth, and genitals still could be affected by antibiotic use.

In 1979 the Food and Drug Administration (FDA) developed five categories for drug labeling on prescription medications to guide drug selection during pregnancy [104–105]. The complete definitions of these categories are found in Table 29-6. Luckily most antibiotics are in generally safe categories, and although none is considered absolutely risk free (category A), none is absolutely contraindicated.

Antibiotic selection in pregnancy must be made by assessing the risk and benefit of a particular drug for a specific infection. Patient education is necessary since long-term effects are not always known.

Monitoring clinical response is important, so that treatment is not unnecessarily prolonged and adequate levels are maintained. A complete reference text on drug dispensing in pregnancy is an important aid. A brief summary of antibiotic safety information is listed in Table 29-7.

Teratogenic Infections in Pregnancy

Congenital syndromes caused by particular infections during pregnancy were first recognized in the 1950s, when congenital rubella syndrome was identified. Today much more is known about the group of infections previously remembered by the pneumonic TORCH, which was penned to remind physicians of the most common teratogenic agents: Toxoplasmosis, Rubella, Cytomegalovirus, and Herpes. These agents were known to literally "create a monster." The definition of teratogenic has been broadened beyond fetal anomalies to include developmental delays and miscarriage. The list of infectious agents producing congenital infections

Table 29-7. Safety data on specific antibiotic

Antibiotic	FDA category
Aminoglycosides	C
Gentamicin Kanamycin/Streptomycin/ Tobramycin	Category D because of eighth-nerve toxicity, nephrotoxicity
Cephalosporins All generations: cephalothin, cephradine, cefaclor, ceftriaxone, cefoxitin, etc.	B: Some of the newer cephalosporins have no reports.
Chloramphenicol	C: Caution when used at term because of gray baby syndrome of cardiovascular collapse and bone marrow depression.
Clindamycin	B
Erythromycin	B: Estolate can induce hepatotoxicity.
Metronidazole	B: Teratogenic in first trimester.
Nitrofurantoin	B: Associated with hemolytic anemia in G-6-PD deficiency.
Norfloxacin/ciprofloxacin	C
Penicillins Pen G, Pen VK, etc., amoxicillin, carbenicillin, Augmentin, Unasyn, methicillin, dicloxacillin, etc.	B
Sulfonamides	B, but D when near term because of the association of jaundice and hemolytic anemia.
Sulfisoxazole	C
Tetracycline/doxycycline	D
Trimethoprim	C: Folate antagonist, so caution is advocated despite the lack of demonstrated abnormalities.
Vancomycin	C
Antifungals	
Clotrimazole, nystatin	B
Miconazole, butaconazole	C
Amphotericin B	B
Antivirals	C

Sources: References 103, 105–106. Used with permission.

also has been expanded. Despite our increased knowledge, many infections, particularly viral infections, have capricious yet potentially devastating outcomes. This section reviews some of the infections acquired during pregnancy that can cause placental or fetal infections. It is important to note that many hotlines exist in cities across the United States for referral, reference, and data collection regarding infections during pregnancy [107].

Toxoplasmosis

Toxoplasmosis is a parasitic infection that occurs in healthy individuals either asymptomatically or as a brief febrile illness consisting of lymphadenopathy, headache, malaise, pharyngitis, and/or myalgias (see Chap. 10) [108,109]. Based on antibody conversion exposure to toxoplasmosis is considered to be 20%–60% in the United States and the United Kingdom [108–110]; in France it is as high as 80% [109, 110].

Toxoplasmosis results from the ingestion of cysts from infected meat or contaminated soil. Cats are the most common domestic vector and shed oocysts in their feces. Infections acquired from water, venison and caribou and seal meat have been reported [108–119, 111]. Lymphadenopathy, hepatitis, pneumonia, or encephalitis can occur. The development of antibodies subsequently limits the active infection. A previous infection provides immunity, but reactivation in the form of retinochoroiditis can occur in healthy individuals. More severe reactivation is seen in immunocompromised individuals, such as CNS disease in AIDS patients. Pregnant women who become immunodeficient could have reactivation of their toxoplasmosis with subsequent spread to the fetus. Congenital infection results when acute toxoplasmosis occurs in a pregnant woman. The frequency of congenital toxoplasmosis in the United States ranges from 1–6.5:1,000 [109, 110] to 1:10,000 births [108]. The risk of transplacental transfer and intrauterine infection is reported to be 20%–25% in the first two trimesters and 65%–70% in the third [108–110]. Only 30%–40% of pregnancies with evidence of acute toxoplasmosis result in an infected infant [108, 110].

The classic congenital toxoplasmosis triad of hydrocephalus, retinochoroiditis, and intracerebral calcifications is considered a rare finding [110]. However, the earlier in pregnancy the infection occurs, the more severe the sequelae [108–110]. Neonatal illness with some evidence of jaundice, hepatosplenomegaly, pneumonia, retinochoroiditis, seizures, nystagmus, microencephaly, and intracerebral calcifications presents in 10% of cases [109]. In the other 90% a slow continued active infection due to the infant's impaired immune status occurs. Retinochoroiditis, mental retardation, palsies, and other neurologic sequelae develop in these infected infants who appear healthy at birth.

Mandatory maternal screening has not been adopted in the United States due to difficulties in the cost, timing, and interpretation of toxoplasmosis testing, given the low incidence [108, 110, 117, 119, 122]. Preventive educative measures are favored that urge the elimination of uncooked food from the diet, careful handling of cats and their feces or contaminated soil, and meticulous hand washing [108–110]. Currently testing for toxoplasmosis in pregnant women with unexplained fever, rash, and adenopathy is recommended [108].

Testing

Many serologic tests that measure IgG and IgM antibodies can be used to diagnose toxoplasmosis. The Sabin-Feldman dye test, indirect immunofluorescence, complement-fixation, enzyme-linked immunosorbent assay (ELISA), direct agglutination, and immunoblot assays all are used [108, 109, 111, 112]. A single high IgG on any test does not assess the time of infection, but a fourfold rise in titer or a positive IgM antibody is considered diagnostic [108, 109]. However, IgM may not absolutely indicate a recent infection [110, 113]. IgA also has been studied with some success in determining acute and congenital toxoplasmosis [115]. Identification of fetal infection can be confirmed by cordocentesis after 20 weeks' gestation with a 1%–2% risk of fetal loss [110, 114, 116] or by amniocentesis [110, 114, 121]. Identification of intracerebral calcification on ultrasound exam are suspect for toxoplasmosis [110, 121].

Therapy

The treatment of acute toxoplasmosis in pregnancy is difficult because of problems with diagnosis and the potential for drug toxicity [108]. Elective abortion is an alternative for those women who have serologic evidence of infection.

Sulfadiazine and pyrimethamine inhibit multiplication of the tachyzoites and bradyzoites and is advocated by some authors, especially if evidence of fetal infection is demonstrated [114, 120, 121]. However, pyrimethamine is teratogenic during the first trimester [108]. Spiramycin, and analogue of erythromycin and a bacterostatic agent, has been used in some countries with success and is considered safe in pregnancy [109, 114, 116]. Clindamycin and trimethoprim-sulfamethazole also have been used, as well as other sulfonamides [108, 109]. The utility of therapy is unclear [110, 116, 117, 118].

Therapy of infected infants with pyrimethamine/sulfadiazine/folinic acid is recommended [108, 109, 120].

The current efforts of a collaborative, randomized, prospective study of congenital toxoplasmosis hopefully will provide better data for screening and treatment [123]. Pregnant patients with suspected toxoplasmosis should be referred to an infectious disease specialist.

Rubella

Rubella (German measles) was the first teratogenic virus to be recognized [124]. Pregnancy does not produce any significant change in the clinical course or cause rubella. Nasopharyngeal exposure is followed by incubation period of 14–21 days. A 1–5-day prodrome of fever, malaise, cough, and conjunctivitis precedes the rash and generalized adenopathy (see Chap. 9). Only 60%–70% of infected individuals develop a rash [125]. The morbilliform eruption also can be mimicked by several other viral illnesses [124].

Aggressive vaccination programs have succeeded in lowering the number of susceptible women of child-bearing age to 10%–20% [124–126]. Congenital rubella disease has been virtually eliminated, with one case reported in 1989 [126]. Since vaccination or a natural infection provides life-long immunity, documentation of antibody titers confirms protection. Reinfection demonstrated by high antibody titers or rubella-specific IgM in a woman previously immune indicates that a fetal infection is possible [124].

Periconceptional exposure earlier than 12 days after the last menstrual period is not known to cause any problems [124]. Thereafter, the period of gestational exposure when maternal viremia occurs is crucial to the type of congenital rubella disease seen.

A maternal rubella infection in the first 2 months of pregnancy has been linked to a 20% spontaneous abortion rate [124]. The classic triad of cataracts, deafness, and congenital heart disease occurs in 20%–80% of first-trimester exposures [107, 125]. A variety of other problems can occur at other stages of gestation. Intrauterine-growth retardation, retinopathy, and deafness all are associated with later gestational exposure [125]. Neurosensory problems are described perhaps due to breast milk transmission or persistent viral replication or reinfection after delivery [124, 125].

Prevention of rubella in pregnancy relies on aggressive attempts to determine the rubella-immune status of all women in the reproductive age group. Pregnancy should be avoided within 3 months of vaccination, but all women should be vaccinated, preferably prior to child-bearing age. Inadvertent vaccination during pregnancy is not considered an absolute reason for elective termination, since the risk of fetal infection after immunization during pregnancy is 1% [126].

Cytomegalovirus

Cytomegalovirus (CMV) is the most common viral infection causing congenital disease, with an incidence of 1%–2% of all live births [107, 124, 125, 127]. A member of the herpesvirus family, CMV is found throughout the world.

CMV is transmitted via infected saliva, urine, cervical secretions, and semen and iatrogenically acquired through infected blood products or transplanted organs. CMV causes a mononucleosis-like illness in 10% of people who have a primary infection. Fever, lymphadenopathy, pharyngitis, polyarthropathy, and chemical liver dysfunction are associated with a primary infection [124] (see Chap. 10). These symptoms can be masked by pregnancy or go undetected. The incubation period for CMV is around 4–8 weeks. Approximately 50% of women in the reproductive age group are seronegative [107, 124]. Despite the 1% risk of primary conversion during pregnancy, a previous infection is not totally protective. IgM-specific antibody implies a recent infection [107]. Reactivation or reinfection can occur, and this is believed to happen more frequently during pregnancy [107].

Viremia during the maternal infection causes placental infection with potential spread to the fetus [125]. Spontaneous abortion is associated with placental infection, most often when the placental involvement is severe and occurs early in gestation [127]. About 40% of infections from CMV actually reach the fetus [127].

Ninety percent of congenital CMV infections are asymptomatic at birth [107]. Five percent of infected infants have cytomegalic inclusion disease (CID), the classic symptomatic presentation with hepatosplenomegaly, jaundice, thrombocytopenia, petechial rash, microcephaly, deafness, chorioretinitis, and cerebral calcifications [125]. Another 5% of infants will have atypical disease with varying neurologic, psychomotor, and behavioral disorders [125]. Late sequelae will develop in another 10%–20% of congenital infections [124]. Maternal antibodies may blunt the damage of reactivation infections, thereby producing less severe fetal infections.

Neonatal infection can result from infected breast milk and from contact with infected cervical secretions during delivery [124]. Interstitial pneumonitis and neurosensory abnormalities may occur.

Screening or prediction of outcome in potentially infected infants is difficult. First, since most primary infections are subclinical, the risk of exposure often is not known. Second, no known treatment exists. Third, since primary infection is not totally protective, prenatal screening for conversion status is not an absolute marker of immunity. One approach is prenatal screening, to identify susceptible patients who are seronegative. Exposed pregnant women could also be tested. If a change in titer or seroconversion occurs, especially in the first 20 weeks of pregnancy, counseling about termination of pregnancy is suggested [128]. The 80% of children who would be normal must be contrasted with the potentially devastating outcome in the others.

Herpes Simplex Virus (HSV)

Herpes simplex virus (HSV, herpes hominus) causes recurrent vesicular mucocutaneous infections (see Chap. 32).

MATERNAL HSV
The identification of a primary HSV infection during pregnancy is crucial; however, 60% of women with HSV-infected infants have no symptoms suggestive of an initial infection [129]. A primary infection does not provide immunity to prevent reinfections, but antibodies appear to blunt the duration and severity of recurrent episodes.

Maternal attacks during pregnancy can increase without an increase in morbidity [107]. Disseminated infection has a greater than 50% mortality rate [129].

FETAL HSV
The frequency of HSV infections during pregnancy is from 1:2500 to 1:10,000 deliveries [129]. HSV infections during pregnancy have different effects depending on the type of maternal infection (primary or recurrent) and the period of gestation in which the infection occurs. Seventy-five percent of neonatal infections are secondary to HSV-2, with 20% attributed to HSV-1 [124, 133]. The routes of infection are hematogenous, ascending, or from contact with HSV virus during delivery.

A primary infection with HSV during pregnancy has tremendous implication for the fetus, since no maternal antibodies exist to modify the intrauterine infection. Viremia during the first 12–20 weeks of gestation is associated with an increased incidence of spontaneous abortion, stillbirth, and congenital malformation [107, 125, 129, 130]. Malformations include hydrencephaly, microcephaly, chorioretinitis, cerebral and cerebellar necrosis, hepatosplenomegaly, bone anomalies, and cutaneous scars and vesicles [125, 129].

A primary infection in the third trimester is associated with perinatal infection, intrauterine-growth retardation, prematurity, and premature labor [130, 131]. Intrauterine infection is usually apparent within the first 24–48 hours of life [131]. Babies surviving an intrauterine primary infection have a 40% morbidity rate with significant neurologic sequelae [125, 130, 131].

Neonates may develop three equally common types of HSV infections: skin or mucous membrane infection, CNS infection, and disseminated HSV [133]. Fifty percent of infected neonates are premature and develop clinical evidence of infection in 5–17 days of life [129]. Left untreated 75% of neonates with localized infection will develop disseminated disease [124, 133], but disease limited to the skin is successfully treated [129]. Over 60% of neonates with CNS or disseminated disease develop skin lesions [133], and despite treatment there is a 50% morbidity and mortality rate in these infants [129].

Neonates with mothers with recurrent HSV lesions have a low attack rate when exposed to genital HSV on delivery, because of the presence of neutralizing antibodies [134].

THERAPY
The management of a primary infection during pregnancy includes counseling about congenital anomalies, intrauterine-growth retardation, prematurity, spontaneous abortion, and neonatal infection. Documenting a primary first episode of HSV is crucial.

Previous protocols called for antepartum cervical and labial culturing at 36 weeks and then weekly to document viral shedding. That approach, however has changed due to the inaccuracy of culture in predicting shedding [135, 136]. Currently it is recommended that if there is a history of genital herpes but no genital lesions, the child be delivered vaginally and cultures obtained on the day of delivery from mother or neonate [137]. If lesions are present when labor or rupture of membranes occurs, C-section should be performed, ideally within 4–6 hours of membrane rupture. Use of a rapid ELISA test for HSV, which has been found to be highly sensitive and specific, could lessen the C-section rate even more [138].

Acyclovir should be considered. Antepartum use, especially in the third trimester, may reduce morbidity and mortality for the child [139, 140].

Varicella-Zoster Virus

Varicella-zoster virus is a herpes family member that results in chickenpox and zoster (see Chap. 9). Since varicella is a childhood disease, 76%–90% of adults are immune [124, 141–144]. Consequently varicella in pregnancy is uncommon, accounting for only 2% of all chickenpox cases, or 5 out of 10,000 pregnancies [141, 142]. Pregnancy may predispose to more serious varicella infections, with reports of increased mortality from maternal varicella pneumonia [142–144]. Maternal infection with varicella usually resolves without complications if pneumonia does not occur.

Acyclovir has been used successfully to treat pneumonia and the other serious complications: pericarditis, encephalitis, and myocarditis [141–143, 145, 146]. Acyclovir's use in pregnancy has not been studied, but no fetal complications have been reported [124, 141]. Aggressive pulmonary management is necessary, and serious maternal illness can precipitate premature delivery.

Varicella infections in pregnancy can produce two distinctly different outcomes, depending on the period of exposure. The fetal varicella syndrome, or varicella embryopathy, is a rare outcome of an early embryonic infection in the first 20 weeks of gestation [124, 129, 141–143]. It consists of limb deformities, skin contractures, mental retardation, bulbar palsy, and ocular defects (chorioretinitis, cataracts, nystagmus) [124, 141–143]. Several large series have revealed no higher incidence of congenital defects in women with varicella as opposed to nonexposed pregnant women, yet in a subset of these women, the specific anomalies described have been identified [124, 141]. One study attributes the defects to a fetal herpes zoster infection with encephalitis [147].

Varicella-zoster immune globulin (VZIG) should be offered to nonimmune pregnant women with close household contacts for varicella, ideally if serologic confirmation of susceptibility can be made [107, 124, 141, 142]. VZIG is best given as soon as possible after exposure, up to 96 hours. Immune globulin is recommended if VZIG is not available [143]. Acyclovir's use is unstudied, and its main effect would be in limiting maternal infection [139–142].

Perinatal varicella, or varicella of the newborn, is a common and serious complication of late gestational infection [124, 141–143]. A fetus whose mother develops varicella 4–5 days before delivery to 2 days after delivery has been exposed to maternal viremia but has no protection from maternal antibodies. 16% of those babies develop varicella, and their mortality rate is 31% [124].

Acyclovir for the mother prior to delivery and for the baby afterward plus VZIG for the baby on delivery is recommended [124, 141–144]. Delaying delivery can maximize passive antibody protection for the baby [142]. Isolation from the mother if delivery occurs during her incubation (prior to viremia and rash) or infectious period helps protect the baby from developing varicella [141]. Breast-feeding by the viremic or infected mother also is discouraged [142]. Potential exposure in the home to neonate and mother should be avoided, or administration of VZIG to the baby could be considered [141].

Varicella virus vaccine soon may be an option for women of child-bearing age [141, 148].

Zoster is more uncommon in pregnancy than varicella and is not believed to cause problems for the newborn or the mother [107, 124, 142].

Beyond TORCH

The list of infectious agents associated with congenital or neonatal infections has grown beyond the TORCH syndrome [149]. Human immunodeficiency virus (HIV-1 and 2), parvovirus, enteroviruses, influenza, Epstein-Barr virus, syphilis, malaria, and listeriosis acquired during pregnancy have been linked to fetal problems, some with clearer evidence than others [149].

HIV has some transplacental spread, but intrapartum and postpartum contact with maternal secretions and breast-feeding are the main route of infection [127]. It is estimated that 13%–35% of infants with HIV-positive mothers are infected. The more advanced the mother's disease, the more likely the child is to be infected. A dysmorphic syndrome has been identified [107]. Maternal screening can help to identify and, it is hoped prevent fetal contamination.

Enteroviruses (echovirus, poliovirus, coxsackievirus) can cause late-pregnancy or neonatal infections, although the risk appears small [128]. Neonatal poliomyelitis has a case fatality rate of 50%; echovirus can produce jaundice and hepatic failure [149]. Some association with spontaneous abortion has been reported.

Parvovirus, the agent of fifth disease, or erythema infectiosum, has been reported to cause hydrops fetalis [128, 149, 150]. Pregnant women with children could often have exposure to parvovirus, yet there is no evidence that gamma globulin use is protective [128].

Hepatitis B can be acquired through contact at delivery [128], and maternal screening is warranted to identify those infants requiring active and passive immunization at birth.

Epstein-Barr virus has been associated with spontaneous abortion, CNS malformation, and congenital heart disease [125, 127].

Congenital syphilis is well recognized. The earliest sign is usually snuffles. Boney abnormalities include a "saddle nose" and anterior bowing of the legs. Rashes include a maculopapular desquamation or vessicles and bullae. Hepatic involvement is evidenced by jaundice, anemia, thrombocytopenia, and hepatosplenomegaly. Inflammatory changes in any other organ may occur.

Listeria monocytogenes infection can result in early neonatal respiratory difficulty, septicemia, and meningitis [149]. Transplacental or ascending infection is believed to be the route of infection.

Group B streptococcus causes early neonatal sepsis in 2–4 infants per 1,000 live births, with a 50% mortality rate [151]. Respiratory distress occurs in the first 3 days [152]. The relationship of vaginal colonization with group B streptococcus, premature rupture of membranes, and premature labor is not clear [151]. Infection from ascending transmission has been seen with and without rupture of membranes, although most infections result from vaginal delivery [152]. Antibiotic prophylaxis has not been entirely successful, although it is hoped that new rapid-identification tests for group B streptococcus will target high-risk groups for treatment [151, 153].

Immunization During Pregnancy

The decision to administer immunizations during pregnancy should be guided by the same judgment used in prescribing any medication during pregnancy: (1) Avoid any drug that is not necessary, and (2) perform a risk-benefit analysis, weighing the immunization complications for the mother and the fetus against the danger of the infection [1, 2]. Providing medical advice after inadvertent immunization in pregnancy requires specific knowledge of the data available of such situations. This section reviews the specific kinds of vaccinations available and their unique applications in pregnancy.

Passive Immunization

The administration of ready-made antibodies to provide instant protection against specific infections is known as passive immunization (Table 29-8). Three types of immunobiologics are available: (1) pooled human immunoglobulin (IG), (2) specific immunoglobulins and (3) antitoxins [156]. An antitoxin is a collection of antibodies acquired from animals immunized with specific antitoxin. Since no active infection occurs, the use of IG and antitoxin in pregnancy provides safe but transient immunity, lasting around 30 days. The main concerns are those concerning contamination with other infective agents and the risk of allergic reactions.

Active Immunization

The use of agents that stimulate the development of protective antibodies in the host is active immunization (Table 29-9). Two kinds of vaccines can be

Table 29-8. Passive immunization

Disease	Antibody source
Black widow spider bite	Antivenom (horse)
Botulism	Polyvalent antitoxin (horse)
Diphtheria	Antitoxin (horse)
Hepatitis A	Pooled human IG
Hepatitis B	Antihepatitis B human IG (HBIG)
Measles	Pooled human IG
Rabies	Antirabies human IG
RH Isoimmunization	Anti–Rh-D human IG
Snake bite	Antivenom (horse)
Tetanus	Antitetanus human IG
Varicella zoster	Anti–V-Z human immunoglobulin

Sources: References 154, 156. Used with permission.

used: live and inactivated vaccines. Attenuated live vaccines consist of bacteria or viruses modified to limit their infectivity. These vaccines cause mild versions of the diseases they protect against, have a greater risk in pregnancy, but provide lifelong protection. A maternal viremia could compromise fetal health or produce intrauterine infection and its sequelae [156, 157]. Inactivated or killed bacteria or virus in inactivated vaccines eliminate the danger of fetal infection but rarely produce a significant or long-lasting antibody response [155].

Whereas vaccines are made from bacteria or viruses, other agents capable of providing protection against infections are toxoids (see Table 29-9). Toxoids are modified bacterial components that can stimulate production of antitoxins [156]. The use of toxoids in pregnancy is safe.

Precautions and Recommendations

The use of live vaccines during pregnancy is to be avoided. Vaccination with measles, mumps, and rubella (MMR) vaccine is specifically contraindicated in pregnancy, and women receiving the vaccine are advised not to get pregnant within 3 months of immunization [156, 158]. Although the vaccine virus can cross the placenta, a CDC registry from 1979 to 1988 found no cases of congenital rubella syndrome after inadvertent vaccination within 3 months of conception [159, 160]. The estimated risk of serious malformation is 0%–1.6% following first-trimester vaccination, as opposed to the greater than 20% risk of congenital rubella syndrome from first-trimester maternal rubella infection [160]. Consequently recommendation for therapeutic termination of pregnancy based only on vaccination is not necessary, but is a decision between the patient and her physician [160].

Table 29-9. Active immunization

Live vaccines[a]	Inactivated vaccines[b]	Toxoids
(Bacterial/Viral)	(Bacterial/Viral)	
BCG (Calmette-Guérin bacillus)	Cholera	Anthrax
Measles	Haemophilus influenza B	Diphtheria
Mumps	Hepatitis B	Tetanus
Oral polio virus	Influenza	
Rubella	Inactivated polio virus	
Yellow fever	Meningococcus	
	Pertussis	
	Plague	
	Pneumococcus	
	Rabies	
	Rickettsia	
	Typhoid	

[a] Potentially harmful if used during pregnancy.
[b] Safe for use during pregnancy.
Sources: References 126, 154, 155. Used with permission.

Administration of yellow fever or oral polio virus vaccine is warranted if the risk of a natural infection outweighs the risk of vaccination [161]. Travel to areas with high risk of exposure should be avoided [157, 161].

Routine use of IG is not recommended after rubella exposure [160], but it is suggested in susceptible pregnant contacts of rubeola (measles) [158].

There is no evidence of risk with inactivated vaccines or toxoids [4]. Td (tetanus toxoid and diphtheria toxoid) is recommended in pregnancy if indicated.

As a precautionary measure based on theoretical risks, vaccinations should be put off until the second or third trimester but not if the danger of infectivity is earlier [156, 162].

Individuals recently immunized with MMR vaccines can shed virus but do not transmit them, so administration is considered safe in the children of pregnant women [155, 156, 159]. Oral polio vaccine also is shed after vaccination, but no risk has been found to the fetus when the household contacts of a pregnant woman are immunized [156]. However, vaccine-induced disease theoretically could be seen in the pregnant woman who has never been vaccinated for polio. In that situation a recommendation would be to immunize the mother with killed/inactivated polio vaccine and her children with live polio vaccine [155].

Rubella is the only vaccine virus isolated from breast milk, but there is no evidence that it is harmful to the breast-feeding infants [156, 157, 160].

Vaccinating post-partum in women known to be susceptible is encouraged [155]. Pregnant women also should be screened for hepatitis surface antigen, to identify babies who may be at risk of acquiring hepatitis B. IG, hepatitis B IG, and hepatitis B vaccine are not contraindicated in pregnancy if their use is warranted [163].

Postpartum Endometritis

"Child-bed fever" is an old-fashioned yet descriptive term that refers to postpartum genital tract infection. Just as it was years ago, the most common infection today in the puerperium or postpartum period is an infection of the uterus [164–168]. Postpartum endometritis is considered to be of two types, depending on the mode of delivery [168]. Following vaginal delivery the incidence of postpartum endometritis is 1%–5% [164, 166, 168]. The frequency following cesarean section prior to antibiotic prophylaxis is 5%–85% [164, 167, 169]; with antibiotic prophylaxis it is 3%–50% [165, 167].

Definition

In postpartum endometritis the lining of the uterus (the endometrium or decidua) is initially infected and the uterine muscle is quickly if not concurrently involved. The infection may spread through the lymphatics to other pelvic tissues. If a cesarean section has been performed, infection may occur initially through the incision, as a cellulitis. Postpartum uterine infection has been indicated by many names besides endometritis, including endomyometritis and endoparametritis [164]. *Metritis with pelvic cellulitis* has been suggested as a more accurate term, since in addition to diffuse infection of the endometrium, involvement of the myometrium and adjacent soft tissue is implied [164, 165].

Clinical Presentation

Presenting symptoms include fever of 38°C or higher, increased afterpains, and abdominal pain. On physical examination unilateral or bilateral abdominal tenderness will be present. Guarding or rebound tenderness indicates that the infection has spread to involve the peritoneum. Bimanual examination of the uterus will demonstrate tenderness. The cul-de-sac should be palpated for fullness, which may indicate an abscess. Any incision or laceration site should be inspected for signs of infection. Leukocytosis from 15,000 to 30,000 WBC/μl will be found, and occasionally foul-smelling or purulent lochia and tachycardia will be noted [164, 168, 170]. The degree of illness may be mild when infection is confined to the endometrium, while women with more extensive infection will appear more ill.

Risk Factors

Intrapartum risk factors of prolonged membrane rupture and labor, multiple cervical exams, and internal fetal monitoring increase the incidence of postpartum endometritis [164, 167]. Young age and low socioeconomic level are also risk factors [167, 171]. Antepartum conditions of malnutrition, anemia, sexual intercourse, prematurely ruptured membranes, and premature labor are presumed but unsubstantiated factors contributing to postpartum endometritis [164].

Pathophysiology

Understanding the postpartum changes in the uterus is necessary to understanding and diagnosing endometritis. Immediately postpartum the uterus is essentially ischemic, as it contracts from its full-term size down to around 16 weeks' size [172, 173]. The uterus consists mostly of myometrium with a thin decidual layer of endometrium composed of irregular, bloody tissue with thrombosed vessels [172]. Most of this lining sloughs off as lochia, and new endometrium forms. By 10 days postpartum rejuvenated endometrium is present everywhere except at the placental site, and vaginal bleeding is minimal. In 2 weeks the uterus shrinks into the pelvis, and by 6 weeks postpartum is near the prepregnant size.

The thin and bloody decidual lining and the more slowly resolving placental site allow a route for two kinds of postpartum infection to occur. Early-onset infection, seen within 48 hours, most often occurs after a cesarean section [165, 169]. Bacteria in the ammniotic fluid infects the incisional site, producing a wound infection that progresses to cellulitis. The ischemic and raw endometrium allows the infection to enter the myometrium, vasculature, and lymphatics [165, 167]. Late endometritis is described from 3 days to 6 weeks after a vaginal delivery and results from placental-site infection [165, 169]. Normal involution of the uterus is effective in removing contaminated lochia, and late postpartum endometritis following vaginal delivery is a localized and hence milder infection [165, 168, 170].

Bacteriology

The organisms causing endometritis are multiple and consist predominantly of bowel and vaginal flora [164, 165, 167]. With an intact amniotic sac the pregnant uterine cavity is considered sterile

[164]. Once the sac has been ruptured, bacteria can ascend through the cervix or invade through an incision. Synergism allows for a mixture of aerobic and anaerobic organisms to multiply, producing polymicrobial culture results in up to 80%–90% of early endometritis [165, 167, 169]. Sixty-three percent of amniotic-fluid cultures obtained at cesarean section more than 6 hours after membrane rupture revealed growth of an average of 2.5 organisms, including anaerobic and aerobic organisms [164]. Anaerobes alone were are found in 30% of cases, and aerobes alone in 7% [164].

The anaerobic organisms recovered include *Peptostreptococcus* and *Peptococcus* species predominantly, *Bacteroides* species (*Bacteroides bivius*, *Bacteroides disiens*), and *Clostridium* species [164, 166, 167, 169]. Aerobic species include enterococcus group B beta-hemolytic streptococci, other *Streptococcus* species, *E. coli*, and *Klebsiella*, and *Proteus* species [164, 166, 167, 169] In early and late postpartum endometritis *M. hominis*, *C. trachomatis*, and *Ureaplasma urealyticum* commonly are cultured [166, 168, 169], but these organisms more frequently are culprits of late postpartum infections [169]. *C. trachomatis* is not always determined to be present at the time of infection, but a positive antepartum culture was found in one-third of women who subsequently developed postpartum infections [164]. Selection for enterococci can result from use of prophylactic antibiotics [169, 173].

However sophisticated the culture techniques, uterine culture results do not always indicate the offending pathogens or their significance. Seventy percent of clinically healthy puerperal women were found to have positive cultures of the uterine cavity [164]. Cervicovaginal flora do not reflect uterine pathogens [174]. The use of cultures is still advocated by some to guide therapy in those cases that clinically do not respond [174]. Blood cultures are positive in 13%–24% [164].

Therapy

The antibiotic therapy of endometritis is generally empiric. Treatment in the past required double or triple antibiotics to provide gram-positive, gram-negative, and anaerobic coverage [164, 173]. The standard has been clindamycin and gentamicin [164, 167, 173], which is curative in over 90% of patients. Penicillin G plus gentamicin results in some treatment failures [167], which may be alleviated by adding metronidazole for aneaerobic coverage [164, 173]. Several single-agent regimens are now available, including the second and third-generation cephalosporins (cefoxitin, cefotetan, cefotaxime, ceftizoxime, moxalactam) and the extended-spectrum penicillins (piperacillin, mezlocillin) [164, 167, 173]. Clavulonic acid or sulbactam combined with ampicillin, amoxicillin, or ticarcillin are more recent single-drug choices [164, 175]. Doxycyline may be added to single-dose regimens to ensure coverage of C. Trachomatis. The use of clindamycin alone [175], the combination of clindamycin with a second-generation cephalosporin like cefoxitin, or clindamycin with aztreonam may provide lower toxicity than if an aminoglycoside is used [164, 167, 173]. Metronidazole with gentamycin or tobramycin could be considered for anerobic coverage, especially in the presence of an abscess, or troublesome diarrhea from clindamycin [164, 167]. Chloramphenicol given with a cephalosporin or penicillin is reserved for pelvic sepsis [164]. Table 29-10 lists dosage regimens.

Table 29-10. IV antibiotic dosages for postpartum endometritis

Antibiotic	Dosage
Cefoxitin	2–3 g q6h
Cefotaxime	2 g q6–8h
Cefotetan	1–3 g q12h
Ceftizoxime	2–4 g q8h
Moxolactam	2 g q8h
Ampicillin-sulbactam	1.5–3 g q6h
Ticarcillin-clavulanate	3.1 g q4–8h
Clindamycin +	900 mg q8h
Gentamicin	1–2 mg/kg load, adjust for renal function
Clindamycin +	900 mg q8h
Cefoxitin	2 g q6–8h
Clindamycin +	900 mg q8h
Aztreonam	2 g q8h
Penicillin +	5 million U q6h
Gentamicin +	1–2 mg/kg load, adjust for renal function
Metronidazole	500 mg q6h

Failure of a patient to respond to antibiotic therapy should initiate a search for pelvic abscess, or phlegmon [164].

Oral therapy with amoxicillin, a cephalosporin, or erythromycin may be indicated for mild symptoms and findings in late postpartum endometritis [168].

Differential Diagnosis

Subinvolution is failure of the postpartum uterus to contract to its original size. Retained products of conception, prolonged lochial discharge, excessive bleeding, and a larger, softer uterus than expected may be found [176]. Treatment with ergotrate or methergine may aid resolution. Antibiotics may be necessary if a concurrent metritis is present. Diagnosis may require a pelvic ultrasound. Dilatation and curettage may be required for treatment.

Infections of the urinary tract and mastitis are common postpartum infections. Five to ten percent of women with endometritis are reported to have a concurrent urinary tract infection [167]. Retained products of conception, venous thromboembolism, septic pelvic thrombophlebitis, wound infection, infected episiotomy site, toxic shock syndrome, and drug fever should all be considered in the febrile patient in the postpartum period [167].

References

1. McCue JD. Evaluations and management of vaginitis. An update for primary care practitioners. Arch Intern Med 149:565–68, 1989.
2. Huggins GR, Preti G. Vaginal odors and secretions. Clin Obstet Gynecol 24:355–77, 1981.
3. Speigel CA. Vaginitis/vaginosis. Clin Lab Med 9:525–33, 1989.
4. Godley MJ. Quantitation of vaginal discharge in healthy volunteers. Br J Obstet Gynecol 92:739–42, 1985.
5. Hanna NF et al. The relationship between vaginal pH and the microbiological status in vaginitis. Br J Obstet Gynecol 92:1267–71, 1985.
6. Larsen B, Galask RP. Vaginal microbial flora: composition and influences of host physiology. Ann Intern Med 96:926–30, 1982.
7. Brown WJ. Variations in the vaginal bacterial flora. A preliminary report. Ann Intern Med 96:931–34, 1982.

8. Hill LVH, Embil JA. Vaginitis: current microbiologic and clinical concepts. *Can Med Assoc J* 134:321–31, 1986.

9. Hammill H. Unusual causes of vaginitis (excluding trichomonas, bacterial vaginosis, and *Candida albicans*). *Obstet Gynecol Clin North Am* 16:337–45, 1989.

10. Riordan T et al. A prospective study of genital infections in a family-planning clinic. *Epidemiol Infect* 104:47–53, 1990.

11. Lefevre JC et al. Lower genital tract infections in women: comparison of clinical and epidemiologic findings with microbiology. *Sex Trans Dis* 15:110–13, 1988.

12. Reed BD, Huck W, Zazove P. Differentiation of *Gardnerella vaginalis*, *Candida albicans*, and Trichomonas vaginalis infections of the vagina. *J Fam Pract* 28:673–80, 1989.

13. Amsel R et al. Nonspecific vaginitis. Diagnosis criteria and microbial and epidemiologic associations. *Am J Med* 74:14–22, 1983.

14. Eschenbach DA et al. Diagnosis and clinical manifestations of bacterial vaginosis. *Am J Obstet Gynecol* 158:819–28, 1988.

15. Hillier S, Holmes KK. Bacterial vaginosis. In KK Holmes et al. (eds.), *Sexually Transmitted Diseases* (2nd ed.). New York: McGraw-Hill, 1984. Pp. 547–59.

16. Landers DV. The treatment of vaginitis: trichomonas, yeast, and bacterial vaginosis. *Clin Obstet Gynecol* 31:437–79, 1988.

17. Swedberg J et al. Comparison of single-dose vs one-week course of metronidazole for symptomatic bacterial vaginosis. *JAMA* 254:1046–49, 1985.

18. Treatment of sexually transmitted diseases. *Med Lett Drugs Ther* 32:5–10, 1990.

19. Greaves WL et al. Clindamycin vs. metronidazole in the treatment of bacterial vaginosis. *Obstet Gynecol* 72:799–802, 1988.

20. Ison CA et al. Local treatment for bacterial vaginosis. *Br Med J* 295:886, 1987.

21. Thompson JL et al. Proline aminopeptidase activity as a rapid diagnostic test to confirm bacterial vaginosis. *Obstet Gynecol* 71:607–11, 1988.

22. Thomason JL, Gelbart SM, James JA. Is analysis of vaginal secretions for volatile organic acids to detect bacterial vaginosis of any diagnostic value? *Am J Obstet Gynecol* 159:1509–11, 1988.

23. Watts DH et al. Bacterial vaginosis as a risk factor for post-cesarean endometritis. *Obstet Gynecol* 75:52–58, 1990.

24. Silver HM et al. Evidence relating bacterial vaginosis to intraamniotic infection. *Am J Obstet Gynecol* 161:808–12, 1989.

25. Sweet RL. Importance of differential diagnosis in acute vaginitis. *Am J Obstet Gynecol* 152:921–24, 1985.

26. Thomason JL, Gelbart SM. *Trichomonas vaginalis*. *Obstet Gynecol* 74:536–41, 1989.

27. Rein MF, Muller M. *Trichomonas vaginalis* and trichomoniasis. In KK Holmes et al. (eds.), *Sexually Transmitted Diseases* (2nd ed.). New York: McGraw-Hill, 1984. Pp. 481–92.

28. Catterall RD, Nicol CS. Is trichomonal infestation a venereal disease? *Br Med J* 1:1177–79, 1960.

29. Bennett JR, Barnes WG, Coffman S. The emergency department diagnosis of trichomonas vaginitis. *Ann Emerg Med* 18:564–66, 1989.

30. Krieger JN et al. Diagnosis of trichomoniasis. Comparison of conventional wet-mount examination with cytologic studies, cultures, and monoclonal antibody staining of direct specimens. *JAMA* 259:1223–27, 1988.

31. Sobel JD. *Vulvovaginal candidiasis*. In KK Holmes et al. (eds.), *Sexually Transmitted Diseases* (2nd ed.). New York: McGraw-Hill, 1984. Pp. 515–23.

32. Monif GR. Classification and pathogenesis of vulvovaginal candidiasis. *Obstet Gynecol* 152:935–39, 1985.

33. Sobel J. Vulvovaginal candidiasis—What we do and do not know. *Ann Intern Med* 101:390–92, 1984.

34. Rigg D, Miller MM, Metzger WJ. Recurrent allergic vulvovaginitis: treatment with *candida allicians* allergen immunotherapy. *Am J Obstet Gynecol* 162:332–36, 1990.

35. Ritter W. Pharmacokinetic fundamentals of vaginal treatment with clotrimazole. *Am J Obstet Gynecol* 152:945–47, 1985.

36. Loendersloot EW et al. Efficacy and tolerability of single-dose versus six-day treatment of candidal vulvovaginitis with vaginal tablets of clotrimazole. *Am J Obstet Gynecol* 152:953–55, 1985.

37. Cokin L. Is more than one application of an antifungal necessary in treatment of acute vaginal candidiasis? *Am J Obstet Gynecol* 152:961–64, 1985.

38. Fleery F, Hughes D, Floyd R. Therapeutic results obtained in vaginal mycoses after single-dose treatment with 500 mg clotrimazole vaginal tablets. *Am J Obstet Gynecol* 152:968–70, 1985.

39. Butoconazole for *vulvovaginal candidiasis*. *Med Lett Drugs Ther* 28:68, 1986.

40. Sobel JD. Recurrent vulvovaginal candidiasis. A prospective study of the efficacy of maintenance

ketoconzole therapy. *N Engl J Med* 315:1455–58, 1986.

41. Burnett LS. Anatomy. In HW Jones, AC Wentz, LS Burnett (eds.), *Novak's Textbook of Gynecology* (11th ed.). Baltimore: Williams & Wilkins, 1988. Pp. 57–58.

42. Graney DO, Vontver LA. Anatomy and physical examination of the female genital tract. In KK Holmes et al. (eds.), *Sexually Transmitted Diseases* (2nd ed.). New York: McGraw-Hill 1990. Pp. 105–15.

43. Word B. Office treatment of cyst and abscess of Bartholin's gland duct. *South Med J* 61:514–18, 1968.

44. Word B. New instrument for office treatment of cyst and abscess of Bartholin's gland. *JAMA* 190:777–78, 1964.

45. Downs MC, Randall HW. The ambulatory surgical management of Bartholin's duct cyst. *J Emerg Med* 7:623–26, 1989.

46. Warden TM. Incision and drainage of cutaneous abscesses and soft tissue infections. In JR Roberts, JR Hedges (eds.), *Clinical Procedures in Emergency Medicine*. Philadelphia: Saunders, 1985. Pp. 986–88.

47. Woodruff JD, Friedrick EG. The vestibule. *Clin Obstet Gynecol* 28:134–41, 1985.

48. Cruikshank SH, Davies J. Anatomy of the female genitalia. In JR Scott (ed.) *Danforth's Obstetrics and Gynecology* (6th ed.). Philadelphia: Lippincott, 1990. Pp. 1–38.

49. Marshall BR, Hepper JK, Zirbel CC. Sporadic puerperal mastitis. An infection that need not interrupt lactation. *JAMA* 233:1377–79, 1975.

50. Wilson ER. The breast. In DC Sabiston (ed.), *Textbook of Surgery* (13th ed.). Philadelphia: Saunders, 1986. Pp. 530–72.

51. Niebyl JR, Spence MR, and Parmley TH. Sporadic (nonepidemic) puerperal mastitis. *J Repro Med* 20:97–100, 1978.

52. Devereux WP. Acute puerperal mastitis. *Am J Obstet Gynecol* 108:78–81, 1970.

53. Stehman FB. Infections and inflammations of the breast. In WH Hindle (ed.), *Breast Disease for Gynecologists*. Norwalk: Appleton & Lange, 1990. Pp. 151–54.

54. Haagensen CD. Infections in the breast. In CD Haagensen (ed.), *Diseases of the Breast*. Philadelphia: Saunders, 1986. Pp. 384–93.

55. Olsen CG, Gorden RE. Breast disorders in nursing mothers. *Am Fam Pract* 41:1509–16, 1990.

56. Landers DV, Sweet RL. Perinatal infections. In HW Jones, AC Wentz, LS Burnet (eds.), *Novak's Textbook of Gynecology* (11th ed). Baltimore: Williams & Wilkins, 1988. Pp. 538–39.

57. Thomsen AC, Hansen KB, Moller BR. Leukocyte counts and microbiologic cultivation in the diagnosis of puerperal mastitis. *Am J Obstet Gynecol* 146:938–41, 1983.

58. Thomsen AC, Espersen T, Maigaard S. Course and treatment of milk stasis, noninfectious inflammation of the breast, and infectious mastitis in nursing women. *Am J Obstet Gynecol* 149:492–95, 1984.

59. Golinger DC, O'Neal BJ. Mastitis and mammary duct disease. *Arch Surg* 117:1027–29, 1982.

60. Isaacs JH. Diagnosis and treatment of benign lesions of the breast. In WH Hindle (ed.), *Breast Disease for Gynecologists*. Norwalk: Appleton & Lange, 1990. Pp. 198–200.

61. Nelson WE, Behrman RE, Vaughan VC (eds.). Breast feeding. In *Nelson Textbook of Pediatrics* (13th ed). Philadelphia: Saunders, 1987. Pp. 124–25.

62. Committee on Drugs. The transfer of drugs and other chemicals into human breast milk. *Pediatrics* 72:375–83, 1983.

63. Kalstone C. Methicillin-resistant staphylococcal mastitis. *Am J Obstet Gynecol* 161:120, 1989.

64. Demey HE et al. Mastitis and toxic syndrome. *Acta Obstet Gynecol Scand* 68:87–88, 1989.

65. Zlatnik RJ. The puerperium: normal and abnormal. In JR Scott et al. (eds.), *Danforth's Obstetrics and Gynecology* (6th ed.). Philadelphia: Lippincott, 1990. Pp. 193.

66. Benson EA. The management of breast abscesses. *World J Surg* 13:753–56, 1989.

67. Scholefield JH, Duncan JL, Rober K. Review of a hospital experience of breast abscesses. *Br J Surg* 74:469–70, 1987.

68. Dixon JM. Repeated aspiration of breast abscesses in lactating women. *Br Med* 297:1517–18, 1988.

69. Haagensen CD. Inflammatory carcinoma. In CD Haagensen (ed.), *Diseases of the Breast* (3rd ed.). Philadelphia: Saunders, 1986. Pp. 808–11.

70. Edmiston CE et al. The nonpuerperal breast infection: aerobic and anaerobic microbial recovery from acute and chronic disease. *J Infect Dis* 162:695–99, 1990.

71. Rosenthal LJ, Greenfield DS, Lesnick GJ. Breast abscess. Management in subareolar and peripheral disease. *NY State J Med* 182–83, 1981.

72. Walker AP et al. A prospective study of the microflora of nonpuerperal breast abscess. *Arch Surg* 123:908–11, 1988.

73. Bundred NJ et al. Are the legions of duct ectasia sterile? *Br J Surg* 72:844–45, 1985.

74. Bennett KW et al. Anaerobic curved rods in breast abscess and vagina. *Lancet* 1:564, 1989.

75. Dixon JM. Breast abscesses. *Br J Surg* 76:655, 1989.

76. Nash AG, Powles T. Review of a hospital experience of breast abscesses. *Br J Surg* 76:103, 1989.

77. Marchant D. The breast. In JR Scott et al. (ed.), *Danforth's Obstetrics and Gynecology* (6th ed.). Philadelphia: Lippincott, 1990. P. 1158.

78. Katzman DK, Wald ER. Staphylococcal scalded skin syndrome in a breast-fed infant. *Pediatr Infect Dis J* 6:295–96, 1987.

79. Bland KI. Inflammatory, infectious and metabolic disorders of the mamma. In KI Bland, EM Copeland (eds.), *The Breast. Comprehensive Management of Benign and Malignant Diseases.* Philadelphia: Saunders, 1991. Pp. 87–112.

80. Hankins GDV, Whalley PJ. Acute urinary tract infections in pregnancy. *Clin Obstet Gynecol* 28:266–78, 1985.

81. Martens MG. Pyelonephritis. *Obstet Gynecol Clin North Am* 16:305–15, 1989.

82. Sweet RL. Bacteriuria and pyelonephritis during pregnancy. *Semin Perinat* 1:25–40, 1977.

83. Cruikshank DP. Cardiovascular, pulmonary, renal and hematologic diseases in pregnancy. In JR Scott et al. (eds.), *Danforth's Obstetrics and Gynecology* (6th ed). Philadelphia: Lippincott, 1990. Pp. 446–48.

84. McNeely SG. Treatment of urinary tract infections during pregnancy. *Clin Obstet Gynecol* 31:480–87, 1988.

85. Gerstner GJ, Muller G, Nahler G. Amoxicillin in the treatment of asymptomatic bacteriuria in pregnancy: a single dose of 3 g amoxicillin versus a 4-day course of 3 doses 750 mg amoxicillin. *Gynecol Obstet Invest* 27:84–87, 1989.

86. Harris RE, Gilstrap LC, Pretty A. Single-dose antimicrobial therapy for asymptomatic bacteriuria during pregnancy. *Obstet Gynecol* 59:546–48, 1982.

87. Harris RE. Acute urinary tract infections and subsequent problems. *Clin Obstet Gynecol* 27:874–90, 1984.

88. Harris RE, Gilstrap LC. Cystitis during pregnancy: a distinct clinical entity. *Obstet Gynecol* 57:578–80, 1981.

89. Stamm WF et al. Diagnosis of coliform infection in acutely dysuric women. *N Engl J Med* 307:463–68, 1982.

90. Whalley PJ, Cunningham FG, Martin FG. Transient renal dysfunction associated with acute pyelonephritis of pregnancy. *Obstet Gynecol* 46:174–77, 1975.

91. Gilstrap LC et al. Renal infection and pregnancy outcome. *Am J Obstet Gynecol* 141:709–16, 1981.

92. VanDorsten JP, Lenke RR, Schifrin BS. Pyelonephritis in pregnancy. The role of in-hospital management and nitrofurantoin suppression. *J Repro Med* 32:895–900, 1987.

93. Angle JL et al. Acute pyelonephritis in pregnancy: a prospective study of oral versus intravenous antibiotic therapy. *Obstet Gynecol* 76:28–32, 1990.

94. Gilstrap LC, Cunningham FG, Whalley PJ. Acute pyelonephritis in pregnancy: an anterospective study. *Obstet Gynecol* 57:409–13, 1981.

96. Lenke RR, VanDorsten JP, Schifrin BS. Pyelonephritis in pregnancy: a prospective randomized trial to prevent recurrent disease evaluating suppressive therapy with nitrofurantoin and close surveillance. *Obstet Gynecol* 146:953–57, 1983.

97. Dunlow S, Duff P. Prevalence of antibiotic-resistant uropathogens in obstetric patients with acute pyelonephritis. *Obstet Gynecol* 76:241–44, 1990.

98. Yost DA, Michalowski E. Adult respiratory distress syndrome complicating recurrent antepartum pyelonephritis. *J Fam Pract* 31:81–82, 1990.

99. Cunningham FG, Lucas MJ, Hankins GD. Pulmonary injury complicating antepartum pyelonephritis. *Am J Obstet Gynecol* 156:797–807, 1987.

100. Krane NK. Acute renal failure in pregnancy. *Arch Intern Med* 148:2347–57, 1988.

101. Blake DA, Niebyl JR. Requirements and limitations in reproductive and teratogenic risk assessment. In JR Niebyl (ed.), *Drug Use in Pregnancy* (2nd ed.). Philadelphia: Lea & Febiger, 1988. Pp. 1–9.

102. Hamod KA, Khouzani VA. Antibiotics in pregnancy. In JR Niebyl (ed.), *Drug Use in Pregnancy* (2nd ed.). Philadelphia: Lea & Febiger, 1988. Pp. 29–36.

103. Gilstrap LC. Antimicrobial agents during pregnancy. In LC Gilstrap, S Faro (eds.), *Infections in Pregnancy*. New York: Wiley-Liss, 1990. Pp. 7–13.

104. Federal Drug Administration. Pregnancy labeling. FDA *Drug Bull* September:23–24, 1979.

105. Briggs GG, Freeman RK, Yaffe SJ. *Drugs in Pregnancy and Lactation* (3rd ed.). Baltimore: Williams & Wilkins, 1990.

106. Wise R. Prescribing in pregnancy. *Br Med J* 294:42–45, 1987.

107. Ellis GL, Melton J, Filkins K. Viral infections during pregnancy: a guide for the emergency physician. *Ann Emerg Med* 19:802–11, 1990.

108. Frenkel JK. Toxoplasmosis in human beings. *JAMA* 196:240–48, 1990.

109. Koshiniemi M, Lappalainen M, Hedman K, Toxoplasmosis needs evaluation. An overview and proposals. *AJDC* 143:724–28, 1989.

110. Antenatal screening for toxoplasmosis in the UK [editorial]. *Lancet* 336:346–48, 1990.

111. McDonald JC et al. An outbreak of toxoplasmosis in pregnant women in northern Quebec. *J Infect Dis* 161:769–74, 1990.

112. Suzuki Y, Thulliez P, Remington JS. Use of acute-stage-specific antigens of *Toxoplasma gondii* for serodiagnosis of acute toxoplasmosis. *J Clin Microbiol* 28:1734–38, 1990.

113. Sever JL. The importance of considering clinical usefulness in the evaluation of medical laboratory tests [letter]. *Am J Obstet Gynecol* 163:678–79, 1990.

114. Daffos F et al. Prenatal management of 746 pregnancies at risk for congenital toxoplasmosis. *N Engl J Med* 318:271–75, 1988.

115. Stepick-Biek P et al. IgA antibodies for diagnosis of acute congenital and acquired toxoplasmosis. *J Infect Dis* 162:270–73, 1990.

116. Teuten B. Antenatal screening for toxoplasmosis. *Lancet* 336:819, 1990.

117. Jeannel D et al. What is known about the prevention of congenital toxoplasmosis? *Lancet* 336:359–61, 1990.

118. Wilson CB. Treatment of congenital toxoplasmosis during pregnancy. *J Pediatr* 115:1003–4, 1990.

119. Frenkel JK. Diagnosis, incidence, and prevention of congenital toxoplasmosis. *AJDC* 144:956–57, 1990.

120. Cook GC. *Toxoplasma gondii* infection: a potential danger to the unborn fetus and AIDS sufferer. *Q J Med* 273:3–19, 1990.

121. Hohlfeld P et al. Fetal toxoplasmosis: outcome of pregnancy and infant follow-up after in utero treatment. *J Pediatr* 115:765–69, 1989.

122. Thorpe JM et al. Prenatal management and congenital toxoplasmosis. *N Engl J Med* 319:372–73, 1988.

123. The Toxoplasmosis Study Group. Congenital toxoplasmosis. *AJDC* 144:619, 1990.

124. Peiris JSM, Madely CR. Viral infections. In WM Barron, MD Lindheumer (ed.), *Medical Disorders in Pregnancy*. St. Louis: Mosby, 1991. Pp. 462–507.

125. Dickinson J, Gonik B. Teratogenic viral infections. *Clin Obstet Gynecol* 33:242–52, 1990.

126. Recommendations of the Immunization Practices Advisory Committee (ACIP). Rubella prevention. *MMWR* 39(RR-15):1–18, 1990.

127. Kaplan C. The placenta and viral infections. *Clin Obstet Gynecol* 33:232–241, 1990.

128. Dascol A et al. Laboratory tests for the diagnosis of viral disease in pregnancy. *Clin Obstet Gynecol* 33:218–31, 1990.

129. Stagno S, Whitley RJ. Herpesvirus infections of pregnancy. *N Engl J Med* 313:1327–30, 1985.

130. Baker D. Herpes and pregnancy: new management. *Clin Obstet Gynecol* 33:253–57, 1990.

131. Baldwin S, Whitley RJ. Teratogen update: intrauterine herpes simplex virus infection. *Teratology* 39:1–10, 1989.

132. Brown ZA et al. Effects on infants of a first episode of genital herpes during pregnancy. *N Engl J Med* 317:1246–51, 1987.

133. Arvin AM. Antiviral treatment of herpes simplex infection in neonates and pregnant women. *J Am Acad Dermatol* 18:200–203, 1988.

134. Prober CG et al. Low risk of herpes simples virus infections in neonates exposed to the virus at the time of vaginal delivery to mothers with recurrent genital herpes simplex virus infections. *N Engl J Med* 316:240–44, 1987.

135. Prober CG et al. Use of routine viral cultures at delivery to identify neonates exposed to herpes simplex virus. *N Engl J Med* 318:887–91, 1988.

136. Arvin AM et al. Failure of antepartum maternal cultures to predict the infant's risk of exposure to herpes simplex virus at delivery. *N Engl J Med* 315:796–800, 1986.

137. Gibbs RS et al. Management of genital herpes infection in pregnancy. *Obstet Gynecol* 71:779–80, 1988.

138. Baker DA et al. Clinical evaluation of a new herpes simplex virus ELISA: a rapid diagnostic test for herpes simplex virus. *Obstet Gynecol* 73:322–25, 1989.

139. Brown ZA, Baker D. Acyclovir therapy during pregnancy. *Obstet Gynecol* 73:526–31, 1989.

140. Brown ZA, Watts DH. Antiviral therapy in pregnancy. *Clin Obstet Gynceol* 33:276–89, 1990.

141. Fox GN, Strangarity JW. Varicella-zoster virus infections in pregnancy. *Am Fam Pract* 39:89–98, 1989.

142. Materns MG. Varicella-zoster infections in pregnancy. In LC Gilstrap, S Faro (eds.), *Infections in Pregnancy*. New York: Wiley-Liss, 1990. Pp. 177–84.

143. Herrman KL. Congenital and perinatal varicella. *Clin Obstet Gynecol* 25:605–9, 1982.

144. Schmidt GA, Hall JB. Pulmonary disease. In WM

Barron, MD Lindheimer (eds.), *Medical Disorders in Pregnancy*. St. Louis: Mosby, 1991. Pp. 216–17.

145. Hankins GD, Gilstrap LC, Patterson AR. Acyclovir treatment of varicella pneumonia in pregnancy. *Crit Care Med* 15:336–37, 1987.

146. Landsberger EJ, Hager WD, Grossman JH. Successful management of varicella pneumonia complicating pregnancy. A report of three cases. *J Repro Med* 31:311–14, 1986.

147. Higa K, Kenjiro D, Manabe H. Varicella-zoster virus infections during pregnancy: hypothesis concerning the mechanisms of congenital malformations. *Obstet Gynecol* 69:214–22, 1987.

148. Weibel RE et al. Live attenuated varicella virus vaccine. Efficacy trial in healthy children. *N Engl J Med* 310:1409–15, 1984.

149. TORCH syndrome and TORCH screening [editorial]. *Lancet* 335;1559–61, 1990.

150. Shmoys S, Kaplan C. Parvovirus and pregnancy. *Clin Obstet Gynecol* 33:268–75, 1990.

151. Watts DH, Eschenbach DA. Treatment of chlamydia, mycoplasma, and group B streptococcal infections. *Clin Obstet Gynecol* 31:435–52, 1988.

152. Hill H. Group B streptococcal infections. In KK Holmes et al. (eds.), *Sexually Transmitted Diseases*. New York: McGraw-Hill, 1984. Pp. 851–60.

153. Tuppurainen N, Hallman M. Prevention of neonatal group B streptococcal disease: intrapartum detection and chemoprophylaxis of heavily colonized parturients. *Obstet Gynecol* 73:583–87, 1989.

154. Amstay MS. Vaccination in pregnancy. *Clin Obstet Gynecol* 10:13–22, 1983.

155. Peiri JSM, Madeley CR. Viral infections. In WM Barron, MD Lindheimer (eds.), *Medical Disorders during Pregnancy*. St. Louis: Mosby, 1991. Pp. 462–507.

156. Blanco JD, Gibbs RS. Immunizations in pregnancy. *Clin Obstet Gynecol* 25:611–18, 1982.

157. Advisory Committee Immunization Practices. General recommendation on immunizations. *MMWR* 38:205–27, 1989.

158. Centers for Disease Control. Rubella vaccination during pregnancy—United States, 1971–1988. *MMWR* 38:289–93, 1989.

159. Advisory Committee Immunization Practices (ACIP) Rubella prevention. *MMWR* 39(RR-15): 1–18, 1990.

160. Advisory Committee Immunization Practices (ACIP). Yellow fever vaccine. *MMWR* 39(RR-6): 1–6, 1990.

161. Advisory Committee Immunization Practices (ACIP). Prevention and control of influenza. *MMWR* 39(RR-7):1–15, 1990.

162. Advisory Committee Immunization Practices (ACIP). Measles prevention. *MMWR* 38(5–9): 1–18, 1989.

163. Advisory Committee Immunization Practices (ACIP). Protection against viral hepatitis. *MMWR* 1–26.

164. Cunningham FG, MacDonald PC, Grant NF (eds.). Abnormalities of the puerpuerium. Puerperal infections. In *William's Obstetrics* (11th ed.). Norwalk, Conn.: Appleton, 1989. Pp. 461–71.

165. Soper DE. Postpartum endometritis. Pathophysiology and prevention. *J Repro Med* 33:97–100, 1988.

166. Newton ER, Prihoda TJ, Gibbs RS. A clinical and microbiologic analysis of risk factors for puerperal endometritis. *Obstet Gynecol* 75:402, 1990.

167. Duff P. Pathophysiology and management of postcesarean endomyometritis. *Obstet Gynecol* 67: 269–76, 1986.

168. Hoyme UB, Kiviat N, Eschenbach DA. Microbiology and treatment of late postpartum endometritis. *Obstet Gynecol* 68:226–32, 1986.

169. Watts DH, Eschenbach DA, Kenny GE. Early postpartum endometritis: the role of bacteria, genital mycoplasmas and *Chlyamydia trachomatis*. *Obstet Gynecol* 73:52, 1989.

170. Gibbs DS et al. Endometritis following vaginal delivery. *Obstet Gynecol* 56:555–58, 1980.

171. Berenson AB et al. Bacteriologic findings of postcesarean endometritis in adolescents. *Obstet Gynecol* 75:627–29, 1990.

172. Cunningham FG, MacDonald PC, Grant NF (eds.). The puerperium. In *William's Obstetrics* (11th ed.). Norwalk, Conn.: Appleton, 1989. Pp. 245–51.

173. Fortunato SJ, Dodson MG. Therapeutic considerations in postpartum endometritis. *J Repro Med* 33:101–6, 1988.

174. Martens MG et al. Transcervical uterine cultures with a new endometrial suction curette: a comparison of three sampling methods in postpartum endometritis. *Obstet Gynecol* 74:273–76, 1989.

175. Martens MG et al. Ampicillin/sulbactam versus clindamycin in the treatment of postpartum endomyometritis. *South Med J* 83:408–13, 1990.

176. Cunningham FG, MacDonald PC, Grant NF, (eds.). Other disorders of the puerperium. In *William's Obstetrics* (11th ed.). Norwalk, Conn: Appleton, 1989. P. 481.

30

Sexually Transmitted Diseases

JOSEPHINE M. WILLIAMS

Patients with sexually transmitted diseases (STDs) are seen in a variety of clinics and practices, including hospital emergency departments. Since many patients with STDs are asymptomatic, the clinician should be alert for those patients who are at risk. These patients include men and women with multiple sexual partners; men and women with new sexual partners within the last several months; men and women with partners infected with a sexually transmitted organism; and sexually active adolescents.

In evaluating a patient for STDs, several factors must be considered [1]. First, the patient may or may not be symptomatic. Second, the patient may be infected with multiple pathogens. Third, the patient's infection may involve more than one site (e.g., gonorrhea infection of the urethra and the rectum or of the cervix and the pharynx). Fourth, sexual contacts should be screened for STDs and treated epidemiologically to prevent development of disease and to prevent further transmission. In light of these factors the patient at risk for an STD should be approached in a systematic manner, with an STD-directed history, physical examination, and screening laboratory studies.

Symptoms of STD in females include change in amount or odor of vaginal discharge; vulvar or vaginal irritation or itching; dysuria, urgency, or frequency; genital lesions; nongenital rash; lower abdominal pain; or abnormal menses. Symptoms in the male include urethral discharge, dysuria, genital lesions, rectal symptoms, or nongenital rash.

All patients should be asked about their last sexual contact, the numbers of partners in the previous two months, their sexual preference, and sites of exposure (vaginal, rectal, oral). They should also be asked about previous STDs and recent antibiotic therapy. IV drug use, needle sharing, sex with IV drug users, exchange of sex for drugs or money, and condom use also should be a part of the STD history.

All patients with suspected STD should have an inspection of the skin, including the palms, inspection of pubic hair for pubic lice and nits, and palpation for inguinal and femoral lymphadenopathy. Women should have inspection of the external genitalia, the perineum, and the anus. Speculum exam of the vagina and the cervix should be done for inspection as well as specimen collection, and a bimanual pelvic exam should be performed.

In men the penis should be inspected, with retraction of the foreskin in uncircumcised individuals. The scrotum should be inspected and the scrotal contents palpated. In men with a history of receptive anal intercourse, anal inspection should be done and in those complaining of rectal symptoms, anoscopy should be performed. All patients with a history of orogenital contact should have inspection of the mouth and pharynx.

Laboratory Studies

Routine screening laboratory studies should be done on all patients suspected of having an STD. (Table 30-1). In women these studies should include the following: (1) cultures for *Neisseria gonorrhoeae* from the endocervix (or from the urethra if the woman has had a hysterectomy), the rectum, and the pharynx if there is a history of orogenital contact; (2) antigen-detection test or culture for *Chlamydia trachomatis* from the endocervix (or urethra); (3) endocervical smear for Gram's stain and (4) potassium hydroxide preparation and saline wet mount of vaginal secretions.

In men the following studies should be performed: (1) urethral culture for *N. gonorrhoeae*; (2) antigen-detection test or culture for *C. trachomatis* from the urethra; (3) rectal and pharyngeal cultures for *N. gonorrhoeae* if there is a history of anogenital or orogenital contact; and (4) urethral smear for Gram's stain.

All patients should have syphilis serology if one has not been done in the previous 3 months, and a human immunodeficient virus (HIV) antibody test should be offered to patients in high-risk groups (gay and bisexual men, IV drug users, prostitutes, female sexual partners of bisexual men, and sexual contacts of IV drug users, prostitutes, and hemophiliacs).

Epidemiologic Treatment of Sex Partners

Epidemiologic treatment of sex partners of individuals proved to have an STD refers to the administration of antibiotics when a diagnosis is considered likely on clinical, laboratory, or epidemiologic grounds but before results of confirmatory tests are known. Table 30-2 lists persons who should receive epidemiologic treatment even if they are asymptomatic. These persons include the sex partners of individuals with gonococcal infection, chlamydial infection, nongonococcal urethritis, mucopurulent cervicitis, and primary, secondary, and early latent syphilis (less than 1 year's duration). *Epidemiologic treatment is not a substitute for interviewing, examining, and testing of partners.* These partners may have other STDs that need treatment, or they may have complicated infections (e.g., a female contact of a patient with gonorrhea may have salpingitis, which would be treated differently from uncomplicated gonorrhea).

STD Reporting

Most states and territories in the United States have some requirement for STD reporting. Gonorrhea, syphilis, chancroid, lymphogranuloma venereum, and granuloma inguinale are notifiable dis-

Table 30-1. Screening laboratory studies for STD patients

Women	Men	All patients
1. Culture for *Neisseria gonorrhoeae* from endocervix, rectum, pharynx (if oro-genital contact), urethra (if cervix absent)	1. Culture for *Neisseria gonorrhoeae* from urethra, rectum (if anogenital contact), pharynx (if orogenital contact)	1. Syphilis serology if not done in the previous 3 months
2. Culture or antigen-detection test for *Chlamydia trachomatis* from endocervix, urethra (if cervix absent)	2. Gram's stain of urethral smear	2. HIV antibody test for high risk patients: gay or bisexual men, IV drug users, prostitutes, female sexual contacts of bisexual men, sexual contacts of IV drug users, hemophiliacs
3. Gram's stain of endocervical smear		
4. KOH preparation of vaginal secretions		
5. Saline wet mount of vaginal secretions		

Table 30-2. Persons who should receive
epidemiologic treatment of STDs

Sexual partners of individuals with any of the
following:
    Gonococcal infection
    Chlamydial infection
    Nongonococcal urethritis
    Mucopurulent cervicitis
    Primary syphilis
    Secondary syphilis
    Early latent syphilis (less than 1 year's duration)
    Chancroid

eases at the federal level. This reporting is an
important part of disease control in that it helps to
identify contacts who may be infected. Finding and
treating those contacts prevents further disease
transmission. Different locales may have different
requirements for reporting. Reporting by clinician,
by laboratory, or by both may be required. Local
health departments should be contacted for the
specific requirements in a particular area.

Referral and Follow-up

It is appropriate to have patients seen in the emergency department with STD cases referred to other
settings for follow-up. The same holds true for referral of sexual partners for evaluation and epidemiologic treatment. Local health departments and
STD clinics usually provide optimal care, since
they are staffed by disease intervention specialists
who can track sexual contacts and counsel patients
on risk-reduction strategies. Other possibilities for
referral include infectious disease specialists, other
physicians specializing in STDs, women's health
clinics, and family practice clinics.

STD Syndromes

The STD syndromes described in this section and
their caustive organisms are listed in Table 30-3.

Urethritis in Men

Urethritis is the inflammation of the urethra and is
the most common STD syndrome seen in men.

ETIOLOGY

Urethritis usually is sexually transmitted and is usually classified as either gonococcal or nongonococcal. Gonococcal urethritis is caused by *N. gonorrhoeae;* nongonococcal urethritis (NGU), which is
estimated to be more than twice as common as
gonococcal urethritis [2], is most commonly caused
by *C. trachomatis,* followed by *Ureaplasma urealyticum.* Several studies have found *C. trachomatis* in
30%–50% of men with nongonococcal urethritis,
and although the evidence is not as convincing for
U. urealyticum, other studies have found that organism in 10%–40% of cases of NGU [3, 4]. Other less
common causes of NGU include herpes simplex
virus and *Trichomonas vaginalis.* Other organisms
that have been implicated as possibly playing a role
in causing NGU are *Bacteroides ureolyticus* [5] and
Mycoplasma genitalium [6].

HISTORY AND CLINICAL FINDINGS

Patients who present to emergency departments are
most likely to be symptomatic, but it must be remembered that significant numbers of men with
urethritis are asymptomatic. The symptoms of
urethritis are urethral discharge, dysuria, and
urethral or meatal itching. Although it is not possible in an individual case of urethritis to make a
distinction between gonococcal and nongonococcal urethritis, on the whole the symptoms of
gonococcal urethritis are more marked than those
of NGU. Patients with gonococcal urethritis are
more likely to have both discharge and dysuria and
to have more copious and purulent discharge; patients with NGU are more likely to have scant
mucoid discharge. Patients with gonococcal
urethritis also are more likely to have a shorter
duration of symptoms at the time of their presentation than those patients with NGU [7]. The usual
incubation period for gonococcal urethritis is 2–6
days, while that for NGU is 7–35 days.

LABORATORY FINDINGS AND CRITERIA
FOR DIAGNOSIS

Every patient suspected of having urethritis should
have a Gram's stain of urethral discharge or of
material collected with a urethral swab. The presence of more than four polymorphonuclear leuko-

Table 30-3. STD syndromes and causative organisms

Syndrome	Organism
Infections in Men	
Urethritis	*Neisseria gonorrhoeae, Chlamydia trachomatis, Ureaplasma urealyticum, Mycoplasma* species, herpes simplex virus, undetermined
Epididymitis	*Neisseria gonorrhoeae, Chlamydia trachomatis*
Infections in Women	
Cervicitis	*Neisseria gonorrhoeae, Chlamydia trachomatis,* herpes simplex virus
Acute urethral syndrome	*Chlamydia trachomatis*
Pelvic inflammatory disease	*Neisseria gonorrhoeae, Chlamydia trachomatis, Mycoplasma* species, anaerobic bacteria, facultative bacteria
Infections in Men and Women	
Genital ulcer disease	
Syphilis	*Treponema pallidum*
Genital herpes	Herpes simplex virus
Chancroid	*Haemophilus ducreyi*
Lymphogranuloma venereum	*Chlamydia trachomatis*
Granuloma inguinale	*Calymmatobacterium granulomatis*
Proctitis	*Neisseria gonorrhoeae, Chlamydia trachomatis,* herpes simplex virus, *Treponema pallidum*

cytes (PMNs) per oil immersion field (magnification of 1000×) in five such fields is usually diagnostic of urethritis [8, 9]. The presence of intracellular gram-negative diplococci is diagnostic of gonococcal urethritis (Fig. 30-1). The diagnosis of NGU is made when there are more than four PMNs per oil immersion field, and no gram-negative diplococci are seen (Fig. 30-2). The sensitivity and specificity of the presence of typical gram-negative diplococci within PMNs in a Gram's stain of urethral exudate or of material collected with a urethral swab in men with urethritis approach 100% for the diagnosis of gonorrhea. However, when only extracellular gram-negative diplococci are seen or when atypical intracellular gram-negative organisms are seen, cultures for *N. gonorrhoeae* are positive in only 21% of cases [7]. The sensitivity of the Gram's stain for detecting gonorrhea in men with asymptomatic urethral infection falls to 50%–70%, although the specificity still approaches 100%.

In men who are symptomatic with no objective evidence of urethritis (no discharge, normal urethral Gram's stain), examination of the spun sediment of the first 5–10 ml of urine may yield a diagnosis. The presence of 15 or more PMNs in five random fields at 400× magnification points to the diagnosis of urethritis [10]. Alternatively these men could be asked to return for an early-morning re-evaluation before first micturition, since this is often the best time to make the diagnosis of urethritis.

Although in symptomatic patients a gram-stained smear of urethral discharge or of material from a urethral swab is usually enough to make a presumptive diagnosis of gonorrhea, isolation of *N. gonorrhoeae* is the standard for definitive diagnosis. Generally, cultures should be done on selective media (e.g., Thayer-Martin's medium). Plates should be inoculated at the time the specimen is

Fig. 30-1. Intracellular *N. gonorrhoeae* on Gram's stain of urethral swab (1000× before reduction)

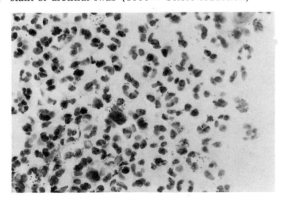

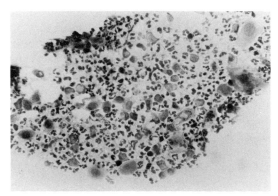

Fig. 30-2. Gram's stain of urethral swab of patient with NGU. Note absence of gram-negative diplococci (1000× before reduction)

collected and ideally should be incubated promptly in an increased carbon dioxide atmosphere (candle jar) at 35°–37°C.

Cultivation of *C. trachomatis* in cell culture is the most sensitive and specific method for diagnosing chlamydial infection, but this method may not be available to many practices. Newer, nonculture antigen-detection techniques have become widely available, including direct fluorescent antibody tests and enzyme immunoassay tests. Men suspected of urethritis should have one of these studies done if possible.

Testing for *U. urealyticum* is not recommended, since the organism can be isolated from many men without urethritis and since facilities for testing for this organism usually are not readily available.

TREATMENT

Treatment of gonococcal urethritis is described in the section "Specific Etiologic Agents," later in this chapter, and summarized in Table 30-4. Treatment of NGU is described in the same section and summarized in Table 30-5.

FOLLOW-UP

For patients with gonorrhea treated with the combined ceftriaxone-doxycycline (or ceftriaxone-tetracycline) regimen, a follow-up (test-of-cure) culture is not necessary, because treatment failure is rare. Patients treated with any other regimen should have test-of-cure cultures done 4–7 days after completion of oral doxycycline or tetracycline therapy.

Table 30-4. Treatment of gonococcal infections

Uncomplicated Gonococcal Infections: Urethritis, Cervicitis, Pharyngeal and Anorectal Infections
Recommended regimen:
    Ceftriaxone 250 mg IM once *plus* doxycycline 100 mg bid PO for 7 days
    Patients unable to take tetracyclines should be treated with erythromycin base 500 mg qid PO for 7 days
Alternative regimen (all followed by doxycycline or erythromycin):
    Spectinomycin[a] 2 g IM once
    Ceftizoxime 500 mg IM once
    Cefotaxime 1 g IM once
    Cefuroxime axetil 1 g PO once with probenecid 1 g PO
    Ciprofloxacin[b] 500 mg PO once
    Norfloxacin[b] 800 mg PO once

Complicated Gonococcal Infections
1. Epididymitis
    Ceftriaxone 250 mg IM once *plus* doxycycline 100 mg bid PO for 10 days
2. Disseminated gonococcal infections (DGI)
    Recommended regimens:
      Ceftriaxone 1 g IM or IV q24h *or*
      Ceftizoxime 1 IV q8h *or*
      Cefotaxime 1 g IV q8h
    Alternative regimen:
    Ampicillin 1 g IV q6h can be used if organism is penicillin sensitive
    Parenteral antibiotics should be continued 24–48 hours after symptoms resolve, then one of the following regimens can be used to complete 1 week of therapy:
    Cefuroxime axetil 500 mg bid PO *or*
    Amoxicillin 500 mg with clavulanic acid tid PO *or*
    Ciprofloxacin 500 mg bid PO
3. Gonococcal endocarditis
    Recommended regimen:
    Ceftriaxone 1–2 q12h IV for at least 4 weeks

[a] Spectinomycin should *not* be used for pharyngeal infection.
[b] Quinolones are contraindicated during pregnancy and in children ≤16 years of age.

Patients treated for NGU usually are not followed up routinely, but they should be asked to seek follow-up evaluation if their symptoms persist or recur.

MANAGEMENT OF SEX PARTNERS

All sexual contacts within the preceding 30 days of patients with gonococcal or nongonococcal urethritis should have a complete STD history

Table 30-5. Treatment of chlamydial infections

Uncomplicated Urethritis, Cervicitis, and Non-LGV Anorectal Infection (and empiric treatment of NGU and mucopurulent cervicitis)
Recommended regimen:
  Doxycycline 100 mg bid PO for 7 days *or*
  Tetracycline 500 mg qid PO for 7 days
  Azithromycin 1 gm PO × 1 dose
Alternative regimen:
  Erythromycin base 500 mg qid PO for 7 days *or*
  Azithromycin 1 gm PO × 1 dose
  Erythromycin ethylsuccinate 800 mg qid PO for
    7 days

Lymphogranuloma Venereum
Recommended regimen:
  Doxycycline 100 mg bid PO for 21 days *or*
  Tetracycline 500 mg qid PO for 21 days
Alternative regimen:
  Erythromycin base 500 mg qid PO for 21 days *or*
  Sulfisoxazole 500 mg qid PO for 21 days

taken and undergo examination and testing. They then should be treated epidemiologically.

Cervicitis

Cervicitis refers to inflammation of the cervical epithelium. The most common cause of cervicitis is infection, usually sexually transmitted, but other causes include physical injury and involvement with neoplasia.

ETIOLOGY
Infection of the endocervix has been termed mucopurulent cervicitis and is most often caused by *C. trachomatis* and *N. gonorrhoeae*. Herpes simplex virus can involve the endocervix as well as the ectocervix with ulcerative lesions, and *T. vaginalis* and *Candida albicans* can cause inflammation of the ectocervix, almost always in association with a vaginitis. This section deals mainly with mucopurulent cervicitis.

HISTORY AND CLINICAL FINDINGS
Many women with cervicitis are asymptomatic and are diagnosed because they are contacts of men with urethritis or because they underwent a routine gynecologic check. However, it is likely that women presenting to an emergency department will be symptomatic. The symptoms of cervicitis are in-creased vaginal discharge, dysuria, intermenstrual bleeding (vaginal spotting), and menorrhagia.

An understanding of the changes that occur in the normal cervix during the menstrual cycle and throughout the reproductive period of a normal woman is necessary to recognize the changes of cervical inflammation [11]. The normal cervix has squamous epithelium covering most of the ectocervix and columnar epithelium lining the endocervical canal. These two types of epithelium meet at the squamocolumnar junction. In young women the squamocolumnar junction may be well out on the surface of the ectocervix, and the columnar epithelium forms a redder, more moist-appearing "area of ectopy" around the cervical os, compared to the more flat-pink appearance of the squamous epithelium. In older women the squamocolumnar junction is well inside the endocervical canal. Ectopic columnar epithelium may persist in the face of oral contraceptive use.

The character and the amount of endocervical mucus also are different during different stages of the menstrual cycle. Generally around the time of ovulation cervical mucus is more copious, thin, and very elastic (i.e., it can be stretched up to 6–8 inches). At other times in the menstrual cycle cervical mucus is less copious, thick, cloudy, and not very elastic.

Clinical findings that suggest cervicitis are the presence of mucopus (yellow exudate) from the cervical os; increased erythema of the cervix; edema of the area of ectopic columnar epithelium; and friability of the cervix (easy bleeding produced by the collection of specimens) [12]. Ulcerative lesions of the cervix suggest herpes simplex virus infection.

LABORATORY FINDINGS AND CRITERIA FOR DIAGNOSIS
Women suspected of having cervicitis should have a Gram-stained smear done of endocervical secretions. To decrease the possibility of contamination of the endocervical specimen with vaginal secretions, the ectocervix first should be cleaned as thoroughly as possible with a large swab. A smear that shows heavy contamination by squamous cells and vaginal flora is unsatisfactory. The presence of 30 or more PMNs in cervical mucus per oil-immersion field in a satisfactory smear supports the diagnosis of

cervicitis [13]. Whereas the urethral Gram's stain sensitivity and specificity for gonorrhea in males symptomatic with urethritis approaches 100%, the same does not hold true for cervicitis. Even in experienced hands, gonococci are identified in only 50%–60% of women with gonococcal cervicitis [13]. Despite the insensitivity of the Gram's stain, specificity is high.

Cultures from the endocervix for *N. gonorrhoeae* as well as cultures or antigen-detection tests for *C. trachomatis* should be performed. The presence of multiple shallow ulcerative lesions on the ectocervix is suggestive of herpes simplex virus infection, and viral isolation should be attempted. Patients with herpetic cervicitis also may have external genital herpetic lesions.

TREATMENT

Gonococcal Cervicitis. Patients with proved gonococcal cervicitis or those with gram-negative intracellular diplococci seen on endocervical Gram's stain should be treated as outlined in Table 30-4.

Chlamydial Cervicitis. Patients with clinical evidence suggestive of mucopurulent cervicitis should be treated empirically for presumed chlamydial infection (Table 30-5). Patients with proved chlamydial infection should be treated with the same regimens.

Herpetic Cervicitis. Patients with ulcerative cervical lesions suggestive of infection with herpes simplex virus should be treated, especially in cases of primary outbreak, as outlined in Table 30-6.

Table 30-6. Treatment of genital herpes simplex virus infections

First Clinical Episode of Genital Herpes
  Acyclovir 200 mg five times daily PO for 10 days

First Clinical Episode of Herpes Proctitis
  Acyclovir 400 mg five times daily PO for 10 days

Complicated Infection Necessitating Hospitalization
  Acyclovir 5 mg/kg IV q8h for 5–7 days

Recurrent Genital Herpes
  Acyclovir 200 mg five times daily PO for 5 days *or*
  Acyclovir 800 mg bid PO for 5 days

MANAGEMENT OF SEX PARTNERS

Sex partners exposed to patients with gonococcal or chlamydial cervicitis and to patients with mucopurulent cervicitis within the previous 30 days should be examined and treated epidemiologically with an appropriate regimen (see Tables 30-4 and 30-5). Epidemiologic treatment of sex partners of women with herpetic cervicitis is not indicated.

Pelvic Inflammatory Diseases

Pelvic inflammatory disease (PID) describes the involvement of the upper genital tract with infection that has spread from the endocervix or vagina. Infection can involve the endometrium, fallopian tubes, ovaries, and pelvic peritoneum to cause endometritis, salpingitis, oophoritis, and peritonitis, respectively. Tubal and tubo-ovarian abscesses can occur, and the process may extend beyond the pelvis to involve the appendix in periappendicitis and the liver capsule in perihepatitis. There are serious sequelae to the syndrome of PID, including tubal-factor infertility, ectopic pregnancy, and chronic pelvic pain [14, 15].

The "typical" patient with PID is a woman under the age of 25; is nulliparous; is using no contraception, neither barrier methods nor oral contraceptives; and has multiple sexual partners. The presence of an intrauterine device (IUD) increases the risk of PID [16].

ETIOLOGY

While *N. gonorrhoeae* and *C. trachomatis* are well established as etiologic agents in PID, other organisms are implicated as possible causes of the syndrome. These organisms include *Mycoplasma hominis, M. genitalium,* mixed anaerobic bacteria, and facultative bacteria [17, 18].

HISTORY AND CLINICAL FINDINGS

Although a woman presenting to the emergency department with PID is likely to be symptomatic, there is a broad range of clinical manifestations of this syndrome from asymptomatic to severely ill. Symptoms of PID include vaginal discharge or bleeding, dysuria, lower abdominal pain, and dyspareunia. Fever, nausea, and vomiting may be present. Because a woman with PID may not have any of these symptoms, all women with an STD should have a routine abdominal and bimanual pelvic exam.

Findings on physical examination include pain on cervical motion, adnexal tenderness, and adnexal swelling. Lower abdominal tenderness, direct or rebound, may be present. The patient with PID may have an elevated temperature, but temperature may be normal.

LABORATORY FINDINGS AND CRITERIA FOR DIAGNOSIS

Positive cultures of cervical specimens for *N. gonorrhoeae* or *C. trachomatis* help to predict the etiology of upper genital tract disease, but they should not be taken as conclusive evidence that the upper genital tract is involved with these organisms. An elevated WBC count greater than 10,000/μl, an erythrocyte sedimentation rate (ESR) greater than 15mm/hr, and elevated acute phase reactants are seen in a majority of patients with PID, but these tests are nonspecific.

Laparoscopy—direct visualization of the pelvic organs—is currently the only method to make the definitive diagnosis of PID. Because laparoscopy requires special skills and training and some surgical risks, in most settings routine laparoscopy to diagnose PID is not feasible. Sweet has proposed a set of criteria for making the diagnosis of PID based on clinical grounds [15] (Table 30-7). Lower abdominal tenderness, cervical motion tenderness, and adnexal tenderness all should be present, as well as one of the seven additional findings outlined in Table 30-7.

DIFFERENTIAL DIAGNOSIS

In the patient with suspected acute PID two important differential diagnoses must be considered: ectopic pregnancy and acute appendicitis. Both of these conditions could have serious adverse outcomes if they are not recognized [19].

The patient with ectopic pregnancy may have missed a menstrual period or may report irregular bleeding. The patient with a very early ectopic pregnancy may not have missed a period at the time of presentation. In patients suspected of having PID those who are not using reliable contraception and those who report irregular or missed menses should have a sensitive pregnancy test to exclude pregnancy. Patients suspected of having an ectopic

Table 30-7. Criteria for the diagnosis of acute PID

All three of the following:
  Lower abdominal tenderness
  Cervical motion tenderness
  Adnexal tenderness (may be unilateral)
plus
One of the following:
  Temperature ≥ 38°C
  WBC count ≥ 10,500/μl
  Purulent material obtained by culdocentesis
  Inflammatory mass present on bimanual pelvic examination or sonography
  Erythrocyte sedimentation rate > 15 mm/hr
  Evidence of the presence of *N. gonorrhoeae* or *C. trachomatis* in the endocervix:
    Gram-negative intracellular diplococci revealed on Gram's stain
  Monoclonal antibody for *C. trachomatis*
  Presence of > 5 WBCs per oil-immersion field on Gram's stain of endocervical discharge

Source: Sweet RL. Pelvic inflammatory disease and infertility in women. *Infect Dis Clin North Am* 1:209, 1987; with permission.

pregnancy or those in whom the diagnosis is unclear should be referred to a gynecologist.

The patient with acute appendicitis generally presents more acutely than the patient with PID, with shorter duration of symptoms. Abdominal pain initially may be generalized but usually localizes to the right lower quadrant. GI symptoms usually are more pronounced in acute appendicitis. Other conditions that may present with similar symptoms and signs to PID include ruptured ovarian cyst and pyelonephritis.

TREATMENT

The Centers for Disease Control (CDC) 1989 STD treatment guidelines summarize both inpatient and outpatient treatment regimens for PID. Hospitalization is recommended whenever possible. As set forth in the guidelines, hospitalization is particularly recommended in the following situations: (1) the diagnosis is uncertain; (2) a surgical emergency such as appendicitis or ectopic pregnancy cannot be excluded; (3) a pelvic abscess is suspected; (4) the patient is pregnant; (5) the patient is an adolescent (the compliance of adolescent patients with therapy is unpredictable, and the long-term sequelae of PID can be particularly severe in this group); (6) severe illness precludes outpatient management; (7) the patient is unable to follow or tolerate an outpatient regimen; (8) the patient has failed to respond to outpatient therapy; and (9) clinical follow-up within 72 hours of starting antibiotic treatment cannot be arranged [20]. Other criteria that have been suggested for hospitalization are fever greater than 39°C and the presence of an IUD [15]. Both inpatient and outpatient treatment of PID are outlined in Table 30-8.

It is recommended that women suffering from PID who have an IUD in place have the IUD removed. Antibiotic therapy should be initiated before the IUD is removed, and contraceptive counseling should be given.

FOLLOW-UP

The follow-up of patients treated for PID should be individualized, but those treated as outpatients should be reevaluated 48–72 hours after treatment is started to document clinical improvement. Patients also should be reevaluated about 1 week after completing treatment and again 2–4 weeks after completing treatment. It is appropriate for those treated as outpatients in the emergency department to be referred to a women's health care clinic or to their gynecologist for evaluation after treatment has been completed.

MANAGEMENT OF SEX PARTNERS

Sex partners of women with PID should be sought and evaluated for STD, regardless of symptoms. They then should be treated epidemiologically with regimens effective against N. gonorrhoeae and C. trachomatis.

Genital Ulcer and Inguinal Lymphadenopathy Disease

ETIOLOGY

Genital ulcer refers to any genital lesion with a defect in the epithelium of either skin or mucosa. Genital ulceration often is associated with regional lymphadenopathy. In the United States genital herpes is the most common form of genital ulceration, followed by syphilis and chancroid. Between 1985 and 1989 the number of reported chancroid cases in the United States steadily increased, with the majority of cases occurring in major metropolitan areas like New York City, Dallas, Boston, and some areas in Florida. In 1990 there was a 43% decrease in the number of reported chancroid cases

Table 30-8. Treatment of pelvic inflammatory disease (PID)

Outpatient Treatment
Recommended regimen:
    Cefoxitin 2 grams IM once plus probenecid
      1 g PO *or*
    Ceftriaxone 250 mg IM once
  plus
    Doxycycline 100 mg bid PO for 10–14 days *or*
    Tetracycline 500 mg qid PO for 10–14 days
Alternative to tetracyclines:
    Erythromycin 500 mg qid PO for 10–14 days
Patients treated for PID as outpatients should be
    reevaluated in 48–72 hours. Those not responding
    to therapy should be hospitalized for parenteral
    treatment.

Inpatient Treatment
Recommended regimen:
    Cefoxitin 2 g q6h IV *or* cefotetan 2 g q12h IV
      or other equivalent cephalosporin
  plus
    Doxycycline 100 mg q12h IV or PO
Alternative regimen:
    Clindamycin 900 mg q8h IV
  plus
    Gentamicin loading dose (2mg/kg) IV or IM followed by maintenance dose (1.5mg/kg) q8h
  plus
    Dioxycydine 100 mg q12h IV or PO
Both regimens should be given for at least 48 hours
    after the patient clinically improves. After
    discharge from hospital continue doxycycline
    100 mg bid PO for a total of 10–14 days

[21] (Fig. 30-3). Lymphogranuloma venereum (LGV) is uncommon, and granuloma inguinale, or donovanosis, is rare. The etiologic agents are herpes simplex virus, Treponema pallidum, Haemophilus ducreyi, C. trachomatis, serovars L₁, L₂, and L₃, and Calymmatobacterium granulomatis (see Table 30-3.) In tropical and subtropical areas of the world, chancroid, LGV, and granuloma inguinale are seen more commonly than they are in the United States and Europe.

There are different incubation periods for the various causes of sexually transmitted genital ulcer disease [22]. For primary genital herpes the incubation period is usually 2–7 days, while that for syphilis is 10–90 days, with most cases occurring 2–4 weeks after exposure. The lesion of chancroid ap-

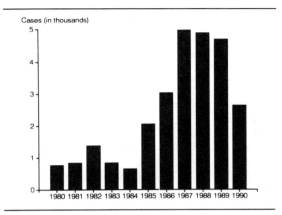

Cases (in thousands)

Fig. 30-3. Chancroid: reported cases, United States, 1980–1990

pears 1–14 days after exposure, and that of LGV appears in 3 days–6 weeks. The initial lesion of granuloma inguinale usually appears after 1–4 weeks but may not appear for up to 6 months.

HISTORY AND CLINICAL FINDINGS
The history elicited from the patient with a genital ulcer can be helpful in defining a specific etiology for the lesion. Table 30-9 lists the different clinical manifestations of genital ulcer. A history of multiple, clustered, painful lesions that began as vesicles and that rapidly ulcerated is highly suggestive of genital herpes. In primary genital herpes there is usually an associated firm, tender lymphadenopathy that is often bilateral. There also may be associated systemic symptoms, such as fever, myalgias, arthralgias, and meningismus.

The lesion of primary syphilis usually begins as a papule that erodes to form the typical indurated chancre with sharply defined borders. The chancre of syphilis usually is not tender (unless superinfected), and the ulcer usually has a smooth clean base. Classically the lesion is single, but multiple lesions do occur. There is often lymphadenopathy associated with the primary chancre, and the involved nodes are enlarged and firm but usually nontender.

The lesion of chancroid usually begins as a papule or pustule that rapidly progresses to a very tender, deeply eroded ulcer with irregular borders and a purulent base. (See color plate 12.) Multiple lesions are often present and may coalesce. There is often an associated tender inguinal lymphadenopathy,

and involved nodes may become fluctuant. In untreated cases involved nodes may rupture spontaneously.

In LGV the most prominent finding is lymphadenopathy, with an ulcerative lesion described in 3%–53% of cases [23]. The lesion may begin as a papule, pustule, or vesicle that ulcerates and may or may not be painful. The lymphadenopathy of LGV is usually unilateral and is usually tender. If femoral and inguinal lymph nodes on the same side are involved, there may be a demarcation between the nodes caused by the inguinal ligament. This is the "groove sign" that is said to be characteristic of LGV. The nodes may become fluctuant and rupture through the skin, usually forming multiple draining sinus tracts. (See color plate 13.)

In granuloma inguinale, also called donovanosis, lesions begin as papules that ulcerate to form beefy red, granulomatous lesions. (See color plate 14.) These lesions usually are painless. Subcutaneous granulomatous nodules in the inguinal area may mimic adenopathy, but the lymph nodes usually are not involved.

LABORATORY FINDINGS
Sometimes the history and the physical examination may be so characteristic the diagnosis of genital herpes can be made accurately on clinical grounds. This is usually the patient who clearly has clustered vesicular lesions on an erythematous base, with perhaps some ulcerations, and tender inguinal lymphadenopathy. However, because the presentations of the various types of genital ulcers may overlap, because presentations may be atypical, and because patients may have several different processes at the same time, in most cases laboratory studies will be needed to aid in making the diagnosis. An algorithm for the diagnosis for genital ulcer disease in sexually active patients is given in Fig. 30-4.

Dark-field examination of ulcer exudate should be done on all ulcerative lesions if dark-field microscopy is available. The demonstration of spirochetes with characteristic motility by dark-field microscopy is enough for a positive diagnosis of primary syphilis (Fig. 30-5). However, if topical antibiotics, antiseptics, and other preparations have been applied to the lesion, the examination may be negative even if the lesion is typical of primary syphilis. In such cases repeating the dark-

Table 30-9. Clinical manifestations of genital ulcers and lymphadenopathy

	Genital herpes	Syphilis	Chancroid	Lymphogranuloma venereum	Granuloma inquinale (Donovanosis)
Organism	Herpes simplex virus	*Treponema pallidum*	*Haemophilus ducreyi*	*Chlamydia trachomatis*	*Calymmatobacterium granulomatis*
Incubation period	2–7 days	10–90 days (2–4 weeks in most cases)	1–14 days	3 days–6 weeks	7–28 days (may be up to 6 months)
Initial lesion	Cluster of vesicles	Papule	Papule or pustule	Papule, pustule, or vesicle (seen in a minority of cases)	Papule
Ulcer	Superficial, nonindurated, painful	Superficial or deep, indurated, usually painless	Deep, nonindurated, purulent, very painful	Superficial or deep, variably painful	Red, "beefy," painless
Lymphadenopathy	Tender, firm	Nontender, firm	Tender, fluctuant, may suppurate	Tender, fluctuant, may suppurate	Pseudolymphadenopathy caused by subcutaneous granulomatous nodules

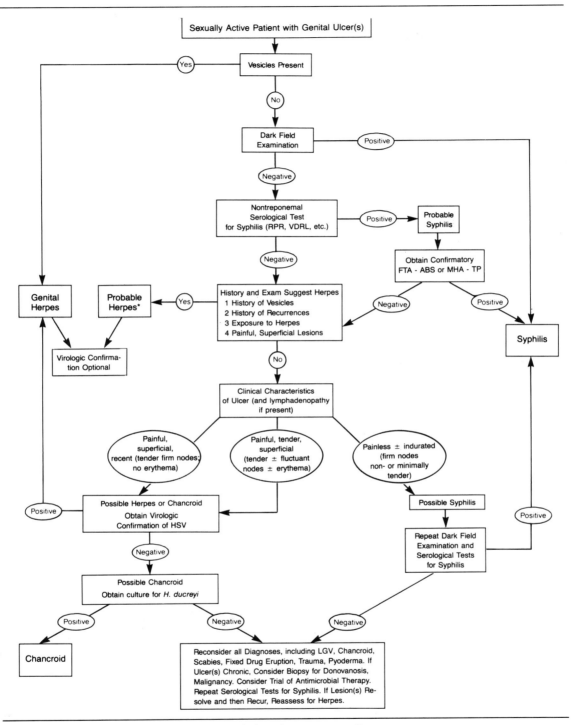

Fig. 30-4. Algorithm for the diagnosis of genital ulcer disease in sexually active patients.
(*Source*: Adapted from Kraus SJ. Genital ulceradenopathy syndrome, in Holmes KK, Mardh PA, Sparling PF et al. (eds): "Sexually transmitted diseases." New York, McGraw-Hill, 1984, pp 706–714)

*Confirmation of probable herpes is desirable. If the confirmation test for herpes is negative, or if the course is atypical, reevaluate the diagnosis, repeat serological test for syphilis in 3 to 4 weeks, consider fixed drug eruption if there is history or recurrent lesions at the same time, and rule out herpes at the next recurrence.
†While awaiting the FTA-ABS test results, mosts clinicians would initiate syphilis therapy for patients having dark-field-negative. RPR-positive ulcers which resemble chancres.

field examination several days later (the patient having been instructed not to use any topicals) may be fruitful.

Serologic tests for syphilis should be done on every patient with genital ulceration. A nontreponemal test, such as the rapid plasma reagin (RPR) test or the Venereal Disease Research Laboratory (VDRL) test, should be done. Though the test may be negative at the time of presentation, it usually turns positive later during the stage of primary syphilis. Because biologic false-positive results of the nontreponemal tests can occur, particularly with acute viral infections, some vaccinations, autoimmune disease, and IV drug abuse, all positive nontreponemal tests should be confirmed by fluorescent treponemal antibody-absorbed (FTA-ABS) test or the microhemagglutination-*Treponema pallidum* (MHA-TP) test. Even the patient with a dark-field positive lesion should have syphilis serology done. If serology is positive, it can serve as a baseline to follow response to therapy.

In all dark-field negative lesions, a culture for herpes simplex virus should be performed. As herpetic lesions progress from the vesicular stage, through the pustular, ulcerative, and crusted stages, the sensitivity falls from greater than 90% to less than 30% [24]. A simple and rapid test for the diagnosis of genital herpes is the Tzanck smear. Material collected from the base of a vesicular lesion or an ulcer is placed on a slide and stained with Wright or Giemsa stain. Multinucleated giant cells are evidence of infection with a herpes virus (Fig. 30-6). This test is not specific for the diagnosis of herpes simplex virus infection, since multinucleated giant cells can be seen with other herpes virus infection, for example, infection with varicella-zoster virus.

In areas where chancroid is prevalent, a Gram-stained smear of ulcer exudate or culture for *H. ducreyi* may yield the diagnosis. Gram-stained smears of chancroidal lesions are reported to show typical gram-negative coccobacilli in a "school of fish" arrangement (Fig. 30-7). *H. ducreyi* is a fastidious organism that requires enriched and selective media for growth, and many laboratories have difficulty isolating the organism. If this organism is suspected, the laboratory should be alerted.

Fluctuant inguinal lymph nodes should be aspi-

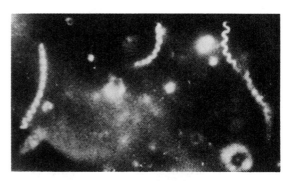

Fig. 30-5. Spirochetes on dark-field microscopy

rated (through uninflamed skin to avoid sinus tract formation), and aspirated material cultured for both *H. ducreyi* and *C. trachomatis*. While specific diagnosis of LGV requires culture of *C. trachomatis*, the diagnosis is most commonly based on complement-fixation serology. Antibody titers of 1:64 or more support the diagnosis of LGV in a patient with compatible clinical presentation [25].

The causative organism of granuloma inguinale, or donovanosis, *C. granulomatis*, is not easily culturable, and the diagnosis usually is based on clinical manifestations together with demonstrating the organism in Wright- or Giemsa-stained crush preparations from genital lesions. The typical "Donovan bodies" are blue or black organisms with a "safety-pin" appearance in the cytoplasm of large mononuclear cells (Fig. 30-8).

DIFFERENTIAL DIAGNOSIS

In addition to the causes of genital ulceration discussed above, there may be other etiologies for this presentation. These include excoriation of skin lesions caused by ectoparasites (e.g., scabies), local trauma, fixed drug eruption, and squamous-cell carcinoma. Careful history and examination should help to eliminate these diagnoses.

With scabies there will be nodular or papular lesions in the genital area as well as lesions involving the buttocks, abdomen, hands, wrists, and elbows. Characteristically the patient complains of intense nocturnal itching. Fixed drug eruptions are most frequently elicited by tetracyclines, and less frequently by barbiturates and phenolphthalein

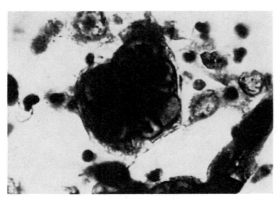

Fig. 30-6. Multinucleated giant cell in HSV cervicitis

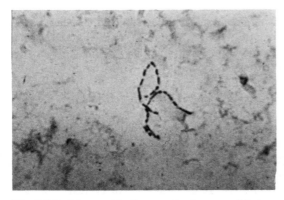

Fig. 30-7. Chancroid. Gram-stained smear of lesion showing the gram-negative *H. ducreyi* in a "school of fish" arrangement

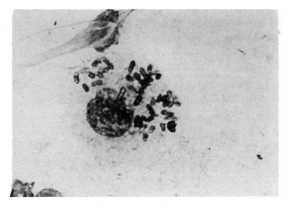

Fig. 30-8. Granuloma inguinale (Donovanosis). Note the "safety-pin" appearance of the organism, *Calymmatobacterium granulomatosis* (Giemsa stain)

laxatives [22, 26]. A very indolent course of a penile ulcer, with enlarged nontender lymph nodes, may point to squamous-cell carcinoma. Genital ulcers associated with nongenital lesions may be seen in erythema multiforme, psoriasis, Behçet's disease, dermatitis herpetiformis, pemphigus, and pemphigoid.

TREATMENT

For effective treatment of genital ulcer disease, a specific diagnosis should be established. The treatment regimens outlined in Tables 30-5, 30-6, 30-10, and 30-11, with the exception of that for

Table 30-10. Treatment of syphilis

Primary, Secondary and Early Latent Syphilis (Less Than 1 Year's Duration)
Recommended regimen:
  Benzathine penicillin G 2.4 million U IM once
Alternative regimen (only in nonpregnant, penicillin-allergic patients):
  Doxycycline 100 mg bid PO for 2 weeks *or*
  Tetracycline 500 mg qid PO for 2 weeks *or*
  Erythromycin base 500 mg qid PO for 2 weeks

Late Latent Syphilis (Greater Than 1 Year's Duration) and Syphilis of Undetermined Duration
Recommended regimen:
  Benzathine penicillin G 2.4 million U IM once weekly for 3 consecutive weeks
Alternative regimen:
  Doxycycline 100 mg bid PO for 4 weeks *or*
  Tetracycline 500 mg qid PO for 4 weeks

Neurosyphilis
Recommended regimen:
  Aqueous crystalline penicillin G 2 million–4 million U IV q4h for 10–14 days
Alternative regimen:
  Procaine penicillin 2.4 million U IM once daily
    plus
  Probenecid 500 mg qid PO for 10–14 days
The following regimens have been shown to have some efficacy:
  Doxycycline 200 mg qid PO for 21 days
  Ceftriaxone 1 g once daily IM for 14 days

Syphilis in Pregnancy
Penicillin regimen appropriate to the stage of disease is the *only* treatment recommended. Penicillin-allergic patients should be desensitized to and then treated with penicillin.

---

granuloma inguinale, are those recommended in the CDC's 1989 STD Treatment Guidelines.

FOLLOW-UP

No routine follow-up of patients diagnosed with genital herpes is necessary unless signs and symptoms do not resolve. The patient treated for primary syphilis should have follow-up nontreponemal serology (RPR or VDRL) 1, 3, 6, and 12 months after treatment. It is appropriate to have the patient followed up in a public health clinic or by a private physician. Antibody titers should have declined fourfold by 3 months, and the tests usually are nonreactive 1 year after treatment [27]. If titers are not decreasing, the patient should be reevaluated.

The patient with chancroid should be reevaluated about 3 days after treatment is initiated, since chancroid ulcers usually start to improve by that time [28]. The patient should be followed until the ulcer is completely healed. The patient with LGV should be followed weekly until adenopathy resolves. Even after antibiotics are started, fluctuant nodes may require aspiration to prevent rupture [23].

Table 30-11. Treatment of chancroid and granuloma inguinale

Chancroid
Recommended regimen:
  Ceftriaxone 250 mg IM once *or*
  Erythromycin base 500 mg qid PO for 7 days
Alternative regimen:
  Trimethoprim-sulfamethoxazole 160/800mg (one double-strength tablet) bid PO for 7 days *or*
  Amoxicillin 500 mg plus clavulanic acid tid PO for 7 days *or*
  Ciprofloxacin* 500 mg bid PO for 3 days

Granuloma Inguinale
Recommended regimen:
  Tetracycline 500 mg q6h PO
Alternative regimens:
  Ampicillin, erythromycin, trimethoprim-sulfamethoxazole, and chloramphenicol have all been used.
Treatment should be continued until lesions have healed completely (usually 3–5 weeks).

---

* Quinolones are contraindicated in pregnancy and in children ≤16 years of age.

MANAGEMENT OF SEX PARTNERS

Symptomatic contacts of patients with genital herpes should be evaluated, but there is little benefit from the evaluation of asymptomatic partners.

Sex partners of patients with primary syphilis should have a routine STD history taken and a physical examination and syphilis serology performed. All contacts in the preceding 3 months should be treated epidemiologically for syphilis.

Sexual contacts of patients with chancroid in the 10 days preceding the onset of symptoms should be examined and treated with one of the regimens recommended for that disease. Partners of patients with LGV in the preceding 2 months should be examined, tested, and treated epidemiologically.

Specific Etiologic Agents

Gonococcal Infections

N. gonorrhoeae is the etiologic agent that causes gonorrhea, a sexually transmitted infection that commonly involves the genitourinary tract, the rectum, and less commonly the oropharynx. In men acute epididymitis may complicate urethritis; in women infection of the endocervix can ascend to involve the uterus and the fallopian tubes in PID. Infection can be spread to neonates from an infected birth canal and is manifested by neonatal conjunctivitis.

The organism *N. gonorrhoeae* is nonmotile and Gram-negative and grows in pairs of cocci (diplococci). The organism is aerobic and grows best at 35°–37°C in a 5% carbon dioxide atmosphere. Since *N. gonorrhoeae* does not tolerate drying, specimens should be immediately plated onto agar media. Chocolate agar is a satisfactory medium for isolation of *N. gonorrhoeae* and should be used for culture of normally sterile material (e.g., blood, cerebrospinal fluid, joint fluid). The presence of high concentrations of other organisms in some of the sites most often cultured for gonococci (rectum, cervix, pharynx) make isolation of *N. gonorrhoeae* difficult due to overgrowth of other organisms. Media that contain antibiotics that inhibit other organisms but permit the growth of gonococci are the answer to this problem. Thayer-Martin medium is chocolate agar that contains vancomycin, colistin, and nystatin, while modified Thayer-Martin medium also has trimethoprim. New York City medium contains vancomycin, colistin, trimethoprim, and either amphotericin-B or nystatin.

Strains of gonococci can be typed primarily by two methods, auxotyping and serotyping. Different gonococcal strains have different requirements for specific nutritional growth factors and will not grow on media that lack these required factors. This requirement for specific nutritional factors is termed auxotrophy and is the basis for auxotyping [29]. Examples of auxotypes are proline-requiring strains, designated Pro-, and strains requiring arginine, hypoxanthine, and uracil and designated AHU. Strains requiring no specific growth factors are referred to as prototrophic or "wild type."

The other method of typing, serotyping, is based on a protein present in the outer membrane, designated protein I, that shows interstrain antigenic variation [29]. These methods of typing are useful in epidemiologic studies looking at transmission or distribution of gonorrhea in communities.

EPIDEMIOLOGY

Incidence.
The number of reported cases of gonorrhea in the United States peaked at slightly over 1 million cases in 1978, then slowly declined over the next several years. In 1990 the number of reported cases was 701,300 [21]. The highest rates are seen in men 20–24 years old, and in women 15–19 years old, with more cases reported in men than in women. In 1990 the male to female ratio was approximately 1.3:1. Reported incidence rates of gonorrhea are more than 30 times higher in blacks than in whites [21]. Some but not all of the higher rates reported in blacks may be due to the fact that blacks are more likely to attend public clinics and case reporting at public clinics is more thorough than in the private sector.

Transmission.
The major risk factor for acquiring gonorrhea is sexual contact with an infected individual. Gonorrhea is not transmitted with 100% efficiency. Studies have shown that the risk for urethritis in a male partner of an infected woman is about 20% per episode of vaginal intercourse [30, 31]. That risk rises to 60%–80% after four or more exposures. The risk of transmission of disease from infected males to females is probably more efficient than from infected females to males, probably about 50%, rising to 90% or more after repeated exposure [32]. Transmission by rectal intercourse is probably quite efficient, but transmission by fellatio is less so, and it is rare following cunnilingus [33].

Antibiotic-Resistant N. gonorrhoeae.
From the time of its introduction in the 1940s until the mid 1970s penicillin was the drug of choice for the treatment of gonorrhea. In 1976 gonorrhea strains with high-level penicillin resistance due to plasmid-mediated penicillinase production were documented in the United States [34]. These strains were imported from Asia and the Philippines. At the same time penicillinase-producing strains of N. gonorrhoeae (PPNG) imported from western Africa were being reported in Europe [35]. The Asian and African strains could be differentiated based on the molecular mass of their respective plasmids [36]. Initially most PPNG isolates could be shown to have been imported into the United States, but after a few years these organisms have become endemic in many parts of the country.

In 1983 an increase in treatment failures, after treatment with penicillin of patients infected with gonococci that did not produce penicillinase, was reported in Durham, North Carolina [37]. This increase was shown to be the result of a strain of N. gonorrhoeae with several antibiotic-resistance loci. Subsequently organisms with chromosomally mediated penicillin resistance have been reported in cities across the United States [38].

Strains of N. gonorrhoeae with high-level resistance to tetracycline were first reported in the United States in 1985. This resistance is plasmid-mediated, and tetracycline-resistant N. gonorrhoeae (TRNG) have been reported in all areas of the country [39].

Since 1976 the number of resistant gonococci isolated in the United States has rapidly increased (Fig. 30-9). By 1990 the number of resistant organisms accounted for more than 9% of reported gonorrhea cases [21]. In some places, such as south Florida, resistant organisms account for more than 30% of the total.

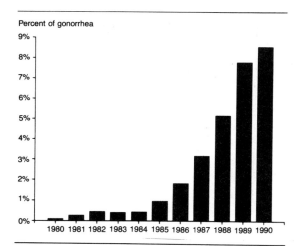

Percent of gonorrhea

Fig. 30-9. Antibiotic-resistant gonorrhea - percentage of reported gonorrhea cases caused by antibiotic-resistant strains: United States, 1980–1990. 1990 cases and rates are projected based on reporting through November 5, 1990. The U.S. totals include the District of Columbia

CLINICAL MANIFESTATIONS

Uncomplicated Gonococcal Infections. Acute urethritis is the most common manifestation of gonorrhea seen in men. This syndrome was discussed in a previous section.

Cervicitis is the most common manifestation of gonorrhea in women and also was discussed in a previous section. Cervicitis commonly is accompanied by infection of the periurethral (Skene's) glands and the Bartholin's gland ducts. Occasionally purulent exudate can be expressed from these areas.

The anorectal mucosa is infected with gonorrhea in about 40% of women with gonococcal cervicitis and in about 45% of homosexual men with gonorrhea [40]. Anorectal infection in women is thought to be a result of perineal contamination with infected cervicovaginal exudate, whereas in homosexual men it is the result of receptive anal intercourse with an infected individual [40]. The majority of patients with anorectal infection are asymptomatic. In symptomatic patients symptoms range from anal pruritus to mucopurulent discharge, tenesmus, and rectal bleeding. Anoscopy in infected individuals may show mucopurulent exudate, erythema, and friability of the rectal mucosa. These symptoms and

signs are not pathognomonic for infection with *N. gonorrhoeae* and can be seen in anorectal infection with other organisms [41].

Gonococcal infection is transmitted to the pharynx by orogenital sexual contact. Transmission by this route is not very efficient, with fellatio carrying a greater risk than cunnilingus [42]. Pharyngeal gonococcal infection occurs in 10%–25% of homosexual men with gonorrhea, in 10%–20% of heterosexual women, and in 3%–7% of heterosexual men [42–44]. Most pharyngeal infections are asymptomatic; however, symptomatic infection with acute pharyngitis and cervical lymphadenitis has been reported [43, 45].

Complicated Gonococcal Infections. EPIDIDYMITIS. Acute epididymitis is the most common complication of gonococcal urethritis in men, and *N. gonorrhoeae* has been shown to cause 21% of cases of epididymitis in men less than 35 years old [46]. Pain in the scrotum, whether of sudden or gradual onset, is the main symptom of epididymitis. A urethral discharge may be present, but up to 50% of patients with epididymitis secondary to *N. gonorrhoeae* may not have a urethral discharge [47]. On examination the scrotum on the involved side is edematous, red, and severely tender. On palpation, the location of swelling is usually posterior to the testis [48]. The presence of urethritis usually can be established by a Gram's stain of a urethral swab specimen or examination of first-void urine [46].

In adolescents and young adults acute epididymitis must be differentiated from testicular torsion, which is a surgical emergency. With torsion the onset of pain is usually sudden, the swelling is in the testis itself, and evidence of urethritis is absent [48]. Doppler-flow studies or radionuclide scanning should be considered if the diagnosis is not clear. Evidence of increased blood flow supports the diagnosis of epididymitis, while decreased blood flow supports that of testicular torsion [49, 50].

PID. PID, the involvement of the upper genital tract with infection that has spread from the endocervix, is estimated to develop in 10%–19% of women with gonococcal cervicitis [14]. The clinical manifestations of PID were discussed in a previous section.

DISSEMINATED GONOCOCCAL INFECTION. Disseminated gonococcal infection (DGI) occurs in 0.5%–3.0% of patients with untreated mucosal infection [51]. It is often termed the "arthritis-dermatitis syndrome" because the most common clinical manifestations are skin lesions, tenosynovitis, and acute arthritis. In sexually active patients under 30 years of age DGI is the most common cause of septic arthritis [52]. Any joint can be involved, but the knees, ankles, wrists, and metacarpal phalangeal joints most often are affected [52].

DGI may have a two-stage presentation, with an earlier bacteremic stage and a later septic-joint stage [53, 54]. In the bacteremic stage patients are more toxic and are likely to have fevers, chills, polyarthritis, and relatively little effusion. Blood cultures are likely to be positive at this stage, and joint-fluid cultures are negative. Skin lesions, usually described as pustules on erythematous bases, are more likely to be seen in the bacteremic stage, and cultures of these lesions may be positive (Fig. 30-10 and color plate 15). In the septic-joint stage there is usually monoarticular disease with positive joint-fluid cultures but negative blood cultures. Skin lesions are less likely in the septic-joint stage.

A definite diagnosis of DGI is based on isolating N. gonorrhoeae from blood, synovial fluid, or skin lesions. Patients with the clinical picture of DGI but negative blood, joint-fluid, or skin-lesion cultures are said to have "probable" DGI if there are positive cultures for N. gonorrhoeae from a mucosal site or from a sex partner. Patients with the typical clinical picture of DGI and the expected response to therapy, but with negative cultures from all sites are said to have "possible" DGI [51].

Any patient suspected of having DGI should have blood, joint-fluid, and skin-lesion (if present) cultures done for the gonococcus as well as cultures from the urethra, cervix, pharynx, and rectum, depending on the history of site of sexual exposure. Factors associated with enhanced risk of DGI include female sex, recent menstruation, and the presence of asymptomatic infection [54, 55]. Patients with recurrent DGI should be screened for complement deficiency, since deficiency of the complement component C5, C6, C7, or C8 predisposes to both gonococcal and meningococcal bacteremia, and about 5% of patients with DGI have such a deficiency [55, 56].

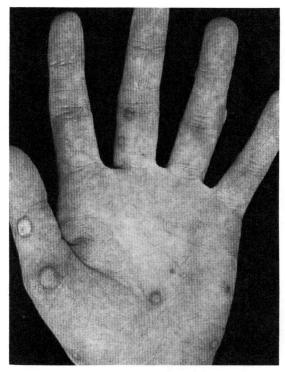

Fig. 30-10. Disseminated N. gonorrhoeae pustules

Gonococcal endocarditis as a result of DGI is uncommon, occurring in about 1%–3% of patients with DGI [54]. Though uncommon recognition of this condition is important, since there can be rapid valvular destruction with possible life-threatening consequences.

LABORATORY DIAGNOSIS

Gram-stained smears of clinical material, especially from the urethra and the cervix, are useful for the diagnosis of gonorrhea (see Fig. 30-1). Sensitivity and specificity of the Gram's stain in urethritis and cervicitis were discussed in previous sections. In patients with gonococcal proctitis, a Gram's stain of rectal smears has a reported sensitivity of 30%–65% [40, 41]. Since most people harbor nonpathogenic Neisseria species in the pharynx, a gram-stained smear of pharyngeal material is not recommended for the diagnosis of pharyngeal gonorrhea [29]. Definitive diagnosis of gonococcal infection is made on the basis of isolation of N. gonorrhoeae. Required growth conditions, as well as selective and nonselective growth media, were discussed in a previous section. Also see Chap. 3.

TREATMENT

Treatment of uncomplicated gonococcal infections is summarized in Table 30-4.

Uncomplicated Urethral, Endocervical, and Rectal Infection. Because of the possibility of co-existing chlamydial infection, it is recommended that patients treated for gonorrhea also be treated for chlamydia.

The recommended regimen for uncomplicated gonococcal infections is ceftriaxone 250 mg IM once *plus* doxycycline 100 mg PO twice daily for 7 days.

An alternative regimen (followed by doxycycline) is ceftizoxime 500 mg IM once *or* cefuroxime axetil 1 g PO once with probenecid 1 g.

For patients unable to take beta-lactam drugs an alternative regimen is spectinomycin 2 g IM once. Ciprofloxacin 500 mg PO once, norfloxacin 800 mg PO once, and ofloxacin 400 mg are other alternatives. These quinolone antibiotics are contraindicated in pregnancy and in children 16 years of age and younger.

For those patients unable to take tetracyclines, erythromycin should be substituted for the treatment of possible chlamydial coinfection. The recommended dosage is erythromycin base 500 mg qid PO for 7 days.

Pharyngeal Infection. Ceftriaxone 250 mg IM once is the recommended treatment for pharyngeal infection. Spectinomycin should *not* be used for pharyngeal gonorrhea. Patients who cannot be treated with ceftriaxone should be treated with ciprofloxacin 500 mg PO once.

PID. The recommended regimen for outpatient treatment of PID is cefoxitin 2 g IM concurrently with probenecid 1 g PO *or* ceftriazone 250 mg IM *or* equivalent cephalosporin, plus doxycycline 100 mg bid PO twice daily for 10–14 days or tetracycline 500 mg PO qid for 10–14 days. Patients who do not tolerate doxycycline can be given erythromycin 500 mg qid PO for 10–14 days. Patients treated as outpatients need to be reevaluated in 72 hours, and those who have not responded to therapy within that time should be hospitalized for parenteral antibiotics.

The CDC 1989 STD treatment guidelines recommend two different regimens for inpatient treatment of PID.

Regimen A includes cefoxitin 2 g q6h IV *or* cefotetan 2 g q12h IV plus doxycycline 100 mg q12h IV or PO.

Regimen B includes clindamycin 900 mg q8h IV plus a gentamicin loading dose (2 mg/kg) IV or IM, followed by a maintenance dose (1.5 mg/kg) q8h.

Both regimens A and B should be given for at least 48 hours after the patient clinically improves. After discharge from the hospital the patient should continue with doxycycline 100 mg bid PO to complete a total of 10–14 days.

Epididymitis. Epididymitis in young (< 35 years of age), sexually active men most likely is sexually transmitted and should be treated with the following regimen: ceftriaxone 250 mg IM once, *plus* doxycycline 100 mg bid PO for 10 days

DGI. Patients with suspected DGI should be hospitalized for initial treatment. Recommended regimens are ceftriaxone 1 g q24h IM or IV *or* cefotaxime 1 g q8h IV or ceftizoxime 1 g q8h IV.

If the organism causing DGI is proved to be penicillin sensitive, treatment may be switched to ampicillin 1 g q6h IV.

Gonococcal Endocarditis. This potentially life-threatening condition should be treated with high-dose IV antibiotics for at least 4 weeks. Ceftriaxone 1–2 g q12h IV or other equivalent therapy should be used.

MANAGEMENT OF SEX PARTNERS

All sex partners in the preceding 30 days of persons diagnosed with gonorrhea should be examined for STDs and treated epidemiologically for gonorrhea.

Chlamydial Infections

C. trachomatis is a bacterium that is an obligate intracellular parasite with a two-stage life cycle [57]. In the elementary body stage the organism has a protective cell wall that allows it to survive extracellularly, though it is metabolically inactive. It is this elementary body stage that is infective. The elementary body enters the cell by endocytosis, loses its cell wall, and replicates by binary fission inside a phagosome. This metabolically active stage is the reticulate body. The phagosome enlarges as the organism replicates and eventually fills the cytoplasm, forming an *inclusion*. As the inclusion enlarges, reticulate bodies acquire cell walls and reorganize into elementary bodies. These elementary bodies are released by rupture of the host cell.

C. *trachomatis* organisms are classified into 15 serovars, with serovars A, B, Ba, and C associated with trachoma; serovars D through K associated with several sexually transmitted diseases, follicular conjunctivitis, and infant pneumonia; and serovars $L_1, L_2,$ and L_3 associated with LGV [57].

EPIDEMIOLOGY

Although chlamydial infections are not reportable at the federal level in the United States, it is estimated that C. *trachomatis* causes between 3 million and 4 million new infections each year [58]. In the United States the major mode of transmission of this organism is sexual with the exception of those acquired by neonates passing through an infected birth canal. Studies in prenatal, family planning, adolescent, and STD clinics have shown that young age, lower socioeconomic status, and unmarried status all increase the likelihood of a woman being infected with C. *trachomatis*. The highest rates of infection (20%–30%) are seen in women attending STD clinics [59].

Studies in men are fewer than those in women, but young age, increased numbers of sex partners, and past history of gonorrhea were predictive of asymptomatic urethral infection with C. *trachomatis* in one study [60]. C. *trachomatis* infections are significantly more common in patients infected with N. *gonorrhoeae* than in those not infected.

CLINICAL MANIFESTATIONS

Urethritis. Urethritis is the most commonly seen syndrome in males caused by C. *trachomatis*, and that organism is the etiologic agent in 30%–50% of men with NGU. The syndrome of urethritis in males was discussed in a previous section.

C. *trachomatis* has been implicated in the acute urethral syndrome (urinary frequency, dysuria, and pyuria without bacteriuria) in young, sexually active women. Studies in STD clinics have shown

that a significant number of women cultured for C. *trachomatis* from the urethra do indeed have the organism at that site [61, 62]. C. *trachomatis* urethritis should be suspected in a young, sexually active woman with acute urethral syndrome, especially if she has a new sex partner or a sex partner with NGU.

Cervicitis. The syndrome of cervicitis was discussed in a previous section. Because many women with chlamydial infection of the cervix have no signs or symptoms, a high index of suspicion is necessary for recognition of this entity [63]. The prevalence of C. *trachomatis* infection appears to be greater in women with cervical ectopy than in those without cervical ectopy [63].

Epididymitis. C. *trachomatis* has been shown to cause most cases of epididymitis in young (< 35 years of age), sexually active men [64]. As with gonococcal epididymitis, patients usually have evidence of an associated urethritis, though the urethritis may be asymptomatic. The signs and symptoms of chlamydial epididymitis are indistinguishable from those of gonococcal epididymitis.

PID. The syndrome of PID was discussed in a previous section. Results of European studies of PID suggest that C. *trachomatis* is the causative agent several times more often than N. *gonorrhoeae* [65, 66]. C. *trachomatis* has been found in the upper genital tract of women with "chronic" PID, whereas this is not the case for N. *gonorrhoeae* [67]. There is also evidence that many cases of PID caused by C. *trachomatis* result in tubal scarring, with subsequent infertility and ectopic pregnancy, even though signs and symptoms of infection may have been absent or mild [67, 68].

Anorectal Infection. Lymphogranuloma venereum (LGV) serovars of C. *trachomatis* can cause a chronic indolent proctocolitis with hyperplastic perirectal lymphatic tissue. Early symptoms are anal itching and mucoid rectal discharge. Patients later develop fever, rectal pain, and tenesmus [23]. Untreated, patients develop perirectal abscesses, rectovaginal fistulas, anal fistulas, and rectal strictures [69]. Non-LGV serovars of *C. trachomatis* have been isolated from male homosexuals with proctocolitis. These serovars produce milder infections, and symptomatic patients present with rectal discharge, bleeding, and pain [70].

DIAGNOSIS

The definitive test for diagnosis of chlamydial infection is isolation of the organism from clinical material by cell culture. This method may be relatively insensitive, and serial passages are needed for isolation of the organism in many cases [71]. Cell culture is both time consuming and expensive and is not uniformly available in many clinical settings.

Nonculture antigen-detection tests for *C. trachomatis* recently have become widely available. These include direct fluorescent antibody (DFA) tests and enzyme immunoassay (EIA) tests. In a DFA test chlamydia-specific monoclonal antibodies conjugated to fluorescein isothiocyanate are used to stain fixed smears of clinical specimens. Smears are then read by fluorescent microscopy. This method is dependent on the skill and the patience of the microscopist, since artifact and cross-reactivity with other organisms can result in false-positive interpretations.

EIA tests are not dependent on the skill of a microscopist, and there are objective cut-off points for a positive test. A summary of several studies that compared antigen-detection methods to cell culture showed that the DFA test had a sensitivity and specificity of 92% and 97%, respectively, in symptomatic men. In a high-prevalence population of women the sensitivity and the specificity were 90% and 95% respectively. Sensitivity was lower (77%) in an intermediate prevalence population of women [72]. EIA tests had a sensitivity of 79% and a specificity of 97% in symptomatic men. In women of both high-prevalence and intermediate-prevalence populations, the sensitivity was 85%–89%, and the specificity was 95%–97% [72].

In some areas resources for chlamydia testing are limited, and patients are treated presumptively based on clinical findings. In cases of limited resources groups that should be given priority for chlamydia testing or emperic treatment include high-risk pregnant women, sexually active adolescents, and women with multiple sexual partners.

TREATMENT

The recommended treatment of uncomplicated chlamydial infections (urethral, cervical, and rectal) (see Table 30-5) is as follows:

doxycycline 100 mg bid PO for 7 days *or*
tetracycline 500 mg qid PO for 7 days *or*
azithromycin 1 g PO as a single dose

Alternative regimens are as follows:

erythromycin base 500 mg qid PO for 7 days *or*
erythromycin ethylsuccinate 800 mg qid PO for 7 days.

Because tetracyclines are contraindicated in pregnancy, pregnant women infected with *C. trachomatis* should be treated with one of the erythromycin regimens or with azithromycin.

The treatment of complicated infections (epididymitis and PID) were covered in a previous section.

Infections due to LGV serovars of *C. trachomatis* should be treated with doxycycline 100 mg bid PO for 21 days.

TREATMENT OF SEX PARTNERS

Sexual contacts in the previous 30 days of patients with chlamydial infection should have complete STD testing and then should be treated epidemiologically.

Syphilis

The causative agent of syphilis is the spirochete *T. pallidum*. The organism's size renders it below the resolution of ordinary light microscopy, and it has to be viewed with dark-field microscopy of serous transudate from primary or secondary lesions or with immunofluorescent or silver staining of biopsy material. *T. pallidum* is spiral in shape, with a characteristic rotary motility. The organism does not grow readily in vitro, though there have been some reports of in vitro replication [73]. It can be maintained in rabbits, and rabbit inoculation has been the standard for documenting infection for research purposes.

EPIDEMIOLOGY

Incidence. With the introduction of penicillin in the 1940s the incidence of primary and secondary syphilis fell from almost 100,000 reported cases in 1940 to about 6,500 cases in 1956 (Fig. 30-11). This number then increased and fluctuated between 19,000 and 26,000 during the period 1961–1978. From the late 1970s to the early 1980s the number of reported cases rose to almost 35,000. Syphilis in homosexual men accounted for most of this increase. The recognition of the acquired immunodeficiency syndrome (AIDS) and the fact that it was predominantly a sexually transmitted disease striking homosexual men most commonly led to a decline in the number of cases of syphilis reported in this population as safer sex practices were adopted.

After 1986, however, there has been a dramatic increase in the number of reported cases of primary and secondary syphilis [74] (Fig. 30-12). This in-

crease has occurred mainly in heterosexual men and women, the highest rates seen in association with illicit drug use, especially "crack" cocaine and prostitution [75, 76]. The number of cases reported to the CDC in 1990 was over 47,000. As a consequence of the increase in syphilis in women there has been an increase in the number of cases of congenital syphilis. In 1989 more than 1,700 cases of congenital syphilis cases were reported, compared to 277 cases in 1980 [77].

The increase in incidence of primary and secondary syphilis is not uniform across the United States, and is highest in major metropolitan areas with large minority populations and serious illicit drug use problems in the inner cities [77, 78].

The increase in the number of cases of syphilis in heterosexual drug users is occurring at the same time that a rapid increase in the rate of HIV infection in that same population is being seen [79]. With reports that currently recommended regi-

Fig. 30-11. Syphilis (primary and secondary) by year, United States, 1941–1989

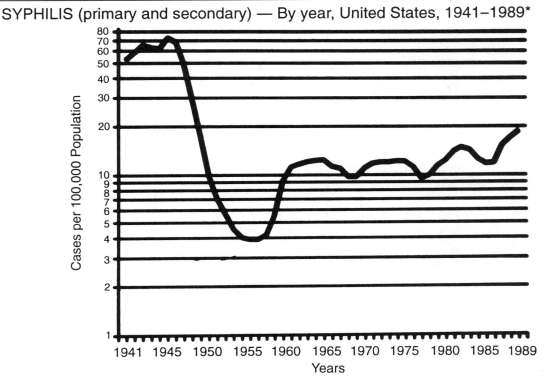

SYPHILIS (primary and secondary) — By year, United States, 1941–1989*

Cases per 100,000 Population

Years

*1941–1946 fiscal years (12-month period ending June 30); 1947–1988 calendar years.

mens may not be adequate to treat syphilis in patients coinfected with HIV, this is potentially a serious problem for the implementation of syphilis control.

Transmission. Syphilis is primarily sexually transmitted, though transmission can occur by other routes, including perinatal transmission and transfusion of infected blood. Transfusion-related syphilis has been effectively eliminated in the United States by routine screening of donated blood. Also blood components rather than whole blood usually are transfused and usually after cold storage for some time. *T. pallidum* does not survive storage at 4°C [80]. Syphilis can be transmitted in utero from an infected mother to a developing fetus. While latent syphilis usually is considered noninfectious for sexual partners, congenital syphilis can occur in babies born to women with latent disease [80].

Syphilis is contracted by physical contact with active primary or secondary lesions in which *T. pallidum* is present. The organism gains access to the body through a break in skin or mucosa and multiplies at the site of entry before the lesion of primary syphilis, the chancre, develops. The incubation period is 10–90 days, with a mean of about 21 days.

CLINICAL MANIFESTATIONS

Primary Syphilis. The lesion of primary syphilis starts off as a papule that rapidly ulcerates to form the classic chancre. (See color plate 11). The chancre is usually a painless ulcer with sharp, well-defined borders and a clean base. Superinfected lesions may be purulent. Classically there is a single lesion, but multiple lesions do occur. The chancre usually is associated with nontender regional adenopathy, which may be bilateral. The lesion of primary syphilis heals spontaneously in 3–8 weeks, even without treatment. The organism then disseminates widely throughout the body.

Secondary Syphilis. Secondary syphilis occurs about 4–10 weeks after the appearance of the primary chancre. With this stage of dissemination patients often have symptoms of systemic illness, with malaise, myalgias, arthralgias, and low-grade fever [81]. The most common findings in secondary syphilis are those of a generalized body rash and

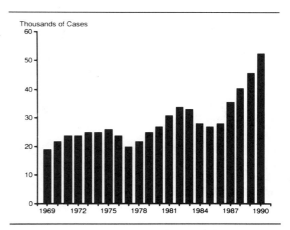

Fig. 30-12. Primary and secondary syphilis - reported cases, United States, 1969–1990. (*Source*: Centers for Disease Control)

generalized lymphadenopathy [81]. The rash may be macular, maculopapular, plaque-like, or pustular, but in adults it is never vesicular. Untreated, lesions progress to involve the entire body, including the palms and the soles. In warm, moist, intertriginous areas, especially the anogenital region, papular lesions coalesce to form large, flat, moist lesions called condylomata lata (Fig. 30-13). Mucous membranes of the mouth and the anogenital region also may be involved with ulcerative lesions called mucous patches. *Skin and mucous membrane lesions of secondary syphilis are teeming with spirochetes and thus are highly infectious.* It is therefore prudent for the physician to examine exanthems of undetermined etiology with gloves.

Other manifestations of secondary syphilis may be seen less commonly. These include patchy alopecia, syphilitic hepatitis, syphilitic glomerulonephritis, synovitis, and gastritis [82]. Headache and meningismus are not uncommon in secondary syphilis, and acute aseptic meningitis may be seen in 1%–2% of patients [83]. Abnormal cerebrospinal fluid (CSF) has been demonstrated in up to 40% of patients with secondary syphilis [84, 85], and spirochetes have been isolated from the CSF of patients with no CSF abnormality [86].

Latent Syphilis. Even without treatment the manifestations of secondary syphilis resolve spontaneously, and the disease enters the latent stage.

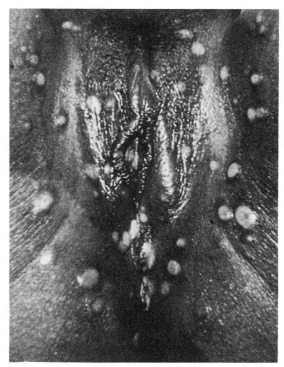

Fig. 30-13. Condylomata lata of secondary syphilis

During the latent stage the patient is free of lesions and symptoms but has reactive serologic tests for syphilis. Latent syphilis usually is divided into early and late latent stages. Early latent syphilis is that stage during which relapses of active secondary syphilis can occur. The majority of these relapses occur during the first year [87]. For treatment purposes early latent syphilis is syphilis of less than 1 year's duration, while late latent syphilis is that of greater than 1 year's duration. Since relapses of secondary syphilis can occur during the early latent stage, patients with this stage of disease are considered potentially infectious for their sexual partners; patients with late latent syphilis are less likely to be infectious. As noted previously, a pregnant woman with late latent syphilis can infect her fetus in utero. Patients with late latent syphilis appear to be resistant to reinfection.

Tertiary Syphilis. Without treatment patients with syphilis can go on to develop a chronic, progressive inflammatory process that produces clini-

cal illness years to decades after the initial infection. This is tertiary syphilis and may manifest itself as gummatous syphilis, cardiovascular syphilis, or neurosyphilis. A study of a large group of patients followed for many years without treatment showed that about one-third of untreated patients went on to develop tertiary syphilis [87]. Gummatous syphilis developed in 15% of patients, cardiovascular syphilis in 10%, and neurosyphilis in 7%. In the antibiotic era tertiary syphilis is recognized less and less.

GUMMATOUS SYPHILIS. The lesions of gummatous syphilis are indolent, granuloma-like lesions that most frequently affect the skin (Fig. 30-14), subcutaneous tissue, bone, and mucous membranes [88]. Although predominantly seen in these areas, any organ system can be involved. Though often described as late benign syphilis, gummatous syphilis can be locally destructive and may in fact be "malignant by position." For example, bony lesions may result in pathologic fractures or joint destruction, lesions of the upper respiratory tract may lead to perforation of the palate, and lesions of the liver may eventually lead to development of cirrhosis.

CARDIOVASCULAR SYPHILIS. The underlying process in cardiovascular syphilis is syphilitic endarteritis of the vasa vasorum of the aorta [89]. This results in medial necrosis, aortitis, and subsequent aneurysm formation. Aneurysms most commonly involve the ascending aorta and the aortic arch. Involvement of the ascending aorta may cause distortion of the aortic valve ring, resulting in aortic valve insufficiency. There may also be ostial stenosis of the coronary arteries [89]. Though the aorta is most often affected, other large arteries may be involved with tertiary syphilis.

NEUROSYPHILIS. The CNS can be involved in all stages of syphilis. As already discussed, abnormal CSF findings have been demonstrated in up to 40% of patients with early syphilis. Not all such patients, however, go on to develop clinical neurosyphilis. Neurosyphilis can be classified as asymptomatic neurosyphilis and clinical neurosyphilis.

In asymptomatic neurosyphilis there are no neurologic signs or symptoms, but CSF abnormalities are seen. Any abnormality in the CSF (pleocytosis, elevated protein level, decreased glucose concentration, reactive CSF VDRL test) in a patient with

Meningovascular syphilis usually occurs 5–10 years following infection and is the result of endarteritis obliterans affecting the small blood vessels of the meninges, brain, and spinal cord. Patients present with signs and symptoms of CNS vascular insufficiency, with resulting stroke syndromes [90]. Even if patients are treated for neurosyphilis, the deficits resulting from meningovascular syphilis may not be reversible.

Parenchymatous neurosyphilis is the end result of widespread parenchymal CNS invasion by *T. pallidum* and usually occurs 15–20 years after initial infection [83, 90]. Tabes dorsalis results from damage to the spinal cord, with demyelinization of the dorsal columns, dorsal roots, and dorsal root ganglia [83]. Patients present with ataxia, paresthesia, incontinence, positive Romberg's sign, and loss of position, vibratory, deep-pain, and temperature sensation. General paresis is the result of involvement of the cerebral cortex [90]. The clinical picture is one of a progressive dementia, with personality changes, changes in sensorium and intellect, hyperflexia, and pupillary disturbances (Argyll Robertson pupils that are small and irregular and that accommodate to near vision but do not react to light) [83].

DIAGNOSIS

Since *T. pallidum* cannot be cultivated in vitro, visualization of the organism in clinical material, by dark-field microscopy or immunofluorescent staining, and serologic testing are the methods available for laboratory diagnosis of syphilis.

Dark-field Microscopy. To establish the diagnosis of primary and secondary syphilis, dark-field microscopy is the quickest method available to clinicians. Lesions to be examined should be cleaned with sterile, nonbactericidal saline, then abraded gently with gauze to provoke oozing but not bleeding. The serous exudate produced is collected on a glass slide, covered with a coverslip, and immediately examined with a dark-field microscope.

T. pallidum is recognized by its characteristic spiral or rotatory motility with flexion about its midpoint (see Fig. 30-5). If the dark-field microscopy of a suspect lesion is negative, the examination should be repeated at least once before the diagnosis of syphilis is ruled out. Reasons for a false-

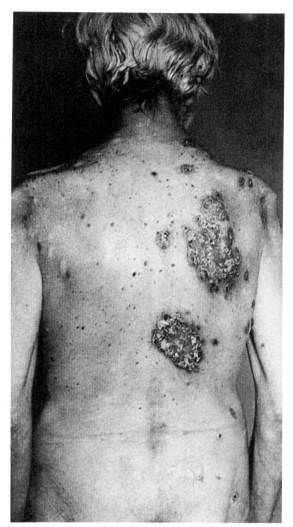

Fig. 30-14. Tertiary syphilis with gummatous lesions of skin

syphilis of greater than 1 year's duration should be considered to be evidence of neurosyphilis [83].

Clinical neurosyphilis may manifest itself as syphilitic meningitis, meningovascular syphilis, or parenchymatous neurosyphilis (tabes dorsalis and general paresis). Syphilitic meningitis occurs early in the course of the disease, usually in the first 2 years following infection [84, 90]. Patients usually present as aseptic meningitis with headache, nausea, vomiting, and photophobia. Patients are usually afebrile and often have cranial nerve abnormalities.

negative dark-field examination include healing lesions with very few organisms present; delay in examining the slides; systemic therapy with some effect against *T. pallidum*; and treatment of lesions with various topical preparations. Examination of oral or rectal lesions may yield false-positive results due to the presence of nonpathogenic treponemes, although experienced microscopists may be able to differentiate between pathogenic and nonpathogenic organisms.

Fluorescent Antibody Microscopy. Fluorescent antibody microscopy is an alternative method for direct detection of *T. pallidum* in clinical material. Clinical material is fixed to a slide, which is then stained with fluorescein-labeled anti–*T. pallidum* antibody. Advantages over dark-field microscopy are (1) immediate examination of slide is not necessary, since motile organisms are not required for the diagnosis; (2) the antibody reagents are highly specific, so there is no confusion with nonpathogenic treponemes; and (3) this method can be used to demonstrate *T. pallidum* in tissue sections as well as lesion exudate [91].

Serologic Tests. The majority of patients with syphilis and certainly all those with latent or late syphilis will be diagnosed based on serologic tests for syphilis. Serologic tests are classified as nontreponemal and specific treponemal.

NONTREPONEMAL TESTS. Nontreponemal serologic tests for syphilis are those tests that measure antibodies to cardiolipin, a lipoidal antigen found in *T. pallidum* [92]. These tests are called nontreponemal because the antibodies are not specific for syphilis. The nontreponemal tests most widely used are the VDRL and the RPR tests. Both tests are based on flocculation reactions between serum and a cardiolipin-cholesterol-lecithin test antigen. In the VDRL test the flocculation is microscopic, whereas in the RPR test the test-antigen preparation contains charcoal particles that become trapped in the lattice formed by antigen-antibody complexes, causing macroscopic clumping to occur on the test card [91].

Nontreponemal tests become positive in early primary syphilis and are present in 70%–80% of patients with primary syphilis by the time they present for medical attention [83, 93]. These tests are positive in virtually every patient who presents with syphilis in the secondary stage [93]. Occasionally patients with secondary syphilis may have false-negative nontreponemal tests due to the "prozone effect." This occurs in patients with very high antibody titers that paradoxically prevent flocculation. This prozone effect can be overcome by dilution of the test serum [93].

A positive nontreponemal test should be quantified, since titers should be followed at regular intervals after treatment. In a study of the serologic response to treatment of early syphilis, Fiumara showed that in successfully treated patients with primary syphilis the RPR was nonreactive by 1 year after therapy, while those with secondary syphilis had negative serology 2 years after therapy [27]. A more recent study of serologic response to treatment showed that only 72% and 56% of patients treated for primary and secondary syphilis, respectively, had negative serology by 3 years [94]. Patients treated for syphilis of longer duration may not have negative serology for up to 5 years [95]. Some patients with documented treatment may have persistently positive nontreponemal serology, usually in a low titer. Patients with persistently positive nontreponemal serology after adequate treatment are said to be serofast. Titers of 1:8 or higher, however, may indicate inadequate treatment, relapse, or reinfection. Even without treatment, the titers of nontreponemal tests will decline over time and may become negative.

A disadvantage of nontreponemal tests is the not uncommon occurrence of false-positive results. False-positive tests may be transient in acute infection, whether viral or bacterial, after immunizations, and in pregnancy [80]. Sustained or persistent nontreponemal tests occur in IV drug users and patients with chronic infections or connective tissue disease, especially systemic lupus erythematosus [80].

SPECIFIC TREPONEMAL TESTS. Since false-positive nontreponemal tests are not uncommon, a reactive RPR or VDRL should be confirmed by a specific treponemal test. The tests most widely used currently are the FTA-ABS, the MHA-TP, and the hemagglutination treponemal test for syphilis (HATTS). These tests detect antibodies that are specific for *T. pallidum* and become reactive during the primary syphilis stage in up to 85% of cases [80, 83]. The FTA-ABS is more sensitive than the hemagglutination test at this stage [83].

Specific treponemal tests usually remain reactive for life, even after treatment, and for this reason should not be used as screening tests for syphilis. False-positive specific treponemal tests, while uncommon, do occur and can be seen in other spirochetal diseases, such as relapsing fever, leptospirosis, and Lyme disease [80]. False-positive tests also can be seen in systemic lupus erythematosus [80].

TREATMENT

The following treatment regimens for syphilis are those recommended by the CDC in their 1989 STD Treatment Guidelines (Table 30-10):

- For primary, secondary, and early latent syphilis (less than 1 year's duration):
    Benzathine penicillin, 2.4 million U IM once
    Alternative regimens for penicillin-allergic individuals include:
        Doxycycline 100 mg bid PO for 14 days or
        Tetracycline 500 mg qid PO daily for 14 days
        (Since compliance with a 14-day oral regimen may be difficult, oral treatment should be used only in penicillin-allergic patients.)
- For late latent syphilis (greater than 1 year's duration) and syphilis of undetermined duration:
    Benzathine penicillin 2.4 million U IM at weekly intervals for 3 weeks, for a total of 7.2 million U
    Alternative regimens for penicillin-allergic patients:
        Doxycycline 100 mg bid PO for 28 days or
        Tetracycline 500 mg qid PO for 28 days
- For neurosyphilis:
    Aqueous crystalline penicillin G 2 million–4 million U q4h IV for 10–14 days or
    Procaine penicillin G 2.4 million U IM once daily, plus probenecid 500 mg qid PO for 10–14 days.
    Doxycycline at a dose of 200 mg bid PO for 21 days has been shown to produce good penetration into the CSF and may have some efficacy in the treatment of neurosyphilis in patients who are allergic to penicillin [96]
    Ceftriaxone 1 g IM once daily for 14 days also

has been shown to have some efficacy in the treatment of neurosyphilis [97].

Treatment in Pregnancy. For pregnant women with syphilis penicillin is the only treatment recommended. Since tetracyclines are contraindicated in pregnancy and since treatment failures in women treated with erythromycin are unacceptably high [98], it is recommended that pregnant women with a history of penicillin allergy be skin tested. If penicillin allergy is documented, patients should be desensitized to penicillin and then treated with the penicillin regimen appropriate to the stage of disease [20].

Jarisch-Herxheimer Reaction. The Jarisch-Herxheimer reaction is a self-limited systemic reaction that may develop a few hours following the initiation of treatment for syphilis. Fever, malaise, myalgias, headache, and postural hypotension are the usual clinical manifestations and usually subside in 24 hours. It is seen most commonly after treatment of primary and secondary syphilis but may be seen at any stage. Patients treated for syphilis should be warned of the possibility of such a reaction. Fluids and aspirin or acetaminophen are usually enough to treat the reaction. The pathogenesis of this reaction remains unclear.

FOLLOW-UP

After treatment patients with primary syphilis should have quantitative nontreponemal tests (VDRL or RPR) at 3-month intervals for the first 12 months. Those patients with secondary syphilis or later-stage disease should also have a repeat test at 24 months. A study of patients treated for primary and secondary syphilis showed that the VDRL titer declined fourfold 3 months after treatment and eightfold 6 months after treatment [99]. After treatment of primary syphilis the VDRL is usually nonreactive by 1 year, and after treatment of secondary syphilis it is nonreactive by 2 years [27]. Treatment failure should be considered if titers of nontreponemal tests do not decrease as expected, or if titers increase. In those cases a CSF examination should be done and the patient retreated appropriately [20]. Patients treated for neurosyphilis should have CSF examination 3 months after treatment and then at 6-month intervals until CSF findings return to normal.

MANAGEMENT OF SEX PARTNERS

All sex partners of patients with early syphilis should be sought and evaluated with history, physical examination, and syphilis serology. For patients with primary syphilis the partners at risk for syphilis would be those in the previous 90 days; for those patients with secondary and early latent syphilis, the at-risk periods are the previous 6 months and 12 months, respectively. In any of these cases if the exposure has been in the previous 90 days, the partner may be infected but as yet seronegative and should be treated epidemiologically with benzathine penicillin 2.4 million U IM once.

SYPHILIS IN THE HIV-INFECTED PATIENT

The presentation, disease progression, serologic responses, and response to therapy of syphilis in the HIV-infected patient may be very different from those seen in the patient who is not HIV infected. Patients with atypical skin lesions have been reported [100], as have been several patients with rapid progression to early neurosyphilis [101]. Seronegative but biopsy-proved secondary syphilis has been identified in HIV-infected patients [100, 102], as well as very high titers of nontreponemal tests in syphilis patients with concurrent HIV infection [100]. There have been several reports of treatment failure in patients who had been treated with standard recommended regimens of benzathine penicillin [101, 103]. These failures have been manifested as neurosyphilis.

Given the situations noted here, a high index of suspicion may be needed to make the diagnosis of syphilis in HIV-infected individuals. Atypical skin lesions should be biopsied and stained for treponemes in those cases with negative serologies, and CSF examination probably should be done on all HIV-infected patients with syphilis, regardless of stage at presentation. (It should be noted that in its 1989 STD Treatment Guidelines the CDC recommends CSF examination in patients with early syphilis only if titers fail to decrease fourfold at 6 months or if titers increase [20].)

There are some arguments for not doing CSF examination in patients with early syphilis and HIV coinfection: a negative CSF may have treponemes and does not entirely rule out neurosyphilis; HIV itself can cause CSF abnormalities like pleocytosis and elevated protein concentration; and other

CNS infections in HIV-infected patients can cause some of the same abnormalities seen in neurosyphilis. However, since syphilis is one of the more readily treatable conditions that may be seen in HIV-infected patients, it would be unfortunate to miss it. Also in case the patient does not respond to therapy as expected, it would be useful to have a baseline CSF examination. Any abnormality in the CSF should be treated with a regimen appropriate for neurosyphilis.

The CDC recommends no change in therapy for early syphilis in HIV-infected patients, though some recommend treatment with a regimen effective against neurosyphilis, especially if CSF examination is not done. After treatment patients should be followed closely, both clinically and with either VDRL or RPR at 1, 2, 3, 6, 9, and 12 months after treatment and beyond, if necessary [20]. If CSF was abnormal before treatment, follow-up CSF exams also should be done.

Genital Herpes Simplex Virus Infections

Herpes simplex virus HSV-1 and HSV-2 are two members of the human herpesvirus family, which also includes varicella-zoster virus, Epstein-Barr virus, cytomegalovirus (CMV), and human herpesvirus 6. They are enveloped, double-stranded DNA viruses that can develop latency. Herpes simplex virus infects mucocutaneous cells and establishes latency in the nuclei of neurons in the sensory nerve ganglia serving those mucocutaneous sites. HSV-1 and HSV-2 are closely related, with large areas of homology in their genomes. In the past it was difficult to differentiate HSV-1 from HSV-2, but with techniques utilizing type-specific monoclonal antibodies [104], for example, typing now can be done.

EPIDEMIOLOGY

Incidence. Since genital herpes is not a reportable disease in the United States and since asymptomatic infections are common, the true incidence of genital herpes is uncertain. However, data reported from the CDC from a survey of private practitioners' office practices showed an almost sevenfold increase in consultations with private physicians for genital herpes infection between 1966 and 1989 [77]. It is estimated that the yearly incidence of genital HSV infection in the United States is 200,000–500,000 cases [77].

Transmission. Genital herpes infection is acquired through contact, usually sexual, of mucosa or abraded skin with contaminated secretions. Since HSV is susceptible to drying and to changes in temperature, aerosol and fomite transmission are unlikely. While the concentration of HSV shed from lesions is 100 to 1000 times higher than the concentration in genital secretions from individuals asymptomatically shedding the virus [105], the risk of acquiring the infections from asymptomatic shedders still is quite substantial. Mertz et al. showed that in patients with first-episode genital herpes 62% of their source contacts had no evidence of orolabial or genital HSV infection in the 3 weeks preceding the onset of first-episode symptoms [106].

Though HSV-1 and HSV-2 usually are isolated from different anatomic sites, both virus types can infect any site. The likelihood that recurrences will occur and the frequency of recurrence, however, are influenced by the virus type and the site of the primary infection. The likelihood of a recurrence after primary genital herpes is 80% with HSV-2, compared to 50% with HSV-1 [107]. The number of genital recurrences is about four times higher with HSV-2 infection than with HSV-1 [108]. The number of genital recurrences also varies widely from one infected individual to another, with some individuals having monthly recurrences, while others have no symptomatic recurrences.

CLINICAL MANIFESTATIONS

First Clinical Episodes. First clinical episodes of genital herpes can be primary or nonprimary. Primary episodes occur in individuals without preexisting anti-HSV antibody. These outbreaks tend to be more severe, with prolonged symptoms, prolonged viral shedding, and higher rates of complication when compared to nonprimary first episodes that occur in individuals with preexisting anti-HSV antibody [107].

Patients usually present with multiple, often bilateral, vesicular, pustular, or ulcerative lesions on the external genitalia. (See color plate 10.) Lesions usually are moderately to severely painful, and there is usually tender inguinal lymphadenopathy,

often bilateral. Often lesions coalesce to form large painful ulcers. In patients with primary disease new lesions may appear in the second week of the course, so lesions in different stages of development will be present. Viral shedding begins just before the appearance of lesions, and virus concentration is at the highest level at the time lesions are first noted. With maturation of lesions virus concentration wanes and is very low by the time lesions are crusted. Figure 30-15 shows the typical course of primary genital herpes.

In women with primary genital herpes, the virus usually can be cultured from the cervix, which is usually abnormal in appearance, ranging from erythema to severe necrosis [107]. Rectal HSV infection may be seen in individuals engaging in receptive anal intercourse. Symptoms include rectal discharge, pain, hematochezia, and tenesmus. Sacral paresthesias, urinary retention, constipation, and impotence help to distinguish HSV proctitis from gonococcal or chlamydial proctitis. Perianal ulcerations may be seen, and lesions of the rectal mucosa may be demonstrated by anoscopy or sigmoidoscopy [109].

Complications of primary genital herpes include aseptic meningitis, autonomic nerve dysfunction, and extragenital lesions. Women are more likely than men to develop aseptic meningitis, which is usually manifested by headache, stiff neck, and photophobia [107]. Sequelae are unusual, and aseptic meningitis does not usually recur with recurrent genital herpes. Autonomic nerve dysfunction, such as sacral paresthesias, constipation, urinary retention, impotence and rarely transverse myelitis, can occur [107].

Extragenital lesions occurring in an immunocompetent host with primary genital disease usually are the result of autoinoculation and not viremic spread. Lesions typically are noted after the appearance of the genital lesions and are seen most frequently on the buttocks, groin, thighs, and fingers [107]. Immunosuppressed individuals with primary genital herpes are at risk for viremia and dissemination. Dissemination may also occur in patients with atopic eczema and has been reported in pregnancy [110].

Recurrent Genital Herpes. The clinical manifestations of recurrent genital herpes are generally

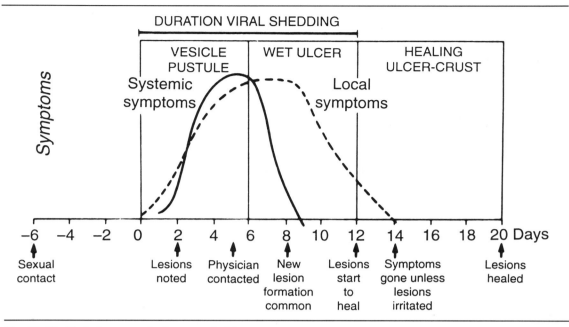

Fig. 30-15. Typical course of primary genital herpes. (*Source:* Adapted from Reference 107)

much milder than those of first episodes. Many patients experience a prodrome, with itching, tingling, or paresthesias occurring from a few hours to 2 days before the appearance of the typical lesions [107]. Recurrent lesions usually are well localized, and the duration of pain, viral shedding, and time to crusting is shorter than in first episodes. Women tend to have more severe and longer-lasting symptoms than men [107]. Systemic symptoms are uncommon, as are any of the complications seen in primary disease.

Immunocompromised Patients. Immunocompromised patients with genital herpes infections have more severe and more prolonged symptoms than normal hosts. Lesions often coalesce to form deep necrotic and painful ulcers, and viral shedding can persist for more than 30 days in bone marrow transplant recipients [111] to indefinitely in patients with AIDS [112]. (See Chap. 16 and Chap. 17.)

DIAGNOSIS

Clinical Diagnosis. The diagnosis of genital herpes usually can be made clinically by recognition of typical vesicular, pustular, or ulcerative lesions in

a sexually active individual. The patient with primary disease will often have lesions in several stages of development. It is important to remember that atypical presentation of genital herpes may occur, with lesions that mimic other causes of genital ulceration, and that patients may have more than one cause of genital ulcer disease. The differential diagnosis of genital ulcer disease was discussed in a previous section.

Laboratory Diagnosis. Laboratory confirmation of a diagnosis of genital herpes can be done by (1) isolation of the virus by tissue cell culture, (2) cytologic techniques, such as Papanicolaou and Tzanck smears, (3) immunologic methods to detect viral antigen, and (4) serology.

VIRAL CULTURE. Viral isolation in tissue-cell culture is the most sensitive and specific test available for the diagnosis of HSV infection and is the gold standard by which other diagnostic methods are measured. Viral isolation rates are dependent on the stage of the lesion being tested, with rates of over 90% from vesicles, decreasing to less than 30% from crusted lesions [24]. Ideally an intact vesicle should be unroofed, and a specimen collected by vigorous rubbing with a cotton or dacron swab. The specimen should be placed immediately in viral transport medium and refrigerated (4°C) until it is inoculated into tissue culture. Eighty percent of positive cultures will be identified by 4 days and 95% within 7 days [113].

CYTOLOGIC DIAGNOSIS. Herpesvirus-induced changes in clinical specimens can be identified by either a Papanicolaou or a Tzanck smear. Multinucleated giant cells will be seen. While these methods are rapid and inexpensive, they are only about 40%–50% as sensitive as culture, so a negative test result cannot exclude HSV infection. These methods do not discriminate among the effects of HSV-1, HSV-2, and the varicella-zoster virus [113].

VIRAL ANTIGEN DETECTION. Several rapid techniques for viral antigen detection currently are available. These include direct immunofluorescence, immunoperoxidase staining, and enzyme-linked immunosorbent assay (ELISA). These tests are only 70%–90% sensitive however, when compared to viral isolation [113].

SEROLOGY. Serologic assays can be useful for differentiating HSV seronegatives from HSV seropositives, for documenting past HSV infection, and for documenting seroconversion in primary genital herpes. The serologic assays that are most widely available, including complement fixation, neutralization, and immunoassays, do not clearly discriminate between HSV-1 and HSV-2 antibodies, however. Recently protein-specific serologic assays using type-specific glycoprotein antigens and a Western blot assay comparing binding of test sera to HSV-1 and HSV-2 antigens have been developed [113].

TREATMENT

Treatment of genital herpes infections is summarized in Table 30-6.

First Clinical Episode. The first clinical episode of genital herpes should be treated with oral acyclovir 200 mg five times daily for 10 days. Oral acyclovir is clearly efficacious for first episodes, shortening the duration of local as well as systemic symptoms, reducing the duration of viral shedding, and decreasing the formation of new lesions [114]. In patients with severe symptoms or complications requiring hospitalization, IV acyclovir 5 mg/kg q8h for 5–7 days or until clinical resolution occurs is the recommended treatment. Although topical acyclovir shortens the duration of local pain and itching in first episodes of genital herpes, it does not prevent the formation of new lesions and seems to be inferior to systemic therapy [114]. First clinical episodes of herpes proctitis should be treated with acyclovir 400 mg five times daily PO for 10 days.

Recurrent Genital Herpes. The duration of lesions and the severity of symptoms of recurrent genital herpes are generally less than in first-episode genital herpes, and the benefit of treatment with oral acyclovir is less clear. Treatment initiated by the patient at the first sign of prodromal symptoms is more effective than treatment initiated by a physician after lesions have appeared [115]. With either type of treatment, while duration of viral shedding and time to crusting of lesions is less than that seen with placebo treatment, duration of pain and itching is not significantly decreased [115]. Those patients with severe or prolonged episodes of recurrent disease or those with prodromal symptoms would probably benefit from treatment with oral acyclovir. The recommended regimen is acyclovir 200 mg 5 times daily PO for 5 days or acyclovir 800 mg bid PO for 5 days.

Suppressive Therapy. Patients who experience six or more recurrences of genital herpes per year are candidates for suppressive therapy with oral acyclovir. Studies have shown that daily acyclovir is effective in preventing recurrence of clinical genital herpes in patients with a history of frequently recurring disease [116, 117]. Those episodes that do occur during suppressive therapy are shorter and less severe. Currently suppressive therapy with acyclovir is approved for use up to 1 year. Recommended regimens are acyclovir 200 mg 2 to 5 times daily PO or acyclovir 400 mg bid PO.

Treatment of the Immunocompromised Patient. While treatment of recurrent genital herpes may not always be warranted in the normal host, immunocompromised patients with recurrent disease should be treated. Acyclovir 400 mg 5 times daily PO for 10 days is the recommended dosage. In those patients needing suppressive therapy the recommended dosage is 400 mg 3 to 4 times daily PO.

In HIV-infected patients who have been treated with long courses of acyclovir, increasing acyclovir resistance has been reported [118]. Acyclovir resistance is usually secondary to thymidine kinase—deficient strains of HSV and is usually manifest by persistent culture-positive lesions despite adequate doses of acyclovir. Studies are ongoing to compare the efficacy of IV treatment with the investigational drug foscarnet with that of vidarabine (adenine arabinoside) for acyclovir-resistant HSV infections. (See Chap. 4.)

MANAGEMENT OF SEX PARTNERS

Sex partners of patients with genital herpes should have routine STD evaluation. Routine treatment is not recommended, however, unless active disease is found. Asymptomatic partners should be informed of the signs and symptoms of genital herpes and encouraged to use latex condoms for sexual intercourse, since there is a real risk of acquiring the infection from asymptomatic viral shedders.

Genital Human Papillomavirus Infections

Human papillomaviruses (HPVs) are unenveloped double-stranded DNA viruses belonging to the papovavirus family. These viruses have not been successfully propagated in cell culture, but through the use of DNA hybridization techniques around 60 types have been identified, with each type generally having a predilection for a particular type of epithelium [119]. HPVs cause benign skin lesions like warts but also have been shown to be strongly associated with epithelial malignancies. Anogenital warts are caused mainly by HPV type 6 (HPV-6) and HPV-11. Viral DNA of other HPV types associated with genital infections like HPV-16, HPV-18, HPV-31, and HPV-35 has been found integrated into cellular DNA in some genital cancers as well as in severely dysplastic tissue [119–121]. Subclinical infection with these viruses is common, and the continued presence of HPV DNA in the epithelium after treatment of visible warts may lead to disease recurrence.

EPIDEMIOLOGY

Incidence. Since HPV can cause subclinical infection and since HPV infections are not reportable in the United States, the true incidence and preva-lence are not known. There is evidence, however, that the incidence and prevalence of HPV infection are increasing. National Disease and Therapeutic Index surveys of private physicians in the United States found an increase in consultations for genital warts from 169,000 in 1966 to 1,150,000 in 1984 [122]. With subclinical infections taken into consideration, HPV infection may well be the most common sexually transmitted disease.

Transmission. Genital HPV infections usually are transmitted by sexual contact. Studies have shown that about two-thirds of sex partners of patients with genital warts themselves develop evidence of infection after an average incubation period of 2–3 months [123, 124] (range 3 weeks to 8 months). Laryngeal and respiratory papillomatosis in infancy is thought to be acquired when neonates pass through infected birth canals. This type of infection is caused primarily by HPV-6 and HPV-11, the types most commonly seen as the cause of maternal genital warts. It is not clear that fomites play any role in the transmission of genital HPV infections.

CLINICAL MANIFESTATIONS

Clinical manifestations of genital HPV infection range from classic genital warts and condylomata acuminata to papular lesions, subclinical lesions, and association with anogenital malignancies.

Anogenital Warts. The classic genital warts are flesh-colored to hyperpigmented exophytic lesions that may be either sessile or pedunculated (Fig. 30-16). The surfaces of these lesions are usually quite rough, with multiple surface projections. These lesions are often described as being "cauliflower-like." Some lesions are more papular with smooth surfaces. Warts can vary greatly in size, from about one millimeter to several centimeters. Lesions are often clustered and may coalesce. Extensive involvement with exophytic warts may be seen in immunosuppressed individuals and in pregnant women [123]. In men overt lesions occur most often on the penile frenulum, corona, and glans, followed by the prepuce, urethral meatus, and penile shaft. In women warts are seen most often at the posterior introitus, followed by the labia minora and majora, the vagina, and the cervix [123]. Perianal warts are seen in both men and women, with the

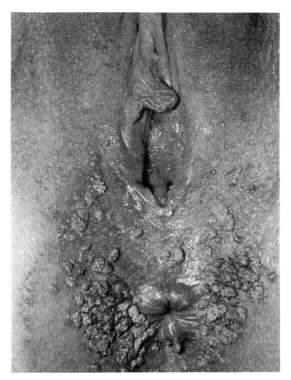

Fig. 30-16. Perianal venereal warts

majority of perianal lesions in men occurring in individuals practicing anal receptive intercourse.

Subclinical HPV Infection. Subclinical HPV infections, often referred to as flat warts or flat condyloma, are not visible to the naked eye but can be identified with the aid of colposcopy or other magnification after application of 3%–5% acetic acid. They are seen most often on the cervix and on vaginal mucosa but may be seen in other areas. With the aid of acetic acid and magnification cervical lesions appear as shiny white patches with irregular surfaces and characteristic capillary loops [125].

Association of HPV with Anogenital Neoplasias. While a conclusive link still has not been found between HPV infection and genital neoplasias, there is strong circumstantial evidence to support such a link. Genital infection with HPV, especially types 16 and 18, is associated with intraepithelial neoplasia of the cervix, vulva, penis, and anus. Associations have been found between cervi-

cal intraepithelial neoplasia (CIN) and the presence of cervical HPV infection and vulvar warts [126, 127]. Similar association has been found between CIN and the presence of HPV infection in sex partners [128]. Buschke-Löwenstein's tumors or giant condylomas are lesions that are locally invasive and may have features of both warts and carcinoma [129].

DIAGNOSIS

HPVs have not been cultivated in vitro, so the diagnosis of HPV infection must be made clinically, through the use of cytology and histology or through DNA-hybridization techniques.

Clinical Diagnosis. In some settings clinical observation is the only method available for the diagnosis of genital HPV infection. Exophytic warts usually are easily recognized by their characteristic appearance. It is important to distinguish anogenital warts from condylomata lata of secondary syphilis. Condylomata lata can be seen on the vulva, under the foreskin, or in the perianal area and are usually associated with other stigmata of secondary syphilis. In addition dark-field microscopy of serous fluid from the condylomata lata shows motile treponemes, and syphilis serology is strongly positive. The more papular wart lesions may be confused with molluscum contagiosum, but the latter can be distinguished by their pearly appearance and central umbilication (Fig. 30-17). A cheesy material often can be expressed from molluscum lesions.

Areas of subclinical infection will not be identified by inspection alone. Examination under magnification by a colposcope after the application of dilute acetic acid for 3–5 minutes will identify areas of subclinical infection with the typical shiny white appearance and characteristic blood vessels. This technique often will demonstrate areas of HPV infection in asymptomatic partners of individuals with proved wart infection [130].

Cytology and Histology. Cytology and histology can aid in the diagnosis of HPV infection, and every woman with a history of anogenital warts in herself or a sex partner should have a cytologic exam of the cervix (Pap smear). The koilocyte, a large cell with a pyknotic nucleus in a cytoplasmic vacuole, is a characteristic feature seen in HPV-infected tissue [131].

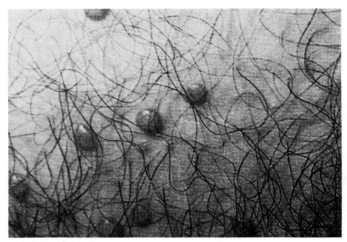

Fig. 30-17. Papules of molluscum contagiosum

Sensitivity of cytology and histology can be increased by the use of immunochemistry techniques that utilize antiserum against bovine papillomavirus to demonstrate the presence of HPV antigens in clinical specimens. Although the sensitivity is increased over routine cytology or histology, immunochemistry often fails to detect HPV infections associated with some dysplasia [132].

DNA Hybridization. DNA-hybridization techniques utilizing DNA probes of known sequence are used widely in research for HPV typing, and some techniques are becoming available for clinical use. It is through hybridization that differentiation of the various HPV types is made possible. The Southern blot assay is quite specific and is the gold standard assay for HPV detection and typing. This test is time consuming and laborious, however, and other less laborious methods of DNA hybridization are now becoming commercially available.

TREATMENT
Of the currently available therapies for genital HPV infection, none has been shown to be completely effective in actually eradicating the virus from underlying tissue. Recurrent disease, which can be seen after any mode of therapy, suggests that there is latent infection with HPV. The goal of treatment, therefore, is to remove visible warts and dysplastic tissue. Treatment regimens include cytotoxic agents, cryotherapy, electrocautery, carbon

dioxide laser, and conventional surgery (Table 30-12).

Cytotoxic Agents. PODOPHYLLIN RESIN. Podophyllin resin, usually as a 10%–25% solution in tincture of benzoin, has been used for many years to treat anogenital warts. Podophyllin acts by arresting mitosis, with subsequent cell death. It is applied to visible warts and allowed to dry. The patient is instructed to wash off the podophyllin 4 hours later. Several treatments usually are necessary, and these are usually done at weekly intervals. With subsequent treatments the medication can be left on for

Table 30-12. Treatment of genital warts

Recommended Regimen
Cryotherapy with liquid nitrogen

Alternative Regimens
Podophyllin resin 10%–25% solution in tincture of benzoin: Apply to visible warts, allow to dry, and instruct patient to wash off in 4 hours. Several weekly treatments usually are necessary. Treat area of less than 2 cm^2 per session. *Not recommended for mucosal warts; contraindicated in pregnancy.*

Trichloroacetic acid (80%–90%): Apply to warts. Treat surrounding area with talc or sodium bicarbonate. Instruct patient to wash off in 4 hours. Several weekly treatments may be necessary.

Surgery: conventional, electrocautery, and laser

longer intervals before washing. Podophyllin may result in clearing of visible warts in up to 75% of patients [133], but relapses may be seen in up to 78% of cases [134].

Local reactions to podophyllin include irritation, ulceration, and scarring. Severe systemic reactions also can occur when large amounts are applied to extensive warts, or when podophyllin is left on the skin for prolonged periods. Neurotoxicity, blood dyscrasia, and hepatotoxicity have been reported [135], as has death [136], after topical application and after oral ingestion. Toxicity of podophyllin to the fetus has been shown in animals, and human fetal death has been reported after podophyllin treatment of a pregnant woman [137], so use of the compound is contraindicated in pregnancy. Animal studies have shown that repeated application to the cervix produced dysplasia, so application to cervical warts is not recommended. *Some authors recommend that podophyllin not be used for any mucosal warts* [138]. It is recommended that an area of less than 2 cm^2 be treated per session [20].

TRICHLOROACETIC ACID. Trichloroacetic acid has been used for the treatment of genital warts. It is applied topically and washed off after 4 hours. Several weekly treatments may be necessary. This treatment can be painful, and care must be taken to avoid normal skin surrounding warts. Treating surrounding skin with talc or sodium bicarbonate (baking soda) protects it from the effect of the acid. This regimen was shown to have an 81% cure rate and a 36% recurrence rate in a comparative study with cryotherapy [139].

Cryotherapy. Cryotherapy, usually with liquid nitrogen, is now the treatment of choice for genital warts in any location. It is also used for the treatment of cervical intraepithelial neoplasia. Liquid nitrogen is applied, either on a cotton swab or with a pressurized spray, directly to lesions, freezing them and resulting in destruction. Several weekly treatments may be necessary. Comparative studies have shown cryotherapy to be more effective than podophyllin [140, 141]. Cryotherapy is not toxic and is safe during pregnancy [142]. The main side effects of this treatment are local pain and ulceration.

Surgery. Conventional surgery, electrocautery, and laser surgery have all been used in the treat-

ment of genital warts. Conventional surgery is used mainly in treatment of perianal warts, while electrocautery is used for treatment of external genital warts on the penile shaft, the labia majora, and the perianal area [143]. Carbon dioxide laser surgery is being increasingly used for the treatment of warts, as well as premalignant lesions. Cure rates with laser treatment range from 60%–90% [144]. Side effects of laser treatment are mainly local pain and swelling.

Interferon. Intralesional interferon alpha has been studied and has been shown to be effective when compared to placebo. After intralesional injections of interferon alpha 3 times weekly for 3 weeks, there was a 62% reduction in wart area compared to a 1% reduction in patients treated with placebo [145]. Flu-like symptoms of fever, chills, myalgias, and headache, as well as leukoplakia, were side effects seen in interferon-treated patients. When compared with other modes of therapy, the high cost and high incidence of toxicity make interferon treatment not as attractive.

MANAGEMENT OF SEX PARTNERS
Sexual partners of patients with HPV infection should be evaluated for the presence of HPV infection as well as other STDs. Female partners of infected men should have cervical cytology (Pap smear) done. Patients and their uninfected partners should be encouraged to use condoms to help reduce the risk of transmission.

References

1. Stamm WE et al. *The Practitioner's Handbook for the Management of STDs*. Seattle: University of Washington, 1988. P. 1.1.
2. Aral SO, Holmes KK. Epidemiology of sexual behavior and sexually transmitted diseases. In KK Holmes et al. (eds.), *Sexually Transmitted Diseases*. New York: McGraw-Hill, 1990. P. 25.
3. Bowie WR. Urethritis in males. In KK Holmes et al. (eds.), *Sexually Transmitted Diseases*. New York: McGraw-Hill, 1990. Pp. 628–29.
4. Bowie WR. Etiology of nongonococcal urethritis. Evidence for *Chlamydia trachomatis* and *Ureaplasma urealyticum*. *J Clin Invest* 59:735, 1977.
5. Fontaine EA et al. Characteristics of a gram nega-

tive anaerobe isolated from men with non-gonococcal urethritis. *J Med Microbiol* 17:129, 1984.

6. Taylor-Robinson D, Furr PM, Hanna NF. Microbiological and serological study of non-gonococcal urethritis with special reference to *Mycoplasma genitalium*. *Genitourin Med* 61:319, 1985.

7. Jacobs NF, Kraus SJ. Gonococcal and nongonococcal urethritis in men. Clinical and laboratory differentiation. *Ann Intern Med* 82:7, 1975.

8. Arya OP et al. Diagnosis of urethritis: role of polymorphonuclear leukocyte counts in gram-stained urethral smears. *Sex Transm Dis* 11:10, 1984.

9. Swartz SL et al. Diagnosis and etiology of nongonococcal urethritis. *J Infect Dis* 138:445, 1978.

10. Bowie WR. Comparison of Gram's stain and first-voided urine sediment in the diagnosis of urethritis. *Sex Transm Dis* 5:39, 1978.

11. Paavonen J, Koutsky LA, Kiviat N. Cervical neoplasia and other STD-related genital and anal neoplasia. In KK Holmes et al. (eds.), *Sexually Transmitted Diseases*. New York: McGraw-Hill, 1990. P. 561.

12. Brunham RC et al. Mucopurulent cervicitis—the ignored counterpart in women of urethritis in men. *N Engl J Med* 311:1, 1984.

13. Holmes KK. Lower genital tract infections in women: cystitis, urethritis, vulvovaginitis, and cervicitis. In KK Holmes et al. (eds.), New York: McGraw-Hill, 1990. Pp. 527–45.

14. Weström L. Incidence, prevalence, and trends of acute pelvic inflammatory disease and its consequences in industrialized countries. *Am J Obstet Gynecol* 138:880, 1980.

15. Sweet RL. Pelvic inflammatory disease and infertility in women. *Infect Dis Clin of N Am* 1:199, 1987.

16. Peterson HB, Galaid EI, Cates W. Pelvic inflammatory disease. *Med Clin of North Am* 74:1603, 1990.

17. Paavonen J et al. Microbiological and histopathological findings in acute pelvic inflammatory disease. *Br J Obstet Gynecol* 94:454, 1987.

18. Weström L. Pelvic inflammatory disease: bacteriology and sequelae. *Contraception* 36:111, 1987.

19. Weström L, Mårdh P-A. Acute pelvic inflammatory disease. In KK Holmes et al. (eds.), *Sexually Transmitted Diseases*. New York: McGraw-Hill 1990. Pp. 593–613.

20. Centers for Disease Control. 1989 sexually transmitted diseases treatment guidelines. *MMWR* 38 (suppl. 8S), 1, 1989.

21. Division of STD/HIV Prevention. *1990 Annual Report*. Washington DC: U.S. Department of Health and Human Services, Public Health Service, Centers for Disease Control, 1991.

22. Piot P, Plummer FA. Genital ulcer adenopathy syndrome. In KK Holmes et al. (eds.), *Sexually Transmitted Diseases*. New York: McGraw-Hill, 1990. Pp. 711–16.

23. Perine PL, Osoba AO. Lymphogranuloma venereum. In KK Holmes et al. (eds.), *Sexually Transmitted Diseases*. New York: McGraw-Hill, 1990. Pp. 195–204.

24. Corey L, Holmes KK. Genital herpes simplex virus infections: current concepts in diagnosis, therapy and prevention. *Ann Intern Med* 98:973, 1983.

25. Schmid GP. Approach to the patient with genital ulcer disease. *Med Clin North Am* 74:1559, 1990.

26. Sehgal VH, Gangwani OP. Genital fixed drug eruptions. *Genitourin Med* 62:56, 1986.

27. Fiumara NJ. Treatment of primary and secondary syphilis. Serological response. *JAMA* 243:2500, 1980.

28. Schmid GP. The treatment of chancroid. *JAMA* 255:1757, 1986.

29. Hook EW, Holmes KK. Gonococcal infections. *Ann Intern Med* 102:229, 1985.

30. Holmes KK, Johnson DW, Trostle HJ. An estimate of the risk of men acquiring gonorrhea by sexual contact with infected females. *Am J Epidemiol* 91:170, 1970.

31. Hooper RR et al. Cohort study of venereal disease. I: The risk of gonorrhea transmission from infected women to men. *Am J Epidemiol* 108:136, 1978.

32. Thin RNT, Williams IA, Nicol CS. Direct and delayed methods of immunofluorescent diagnosis of gonorrhea in women. *Br J Vener Dis* 47:27, 1970.

33. Handsfield HH. *Neisseria gonorrhoeae*. In GL Mandell, RG Douglas, JE Bennett (eds.), *Principles and Practice of Infectious Diseases*. New York: Churchill-Livingstone, 1990. Pp. 1613–31.

34. Ashford WA, Golash RG, Hemming VG. Penicillinase-producing *Neisseria gonorrhoeae*. *Lancet* 2:657, 1976.

35. Phillips I. Beta-lactamase-producing penicillin-resistant gonococcus. *Lancet* 2:656, 1976.

36. Perine PL et al. Epidemiology and treatment of penicillinase-producing *Neisseria gonorrhoeae*. *Sex Transm Dis* 6(suppl.):152, 1979.

37. Centers for Disease Control. Penicillin-resistant gonorrhea—North Carolina. *MMWR* 32:273, 1983.

38. Rice RJ et al. Chromosomally mediated resistance in *Neisseria gonorrhoeae* in the United States: results

of surveillance and reporting: 1983–1984. *J Infect Dis* 153:340, 1986.

39. Centers for Disease Control. Tetracycline-resistant *Neisseria gonorrhoeae*—Georgia, Pennsylvania, New Hampshire. *MMWR* 34:563, 1985.

40. Klein EJ et al. Anorectal gonococcal infection. *Ann Intern Med* 86:340, 1977.

41. Quinn TC et al. The polymicrobial origin of intestinal infections in homosexual men. *N Engl J Med* 309:576, 1983.

42. Wiesner PJ et al. Clinical spectrum of pharyngeal gonococcal infection. *N Engl J Med* 288:181, 1973.

43. Bro-Jørgensen A, Jensen T. Gonococcal pharyngeal infections: report of 110 cases. *Br J Vener Dis* 49:491, 1973.

44. Kinghorn GR, Rashid S. Prevalence of rectal and pharyngeal infection in women with gonorrhea in Sheffield. *Br J Vener Dis* 55:408, 1979.

45. Tice AW, Rodriguez VL. Pharyngeal gonorrhea. *JAMA* 246:2717, 1981.

46. Berger RE et al: Etiology, manifestations and therapy of acute epididymitis: prospective study of 50 cases. *J Urol* 121:750, 1979.

47. Watson RA. Gonorrhea and acute epididymitis. *Milit Med* 144:785, 1979.

48. Berger RE. Acute epididymitis. In KK Holmes et al. (eds.), *Sexually Transmitted Diseases*. New York: McGraw-Hill, 1990. Pp. 641–51.

49. Perri AJ et al. The Doppler stethoscope and the diagnosis of the acute scrotum. *J Urol* 116:598, 1976.

50. Holder LE et al. Testicular radionucleide angiography and static imaging: anatomy, scintigraphic interpretation, and clinical indications. *Radiology* 125:739, 1977.

51. Hook EW, Handsfield HH. Gonococcal infections in the adult. In KK Holmes et al. (eds.), *Sexually Transmitted Diseases*. New York: McGraw-Hill, 1990. Pp. 149–65.

52. Masi AT, Eisenstein BI. Disseminated gonococcal infection (DGI) and gonococcal arthritis (GCA). II. Clinical manifestations, diagnosis, complications, treatment, and prevention. *Semin Arthritis Rheum* 10:173, 1981.

53. Keiser H et al. Clinical forms of gonococcal arthritis. *N Engl J Med* 279:234, 1968.

54. Holmes KK et al. Disseminated gonococcal infection. *Ann Intern Med* 74:979, 1971.

55. O'Brien JP, Goldenberg DL, Rice PA. Disseminated gonococcal infection: a prospective analysis of 49 patients and a review of pathophysiology and immune mechanisms. *Medicine* 62:395, 1983.

56. Petersen BH et al. *Neisseria meningitidis* and *Neisseria gonorrhoeae* bacteremia associated with C6, C7, or C8 deficiency. *Ann Intern Med* 90:917, 1979.

57. Schachter J. Chlamydial infections. *N Engl J Med* 298:428, 1978.

58. Centers for Disease Control. *Chlamydia trachomatis* infections: policy guidelines for prevention and control. *MMWR* 34(suppl. 3S):53S, 1985.

59. Thompson SE, Washington AE. Epidemiology of sexually transmitted *Chlamydia trachomatis* infections. *Epidemiol Rev* 5:96, 1983.

60. Karam G et al. Asymptomatic *Chlamydia trachomatis* infections among sexually active men. *J Infect Dis* 154:900, 1986.

61. Paavonen J. *Chlamydia trachomatis*–induced urethritis in female partners of men with nongonococcal urethritis. *Sex Transm Dis* 6:69, 1979.

62. Stamm WE et al. Causes of the acute urethral syndrome in women. *N Engl J Med* 303:409, 1980.

63. Harrison HR et al. Cervical *Chlamydia trachomatis* infection in university women: relationship to history, contraception, ectopy, and cervicitis. *Am J Obstet Gynecol* 153:244, 1985.

64. Berger RE et al. *Chlamydia trachomatis* as a cause of acute "idiopathic" epididymitis. *N Engl J Med* 298:301, 1978.

65. Svensson L et al. Differences in some clinical and laboratory parameters in acute salpingitis related to culture and serologic findings. *Am J Obstet Gynecol* 138:1017, 1980.

66. Henry-Suchet J et al. Microbiology of specimens obtained by laparoscopy from controls and from patients with pelvic inflammatory disease or infertility with tubal obstruction: *Chlamydia trachomatis* and *Ureaplasma urealyticum*. *Am J Obstet Gynecol* 138:1022, 1980.

67. Henry-Suchet J et al. Microbiologic study of chronic inflammation associated with tubal factor infertility: role of *Chlamydia trachomatis*. *Fertil Steril* 47:274, 1987.

68. Sellors JW et al. Tubal factor infertility: an association with prior chlamydial infection and asymptomatic salpingitis. *Fertil Steril* 49:451, 1988.

69. Levine JS, Smith PD, Brugge WR. Chronic proctitis in male homosexuals due to lymphogranuloma venereum. *Gastroenterology* 79:563, 1980.

70. Quinn TC et al. *Chlamydia trachomatis* proctitis. *N Engl J Med* 305:195, 1981.

71. Jones RB et al. Effect of blind passage and multiple sampling on recovery of *Chlamydia trachomatis* from urogenital specimens. *J Clin Microbiol* 24:1029, 1986.

72. Stamm WE. Diagnosis of *Chlamydia trachomatis*

genitourinary infections. *Ann Intern Med* 108:710, 1988.

73. Fieldsteel AH, Cox DL, Moeckli RA. Cultivation of virulent *Treponema pallidum* in tissue culture. *Infect Immun* 32:908, 1981.

74. Centers for Disease Control. Increases in primary and secondary syphilis—United States. *MMWR* 36:393, 1987.

75. Centers for Disease Control. Relationship of syphilis to drug use and prostitution—Connecticut and Philadelphia, Pennsylvania. *MMWR* 37:755, 1988.

76. Rolfs RT, Goldberg M, Sharrar RG. Risk factors for syphilis: cocaine use and prostitution. *Am J Public Health* 80:853, 1990.

77. Division of STD/HIV Prevention. *Sexually Transmitted Disease Surveillance 1989*. Washington DC: U.S. Department of Health and Human Services, Public Health Service, Centers for Disease Control, 1990.

78. Rolfs RT, Nakashima AK. Epidemiology of primary and secondary syphilis in the United States. *JAMA* 264:1432, 1990.

79. Quinn TC et al. The association of syphilis with risk of human immunodeficiency virus infection in patients attending sexually transmitted disease clinics. *Arch Intern Med* 150:1297, 1990.

80. Hutchinson CM, Hook EW. Syphilis in adults. *Med Clin North Am* 74:1389, 1990.

81. Chapel TA. The signs and symptoms of secondary syphilis. *Sex Transm Dis* 7:161, 1980.

82. Thin RN. Early syphilis in the adult. In KK Holmes et al. (eds.), *Sexually Transmitted Diseases*. New York: McGraw-Hill, 1990. P. 221.

83. Tramont EC. *Treponema pallidum* (syphilis). In GL Mandell, RG Douglas, JE Bennett (eds.), *Principles and Practice of Infectious Diseases*. New York: Churchill-Livingstone, 1990. P. 1794.

84. Merritt HH, Moore M. Acute syphilitic meningitis. *Medicine* 14:119, 1935.

85. Lukehart SA et al. Invasion of the central nervous system by *Treponema pallidum*: implications for diagnosis and treatment. *Ann Intern Med* 109:855, 1988.

86. Chesney AM, Kemp JE. Incidence of *Spirochaeta pallida* in cerebrospinal fluid during early stage of syphilis. *JAMA* 83:1725, 1924.

87. Clark GE, Danbolt N. The Oslo Study of the Natural Course of Untreated Syphilis: an epidemiologic investigation based on a re-study of the Boeck-Bruusgaard material. *Med Clin North Am* 48:613, 1964.

88. Kampmeier RH. Late benign syphilis. In KK Holmes et al. (eds.), *Sexually Transmitted Diseases*. New York: McGraw-Hill, 1990. P. 251.

89. Heggtveit HA. Syphilitic aortitis: a clinicopathologic autopsy study of 100 cases, 1950 to 1960. *Circulation* 29:346, 1964.

90. Simon RP. Neurosyphilis. *Arch Neurol* 42:606, 1985.

91. Larsen SA, Hunter EF, Creighton ET. Syphilis. In KK Holmes et al. (eds.), *Sexually Transmitted Diseases*. New York: McGraw-Hill, 1990. P. 927.

92. Matthews HM, Yang T-K, Jenkin HM. Unique lipid composition of *Treponema pallidum* (Nichols virulent strain). *Infect Immun* 24:713, 1979.

93. Musher DM. Syphilis. *Infect Dis Clin North Am* 1:83, 1987.

94. Romanowski B et al. Serologic response to treatment of infectious syphilis. *Ann Intern Med* 114:1005, 1991.

95. Fiumara NJ. Serologic responses to treatment of 128 patients with late latent syphilis. *Sex Transm Dis* 6:243, 1979.

96. Yim CW, Flynn NM, Fitzgerald FT. Penetration of oral doxycycline into the cerebrospinal fluid of patients with latent or neurosyphilis. *Antimicrob Agents of Chemother* 28:347, 1985.

97. Hook EW et al. Ceftriaxone therapy for asymptomatic neurosyphilis. *Sex Transm Dis* 13:185, 1986.

98. Centers for Disease Control. Congenital syphilis—United States, 1983–1985. *MMWR* 35:625, 1986.

99. Brown ST et al. Serologic response to syphilis treatment: a new analysis of old data. *JAMA* 253:1296, 1985.

100. Gregory N, Sanchez M, Buchness MR. The spectrum of syphilis in patients with human immunodeficiency virus infection. *J Am Acad Dermatol* 22:1061, 1990.

101. Johns DR, Tierny M, Felsenstein D. Alteration in the natural history of neurosyphilis by concurrent infection with the human immunodeficiency virus. *N Engl J Med* 316:1569, 1987.

102. Hicks CB et al. Seronegative secondary syphilis in a patient infected with the human immunodeficiency virus (HIV) with Kaposi's sarcoma. *Ann Intern Med* 107:492, 1987.

103. Berry CD et al. Neurologic relapse after benzathine penicillin therapy for secondary syphilis in a patient with HIV infection. *N Engl J Med* 316:1587, 1987.

104. Goldstein LC et al. Monoclonal antibodies to herpes simplex viruses: use in antigenic typing and rapid diagnosis. *J Infect Dis* 147:829, 1983.

105. Corey L, Spear PG. Infections with herpes simplex virus. Parts 1 and 2. *N Engl J Med* 314:686, 749, 1986.

106. Mertz GJ et al. Frequency of acquisition of first-episode genital infection with herpes simplex virus

from symptomatic and asymptomatic source contacts. *Sex Transm Dis* 12:33, 1985.

107. Corey L et al. Genital herpes simplex virus infections: clinical manifestations, course and complications. *Ann Intern Med* 98:958, 1983.

108. Reeves WC et al. Risk of recurrence after first episodes of genital herpes: relation to HSV type and antibody response. *N Engl J Med* 305:315, 1981.

109. Goodell SE et al. Herpes simplex proctitis in homosexual men: clinical, sigmoidoscopic and histopathological features. *N Engl J Med* 308:868, 1983.

110. Lagrew DC et al. Disseminated herpes simplex virus infection in pregnancy: successful treatment with acyclovir. *JAMA* 252:2058, 1984.

111. Meyers JD, Flournay N, Thomas ED. Infection with herpes simplex virus and cell-mediated immunity after marrow transplant. *J Infect Dis* 142:338, 1980.

112. Siegal FP et al. Severe acquired immunodeficiency in male homosexuals, manifested by chronic perianal ulcerative herpes simplex lesions. *N Engl J Med* 305:1439, 1981.

113. Fife KH, Corey L. Herpes simplex virus. In KK Holmes et al. (eds.), *Sexually Transmitted Diseases*. New York: McGraw-Hill, 1990. P. 941.

114. Corey L et al. Treatment of primary first-episode genital herpes simplex virus infections with acyclovir: results of topical, intravenous and oral therapy. *J Antimicrob Chemother* 12(suppl. B):79, 1983.

115. Reichman RC et al. Treatment of recurrent genital herpes simplex infections with oral acyclovir: a controlled trial. *JAMA* 251:2103, 1984.

116. Douglas JM et al. A double-blind study of oral acyclovir for suppression of recurrences of genital herpes simplex virus infection. *N Engl J Med* 310:1551, 1984.

117. Mertz GJ et al. Long-term acyclovir suppression of frequently recurring genital herpes simplex virus infection: a multicenter double-blind trial. *JAMA* 260:201, 1988.

118. Erlich KS et al. Acyclovir-resistant herpes simplex virus infections in patients with the acquired immunodeficiency syndrome. *N Engl J Med* 320:293, 1989.

119. de Villiers E-M. Heterogeneity of the human papillomavirus group. *J Virol* 63:4898, 1989.

120. Dürst M et al. The physical state of human papillomavirus type 16 DNA in benign and malignant genital tumors. *J Gen Virol* 66:1515, 1985.

121. Yee C et al. Presence and expression of human papillomavirus sequences in human cervical carcinoma cell lines. *Am J Pathol* 119:361, 1985.

122. Becker TM, Stone KM, Alexander ER. Genital human papillomavirus infection: a growing concern. *Obstet Gynecol Clin North Am* 14:389, 1987.

123. Oriel JD. Natural history of genital warts. *Br J Vener Dis* 47:1, 1971.

124. Sand PK et al. Evaluation of male consorts of women with genital human papilloma virus infection. *Obstet Gynecol* 68:679, 1986.

125. Reid R et al. Noncondylomatous cervical wart virus infection. *Obstet Gynecol* 55:476, 1980.

126. Syrjänen K. Human papillomavirus lesions in association with cervical dysplasias and neoplasias. *Obstet Gynecol* 62:617, 1983.

127. Walker PG et al. Abnormalities of the uterine cervix in women with vulval warts. A preliminary communication. *Br J Vener Dis* 59:120, 1983.

128. Campion MJ, Singer A, Clarkson PK. Increased risk of cervical neoplasia in consorts of men with penile condylomata acuminata. *Lancet* 1:943, 1985.

129. Boxer RJ, Skinner DG. Condylomata acuminata and squamous cell carcinoma. *Urology* 9:72, 1977.

130. Krebs H-B, Schneider V. Human papillomavirus-associated lesions of the penis: colposcopy, cytology and histology. *Obstet Gynecol* 70:299, 1987.

131. Meisels A, Fortin R. Condylomatous lesions of the cervix and vagina: I. Cytologic patterns. *Acta Cytologica* 20:505, 1976.

132. Guillet G et al. Papillomavirus in cervical condylomas with and without associated cervical intraepithelial neoplasia. *J Invest Dermatol* 81:513, 1983.

133. Jensen SL. Comparison of podophyllin application with simple surgical excision in clearance and recurrence of perianal condylomata acuminata. *Lancet* 2:1146, 1985.

134. Simmons PD. Podophyllin 10% and 25% in the treatment of ano-genital warts: a comparative double-blind study. *Br J Vener Dis* 57:208, 1981.

135. Slater GE, Rumack BH, Peterson RG. Podophyllin poisoning: systemic toxicity following cutaneous application. *Obstet Gynecol* 52:94, 1978.

136. Cassidy DE, Drewry J, Fanning JP. Podophyllin toxicity: a report of a fatal case and a review of the literature. *J Toxicol Clin Toxicol* 19:35, 1982.

137. Chamberlain MJ, Reynolds AL, Yeoman WB. Toxic effect of podophyllin application in pregnancy. *Br Med J* 3:391, 1972.

138. Brown DR, Fife KH. Human papillomavirus infections of the genital tract. *Med Clin North Am* 74:1455, 1990.

139. Godley MJ et al. Cryotherapy compared with trichloroacetic acid in treating genital warts. *Genitourin Med* 63:390, 1987.

140. Bashi SA. Cryotherapy versus podophyllin in the treatment of genital warts. *Int J Dermatol* 24:535, 1985.

141. Ghosh AK. Cryosurgery of genital warts in cases in which podophyllin treatment failed or was contraindicated. *Br J Vener Dis* 53:49, 1977.

142. Matsunaga J, Bergman A, Bhatia NN. Genital condylomata acuminata in pregnancy: effectiveness, safety and pregnancy outcome following cryotherapy. *Br J Obstet Gynecol* 94:168, 1987.

143. Oriel D. Genital human papillomavirus infection. In KK Holmes et al. (eds.), *Sexually Transmitted Diseases*. New York: McGraw-Hill, 1990. P. 433.

144. Baggish MS. Improved laser techniques for the elimination of genital and extragenital warts. *Am J Obstet Gynecol* 153:545, 1985.

145. Eron LJ et al. Interferon therapy for condylomata acuminata. *N Engl J Med* 315:1059, 1986.

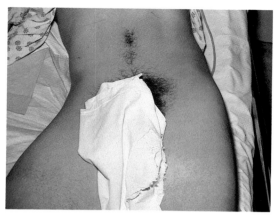

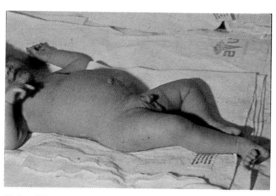

Color Plate 1. Toxic shock syndrome: note erythematous sunburn type rash on perineum. (Courtesy of Frederick Koster, M.D.)

Color Plate 2. Staphylococcal scalded skin syndrome: note sunburn-type rash. (Courtesy of Upjohn Pharmaceuticals)

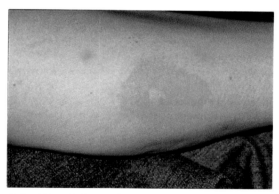

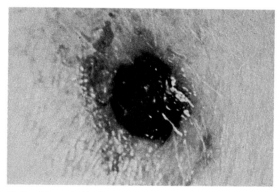

Color Plate 3. Lyme disease. Plaque of erythema chronicum migrans. (Courtesy of Upjohn Pharmaceuticals)

Color Plate 4. Ecthyma gangrenosum—note erythematous macule with necrotic center

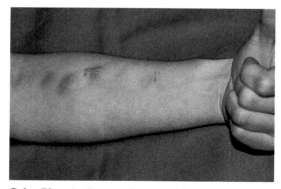

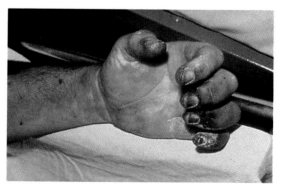

Color Plate 5. Sporotrichosis nodules along lymph channels. (Courtesy of Upjohn Pharmaceuticals)

Color Plate 6. Purpura, echymosis, and gangrene of septicemic plaque. (Courtesy of Upjohn Pharmaceuticals)

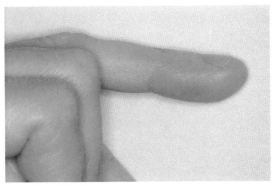

Color Plate 7. Osler's node of the finger

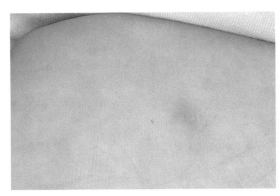

Color Plate 8. Janeway lesion of heel

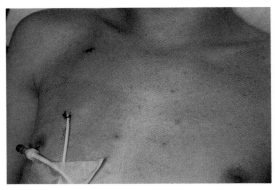

Color Plate 9. Cellulitis surrounding central line exit site

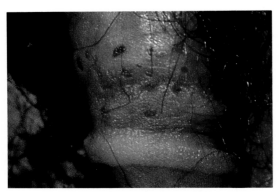

Color Plate 10. Grouped ulcers of genital herpes. (Courtesy of Upjohn Pharmaceuticals)

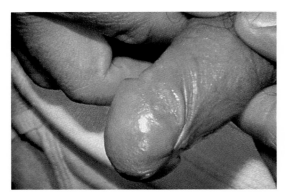

Color Plate 11. Chancre of primary syphilis. (Courtesy of Upjohn Pharmaceuticals)

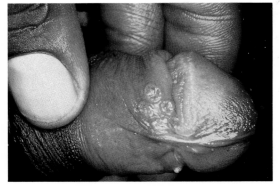

Color Plate 12. Chancroid lesion characterized by tender, eroded ulcer. (Courtesy of Upjohn Pharmaceuticals)

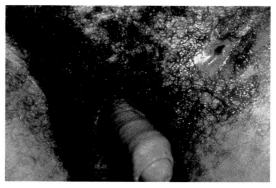

Color Plate 13. Suppurating lymph nodes of lymphogranuloma venereum. (Courtesy of Upjohn Pharmaceuticals)

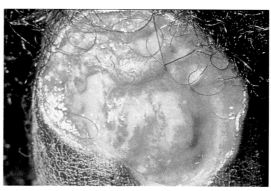

Color Plate 14. Genital ulcer of granuloma inguinale. (Courtesy of Upjohn Pharmaceuticals)

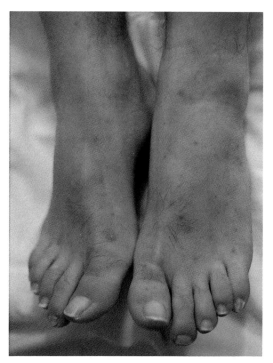

Color Plate 15. DGI. Lesions of *N. gonorrhoeae* more commonly found on the distal extremities

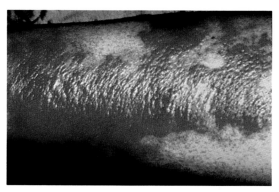

Color Plate 16. Raised red lesion of erysipelas on the lower extremity. (Courtesy of Upjohn Pharmaceuticals)

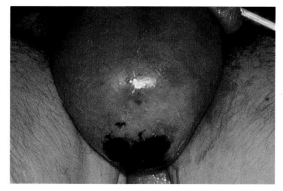

Color Plate 17. Synergistic necrotizing cellulitis: note discoloration of overlying dependent skin. (Courtesy of Upjohn Pharmaceuticals)

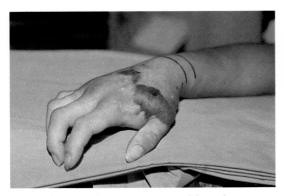

Color Plate 18. Acute streptococcal hemolytic gangrene: note cellulitic lesion with hemorrhagic bleb and cellulitic edge demarcated on wrist, advancing within 24 hours

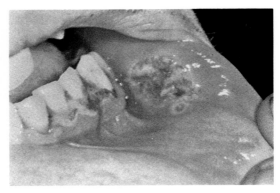

Color Plate 19. Clinical appearance of periapical abscess

THE NERVOUS SYSTEM

31

Nervous System Infections

WILLIAM P. REED
DAVID R. JOHNSON
LARRY E. DAVIS

Infectious agents reach the CNS by many routes, including the bloodstream as in viral encephalitis and many forms of meningitis. They also can spread from adjacent foci of infection, such as anaerobic brain abscess from chronic otitis media, *Streptococcus pneumoniae* meningitis from cribriform plate fracture [1], congenital dermal sinus tracts leading to recurrent *Staphylococcus epidermidis* meningitis, and the olfactory pathway with *Naegleria fowleri* amebic meningitis [2]. Peripheral nerves can carry rabies virus to the brain [3], and ventricular peritoneal shunts can lead to ventriculitis caused by many organisms, often of low virulence [4]. Many infections of the nervous system are due to agents that have initially colonized or caused infections in other parts of the body. For example, staphylococcal meningitis is frequently accompanied by or preceded by manifestations of *Staphylococcus aureus* infection elsewhere in the body, such as the endocardium. Organisms that have colonized or infected distant sites most commonly reach the nervous system through the bloodstream. Therefore, when the nervous system is involved with an infection, it is important to look for adjacent or sometimes distant foci from which the infection may have spread to the CNS. However, most distant infections, even with bacteremia, do not involve the CNS [5, 6]. This sparing of the CNS is at least in part due to

a number of barriers and host defenses, including the reticulo-endothelial system, humoral and cellular immune responses, and the blood-brain barrier [7, 8]. Even though infections of the CNS are relatively uncommon, they can progress rapidly when they do occur, and the consequences may be devastating to the affected individual. As a result of this potentially rapid progress, any time an infection of the CNS is suspected, the situation should be regarded as a medical emergency with diagnostic studies performed rapidly and treatment started at the earliest possible time.

In contrast to the frequently rapid progression of infections involving the CNS, some agents cause manifestations of disease only after they have been present for longer periods of time. For instance, tuberculosis and many fungi typically cause a subacute illness with manifestations appearing only after they have been present for weeks or months. Other agents cause illness years after they have been acquired. Examples include shingles resulting from prior *varicella-zoster* virus infection, subacute sclerosing panencephalitis following prior *rubeola* (measles) virus, and Creutzfeldt-Jakob disease due to infection many years previously with a slow virus or prion.

Most signs and symptoms of infections of the CNS are caused by pathologic changes that occur at the site of the infection. For example, nuchal rigidity that occurs in patients with meningitis is not caused by the responsible bacteria or virus but rather by irritation and inflammation that occur in the cervical leptomeninges and adjacent pain-sensitive spinal nerves and roots. Many tests used to evaluate the CNS for infection are aimed at identifying the site of pathological changes rather than the responsible organism. For instance, CT or MRI scans may indicate that a brain abscess is present but will not identify the responsible organism. Cultures or serologic studies are required to identify infecting organisms. The specific organism may determine the time course of the disease and should determine the treatment that will be administered.

Generalized Infections of the Brain

Encephalitis occurs when an infectious agent invades the brain and spreads widely throughout the brain parenchyma. The infectious organism may also infect selected cell types, as in poliomyelitis, or it may produce a localized brain infection, as in a brain abscess. The type of brain involvement is determined mainly by the class of infecting organism. Thus, viruses tend to cause encephalitis, while many bacteria, fungi, and parasites cause brain abscesses and more localized brain infections. In addition, the infectious agent determines the time course of the brain infection. Viruses tend to have a rapid time course, causing an acute encephalitis, while most fungi and parasites cause a subacute or chronic CNS infection.

Acute Encephalitis

An acute encephalitis has an abrupt onset, and the symptoms may reach their peak within several days. The majority of infectious agents that cause an acute encephalitis are viruses. It is important that the patient with an acute encephalitis be recognized promptly since early treatment is often important. In addition the signs and symptoms of encephalitis can rapidly progress to coma, so patients should be placed in intensive care units.

PATHOGENESIS AND PATHOPHYSIOLOGY

Most infectious agents that cause an acute encephalitis reach the brain via a hematogenous route. Rabies virus, which reaches the brain via peripheral nerves [9], or *Naegleria* organisms, which enter through the cribriform plate [10], are exceptions to this rule. Once the infectious agent has reached the brain parenchyma, a widely disseminated infection involving both neurons and glia ensues. Neuronal necrosis and death of glia cells result in secondary cerebral edema. Because the primary infection began elsewhere in the body and then progressed to involve the brain, immune inflammatory cells appear early in an encephalitis. The typical inflammatory response is a perivascular cuffing, with infiltration of lymphocytes and macrophages into the adjacent brain parenchyma [11]. In the case of many viral encephalitides these immune cells are responsible for terminating the infection. Degenerating neurons and glia are removed by phagocytic cells. In their place is a glial nodule comprised of glial cells, microglia, and glial fibers. Some viruses, such as herpes simplex, cytomegalovirus, varicella-zoster, and measles viruses produce Cowdry-type A intranuclear inclusion bodies in infected cells. Rabies virus produces cytoplasmic inclusions. Many infectious agents, however, produce no characteristic pathologic findings in the brain.

In the majority of viral encephalitides maximum pathologic involvement develops rapidly, and the disease runs its acute course in 2 weeks. Recovery from acute encephalitis, however, may be slow, often requiring months.

EPIDEMIOLOGY AND PREDISPOSING FACTORS

The majority of cases of acute encephalitis in the United States result from infection with an arbovirus or a herpes simplex virus. The term arbovirus is derived from *arthropod-borne virus*. These viruses belong to the togavirus, bunyavirus, and reovirus families and are usually transmitted to humans by hematophagous arthropods such as mosquitoes or ticks. Worldwide there are more than 250 strains but in the United States fewer than 15 are important. Arboviruses are maintained in nature by a complex zoonosis of apparent infections between small animals (mainly birds) and mosquitoes or ticks. Human infections occur when a person is

Table 31-1. Important causes of acute encephalitis

Organism	Vector	Geographic distribution
Togavirus		
Western equine	Mosquito	United States, Canada
St. Louis	Mosquito	United States, Canada
Eastern equine	Mosquito	Eastern United States, Caribbean
Venezuelan equine	Mosquito	Central America, southwestern United States
California	Mosquito	United States
Colorado tick fever	Tick	United States, Canada
Japanese B	Mosquito	Eastern Asia, Pacific Islands
Louping ill	Tick	Great Britain
Murray Valley	Mosquito	Australia, New Guinea
Russian spring-summer	Tick	Eastern Europe, Asia
West Nile	Mosquito	Africa, India, Middle East
Mumps virus	—	Worldwide
Herpes simplex virus	—	Worldwide
Rickettsiae rickettsii	Tick	United States, Canada, South America
Plasmodium falciparum	Mosquito	Asia, Africa, South America
Rabies virus	Dog, wolf, skunk, fox, bat, raccoon	Worldwide except islands such as England and Japan

bitten by an infected arthropod. The majority of human infections are asymptomatic, with only 1%–5% causing an encephalitis. Because arbovirus encephalitis is transmitted by a vector, the incidence in humans is seasonal and occurs mainly in the summer and early fall. While cases may be solitary, clusters or epidemics of encephalitis from a specific arbovirus are more common. The incidence of viral CNS infections is not uniform throughout the United States, with areas heavily infested by mosquitoes experiencing a greater frequency of arbovirus encephalitis. In addition, the strains of arbovirus that cause encephalitis vary regionally (Table 31-1).

In contrast herpes simplex encephalitis never occurs in epidemics. It is the most common cause of sporadic fatal endemic encephalitis. Herpes simplex virus type 2 is the most common form of encephalitis in the neonatal period, and type 1 is usually responsible for encephalitis acquired after the neonatal period. The majority of children and adults with herpes simplex encephalitis have antibodies to type 1 virus on admission to a hospital. This implies that the encephalitis is not the result of a primary viral infection, but rather the result of an exacerbation of a latent viral infection. It is

poorly understood how the virus travels from its latent site in a sensory ganglion to the brain. However, the incidence of this encephalitis does not appear to increase significantly in individuals who are immunosuppressed, suggesting that a defect in the immune system is not the primary factor in determining whether an encephalitis develops.

PRESENTATION
The hallmarks of an acute encephalitis are fever with the abrupt onset of headache and mental obtundation [12, 13]. Thus, encephalitis differs from meningitis, in which patients present with a prominent stiff neck, headache, and less mental obtundation. Patients with encephalitis often have a prodromal illness that lasts for several days. The prodrome varies with the organism and may include symptoms such as parotitis (mumps) or malaise and myalgia (togavirus). Patients with herpes simplex encephalitis seldom have a prodromal illness.

As encephalitis progresses, mental changes may include delirium, stupor, and even coma. Papilledema is uncommon on admission to the hospital but may develop later in the clinical course. Seizures (generalized or focal) may develop. Focal neurologic signs may also develop but are uncom-

Table 31-2. Signs and symptoms of acute encephalitis

Common Signs and Symptoms
Fever
Headaches, nausea, vomiting
Mental changes: confusion, delirium, lethargy, stupor, coma
Seizures: generalized or focal
Hyperreflexia, Babinski's sign, spasticity
Mild stiff neck

Less Common Signs and Symptoms
Tremors of arm or face, dysarthria
Hemiparesis, cranial nerve palsies
Aphasia, ataxia, blindness

mon (Table 31-2). The severity of clinical signs depends on the infectious organism, the age of the patient, and other biologic factors that are poorly understood. In general very young and very old persons have the most serious encephalitis.

Patients infected with rabies virus frequently have a prodromal illness of several days consisting of fevers, aches, hydrophobia, and a burning numbness or paresthesia around the original wound site. Most patients develop "furious" rabies, which is characterized by agitation, confusion, excessive motor movements, muscle spasms, vocal cord paralysis, seizures, focal limb paralysis, and coma [14, 15]. Early in the course of rabies encephalitis, patients may experience periods of agitation and confusion, followed by brief periods of lucidity. Hydrophobia occurs in only one-half of patients and is characterized by violent jerking contractions of the diaphragm and accessory muscles of the inspiration that is triggered by an attempt to swallow liquids. Abnormalities of the autonomic nervous system are common and include dilated irregular pupils, increased lacrimation and salivation, and diffuse sweating. About 20% of patients experience "dumb rabies" [14]. These patients present with an ascending motor paralysis that resembles the Guillain-Barré syndrome.

Patients with acute cerebral malaria are usually infected with *Plasmodium falciparum* [16]. The cerebral signs appear to develop from brain hypoxia and metabolic activities of the parasites in erythrocytes that become packed in cerebral vessels. The clinical features vary considerably but usually include

headache, delirium, confusion, seizures, and often coma. Patients may develop Cheyne-Stokes respirations and focal neurologic signs.

There are no pathognomonic features of the encephalitis that allow one to determine the etiology based on signs and symptoms. Thus, herpes simplex encephalitis cannot reliably be distinguished on clinical grounds alone from other causes of encephalitis [17–19].

LABORATORY STUDIES

The cerebrospinal fluid (CSF) is usually abnormal (Table 31-3). A normal CSF does not rule out viral encephalitis, but it should raise suspicion of a toxic or metabolic encephalopathy. The opening pressure may be normal, mildly elevated, or severely elevated. The CSF is usually clear and colorless and contains five to several hundred WBCs per cubic millimeter. Generally the WBCs are predominantly lymphocytic. The CSF glucose is usually normal, while the protein level is mildly elevated (45–200 mg/dl). The EEG is always abnormal in encephalitis and usually shows diffuse bilateral slowing with occasional spikes. Patients will require a CT or an MRI to rule out structural causes of the neurologic symptoms. Diffuse or focal abnormalities on imaging are consistent with encephalitis.

Early in the illness MRI scans show areas of increased signal intensities on T2-weighted scans that represent cerebral vascular permeability. When the abnormality is located in only one or both temporal lobes, the possibility of herpes simplex encephalitis is somewhat increased. Later in the clinical course the CT and MRI scans may demonstrate areas of brain necrosis and hemorrhage. Cerebral arteriograms are seldom helpful in establishing the diagnosis. In the first week of the illness there is usually no evidence of intrathecal immunoglobulin synthesis or oligoclonal bands. However, these often appear later in the illness and during convalescence. CSF bacterial and fungal cultures are sterile, and CSF viral cultures are usually sterile. Exceptions include CSF from patients with meningoencephalitis from mumps virus or lymphocytic choriomeningitis virus. Isolation of herpes simplex virus from the mouth or the lip does not aid in the diagnosis of herpes simplex encephalitis [17]. In most instances, including herpes sim-

Table 31-3. Spinal fluid profiles in CNS infections

Infection	Opening pressure	WBCs	Protein	Glucose	Bacterial or fungal culture
Bacterial meningitis	Elevated	50–10,000 PMNs	Elevated	Depressed	Positive
Viral meningitis	Normal or slightly elevated	20–1000 lymphocytes	Slightly elevated	Normal	Negative
Viral encephalitis	Slightly elevated	10–200 lymphocytes	Normal or slightly elevated	Normal	Negative
Brain abscess	Elevated	0–500 lymphocytes and PMNs	Elevated	Normal	Negative
Fungal or tuberculous meningitis	Elevated	50–10,000 PMNs and lymphocytes	Elevated	Depressed	Positive
Subdural empyema	Elevated	10–1000 PMNs	Slightly elevated	Normal	Negative
Epidural abscess	Normal or elevated	0–200 lymphocytes	Slightly elevated	Normal	Negative
Lyme disease	Normal	0–200 lymphocytes	Slightly elevated	Normal	Negative

plex encephalitis, the infectious agent can be isolated from a brain biopsy taken from an area of involvement.

DIAGNOSIS

The diagnosis of acute encephalitis is based on the clinical signs and symptoms, an abnormal CSF, and an abnormal EEG. The etiology of the encephalitis is usually established from serologic tests. The infectious agent is only rarely isolated from CSF. The immunoglobulin M (IgM) antibody-capture enzyme-linked immunosorbent assay (MAC ELISA) can be used to detect serum antibody to most arbovirus infections during the first few days of the encephalitis [20]. This test is available in many, but not all, state virus diagnostic laboratories and some private reference laboratories. Acute and convalescence viral antibody titers also are available in many virus laboratories. Complement-fixation and hemagglutination-inhibition antibodies tests are available for all arbovirus strains found in the United States.

The diagnosis of rabies encephalitis is based on serologic identification of rabies antibodies during the acute infection, identification of rabies viral antigen by fluorescent antibody staining of corneal impression smears, skin biopsies or brain tissue, identification of Negri bodies (cytoplasmic inclusion bodies) in human brain tissue, or isolation of rabies virus from infected saliva, CSF, or brain. In patients who have not received antirabies immunization, serum neutralizing antibodies seldom are present, before the onset of the encephalitis but can be detected within 7–10 days of clinical onset. The immunoadherence hemagglutination technique has become popular since it is rapid and inexpensive [21]. Rabies antibodies usually rise fourfold over several days to a week. If the patient has received rabies vaccination, use of the CSF rabies-neutralizing antibody test may be helpful. In immunized patients the CSF titer is low (< 1:64), whereas patients with rabies encephalitis often develop high CSF titers of 1:200 or greater. The use of immunofluorescent staining of corneal impression smears or nuchal-skin biopsy specimens for evidence of rabies antigen can be helpful if done by qualified, experienced laboratories, such as the Centers for Disease Control (CDC), in Atlanta, Georgia. The CDC has physicians available by telephone to assist in establishing the diagnosis.

The diagnosis of herpes simplex encephalitis is difficult because there are no pathognomonic clinical signs or symptoms or common laboratory tests. The presence of active herpes simplex cold sores or a history of recurrent herpes labialis does not help in establishing the diagnosis [17]. Herpes simplex virus (HSV) type 1 is only rarely isolated from CSF. Most patients have preexisting herpes simplex antibodies, so no specific serologic test is currently available for the diagnosis of herpes simplex encephalitis. At present the diagnosis of an acute infection can be made only by examination of cerebral biopsy specimens. A cerebral cortex biopsy should be seriously considered in patients with an acute unknown sporadic encephalitis when a neurosurgeon and a diagnostic virology laboratory are available. Experience from the National Institute of Allergy and Infectious Diseases Cooperative Study has shown that only 45% of patients clinically suspected of having herpes simplex encephalitis have HSV isolated from the cerebral biopsy specimen (22). If a cerebral biopsy is to be performed, it should be taken from an area of pathologic involvement, usually from the posterior frontal and temporal lobes [17]. Few complications develop from a properly performed biopsy [23]. Once the specimen has been obtained, tissue should be inoculated into tissue-culture cell lines that will replicate HSV. Elevated CSF titers to HSV do not appear until convalescence [17].

The diagnosis of cerebral malaria is made by the identification of malarial parasites on thick or thin blood smears. As polymerase chain reaction tests to detect fragments of nucleic acids from infectious agents in CSF become better and more standardized, they should be helpful in establishing the etiology of many encephalitides, including HSV [24].

SYMPTOMATIC THERAPY

The patient should be placed in an intensive care unit early in the illness, because the encephalitis may progress rapidly. All patients should receive care to prevent decubitus ulcers, corneal abrasions, and contractures. If seizures develop, phenytoin usually is given since it does not cloud the sensorium. A loading dose of phenytoin usually is given slowly as an IV infusion at a rate not exceeding 50 mg per minute. A total dose of 15 mg/kg should be given. Blood pressure and an ECG may be checked during the phenytoin infusion. If hypotension develops, the infusion rate should be slowed. If cardiac arrhythmias appear, the infusion should be

stopped temporarily and restarted at a slower rate. If the phenytoin fails to stop seizures, use of IV phenobarbital should be considered.

Increased intracranial pressure may develop as a consequence of vascular engorgement and cerebral edema. If this develops, placement of an intracranial pressure monitor should be considered to monitor accurately the intracranial pressure. Treatment of increased intracranial pressure consists of nasotracheal intubation with hyperventilation from a mechanical ventilator. Arterial PCO_2 should be maintained at 25–30 mm Hg. IV mannitol at a dose of 0.25–0.50 g/kg also should be given intermittently as a bolus to control intracranial pressure. Serum osmolarity should be monitored to ensure that it is maintained below 320 mOsm/l. IV fluids initially should be restricted to about 75% of the calculated daily requirement. Care should be taken to ensure that the patient does not become hypovolemic, since that can cause arterial hypotension and decrease cerebral blood perfusion. Use of corticosteroids is controversial since much of the cerebral edema is of the cytotoxic type, which often does not respond to corticosteroids.

SPECIFIC THERAPY

Herpes simplex and varicella-zoster encephalitis can be treated with the antiviral drug acyclovir (Zovirax). In the treatment of herpes simplex encephalitis this drug has maximum benefit when given early in the course of the encephalitis [25]. Acyclovir should be given at a dose of 30 mg/kg/day IV, divided into three infusions. The drug should be given slowly over 1 hour because rapid administration can cause renal toxicity. It should be given for at least 10 days, but if a brain biopsy is obtained and is culture negative after 5 days and the clinical picture does not suggest herpes simplex encephalitis, administration of the drug may be discontinued. Some clinicians empirically treat possible cases of herpes simplex encephalitis with acyclovir without obtaining a brain biopsy. In that situation the drug must be continued for the full 10 days. Limited studies suggest that Epstein-Barr and cytomegalovirus encephalitis may respond to ganciclovir [26]. Ganciclovir is given at a dose of 2.5–7.5 mg/kg q8h IV or 5 mg/kg q12h IV. The optimal duration of therapy is unknown. Currently there is no specific antiviral treatment for RNA viruses such as arboviruses, rabies, or mumps [15].

The treatment of cerebral malaria has become more difficult with the appearance of strains resistant to chloroquine. In the treatment of acute malaria use of a schizonticidal drug is essential to remove parasites from the blood [27]. In adults chloroquine hydrochloride 250 mg q6h for 3 days or oral chloroquine phosphate 1 g initially and then 500 mg q6h for 3 days is commonly administered to treat chloroquine-sensitive strains. For chloroquine-resistant strains a loading dose of 10 mg/kg of quinidine gluconate (equivalent to 6.2 mg quinidine base) is given over 1–2 hours, followed by a constant infusion of 0.02 mg/kg quinidine gluconate per minute [28]. Tetracycline 250 mg qid for 10 days or a sulfonamide such as sulfadiazine or sulfisoxazole and pyrimethamine 25 mg q8h may be added. The use of dexamethasone 10 mg q4h IV has been thought to be beneficial by some authors, but it was of no value in a double-blind study [29].

OUTCOME

The prognosis of acute encephalitis depends on the etiologic agent. Rabies encephalitis normally is fatal. Eastern equine, Japanese B, Murray Valley, and Russian spring-summer encephalitides usually are severe with mortality rates as high as 20%–40% and permanent neurologic sequelae in up to 50% of cases [30]. Herpes simplex encephalitis when treated with acyclovir has a mortality rate of about 30% and a morbidity rate of 50%. About 30% of patients with cerebral malaria die and about one-third are left with neurologic sequelae. Western equine, St. Louis, California, and mumps encephalitides have mortality rates of 2%–10% [31]. Five to 10% of survivors are left with neurologic sequelae. Venezuelan and equine encephalitides and Colorado tick fever viruses cause a mild encephalitis from which full recovery usually occurs [32]. Recovery from encephalitis is slow and often takes several months. Neurologic sequelae from acute encephalitis include mental retardation or dementia, seizures, hemiparesis, aphasia, postencephalitic Parkinson's disease, and ataxia.

IMMUNOPROPHYLAXIS
AND CHEMOPROPHYLAXIS

Vaccines are not available for viruses that cause most forms of encephalitis in the United States. In Asia a vaccine for Japanese B encephalitis virus is available. The long incubation period of rabies allows for a unique postexposure immunization period. In determining whether an individual should receive postexposure rabies prophylaxis, it is important to determine whether the individual is actually at risk. A useful algorithm (Fig. 31-1) is recommended by the CDC [33].

Not all animal bites carry a risk of transmitting rabies. In the United States raccoons, foxes, skunks, and bats are the primary wild animals that are infected. In other areas of the world mongooses, weasels, wolves, and coyotes also may be infected. Dogs are the primary domestic animals that may be infected, but pet cats and skunks also have transmitted the disease. Small animals such as rodents and squirrels do not transmit rabies. Physicians should know which animals in their area are potentially infected with rabies virus. Once the decision has been made to undertake postexposure prophylaxis, the following regimen should be started. The wound should be thoroughly cleaned and generously flushed with soap and water, a procedure that has been shown to significantly reduce the incidence of rabies. Both active and passive immunization for rabies should be given. Individuals should receive a rabies vaccine produced from human diploid cells (IMOVAX-rabies), 1 ml IM on days 1, 3, 7, 14, and 28. Human rabies immunoglobulin 20 IU/kg should be administered on day 1, one-half at the wound site and one-half IM (in the deltoid muscle). The vaccine has been shown to produce rapid excellent antibody responses, with some minor local reactions and only rare systemic anaphylactic reactions [34].

Chemoprophylaxis for individuals traveling into malaria-endemic areas should follow the CDC guidelines [35]; this topic is discussed in Chap. 19.

Subacute Encephalitis

In subacute encephalitis signs and symptoms appear over several weeks. Because of the subacute onset these patients present less often to emergency departments. Bacteria (*Treponema pallidum* and *Borrelia burgdorferi*), parasites (*Toxoplasma gondii* and *Trypanosoma brucei gambiense*), and viruses (rubeola and JC papovavirus, or the virus of progressive multifocal leukoencephalitis) can cause a subacute

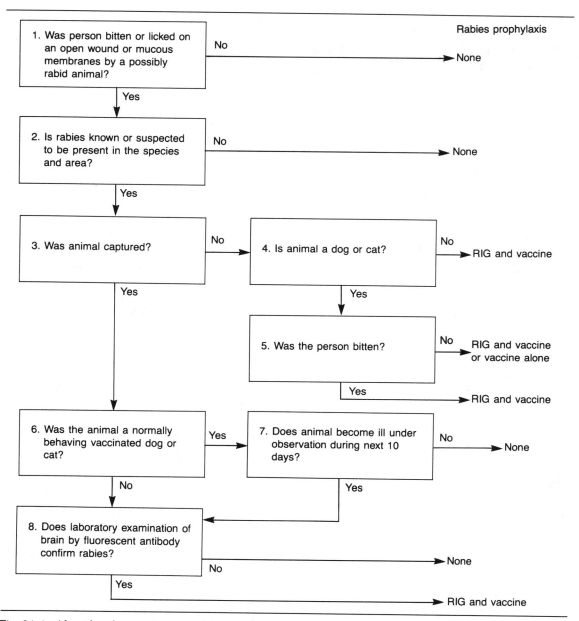

Fig. 31-1. Algorithm for postexposure rabies prophylaxis. RIG = rabies immune globulin. (*Source*: From reference 33. Used with permission)

encephalitis. These infections can occur in healthy individuals, but their incidence increases in immunodeficient individuals.

PATIENT PRESENTATION

Patients with subacute encephalitis present with progressive confusion, disorientation, obtundation, and focal neurologic signs such as hemiparesis and aphasia. Seizures occur in approximately one-half of the patients. The disease progresses over days to weeks. The CSF is abnormal and contains a mild lymphocytosis, elevated protein level, and normal glucose level (see Table 31-3). Patients with meningoencephalitis often complain of a headache and stiff neck and have a more dramatic CSF pleocytosis.

Patients with CNS toxoplasmosis may have a prodromal illness with cervical lymphadenopathy, fever, myalgia, and atypical lymphocytosis [36]. Occasionally chorioretinitis may be present. CNS manifestations may present as a subacute encephalitis, meningoencephalitis, or space-occupying lesions. Multiple space-occupying lesions are common in persons who have underlying immunodeficiency diseases such as AIDS. Patients with human African trypanosomiasis, or sleeping sickness, acquire their infection following a bite of an infected tsetse fly weeks to a few years earlier in Africa. Clinically the patients present with a generalized adenopathy, intermittent fevers, splenomegaly, and headaches [37]. The patient develops a slowly progressive apathy, increased daytime sleepiness, abnormal limb movements, personality changes, and occasionally psychosis. Eventually seizures and dementia develop.

Patients previously infected with rubeola (measles virus) may develop subacute sclerosing panencephalitis (SSPE) 4–10 years later [38]. These individuals, who are usually children, experience subtle progressive deterioration of school performance, personality changes, and progressive dementia [39–41]. Myoclonal jerks, dysarthria, and seizures can develop. The end stage is a severe dementia with quadraparesis. The course of disease is slow and relentlessly progressive over 1–2 years. In the interim between the primary measles infection and the onset of SSPE, the child appears normal.

DIAGNOSIS
The diagnosis of subacute encephalitis usually can be made in the emergency department from CSF, EEG, and MRI results. Patients with subacute encephalitis have an abnormal EEG with diffuse slowing. The CSF is abnormal and usually characterized by lymphocytic pleocytosis, elevated protein, and normal glucose. The MRI scan is usually abnormal, showing multiple areas of increased signal intensity on T2 weighted scans. The diagnosis of toxoplasma encephalitis is usually made serologically. These patients have an elevated indirect fluorescent antibody test, Sabin-Feldman die test, and indirect hemagglutination (IHA) test [42]. Unless the individual is immunosuppressed (such as with a concomitant human immunodeficiency virus [HIV] in-

fection), titers are usually markedly elevated at the time of the subacute encephalitis. The diagnosis of trypanosomiasis can be suspected in individuals who have subacute encephalitis and markedly elevated IgM levels in their CSF [37]. Trypanosomes frequently are identified in peripheral blood smears, and antibody tests for trypanosomiasis are available from the CDC. The diagnosis of SSPE is made by finding markedly elevated rubeola virus titers in CSF and serum. Patients with SSPE frequently have an EEG with periodic bursts of stereotypic slow and sharp waves that occur at intervals of 3–10 seconds and that may be associated with the patient's myoclonic jerks [39].

TREATMENT
Treatment of CNS toxoplasmosis involves pyrimethamine (0.5 mg/kg/day) combined with sulfadiazine (30–50 mg/kg/day) for 4–6 weeks [36]. Patients who are immunosuppressed require longer treatment. Folinic acid (Leukovorin) can be given, 5 mg IM every other day, to minimize the toxicity of pyrimethamine [43]. Spiramycin, which is available in Canada and Europe but not in the United States, also has been shown to be beneficial. Human African trypanosomiasis requires treatment with melarsoprol (Mel B) once the infection has entered the brain [44]. Suramine and pentamidine are useful drugs, but they do not cross the blood-brain barrier. Recently difluoromethylornithine has been found useful in the treatment of gambiense encephalitis [45–47]. There is no proved antiviral treatment for SSPE, but systemic or intrathecal interferon alpha has induced remissions [48].

Meningitis

Acute Meningitis

VIRAL MENINGITIS
Each year more than 10,000 cases of aseptic meningitis are reported to the CDC, and many additional ones undoubtedly occur [49]. The terms *aseptic meningitis* and *viral meningitis* frequently are used interchangeably, since viruses are responsible for the majority of cases of meningitis not caused by identifiable bacterial, mycobacterial, or fungal agents.

The enteroviruses, including echovirus and coxsackievirus, together with the mumps virus cause the majority of cases of aseptic meningitis [11, 50], but HSV-2, cytomegalovirus, arboviruses, poliovirus, HIV, and lymphocytic choriomeningitis virus may also cause similar disease. There are about 75 strains of echoviruses and coxsackieviruses. These enteroviruses can be isolated from sewers and other sources of water, especially during the summer months. Infection occurs by the fecal-oral route, with the primary infection occurring in the GI and upper respiratory tracts. Most of the initial infections are asymptomatic, although there may be mild symptoms of gastroenteritis or upper respiratory disease. When the virus reaches the leptomeninges, it does so by the hematogenous route and elicits a lymphocytic inflammatory reaction.

Epidemiology. Cases may occur at any time of the year, but they most frequently are identified during summer and early fall. Most cases occur sporadically without an identifiable source for the infection, but there may be some clustering of cases in both time and location. Most clinically apparent viral meningitis occurs in children and young adults [51].

Presentation. The onset is commonly abrupt with fever, headaches, nuchal rigidity, and occasionally vomiting. Some patients complain of eye pain, particularly with eye movement. There may be irritability and lethargy but the patient is seldom confused or obtunded [52, 53]. There may be associated rashes, parotitis, diarrhea, myalgia, herpangina, or sore throat. With mumps meningitis the parotitis occasionally fails to occur until after the meningitis has appeared [54]. With mumps virus, arbovirus, and lymphocytic choriomeningitis virus infections there may be encephalitic as well as meningeal signs. Since the virus is cleared from the CSF by the host's immune system in 1 or 2 days, the symptoms gradually subside after 3–4 days of acute discomfort.

Physical examination typically reveals a patient in acute discomfort, with a fever of 37.8°–40°C, irritability or lethargy, with nuchal rigidity and Kernig's sign (inability to fully extend the knee with the hip flexed to 90°) or Brudzinski's sign (flexion of the hips with passive flexion of the neck) [55]. The patient's mentation usually is normal.

The venous white blood count usually is normal or mildly elevated, and the CSF has a normal or slightly elevated opening pressure. The CSF has a pleocytosis in the range of 20–1000 WBCs per microliter (see Table 31-3). Polymorphonuclear neutrophils (PMNs) may be abundant when the CSF is first obtained (Fig. 31-2), but lymphocytes rapidly become the predominant cell. The CSF glucose commonly is normal, and protein may be normal or slightly elevated. The CSF glucose may be mildly depressed in patients with mumps, lymphocytic choriomeningitis, varicella-zoster, or herpes simplex type 2 infection [56]. If the CSF glucose is below 25 mg/dl, bacterial or fungal meningitis should be a major consideration. Viruses may be isolated from the CSF during the first day of illness but are seldom found later. There may be a significant rise in the serum antibody titer due to the responsible agent, but serologic tests to establish the diagnosis often fail to do so because of the impracticability of testing for the many possible agents that may be responsible for the disease. The EEG usually is normal, although there may be mild background slowing, and CT or MRI scans of the head are normal.

Differential Diagnosis. The diagnosis is usually made when a person presents with fever, headache, and nuchal rigidity and has CSF findings characteristic of viral meningitis. Bacteria or fungi cannot be isolated from the CSF, and there are no signs or x-ray evidence of parameningeal infection such as sinusitis, otitis media, or trauma. Although the initial CSF laboratory findings are frequently characteristic, it can be seen from Fig. 31-2 that there is considerable overlap of the percentage of neutrophils and the levels of protein and glucose in patients with viral or bacterial meningitis. In the case of aseptic meningitis a repeat lumbar puncture performed 6–24 hours later frequently will show lymphocytic predominance in the majority of patients.

Therapy. Most patients do not require hospitalization but get hospitalized because bacterial meningitis cannot be ruled out. No specific therapy is indicated. Currently available antiviral drugs have no activity against the majority of agents that cause viral meningitis.

BACTERIAL MENINGITIS

Bacterial meningitis is a life-threatening medical emergency, and its prompt diagnosis and treatment is one of the true challenges to the emergency physician. The overall incidence of bacterial meningitis in the United States is about 10 cases per 100,000 persons, with approximately 20,000 to 25,000 new cases per year [57, 58]. Since the disease is relatively uncommon, the diagnosis is often delayed with a resulting increase in morbidity and mortality [59–62]. In fact, cases of meningitis are a leading cause of malpractice suits against emergency physicians [63]. The introduction of antibiotics led to a decrease in mortality rates from bacterial meningitis, but 14% of patients still die [64]. In addition, survivors may suffer from long-term neurologic sequelae [65–67].

Pathogenesis and Pathophysiology. Meningitis is characterized by inflammation of the pia-arachnoid and surrounding CSF. The first step in a sequence of events leading to meningitis is nasopharyngeal mucosal colonization by potentially pathogenic bacteria. [68]. Once adherent to the mucosa, bacteria infect by crossing through the host cell into tissue and the bloodstream. The organism then reaches the CNS by one of several mechanisms: (1) from nasopharyngeal venules (pharyngeal infection or colonization), (2) via the bloodstream (bacteremia), or (3) through direct contiguous spread from an adjacent intracranial focus or skin surface (congenital dural defect, skull fracture, sinusitis, brain abscess). Alternatively the organism may be inoculated by trauma or at the time of a neurosurgical or diagnostic procedure. These events may occur in any person, but certain individuals are especially susceptible, including those who are asplenic (sickle cell disease or past splenectomy), who congenitally lack terminal complement components, or who have poor antibody responses to bacterial polysaccharides (young children or persons with multiple myeloma) [68, 69].

Once access has been gained to the CSF, bacterial replication takes places relatively unimpeded [70]. Low levels of antibody and complement in the

CSF lead to poor organization and phagocytosis of the organisms, even though polymorphonuclear cells are usually present in bacterially infected CSF. The most frequent infecting bacteria are highly encapsulated species, which further impede phagocytosis. As the infection proceeds, pus accumulates in the subarachnoid space and leads to cerebral edema, increased intracranial pressure, obstruction of CSF flow, and compression of cranial nerves [70, 71].

Epidemiology and Predisposing Factors. Because antibiotic therapy should be initiated before definitive bacteriologic information is available, it must be based on knowledge of epidemiologic and predisposing host factors, as well as on clues obtained during the clinical examination. *Haemophilus influenzae, Neisseria meningitidis,* and *S. pneumoniae* are responsible for 75%–80% of all cases of meningitis, with the incidence of each organism being dependent on patient age [72–75]. Fig. 31-3 shows the predominant organisms in each age group [72]. Neonatal meningitis is usually caused by gram-negative bacteria, especially *Escherichia coli,* or by group B streptococci [76, 77]. In infants and children the most common cause of bacterial meningitis is *H. influenzae* type B [73, 76]. Adult meningitis is most often caused by *N. meningitidis* and *S. pneumoniae.* Meningococcal meningitis is unique in that it may occur in outbreaks or cyclical waves about every 10 years and should be suspected especially during epidemics. Adults may rarely acquire *H. influenzae* meningitis as a consequence of contact with infected children [73]. The aged patient is predisposed to *S. pneumoniae* and *Neisseria meningitidis,* as well as to gram-negative enteric bacilli [74, 78].

Special clinical circumstances predispose individuals to meningeal infection with certain bacteria, as outlined in Table 31-4 [79–88]. When a patient with meningitis has a preexisting disease or medical condition, it may be possible to predict which organisms are most likely to be recovered in cultures, and such predictions should guide initial therapy.

Presentation. When all the features of a classic case of bacterial meningitis are present, the diagnosis may not be difficult. In one study, however,

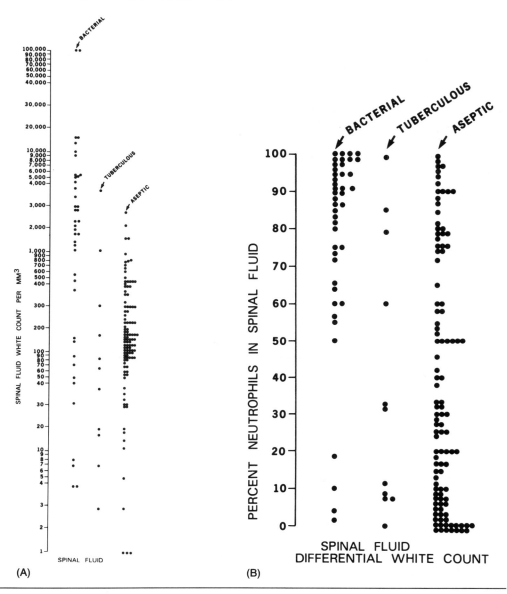

Fig. 31-2. Bacterial, tuberculous, and aseptic meningitis: CSF white counts (A), differential cell counts (B), glucose (C), and protein values (D) for a large series of patients. (*Source:* Modified from reference 51 with permission)

emergency department physicians failed to suspect the diagnosis in 23% of patients with bacterial meningitis [89]. Failure to recognize the disease occurs especially when it is in its early stages, when another condition such as pneumonia is more prominent, or when it has an atypical presentation,

as is common in the very young and the very old. The four common presenting clinical features of bacterial meningitis are fever, headache, altered mental status, and stiff neck. No single symptom or sign is specific for meningitis, and the presentation in neonates and infants commonly is nonspecific

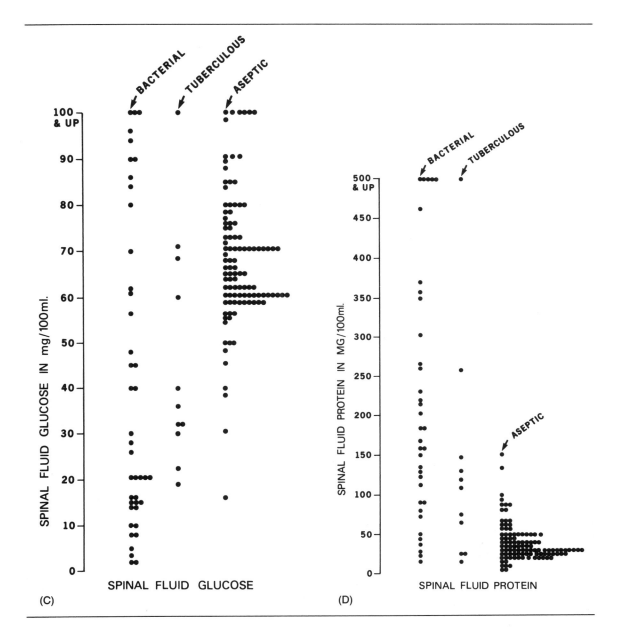

(C)   SPINAL FLUID GLUCOSE

(D)   SPINAL FLUID PROTEIN

[82, 90]. In general fever is the most common presenting symptom, but in one series fever was present in only two-thirds of patients [82]. The mental status may range from an alert state to deep coma, with an altered mental status occurring in 50%–80% of patients [82, 66]. A variety of other nonspecific symptoms may be present, including chills, sore throat, cough, rhinorrhea, earache, leg weakness, dizziness, myalgias, and arthralgias. It can be particularly difficult to distinguish meningitis from influenza, which may present with fever, headache, and myalgias. The diagnosis of meningitis often is delayed in the elderly because of an atypical presentation. These individuals are prone to other diseases that may be mistakenly diagnosed when the patient actually has men-

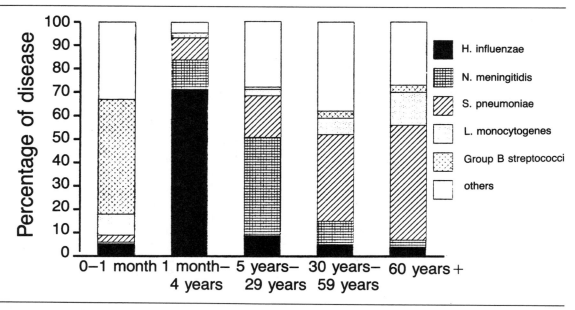

Fig. 31-3. Bacterial pathogens responsible for meningitis in different age groups in survey population of 1 million in the United States in 1986. (*Source*: Modified from reference 72, with permission)

ingitis. These other diseases include subdural or subarachnoid hemorrhage, dementia, stroke, non-ketotic hyperosmolar coma, drug-induced delirium, and sepsis from other sources. The fact that the elderly may not mount a febrile response to infection further complicates matters [91].

The classic meningeal sign is pain and stiffness with passive flexion of the neck. Other less frequently found meningeal manifestations include Kernig's sign and Brudzinski's sign [55]. Abnormal meningeal manifestations usually are elicited on initial presentation, but they are not necessary to suspect the diagnosis of bacterial meningitis. These manifestations are not reliably found in infants under the age of 1 year [92] and may occasionally be absent in older children and adults. In one review of 1064 pediatric cases of meningitis beyond the neonatal period, 16 [1.5%], including 8 children over the age of 2, had no meningeal signs throughout the entire hospitalization [93]. Occasional nonelderly adults [82, 90, 94] and nearly 20% of elderly patients [74] may fail to have meningeal signs. A petechial or purpuric rash in a patient with meningitis suggests *N. meningitidis* as the cause, although similar rashes rarely occur with *S. pneumoniae*, *H. influenzae*, and viral meningitis.

Patients with meningitis following head trauma or a neurosurgical procedure may present with an occult fever, change in mental status, or frank sepsis and meningeal findings. A malfunctioning ventriculoperitoneal or ventriculoatrial shunt in a patient with any symptoms of CNS infection should suggest ventriculitis. In that case CSF must be recovered from the shunt itself. The most common infecting organism is *S. epidermitidis*, which may cause a subacute or chronic infection with immune complex mediated glomerulonephritis as a major manifestation.

The course of bacterial meningitis is frequently rapid with progressive deterioration of neurologic function [90], but the illness occasionally may evolve over 1–7 days, with systemic symptoms such as low-grade fever, myalgias, arthralgias, or headache without initial typical signs of meningeal irritation. Meningitis caused by gram-negative enteric bacilli is more likely to progress in a less rapid manner.

Neonatal and Infant Presentation. In the neonatal period the signs and symptoms of meningitis are often nonspecific and the diagnosis may be difficult. Fever, irritability, seizures, and a bulging

Table 31-4. Organisms that cause meningitis in select groups

Setting	Likely etiologic agent
Neonate (0–1 month)	Group B streptococci *Escherichia coli* *Listeria monocytogenes* Other gram-negative bacilli
1 month–4 years	*Haemophilus influenzae* *Streptococcus pneumoniae* (pneumococcus) *Neisseria meningitidis*
5–29 years	*N. meningitidis* *S. pneumoniae* *Haemophilus influenzae*
30–59 years	*S. pneumoniae* *N. meningitidis*
Over 60 years	*S. pneumoniae* *L. monocytogenes* Gram-negative bacilli
Acute otitis media or sinusitis	*S. pneumoniae* *H. influenzae*
Chronic otitis, sinusitis, mastoiditis	Anaerobes Gram-negative bacilli
Pneumonia	*S. pneumoniae* *N. meningitidis*
Acute endocarditis	*Staphylococcus aureus* *S. pneumoniae*
IV drug use	*S. aureus* Gram-negative bacilli Fungi
Penetrating trauma or recent neurosurgery	Staphylococci Gram-negative bacilli
CSF rhinorrhea	*S. pneumoniae*
Hyposplenism	*S. pneumoniae* *H. influenzae* *N. meningitidis*
Ventriculoatrial shunt	*Staphylococcus epidermitidis*
Alcoholic	*S. pneumoniae* *L. monocytogenes*
Immunosuppression	Gram-negative bacilli Fungi *L. monocytogenes* Unusual organisms

fontanelle are considered characteristic, and when these symptoms are present the diagnosis is easy for an experienced clinician. However, findings often include only fever or hypothermia, cyanosis, lethargy, irritability, and vomiting without a stiff neck or a bulging fontanelle [95]. Because of this frequent nonspecific presentation the only reliable way to establish the diagnosis in neonates is with a lumbar puncture, which necessarily leads to a large number of negative lumbar punctures [96]. Emergency physicians are encouraged to obtain CSF for examination in patients of this age group who present with a significant fever.

Infants 2 months to 2 years of age also present a challenge. These patients will usually present with fever, altered mental status, a bulging fontanelle, and seizures [92]. Nonspecific findings include vomiting, ataxia, and irritability. The lack of meningeal signs, however, does not exclude meningitis in this age group [93]. The febrile child who is lethargic, disinterested, and inconsolable but who has no focal neurologic signs may need a lumbar puncture even in the absence of meningeal signs.

There is some disagreement in the literature as to which children with an apparent febrile seizure need a lumbar puncture since a small percentage will have meningitis. Certain characteristics suggest a febrile seizure. These include (1) age of 6 months to 6 years, (2) onset of seizure 2–6 hours from the onset of fever, (3) generalized seizure, (4) seizure duration of less than 20 minutes, (5) single seizure, and (6) normal neurologic exam following the seizure [97, 98]. Unfortunately retrospective studies of children with meningitis have shown that 13%–18% of these patients present with a seizure, and in most the seizure was indistinguishable from a classic febrile seizure [99, 100]. It is not unreasonable for the emergency physician to obtain CSF on all children with a fever and a seizure who are under 2 years of age [98, 101]. In older children meningeal signs are more reliable, and the physician can proceed primarily on clinical findings.

Laboratory Studies. Lumbar puncture and examination of the CSF is the definitive procedure for making the diagnosis of meningitis and should be accomplished as soon as the diagnosis is entertained. The procedure should be performed carefully [102], keeping in mind the major concerns that relate to possible adverse consequences, including uncal herniation, spread of infection to the CSF, and bleeding, which can lead to spinal cord compression. The possibility of uncal herniation as a consequence of lumbar puncture should be suspected if initial examination reveals papilledema, coma, or major focal neurologic defects, all of which are uncommon manifestations of meningitis.

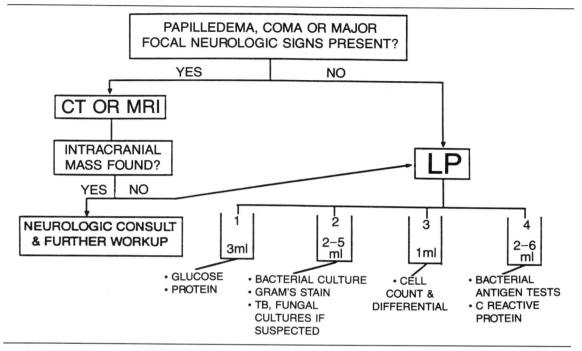

Fig. 31-4. Algorithm for determining need for CT scans and neurological consultation prior to performing lumbar puncture in suspected meningitis

Although lumbar puncture may be accomplished without adverse consequences in this circumstance [103], it would be reasonable to obtain a CT or an MRI scan prior to lumbar puncture, following the scheme outlined in Fig. 31-4. However, when bacterial meningitis is suspected, antibiotic treatment should be initiated prior to sending the patient for a scan. When a CT or an MRI scan is not immediately available and there is a significant chance (as in suspected meningitis) that CSF analysis will affect treatment, then lumbar puncture should be performed without delay.

Lumbar puncture should not be performed through an area of cellulitis or abscess, to avoid spreading infection to the CSF. A bleeding diathesis is a relative contraindication [104]. When meningitis is suspected in a patient with a coagulopathy, rapid correction of the bleeding disorder prior to lumbar puncture is desirable. When that is not possible, lumbar puncture may still be performed, but careful attention subsequently should be paid to signs of an expanding spinal hematoma, which include the appearance of paraplegia, bladder incontinence, or pain following the procedure. Vagal cardiac arrests also have been reported following lumbar puncture. The most commonly reported complication of lumbar puncture is headache, which follows 10%–25% of the procedures and has been related to the size of the needle and the number of attempts [103].

Patients with bacterial meningitis usually have elevated opening CSF pressures during lumbar puncture (see Table 31-3). Normal opening pressures are 80–100 mm of water with 5–10 mm respiratory variation, but in meningitis the pressures commonly are 200–300 mm of water and may reach 600 mm even in the absence of a mass lesion [104]. CSF pressures are related to venous intracranial pressure and may also be elevated by intracranial venous sinus thrombosis, obstruction of the jugular veins or the superior vena cava, and congestive heart failure. Severe dehydration or circulatory collapse may decrease CSF pressure [104].

Sufficient CSF should be removed to obtain all the necessary tests to make a diagnosis. The fluid should be collected in four tubes in approximately the quantities shown in Fig. 31-4 and inspected for clarity. Normal CSF is crystal clear when viewed against a white background, but it may appear turbid with as few as 200–400 WBCs per microliter. Xanthochromia often indicates lysis of RBCs from previous subarachnoid hemorrhage. Clotting of the CSF is clearly abnormal and may be seen when the protein level is very high or with a traumatic tap.

A gram-stained specimen of CSF should be examined in the emergency department or the laboratory within a few minutes. A turbid specimen can be examined without centrifugation, while clear specimens should be spun down before staining. By the time most patients present with meningitis, more than 10^6 organisms per milliliter frequently are present, and this number can readily be seen on a gram-stained smear. An etiologic agent is revealed by Gram's stain in 60%–90% of cases [103]. Some laboratories use an acridine orange stain when a Gram's stain of CSF is negative, since that test may have increased sensitivity [105, 106]. Two-to-5-ml sample of CSF should be transported promptly to the laboratory for culture to facilitate diagnosis and document antibiotic sensitivities [107]. In cases of partially treated meningitis the laboratory should be notified so that methods, including prolonged incubation, can be used to improve culture yield.

The CSF glucose is usually low in bacterial meningitis, but it may be normal (see Fig. 31-2). The normal value for CSF glucose is 60%–70% of the serum glucose. This relationship holds until the CSF glucose reaches approximately 300 mg/dl, at which point the CSF concentration does not rise further. In a pediatric series a CSF-blood glucose ratio of 0.4 or less gave an 80% sensitivity and a 97% specificity for the diagnosis of bacterial meningitis [108]. In cases where exogenous glucose has been given intravenously, approximately 2 hours are required for equilibration across the blood-brain barrier. CSF glucose also may be reduced in nervous system involvement by *Mycoplasma pneumoniae*, viruses (e.g., mumps, herpes simplex), syphilis, mycobacteria, sarcoid, and subarachnoid hemorrhage. CSF protein is typically elevated in cases of bacterial meningitis (see Fig. 31-2) but the finding is nonspecific and may be seen in a variety of conditions. Infants under the age of 1 year will have higher normal values than adults. In cases of a traumatic lumbar puncture CSF protein is elevated

by approximately 1 mg/dl for each 1000 RBCs present [104].

CSF cell counts are helpful in the diagnosis of meningitis. Normally adults have 0–5 mononuclear cells per microliter and 0–2 PMNs per microliter [109]. The neonate may normally have up to 30 cells per microliter with 60% PMNs [110], while infants and small children may occasionally have up to 3 PMNs in the CSF in the absence of disease [111]. It is still useful, however, to set the normal value at zero for persons other than neonates and consider other factors such as the CSF Gram's stain, protein, and glucose in addition to the clinical setting when evaluating a patient for meningitis. In approximately 4% of patients with bacterial meningitis the CSF will show 0–25 polymorphonuclear cells per microliter [112–115]. This may occur when the lumbar puncture is performed early in the course of bacterial meningitis before an inflammatory response can develop, or when the patient is immunosuppressed from disease or drugs [116].

Immunologic tests are available to aid in the diagnosis and early treatment of bacterial meningitis. Tests such as latex agglutination, ELISA, and counterimmunoelectrophoresis can be performed on CSF, blood, or urine to identify soluble antigens from *S. pneumoniae*, *H. influenzae*, and *N. meningitidis* [117–121]. The main advantage to these tests is that they may be able to identify an organism within hours or when the patient is partially treated and the culture negative. Both false-negative and false-positive results can be a problem with these tests [105, 116, 117], resulting in some laboratories being reluctant to employ them.

Nonspecific tests have been described that may help distinguish bacterial from viral meningitis. These tests include elevated levels of CSF lactic acid, lactate dehydrogenase, amino acids, and C-reactive protein (CRP) [104]. The CRP may be elevated in both CSF and serum in pediatric patients with bacterial meningitis. Its main usefulness may be in the distinction between bacterial and viral meningitis in children [122, 123], but its usefulness in adults has been questioned [124].

Therapy. Despite the common acknowledgment that antibiotics should be given as early as possible in bacterial meningitis, there is often a significant delay before they are administered. In one study the time from presentation in the emergency department until antibiotics were administered in community acquired bacterial meningitis was 2.1 hours in pediatric cases and 4.9 hours in adult cases. The relative infrequency of meningitis in adults and the practice of getting CT scans before lumbar puncture were cited as reasons for the delay in treatment [125]. A CT scan is rarely needed in a patient presenting with fever and meningeal signs and should be performed only in the uncommon situation where there is also papilledema, coma, or focal signs. CT scanning, blood work, and other diagnostic procedures should never significantly delay treatment in cases where there is a clear diagnosis of bacterial meningitis. When there is a strong suspicion of meningitis, antibiotics should be ready for infusion as soon as the clinician has finished with the lumbar puncture, especially if the CSF is turbid. Antibiotics always should be initiated prior to the patient leaving the emergency department, since delays often occur during the admissions process.

Some patients will present to the emergency physician after previously receiving antibiotics or may need to be given antibiotics prior to a lumbar puncture being performed. Prior oral antibiotics can decrease the positive yield of CSF cultures by 4%–33% and of CSF Gram's stains 7%–41% [126]. CSF cell counts, glucose, and protein usually are not affected by pretreatment with antibiotics, but an occasional patient with bacterial meningitis and partial treatment will present with parameters suggestive of viral or aseptic meningitis [127]. After only 1–2 hours of intravenous antibiotics the majority of CSF cultures are still positive [126], but cultures obtained 24 hours after initial antibiotic administration are positive in only about 20% of cases. Periods of treatment shorter than 24 hours yield positive cultures somewhat more frequently [128, 129].

Another dilemma sometimes encountered by the emergency physician is when the CSF does not clearly indicate either a viral or a bacterial etiology. Although the majority of cases are fairly clear cut, there is some overlap between the two groups in the cell counts, glucose, and protein (see Fig. 31-2), especially when there is lymphocyte predominance in a patient who otherwise appears to have bacterial meningitis. Given the gravity of this disease, it is reasonable to initiate antibiotic treatment in questionable cases and observe the clinical course of the patient while awaiting final culture results. A repeat lumbar puncture in 8–12 hours may be useful in these cases to show if there is a persistent lymphocyte predominance and thus a likely viral etiology. When a viral etiology is demonstrated, the antibiotics may be stopped without a full course having been administered.

When the initial studies of the CSF permit the clear-cut identification of an organism, then antibiotic therapy should be directed at the offending bacteria. In most cases the causative organism initially will not be known to the emergency physician, and empiric antibiotic treatment will be necessary. The choice of antibiotics depends on the age of the patient, the presence of predisposing factors or underlying disease, and epidemiologic factors (see Table 31-4). Therapy should be bacteriocidal in the CSF, not bacteriostatic, when possible.

Many antibiotics penetrate the blood-brain barrier poorly under normal circumstances (Table 31-5). A few antibiotics achieve good CSF concentration with or without inflammation (chloramphenicol, trimethoprim-sulfamethoxazole, rifampin, metronidazole, and possibly some of the quinolones). Chloramphenicol and trimethoprim-sulfamethoxazole are present in concentrations of 30%–50% of serum. When the meninges are inflamed, the penetration of many antibiotics is improved. This is particularly true of penicillins and selected cephalosporins. Several third-generation cephalosporins, penicillins, vancomycin, erythromycin, and tetracycline penetrate fairly well into the CSF in meningitis (See Table 31-5). Aminoglycosides occasionally are given intraventricularly to be effective since they do not predictably penetrate into the CSF (except in the neonate).

Treatment of meningitis in the neonate and infant up to 1 month old is directed toward organisms that generally are acquired during delivery. These organisms include group B streptococcus, *E. coli*, *Listeria monocytogenes*, and miscellaneous gram-negative organisms (*Klebsiella* species, *Serrata* species, *Proteus* species, and *Enterobacter* species). Empiric therapy in this group (Table 31-6) could include ampicillin plus either an aminoglycoside or a

Table 31-5. Penetration of antibiotics into the CNS

| | Penetration | | | |
| | CSF | | | |
Antibiotic	Normal meninges	Meningitis	Brain tissue	Brain abscess
Penicillins				
Penicillin G	Poor	Fair–good	Poor–good	Poor–good
Ampicillin	Poor	Fair–good	Poor	Poor–fair
Carbenicillin	Poor	—	—	—
Methicillin	Poor	—	—	Fair–good
Nafcillin	—	Fair	—	—
Cephalosporins				
Cephalothin	Poor	Poor–fair	Fair	—
Cefazolin	Poor	Fair–good	—	—
Cefotaxime	Good	Good	—	—
Ceftriaxone	Good	Good	—	—
Ceftazidime	Good	Good	—	—
Aminoglycosides				
Gentamicin	Poor	Fair	—	—
Amikacin	—	Poor	—	—
Tetracyclines				
Tetracycline	—	Fair	—	—
Oxytetracycline	—	Poor	Poor	—
Chlortetracycline	—	Poor	Poor	—
Doxycyaline	Fair–good	—	—	—
Dimethylchlortetracycline	Poor	—	—	—
Miscellaneous antibacterials				
Chloramphenicol	Good	Good	Good	Fair
Clindamycin	Poor	Fair	—	Good
Metronidazole	—	Good	—	Good
Trimethoprim	Good	Good	Poor	Good
Sulfonamides	Fair–good	Good	Poor	—
Rifampin	Fair	Good	—	—
Polymyxin B	Poor	Poor	—	—
Vancomycin	Poor	Good	—	—
Erythromycin	Poor	Poor–fair	—	—
Ciprofloxacin	Fair	Fair	—	—

third-generation cephalosporin such as ceftazidime, cefotaxime, or ceftriaxone [95]. If an aminoglycoside is selected, it should be given intravenously because of a higher mortality rate with intrathecal therapy in this age group [130]. Gentamicin is often the first-line aminoglycoside, but amikacin or tobramycin may be substituted if resistance is a problem in the environment [95]. Third-generation cephalosporins should not be used alone in this age group because of their poor activity against *L. monocytogenes* and enterococcus [131]. Ampicillin should be added to cover those organ-

isms. In the 1-month to 3-month age group similar organisms need to be covered. *H. influenzae*, *S. pneumoniae*, and *N. meningitidis*, however, also become a possibility. An appropriate regimen would be the combination of ampicillin plus cefotaxime or ceftriaxone. An alternative in this group might be ampicillin plus chloramphenicol. It should be remembered, however, that chloramphenicol is bacteriostatic for only gram-negative enteric bacilli [78]. For children 3 months to 10 years of age treatment is directed at *H. influenzae*, *S. pneumoniae*, and *N. meningitidis*. Traditional therapy for

Table 31-6. Initial treatment of bacterial meningitis in selected groups

Setting	First choice	Alternative
0–1 month	Ampicillin, first week of life: 50–100 mg/kg/day; age 1 week to 1 month: 150–200 mg/kg/day *plus* aminoglycoside (dose to be determined by renal function)	Ampicillin *plus* cefotaxime 100 mg/kg/day or ceftazidime 60 mg/kg/day
1–3 months	Ampicillin 300–400 mg/kg/day *plus* cefotaxime 150 mg/kg/day or ceftriaxone 100 mg/kg/day	Ampicillin *plus* chloramphenicol 50–100 mg/kg/day; aminoglycoside if gram-negative bacillus suspected.
3 months–5 years	Ceftriaxone 100 mg/kg/day or cefotaxime 150–180 mg/kg/day	Ampicillin 300–400 mg/kg/day *plus* chloramphenicol 50–100
> 5 years	Ampicillin 300–400 mg/kg/day or penicillin 100,000–500,000 U/kg/day	Ceftriaxone 100 mg/kg/day or cefotaxime 150–180 mg/kg/day
> than 60 years Alcoholic	Ampicillin (some physicians would add ceftriaxone 4 gm/day or cefotaxime 8 gm/day or ceftazidime 6 gm/day)	Aztreonam 6–8 gm/day plus TMP/SMX 10 mg/kg/day (based on trimethoprim component)
Penetrating injury	Methicillin 250–300 mg/kg/day or nafcillin 150–200 mg/kg/day *plus* aminoglycoside 3–5 mg/kg/day	Vancomycin 2 gm/day in adult with normal renal function plus ceftazidime or ceftriaxone
Infected intra-ventricular device	Vancomycin 40–60 mg/kg/day (in infant) or 2 gm/day (in adult) plus rifampin at 10 mg/kg/day to maximum of 600 mg/day	None Vancomycin *plus* ceftriaxone or ceftazidine or cefotaxime (at above dosages)
Immunosuppressed individual	Ceftriaxone or ceftazidine plus aminoglycoside (at above dosages)	
Penicillin and cephalosporin allergy	Chloramphenicol 50–100 mg/kg/day can be substituted for penicillin, ampicillin, methicillin, nafcillin, ceftriaxone, ceftazidime or cefotaxime in allergic individuals	Aztreonam, vancomycin *plus* TMP/SMX at above dosages

this age group has been ampicillin plus chloramphenicol. Treatment with selected second- or third-generation cephalosporins, however, is just as effective [132]. Cefuroxime, cefotaxime, and ceftriaxone are all appropriate, although cefuroxime is less active on a weight basis against *H. influenzae* [95]. The use of one of these agents avoids the toxicity of chloramphenicol. In addition chloramphenicol-resistant and ampicillin-resistant *H. influenzae* have been reported [133].

In older children and young adults (10 to 50 years of age) empiric therapy should be directed at *S. pneumoniae* and *N. meningitidis*. Ampicillin or penicillin G will adequately cover those organisms, although approximately 2% of them are resistant to penicillin. *H. influenzae* meningitis is rare in adults but is thought to be increasing. For that reason ampicillin may have a slight advantage. Third-generation cephalosporins are also an alternative in

this population and would be considered by some clinicians as appropriate primary therapy [134]. Although *S. pneumoniae* is the most common cause of meningitis in the elderly, *Listeria* organisms and enteric gram-negative bacilli are also a concern [74]. Ampicillin alone or ampicillin plus a third-generation cephalosporin (cefotaxime, ceftriaxone, or ceftazidime) is the treatment of choice [131]. Gram-negative meningitis acquired in the hospital or after neurosurgery may involve resistant organisms [75, 78]. Reasonable coverage would be a third-generation cephalosporin combined with trimethoprim-sulfamethoxazole or an aminoglycoside [78]. The aminoglycoside should be given both intravenously and intrathecally. If available a preservative-free aminoglycoside should be used for intrathecal administration. If staphylococcal coverage is deemed necessary, for example, in IV drug abusers or situations following CNS trauma or surgery, nafcillin or vancomycin may be combined with a third-generation cephalosporin. Empiric treatment strategies of patients with immunosuppression, ventriculo-peritoneal shunts, and other conditions are summarized in Table 31-6.

It is thought that inflammation continues to involve the CNS even after and sometimes as a result of antibiotic administration. Bacterial lysis and death releases inflammatory endotoxins and cell-wall debris, which results in continued tissue damage. This continuing damage may be limited in certain circumstances by the use of corticosteroids [135]. A recent study has suggested that dexamethasone in dosage of 0.15 mg/kg q6h during the first 4 days may reduce the severity of hearing loss in children with *H. influenzae* meningitis [132]. Other ways that have been proposed to reduce inflammation include the development of (1) nonlytic antibiotics, (2) products to capture the cell wall, such as polymyxin B and antibodies, and (3) antibodies to block leukocyte adherence to endothelia [135]. None of these is well enough developed for general use at the present time.

Disposition. Patients with bacterial meningitis must always be admitted to a hospital ward for IV antibiotics, observation, and supportive care. There is no role for oral or intramuscular antibiotics in the treatment of this disease in the United States. Intensive care frequently is required for management of hemodynamic instability, altered mental status, seizures, increased intracranial pressure, or threatened airway. The decision to transfer a patient to another facility should be made solely on the basis of the existence of capabilities at the receiving hospital that are not available at the referring institution. In general that means intensive care unit facilities (neonatal, pediatric, or adult). Lumbar puncture should be obtained prior to transfer when possible, and samples of CSF should be cultured and sent with the patient. Appropriate doses of antibiotics always should be given prior to transfer, even if lumbar puncture cannot be obtained [134]. Serious consideration should be given to endotracheal tube placement prior to transfer in a comatose patient. At least one IV line should be established and another may be necessary if several medications are to be given en route. If the patient has had one or more seizures, it is appropriate to give a loading dose of phenytoin prior to transfer, and plans for treatment of recurrent seizures should be discussed with the accompanying personnel. The out-of-hospital time should be minimized, which may mean using a helicopter or fixed-wing air transport. Critically ill or intubated patients and those receiving IV medications will need a paramedic, nurse, or physician present during transport.

Complications. In general the course of untreated bacterial meningitis is rapid, with progressive deterioration of neurologic function. With progression the brain swells, intracranial pressure increases, and coma, hypertension, bradycardia, third-nerve palsy, and seizures may be observed [66]. Focal cerebral signs such as hemiparesis also may occur in a small percentage of patients. Papilledema is unusual in this setting. Patients presenting with signs and symptoms of increased intracranial pressure should be considered for endotracheal intubation and hyperventilation. Twenty percent mannitol may also be given intravenously (1–2 gm/kg) over 20–60 minutes. IV dexamethasone may also be appropriate in this setting. An intracranial pressure monitoring device may be necessary.

Seizures complicate the course of meningitis in 20%–30% of cases. Seizures are particularly common in the pediatric age group [66]. Generalized seizures presenting after the first 72 hours or focal seizures presenting at any time may represent underlying cerebral damage [68]. In the acute setting seizures are treated with appropriate doses of diazepam, lorazepam, phenobarbital, and/or phenytoin. Cranial nerve abnormalities occur in 10%–20% of patients. Cranial nerves III, IV, VI, and VII most commonly are involved [68, 82]. Sensorineural hearing loss is common in children over 3 years and may be bilateral [67, 132]. Subdural effusions can occur in children under 18 months of age. In general they resolve spontaneously but should be drained if there is a suspicion that they are infected, the head circumference is rapidly enlarging, or there is evidence of increased intracranial pressure. CT scanning may be helpful in evaluating these collections. The syndrome of inappropriate antidiuretic hormone (SIADH) secretion may also occur, and fluid intake is generally restricted the first few days while electrolytes are monitored. Neonates are particularly prone to this complication [95].

Chemoprophylaxis. Secondary cases of meningitis may occur with *N. meningitidis* and *H. influenzae* meningitis. Chemoprophylaxis may be indicated for those exposed to a patient with meningitis from either organism. The goal of prophylaxis is to eliminate the nasopharyngeal carrier state. The antibiotics commonly used to treat infections caused by these organisms may not be effective in eliminating the carrier state. Following a case of meningococcal meningitis, prophylaxis is indicated for the following individuals: (1) hospital personnel with contact with respiratory secretions from the index case, (2) day-care or school contacts, (3) household contacts, and (4) the index case on completion of parenteral therapy for invasive disease. Generally rifampin is used, although sulfadiazine and minocycline are alternatives [136]. The dosages of these antibiotics are listed in Table 31-7.

Rifampin is also used to eradicate the carrier state of *H. influenzae* type B. If a household includes one child under the age of 4 years other than the index case, then prophylaxis for all household contacts (children and adults) is indicated [137]. The index case should also receive rifampin upon completion of parenteral therapy. Ultimately vaccination of infants against *H. influenzae* type B may provide the best protection against bacterial meningitis [138].

AMEBIC MENINGOENCEPHALITIS

A fatal form of meningoencephalitis may be caused by amebae classified as *N. fowleri* and *Acanthamoeba* (previously called *Hartmannella*). There have been well over 100 reported cases of *Naegleria* brain infection and somewhat fewer cases of disease due to *Acanthamoeba* organisms [139].

Naegleria organisms cause an illness referred to as primary amebic meningoencephalitis (PAM) [10]. Many of the individuals with *Naegleria* infection have reported swimming in fresh or brackish water 5–15 days preceding the onset of symptoms. A number of these people have been healthy young individuals who dived deeply into the water [140]. It is thought that the organisms entered the brain by following olfactory nerves through the cribriform plate. *Acanthamoeba* infection is not preceded by swimming, and the disease typically progresses more slowly over several weeks. Granulomatous amebic encephalitis (GAE) due to *Acanthamoeba* infection seems to be caused by hematogenous spread to the brain as well as other organs of the body [2, 141, 142].

Presentation. With *Naegleria* infection there may be severe persistent bifrontal headache, fever, nausea, and vomiting. There also may be an associated rhinitis or pharyngitis. These initial non-specific symptoms may be replaced by seizures, ataxia, diplopia, bizarre behavior, and coma [143]. Some patients have complained of abnormalities in taste and smell. The disease tends to progress over days in a moderately acute manner. *Acanthamoeba* infections progress more insidiously without preceding rhinitis or pharyngitis and with no abnormalities in taste or smell [144]. With *Naegleria* infections there may be redness or necrosis of the nasal mucosa. Nucal rigidity is common, and there may be focal neurologic signs or a depressed state of consciousness.

Table 31-7. Chemoprophylaxis of close contacts

Organism	Drug	Age	Dosage
N. meningitidis	Rifampin	<1 month	5mg/kg q12h for 2 days
		1 month–12 years	10 mg/kg q12h for 2 days
		> 12 years	600 mg q12h for 2 days
	Sulfadiazine	<1 year	500 mg q24h for 2 days
		1–12 years	500 mg q12h for 2 days
		> 12 years	1 g q12h for 2 days
	Minocy-cline	>12 years	100 mg q12h for 5 days
H. influenzae	Rifampin	0–12 years	20 mg/kg (max. 600 mg) q24h for 4 days
		>12 years	600 mg q24h for 4 days

Peripheral leukocytosis is common. The CSF may have an elevated opening pressure, increased protein, variably decreased glucose, and several thousand WBCs that are predominantly PMNs. The fluid also may contain RBCs. The diagnosis usually is made by identifying amebae in the CSF by high-power microscopic examination [140]. Unless the disease is carefully considered, the organisms may be misinterpreted as WBCs, although if carefully observed they have ameboid movements even at room temperature. Their movement is more apparent on warming of the slide. The amebae can be identified when stained with hematoxylin and eosin, Wright's stain, or Gram's stain [139, 140].

Differential Diagnosis. The disease has commonly been initially misdiagnosed as bacterial, fungal, tuberculous, or viral meningitis.

Therapy. The disease has a high mortality rate, and treatment usually has been ineffective. Studies in experimental animals and experience in a few human patients have shown that amphotericin B alone or a combination of amphotericin B and either tetracycline or miconazole may be effective against *Naegleria* [144, 145]. No treatment has been curative in *Acanthameba* CNS infections [146]. Treatment has been successful in a human when combined IV and intrathecal therapy with amphotericin B, miconazole, and rifampin has been administered [139, 144]. Antiparasitic therapy has been disappointing.

Subacute Meningitis

Meningitis may occasionally follow a subacute or indolent course, with the person being ill for weeks or months before the disease is sufficiently advanced to lead to diagnostic evaluation [147, 148]. These patients typically have fever and stiff neck and may have headache, lethargy, confusion, nausea, or vomiting. Although an infectious agent is most commonly responsible for subacute meningitis, a large variety of organisms and noninfectious causes need to be considered (Table 31-8). In most instances, the CSF shows pleocytosis, elevated protein, and decreased glucose. Mononuclear cells are likely to predominate, although some patients have large numbers of polymorphonuclear leukocytes in the CSF. The organisms commonly

Table 31-8. Causes of subacute meningitis

Bacteria
  Pyogenic (partially treated)
  Tuberculosis
  Syphilis
  Brucellosis
  Leptospirosis
  Lyme disease
Higher Bacteria
  Actinomycosis
  Nocardiosis
Fungus
  Cryptococcosis
  Coccidioidomycosis
  Histoplasmosis
  Blastomycosis
Protozoa and helminthic meningitis
  Toxoplasmosis
  Cysticercosis
  Echinococcosis
Neoplastic
  Primary CNS tumors
  Metastatic tumors to meninges
Unknown etiologies
  Vogt-Koyanagi-Harada syndrome
  Behçet's disease
  Granulomatous angiitis
  Chronic benign lymphocytic meningitis
  Mollaret's meningitis
  Sarcoidosis
  Epidermoid cyst

grow slowly on culture, but some of the diseases may be diagnosed more rapidly by the use of serologic tests to identify soluble antigen or antibody to the organisms.

Evaluation of a patient for the cause of subacute meningitis involves a variety of studies. Chest x-ray and a CT or an MRI scan of the head usually are indicated. Skin tests should be performed with purified protein derivative (PPD) for tuberculosis, and other control tests should be applied to identify anergy if present. Serologic studies of serum should include measuring antibody to brucella, syphilis, toxoplasma, *Coccidioides immitis*, Lyme disease, and HIV. CSF should have the opening pressure determined, cells enumerated, protein and glucose levels measured, and a VDRL serologic test for syphilis performed. The fluid should be examined for malignant cells by cytology. Cryptococcal antigen should be looked for, and coccidioides and Lyme disease antibody should be sought. Cultures should be performed for bacteria, brucella, tuberculosis, and fungi. Repeat examinations of the CSF commonly are required. Blood and urine should be examined routinely, and it may be necessary to culture sputum and gastric aspirate for tuberculosis and to perform bone marrow biopsy or biopsy of lesions identified elsewhere in the body.

TUBERCULOUS MENINGITIS

Most tuberculous infections originally are acquired through a respiratory route. A brief bacillemia frequently occurs, and many parts of the body are seeded. Seeding of the brain may lead to the development of small granulomas called Rich's foci [149]. The organisms contained in these foci may remain inactive for life or they may rupture, discharging living mycobacteria into the CSF, which then cause meningitis. Tuberculous infection of the brain usually involves the leptomeninges and occasionally the ventricular system and choroid plexus. The exudate is most intense in the basal cisterns and may also spread along the sylvian fissures. An initial semipurulent exudate may become thick or fibrotic, which protects organisms harbored therein from antibiotics. The exudate may also lead to hydrocephalus. Tuberculous meningitis continues to occur with disturbing frequency, and the diagnosis is complicated by the fact that organisms grow slowly and may take as long as 6 weeks to grow.

Predisposing Factors. Persons at high risk include those who are at risk for developing other forms of tuberculosis, including alcoholics and individuals immunosuppressed by malignancy, immunosuppressive therapy, or HIV infection. The disease also appears to be more common in Native Americans. The occurrence of tuberculous meningitis in childhood used to be very common, but it is now rare [150–152]. Cases often occur many years after the primary infection and are due to late breakdown of granulomas resulting from the waning cellular immunity of aging or other immunosuppressive conditions [153].

Presentation. The onset of symptoms is frequently insidious over 1–3 weeks or even longer [147, 149]. Neck stiffness is not initially prominent but the person may become listless and irritable and fatigue easily. Anorexia, vomiting, malaise, and

headache are frequent. The fever is commonly low grade and may not be accompanied by night sweats, as is typical of active pulmonary tuberculosis. Meningeal signs gradually become prominent, and eventually confusion, coma, seizures, and focal neurologic signs may develop. Examination of the fundi may reveal choroidal tubercules. There may be signs of hyponatremia due to inappropriate antidiuretic hormone secretion.

The CSF usually has leukocytes present, but there are seldom more than a few hundred WBCs per microliter. Lymphocytes commonly predominate, although there is often a mixture of lymphocytes and neutrophils, with neutrophils occasionally predominating [51, 154] (see Fig. 31-2). The CSF protein is typically elevated and glucose depressed. CSF chloride used to be measured, but it is seldom helpful. Positive acid-fast organisms are found on smears of the CSF in only 10%–20% of proved cases [154–157]. Culture using specialized media requires 2–6 weeks, and not all individuals who respond clinically to antituberculosis therapy prove to have positive CSF cultures. Due to the slowness with which the organisms grow in culture and the fact that as many as 40% of patients with clinical evidence of tuberculous meningitis have negative cultures [158, 159], there has been a great deal of interest in developing techniques to identify tuberculous antigens on DNA or to detect antibody to components of the organism in CSF [160]. Currently the leading candidate for a clinically useful test appears to be examination of CSF for tuberculostearic acid, which is performed by the CDC [161]. Chest x-rays should be performed; they suggest old or active tuberculosis in 50% or more of cases. Tuberculin skin tests with PPD are positive in 80%–85% of cases, but the results may be negative in persons with disseminated or overwhelming tuberculosis and in persons who are malnourished or who have had recent viral infections such as measles and influenza [151, 153, 155].

Therapy. The results of therapy for tuberculous meningitis are superior when treatment is started at an early stage. Due to the slowness of currently available diagnostic tests and the frequency with which they may be falsely negative, it seems prudent to start therapy when the diagnosis is suspected and when the appropriate diagnostic studies have been obtained for cultural purposes and to rule out other diagnoses. Tuberculous infections require the use of more than one drug for treatment, since the use of single drugs frequently induces resistance in the organism. Current therapy for tuberculous meningitis usually consists of at least isoniazid and rifampin, both of which cross the blood-brain barrier quite well. Streptomycin or pyrazinamide are often added, although they may pass the blood-brain barrier poorly. Other drugs that may be used include ethambutol and ethionamide. These drugs and their dosages are listed in Table 31-9. The use of corticosteroids has been reported in several studies, but conclusions about their value are not uniform [162–164]. Their use in low dosages may help in patients with cerebral edema, but the value otherwise is questionable. Traditionally therapy is continued for 18–24 months, but some regimens using multiple drugs may be curative after as short a time as 9 months of treatment.

The outcome of tuberculous meningitis depends on how early in the course of disease treatment is begun. Death is common when the disease is advanced and major neurologic deficits are present [152]. Hyponatremia, seizures, hemiplegia, and ophthalmoplegia are not uncommon during treatment. There may also be facial paralysis, blindness, or deafness. Complete resolution of all manifestations occurs in less than one-half of those who are treated. Residual neurologic abnormalities may include cranial nerve deficits, hemiplegia, cerebellar dysfunction, hydrocephalus, and psychomotor retardation [165]. Hydrocephalus may be treatable by surgical placement of a shunt to drain the CSF into the atrium or the peritoneum [166]. Relapses after adequate treatment are uncommon.

CRYPTOCOCCAL MENINGITIS

Cryptococcus neoformans are encapsulated yeasts that inhabit soil, particularly soil contaminated by pigeon droppings. Pigeons carry the organisms on their beaks and feet and may contaminate their excreta during defecation. Although now commonly referred to as cryptococci, the organisms used to be called *Torula*. The infection is usually acquired through the lung, but the lung is seldom a site of major pathology [167, 168]. Dissemination to other sites may occur, and in most organs other than the CNS the cryptococci are relatively well

contained. In the CNS, however, the organisms produce a large protective capsule that induces little inflammatory reaction, so they are able to proliferate quite freely. The initial reaction that occurs is a lymphocytic leptomeningitis with free capsular polysaccharide being liberated into the CSF. The organisms may penetrate into the brain substance, where they form cysts containing mucoid material and intact organisms.

Predisposing Factors. Cryptococcal meningitis occurs more often in men than women, and most of the patients are over 40 years of age. Infection of the CNS is more likely to occur in renal transplant recipients, patients with leukemia, malignant lymphoma, or Hodgkin's disease, and in immunosuppressed persons, especially those treated with large doses of steroids and those who have AIDS [167, 168].

Presentation. The onset of the disease is slower than that of tuberculous meningitis and may follow a course with wide fluctuation in intensity of symptoms [167]. The most common complaint is headache, but nausea, vomiting, disturbances of consciousness and orientation, signs of meningeal irritation, cranial nerve involvement, pathologic reflexes, and loss of hearing are also common. About one-half of the patients are febrile. Severely immunocompromised individuals may have a rapid onset of the disease.

The disease should be suspected in patients with a subacute course of meningitis, especially if they are immunocompromised. Lumbar puncture usually reveals an elevated opening pressure, elevated protein, and lymphocytic pleocytosis. Glucose is decreased in 50% of patients. The organisms may be seen on direct microscopic examination, but they are often misinterpreted as lymphocytes. If India ink is added to the CSF, budding encapsulated yeasts may be found in over one-half of the cases. Cytologic stains, including Papanicolaou's stain, may give positive results [169]. Cultures from the CSF may also be positive. There are reports of the organisms being found in cisternal CSF when they were not present in the lumbar CSF [170]. The laboratory must be warned that fungi may be present, or the cultures otherwise may not be held long enough. The organisms may often be found in the

Table 31-9. Antituberculous drugs useful in treatment of tuberculous meningitis

Drug	CSF penetration	Dosage	Route	Toxicity
Used Frequently				
Isoniazid	Good	20 mg/kg/day (max. 600 mg/day)	PO	Hepatic
Rifampin	Good	15 mg/kg/day (max. 600 mg/day)	PO	Hepatic
Streptomycin	Poor	20 mg/kg/day (max. 1 g/day)	IM	Renal and vestibular
Used Less Often				
Ethambutol	Fair with meningitis	15–25 mg/kg/day for the first month, then 15 mg/kg/day	PO	Optic nerve
Ethionamide	Good	250 mg bid, then increase to 1 g/day maximum	PO	Varied, involving GI tract, postural hypotension, peripheral neuropathy, seizures
Cycloserine	Good	250 mg bid	PO	CNS

urine and blood or sputum of patients with meningitis. Serologic studies to examine spinal fluid, blood, and urine for cryptococcal antigen can be extremely useful. Latex agglutination or complement-fixation tests can be performed in a day, and serum or CSF antigen demonstrated in over 90% of persons with active cryptococcal meningitis [171, 172].

Therapy. The disease was regularly fatal prior to the introduction of antifungal therapy, but now more than one-half of patients survive [168, 170, 173]. Amphotericin B has been the traditional mainstay of therapy, but it is difficult to use since it predictably decreases renal function and frequently causes nausea, vomiting, chills, fever, and phlebitis [174–178]. The addition of 5-fluorocytosine has improved survival but adds additional complications, including leukopenia, thrombocytopenia, and enterocolitis [179, 180]. Because the drug is renally excreted, high levels may accumulate when amphotericin B leads to renal impairment. Frequent monitoring of blood levels of 5-fluorocytosine is desirable for reducing the frequency of this complication. Some studies have suggested that intravenous and intraventricular miconazole or oral fluconazole may be effective. Oral fluconazole appears to be as effective as intravenous amphotericin B. The CSF cells, proteins, and glucose return to normal, and the organisms and cryptococcal antigen are cleared slowly with successful treatment. Table 31-10 summarizes the treatment of fungal meningitis.

Advanced or disseminated disease at the initiation of therapy is a sign of poor prognosis. Other patients who are less likely to do well include those with AIDS, lymphoreticular malignancy, corticosteroid therapy, high opening pressure on lumbar puncture, markedly depressed CSF glucose level, many cryptococci seen on smear, cryptococci isolated from extraneural sites, or a high titer of cryptococcal antigen in CSF or serum [181]. Of persons who survive, some will experience relapse after completion of therapy.

COCCIDIOIDAL MENINGITIS

C. immitis is a fungus found in the southwestern United States, northern Mexico, Central America, and South America [182]. The fungus lives in soil in the "lower Sonoran life zone" in a mycelial-

Table 31-10. Treatment of fungal meningitis

Amphotericin B
IV 0.5–1.0 mg/kg/day:
   Begin with 1 mg/day and slowly increase dose to 50–100 mg every other day.
   Try to achieve plasma amphotericin B level twice the minimum serum killing level of the cultured fungus.
   Monitor BUN and creatinine clearance.
   Premedication with aspirin, benadryl, thorazine, and hydrocortisone IV may help minimize side effects.
   Therapy should last 1–3 months with total dose 1–3 g.
Intrathecal 0.2–0.5 mg three times a week:
   Use a cisternal reservoir, if possible. Intrathecal injection allows for lower dosage, but CNS side effects are worse.
Major toxicity:
   Immediate reactions of chills, fever, nausea, and phlebitis at site of injection; nephrotoxicity; normocytic, normochromic anemia; shock, seizures, cardiac arrhythmias may occur.

5-Fluorocytosine
Oral: 150 mg/kg/day in four divided doses.
Major toxicity: Diarrhea, hallucinations, SGOT elevation, bone marrow suppression.

Fluconazole
Oral or intravenous: In adults 400 mg initially, followed by 200 mg once daily for acute disease. Oral absorption excellent. Long-term maintenance with 200 mg PO each day for preventing relapse of cryptococcal meningitis in AIDS.
Major toxicity: Hepatic dysfunction, skin rash.

arthrospore form that is highly infectious to nonimmune individuals. There is also a spherule-endospore form, which is isolated from infected persons but is not infectious to others.

Predisposing Factors. Humans may inhale the arthrospores, especially when dry late-summer winds lead to airborne dust or when construction has disturbed the soil. Infection, which is often asymptomatic, is common in persons who live in heavily contaminated areas such as the San Joaquin Valley in California and portions of Arizona. Even transient exposure while traveling through such areas may result in clinically apparent disease. There appears to be increased susceptibility to disseminated disease in blacks, Filipinos, and pregnant women [182].

Presentation. The initial infection of the pulmonary tract is asymptomatic in over one-half of infected individuals, but others may develop various manifestations referred to as "valley fever" [182]. This form of the disease is characterized by mild influenza-like symptoms, or there may be severe pneumonia. Erythema nodosum is common, but other manifestations may include erythema multiforme, arthralgias, and meningismus. Most patients recover spontaneously, but a few develop chronic pulmonary forms of the disease with residual nodules or cavities. Rarely the disease may disseminate to the meninges with the resulting meningitis characterized by headaches, mild nuchal rigidity, lethargy, malaise, confusion, personality changes, and cranial nerve palsies, which may be present in various degrees for 1–6 months before the diagnosis is made [183, 184]. Hydrocephalus, which may be noncommunicating or communicating, may lead to obtundation, papilledema, and other neurologic findings. There may be various skin manifestations such as verrucous granulomas, subcutaneous abscesses, or indolent ulcers.

Eosinophilia is common in the blood or in tissue biopsies. Lumbar CSF shows pleocytosis, which usually has a predominance of mononuclear cells, but occasionally eosinophiles are also present. The protein is elevated and glucose depressed. Skin tests for coccidioidomycosis, which are customarily positive early in the infection, usually become negative with meningitis and other disseminated disease. This anergy may be specific only for *Coccidioides* antigens. Two available skin-testing antigens include coccidioidin and the more reactive spherulin. Lack of reactivity to 1:100 coccidioidin is the standard for determining anergy [182]. Several serologic tests are available, but the serum complement-fixation test for measuring IgG antibody to coccidioidomycosis usually shows a titer higher than 1:16 with meningitis or other disseminated disease due to the organism. Patients with meningitis also frequently have a positive CSF complement-fixation test. The height of the titer corresponds roughly with the extent of disease, and titer decreases during treatment suggest therapeutic success. It is important to culture the CSF for the organism, but it is recovered in only 20%–40% of cases with meningitis, thus indicating a need for biopsy and culture of any other site where the organism may be found, including urine, in all individuals in whom the diagnosis is suspected, and sputum or lung biopsies in persons with pulmonary lesions and any skin lesions.

Therapy. Treatment is important since untreated individuals usually die within 2 years. IV amphotericin B is considered by many to be the drug of choice, although toxicity with this drug presents serious constraints to its use [174–178]. Treatment is begun with 1 mg IV, which is increased on a daily basis until 40–60 mg is being administered daily or every other day (see Table 31-10). Chills, fever, and phlebitis may occur, but renal toxicity is the major factor preventing administration of quantities that might be curative. Intrathecal administration of amphotericin B is often added to IV therapy. The decision to use intrathecal therapy commonly is based on an inadequate response to IV therapy. The drug may be injected into the cisterna magna or placed in an Ommaya reservoir that allows injection of the drug directly into a lateral ventricle. The initial intraventricular dose is usually about 0.025 mg/day, which can be increased until 0.5 or 1 mg is administered several times per week. Intrathecal use of the drug may lead to seizures, elevated CSF protein and cells, and a decrease in glucose levels. After several weeks of treatment the IV drug may be stopped and the frequency of intrathecal injections decreased to once every week or two. One guide for determining the frequency of intrathecal injections can be following the CSF complement-fixation titer. Intrathecal treatment given weekly, biweekly, or monthly may be necessary for the remainder of the patient's life.

Recently available imidazole drugs are effective against the organism and may have a role in the treatment of coccidioidal meningitis. These drugs, including miconazole, ketoconazole, and fluconazole, are all less toxic than amphotericin B.

OTHER FUNGAL MENINGITIDES
Histoplasma capsulatum occurs in the soil of central and southeastern United States, particularly near the great river basins. The organism commonly infects individuals living in the area but usually in an asymptomatic pulmonary form. Dissemination

involving the CNS is not common [185] and may be in the form of meningitis, focal cerebritis, or spinal cord compression [186, 187]. Clinical features of *Histoplasma* meningitis do not differ greatly from those due to cryptococcus. The organism is not readily recovered from the CSF, and serologic studies are only variably helpful. Recently *Histoplasma* antigen has been found in the CSF in several infected individuals, and this test together with antibody studies of the CSF may prove to be the most valuable diagnostic study [187]. Because histoplasmosis of the CNS can progress, it should be treated with amphotericin B when diagnosed (see Table 31-10). Treatment has the potential for being curative.

Candida albicans and other candida are commonly found worldwide and are frequent causes of candidemia, especially in immunosuppressed patients receiving prolonged IV therapy. Meningitis occurs infrequently during candidemia and is more common in immunocompromised persons [188]. The manifestations are usually subacute but may be more acute in severely immunocompromised individuals. The CSF usually has a pleocytosis with less than 500 WBCs per microliter, and in one-half of the cases the glucose is low and the protein high. Candida may be seen on a smear of the CSF in about one-half of the cases, but cultures are usually positive, with the organism growing in 24–72 hours. Amphotericin B is the standard treatment for disseminated candidiasis with meningitis. The addition of 5-fluorocytosine, which penetrates well into the CSF, has been successful. Miconazole, ketoconazole, and fluconazole may have roles in treating this disease [189] (see Table 31-10).

Other fungi reported to cause meningitis include *Torulopsis glabrata, Blastomyces dermatitidis, Paracoccidioides brasiliensis, Aspergillus* species, and *Sporothrix schenckii.*

LEPTOSPIROSIS

Leptospira is a common organism found in dogs, rodents, cattle, and swine, where it may be present without causing apparent illness. It is relatively infrequent for the organism to cause disease in humans, but when it does cause disease several organ systems, including the CNS, are involved [190]. There are several serogroups, which include *Leptospira icterohaemorrhagica, Leptospira canicola,* *Leptospira pamona, Leptospira autumnalis,* and *Leptospira australis.*

Leptospirosis has two phases, which may merge or be distinct [191]. In the first phase the organisms are present in the blood and the CSF without a detectable host response [192]. In the second, more symptomatic phase there is a major host inflammatory response, but the organisms may no longer be found.

Epidemiology. Human leptospirosis in the United States usually occurs in the summer and autumn months following contact with infected urine or ingestion of urine-contaminated water. Persons at risk include those whose occupation or recreational activities bring them in contact with such a source of infection.

Presentation. The first manifestations of disease occur 7–13 days after infection. The first phase of the illness, which lasts approximately a week, is characterized by fever and malaise with nonspecific systemic symptoms [192]. The second phase may follow immediately or after a delay of several days and is characterized by fever, headache, muscular pain or tenderness, nausea, vomiting, anorexia, meningeal signs, and uveitis [193]. Conjunctival suffusion occurs in one-third of cases, and meningeal signs are present in two-thirds. Jaundice is common. Clinical manifestations may be absent even when there is spinal fluid pleocytosis.

Laboratory studies commonly show pyuria, hematuria, and abnormal liver function tests. CSF findings resemble those of viral meningitis with normal pressure and glucose and increased protein and cells, predominantly lymphocytes. Early in the disease polymorphonuclear leukocytes may predominate in the CSF. The CSF also may be xanthochromic. Attempts to isolate the organism by culture are not useful in the clinical setting. IgM antibodies to the infecting organism may be present at the time when meningeal symptoms appear. A macroscopic slide agglutination and microscopic agglutination tests are available, and a fourfold or greater increase in titer establishes the diagnosis. Since an initial titer is not usually available, a presumptive diagnosis may be made when the slide test is positive and the microscopic agglutination titer is 1:200 or greater.

Therapy. Either penicillin G 2.4 million–3.6 million U/day parenterally) or tetracyclines (2 g/day PO in divided doses) are used in acute stages of the disease, but it is doubtful that antibiotic therapy significantly alters the disease course [190]. This may be because the organisms largely have disappeared by the time the clinical manifestations occur. Full recovery without sequelae is expected in patients who do not have jaundice, but in jaundiced individuals mortality rates may be as high as 17%.

Chronic Meningitis

NEUROSYPHILIS
Syphilis is caused by a spiral bacterium, *T. pallidum* [194]. This spirochete produces its CNS manifestations as a consequence of a chronic meningitis (meningovascular syphilis), low-grade encephalitis (general paresis), and chronic arachnoiditis (tabes dorsalis).

Pathogenesis and Pathophysiology. Syphilis is acquired primarily by sexual contact. The initial site of infection is usually the vagina or the penis. About 3 weeks after the initial infection, genital chancres develop as the major manifestation of primary syphilis. Two to 6 weeks later the spirochetes disseminate throughout the body and produce secondary syphilis. At this stage, spirochetes invade the CNS and meninges in approximately 25% of patients [195]. In most circumstances the CNS invasion is asymptomatic, but occasional patients may develop an acute syphilitic meningitis that clinically appears to be an acute aseptic meningitis. In the absence of treatment this stage usually resolves spontaneously. A latent period (latent neurosyphilis) then ensues, in which the patient is asymptomatic but has a low-grade meningitis. Two to 8 years after the CNS invasion, the chronic meningitis may become symptomatic [195]. In meningovascular syphilis the meningeal inflammation damages meningeal blood vessels (Huebner's arteritis). The arteritis may cause stenosis or thrombosis of blood vessels with subsequent brainstem or cerebral cortex infarctions. In addition the chronic meningitis may directly damage cranial nerves.

Eight to 20 years after the initial CNS infection, spirochetes that invaded the brain may cause a low-grade bacterial encephalitis [195]. If untreated for

several years the brain infection produces widespread neuronal loss and cerebral atrophy. Histologically one sees the picture of an encephalitis with perivascular cuffing, granular ependymitis, and increased tissue gliosis. Under rare circumstances the spirochetes may form a localized abscess (gumma) in the brain.

Fifteen to 20 years after the initial CNS infection, the chronic meningitis may become transformed into an arachnoiditis with invasion of fibroblasts into the meninges. The chronic arachnoiditis may result in ischemic damage to the posterior spinal cord and optic nerves.

Epidemiology and Predisposing Factors. Syphilis occurs worldwide. Primary syphilis typically involves young adults who are sexually promiscuous. Historically in the sixteenth, seventeenth, and eighteenth centuries the organism appeared to be more virulent and often caused widespread organ involvement and death within a few years. Since 1900 the organism appears to invade the CNS less commonly. However, in patients with immunosuppressive diseases such as AIDS, the course of syphilis appears to be faster and more severe than syphilis in immunocompetent individuals [196].

Presentation. Signs of acute syphilitic meningitis may occur at the time of secondary syphilis or be delayed for up to a year [197]. Patients usually complain of headache, fever, photophobia, and a stiff neck. Only 10% of patients have a secondary syphilitic rash at the time of the meningitis. A generalized lymphadenopathy also may be present. Occasional patients develop cranial nerve palsies (especially the facial and auditory nerves). Sensorineural deafness may occur and is often associated with tinnitus and vertigo. Seizures, aphasia, or hemiplegia rarely occur. The meningitis usually lasts several weeks and spontaneously subsides even in the absence of treatment.

The onset of meningovascular syphilis is usually abrupt, although preceding headache, dizziness, and memory loss can occur. In 25% of patients the neurologic signs progress over several days [195, 198]. The most common clinical manifestations include hemiparesis (80%), aphasia (30%), and seizures (14%) [195]. Involvement of small branches of brainstem arteries may produce vomiting, vertigo, nystagmus, ataxia, and impaired pain sense over the face.

Parenchymatous neurosyphilis, also known as general paresis or lues, usually has an insidious onset. The early signs are neuropsychiatric and include irritability, forgetfulness, nervousness, impaired concentration ability, carelessness in appearance, insomnia, and subtle personality changes [195]. As the disease progresses, patients lose insight, have impaired recent memory, and display periods of confusion and disorientation. Patients often have difficulties in judgment and may develop changes in affect with periods of elation or depression. Psychosis occasionally appears. A few patients also develop seizures, aphasia, and motor disturbances such as tremors or spasticity. Pupillary abnormalities are common and an Argyll-Robertson pupil may be seen. The Argyll-Robertson pupil has the following characteristics: (1) the pupils are small and fixed and do not react to light; (2) the pupils react normally to accommodation; (3) mydriates (atropine) fail to dilate pupils fully; and (4) the person can see. Pupillary abnormalities not always meeting the full criteria for Argyll-Robertson pupils are seen in approximately one-half of patients with general paresis.

Tabes dorsalis, a manifestation of neurosyphilis, is now less common than it used to be. Signs of tabes dorsalis develop slowly and include a sensory ataxia and an inability to perceive joint movements [195]. As the disease progresses, the gait becomes broad based and slapping. Over one-half of the patients develop painful paresthesias, often described as lightning pains or shooting sensations in the legs, abdomen, or arms. Pupillary abnormalities are common, and Argyll-Robertson pupils are seen in approximately 50% of patients. Deep tendon reflexes are frequently absent at the ankles. There is often a decreased ability to appreciate deep pain sensation in the legs. In the absence of normal pain appreciation, the patient may repeatedly traumatize knee or ankle joints (Charcot's joints). Optic atrophy occasionally develops, with subsequent loss of vision.

Laboratory Studies. Invasion of the meninges by *T. pallidum* results in characteristic changes in the CSF. These changes are present in all stages of neurosyphilis, including the asymptomatic (latent) stage [199]. The CSF usually has a normal opening pressure. There is a low-grade CSF pleocytosis, with lymphocytes predominating. The cell count ranges from 10 to several hundred lymphocytes per microliter, depending on how active the infection is. The CSF protein typically is elevated above 40 mg/dl but is seldom greater than 200 mg/dl. There is an increased synthesis of CSF IgG [200], and electrophoresis of CSF typically shows several oligoclonal bands in the gamma globulin region [201].

In general paresis the EEG frequently shows diffuse slowing. CT and MRI scans are frequently abnormal in meningovascular syphilis and general paresis [202]. In meningovascular syphilis the brain abnormalities give the appearance of a stroke. In general paresis one often sees ventricular dilatation and brain atrophy.

CSF Serologic Tests for Syphilis. The CSF VDRL test is the standard CSF diagnostic test for neurosyphilis. In this nontreponemal test CSF is evaluated for its ability to flocculate a suspension of cardiolipin-cholesterol-lecithin antigen [203]. While false-positive nontreponemal tests may occur occasionally in serum, false-positive CSF VDRL tests are rare. Thus, the presence of a reactive or positive CSF VDRL test is virtually diagnostic of active neurosyphilis [204]. The VDRL test can be quantitated and used to follow response to treatment. Following successful treatment for neurosyphilis, the CSF VDRL titer falls to low levels or zero.

A specific treponemal test, the fluorescent treponemal antibody absorption (FTA-ABS) test can be used to evaluate CSF. Controversy exists, however, about its usefulness for diagnosing active neurosyphilis [205]. The CSF FTA-ABS test is extremely sensitive and, like the serum FTA-ABS test, once the test becomes reactive, it remains so for life. Thus, a reactive CSF FTA-ABS test can indicate several things: (1) active neurosyphilis; (2) asymptomatic neurosyphilis; (3) treated neurosyphilis; and (4) false-positive reaction. False-positive reactions may occur when serum treponemal antibody leaks into CSF through a break of the blood-brain-CSF barrier or when a small amount of blood containing the treponemal antibody contaminates the CSF at the time of a lumbar puncture [206].

Diagnosis. A diagnosis of neurosyphilis can be made in a patient with signs and symptoms of neurosyphilis who has a reactive CSF VDRL test. It is currently unknown how often neurosyphilis occurs with a nonreactive CSF VDRL test, but there has been some concern that this test is not sensitive enough to detect all cases of active neurosyphilis [205]. A nonreactive blood FTA-ABS test or a nonreactive CSF FTA-ABS test rules out chronic neurosyphilis in the immunocompetent patient.

Therapy. Penicillin remains the drug of choice to treat all forms of syphilis, including neurosyphilis [204]. To date no penicillin-resistant *T. pallidum* strains have been recognized. To achieve adequate antibiotic levels in the brain and CSF following systemic therapy, the blood-brain barrier must be overcome. It has been found that some of the older penicillin regimens employing benzathine penicillin in standard doses or procaine penicillin (with or without 2% aluminum monostearate) in doses under 2.4 million units daily do not consistently provide treponemicidal levels of penicillin in the CSF [207, 208]. Therefore, in 1989, the CDC altered their recommendations for the treatment of neurosyphilis (Table 31-11).

T. pallidum spirochetes divide at very slow rates, with a division time of at least 30 hours. Thus, for drugs such as penicillin that kill organisms during cell division, treatment should continue for 2–4 weeks. Occasional patients may develop a Jarisch-Herxheimer reaction in the first 24 hours after starting penicillin. These patients develop a fever with transient worsening of their psychosis or neurologic signs. If these signs develop, 2–3 days of prednisone 5 mg qid PO with gradual reduction of dosage may be beneficial. If a patient is allergic to penicillin, efforts should be made to desensitize the patient to penicillin [204]. As an alternative drug ceftriaxone has been shown to successfully treat primary and secondary syphilis, and it will cross the blood-brain barrier [209]. Ceftriaxone is usually given for several weeks in the doses that are normally given in treatment of bacterial meningitis.

Over 90% of patients with neurosyphilis are cured with a full course of penicillin. However, the patient should be followed for 1–2 years to ensure that the treatment was effective. A lumbar puncture with CSF examination should be repeated at 2 weeks, 4 weeks, 6 months, 1 year, and possibly 2 years later. With effective therapy the CSF pleocytosis should resolve within 6 months. The CSF protein level should fall to normal or near normal by 6 months to 1 year. The CSF VDRL titer should head toward zero by 1 year, but it may not always become nonreactive. An increase in pleocytosis, protein level, or VDRL titer in CSF is an indication for retreatment. All recognized sexual partners should be tested for syphilis and treated if the test is reactive.

Outcome and Complications. It is considered that all patients with neurosyphilis can be cured with appropriate antibiotic treatment. Neurologic sequelae depend on how early the disease was diagnosed. Patients with latent or asymptomatic neurosyphilis have an excellent prognosis. Patients with meningovascular syphilis may be left with neurologic residuals similar to those seen following a stroke. Patients with general paresis who are treated early in the course of the dementia may show a remarkable improvement in cognition. Unfortunately patients whose dementia has been present longer than 1 year frequently have only mild to moderate improvement. Patients with tabes dorsalis frequently do not improve and may worsen in spite of appropriate antibiotic treatment.

MYELOPATHY ASSOCIATED WITH HUMAN T-LYMPHOTROPHIC VIRUS TYPE 1

Human T-lymphotrophic virus type 1 (HTLV-1) is a retrovirus that is distinct from the HIV-1 and HIV-2. HTLV-1 virus has been associated with both adult T-cell leukemia and a form of spastic paraparesis. Fortunately patients with the spastic paraparesis seldom develop leukemia.

Table 31-11. Treatment of neurosyphilis

Aqueous crystalline penicillin G 12 million–24 million U/day (2 million–4 million U q4h) IV for 10–14 days, followed by benzathine penicillin G, 2.4 million U weekly IM for three doses

or

Aqueous procaine penicillin G 2.4 million U daily IM plus probenecid 500 mg qid PO, both for 10–14 days, followed by benzathine penicillin G 2.4 million U weekly IM for three doses

Pathophysiology and Epidemiology. The neurologic illness clusters in tropical areas, especially in India, Africa, the Seychelles, the Caribbean, and southern Japan [210, 211]. In these areas many individuals who appear healthy harbor the virus and have antibodies to the virus in their blood. A small percentage of these individuals subsequently develop a progressive spastic paraparesis. The disease occurs more often in women than in men. The age of onset ranges from 10 to 70 years, with the mean onset being at about 40 years.

Limited pathologic studies show a chronic meningoencephalomyelitis primarily involving the spinal cord [211]. Inflammatory changes include perivascular lymphocytic cuffing, fibroblastic thickening of meninges, reactive gliosis, and perivascular fibrosis of small blood vessels. Demyelination and axonal loss occur in spinal cord tracts, especially the posterior columns and pyramidal tracts. On occasion the intensity of myelin destruction may be severe enough to produce a vacuolar myopathy. Like HIV the virus can be spread sexually, via exposure to blood products, and congenitally.

Presentation. Initial signs are usually a slowly progressive gait disturbance, which may be accompanied by dysesthesias in the legs. The signs are usually bilateral and slowly progress over months to years. The full-blown syndrome is characterized by a paraparesis or paraplegia with spasticity of legs and occasionally arms. There also is an associated bladder dysfunction and penile impotence [210, 212]. Individuals have sensory loss in the legs, but a sensory level is seldom identified.

Laboratory. The CSF usually demonstrates a mild lymphocytic pleocytosis with elevated protein, but on occasion it is entirely normal. Oligoclonal bands and elevated gamma globulin in the CSF may be seen in up to 50% of cases. Leg and arm nerves usually show normal motor conduction velocities and normal sensory latency. Posterior tibial nerve somatosensory evoked potentials usually show abnormal latencies, suggesting spinal cord abnormalities. However, the median nerve somatosensory evoked potentials are usually normal. MRI studies of the spinal cord demonstrate diffuse lesions within the spinal cord, particularly in the

thoracic region. The patients have antibodies to HTLV-1 virus in both serum and CSF. HTLV-1 virus has been isolated from patients' blood and CSF [213].

Diagnosis. The diagnosis is made in a patient with progressive spastic paraparesis who has antibodies to HTLV-1 virus. The differential diagnosis usually considered in this illness includes neuromyelitis optica, multiple sclerosis, adrenomyeloneuropathy, primary lateral sclerosis, HIV myelopathy, and other infections of the spinal cord such as syphilis (tabes dorsalis).

Treatment. At present there is no proven treatment for this disease. Trials are under way to determine whether zidovudine, an antiretroviral drug that has been useful in the treatment of HIV infection, will be of benefit. Symptomatic treatment, including rehabilitation with the use of walkers and other gait assistance devices, should be of help.

Outcome. In most cases the disease is slowly progressive and produces an increasingly severe spastic quadriparesis. Over years the patient becomes unable to walk. Unlike HIV infection, which can damage the brain and the spinal cord, HTLV-1 virus does not produce dementia.

NEUROLOGIC ASPECTS OF LYME DISEASE
Lyme disease, or Lyme borreliosis, is due to the spirochete *B. burgdorferi* [214]. The disease was initially described in Europe in the early 1900s but was not recognized in the United States until 1975. It has now become the most common vector-borne disease in the United States.

Pathogenesis and Pathophysiology. Approximately 10%–50% of individuals become infected following a bite by a *B. burgdorferi*–infected *Ixodes* tick. The initial spirochetal replication occurs locally in the skin. Several weeks later the spirochetes disseminate to infect multiple organs, including joints and the nervous system [215]. Several weeks after the primary infection patients commonly develop a migrating arthritis that primarily involves large joints. Spirochetes may also invade the meninges to give rise to a subacute meningitis. Subsequent damage to the seventh cranial nerve, resulting in a facial palsy, is common. In addition there is often damage to peripheral nerves. The damage is primarily to axons with some demyelination in the proximal and distal nerve segments [216]. In occasional patients spirochetes infect the brain to produce a low-grade meningoencephalitis several months to years after the primary infection [217].

Presentation. Neurologic signs and symptoms occur primarily in stage 2 of Lyme disease, which is the stage of early disseminated infection. It has been estimated that 15% of untreated patients develop neurologic involvement [218, 219]. The classical features include a radicular neuritis, aseptic meningitis, and cranial neuritis [220]. In Europe this syndrome is called Bannwarths's syndrome. The radicular pain may be either unilateral or bilateral and frequently involves the same dermatome as the tick bite. On formal testing, touch and pain sensation may be slightly decreased in the affected dermatome. The hypesthesia is similar to that seen in patients with recovered herpes zoster. Patients with meningitis experience headache, meningismus, photophobia, nausea, and vomiting but may not be febrile [221]. Up to one-half of patients develop some degree of facial-nerve involvement. The resulting Bell's palsy may be either unilateral or bilateral [222]. Occasionally the third, fourth, fifth, sixth, and eighth cranial nerves also are involved. Occasional patients may also develop mononeuritis multiplex, carpal tunnel syndrome [223], or Guillain Barré–like syndrome. The Guillain Barré–like syndrome differs from the classical disease in that CSF pleocytosis typically is present and a sural nerve biopsy does not show classic demyelinating lesions.

In occasional individuals the disease will progress from early disseminated stage 2 to late persistent stage 3 infection, and a chronic arthritis of large joints may reappear. In addition some patients develop CNS involvement with a progressive encephalopathy or meningoencephalitis [219, 224–226]. These patients may develop spastic paraparesis, hemiparesis, transverse myelitis, or a dementia-like syndrome. Patients who develop dementia-like syndromes develop lethargy, poor concentration, fatigue, memory loss, irritability, and even episodes of frank psychosis.

Laboratory. Patients with the early disseminated stage 2 disease usually have an abnormal CSF. The opening pressure usually is normal, but the CSF shows a lymphocytic pleocytosis, mildly elevated protein, and normal glucose. If peripheral nerve involvement is present, electromyograms of involved limbs have generally suggested axonal nerve involvement [216].

Laboratory abnormalities also have been reported in the late persistent stage 3 infections. CSF pleocytosis and elevated protein levels are found in fewer than one-half of the patients. Oligoclonal bands usually are not present in patients from the United States. Neuropsychological tests may show abnormalities in memory but usually there is no change in IQ score. The MRI scans occasionally show small foci of increased signal intensity, usually in the white matter on T2 weighted images [223, 226]. CT scans have usually been normal.

Diagnosis. Several serologic tests have been developed for diagnosing Lyme disease, but none is ideal. The immunofluorescent antibody test detects antibody to whole B. burgdorferi spirochetes but antibodies directed against other spirochetes may cross-react. Therefore, serum immunofluorescent antibody titers should be greater than or equal to 1:128 before the test is considered positive. The ELISA antibody test is felt to be more specific than the immunofluorescent test and is now widely used. However, false-positive immunofluorescent and ELISA antibody tests have been reported in patients with other spirochetal diseases such as syphilis, yaws, and pinta, as well as in patients with systemic lupus erythematosus and rheumatoid arthritis. Up to 4% of normal individuals may also have low ELISA antibody levels. A variation of the ELISA test using a preparation of only the 41KD flagella antigen appears to be more sensitive and specific than previous ELISA tests [227]. The immunoblot or Western blot test for B. burgdorferi appears to be the most specific of the available tests but is not widely available. Since no serologic test for Lyme disease is yet ideal, test results must always be interpreted along with the patient's history and examination [228].

The diagnosis of neurologic Lyme disease usually is based on serologic tests. The earliest immune response usually is directed against the 41KD antigen of the spirochetal flagella [229]. Serum IgM antibody is usually detectable 3–4 weeks following infection, peaks at 6–8 weeks, and declines after 4 months [215]. Serum IgG antibody, which is directed against multiple spirochetal antigens, usually is first detectable at 8 to 12 weeks, peaks by 6 months, and persists for many years.

Therapy. Patients with neurologic Lyme disease have shown clinical improvement following parenteal courses of penicillin [230] and ceftriaxone [231]. In one study ceftriaxone was shown to be slightly superior to penicillin [231]. The usual adult dose of ceftriaxone is 2 g/day IV for 14–28 days. The pediatric dose of ceftriaxone is 50–80 mg/kg per day IV for 10–20 days [232]. The adult dosage of penicillin G is usually 20 million–24 million U/day IV for 10–21 days. The pediatric dose of penicillin G is 250,000–400,000 units/kg per day IV for 10–21 days [232]. Adverse effects of both drugs include diarrhea, pseudomembranous colitis, and a Jarisch-Herxheimer reaction.

Outcome. Most patients with early disseminated infection and neurologic disease respond well to treatment and make a good to excellent recovery [223, 231]. The outcome of patients with late persistent stage 3 infection and CNS involvement has been somewhat less successful. Following antibiotic treatment many patients do make a slow clinical improvement over several months.

Localized Disease

The Dura

INFECTIONS OF THE CRANIAL DURA

The cranial meninges isolate the brain from surrounding bony structures, including the mastoids and the sinuses. The outer layer of the meninges is the dura, which forms the inner layer of the cranial periosteum. Beneath this is the arachnoid, which is a distinct layer surrounding the subarachnoid space, which contains the CSF. The third layer is the pia, which is adherent to the brain and the spinal cord. Infections of the cranial dura commonly are initiated by infections in the sinuses, the mastoids, or the middle ear [1]. Occasionally infections occur in this region by hematogenous dissemination or from penetrating wounds. The dura functions as a barrier and may restrict infections to the epidural space in areas where the dura is not adherent to the periosteum. Penetrating veins may carry microorganisms into the subdural space, producing subdural empyema, or the infection may extend deeper, producing meningitis or brain abscess. Although all of these structures may occasionally be infected, it is relatively uncommon to have meningitis occur as a consequence of subdural empyema [233].

The most common bacterial species infecting these structures are those that cause sinusitis, mastoiditis, and otitis. These include aerobic and anaerobic streptococci, *Bacteroides fragilis*, *S. aureus*, and a wide variety of less frequently occurring organisms [234]. Gram-negative bacilli may infect previously existing subdural hematomas.

Presentation. The onset is commonly insidious, following acute sinusitis or otitis, or the symptoms may develop more rapidly following surgery or trauma. Fever, headache, meningismus, and disturbed consciousness are early manifestations, but there also may be evidence of an associated sinusitis, otitis, or osteomyelitis. As the infection extends, it may cause increased intracranial pressure and irritate underlying meninges or brain, producing focal neurologic signs. These focal signs may include hemiparesis, aphasia, focal seizures, and unilateral third-nerve palsy [1, 233, 235].

Peripheral leukocytosis is common. Radiologic studies or bone scans may reveal infections of the adjacent sinuses or mastoids or cranial osteomyelitis. Lumbar puncture may be dangerous because of increased intracranial pressure [236, 237]. The CSF may contain WBCs, which seldom exceed a few hundred and which are most commonly PMNs, although lymphocytes may predominate. CSF glucose is usually normal, but protein may be high. There is usually no growth on CSF culture. CT or MRI scans and angiography may identify the location and the extent of infection [238, 239].

Differential Diagnosis. The presence of meningismus together with spinal fluid pleocytosis may lead to an initial incorrect diagnosis of acute bacterial or chronic meningitis. Also the diagnosis of sinusitis, otitis, or mastoiditis may be made without associated involvement of the dura being recognized. Infections of the frontal sinuses associated with neurologic manifestations are more likely to be due to dural infections than to meningitis [240]. Thus, patients who have focal neurologic signs together with minimal spinal fluid abnormalities may have subdural empyema rather than meningitis. Encephalitis, brain abscess, and intracranial thrombophlebitis may all have similar presentation.

Therapy. Early surgical drainage and antibiotic therapy are important for relieving pressure symptoms from the collection of pus. The drainage and any surgical specimens removed should be cultured aerobically and anaerobically, and therapy should depend on the antibiotic sensitivity of organisms that are isolated. IV penicillin in high doses is reasonable initial therapy because of the frequent occurrence of streptococci and because most anaerobes that cause infections in this area will respond to doses of 20 million U/day in adults and 320,000–480,000 U/kg/day in children. All isolated bacteria should be treated, and treatment should be continued for 2–4 weeks. Longer therapy is indicated if osteomyelitis is present.

SPINAL EPIDURAL ABSCESS

Spinal epidural abscess is an uncommon disorder that is important, however, in that the diagnosis is commonly missed, leading to inappropriate therapy [241]. The spinal dura is not attached to the overlying bony structures, as in the cranium, and this feature allows infection to spread extensively in either cephalad or caudad direction. Most epidural abscesses are in the posterior epidural space and in midthoracic or lower lumbar locations, where the epidural space is most prominent [242]. Epidural abscesses seldom penetrate the theca, and so purulent meningitis is rare. Organisms that infect the epidural spinal cord space usually are acquired from hematogenous spread and differ from those causing cranial dural infections. They are likely to include staphylococci and gram-negative bacilli, both of which tend to cause a relatively acute illness. Chronic abscesses may result from contiguous chronic foci, such as vertebral osteomyelitis, pharyngeal infection, psoas abscesses, or decubitus ulcers.

Presentation. There are four clearly defined sequential symptomatic stages: spinal ache, root pain, weakness, and paralysis [243]. In the initial stage fever and tenderness over the affected area of the spine are common. Spinal root pain radiates from the spinal area and there may be reflex changes consistent with the anatomical level of the lesion. The weakness may be associated with ascending numbness and impaired bladder and bowel control. The appearance of paralysis may be rapid or may require several weeks.

The peripheral WBC count is variable. Vertebral osteomyelitis may be apparent by x-ray or bone scan. Lumbar puncture may spread the infection into the spinal fluid and should be performed only with the needle being frequently removed to check for the presence of pus. The CSF commonly has a predominantly lymphocytic pleocytosis, of up to 200 cells per microliter. Glucose usually is normal, and bacteriologic studies negative. Manometric studies and myelograms are consistent with obstruction of the spinal canal. CT or MRI scans may delineate the abscess. Blood cultures are positive in one-half of the cases.

Differential Diagnosis. When a patient has an acute epidural abscess, the initial diagnosis is incorrect about three-fourths of the time [241–243]. Incorrect initial diagnoses include meningitis, perinephric abscesses, rheumatoid spondylitis, acute back strain, acute poliomyelitis, subcutaneous extradural hematoma, hematomyelia, polyneuritis, uncomplicated vertebral osteomyelitis, and transverse myelitis. Transverse myelitis is characterized by neurologic impairment that appears rapidly in the absence of back pain, while epidural abscess is more likely when there is associated vertebral osteomyelitis or remote pyogenic infection and blood cultures are positive. Common initial diagnoses for chronic epidural abscess include poliomyelitis, spinal cord tumor, embolus, spinal vessel thrombosis, vertebral osteomyelitis, chronic meningitis, or

Pott's disease with compression myelitis. Other diagnoses that may be confused with spinal epidural abscess include extruded intravertebral disc, cholecystitis, pyelonephritis, cerebrovascular accident, hysteria, infected disc, and herpes zoster.

The most useful findings for identifying the disease and defining its extent include CT and MRI scans. The presence of positive blood cultures when any of the above mentioned disorders is considered should raise a question of spinal epidural abscess. Encountering pus at lumbar puncture or surgery is diagnostic.

Therapy. Rapid surgical drainage of the abscess is essential. The abscess may commonly extend over four or five segments of the spine but can affect up to 26 segments [241]. Therapy should be directed at any isolated organisms, which include *S. aureus* in over one-half of the cases, or gram-negative bacilli such as *E. coli* and *Pseudomonas aeruginosa*, which also are frequently encountered [241–243]. When no agent is isolated, penicillin-resistant staphylococci should be suspected, with therapy directed at them and at gram-negative bacilli. Therapy should be continued for 2–4 weeks, or longer if osteomyelitis is present.

SEPTIC THROMBOPHLEBITIS OF SINUSES AND CEREBRAL VEINS

Cerebral venous or sinus thrombophlebitis is usually preceded by adjacent infection such as meningitis, epidural or subdural abscess, or infections involving the face, sinuses, ears, or mastoids. The most frequently involved venous structures are the cavernous, lateral, and superior sagittal sinuses and the cortical vessels [244]. Meningitis may lead to cortical thrombophlebitis. Infected lesions on the upper half of the face, as well as sphenoid or ethmoid sinusitis may lead to cavernous sinus thrombosis and phlebitis. Ear or mastoid infections may lead to lateral sinus thrombosis.

Presentation. A patient who is already ill with one of the preceding adjacent infections may experience new chills, fever, headache, and lethargy. These symptoms may progress to seizures and focal neurologic deficits in the case of cortical thrombophlebitis. With cavernous sinus disease ophthalmic vein obstruction may produce facial edema,

proptosis, and chemosis. Distention of retinal vessels and superficial veins of the forehead also may occur. Lateral sinus thrombosis may produce edema and venous engorgement behind the ear. Signs of increased cranial pressure also may appear.

Blood cultures commonly are positive. The CSF pressure is elevated, and there may be pleocytosis and elevated protein, but the glucose usually is normal and no bacteria are likely to be found. Cerebral arteriograms may show obstruction in the superior sagittal or lateral sinuses during the late venous phase. CT or MRI scans may show areas of infarction following a venous distribution pattern, and there may be a high-signal intensity from the thrombus within the sinus or vein.

Therapy. Surgical drainage and removal of any infected adjacent foci are essential. High-dose IV antimicrobial drugs should be selected by antibiotic sensitivity testing of the organism. Before results are known, therapy should be broad in spectrum and should include antistaphylococcal drugs. Anticoagulants should be avoided.

Brain Parenchyma

Certain infections of the nervous system are typically localized and cause focal manifestations. Thus, in contrast to viral encephalitis, which is more likely to be generalized and involve many areas of the brain, bacterial infections are more likely to be localized, causing meningitis, dural abscesses, or localized brain abscess. Most fungi and parasites behave in a similar manner. Such localized infections may arise directly by extension from other foci, such as mastoiditis and sinusitis, or may follow skull fracture or craniotomy. The organisms may also be carried to the CNS by the bloodstream. These infections commonly begin as a localized form of encephalitis that then softens and becomes necrotic, with formation of a capsule and surrounding inflammation and edema. These localized space-occupying lesions may slowly expand, leading to focal neurologic deficits or to increased intracranial pressure. The onset of focal brain infections is typically subacute, with the patient having headache, lethargy, focal or generalized seizures, and fever. Focal neurologic signs are not always present but may develop when the lesion is in a location that interferes with specific neural functions.

BACTERIAL BRAIN ABSCESS

Organisms that cause brain abscess may reach the brain hematogenously or by extension from contiguous infected foci. Hematogenously acquired bacterial brain abscesses tend to originate at the junction of white and gray matter, which is a relatively poorly vascularized area supplied by end arterioles without an extensive anastomosing capillary network [245]. Although hematogenously acquired brain infection is uncommon, brain abscesses may occur in patients who have congenital cyanotic heart disease or pulmonary, dental, tonsilar, or uterine infection. Brain abscesses also occur in patients with *Nocardia asteroides* infection. The lung appears to be an important filter that prevents many bacteria from reaching the brain, since patients with cyanotic congenital heart disease are not particularly prone to the development of cerebral abscess until after the age of 2 years, when right-to-left shunting of blood occurs, thus allowing the blood to bypass the lung. Subsequently as many as 10% of children with cyanotic heart disease may develop brain abscesses. It is common for abscesses of hematogenous origin to be multiple. Brain abscesses originating from infected sinuses or ears are located adjacent to those structures. Abscesses may also be associated with infections of the bone, dura, subdural space, arachnoid, and subarachnoid space [246–248]. Infections may also occur when septic thrombophlebitis propagates retrogradely into the brain parenchyma. Brain abscess may follow penetrating trauma or surgery [249–251].

When bacteria grow in a localized area in the brain, they cause tissue death and liquefaction of the center, leaving an unencapsulated abscess with surrounding inflammation. As the lesion matures, a capsule forms. The lesion may rupture into a ventricle, causing catastrophic ventriculitis.

Presentation. The patient is likely to have had several days or weeks of headache, focal or generalized seizures, signs of increased intracranial pressure, and possibly signs of localized neurologic deficit [252]. Fever is common but not always present. There may be evidence of an underlying predisposing disease, such as congenital cyanotic heart disease, mastoiditis, sinusitis, or lung infection.

When a brain abscess is suspected, a CT scan should be performed before a lumbar puncture is attempted, since there is a high frequency of temporal lobe or cerebellar herniation. If fluid is obtained, it is usually under increased pressure and has minimal pleocytosis and elevated protein. Glucose levels are normal and cultures usually sterile. EEGs are quite sensitive and are often abnormal, with focal delta waves which can localize cerebral but not cerebellar abscesses. Radionuclide brain scans and MRI scans may show abnormalities early in the disease during the encephalitic stage, but CT scans may not show an abnormality until the abscess has formed and encapsulated [238, 253]. Early in the disease cerebritis appears as a low-density area and does not enhance. Later in the disease a peripheral enhancing ring indicates formation of a capsule [254]. Angiography commonly reveals a space-occupying lesion.

Pus obtained at surgery or by stereotactic biopsy should be inoculated immediately into anaerobic, fungal, and routine microbiological media, and the laboratory should be alerted since prolonged incubation may be necessary for the identification of *N. asteroides*. This organism should be particularly suspected in compromised hosts or those with a nodular or cavitary pulmonary lesion or from whom a *Nocardia* organism has been recovered in the sputum. Anaerobic cultures are particularly important since anaerobes may be found in 35%–89% of brain abscesses [245, 255–259]. When anaerobic culturing technique is not optimal, the abscess may mistakenly be called sterile.

Differential Diagnosis. The above mentioned studies may not differentiate among bacterial brain abscess, necrotic foci from localized herpetic encephalitis, necrotic infarcts, and primary or metastatic tumor. Brain abscess should be particularly suspected in patients who have chronic infected foci and who develop persistent headache, fever, lethargy, focal neurologic signs, or seizures. The meningeal irritation may lead to major manifestations of meningitis, in which case a lumbar puncture should be done following a CT or MRI scan to rule out a space-occupying lesion. A firm diagnosis is frequently made only when pus is encountered at surgery.

Therapy. Surgical drainage should be considered in every patient, because it may prevent herniation and speed healing. Surgery is impractical, however, early in the infection when only cerebritis is present, when abscesses are located so deeply that drainage would be impossible without causing severe cerebral damage, when they are multiple and widely spaced, or occasionally when they are in areas such as the motor cortex, where surgical damage could be of major consequence. It is also important to perform surgery or to obtain organisms through a stereotactically guided biopsy to help direct antibiotic therapy. Cures may be accomplished in some cases through antibiotic administration alone, particularly when the infecting organisms are known and are available for antibiotic-sensitivity testing.

Antimicrobial therapy is essential, and whenever possible it should be designed to treat all isolated organisms. The blood-brain barrier is broken in the presence of an abscess, so most antimicrobial drugs initially may penetrate into the abscess. As healing occurs the blood-brain barrier may obstruct entry of antibiotics, but there are few data relating to the penetration of drugs into brain abscesses (see Table 31-5) [247, 256, 260, 261]. Chloramphenicol penetrates well into brain tissue and frequently achieves concentrations higher than those in serum, but it penetrates erratically into pus found in brain abscesses [256]. The drug nevertheless is used frequently since it is effective against most gram-positive aerobes, many gram-negative aerobes, and most anaerobic bacteria, including B. fragilis. Penicillin penetrates erratically into both brain and pus in brain abscesses and also is used commonly since it is effective against most gram-positive organisms, both aerobic and anaerobic, when given in high concentration. It is generally not useful when S. aureus or Nocardia organisms are suspected. Methicillin has fair to good penetration into brain abscesses, and cephalothin and other first-generation cephalosporins have fair penetration into brain. Sulfa compounds are the drug of choice for treating nocardial infections [262]. Metronidazole has excellent penetration into brain abscesses and is highly effective against most anaerobes but ineffective against all aerobes [256].

Antibiotic therapy is more difficult when surgery or a biopsy cannot be performed, since the therapy must be directed at many possible pathogens [263–266]. In those circumstances a combination of chloramphenicol or metronidazole and either a penicillin or a cephalosporin is generally used. Treatment must be continued for a minimum of 6 weeks if surgical drainage is not performed.

CYSTICERCOSIS

Cysticercosis is caused by tissue invasion by the pork tapeworm *Taenia solium*. Humans acquire the more common tapeworm or intestinal form of the disease from eating pork or other meat containing cysts that have not been killed by adequate heating. In the form of human disease, called cysticercosis, humans become an intermediate host by ingesting eggs (fecal-oral transmission). The embryos disseminate hematogenously and form larval cysts in the brain and meninges, and occasionally in subcutaneous tissue, muscles, or the eye. The brain cysts may grow to 0.5–2.0 cm in diameter [267–269]. They remain viable for periods of up to 5 years with little inflammatory response until they die. Degenerating cysts may be surrounded by plasma cells, lymphocytes, eosinophiles, and macrophages, and eventually a surrounding fibrous capsule may calcify. Parenchymal cysts may irritate, compress, or destroy brain tissue. In addition to causing parenchymal cysts, the organisms may float in the subarachnoid space and attach to the pia, where they form grape-like clusters of cysts around the basal cisterns. Intraventricular cysts may obstruct the flow of CSF, producing intracranial hypertension.

Epidemiology. The disease occurs worldwide but is most prevalent in Latin America, Eastern Europe, China, India, and South Africa. Cysticercosis is the most common cause of space-occupying lesions of the brain in some areas of Latin America. The disease is not uncommon in areas of the United States where there are recent immigrants from Latin America.

Presentation. Initial symptoms of cysticercosis occur several years following infection, when the cysts degenerate and inflammation develops. The manifestations depend on the CNS location of the lesions and on the degree of associated inflammation [267–269]. The manifestations are extremely varied and result from meningeal inflammation, or intracranial hypertension. Focal symptoms may result from cerebral cysts or rarely spinal cord mass lesions. Seizures, either generalized or focal, are particularly common initial presentations. In many instances the presence of cysts is asymptomatic.

Peripheral eosinophilia is rare. In about 50% of the cases the CSF contains a lymphocytic pleocytosis, and eosinophiles are found in 15%. Protein may be elevated, and occasionally glucose may be slightly low. Serum ELISA tests are frequently positive for antibodies in the presence of the disease, and there is an immunoblot test that is highly sensitive (90%) and specific (99%) in both serum and CSF [270, 271, 272]. Radiographs may show intracerebral calcification, and CT or MRI scans often demonstrate one or more cysts 5–20 mm in diameter located near the white and gray junction in the cerebral cortex [272]. If the cyst is degenerating, surrounding cerebral edema is commonly seen. With the administration of gadolinium, the cyst wall enhances on MRI scans.

Differential Diagnosis. Cysticercosis may resemble any space-occupying lesion in the head, such as brain abscess or cystic tumor, but it should be suspected particularly in persons from an endemic area or who have a chronic or relapsing meningitis.

Therapy. Treatment may not be necessary in asymptomatic patients and must be individualized. In symptomatic patients praziquantal 50 mg/kg/day PO in three divided doses can be given for 15 days [273]. The drug acts by killing live cysts and causing them to degenerate, so some patients experience increased signs during treatment. If that occurs, oral prednisone 40–60 mg/day or dexamethasone 12–24 mg/day can be used. Albendazole is another drug that shows promise in the treatment of neurocysticerosis [274]. Surgical removal of the cyst is often indicated if it is intraventricular or in the spinal cord.

ECHINOCOCCOSIS

Echinococcosis is sometimes referred to as unilocular hydatid disease. It is worldwide in distribution but most prevalent in cattle- and sheep-raising areas. Cases in the United States are fairly common in Alaska and have also occurred in Arizona, New Mexico, and Utah. The disease most often involves the liver, but cysts may also be found in the brain. The diagnosis can be made by a serum ELISA test. Treatment is surgical excision.

Infections Associated with Motor Dysfunction

BOTULISM

Clostridium botulinum is a gram-positive, rod-shaped, spore-forming, obligate anaerobic bacterium that is widely distributed in soil and water. Six strains of *C. botulinum* exist, with type A being more common west of the Mississippi and type B more common to the east. Type E is found mainly in Alaska and around the Great Lakes. The spores are capable of surviving 100°C (boiling) for at least 6 hours but are killed at temperatures of 120°C for 5 minutes. The temperature required to kill spores is important to the canning industry and was responsible for the emergence of the pressure cooker in canning foods. Foods canned at home without a pressure cooker may contain viable spores, which can germinate and produce toxin under anaerobic conditions. Home-canned foods account for 90% of botulism cases.

Pathogenesis. Botulinum toxin is one of the most potent toxins involving humans. It is odorless and tasteless. Unlike *C. botulinum* spores the toxin is heat labile and is denatured by heating above 60°C. Thus, botulinum toxin–contaminated food that is well cooked does not cause disease. There are three forms of botulinum poisoning. The most common is food-borne botulism, in which the individual ingests preformed toxin. Wound botulism occurs when *C. botulinum* spores are inoculated into skin following trauma or via subcutaneous injection with contaminated needles ("skin popping"). The spores germinate in anaerobic conditions and subsequently produce toxin. The third type occurs in infants 2–9 months of age [275]. These infants ingest *C. botulinum* spores that germinate and grow in the GI tract. The toxin then passes through the intestinal mucosa to reach the bloodstream. In older children and adults *C. botulinum* only rarely replicates in the intestinal tract, because its growth is inhibited by normal intestinal microflora [276].

Botulinum toxin resists denaturation by stomach

acid and most intestinal enzymes. After absorption from the upper intestinal tract it then circulates in the blood until it reaches cholinergic synapses. The toxin does not cross the blood-brain barrier, so brain cholinergic synapses are not involved. Botulinum toxin binds to a specific receptor on the presynaptic side of the cholinergic synapse and is internalized into the presynaptic nerve terminal. After this stage the toxin can no longer be neutralized by antibody. Once inside the cell, the short chain of the di-chain molecule separates and initiates a sequence of events that blocks release of stimulus-induced quantal acetylcholine into the synaptic cleft, which results in failure of signal transmission from nerve to muscle.

Clinical Presentation. The mean incubation period for food-borne botulism is 2 days (range 0.5–8.0 days) after ingestion of the toxin. The classic presentation and progression of botulism involves eight terms all beginning with the letter D: descending paralysis, diplopia, dyspnea, dysarthria, dizziness, dysphagia, dry mouth, and death. The descending paralysis is usually symmetrical and involves all skeletal muscles and many smooth muscles. Bulbar and limb muscles become weak and progress to paralysis over 1–2 days. Smooth-muscle paralysis of the GI tract and urinary bladder results in constipation, occasional paralytic ileus, and urinary retention. Patients do not have sensory loss, decreased mentation, memory loss, fever, blood pressure fluctuations, or abnormal heart rate.

Laboratory. Most laboratory tests are normal in botulism, including blood counts and CSF analysis. MRI and CT scans of the head are normal. Repetitive motor nerve stimulation at 20 or 50 hertz usually shows incremental responses in the compound muscle action potentials of innervated muscles. The diagnosis is made by a state health laboratory or reference laboratory that detects botulinum toxin in stool (25 gm), serum (10–20 ml), and suspected food samples.

Therapy. The treatment of botulism should begin as soon as the clinical diagnosis is made. When there is a cluster of cases, a firm clinical diagnosis can be made even before laboratory confirmation. Treatment includes three steps: (1) neutralizing

circulating toxin, (2) supporting the patient's respiration and other bodily functions, and (3) removing any possible remaining toxin from the GI tract. Since most cases of botulism belong to types A, B, and E, it is possible to give equine anti-A, -B, -E botulinum serum to most patients. One vial (10 ml) should be given IV and a second IM. If botulism is suspected, the botulism officer at the CDC (telephone 404-639-3753 days; 404-639-2888 evenings and weekends) should be contacted to have the antitoxin sent by airline from the nearest regional branch. Antitoxin may prevent progression of the disease, but it will not reverse paralysis that has already developed, since toxin that has already been internalized into the synapse cannot be neutralized. Since the antitoxin is of equine origin, there is approximately a 4% incidence of subsequent serum sickness.

Weakness may progress for several days, so it is important to have the patient placed in an intensive care unit and monitored for the possible need of intubation and assisted ventilation. When the intoxication is severe, the respiratory weakness may last for weeks and necessitate tracheostomy. An ileus may last for several days, so feeding via nasogastric tube should not begin until bowel sounds have returned. Urinary retention may require the use of a urinary catheter. In food-borne botulism laxatives may be given to remove unabsorbed toxin from the GI tract if GI paralysis has not occurred.

Treatment of infant botulism is primarily supportive and neither antitoxin nor antibiotics appears to be of value in hastening recovery [275]. In addition clinical recovery may occur in spite of the fact that the infant is still shedding C. botulinum bacteria and botulinum toxin in the stool [277]. In wound botulism the wound should be debrided and cleaned with 3% hydrogen peroxide to produce aerobic conditions, which inhibit growth of the bacteria. Antitoxin should be injected into the wound site, and penicillin (10 million U/day IV in adults) should be given to kill any C. botulinum.

Outcome. Patients with severe intoxications are usually hospitalized for 1–6 months, with weeks to months of respiratory assistance, and often complain of fatigue for a year. The mortality from food-borne botulism is 10%–20%; from infant botulism it is less than 5%.

Tetanus

Tetanus, like botulism, is not a true infection of the nervous system. The disease results from a toxin, tetanospasmin, that acts on spinal cord and brain stem neurons. The toxin, which has a molecular weight of 160,000 daltons, is produced by a gram-positive anaerobic bacillus, *Clostridium tetani*, that is found in superficial layers of soil around the world.

Pathogenesis and Epidemiology. Fewer than 200 cases of tetanus are reported annually from the United States, but there are approximately 300,000 cases worldwide. The U.S. cases occur primarily in nonimmunized individuals, such as newborn infants and elderly persons. Bacterial spores enter the skin following trauma, such as a puncture wound or laceration, but may also enter the body following obstetric delivery, surgery, and dental extraction or with middle ear infections. Tetanus may occur in heroin addicts. Neonatal tetanus results from infection of the umbilical stump.

The spores germinate under anaerobic conditions, and the bacteria produce tetanospasm. The toxin is picked up locally by axon terminals at neuromuscular junctions and is transported in a retrograde fashion toward the motor neuron cell body located in the spinal cord [278]. At that point the toxin passes transsynaptically, to be taken up by nerve terminals of predominantly inhibitory neurons that release glycine as their neurotransmitter (Renshaw cells). The toxin then appears to inhibit the inhibitory neurons. The consequence of this unique inhibition is an increase in firing volleys of motor neurons, resulting in uncontrolled muscle spasms [279]. Once the toxin is bound to neurons and internalized it no longer can be inactivated by antibody. The incubation period of tetanus usually is 1–2 weeks [280].

Presentation. A wound site may or may not be obvious when the first clinical manifestations appear. Early symptoms consist of irritability, restlessness, headaches, and a low-grade fever and are followed by muscle spasms in 1–3 days [281]. In most patients the illness progresses to involve painful reflex spasms of many muscle groups, but occasional patients develop localized tetanus, consisting of spasms of muscles near the wound site without generalized muscle spasms. Other patients may develop rigidity in jaw muscles (lockjaw). At times patients may assume an opisthotonic posture. Respirations may be impaired by laryngeal spasms or tonic contractions of respiratory muscles. Patients are invariably conscious and usually mentally alert early in the clinical course. Sympathetic overactivity may be present, with increased sweating, tachycardia, and blood pressure fluctuations. During the acute phase patients are subject to hypoxia, pneumonia, vertebral fractures, and life-threatening cardiac arrhythmias. The spasms of tetanus increase in severity for about 3 days, remain stable over the next week, and then slowly subside over the following two weeks.

Neonatal tetanus usually occurs in the first 10 days of life with *C. tetani* infecting the umbilical stump. It is characterized by difficulty in sucking, increased irritability, increased muscular rigidity, opisthotonus, and intermittent total muscular spasms [282].

Laboratory. There may be a mild increase in total white blood count. The CSF is usually normal. Sinus tachycardia is common on ECG. MRI and CT scans of the head and spinal cord are usually normal. In 30% of patients *C. tetani* can be isolated by anaerobic culture from a wound. No serologic tests are available.

Differential Diagnosis. The clinical diagnosis of tetanus is made in a patient who over 1–2 days has had the onset of repeated focal or generalized muscle spasms. A suspicious wound may be present or absent. The differential diagnosis includes neuroleptic drug reactions, focal seizures, strychnine poisoning, rabies, peritonitis, atypical muscle cramps, and hysteria. In lockjaw, dislocation of the mandible, alveolar abscess, or other mandibular abnormalities must be considered.

Therapy. Treatment is aimed at removing excess tetanospasmin from any wound, supporting the patient, and administering drugs to decrease the intensity of the muscle spasms. The wound should be thoroughly débrided and irrigated with 3% hydrogen peroxide to produce aerobic conditions, which help prevent growth of the organisms. Penicillin

(10 million U/day IV) should be given to eliminate *C. tetani.* Human tetanus–immune globulin (3,000–10,000 U) may be injected IM and around the wound site. Although this antitoxin will not reverse toxin already fixed to the lower motor neurons, it will inactivate toxin in the wound.

The patient should be placed in an intensive care unit and stimulation avoided, since it frequently increases the severity of muscle spasms. Oxygen should be administered nasally. If respiratory embarrassment develops from the spasms, a tracheostomy should be performed and the patient placed on intermittent positive pressure breathing with a volume-cycle respirator.

Muscle-relaxant drugs are helpful in preventing painful muscle spasms. Diazepam is usually the drug of choice, 10–30 mg q1–3h IV as needed. The dose should be titrated so that the patient has minimal spasms. Alternatively chlorpromazine 75–100 mg IV q3–4h may be given. Occasionally curare-like drugs may be helpful. When these drugs are given, blood pressure should be monitored and intubation with assisted ventilation is often necessary. If sympathetic overactivity is severe, propranolol may be required for control of hypertension and tachycardia. In addition pulmonary artery catheterization for measurement of cardiac output and wedge pressure is helpful [281].

Outcome. The case mortality rate is approximately 60% without intensive care but may be reduced to as low as 10% if the patient is placed in an intensive care unit. Those who survive usually make a full recovery unless they have experienced hypoxic damage to the brain [283].

Paralytic Poliomyelitis

Polio viruses are found worldwide. In temperate zones poliomyelitis has a seasonal incidence, with most cases occurring in late summer or early fall. In tropical regions infections occur throughout the year. In the United States the use of polio virus vaccines has reduced the number of cases of acute poliomyelitis to less than 10 per year, with most of these cases being a complication of the live polio virus vaccine. Worldwide, however, poliomyelitis still represents a serious childhood illness. The older the infected individual is, the greater the probability that paralysis will develop and that the paralysis will be severe.

Presentation. The infection may be asymptomatic, but in patients developing paralysis the incubation period is usually 4–10 days. The illness begins with fever, malaise, and headache, followed 1 day later by neck and back stiffness [5]. In some patients the illness stops at this point, leaving them with only aseptic meningitis. In others the major illness begins 2–5 days later, with muscle weakness and tenderness. The leg and arm muscles are unusually sensitive, stiff, and somewhat painful, and there may be a brief period of hyperreactive deep-tendon reflexes. Soon, however, a progressive asymmetrical weakness begins, usually greater in proximal than distal muscles. Legs are usually weaker than arms, and occasionally muscles of the thorax and trunk are severely involved. During the acute phase of the illness sensory complaints may be noted, but objective changes in sensation do not occur. Within 1 week the muscle tone becomes flaccid. Atrophy of muscles develops 5–7 days after the onset of the weakness and progresses over several weeks. In 10% of patients there is clinical involvement of bulbar muscles, particularly the ninth and tenth cranial nerves, resulting in pharyngeal and laryngeal muscular weakness. Facial weakness also may develop.

Laboratory. The blood is usually normal or has a mild leukocytosis. The CSF typically contains 20–300 lymphocytes per microliter. Early in the clinical course, however, polymorphonuclear leukocytes may predominate. CSF protein usually is mildly elevated, and the glucose is normal. The diagnosis can be confirmed by isolation of poliovirus from the throat or the stool. Poliovirus is seldom isolated from CSF. The poliovirus isolates should be sent to reference laboratories to determine whether the virus is wild-like or vaccine-like [284]. Patients with poliomyelitis will develop a fourfold or greater rise in serum-neutralizing antibodies or complement-fixing antibodies over several weeks.

Differential Diagnosis. The diagnosis should be suspected in any person who presents with a rapidly progressive asymmetrical paralysis and a CSF that has pleocytosis. The major differential diagnosis includes Guillain-Barré syndrome, diphtheritic polyneuropathy, botulism, and tick paralysis, all of which have an acellular CSF. However, the acute inflammatory polyneuropathy of Lyme disease may have a similar CSF pleocytosis.

Therapy. Although there is no antiviral treatment for poliomyelitis, symptomatic treatment is important. Patients should be hospitalized and placed in an intensive care unit, since the disease may progress rapidly. If bulbar and cervical involvement is severe, breathing and swallowing problems may be severe enough to require intubation. Mechanical ventilation should be used if the vital capacity falls below 30%–50% of predicted volume, if respirations become irregular or labored, or if arterial oxygen tension decreases. Mild analgesics may be necessary for the limb pain, and hot packs may provide comfort to painful muscles. Patients with severe paralysis often experience rapid resorption of bone, with increased serum and urinary calcium, which may result in nephrolithiasis or bladder calculi. Hydration and acidification of the urine can prevent urinary stone formation. Patients with severe muscle weakness require extensive physical therapy and possible bracing.

Outcome. Death occurs in approximately 5% of affected patients and is usually due to severe bulbar and respiratory involvement. In survivors strength begins to increase several weeks after the acute illness. By 6 months 80% of patients have made a good or full recovery.

A postpolio syndrome has been recognized in individuals 20–50 years after the primary poliomyelitis. Usually the acute illness was severe and left the patient with residual weakness that was stable for over 10 years. These patients then develop progressive muscular weakness, muscle atrophy, and occasionally respiratory insufficiency [285]. Muscle biopsies have found both remote atrophy and recent denervation. The electromyogram often shows evidence of active denervation, with fibrillation potentials and positive sharp waves [286]. There is no evidence for persistence of the poliovirus. Rather it appears that some surviving motor neurons begin dying many years after the acute infection [286]. Currently there is no specific therapy to prevent progression, but muscle exercise programs appear to slow the progression of weakness.

Rehabilitation therapy and bracing may be of benefit to help the patient ambulate.

Infections Associated with Sensory Dysfunction

Herpes Zoster

(See Chap. 32 for a complete discussion of herpes zoster.)

Leprosy

Leprosy remains a major infectious disease on a worldwide basis, with over 12 million estimated cases [287]. However, it is uncommonly recognized in the United States, due in part to the fact that many physicians' knowledge of the disease is inadequate for recognition of disease cases. The spectrum of clinical manifestations is broad, ranging from the lepromatous form, in which clinical manifestations are associated with the growth of large numbers of organisms, to the tuberculoid form, in which the clinical manifestations are related primarily to the immunological response to the organism.

Epidemiology. From 1985 through 1987 1139 cases of leprosy were reported in the United States; more than three-quarters of them occurred in foreign-born persons, particularly persons from Mexico, the Philippines, Kampuchea, American Samoa, Vietnam, Laos, and India. The only known source for the disease is infected humans discharging the organism, although other sources seem likely [288, 289]. Thus, cases occur much more commonly in household contacts than in those with no known contacts. Persons of all races may be infected.

Presentation. Leprosy is most commonly manifested by either cutaneous lesions or neurological involvement of peripheral nerves. In the lepromatous form of the disease there is skin involvement, which is bilateral and symmetrical with erythematous macules, papules, or nodules. Extensive diffuse infiltration of the skin by organisms and host response cells may lead it to appear smooth and shiny but otherwise normal [290]. In the tuberculoid form, which has few detectable organisms but a prominent host immunological response, there may be large erythematous plaques with sharply demarcated and raised outer edges. The center, which may be flattened, dry, and hairless, is anesthetic. Peripheral nerves may be visibly swollen.

Emergency physicians may see leprosy patients with complications that include erythema nodosum leprosum (ENL). ENL occurs in patients with lepromatous forms of the disease. The erythematous nodular lesions characteristic of this disorder may persist for months and be associated with high fever and a leukemoid reaction. There also may be polyarthralgia and an excruciatingly painful neuritis associated with sudden loss of peripheral nerve function, such as a complete foot drop. An immune-type glomerulonephritis also may be present. Nerve abscesses may occur and require surgical drainage. Patients receiving antilepromatous therapy may have a "reversal reaction," with nerve swelling that may be associated with neuritis or loss of motor function. Patients with the lepromatous form of the disease may also develop conjunctivitis, superficial punctate keratitis, and leprotic iridocyclitis.

The diagnosis of leprosy is suspected on clinical grounds and confirmed by skin biopsy or microscopic examination of skin scrapings for bacteria [291]. The laboratory must be alerted to the possible diagnosis so it will use the specialized stains required for identification of the microorganisms.

Therapy. Antibacterial treatment for the disorder is beyond the scope of this chapter but includes dapsone, clofazimine, and rifampin [292, 293]. Severe ENL and reversal reactions are treated with corticosteroids. Prednisone 60–80 mg/day may lead to some improvement within 48 hours. Subsequently the dose may be tapered to avoid a rebound reaction. In areas of the world where it is available thalidomide may be used for control of ENL in patients in whom pregnancy is not a consideration. An initial dosage of 300 mg/day may be slowly decreased to 100 mg given at bedtime.

References

1. Kubik CS, Adams RD. Subdural empyema. *Brain* 66:18–42, 1943.

2. Martinez AJ et al. Experimental Naegleria meningoencephalitis in mice. Penetration of the olfactory mucosal epithelium by Naegleria and pathologic changes produced: a light and electron microscopy study. *Lab Invest* 29:121–33, 1973.

3. Murphy FA et al. Comparative pathogenesis of rabies and rabies-like viruses. Viral infection and transit from inoculation site to the central nervous system. *Lab Invest* 28:361–76, 1973.

4. Schoenbaum SV, Gardner P, Shillito J. Infections of cerebrospinal fluid shunts: epidemiology, clinical manifestations, and therapy. *J Infect Dis* 131: 543–52, 1975.

5. Price RW, Plum F. Poliomyelitis. In PJ Vinken (ed.), *Handbook of Clinical Neurology* (Vol. 34). Amsterdam: North-Holland, 1978 Pp. 93–132.

6. Mims CA. Aspects of the pathogenesis of virus diseases. *Bacteriol Rev* 28:30–71, 1964.

7. Johnson RT, Mims CA. Pathogenesis of viral infections of the nervous system. *N Engl J Med* 278: 23–30, 1968.

8. Sissons JBP, Oldstone MBA. Killing of virus-infected cells: the role of antiviral antibody and complement in limiting virus infection. *J Infect Dis* 142: 442–48, 1980.

9. Rupprecht CE. Perspectives on rabies virus pathogenesis [editorial]. *Lab Invest* 57:603, 1987.

10. Ma P et al. Naegleria and acanthamoeba infections: review. *Rev Infect Dis* 12:490–513, 1990.

11. Adams RD, Weinstein L. Clinical and pathological aspects of encephalitis. *N Engl J Med* 239:865–76, 1948.

12. Kennard C, Swash M. Acute viral encephalitis, its diagnosis and outcome. *Brain* 104:129–48, 1981.

13. Rennels MB. Arthropod-borne virus infections of the central nervous system. *Neurol Clin* 2:241–45, 1984.

14. Miller A, Nathanson N. Rabies: recent advances in pathogenesis and control. *Ann Neurol* 2:511–19, 1977.

15. Warrell DA, Warrell MJ. Human rabies and its prevention: an overview. *Rev Infect Dis* 10(4): S726–31, 1988.

16. Macpherson GG et al. Human cerebral malaria. A quantitative ultrastructural analysis of parasitized erythrocyte sequestration. *Am J Pathol* 119(3): 385–401, 1985.

17. Wolinsky JS. Herpes simplex encephalitis. *Johns Hopkins Med J* 147:157–66, 1980.

18. Whitley RJ et al. Adenine arabinoside therapy of biopsy-proved herpes simplex encephalitis. *N Engl J Med* 297:289–94, 1977.

19. Whitley RJ et al. Herpes simplex encephalitis: clinical assessment. *JAMA* 247:317–20, 1982.

20. Monath TP et al. Immunoglobulin M antibody capture enzyme-lined immunosorbent assay for diagnosis of St. Louis encephalitis. *J Clin Microbiol* 20:784–90, 1984.

21. Smith JS et al. Demonstration of antigenic variation among rabies virus isolates by using monoclonal antibodies to nucleocapsid proteins. *J Clin Microbiol* 24:573–80, 1986.

22. Whitley RJ et al. Diseases that mimic herpes simplex encephalitis. *JAMA* 262:234–39, 1989.

23. Whitley RJ et al. Vidarabine versus acyclovir therapy in herpes simplex encephalitis. *N Engl J Med* 314:144–49, 1986.

24. Rodu B. Molecular biology in medicine. The polymerase chain reaction: the revolution within. *Am J Med Sci* 299:210–16, 1990.

25. Whitley RJ. Herpes simplex virus infections of the central nervous system. *Am J Med* 85(2A):61–67, 1988.

26. Faulds D, et al. Ganiclovir. A review of its antiviral activity, pharmacokinetic properties and therapeutic efficacy in cytomegalovirus infections. *Drugs* Apr 39(4):597–638, 1990.

27. Centers for Disease Control. Chemoprophylaxis of malaria. *MMWR* 27:10–15, 1978.

28. Centers for Disease Control. Treatment of severe plasmodium falciparum malaria with quinidine gluconate: discontinuation of parenteral quinine from CDC drug service. *MMWR* 40:240, 1991.

29. Hoffman SL et al. High-dose dexamethasone in quinine-treated patients with cerebral malaria: a double-blind, placebo-controlled trial. *J Infect Dis* 158:325–31, 1988.

30. Przelomski MM et al. Eastern equine encephalitis in Massachusetts: a report of 16 cases, 1970–1984. *Neurology* 38:736–39, 1988.

31. Balfour HH et al. California arbovirus (La Crosse) infections. I. Clinical and laboratory findings in 66 children with meningoencephalitis. *Pediatrics* 52:680–91, 1973.

32. Ehrenkranz NJ, Ventura AK. Venezuelan equine encephalitis virus infection in man. *Ann Rev Med* 25:9–14, 1974.

33. Fishbein DB, Arcangeli S. Rabies prevention in primary care. A four-step approach. *Postgrad Med* 82:83–95, 1987.

34. Anderson LJ et al. Clinical experience with a human diploid cell rabies vaccine. *JAMA* 244:781–84, 1980.

35. Centers for Disease Control. Change of dosing regimen for malaria prophylaxis with mefloquine. *MMWR* 40:72–73, 1991.

36. Townsend JJ et al. Acquired toxoplasmosis. A ne-

glected cause of treatable nervous system disease. *Arch Neurol* 32:335–43, 1975.

37. Spencer HC et al. Imported African trypanosomiasis in the United States. *Ann Intern Med* 82:633–38, 1975.

38. Modlin JF et al. Epidemiologic studies of measles, measles vaccine, and subacute sclerosing panencephalitis. *Pediatrics* 59:505–12, 1979.

39. Ohya T et al. Subacute sclerosing panencephalitis. *Neurology* 24:211–18, 1974.

40. Dyken PR. Subacute sclerosing panencephalitis. Current status. *Neurol Clin* 3:179–96, 1985.

41. Graves ML. Subacute sclerosing panencephalitis. *Neurol Clin* 2:267–80, 1984.

42. Krick JA, Remington JS. Current concepts in parasitology. Toxoplasmosis in the adult—an overview. *N Engl J Med* 298:550–53, 1978.

43. TenPas A, Abraham JP. Hematological side-effects of pyrimethamine in the treatment of ocular toxoplasmosis. *Am J Med Sci* 249:448–53, 1965.

44. Drugs for parasitic infections. *Med Lett Drugs Ther* 21:105–12, 1979.

45. Doua F et al. Treatment of human late stage gambiense trypanosomiasis with α-difluoromethylornithine (eflornithine): efficacy and tolerance in 14 cases in Cote D'Ivoire. *Am J Trop Med Hyg* 37:525–33, 1987.

46. Pepin J et al. Difluoromethylornithine for arseno-resistant *Trypanosoma brucei gambiense* sleeping sickness. *Lancet* 2:1431–33, 1987.

47. Taelman H et al. Difluoromethylornithine, an effective new treatment of Gambian trypanosomiasis. *Am J Med* 82:607–14, 1987.

48. Miyazaki M. Apparent response of subacute sclerosing panencephalitis to intrathecal interferon alpha. *Am Neurol* 29:97–99, 1991.

49. U.S. Department of Health and Human Services. Summary of Notifiable Diseases, United States 1989. *MMWR* 38, 1990.

50. Lepow ML et al. A clinical, epidemiologic and laboratory investigation of aseptic meningitis during the four-year period, 1955–1958. I. Observations concerning etiology and epidemiology. *N Engl J Med* 266:1181–87, 1962.

51. Karandanis D, Shulman JA. Recent survey of infectious meningitis in adults: review of laboratory findings in bacterial, tuberculous, and aseptic meningitis. *South Med J* 69:449–57, 1976.

52. Lepow ML A clinical epidemiologic and laboratory investigation of aseptic meningitis during the four-year period, 1955–1958. II. The clinical disease and its sequelae. *N Engl J Med* 266:1188–93, 1962.

53. Sullivan RJ et al. Viral aseptic meningitis: 12 years experience. *Missouri Med* Sept:11–15, 1971.

54. Sells CJ, Carpenter RL, Ray CG. Sequelae of central-nervous-system enterovirus infections. *N Engl J Med* 293:1–4, 1975.

55. Verghese A, Gallemote G. Kennig's and Brudzinski's signs revisited. *Rev Infect Dis* 9:1187–92, 1987.

56. Wilfret CM. Mumps meningoencephalitis with low cerebrospinal-fluid glucose, prolonged pleocytosis and elevation of protein. *N Engl J Med* 280:855–58, 1969.

57. McCabe WM. Empiric therapy for bacterial meningitis. *Rev Infect Dis* 5(suppl.):S74, 1983.

58. Bolan G, Barza M. Acute bacterial meningitis in children and adults. *Med Clin North Am* 69:231, 1985.

59. Romer FK. Difficulties in the diagnosis of bacterial meningitis. *Lancet* 2:345, 1977.

60. Smales OR, Rutter N. Difficulties in diagnosing meningococcal meningitis in children. *Br Med J* 278:588, 1979.

61. Brahams D. The evils of delay. *Lancet* 2:51, 1987.

62. Valmari P. Primary diagnosis in a life-threatening childhood infection. A nationwide study on bacterial meningitis. *Ann Clin Res* 17:310, 1985.

63. Britten RM, Magen BS. Preventive measures to limit legal liability in pediatric emergencies: an analysis through cases concerning failure to diagnose meningitis. *Pediatr Emerg Care* 2:109, 1986.

64. Centers for Disease Control. Bacterial meningitis and meningococcemia—United States. *MMWR* 28:277, 1979.

65. Kresky B, Buchbinder S, and Greenberg IM. The incidence of neurologic residua in children after recovery from bacterial meningitis. *Arch Pediatr* 79:63, 1962.

66. Dodge PR, Swartz MN. Bacterial meningitis—a review of selected aspects. II. Special neurologic problems, postmeningitis complications and clinicopathological correlations. *N Engl J Med* 272:954, 1965.

67. Dodge PR et al. Prospective evaluation of hearing impairment as a sequela of acute bacterial meningitis. *N Engl J Med* 311:869, 1984.

68. Goldschneider I, Gotschlich E, Artenstein M. Human immunity to meningococcus. *J Exp Med* 129:1307, 1969.

69. Ellison R et al. Prevalence of congenital or acquired complement deficiency in patients with sporadic meningococcal disease. *N Engl J Med* 308:913, 1983.

70. Quagliarello VJ, Scheld WM. Review—recent advances in the pathogenesis and pathophysiology of bacterial meningitis. *Am J Med Sci* 292:306–9, 1986.

71. McMenanin J, Volpe J. Bacterial meningitis in infancy: effects on intracranial pressure and cerebral blood flow velocity. *Neurology* 34:500, 1984.

72. Wenger JD et al. Bacterial meningitis in the United States, 1986: report of a multistate surveillance study. *J Infect Dis* 162:1316–23, 1990.

73. Ward JI et al. *Haemophilus influenzae* meningitis: a national study of secondary spread in household contacts. *N Engl J Med* 301:122, 1979.

74. Gorse GJ et al. Bacterial meningitis in the elderly. *Arch Intern Med* 144:1603, 1984.

75. Mangi RJ, Quintilami R, Andriole VT. Gram-negative bacillary meningitis. *Am J Med* 59:829, 1975.

76. Reed MD. Current concepts in clinical therapeutics: bacterial meningitis in infants and children. *Clinical Pharmacy* 5:798, 1986.

77. McCracken GH Jr, Mize SG. A controlled study of intrathecal antibiotic therapy in gram-negative enteric meningitis of infancy: a report of the Neonatal Meningitis Cooperative Study Group. *J Pediatr* 89:66, 1976.

78. Gower DJ et al. Gram-negative bacillary meningitis in the adult: review of 39 cases. *South Med J* 79:1499, 1986.

79. Molavi A, Blumberg EA. Infections of the central nervous system. In D. Schillinger, A. Harwood-Nuss (eds.), *Infections in Emergency Medicine* (Vol. 1). New York: Churchill-Livingstone, 1989.

80. Heerema MS et al. Anaerobic bacterial meningitis. *Am J Med* 67:219, 1979.

81. Schlesinger LS, Ross SC, Schaberg DR. Staphylococcus aureus meningitis: a broad-based epidemiologic study. *Medicine* 66:148, 1987.

82. Carpenter RR, Petersdorf RG. The clinical spectrum of bacterial meningitis. *Am J Med* 33:262, 1962.

83. Hand WL, Sanford JP. Posttraumatic bacterial meningitis. *Ann Intern Med* 72:869, 1970.

84. Griesemer DA, Winkelstein JA, Luddy R. Pneumococcal meningitis in patients with a major sickle hemoglobinopathy. *J Pediatr* 92:82, 1978.

85. Chernik NL, Armstrong D, Pasner JB. Central nervous system infections in patients with cancer. *Medicine (Baltimore)* 52:563, 1973.

86. Nieman RE, Lorber B. Listeriosis in adults: a changing pattern. Report of eight cases and review of the literature, 1968–1978. *Rev Infect Dis* 2:207, 1980.

87. Schoenbaum SC, Gardner P, Shillito J. Infections

of cerebrospinal fluid shunts: epidemiology, clinical manifestations, and therapy. *J Infect Dis* 131:543, 1975.

88. Downs NJ, Hodges GR, Taylor SA. Mixed meningitis. *Rev Infect Dis* 4:693, 1987.

89. Ansari A, Lipsey A, Nachum R. Cerebrospinal fluid muramidase levels in meningitis. *J Pediatr* 94:752–55, 1979.

90. Swartz MN, Dodge PR. Bacterial meningitis—a review of selected aspects. *N Engl J Med* 272:725, 1965.

91. Norman DC, Grahn D, Yoshikawa TT. Fever and aging. *J Am Geriatr Soc* 33:859, 1985.

92. Singer JI. Acute bacterial meningitis. In P Rosen et al. (eds.), *Emergency Medicine Concepts and Clinical Practice* (2nd ed.). St. Louis: Mosby, 1988.

93. Geiseler PJ, Nelson KE. Bacterial meningitis without clinical signs of meningeal irritation. *South Med J* 75:448, 1982.

94. Callaham M. Fulminant bacterial meningitis without meningeal signs. *Ann Emerg Med* 18:90, 1989.

95. Meade RH. Bacterial meningitis in the neonatal period. *Med Clin North Am* 69:257, 1985.

96. Groover RV, Sutherland JM, Landing BH. Purulent meningitis of newborn infants. *N Engl J Med* 264:1115, 1961.

97. Ouellette EM. The child who convulses with fever. *Pediatr Clin North Am* 21:467, 1974.

98. Rosman NP. Febrile seizures. *Emerg Med Clin North Am* 5:719, 1987.

99. Samson JH, Apthorp J, Finley A. Febrile seizures and meningitis. *JAMA* 210:1918, 1969.

100. Ratcliffe JC, Wolf SM. Febrile convulsions caused by meningitis in young children. *Ann Neurol* 1:285, 1977.

101. Lorber J, Sunderland R. Lumbar puncture in children with convulsions associated with fever. *Lancet* 1:785, 1980.

102. Kooiker JC. Spinal puncture and cerebrospinal fluid examination. In JR Roberts, JR Hedges (eds.), *Clinical Procedures in Emergency Medicine*. Philadelphia: Saunders, 1985.

103. Marton KI, Gean AD. The spinal tap: a new look at an old test. *Ann Intern Med* 104:840, 1986.

104. Dougherty JM, Roth RM. Cerebral spinal fluid. *Emerg Med Clin North Am* 4:281, 1986.

105. Laner BA. Comparison of acridine orange and Gram stains for detection of micro organisms in cerebrospinal fluid and other clinical specimens. *J Clin Microbiol* 14:201, 1981.

106. Kleiman MB, Reynolds JK, Watts NH. Superiority of acridine orange stain versus gram stain in par-

tially treated bacterial meningitis. *J Pediatr* 104: 401, 1984.

107. Dougherty JM, Jones J. Cerebrospinal fluid cultures and analysis. *Ann Emerg Med* 15:317, 1986.

108. Donald PR et al. Simultaneous determination of cerebrospinal fluid glucose and blood glucose concentrations in the diagnosis of bacterial meningitis. *J Pediatr* 103:413, 1983.

109. Haywood RA, Oye RK. Are polymorphonuclear leukocytes an abnormal finding in cerebrospinal fluid? *Arch Intern Med* 148:1623, 1988.

110. Sarff LD, Platt LH, McCracken GH. Cerebrospinal fluid evaluation in neonates. Comparison of high risk infants with and without meningitis. *J Pediatr* 88:473, 1976.

111. Portnoy JM, Olson LC. Normal cerebrospinal fluid values in children: another look. *Pediatrics* 75:484, 1985.

112. Polk DB, Steele RW. Bacterial meningitis presenting with normal cerebrospinal fluid. *Pediatr Infect Dis* 6:1040, 1987.

113. Onorato IM, Wormser GP, Nicholas P. "Normal" CSF in bacterial meningitis. *JAMA* 244:1469, 1980.

114. Fishbein DB et al. Bacterial meningitis in the absence of CSF pleocytosis. *Arch Intern Med* 141: 1369–72, 1981.

115. Greiseler PJ et al. Community acquired purulent meningitis: a review of 1,316 cases during the antibiotic era, 1954–1976. *Rev Infect Dis* 2:725, 1980.

116. Sande MA, Tierney LM Jr. Meningitis—Medical Staff Conference, San Francisco General Hospital Medical Center and VA Medical Center, San Francisco. *West J Med* 140:443, 1984.

117. Ward JI et al. Rapid diagnosis of hemophilus influenza type B infections by latex particle agglutination and counterimmunoelectrophoresis. *J Pediatr* 93:37, 1978.

118. Abramowicz M (ed.). Counterimmunoelectrophoresis (CIE) for the rapid diagnosis of bacteremia and bacterial meningitis. *Med Lett Drugs Ther* 23:43, 1981.

119. Wilson CB, Smith AL. Rapid tests for the diagnosis of bacterial meningitis. In JS Remington, MN Swartz (eds.), *Current Clinical Topics in Infectious Diseases*, vol. 7. New York: McGraw-Hill, 1986.

120. Daum RS et al. Evaluation of a commercial latex particle agglutination test for rapid diagnosis of *Haemophilus influenzae* type B infection. *Pediatrics* 69:466, 1982.

121. Russel R et al. Value of antigen quantitation in

haemophilus influenzae type B meningitis. *J Pediatr* 104:23, 1984.

122. Valmari P, Peltola H. Serum C-reactive protein: a valuable differentiation between viral and bacterial meningitis. *Infect Med* 4:308–59, 1987.

123. Eiden J, Yolken RH. C-reactive protein and limulus amebocyte lysate assay in diagnosis of bacterial meningitis. *J Pediatr* 108:423, 1986.

124. Komorowski RA, Farmer S, Knox KK. Comparison of cerebrospinal fluid C-reactive protein and lactate for diagnosis of meningitis. *J Clin Micro* 24:982, 1986.

125. Bryan CS, Reynolds KL, Crout L. Promptness of antibiotic therapy in acute bacterial meningitis. *Ann Emerg Med* 15:544, 1986.

126. Talan DA et al. Role of empiric antibiotics prior to lumbar puncture in suspected bacterial meningitis: state of the art. *Rev Infect Dis* 10:365, 1988.

127. Converse GM et al. Alteration of cerebrospinal fluid findings by partial treatment of bacterial meningitis. *J Pediatr* 83:220, 1973.

128. Barson WJ et al. Prospective comparative trial of ceftriaxone vs. conventional therapy for treatment of bacterial meningitis in children. *Pediatr Infect Dis* 4:362–68, 1985.

129. Del Rio MA et al. Ceftriaxone versus ampicillin and chloramphenicol for treatment of bacterial meningitis in children. *Lancet* 1:1241–44, 1983.

130. McKracken GH, Mize SG, Threlkeld N. Intraventricular gentamicin therapy in gram-negative bacillary meningitis of infancy. *Lancet* 1:787, 1980.

131. McGee ZA, Baringer JR. Acute meningitis. In GL Mandell, RG Douglas, JE Bennett (eds.), *Principles and Practice of Infectious Disease* (3rd ed.). New York: Churchill-Livingstone, 1990.

132. Lebel MH et al. Dexamethasone therapy for bacterial meningitis. *N Engl J Med* 319:964, 1988.

133. Williams JD, Moosdeen F. Antibiotic resistance in *Haemophilus influenzae*: epidemiology, mechanisms, and therapeutic possibilities. *Rev Infect Dis* 8(suppl.):S555, 1986.

134. Lauter CB. Antibiotic therapy of life-threatening infectious diseases in the emergency department. *Ann Emerg Med* 18:1339, 1989.

135. Tuomanen E. Partner drugs: a new outlook for bacterial meningitis [editorial]. *Ann Intern Med* 109:690, 1988.

136. Shapiro ED. Prophylaxis for bacterial meningitis. *Med Clin North Am* 69:269–70, 1985.

137. Band J, Fraser DW, Ajello G. Prevention of *Haemophilus influenzae* type B disease. *JAMA* 25:2381, 1984.

138. Eskola J, Peltola H, Takala AK. Efficacy of *Haemophilus influenzae* type B polysaccharide-diphtheria toxoid conjugate vaccine in infancy. *N Engl J Med* 317:717, 1987.

139. Thong YN. Primary amoebic meningoencephalitis: fifteen years later. *Med J Aust* 1:352–54, 1980.

140. Duma RJ et al. Primary amebic meningoencephalitis. *N Engl J Med* 281:1315–24, 1969.

141. Carter RF. Primary amoebic meningo-encephalitis. An appraisal of present knowledge. *Trans R Soc Trop Med Hyg* 66:193–213, 1972.

142. Martinez AJ, Markowitz SM, Duma RJ. Experimental pneumonitis and encephalitis caused by acanthamoeba in mice: pathogenesis and ultrastructural features. *J Infect Dis* 131:692–99, 1975.

143. Duma RJ et al. Primary amoebic meningoencephalitis caused by *Naegleria*. Two new cases, response to amphotericin B and a review. *Ann Intern Med* 74:861–69, 1971.

144. Seidel J. Primary amebic meningoencephalitis. *Pediatr Clin North Am* 32:881–92, 1985.

145. Stevens AR et al. Primary amoebic meningoencephalitis: a report of two cases and antibiotic and immunologic studies. *J Infect Dis* 143:193–99, 1981.

146. Martinez AJ. Infection of the central nervous system due to acanthamoeba. *Rev Infect Dis* 13 (suppl. 5):S399–402, 1991.

147. Ellner JJ, Bennett JE. Chronic meningitis. *Medicine* 55:341–69, 1976.

148. Wilhelm C, Ellner JJ. Chronic meningitis. *Neurol Clin* 4:115, 1986.

149. Smith HV. Tuberculous meningitis. *Int J Neurol* 4:134–57, 1963.

150. Mintz AA. Tuberculosis meningitis in children before and since isoniazid. *South Med J* 69:1061–62, 1976.

151. Smith AL. Tuberculous meningitis in childhood. *Med J Aust* 1:57–60, 1975.

152. Sumaya CV et al. Tuberculosis meningitis in children during the isoniazid era. *J Pediatr* 87:43–49, 1975.

153. Haas EJ et al. Tuberculous meningitis in an urban general hospital. *Arch Intern Med* 137:1518–21, 1977.

154. Mackay JB. Tuberculous meningitis: a 25 year survey in the Wellington area. *NZ Med J* 66:82–89, 1966.

155. Hinman AR. Tuberculous meningitis at Cleveland Metropolitan General Hospital 1959 to 1963. *Am Rev Respir Dis* 95:670–73, 1967.

156. Illingworth RS. Miliary and meningeal tuberculosis. *Lancet* 2:646–49, 1956.

157. Stewart SM. The bacteriological diagnosis of tuberculosis meningitis. *J Clin Pathol* 6:241–42, 1953.

158. Molavi A, LeFrock JL. Tuberculous meningitis. *Med Clin North Am* 69:315–19, 1985.

159. Alvarez S, McCabe WR. Extrapulmonary tuberculosis revisited: a review of experience at Boston City and other hospitals. *Medicine* 63:25–55, 1984.

160. Daniel TM. New approaches to the rapid diagnosis of tuberculous meningitis. *J Infect Dis* 155:599–602, 1987.

161. Brooks JB et al. Rapid diagnosis of tuberculous meningitis by frequency-pulsed electron-capture gas-liquid chromatography detection of carboxylic acids in cerebrospinal fluid. *J Clin Microbiol* 28:989–97, 1990.

162. Weiss W, Flippin HF. The changing incidence and prognosis of tuberculous meningitis. *Am J Med Sci* 250:46–59, 1965.

163. Escobar JA et al. Mortality from tuberculous meningitis reduced by steroid therapy. *Pediatrics* 56:1050–55, 1975.

164. O'Toole RD et al. Dexamethasone in tuberculous meningitis. Relationship of cerebrospinal fluid effects to therapeutic efficacy. *Ann Intern Med* 70:39–48, 1969.

165. Kocen RS, Parsons M. Neurological complications of tuberculosis: some unusual manifestations. *Q J Med* 153:17–30, 1970.

166. Stevens DL, Everett ED. Sequential computerized axial tomography in tuberculous meningitis. *JAMA* 239:642, 1978.

167. Lewis JL, Rabinovich S. The wide spectrum of cryptococcal infections. *Am J Med* 53:315–22, 1972.

168. Littman ML, Walter JE. Cryptococcosis: current status. *Am J Med* 45:922–32, 1968.

169. Saigo P et al. Identification of *Cryptococcus neoformans* in cytologic preparations of cerebrospinal fluid. *Am J Clin Pathol* 67:141–45, 1977.

170. Berger MP, Paz J. Diagnosis of cryptococcal meningitis. *JAMA* 236:2517–18, 1976.

171. Goodman JS, Kaufman L, Koenig MG. Diagnosis of cryptococcal meningitis. Value of immunologic detection of cryptococcal antigen. *N Engl J Med* 285:434–36, 1971.

172. Snow RM, Dismukes WE. Cryptococcal meningitis. Diagnostic value of cryptococcal antigen in cerebrospinal fluid. *Arch Intern Med* 135:1155–57, 1975.

173. Sarosi GA et al. Amphotericin B in cryptococcal meningitis. Long-term results of treatment. *Ann Intern Med* 1:1079–82, 1969.

174. Abernathy RS. Treatment of systemic mycosis. *Medicine* 52:385–94, 1973.

175. Bennett JE. Chemotherapy of systemic mycoses [first of two parts]. *N Engl J Med* 143:30–32, 319–22, 1974.

176. Bindschadler DD, Bennett JE. Pharmacologic guide to the clinical use of amphotericin B. *J Infect Dis* 120:427–36, 1969.

177. Drutz DJ et al. Treatment of disseminated mycotic infections. A new approach to amphotericin B therapy. *Am J Med* 45:405–18, 1968.

178. Winn WA. The use of amphotericin B in the treatment of coccidioidal disease. *Am J Med* 27:617–35, 1959.

179. Bennett JE et al. A comparison of amphotericin B alone and combined with flucytosine in the treatment of cryptococcal meningitis. *N Engl J Med* 301:126–31, 1979.

180. Utz JP et al. Therapy of cryptococcosis with a combination of flucytosine and amphotericin B. *J Infect Dis* 132:368–74, 1975.

181. Diamond RD, Bennett JE. Prognostic factors in cryptococcal meningitis. A study of 111 cases. *Ann Intern Med* 80:176–81, 1974.

182. Drutz DJ, Catanzaro A. Coccidioidomycosis. Part I. *Am Rev Respir Dis* 117:559–84, 1978.

183. Caudill RG, Smith CD, Reinarz JA. Coccidioidal meningitis. A diagnostic challenge. *Am J Med* 49:360–65, 1970.

184. Colwell JA, Tillman SP. Early recognition and therapy of disseminated coccidioidomycosis. *Am J Med* 31:676–89, 1961.

185. Goodwin RA, Des Prez RM. Histoplasmosis. *Am Rev Respir Dis* 117:929–56, 1978.

186. Goodwin RA et al. Disseminated histoplasmosis: clinical and pathologic correlations. *Medicine* 59:1–33, 1980.

187. Wheat LJ et al. Disseminated histoplasmosis in the acquired immune deficiency syndrome: clinical findings, diagnosis and treatment, and review of the literature. *Medicine (Baltimore)* 69:361–374, 1990.

188. Bayer AS et al. Candida meningitis. *Medicine* 55:477–86, 1976.

189. Edwards JE et al. Severe candidal infections. Clinical perspective, immune defense mechanisms, and current concepts of therapy. *Ann Intern Med* 89:91–106, 1978.

190. Pierce JR, Jabbari B, Shraberg D. Leptospirosis: a neglected cause of nonbacterial meningoencephalitis. *South Med J* 70:150–52, 1977.

191. Edwards GA, Domm BM. Human leptospirosis. *Medicine (Baltimore)* 39:117–56, 1960.

192. Cargill WH Jr, Beeson PB. The value of spinal fluid

examination as a diagnostic procedure in Weil's disease. *Ann Intern Med* 27:396–400, 1947.

193. Heath CW Jr, Alexander AD, Galton MM. Leptospirosis in the United States. Analysis of 483 cases in man. 1949–1961. *N Engl J Med* 273:915–22, 1965.

194. Musher DM. Biology of *Treponema pallidum*. In KK Holmes et al. (eds.), *Sexually Transmitted Diseases*. New York: McGraw-Hill, 1990. Pp. 205–11.

195. Merritt HH, Adams RD, Solomon HC. Neurosyphilis. New York: Oxford University Press, 1946.

196. Davis LE. Neurosyphilis in the patient infected with human immunodeficiency virus [editorial]. *Ann Neurol* 27:211–12, 1990.

197. Merritt HH, Moore M. Acute syphilitic meningitis. *Medicine* 14:119–83, 1935.

198. Holmes MD, Brant-Zawadzki MM, Simon RP. Clinical features of meningovascular syphilis. *Neurology* 34:553–56, 1984.

199. Simon RP. Neurosyphilis. *Arch Neurol* 42:606–13, 1985.

200. Kabat EA, Moore DH, Landow H. An electrophoretic study of the protein components in cerebrospinal fluid and their relationship to the serum proteins. *J Clin Invest* 21:571–80, 1942.

201. Vartdal F et al. Neurosyphilis: intrathecal synthesis of oligoclonal antibodies to *Treponema pallidum*. *Ann Neurol* 11:35–40, 1982.

202. Ganti SR et al. Computed tomography in cerebral syphilis. *J Comput Assist Tomogr* 5:345–47, 1981.

203. Jordon KG. Modern neurosyphilis—a critical analysis. *West J Med* 149:47–57, 1988.

204. Centers for Disease Control. 1989 sexually transmitted diseases treatment guidelines. *MMWR* 38(no. S-8)5–15, 1989.

205. Davis LE, Schmidt JW. Clinical significance of cerebrospinal fluid tests for neurosyphilis. *Ann Neurol* 25:50–55, 1989.

206. Davis LE, Sperry S. The CSF-FTA test and the significance of blood contamination. *Arch Neurol* 6:68–69, 1979.

207. Mohr JA et al. Neurosyphilis and penicillin levels in cerebrospinal fluid. *JAMA* 236:2208–9, 1976.

208. Dunlop EMC, Al-Egaily SS, Houang ET. Penicillin levels in blood and CSF achieved by treatment of syphilis. *JAMA* 241:2538–40, 1979.

209. Hook EW, Roddy RE, Handsfield HH. Ceftriaxone therapy for incubating and early syphilis. *J Infect Dis* 158:881–84, 1988.

210. Jacobson S et al. Isolation of an HTLV-1-like retrovirus from patients with tropical spastic paraparesis. *Nature* 331:540–43, 1988.

211. Roman GC. The neuroepidemiology of tropical

spastic paraparesis. *Ann Neurol* 23:S113–S120, 1988.

212. Shibasaki H et al. Clinical picture of HTLV-1 associated myelopathy. *J Neurol Sci* 87:15–24, 1988.

213. Vernant JC et al. Endemic tropical spastic paraparesis associated with human T-lymphotropic virus type I: a clinical and seroepidemiological study of 25 cases. *Ann Neurol* 21:123–30, 1987.

214. Barbour AG, Hayes SF. Biology of *Borrelia* species. *Microbiol Rev* 50:381–400, 1986.

215. Steere AC. Lyme disease. *N Engl J Med* 321:586–96, 1989.

216. Vallat JM et al. Tick-bite meningoradiculoneuritis: clinical, electrophysiologic, and histologic findings in 10 cases. *Neurology* 37:749–53, 1987.

217. Logigian EL, Kaplan RF, Steere AC. Chronic neurologic manifestations of Lyme disease. *N Engl J Med* 323:1438–44, 1990.

218. Burgdorfer W, Hayes SF, Corwin D. Pathophysiology of the Lyme disease spirochete, *Borrelia burgdorferi*, in ixodid ticks. *Rev Infect Dis* 11(suppl. 6):1442–50, 1989.

219. Pachner AR, Duray P, Steere AC. Central nervous system manifestations of Lyme disease. *Arch Neurol* 47:790–95, 1989.

220. Pachner AR, Steere AC. The triad of neurologic manifestations of Lyme disease. *Neurology* 35:47–53, 1985.

221. Finkel MF. Lyme disease and its neurologic complications. *Arch Neurol* 45:99–104, 1988.

222. Clark JR et al. Facial paralysis in Lyme disease. *Laryngoscope* 95:1341–45, 1985.

223. Halperin JJ. Abnormalities of the nervous system in Lyme disease response to antimicrobial therapy. *Rev Infect Dis* 11(suppl. 6):1499–1504, 1989.

224. Halperin JJ et al. Lyme borelliosis-associated encephalopathy. *Neurology* 40:1340–43, 1990.

225. Halperin JJ et al. Lyme neuroborreliosis: central nervous system manifestations. *Neurology* 39:753–59, 1989.

226. Reik L et al. Demyelinating encephalopathy in Lyme disease. *Neurology* 35:267–69, 1985.

227. Hansen K, Hindersson P, Pedersen NS. Measurement of antibodies to the *Borrelia burgdorferi* flagellum improves serodiagnosis in Lyme disease. *J Clin Microbiol* 26:338–46, 1988.

228. Duffy J et al. Diagnosing Lyme disease: the contribution of serologic testing. *Mayo Clin Proc* 63:1116–21, 1988.

229. Craft JE et al. Antigens of *Borrelia burgdorferi* recognized during Lyme disease. *J Clin Invest* 78:934–39, 1986.

230. Steere AC, Pachner AR, Malawista SE. Neurologic abnormalities of Lyme disease: successful treatment

with high-dose intravenous penicillin. *Ann Intern Med* 99:767–72, 1983.

231. Dattwyler RJ et al. Treatment of late Lyme borreliosis—randomized comparison of ceftriaxone and penicillin. *Lancet* 1:1191–94, 1988.

232. Treatment of Lyme disease. *Med Lett Drugs Ther* 31:57–59, 1989.

233. Courville CR. Empyema secondary to purulent frontal sinusitis. A clinicopathologic study of 42 cases verified at autopsy. *Arch Otolaryngol* 39:211–30, 1944.

234. Yoshikawa TT, Chow AW, Guze LB. Role of anaerobic bacteria in subdural empyema. Report of four cases and review of 327 cases from the English literature. *Am J Med* 58:99–103, 1975.

235. Coonrod JD, Dans PE. Subdural empyema. *Am J Med* 53:85–91, 1972.

236. Duffy GP. Lumbar puncture in the presence of raised intracranial pressure. *Br Med J* 1:407–09, 1969.

237. Garfield J. Management of supratentorial intracranial abscess: a review of 200 cases. *Br Med J* 2:7–11, 1969.

238. Kaufman DM, Leeds NE. Computed tomography (CT) in the diagnosis of intracranial abscesses. *Neurology* 27:1069–73, 1977.

239. Lott T et al. Evaluation of brain and epidural abscesses by computed tomography. *Radiology* 122:371–76, 1977.

240. Biehl JP. Subdural empyema secondary to acute frontal sinusitis. *JAMA* 158:721–24, 1955.

241. Baker AS et al. Spinal epidural abscess. *N Engl J Med* 293:463–68, 1975.

242. Hulme A, Dott NM. Spinal epidural abscess. *Br Med J* 1:64–65, 1954.

243. Heusner AP. Nontuberculous spinal epidural infections. *N Engl J Med* 239:845–54, 1948.

244. Krayenbuhl H. Cerebral venous and sinus thrombosis. *Clin Neurosurg* 14:1–10, 1967.

245. Heineman HS, Bradue AI. Anaerobic infection of the brain. Observations on 18 consecutive cases of brain abscess. *Am J Med* 35:682–97, 1963.

246. De Louvois J, Gortvai P, Hurley R. Bacteriology of abscesses of the central nervous system: a multicenter prospective study. *Br Med J* 2:981–84, 1977.

247. De Louvois J, Gortvai P, Hurley R. Antibiotic treatment of abscesses of the central nervous system. *Br Med J* 2:985–87, 1977.

248. Brewer NS, MacCarty CS, Wellman WE. Brain abscess: a review of recent experience. *Ann Intern Med* 82:571–76, 1975.

249. Wood PH. Diffuse subdural suppuration. *J Laryngol* 66:496–515, 1952.

250. Berk SL, McCabe WR. Meningitis caused by gram-negative bacilli. *Ann Intern Med* 93:253–60, 1980.

251. Crane LR, Lerner AM. Non-traumatic gram-negative bacillary meningitis in the Detroit Medical Center, 1964–1974. *Medicine* 57:197–209, 1978.

252. Samson DS, Clark K. A current review of brain abscess. *Am J Med* 54:201–10, 1973.

253. Crocker EF et al. Technetium brain scanning in the diagnosis and management of cerebral abscess. *Am J Med* 56:192–201, 1974.

254. Weisberg LA. Computed tomography in the diagnosis of intracranial disease. *Ann Intern Med* 91:87–105, 1979.

255. Beller AJ, Sahar A, Praiss I. Brain abscess. Review of 89 cases over 30 years. *J Neurol Neurosurg Psychiatry* 36:757–68, 1973.

256. Ingham HR, Selkon JB, Roxby CM. Bacteriological study of otogenic cerebral abscesses: chemotherapeutic role of metronidazole. *Br Med J* 2:991–93, 1977.

257. McFarlan AM. The bacteriology of brain abscess. *Br Med J* 2:643–52, 1943.

258. Morgan H, Wood M, Murphey F. Experience with 88 consecutive cases of brain abscess. *J Neurosurg* 38:698–706, 1973.

259. Swarz MN, Karchner AW. Infections of the central nervous system. In A Balows, RM Dehaan, VR Dowell Jr (eds.), *Anaerobic Bacteria: Role in Disease.* Springfield, IL: Thomas, 1974. Pp. 309–50.

260. Black P, Graybill JR, Charache P. Penetration of brain abscess by systemically administered antibodies. *J Neurosurg* 38:705–16, 1973.

261. Norrby R. A review of the penetration of antibiotics into CSF and its clinical significance. *Scand J Infect Dis* 14: (suppl.) 296–309, 1978.

262. Greene BM. Trimethoprim-sulfamethoxazole and brain abscess. *Ann Intern Med* 82:812–13, 1975.

263. Berg B. Nonsurgical cure of brain abscess: early diagnosis and follow-up with computerized tomography. *Ann Neurol* 3:474–78, 1978.

264. Heineman HS, Bradue AI, Osterholm JL. Intracranial suppurative disease. Early presumptive diagnosis and successful treatment without surgery. *JAMA* 218:1542–47, 1971.

265. Kaplan K. Brain abscess. *Med Clin North Am* 69:345–60, 1985.

266. Bloom WH, Tuazon CU. Successful treatment of multiple brain abscesses with antibiotics alone. *Rev Infect Dis* 7:189–99, 1985.

267. Earnest MP et al. Neurocysticercosis in the United States: 35 cases and a review. *Rev Infect Dis* 9:961–79, 1987.

268. Del Brutto OH, Sotelo J. Neurocysticercosis: an update. *Rev Infect Dis* 10:1075–87, 1988.

269. McCormick GF, Zee C-S, Heiden J. Cysticercosis cerebri: review of 127 cases. *Arch Neurol* 39:534–39, 1982.

270. Larralde C et al. Reliable serology of *Taenia solium* cysticercosis with antigens from cyst vesicular fluid: ELISA and hemagglutination tests. *Am J Trop Med Hyg* 35:965–73, 1986.

271. Tsang VCW, Brand JA, Boyer AE. An enzyme-linked immunoelectrotransfer blot assay and glycoprotein antigens for diagnosing human cysticercosis (*Taenia solium*). *J Infect Dis* 159:50–59, 1989.

272. Byrd SE et al. The computed tomographic appearance of cerebral cysticercosis in adults and children. *Radiology* 144:819–23, 1982.

273. Sotelo J. Therapy of parenchymal brain cysticercosis with praziquantel. *N Engl J Med* 310:1001–07, 1984.

274. Escobedo F et al. Abendazole therapy for neurocysticercosis. *Arch Intern Med* 147:738–41, 1987.

275. Arnon SS. Infant botulism. *Ann Rev Med* 31:541–60, 1980.

276. Arnon SS. Infant Botulism: anticipating the second decade. *J Infect Dis* 54:201–06, 1986.

277. Thompson JA. Infant botulism. *Sem Neurol* 2:144–50, 1982.

278. Kryzhanovsky GN. Present data on the pathogenesis of tetanus. *Prog Drug Res* 19:301–13, 1975.

279. Griffin JW. Bacterial toxins. Botulism and tetanus. In PGE Kennedy, RT Johnson (eds.), *Infections of the Nervous System*. London: Butterworths, 1987. Pp. 76–92.

280. Weinstein L. Tetanus. *N Engl J Med* 289:1293–1296, 1973.

281. Bleck TP. Review: pharmacology of tetanus. *Clin Neuropharmacol* 9:103–20, 1986.

282. Adams JM, Kenny JD, Rudolph AJ. Modern management of tetanus neonatorum. *Pediatrics* 64:472–77, 1979.

283. Flowers MW, Edmondson RS. Long-term recovery from tetanus: a study of 50 survivors. *Br Med J* 42:303–9, 1980.

284. Kew OM, Nottay B. Molecular epidemiology of polioviruses. *Rev Infect Dis* 6(suppl.):S499–504, 1984.

285. Howard RS, Wiles CM, Spencer GT. The late sequelae of poliomyelitis. *Q J Med* 66:219–32, 1988.

286. Cashman NR et al. Late denervation in patients with antecedent paralytic poliomyelitis. *N Engl J Med* 317:7–12, 1987.

287. Neill MA, Hightower AW, Broome CV. Leprosy in the United States, 1971–1981. *J Infect Dis* 152:1064–69, 1985.

288. Blake LA et al. Environmental nonhuman sources of leprosy. *Rev Infect Dis* 9:562–77, 1987.

289. Reich CV. Leprosy: cause, transmission, and a new theory of pathogenesis. *Rev Infect Dis* 9:590–94, 1987.

290. Van Voorhis WC et al. The cutaneous infiltrates of leprosy. Cellular characteristics and the predominant T-cell phenotypes. *N Engl J Med* 307:1593–97, 1982.

291. Jacobson RR, Trautman JR. The diagnosis and treatment of leprosy. *South Med J* 69:979–85, 1976.

292. Shepard CC. Leprosy today. *N Engl J Med* 307:1640–41, 1982.

293. World Health Organization. Chemotherapy of leprosy for control programmes. Geneva: WHO, 1982. WHO Technical Report Series, no. 675.

THE SKIN, SOFT TISSUE, BONES, AND JOINTS

32

Skin and Soft-Tissue Infections

J. STEPHAN STAPCZYNSKI

Skin and soft-tissue infections cover a wide clinical spectrum, from those that are superficial, localized, and sometimes self-limited to those that are deep, rapidly spreading, and potentially life threatening [1–7]. While these infections may be due to a variety of infectious agents—viruses, bacteria, or fungi—those caused by bacteria represent the clinical challenge for early diagnosis and treatment. The majority of patients with superficial infections can be treated as outpatients, but compliance with treatment and appropriate follow-up are crucial to a successful result. Patients with deep and spreading infections require immediate resuscitation, broad-spectrum antibiotics, and rapid surgical exploration.

Normal epithelium is resistant to most bacteria. In addition this barrier is enhanced by the presence of coagulase-negative staphylococci, which inhibit the growth of most other organisms [1, 2]. Except when exposed to other infected individuals, normal skin does not usually harbor streptococci [1, 2]. Colonization with *Staphylococcus aureus* is limited to neonates (because of their minimal cutaneous flora), the anterior nares, or perineal skin [1, 2]. Therefore, skin or soft-tissue infections usually are seen in states where the epithelial barrier has been damaged by trauma, overhydration, vascular insufficiency, or preexisting skin diseases [1]. The microbiology of bacterial skin and soft-tissue infections usually reflects the indigenous skin flora or that of adjacent mucous membranes. The major exception is when systemic immunologic impairments render the patient susceptible to a wider array of potential pathogens; in those circumstances opportunistic organisms can produce serious infections [1].

For the purposes of discussion and classification, these infections will be divided into two major groups: (1) superficial, usually localized infections and (2) deep, often rapidly spreading infections.

Superficial, Localized Infections

Superficial, localized infections are usually found in otherwise healthy individuals [5–7]. By nature, they tend to remain superficial and localized or spread to only a limited extent. Some infections may resolve by themselves, provided local and systemic host defenses are intact. While definitive microbiologic diagnosis can be made by appropriate stains, cultures, or immunologic techniques, diagnosis is based predominantly on clinical appearance

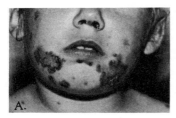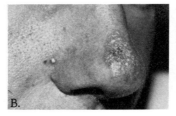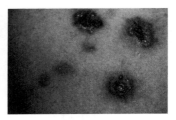

Fig. 32-1. Impetigo. Note characteristic crusted erosions around the mouth. A. Characteristic erosions of impetigo; B. Crusts of impetigo; C. Vesicles of bullous impetigo. (Courtesy of Upjohn Pharmaceuticals. Used with permission)

and circumstances [6, 7]. In general clinical diagnosis and presumptive treatment are overwhelmingly successful, and the majority of these patients can be treated as outpatients. Patient compliance and adequate follow-up, however, are key to a successful outcome.

While the majority of superficial bacterial skin and soft-tissue infections can be cured with oral antibiotics, there are three high risk situations in which inpatient treatment with IV antibiotics may be required: (1) infections around the eyes or on the face, because of the potential for intraorbital or intracranial spread, (2) infections in the presence of impaired local host defenses, such as edema, lymphedema, or arterial insufficiency, and (3) infections in the presence of a defective immune system.

Vesicular, Weeping Infections

IMPETIGO
Impetigo is a vesicular, weeping superficial skin infection produced by *Streptococcus pyogenes* (group A streptococci), although *S. aureus* also may be found to varying degrees [3, 6–9]. In fact some recent series report isolation of *S. aureus* more than streptococci [10–14]. A variant form of impetigo forms medium-sized bullae and is commonly associated with *S. aureus*, often group II phage type 71 strains [3, 6–9].

Impetigo typically is found in children and young adults, usually located on the arms, legs, or face [6–9] (see Fig. 32-1). In the nonbullous variety the lesions start as small breaks in epidermal barrier, followed by erythematous macules that develop into small vesicles, eventually breaking open to yield a clear exudate that dries into a honey-colored crust [6–9]. In the bullous form the vesicles slowly enlarge into flaccid bullae, typically 2–5 cm in diameter, before breaking open and leaving a raw red base [6–9]. Regional lymphadenitis is found in 80%–90% of the nonbullous variety and in about 30% of the bullous form. Because impetigo is a superficial infection, fever or systemic toxicity is unusual.

Impetigo is contagious and easily spread among infants and preschool children. Predisposing factors are thought to include prior skin lesions (such as dermatitis, varicella, scabies, or trauma), poor hygiene, and malnutrition [3, 6, 7].

Diagnosis is based on clinical appearance; routine culture is not necessary. While endemic cases of impetigo have a low rate (less than 2%) of poststreptococcal glomerulonephritis, a urinalysis is recommended on clinical diagnosis of impetigo. There are no reports of acute rheumatic fever following streptococcal impetigo.

Systemic antibiotics are traditionally recommended because they are effective, treat the skin involvement, eradicate the pathogenic bacteria from potential sites of colonization (e.g., nasopharynx), and reduce secondary spread of the infection (Table 32-1) [8, 9, 15, 16]. Studies from the 1950s to the 1970s documented that for treatment of nonbullous impetigo, penicillin V PO for 10 days or benzathine penicillin IM once was effective. More recent studies from the 1980s found dominant isolation of *S. aureus* and correspondingly lower treatment success rate with penicillin [5, 10, 11]. Those authors recommended a drug with activity against *S. aureus*, such as a semisynthetic penicillinase-resistant penicillin, cephalosporin, or erythromycin PO at standard doses for 10 days (see Table 32-1) [5, 10, 11]. Additionally because of the strong association of *S. aureus* with bullous impetigo, such agents are recommended for the treatment of this form of impetigo. For penicillin-allergic patients, erythromycin 250–500 mg q6–8h PO for 10 days is effective. In endemic cases these antibiotics have over a 90%–95% clinical and bacteriologic cure rate [10–14]. There is no evidence that prompt antibiotic treatment of impetigo prevents or reduces the incidence of poststreptococcal glomerulonephritis.

Heretofore topical therapy has not been considered appropriate for the treatment of impetigo because of the low response rate to the previously available agents [15]. The recent availability of 2% mupirocin topical ointment may offer an alternative to systemic therapy. When applied three times a day to the affected area, the clinical and bacteriologic cure rates have been reported to be over 95% in the studies published to date [17–22]. There is about a 3% occurrence of local side effects (burning or stinging), which appear to be related to the vehicle (polyethylene glycol) rather than the active agent [23]. The major drawback to mupirocin is that sites of colonization are not affected by such topical treatment; therefore, the effect of mupirocin treatment of impetigo on the secondary spread of this disease within families is uncertain.

While it may be tempting to scrub the crusted impetigo lesions with soaps, animal and clinical studies have found that such treatment does not add to antibiotic therapy and may spread the infection further or delay healing [24]. Impetigo usually heals without a scar.

An inciting factor for impetigo in warm climates is often the minor skin damage from insect bites or traumatic abrasions. Prophylactic treatment with topical antibiotics may be useful in preventing this infection [25].

Follow-up is necessary only if the patient fails to improve.

ECTHYMA

Ecthyma is an uncommon ulcerative form of impetigo caused by *S. pyogenes*, almost always in concert with *S. aureus* [6, 7, 26, 27]. This distinctive cutaneous infection is seen primarily in children with poor hygiene. Ecthyma starts as a superficial vesicle that spreads deeper, producing a crust-covered ulcer. Ecthyma lesions may be multiple and are usually found on the lower extremities. Antibiotic therapy is the same as for impetigo, but unlike impetigo, ecthyma usually heals with a scar [28]. Mupirocin ointment can also be used to treat ecthyma [17, 18, 20–22].

HERPETIC SKIN INFECTIONS

Herpes Simplex. Herpes simplex virus (HSV) is a DNA virus that comes in two forms: HSV-1, which causes predominantly oral-labial and nongenital infections, and HSV-2, which typically pro-

Table 32-1. Oral antibiotics for treatment of soft-tissue infections

Antibiotic	Pediatric dosage	Adult dosage	Frequency
Penicillin V	25–50 mg/kg/day	1–2 g/day	q6h
Dicloxacillin	12.5–25.0 mg/kg/day	1–2 g/day	q6h
Amoxicillin-clavulanate	20–40 mg/kg/day	0.75–1.50 g/day	q8h
Cephalexin	25–50 mg/kg/day	1–2 g/day	q6–12h
Cephradine	25–50 mg/kg/day	1–2 g/day	q6–12h
Erythromycin	30–50 mg/kg/day	1–2 g/day	q6h
Trimethoprim-sulfamethoxazole	1 ml/kg/day suspension[a]	4 regular tabs/day[b]	q12h

[a] 1 ml = 8 mg trimethoprin (TMP) + 40 mg sulfamethoxazole (SMZ)
[b] 1 regular tablet = 80 mg TMP + 400 mg SMZ

duces genital infections [29–31]. Either type can cause infection in each location. While related, the HSV types are sufficiently immunologically distinctive that prior infection with one does not provide complete immunity to subsequent infection with the other. This chapter discusses cutaneous HSV infections in otherwise healthy individuals; disseminated infections in immunocompromised patients are considered in Chap. 16 and Chap. 17.

Cutaneous HSV infections are classified as (1) primary infections, afflicting previously uninfected individuals; (2) first-episode infection, a less severe, first-time infection, usually with HSV-2, in patients with neutralizing antibodies directed against the other type, usually HSV-1, that confers partial protection; and (3) recurrent, clinical relapses in those previously infected [29–31]. Recurrent episodes occur because HSV appears able to reside in latent fashion in sensory ganglia. Under the stimulus of a variety of well-described but poorly understood conditions, the latent virus is reactivated and travels down the peripheral sensory nerves to produce the recurrent lesions [29–32].

The incubation period for primary HSV-1 infection is 3–10 days [29]. Initial symptoms usually are mucosal pain and tenderness for a few days, followed by extensive involvement of the oral mucosa with vesicles and superficial erosions [30]. The gingiva are usually involved with swelling and redness, giving rise to the term often applied to this primary infection, *herpetic gingivostomatitis* (see Figure 9-4). These lesions are painful, making it difficult for the patient to eat or drink. Fever and submandibular adenopathy are common. Recovery and healing of this primary infection typically takes 1–3 weeks. HSV-1 is ubiquitous; by late adolescence over half the general U.S. population will have serologic evidence of previous HSV-1 infection [29, 33].

Recurrent HSV-1 infections typically appear as a cluster of vesicles, 5 to 15 mm in size and on an erythematous base, preceded by several hours of local pain or paresthesia [29, 30]. The vesicles persist for a few days, then crust over, dry up, and heal, usually in 7–10 days [29, 30, 33]. Common sites for recurrent HSV-1 are the lips, face, and neck, although recurrences can affect any part of the body [29, 30, 33]. Regional adenopathy is common with recurrences.

The incubation period for primary HSV-2 infection averages about 6 days, with a reported range of 1–45 days [29, 31, 32]. Primary HSV-2 infection typically is more severe in females, with extensive vesicles, erosions, erythema, and swelling of the labia and vaginal opening, a process termed *herpetic vulvovaginitis* [29–32]. Fever, purulent discharge, and inguinal adenopathy are usually present [31, 32]. Primary HSV-2 infection in males tends to be less severe, usually with a confined cluster of herpetic vesicles on the penis, bilateral inguinal adenopathy, and sometimes urethritis with lesions around the urethral meatus [30]. Since antibodies to HSV-1 are found in the majority of adolescents or adults before they begin sexual activity, severe, primary infections with HSV-2 are uncommon; most initial infections with HSV-2 are the less severe first-episode infections [30]. Initial infections with HSV-2 typically last 2–3 weeks before lesions heal.

Recurrent HSV-2 infections typically are preceded by local pain or paresthesia, followed by the development of a cluster of small vesicles situated on an erythematous base [31, 32]. Inguinal lymphadenopathy is seen in 25%–30% [32]. Dysuria and urethral discharge are seen in 10% and 4% of men, respectively [32]. Dysuria and vaginal discharge are reported in 25% and 45% of women, respectively [32].

The frequency of recurrences varies greatly from patient to patient [29, 30]. In general genital HSV infections recur more often than oral-labial HSV infections [34]. There is also some difference between HSV-1 and HSV-2 [34]. For nongenital HSV infections, HSV-1 is more likely to recur than HSV-2. For genital HSV infections the opposite is true: HSV-2 is more likely to recur than HSV-1. The great individual variation in recurrence rates makes it difficult to analyze the efficacy of proposed treatment regimens to decrease the frequency of relapses [29, 30].

The characteristic appearance of HSV lesions usually leaves little doubt in the diagnosis. When appropriate, HSV infection can be documented by several techniques [29]. Cytologic examination (Tzanck test; see Chap. 3) of material obtained by scraping the base of the vesicles usually is positive in oral-labial infection but positive in only about half of genital lesions. Cytologic examination is positive when multinucleated giant cells with intranuclear inclusion bodies are seen, but this appearance is not specific for HSV; the same will be seen with varicella-zoster infections. Indirect immunofluorescent microscopic examination with monoclonal antibodies appears to be more sensitive (overall 75%) than cytologic examination alone. The enzyme-linked immunosorbent assay (ELISA) test for HSV antigens in specimens collected by scraping the lesions is reported to be quite sensitive, but this high value falls off quickly unless the specimen is analyzed quickly. The virus can be readily isolated by cell-culture techniques from the vesicle fluid in primary or secondary lesions; this is the diagnostic test against which others are compared [29]. Antibody titers against HSV-1 and HSV-2 rise within a week after a primary infection but do not change significantly with recurrences. In general, diagnosis is clinical, with cytologic examination or viral-culture techniques being reserved for cases when precise diagnosis is important.

General treatment measures are often used to treat the pain of the herpetic lesions, but effectiveness is variable and response is generally less than satisfactory [30]. For primary infections systemic analgesics may be required. Cool compresses with tap water or Burow's solution or sitz baths with colloidal oatmeal may have some benefit. Topical anesthetics, such as viscous lidocaine, dibucaine ointment, diphenhydramine elixir, and dyclonine solution, may be useful when applied frequently to relieve pain. Mouthwashes used in oral HSV infections may have some role to decrease irritation on the mucous membranes and prevent secondary infection. Topical antibiotics, applied as liquids or ointments, may also decrease secondary infection.

Acyclovir is the only currently available anti-infective agent useful in the treatment of mucocutaneous HSV infections [29, 30, 33]. Because genital HSV is a sexually transmitted disease, can cause serious neonatal infections, and may have a possible role in cervical dysplasia and carcinoma, studies with acyclovir have tended to concentrate more on treating genital HSV infections rather than oral-labial infections. For primary and first-episode HSV genital infections, acyclovir 200 mg PO five times a day, begun within 3 days after the appearance of lesions and continued for 5 days, hastens healing of the lesions and shortens the duration of discomfort [35, 36]. For recurrent genital HSV infections treatment with acyclovir 800 mg bid PO or 200 mg PO five times a day, initiated

within 2 days and continued for 5 days, may shorten the clinical course [37]. The same study suggests that patient-initiated treatment started during the prodromal phase may abort the development of lesions [37]. For patients with frequent genital HSV recurrences, prophylactic treatment with acyclovir 200 mg tid will reduce or prevent relapses [38]. Topical 5% acyclovir is of low efficacy in shortening primary and first-episode genital HSV infections. Topical acyclovir has no proven benefit for recurrent genital HSV infections [39].

Because primary and recurrent oral-labial HSV infections are self-limited, do not have serious complications in otherwise immunocompetent hosts, and do not possess public health hazards, the benefits of acyclovir treatment of nongenital HSV infections is less clear [29, 30, 33]. Currently acyclovir treatment of nongenital HSV infections in otherwise healthy individuals is not recommended [30, 33].

Herpes Zoster. Varicella-zoster virus (VZV) is a DNA virus that produces two distinct diseases: (1) a primary infection (varicella or chickenpox; see Chap. 9) with systemic manifestations and a generalized rash, and (2) recurrent infection (zoster) with a localized rash and few systemic symptoms [40, 41]. Following resolution of the primary infection, varicella-zoster virus becomes latent in the sensory ganglia of the dorsal root or cranial nerves. For reasons not fully understood, the immune mechanisms that function to keep VZV controlled may break down, allowing the virus to travel down the sensory nerves to the skin and produce the characteristic vesicular lesions along a dermatomal pattern [40, 41].

Less than 10% of the cases occur in children, and 40% occur in individuals age 50–70. The incidence increases in older patients and reaches 10 cases per 100 person-years in those aged 80 years or older. Patients who have deficits in their cellular immune system have increased risk. Cancer patients have a risk of approximately 2%, but 15% of those with Hodgkin's disease develop herpes zoster. A history of chickenpox commonly is present, but some patients have had unrecognized prior infection with the virus.

Many patients with herpes zoster report pain, pruritus, or discomfort for several days prior to the eruption of the vesicular rash [40, 41]. The lesions tend to stay confined to one or a few contiguous dermatomes. The rash first appears as erythematous macules or papules that usually develop into vesicles in 1 day. The vesicles usually have an erythematous base and can be scattered throughout the dermatome or become confluent. The vesicles typically resolve in 2 weeks by first becoming purulent, then breaking open and crusting over, before healing. Herpes zoster most often affects the face, neck, and chest dermatomes. The prodromal discomfort of herpes zoster may evolve into a variety of bothersome sensory abnormalities in the affected dermatome. These sensory changes, especially persistent pain, are quite distressing to patients. The elderly are more likely to have persistent sensory abnormalities with herpes zoster [40, 41].

Complications include spread of the virus to the eye to the anterior root or motor nerves, to the spinal cord and brain, or to the entire body, causing disseminated zoster. There also may be involvement of the motor fibers to the facial nerve, which causes facial weakness as well as pain and vesicles. Ascending myelitis or encephalomyelitis may occur but only rarely. Postherpetic pain may persist a month or longer in 9%–14% of patients; in one-third of those patients the pain may last a year or longer. This complication increases with age and occurs in at least one-half of patients past age 60. The pain may be steady, burning, boring, tearing, or aching, or it may take a form characterized by paroxysmal jabbing or lancinating pains or have a tic-like nature.

The diagnosis is usually made on the basis of a typical dermatomal rash in a patient with or without manifestations of pain. The vesicles are indistinguishable from those that occur in primary chickenpox.

Confirmation of herpes-zoster infection can be obtained from cytologic examination (Tzanck test), viral culture, biopsy, direct immunofluorescence of material obtained from a vesicle, or detection of neutralizing antibodies in the serum, similar to the techniques used in herpes simplex infections [40, 42]. For practical reasons cytologic examination is the most sensitive and readily available test used in the emergency department [42].

Most patients with localized zoster do not require hospitalization, even if they are immunocompromised. However, such patients are contagious and

should be kept away from those who have hematologic malignancies or who are on immunosuppressive drugs. Patients with ophthalmic zoster must be treated aggressively. A clue to ophthalmic involvement is involvement of the nasociliary branch of the facial nerve.

Because zoster lesions are painful, analgesics may be required, including tricyclic antidepressants [43, 44]. A variety of topical agents have been used to provide symptomatic relief from the painful lesions: Burow's solution, collodion, phenol shake solutions, and occlusive dressings.

Most cases of localized herpes zoster in otherwise healthy individuals do not require antiviral treatment [40, 41]. However, because this acute disease and the postherpetic symptoms are more severe in the elderly, some consideration may be given to treating those patients. Patients with trigeminal nerve involvement also should be treated. High-dose oral acyclovir (800 mg five times a day for 7 days) administered within 48 hours after onset of the rash may shorten the course and reduce the pain of postherpetic neuralgia [45]. Ophthalmologic dosing is up to 8 g daily. Liquid acyclovir may be more convenient for high-dose regimens. However, there is no reduction in postherpetic neuralgia. The benefits of this large dose are not sufficiently profound to justify the cost for most patients. Intravenous acyclovir (500 mg/m^2 q4h for 7 days or 10 mg/kg q8h for 7 days) reduces pain, inhibits dissemination, and promotes healing in immunocompromised patients [46]. Lesser doses or topical treatment with acyclovir do not appear beneficial in immunocompetent individuals.

Oral steroids are commonly believed to decrease the severity of the acute attack (local pain and swelling) and to reduce the incidence of postherpetic neuralgia, especially in the elderly [40, 41]. This belief is based on the results of three small studies published between 1964 and 1980 [40]. A more recent study failed to show a benefit from systemic steroids [47]. Until further information is available, it seems prudent to restrict steroid therapy to elderly patients without contraindications to such treatment. A typical regimen is to use prednisone 40–60 mg a day, slowly tapered over 3–4 weeks. Such doses do not enhance the rate of healing or increase the risk of dissemination.

Postherpetic neuralgia has been reported to be

helped by a wide variety of agents, reflecting the difficulty in providing relief to patients with this syndrome [43, 44, 48]. The use of low doses of tricyclic antidepressants (amitriptyline 50–150 mg/day in divided oral doses) with or without phenothiazines appears to be the most effective therapy [44, 48]. Treatment for at least 1 week is necessary to determine benefit, and the duration of therapy may be several months [44, 48]. Carbamazepine (100 mg bid with doses increased to reach anticonvulsant levels) may be helpful in treatment of lancinating pain. A wide variety of topical, intramuscular, and oral agents also have had reported success in selected patients [43, 44, 48, 49]. Transcutaneous electrical nerve stimulation (TENS) is also sometimes used. Surgical ablative approaches have not been beneficial.

Erythematous, Spreading Infections

SIMPLE CELLULITIS

Cellulitis is an inflammatory process of the deep dermis that occurs when bacteria breach the protective epithelium and gain access to the subcutaneous tissues [1, 2, 6]. The majority of cases are due to streptococci, staphylococci, and *Haemophilus influenzae* (usually in children) [2, 3, 6, 50–57]. Other bacteria may be isolated in certain clinical situations (Table 32-2) [54–57]. In immunocompromised individuals a wide variety of bacteria (*Enterobacteriaceae and Pseudomonas* species) and fungi (*Candida and Cryptococcus* species) may produce cellulitis.

Cellulitis appears as a spreading inflammation with local warmth, erythema, and sometimes induration [6, 58]. If untreated, induration and suppuration can develop [3]. In severe cases vesicles, bullae, and abscesses may occur. Lymphangitis and regional lymphadenopathy are common. In adults and children with truncal or extremity involvement, fever and systemic toxicity are uncommon [6, 7, 50, 51, 58–60].

Because cellulitis due to H. influenzae can be associated with bacteremia or disseminated infection, clinical clues that suggest infection with this organism are important to note: (1) facial cellulitis, especially in a child less than 2 years old, with otitis media or rhinitis without an obvious portal of entry, (2) extremity cellulitis in a child accompanied by fever and leukocytosis, (3) a violaceous hue to the erythema, and (4) multiple separate sites of involvement [50–53].

Microbial evaluation of cellulitis can be done by a number of techniques: (1) swab stains or cultures of open wounds or drainage [58–61], (2) stains or cultures of fluid obtained by subcutaneous aspiration [60–70], (3) blood cultures [59–61, 63, 68, 69], (4) stains or cultures of punch biopsy of the cellulitis, or (5) immunologic evidence of bacterial infection [71, 72]. The yield from such methods varies with the clinical technique utilized (Table 32-3). Because the majority of cases in previously healthy individuals are due to either streptococci or staphylococci, routine culture in adults is not required, and empiric therapy is usually successful [64, 66, 68–70]. In immunocompromised individ-

Table 32-2. Clinical syndromes of cellulitis associated with bacteria other than staphylococci or streptococci

Clinical syndrome	Causative agent
Facial cellulitis in children, especially without a portal of entry	H. influenzae
Facial cellulitis with exterior trauma	S. aureus
Facial cellulitis from a dental abscess or intraoral laceration	Anaerobic mouth flora
Infants, especially with face or neck involvement	Group B streptococci
Cellulitis within 24 hours after cat or dog bite	P. multocida
Cellulitis at a vein donor site (e.g., after saphenous venectomy for coronary bypass graft)	Group A streptococci
Cellulitis associated with venous insufficiency or lymphatic compromise	Beta-hemolytic streptococci (groups A, B, C, and G reported)

Table 32-3. Approximate incidence of pathogen isolation in previously healthy patients with cellulitis

Clinical syndrome	Percentage of positive cultures	
	Aspiration	Blood
Extremity or truncal cellulitis with intact skin	10–40	< 5
Extremity or truncal cellulitis with broken skin or pur-ulence	80–90	< 5
Facial cellulitis in children	40	40–80

uals, the range of potential pathogens is greater, and microbiologic diagnosis is recommended.

Most cases of cellulitis in adults and many cases in children can be adequately treated with oral antibiotics for 10 days (see Table 32-1) [3–7, 12]. The following patients should be considered for admission and treatment with IV antibiotics: (1) children and adults with facial cellulitis (because of the risk of intracranial or intraorbital spread) [3, 4, 6, 7], (2) children and adults with high fever and systemic toxicity [6, 7, 51, 52], (3) infants with

cellulitis [6, 7, 51, 56], and (4) patients with immu-nodeficiencies or local host defense impairments [3] (Table 32-4). With the advent of long-acting, broad-spectrum antibiotics, such as ceftriaxone, more patients with facial cellulitis are being treated on an outpatient basis. These patients must be carefully selected and followed up.

ERYSIPELAS

Erysipelas is a distinctive type of cellulitis that in-volves the superficial dermis. It most commonly is caused by S. pyogenes, although other beta-hemoly-tic streptococci and S. aureus may produce a similar picture [3, 6, 7, 72–74]. This disease is uncommon in developed countries and is most often found at the extremes of age, that is, in infants and the elderly [73, 75]. In the preantibiotic era the face was the most common location for involvement, but a recent report from Israel documents a prepon-derance of cases involving the legs, presumably owing to walking in sandals or being barefoot [76].

Erysipelas starts off as a small, raised, painful plaque that spreads with a distinct advancing edge over several days to reach a maximum size, if un-treated, of 10–15 cm in diameter (see Color Plate

Table 32-4. IV antibiotics for treatment of serious soft-tissue infections

Antibiotic	Pediatric dosage	Adult dosage	Frequency
Penicillin G	50,000 U/kg/day	20 million U/day	q6h
Ampicillin	100–200 mg/kg/day	6–12 g/day	q6h
Nafcillin	25–50 mg/kg/day	8–12 g/day	q8h
Oxacillin	150 mg/kg/day	8–12 g/day	q6h
Ampicillin-sulbactam	—	6–12 g/day	q6h
Ticarcillin-clavulanate	—	12–18 g/day	q6–8h
Cefazolin	25–50 mg/kg/day	4–8 g/day	q8h
Cefuroxime	50–100 mg/kg/day	3–6 g/day	q8h
Cefotaxime	50–150 mg/kg/day	6–8 g/day	q6h
Ceftriaxone	50–75 mg/kg/day	1–4 g/day	q12–24h
Erythromycin	40 mg/kg/day	2–4 g/day	q6h
Vancomycin	40 mg/kg/day	1–2 g/day	q6–12h
Chloramphenicol	50–100 mg/kg/day	3–6 g/day	q6h
Clindamycin	20–40 mg/kg/day	2–3 g/day	q6–8h
Metronidazole	—	30 mg/kg/day	q6h
Gentimicin	6.0–7.5 mg/kg/day	3–6 mg/kg/day	q8h
Amikacin	15 mg/kg/day	15 mg/kg/day	q8h
Aztreonam	—	6–8 g/day	q6–8h

16., [3, 6, 7, 73]. The involved area is typically elevated. In erysipelas, as opposed to simple cellulitis, high fever, systemic toxicity, and leukocytosis are common, especially at the extremes of age [3, 6, 7, 73, 75]. Bacteremia previously was seen in up to 30% of patients, but now it is relatively rare [3]. During convalescence, desquamation of the involved skin occurs. In untreated cases of erysipelas mortality can be as high as 40%.

Most patients with erysipelas, particularly infants and the elderly, should be treated with parenteral penicillin [3, 6, 7]. Where possible the affected part should be elevated to reduce swelling. Clinical improvement usually is seen within 24 hours after antibiotics are initiated. The Israeli study found that older children and young adults with erysipelas involving their legs had a lower incidence of systemic manifestations and could be adequately treated with oral antibiotics as outpatients [76].

ERYSIPELOID

Erysipeloid is a distinctive, local cellulitis due to *Erysipelothrix rhusiopathiae*, a gram-positive bacillus that can be found in saltwater fish, shellfish, and occasionally poultry, beef, and animal hides [77, 78]. Most human infections are occupational in nature, since the bacteria are inoculated through a break in the skin, typically the hands [78]. With hand infections, the web spaces often are affected, while the distal phalanges tend to be spared. Within a week after inoculation a painful violaceous lesion develops that slowly spreads with distinct raised edges. In large erysipeloid lesions, often as the rash expands, the central portion clears [77]. Erysipeloid tends to be self-limited in spread and may spontaneously heal, but if untreated, relapse has been reported 4 to 14 days after complete healing [77]. Diffuse cutaneous infections with E. rhusiopathiae are rare and present as violaceous lesions involving multiple areas of the body [77, 78]. Although systemic infections with E. rhusiopathiae are rare, an overwhelming number of these serious infections have been reported to be endocarditis involving the aortic valve [79].

E. rhusiopathiae is difficult to culture from erysipeloid lesions, and the organism cannot be detected by gram-staining of aspirates or biopsies; therefore, skin biopsy is necessary to isolate the organism [78].

Erysipeloid responds well to penicillin, cephalosporin, and erythromycin in standard doses (see Tables 32-1 and 32-4).

UNUSUAL ORGANISMS THAT PRODUCE CELLULITIS

Vibrio Species. Various Vibrio species (e.g., *Vibrio vulnificus, Vibrio alginolyticus,* and *Vibrio parahaemolyticus*) may produce acute cellulitis, most typically when a wound is contaminated by seawater [80, 81]. *V. vulnificus* typically causes severe cellulitis because of its ability to produce an exotoxin [80, 82–84], while V. *parahaemolyticus*, a common cause of gastroenteritis, may produce cellulitis but rarely causes skin or subcutaneous-tissue necrosis [80]. These infections also are reported to occur after ingestion of raw oysters or even without any discernable preexisting injury [80]. *Vibrio* infections may progress beyond cellulitis, with the development of bullous lesions, soft-tissue necrosis, and bacteremia [80, 82]. Patients with compromised host defenses are at risk for these serious complications from Vibrio infections. The most commonly reported predisposing illness has been cirrhosis of the liver [80, 84]. Although a *Vibrio* infection is an uncommon condition, it should be suspected in a cirrhotic patient with skin lesions who has been in coastal waters. Death has been reported in up to 25% of patients, usually older individuals with underlying illnesses and soft-tissue necrosis [80]. These organisms are sensitive to a wide variety of antibiotics, including chloramphenicol, tetracycline, erythromycin, cephalosporins, and broad-spectrum penicillins [80]. Débridement of necrotic tissue may be required in serious cases [80, 82–84].

Aeromonas Hydrophila. *Aeromonas hydrophila* is a gram-negative bacillus found in freshwater lakes, rivers, and soil [85, 86]. An acute cellulitis may develop if this organism is inoculated into abraded or lacerated skin [85]. Serious infection with bullae and subcutaneous-tissue necrosis have been reported. Ciprofloxacin, trimethoprim-sulfamethoxazole, and cephalosporins are effective against Aeromonas species.

Pasteurella Multocida. *Pasteurella multocida*, a small gram-negative coccobacillus, is a resident organism in the normal oral flora of dogs and cats [87, 88]. After a bite from either animal a cutaneous infection can rapidly develop. While a wide spectrum of bacteria have been isolated from infected wounds due to dog or cat bites *P. multocida* is distinct for its ability to cause intense cellulitis within 24 hours after the injury [87, 88]. Cat bites, especially puncture wounds on the hand, wrist, or foot, appear particularly high risks for this infection [88]. Penicillin is the drug of choice for established *P. multocida* infections. The use of prophylactic antibiotics to prevent infection after mammalian bites is controversial, and antibiotic choices are not clear (see Chap. 13) [89].

CANDIDAL SKIN INFECTIONS

Candida albicans is a commensal yeast, commonly found on the mucosal surfaces of the GI tract, the vagina, and the oropharynx and on the skin [90, 91]. Normally the epidermal or mucosal barrier is resistant to candidal infection, and the indigenous flora also serve to keep candidal growth in check. Under predisposing conditions, a *Candida* organism may change from a commensal organism into a pathogen, producing mucocutaneous infections. Predisposing conditions include the following: (1) increased local moisture or warmth, (2) damage to the epithelial barrier, as seen in seborrheic dermatitis or after radiation therapy, (3) suppression of the normal bacterial flora, as seen during the use of broad-spectrum antibiotics, (4) changes in the hormonal milieu, as seen during pregnancy and the use of oral contraceptives or corticosteroids, (5) hyperglycemia, and (6) depression of systemic host defenses, as seen with hematological malignancies or immunosuppressive agents [90, 91].

Cutaneous candidal infections usually are found in intertriginous skin folds (axillary, perineal, inframammary, abdominal), where warmth and moisture predispose to the growth of *Candida* species [90]. Most patients report pruritus and pain. The rash is beefy red and moist, often with distinct edges and papular satellite lesions. A "cheesy" discharge is sometimes present.

Candidal infections of the female genital tract usually present with a white discharge in the vaginal canal with variable degrees of vulvar redness and swelling [92].

Oropharyngeal candidal infections usually start as small, punctate lesions that spread into white plaques loosely adherent to an underlying inflamed mucosa [93]. When severe a *Candida* infection can extend into the esophagus. Candida can infect the corners of the mouth (perleche), appearing as erythematous, moist fissures.

The diagnosis of candidal infections can be made by finding budding yeast cells on microscopic examination of the exudate or a scraping obtained from the rash. Potassium hydroxide is useful to reduce the interference from epithelial cells and to make it easier to see the candidal organisms [90]. Mucousmembrane infections usually have hyphal elements, but infections on the skin usually do not. *Candida* can be easily cultured on routine bacterial or fungal media.

An important aspect in the treatment of mucocutaneous candidiasis is the reduction or elimination of predisposing factors for candidal growth whenever possible: a decrease in moisture, discontinuing of antibiotics or steroids, and control of hyperglycemia.

Several topical antifungal agents are effective in candidal infections (Table 32-5). It generally is best to start with topical therapy for acute candidiasis. Systemic therapy with orally absorbable antifungal agents should be reserved for chronic, persistent, and recurrent infections. Intertriginous candidal infections should be treated by a cleaning of the lesions with water to remove the irritating exudate, followed by a thorough drying, and then application of a topical cream or powder (clotrimazole or miconazole) three or four times a day. Topical steroids added to antifungal agents may hasten symptomatic relief and are useful agents because they will also treat concomitant seborrhea. Acute vulvovaginal candidiasis can be treated with vaginal tablets, suppositories, or creams installed nightly for 3–7 days [92]. Vaginal candidiasis can also be treated with a short oral course of antifungal agents from the azole group (ketoconazole, fluconazole, itraconazole) [92]. The additional use of a topical steroid-antifungal cream is useful in severe vulvitis (see Chap. 29). Oral thrush can be treated with nystatin suspension four times a day [93]; clotrimazole buccal troches 10 mg used five times a day also are effective for oropharyngeal infections [93].

Pustular, Purulent Infections

FOLLICULITIS

Simple common folliculitis is a superficial infection of hair follicles and is usually precipitated by one of

Table 32-5. Topical therapy for cutaneous fungal infections

Agent	Candidiasis	Dermatophytes	Tinea Versicolor
Amphotericin B	Yes	No	No
Ciclopirox olamine	Yes	Yes	Yes
Clotrimazole	Yes	Yes	Yes
Econazole	Yes	Yes	Yes
Haloprogin	Yes	Yes	Yes
Ketoconazole	Yes	Yes	Yes
Miconazole	Yes	Yes	Yes
Naftifine	No	Yes	Yes
Nystatin	Yes	No	No
Tioconazole	Yes	Yes	No
Tolnaftate	No	Yes	No

the following conditions: (1) trauma to the skin, (2) traction to the hair, (3) overhydration and maceration, or (4) occlusion of the sebaceous glands by application of chemicals, oils, or topical steroids [3, 4, 6, 7]. The bacteria most commonly implicated in folliculitis is *S. aureus* [4], with streptococci, *Proteus* organisms, and *Pseudomonas* organisms occasionally being isolated.

The individual lesions are dome-shaped pustules, pierced by a strand of hair and sometimes surrounded by a thin rim of erythema.

Acute cases of folliculitis can be treated by topical use of general soaps or detergents or by the application of mupirocin [3, 6, 7, 18, 20, 21]. Oral antibiotics sometimes are required in extensive or resistant cases. Drying agents (Xeric AC, 6.25% solution of aluminum chloride in anhydrous ethyl alcohol) are especially helpful in chronic cases.

Pityrosporum Folliculitis. Recently a distinct variety of folliculitis due to the yeast *Pityrosporum orbicular* has been described [94]. It was found to be more common in women than in men and to typically affect the upper trunk or arms with papular or pustular lesions 2–4 mm at the base of hair follicles [94]. Episodic pruritus, sometimes with a stinging sensation, is common. Predisposing factors appear to be excessively oily skin or occlusion of pores with sunscreens or emollients. Because the fungal etiology of this disorder is not commonly appreciated, patients are often misdiagnosed as having bacterial folliculitis, acne, idiopathic pruritus, or neurodermatitis (neurotic excoriations) [94]. Diagnosis is

best made by microscopic examination, which demonstrates budding yeast cells inside the dilated follicle. Culture of *P. orbicular* requires lipid-enriched media. Treatment is effective with a number of agents: selenium sulfide shampoo, 50% propylene glycol in water, topical erythromycin, and topical antifungal creams [94]. Improvement is usually seen in 3–4 weeks, but further intermittent treatment is sometimes required to prevent relapses.

Hot-Tub Folliculitis. A specific form of folliculitis due to prolonged immersion in hot tubs has been reported a number of times since 1975 [95–97]. This syndrome also has been reported related to home shower and bath use [98]. The bacteria responsible is *Pseudomonas aeruginosa*, with reported serotypes O-7, O-8, and O-11 [96, 97]. Normal dry skin is usually impervious to *Pseudomonas* organisms, but under conditions of superhydration of the stratum corneum, these organisms may proliferate in the hair follicles. Cases may occur sporadically or in epidemics. Predisposing factors appear to be prolonged immersion, insufficient chlorination, and high levels of organic debris in the water [96, 97, 99].

This syndrome usually presents 8–48 hours after immersion in the hot tub, although the reported time ranges between 6 hours and 5 days [95–97, 99]. The rash most commonly is papulovesicular, with individual lesions 2–5 mm in diameter. A variety of other lesions may be seen: macules, papules, papulopustules, nodules, and urticaria [96].

The rash can be found on any portion of the body that was submerged in water but is most common on the trunk, buttocks, and proximal limbs. It usually spares the face, neck, palms, soles, and mucous membranes. The rash is often pruritic. Associated symptoms reported in up to 50% of cases include weakness, myalgia, chills, fever, headache, earache, sore throat, adenopathy, rhinitis, and vomiting [99].

Treatment with antibiotics is not necessary or useful; the rash usually resolves spontaneously in 8–10 days (although it may last up to 4 weeks) [95–97, 99]. Serious infections can now be treated on an outpatient basis with ciprofloxacin. The syndrome may recur with exposure to the same hot tub. The disorder can be prevented by effective chlorination, routine periodic hyperchlorination, and reduction in organic debris [96, 97, 99].

FURUNCLE (BOIL)

A furuncle results when a superficial follicular infection extends deeper into the hair follicle and forms an inflammatory subcutaneous nodule that often suppurates [3, 4, 6, 7, 100]. The same bacteria that are found in folliculitis have been implicated in furuncles [4, 6, 7, 100].

Furuncles present as subcutaneous nodules that are occasionally fluctuant [3, 4, 6, 7]. It has been estimated that the typical adult has 5 or 6 minor furuncles per year.

Small furuncles in the nodular stage are treated with local heat to induce spontaneous drainage or regression [101]. Systemic antibiotics are useful if the furuncle is large, located on the face, or associated with cellulitis or lymphangitis, or if the patient has a significant underlying disease affecting host defenses [2, 3, 101, 102]. It usually is best to avoid premature incision and drainage, especially if the lesion is on the face [102]. When a furuncle suppurates, it may spontaneously drain, but sometimes additional incision and drainage may be necessary for large lesions [101].

An intensive regimen of hygiene and topical nasal antibiotics to prevent staphylococcal colonization may be useful in cases of recurrent furunculosis, especially in families [102–104].

CARBUNCLE

A carbuncle is the lesion formed when multiple furuncles become interconnected and drain through several skin openings [2–4, 6, 7]. Carbuncles usually are found where overlying skin is thick, which allows the infection to tract between the cutaneous openings [6, 7]. Common locations include the chin, the back of the neck, and the scalp. S. aureus is the most common bacterial isolate [2–4].

When patients present, the carbuncle usually is spontaneously draining, and further incision may not be required. The key concept is patience, with a prolonged course of antibiotics and wound care before extensive surgery [105]. Large, necrotic areas should be minimally débrided, purulent collections drained, and the wound packed open to allow for healing by granulation.

CUTANEOUS ABSCESS

Cutaneous abscesses are soft-tissue infections that are commonly seen in the emergency department [106–108]. The pathogenesis of a typical cutaneous abscess is that bacterial flora from the overlying skin or adjacent mucous membrane gain entry into the subcutaneous tissues via breaks or pores in the epithelial covering [108]. Localized suppuration occurs, but overall host defenses contain the bacteria and prevent systemic spread. Such an abscess therefore tends to be superficial, well localized, single, and without systemic toxicity. Rarely a patient with an abscess may have a deeper, spreading infection, such as necrotizing fasciitis or myositis. Such infections can be recognized by their widespread involvement of soft tissue and systemic manifestations.

Cutaneous abscesses are common; many adults will develop at least one during their lifetimes. Some systemic diseases predispose to frequent or recurrent cutaneous abscesses. Between one-fourth and one-half of patients with inflammatory bowel disease will experience cutaneous abscesses. Patients with various immune deficiencies (e.g., chronic granulomatous disease) also are predisposed to cutaneous abscesses.

Cutaneous abscesses can be found in any location but tend to be concentrated on the head, neck, extremities, or perineal region [108]. Involvement of the head or neck generally is due to obstruction of sebaceous glands or occasionally cystic acne. Abscesses in the axilla are usually caused by infection of the apocrine sweat glands. Recurrent infection of apocrine glands with scarring and persistent inflammation is termed *hidradenitis suppurative*. This disorder is most common in postpubescent females. Abscesses on the extremities usually are due to needle puncture wounds, cuts, and abrasions. Extremity abscesses due to IV drug abuse tend to be found in patients with sclerotic veins who either miss an attempted IV injection or resort to subcutaneous injection ("skin popping").

Occasionally these abscess are sterile, due to an inflammatory reaction from the foreign material injected. An abscess in the buttock crease is often associated with a pilonidal tract or sinus. Abscesses about the vaginal opening generally are due to infection of Bartholin's glands. Abscesses around the rectum usually originate from infection in the anal crypts that burrows outward to point on the skin. Recurrence or persistence of perirectal abscesses is due to the presence of the fistulous tract connecting the anal crypt with the subcutaneous abscess cavity. Inflammatory bowel disease with anorectal involvement is a predisposing factor in recurrent perirectal fistulae and abscesses.

A cutaneous abscess presents as a painful, fluctuant, subcutaneous nodule, often with overlying or surrounding inflammation. Usually the patient has experienced symptoms for several days before seeking medical attention. Systemic toxicity and fever are rare. Sometimes the patient has attempted to drain the abscess by squeezing or using a sharp instrument.

The most effective treatment for cutaneous abscesses is incision and drainage [108]. An all too common error is that patients are treated with antibiotics and warm soaks for a period of time before incision and drainage. Such a course at best only delays resolution of the infection and at worst may allow progression to systemic sepsis. It is best to drain abscesses during the first medical contact. Sometimes a subcutaneous fullness is felt but without demonstrable fluctuance. In those cases purulence can be sought with a needle aspiration. If pus is obtained, then a formal incision and drainage can follow.

Adequate analgesia is both humane and usually required for complete exploration of the abscess cavity. Local infiltration of anesthetics is the most commonly used method for analgesia, but by themselves local anesthetics often produce inadequate analgesia for incision and drainage of abscesses. This may be because of the reduced effectiveness of these local agents in areas of inflammation and increased tissue pressure. Premedication with a 50-50 mixture of nitrous oxide and oxygen (Nitronox) via inhalation, followed by a short-acting IV narcotic (fentanyl 50–100 µg) and benzodiazepine (midazolam 2–3 mg) before infiltration of local anesthetics makes this procedure much less painful and often renders the patient amnesic for the event. It requires the physician's judgment to select those patients who can safely receive these drugs in the emergency department. It is important for the emergency physician to realize which patients are not appropriate for incision and drainage in the emergency department. In general for the elderly, patients with underlying cardiopulmonary disorders, patients with large or difficult-to-evacuate abscesses (such as rectal abscesses), or immunodeficient individuals, incision and drainage in the operating room with appropriate regional, spinal, or general anesthesia is often best.

The incidence of bacteremia following incision and drainage of cutaneous abscesses is about 30% [109]. In the vast majority of patients such bacteremia is transient and does not lead to systemic infection or spread. However, patients at risk for endocarditis and those with indwelling vascular devices should receive antibiotic prophylaxis prior to incision and drainage of cutaneous abscesses (see Chap. 24 and Table 24-7 for prophylaxis regimens for endocarditis).

The incision can be made with almost any scalpel, but a No. 11 blade has the advantage that the point can be used to puncture the roof of the abscess cavity and the blade then used to make the incision with an upward motion. This procedure avoids a blind downward cut that may inadvertently injure vessels, nerves, or tendons. The incision should be made the length of the abscess cavity. For abscesses deep in soft tissue the incision should enter as much of the cavity as possible. To achieve complete drainage, it may be necessary to cut an ellipse out of the roof of the abscess.

An abscess is usually not a hollow sphere containing liquid pus but instead is an irregularly shaped cavity divided by septae of granulation tissue into many loculated areas of purulence, which must be broken up and removed to achieve complete drainage. These loculations are best broken up by a soft, blunt instrument inserted into the abscess cavity. A fingertip often works well, but a blunt tipped clamp or even cotton-tipped swab can also be effective. This activity should be done gently but thoroughly. The remaining tissue and pus should be removed by irrigation with normal saline under pressure (e.g., from a syringe) through a plastic catheter. Complete drainage is the key to effective treatment; there is no proved benefit to irrigation with antibiotic or antiseptic agents.

Following incision and drainage, it is common practice that the abscess cavity and incision be packed open for 24–48 hours to allow for continued drainage. Repacking may be required, and the abscess cavity and incision should be allowed to heal by secondary intention. Obviously packing the incision open its entire length leads to a scar of similar size. Smaller scars would occur if, following adequate drainage, the incision could be closed. Prospective studies found, however, that primary suturing following incision and drainage has a recurrence rate of over 20%–30%, even with antibiotic coverage [106, 108]. A few recent studies from Britain have found that incision, drainage, curettage, irrigation with hydrogen peroxide, primary closure of the incision with interrupted monofilament nylon sutures, and the use of a small-bore drain when necessary yielded a reaccumulation rate of less than 5% [110]. Such a method also reduces the time to skin healing and time lost from work from cutaneous abscesses. Primary closure of abscesses is not a common practice in the United States.

Packing should be loosely placed into all recesses of the abscess cavity and then out through the incision. The purpose of packing is to allow for free drainage; excessively tight packing defeats this purpose and traps purulence inside the cavity. Plain ribbon gauze, one-quarter to one-half inch in width is adequate; antiseptic gauze is not required. Packing should be removed in 24–48 hours. If purulence recurs, the wound should be explored, irrigated, and packed again. When the wound is dry and without pus, packing is not necessary.

For the vast majority of otherwise healthy patients with normal host defenses, antibiotics have no proved benefit following incision and drainage of localized cutaneous abscesses [108, 111]. There is also no indication for routine culture or Gram's stain [108].

Some physicians may want to use antibiotics as adjunctive therapy following incision and drainage

in certain types of patients: 1) those with evidence of systemic toxicity, 2) those with extensive surrounding cellulitis, 3) those with underlying immunodeficiencies or poor host responses (e.g., diabetes mellitus), 4) those with involvement in high-risk areas (e.g., central facial triangle), and 5) those who fail to respond to incision and drainage.

Adjunctive antibiotics should be selected according to the most likely bacterial pathogen(s). The organisms found in abscesses tend to reflect the flora found on the overlying skin or adjacent mucous membrane [112–114]. Abscesses on the trunk or extremity usually are due to staphylococci or streptococci. In either location the most appropriate adjunctive antibiotic would be a semisynthetic penicillinase-resistant penicillin (e.g., dicloxicillin), a first-generation cephalosporin (e.g., cephalexin), or erythromycin at standard doses (see Table 32-1). Abscesses near the mouth usually contain bacteria commonly found in the oral flora. In that location an appropriate adjunctive antibiotic would be penicillin or erythromycin (see Table 32-2). Perirectal abscesses contain bacteria from the large intestine: the gram-negative bacilli and fecal anaerobes. In that location appropriate adjunctive antibiotics would be cefoxitin, cefotetan, ticarcillin-clavulanate, or ampicillin-sulbactam. For some patients, for example, IV drug abusers and persons with immunodeficiencies or recurrent infections, it might be more difficult to predict the bacteria found in the abscess. For those patients, the Gram's stain can be used to guide initial antibiotic selection. The mainstay of treatment, however, is incision and drainage; antibiotics will not make up for an inadequate procedure [108].

The Gram's stain is usually better than culture in disclosing the range of bacteria found in an abscess [112, 114]. Most abscesses are polymicrobial, often containing organisms or anaerobes that are not easily cultured. The Gram's stain often shows a wider range of organisms than those that grow on culture [112, 114]. However, a routine Gram's stain or culture is not indicated in the vast majority of patients with simple cutaneous abscesses.

A Bartholin's gland abscess presents as a painful swelling posterolateral to the vaginal orifice. These abscesses are best drained from the mucosal (or vaginal) side of the labia. Because these abscesses have a high rate of recurrence after simple incision and drainage, marsupialization (where the wall of the cyst is sutured to the mucosal surface) is recommended. Commercially available short, balloon-tipped (Word) catheters are also available for insertion after drainage of Bartholin's gland abscesses and are reported to have as low a rate of recurrence as marsupialization. Placement of a Word catheter avoids the need for packing. Marsupialization does not have to be done as part of the initial incision and drainage in the emergency department (see Chap. 29).

Hidradenitis suppurative is a chronic, recurrent inflammation of the apocrine sweat glands. It presents after puberty, when the function of these glands is stimulated by the sex steroid hormones. The axilla is the most commonly involved area, but the infection may also develop in the inguinal and perianal regions. Incision and drainage is indicated for acute abscesses, but extensive incisions should be avoided. Antistaphylococcal antibiotics, heat, and good local skin care also are recommended. Shaving and deodorants are contraindicated. Because of the recurrent nature, cure usually requires surgical excision of skin from the involved areas.

Perirectal abscesses start in the anal crypts, penetrate the rectal wall, track through the ischiorectal space, and point to the skin surface around the anal opening. Occasionally the infection stays localized to the anal crypts, developing into a submucous abscess, and presents as a tender mass protruding from the rectal mucosa. Sometimes the infection tracks superiorly into the ischiorectal or supralevator space and does not point on the skin. Small perirectal abscesses can be drained in the emergency department, but because of their development from the anal crypts, the recurrence rate is high unless the fistulous connection is also excised or closed. However, such excision can wait until follow-up and should not be attempted in the emergency department on the initial visit. Patients with perirectal abscesses that are large, submucosal, or track superior with involvement into the ischiorectal space should be drained in the operating room with adequate anesthesia (see Chap. 24).

Pilonidal abscesses occur in the buttock crease and are the result of infection of a preexisting sinus tract leading into a cavity; both are lined with stratified squamous epithelium. There is controversy whether these tracts are congenital remnants or acquired from ingrowth of hair follicles. These tracts and cavities often contain hair and keratin. Since these cavities communicate with skin that is easily contaminated by feces, the most common bacteria are fecal in origin. These abscesses usually are localized and usually can be drained in the emergency department. A definitive operation to remove the sinus tract and the cavity 7–10 days later is often recommended. Rarely the sinus tract may burrow deep and a more extensive surgical procedure is required.

Most patients can be discharged after the incision and drainage [107, 108]. All patients should receive instructions to return immediately if fever, chills, or evidence of worsening infection develops. All patients should be rechecked in 24–48 hours. If the wound is no longer purulent, further repacking is not required. The patient can start warm soaks and cleaning two or three times a day. Following the soaking, the wound should be dried and covered only loosely with gauze. The patient should receive the same instructions to return should infection recur.

Patients with any type of abscess and evidence of extensive systemic involvement or who are immunodeficient should be admitted to the hospital because they will require antibiotics before incision and drainage and close observation following the procedure. Other patients may require admission because of their age or underlying medical disorders that make it appropriate that incision and drainage be done on an inpatient basis. Some patients have large abscesses or have them in difficult areas and require general anesthesia or extensive postoperative wound care; such patients also should be admitted. It is the wise physician who understands the limitations of the emergency department and knows when it is appropriate to have a patient admitted for incision and drainage of an abscess.

Lymphangitic Infections

LYMPHANGITIS

Lymphangitis describes the process whereby inflammation from a cutaneous infection ascends the lymphatic channels toward the regional lymph nodes. Lymphangitis usually is found in infections produced by streptococci: cellulitis and erysipelas [2, 3]. It appears as ascending streaks of erythema, following lymphatic channels, usually with regional lymphadenopathy. Antibiotic treatment is the same as for the initial infection, but because the infection is more extensive, the patient is generally admitted for IV therapy and close observation.

CAT-SCRATCH DISEASE

Cat-scratch disease is a self-limited syndrome that appears to follow exposure to cats. Presumably a scratch inoculates an infectious organism onto the patient [115]. The cat is commonly immature and the patient is usually a child or an adolescent. At the primary site an erythematous papule develops, and within 2 weeks regional lymphadenopathy occurs [115]. The primary lesion may persist for weeks and the lymphadenitis may last for months. The lymph nodes become fluctuant in 10%–20% of cases. Fever may be noted, but systemic manifestations are rare [116, 117]. Fewer than 3% of patients with cat-scratch disease have systemic involvement, presenting as encephalitis, neuropathies, various rashes, pleurisy, arthritis, osteomyelitic lesions, splenic abscesses, or thrombocytopenic purpura [116].

Until recently the cause of cat-scratch disease was considered unknown. However, through special microbiologic techniques a gram-negative, non-acid-fast coccobacillus has been isolated that appears to be the etiologic agent [118].

Currently diagnosis is based on clinical history and exclusion of other causes of lymphadenitis. A skin test for cat-scratch disease is available that appears to be safe and sensitive, but it has not been standardized [115].

Despite the apparent bacterial nature of cat-scratch disease, no antibiotic treatment has proved effective in shortening the course of the disease [119].

SPOROTRICHOSIS

Sporothrix schenckii is a fungus found on plants and in soil. If inoculated into a wound, most often the hand, an infection may slowly develop, producing a small painless papule with some exudate [120]. Secondary nodules develop along the path of ascending lymphatic channels, but regional lymphadenopathy is rare. Ulceration is common in the primary lesion and sometimes is seen in the secondary

lymphangitic spread. Sporotrichosis is diagnosed by the clinical appearance, fungal culture, or direct immunofluorescence [120]. It also should be considered when a patient fails to respond to topical or oral antibiotics used to treat presumptive bacterial ulcerations. Current recommended therapy for cutaneous and lymphatic sporotrichosis consists of oral saturated solution of potassium iodide and local heat [120]. Therapy may be required for several months to a year, and relapses are occasionally seen. Recent experience with itraconazole, a new orally absorbable triazole, indicates that an oral dose of 100 mg per day is effective and reduces both the length of treatment and the relapse rate [120, 121].

Macular, Scaling Infections

INFECTIONS CAUSED BY DERMATOPHYTES

Dermatophytes are a saprophytic group of fungi adapted to living on keratin found in the superficial epidermis, hair, and nails [122–124]. These fungi, which belong to the genera *Trichophyton*, *Microsporum*, and *Epidermophyton*, are widespread and can be found in the soil, on animals, and on humans. These organisms are not invasive; the living epidermal layers are able to resist infection. In addition cell-mediated immunity that develops after the initial infection helps prevent subsequent involvement.

Similar to candidal skin infections, predisposing factors for dermatophytid infections include local skin changes (increased warmth, moisture, poor hygiene, preexisting dermatitis) and systemic host defense impairments (immunodeficiencies, hormonal changes, malnutrition) [122, 123].

Dermatophyte infections are categorized according to the area or pattern of involvement rather than the specific organism, because different fungi may produce similar clinical pictures.

Tinea capitis is a relatively common infection of school-aged children, caused primarily by *Trichophyton tonsurans* and *Microsporum* species [123]. Patients usually report no pain or discomfort but seek medical attention when patchy hair loss, broken hairs, erythema, or scaling is noted. In ectothrix infections due to *Microsporum canis* or *Microsporum audouinii* spores are deposited on the outside of the hair shaft. This enables a green phosphorescence to be seen when viewed under 360-nm light (Wood's light). In endothrix infections due to *T. tonsurans*, the spores are nonfluorescent and are deposited within the hair shaft. This produces brittle hair, and the individual shafts are easily broken off just above the scalp. Involvement of multiple areas leads to patchy hair loss.

Unfortunately the value of Wood's-light examination in the diagnosis of tinea capitis has been reduced, because *Trichophyton* species have replaced *Microsporum* species as the dominant pathogens [122]. The diagnosis can be substantiated by finding branching, septated hyphae under microscopic examination. Care should be taken to select hairs that appear to be infected and allow 10–20 minutes for the potassium hydroxide to partially dissolve the collagen fibrils of the hair shaft. In most cases microscopic examination is adequate; if not, fungal cultures can be done.

Tinea capitis is treated with microsized griseofulvin once a day for 6–8 weeks [124]. The dose needs to be adjusted according to body weight (Table 32-6). Treatment should be continued for 2 weeks past clinical healing. There is no reason to cut or shave the hair. Topical antifungals are not useful. Tinea capitis is a contagious disease and is easily spread through schools or families. Two-percent selenium sulfide shampoo used twice a week may reduce the number of secondary cases of tinea capitis.

Tinea corporis is the dermatophytid infection of the trunk or extremities [122, 123]. Tinea corporis is found more in hot, humid climates and is more common in children. The rash begins as an erythematous macule that slowly enlarges with a clearing center, an appearance termed "ringworm." The advancing edge is typically scaling and may be slightly pruritic or vesicular. Acute fungal infection may be bullous at onset and must be considered in the differential diagnosis of pyoderma. Diagnosis is made by scraping the advancing edge, dissolving the debris with potassium hydroxide, and finding hyphae upon microscopic examination.

Topical treatment applied twice a day for 4 weeks is usually effective (see Table 32-6). The rash may resolve within one week, but treatment should be continued for the full course to prevent relapse.

Table 32-6. Treatment of dermatophyte infections

Tinea Capitis
Griseofulvin for 6–8 weeks
  Children: 10 mg/kg/day as single dose
  Adults: 500 mg/day as single dose
  Supplied as: suspension 125 mg/5 ml; tablets
    250 mg and 500 mg

Tinea Corporis
Topical antifungal agents bid for 4 weeks

Tinea Cruris
Daily cleaning and use of drying agents
Topical antifungal agents bid for 4 weeks

Tinea Manum
Topical antifungal agents bid for 4 weeks (useful for
  superficial infection of palms)

Tinea Pedis
Daily cleaning
Use of drying agents (e.g., aluminum chloride hexa-
  hydrate bid for 7–10 days)
Topical antifungal agents bid for 4 weeks (useful for
  superficial infection of soles)
Keratolytic agents bid (as needed for hyperkeratotic
  lesions)
Griseofulvin 500 mg/day as single dose for 12 weeks
  (useful in severe or resistant cases)

Tinea Unguium
Surgical removal of nail
Griseofulvin 500 mg/day as single dose for an ex-
  tended period of time
Topical therapy rarely effective

Tinea cruris is dermatophyte infection of the groin and is found most often in obese men [122, 123]. Heat and moisture are important predisposing factors. Tinea cruris often starts in the inguinal crease, affects both the groin and the inner thigh area and sometimes produces a symmetrical, raised, erythematous rash. Unlike *Candida* species, tinea cruris does not infect the scrotum, vulva, or vagina.

Tinea cruris is diagnosed by fungal scrapings or culture. An important aspect of treatment is daily cleaning, thorough drying, and the use of a moisture-absorbing powder (like baby powder) twice a day. Topical antifungal agents usually are effective [125, 126].

Tinea manum is dermatophyte infection of the

hands and usually involves the palmar surface; one hand and both feet are usually involved. The rash is slightly erythematous and scaling. Tinea manum usually occurs in association with tinea pedis. The hypersensitivity ("id") reaction to tinea infection elsewhere on the body produces sterile vesicles on the fingers and should not be confused with primary fungal infection. Tinea manum is treated with topical antifungal agents [124, 125].

Tinea pedis is probably the first or second most common fungal infection of the adult population [122]. It has been estimated that at least one-third of adults will have tinea pedis at least once during their lifetime. Tinea pedis has three different clinical appearances [122–124]. The most common variety presents with interdigital involvement, usually with vesicles on an erythematous or scaling base. Maceration and fissures are common. Local trauma and persistent moisture usually are necessary for these fungi to initiate an infection. Severe interdigital infection may become secondarily infected with aerobic bacteria and produce an exudative, macerated, pruritic infection.

The "moccasin-foot" variety of tinea pedis presents with a scaling eruption that involves the entire plantar surface and extends up the sides of the foot and the heel [127]. *Trichophyton rubrum* is the dermatophyte most commonly associated with the moccasin-foot form. The least common variety of tinea pedis is that rare case with an extensive vesicular or bullous eruption.

Tinea pedis requires local measures for effective treatment: daily cleaning, thorough drying, use of nonocclusive footwear, absorbent cotton socks, and astringent (antimoisture) powders [124]. Topical antifungal agents applied to the involved area twice a day is the mainstay for treatment. For interdigital infections that are suprainfected, 20% aluminum chloride hexahydrate solution applied twice a day has both antibacterial and drying properties. When there is thick, hyperkeratotic involvement, keratolytic agents may be required in addition to antifungal therapy. Available agents such as salicylic acid (e.g., Keralyt) or benzoic and salicylic acids (e.g., Whitefield's ointment and Actinea cream) should be applied twice a day along with the antifungal agents or alternated with their application. For severe cases oral griseofulvin for an extended period may be required. Unless the predisposing conditions are eliminated, relapses of tinea pedis are common.

Treatment for tinea pedis is involved, time consuming, and often unsuccessful [122, 124]. It is best to refer the patient to a physician or dermatologist who can undertake the commitment required to successfully treat this disorder.

Tinea unguium (onychomycosis) is a chronic dermatophyte infection of the nails [122, 123]. The fungi usually live in the proximal nail, where the soft keratin is most favorable to their growth. Over time the nail becomes thickened, deformed, and friable. Severe infections may destroy the nail, leaving only a few fragments protruding out from under the cuticle. Samples for potassium-hydroxide examination or fungal culture should be obtained by first scraping away the superficial layers of the proximal nail and analyzing samples from the deeper layers.

TINEA VERSICOLOR

Tinea versicolor is an infection of the keratinized epidermis caused by *P. orbicular* (previously identified as *Malassezia furfur*) [128]. The infection is usually asymptomatic but may on occasion become pruritic after exposure to sunlight. *P. orbicular* is a normal skin resident, and human infections usually result from a change in host resistance. Identifiable factors include increase in skin temperature or moisture, pregnancy, and corticosteroid therapy.

Tinea versicolor presents with hyper- or hypopigmented macular patches, sometimes scaling and usually located on the trunk, shoulders, or arms (Fig. 32-2). The diagnosis is confirmed by scraping the macular patches, dissolving the debris with potassium hydroxide, examining the mixture with a microscope, and finding budding yeast or short, angular hyphae [128]. *P. orbicular* is not easily cultured, and routine fungal cultures are usually negative.

Examination of the rash with a Wood's light may show a golden or orange fluorescence [128]. Even if absent Wood's light will make the faint pigmentary changes easier to see and allow the margins to be more easily identified.

Tinea versicolor can be treated with a wide variety of topical agents, provided they are used for a sufficient length of time and applied to all areas of involvement (Table 32-7). Two to four weeks of

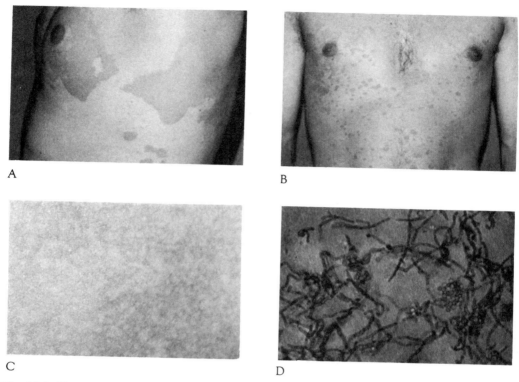

Fig. 32-2. Tinea versicolor. Note irregular plaques. A. Pink tinea versicolor lesions; B. Tinea versicolor resembling pityriasis rosea; C. Abnormal suntan of a patient with tinea versicolor; D. Methylene-blue-stained hyphae of *Malassezia furfur*. (Courtesy Upjohn Pharmaceuticals. Used with permission)

treatment is usually required. Because of clinically inapparent involvement it is recommended that entire trunk and proximal extremities be treated. The requirement for such a large treatment area makes the use of topical antifungals prohibitively expensive. Fortunately a number of less expensive alternatives exist. Recent experience with the new orally active triazole antifungal agents has found them to be extremely effective when administered at low doses (fluconazole 100 mg/day or itraconazole 200 mg/day) for 5–7 days [129]. Itraconazole is as effective as topical agents and does not have the irritant side effects associated with selenium sulfide or the keratolytic agents so it is well tolerated by patients.

Treatment usually eliminates scaling and itching in a few days, but the pigmentary changes may require several months to resolve. Relapse is com-

mon but can be minimized by adequate initial treatment.

ERYTHRASMA

Erythrasma is a superficial infection of the intertriginous skin caused by *Corynebacterium minutissimum* [3, 4, 130]. *C. minutissimum* is part of the resident cutaneous flora but under conditions of heat, humidity, or changes in host defense may produce a desquamative infection. Other than occasional itching, erythrasma usually is asymptomatic [130, 131].

Erythrasma appears as patches in the intertriginous skin creases. The patches may be smooth to sometimes slightly raised, are a light brownish-red in color, and are sharply demarcated from noninvolved skin [3, 4]. Interdigital erythrasma produces scaling and fissures between the toes [130].

Table 32-7. Treatment of tinea versicolor

Zinc pyrithione
  Available in shampoos: Breck, Danex, DHS-Zinc,
    Head & Shoulders, Zincon
  Apply to rash, leave on for 5 minutes, then wash
    off; use nightly for 2 weeks.
Selenium sulfide suspension
  Available in shampoos: 2.5%, Exsel, Selsun (by
    prescription), Iosel; 1%, Selsun-Blue (OTC)
  Apply to rash, leave on for 5 minutes, then wash
    off; use nightly for 2 weeks.
Salicylic acid-sulfur
  Available in shampoos: Ionil, Sebulex, TiSeb,
    Vanseb
  Apply to rash, leave on overnight, wash off in
    morning; use for 1–2 weeks.
Propylene glycol 50% in water:
  Apply twice a day to rash; use for 2 weeks.
Benzoyl peroxide 5%–10%
  Available in lotions, Benoxyl; gels, Benzasel, Pan
    Oxyl, Pera Gel, Desquam-X; cleaner, Desquam-X
    wash
  Apply daily to rash; use for 3 weeks.
Topical antifungals
  Apply twice a day to rash; use for 2–4 weeks.
Itraconazole
  200 mg (adults) per day PO for 5–7 days
Ketoconazole
  200 mg (adults) per day PO for 5 days
  or
  400 mg (adults) PO as one-time dose
Fluconazole
  100 mg (adults) per day PO for 5–7 days

Rare patients may have generalized involvement. Individuals with persistent or widespread infection usually have a defect in cell-mediated immunity.

Erythrasma may be misdiagnosed as a dermatophyte infection. An important diagnostic characteristic of erythrasma is that it fluoresces coral-red when exposed to Wood's light [3, 4, 130, 131]. The color is due to a water-soluble porphyrin produced by C. *minutissimum*, which may not be present if the area has been recently washed.

A Gram's stain of scrapings taken from the affected patches may show the causative bacteria as gram-positive coccobacillary or filamentous forms. Culture requires special media.

Erythrasma is best treated with a 10–21-day course of oral erythromycin or tetracycline [3, 130].

Topical therapy with a variety of antifungal (e.g., clotrimazole) or keratolytic (e.g., salicylic acid) agents may produce clinical resolution, but the recurrence rate is higher than when oral antibiotics are used.

Exophytic Skin Infections (Warts)

Since the 1800s warts have been considered infectious, but it wasn't until 1949 that virus particles were identified in specimens taken from human warts [132, 133]. It is now known that warts are benign intraepidermal tumors produced by a double-stranded DNA virus, the human papillomavirus (HPV). Recent research has discovered wide variation in the DNA sequence of HPV; based on these differences 55 distinct HPV types have been isolated to date [133]. Undoubtedly more will be identified.

Each HPV type has a preference for a particular location and tends to produce a characteristic clinical appearance. A few HPV types have been implicated in the development of premalignant and malignant conditions: cervical dysplasia and carcinoma, laryngeal papillomas, laryngeal cancer, and Bowen's disease [133]. This is not surprising since HPVs are considered part of the *Papovaviridae* family, which contains two well-known oncogenic viruses: polymaviruses and simian virus 40 (SV40).

Because warts are due to infectious agents, they are contagious and can spread from person to person or be autoinoculated from one part of the body to another. The incubation period from exposure to HPV until the clinical appearance of warts varies widely, but averages 2–3 months. Both humoral and cellular immunity are stimulated by the growth of these benign tumors and will produce spontaneous regression of common warts in about half of patients by 1 year.

Warts usually are characterized by their appearance, which is determined by the interaction between the HPV type and the site of infection [133, 134]. Common warts are rough, hyperkeratotic papular lesions of varying color and are found most commonly on the hands. These lesions are vascular and bleed easily when traumatized. Flat (juvenile) warts are smooth, small papules of varying color, usually occurring as multiple lesions on children. Filiform warts are thin lesions that project off the epithelial surface, commonly found on the neck or face.

Plantar warts are rough, hyperkeratotic lesions found commonly over pressure points on the sole of the foot. Punctate black dots due to thrombosed capillaries may be seen. As opposed to simple calluses, warts distort the natural skin lines. The coalescence of multiple plantar warts into one large lesion is called a mosaic wart.

Genital (venereal) warts, or condylomata acuminata, are the soft, cauliflower-like warts that develop in the intertriginous and perineal areas. In women these warts usually are found on the labial surfaces. In men genital warts are usually seen on the glans, foreskin, or ureteral meatus.

Anal warts are soft, friable warts found on the perianal skin or growing from the anal mucosa.

Molluscum contagiosum is spread by contact with children. Lesions of 1–5 mm are most prominent around the genitalia, thighs, and buttocks. They are painless, skin-colored, and contain a central umbilication.

The treatment of warts should be based on several principles [134–136]. Warts are usually asymptomatic, and most patients seek treatment for cosmetic reasons. Warts are benign, and treatment is not mandatory because of the fear of malignant transformation [137]. Anogenital warts may be spread during sexual contact, so treatment does have a role in reducing their spread. A sizable number of common warts will regress with time; sometimes the best treatment is a period of observation. Most treatment regimens require repeated application over a period of 3–4 months; it is best that patients be referred to a physician with the expertise to properly treat and follow them during this prolonged interval.

The various treatment options are categorized in Table 32-8. In general keratolytics, caustics, and cantharidin do not produce pain on application, and their use can be recommended for most cases of common warts. Keratolytics, liquid nitrogen, and cantharidin are the treatments associated with the least amount of scarring. Liquid nitrogen is highly effective but may be painful during use. Podophyllin resin is also effective, but it can be very irritating to normal skin if left on for extensive periods of time (> 12 hours). Podophyllotoxin is a purified active agent from podophyllin resin and

Table 32-8. Treatment options for warts

Keratolytics
Salicylic acid
Cellular poisons
25% podophyllin resin
0.5% podophyllotoxin
Cantharidin
Dinitrochlorobenzene
Formaldehyde
Glutaraldehyde
Bleomycin
5-fluoracil
Caustics
Trichloroacetic acid
Acetic acid
Cryotherapy
Liquid nitrogen
Surgical removal
Electrosurgical
Sharp curettage
Blunt dissection (plantar warts)
Laser surgery

offers the advantages of a consistent concentration and reduced incidence of side effects. Despite initial success with chemical treatments, relapses are common, perhaps secondary to failures in instructions of home treatment. Twenty to 50% of simple warts are resistant to complete elimination [134–136].

Deep, Rapidly Spreading Infections

In general these infections have a deeper involvement than the skin; the subcutaneous fat, fascia, or muscle is infected [138–140]. A common characteristic of these infections is the necessity of surgery for successful treatment; some require extensive incision and drainage of pus, while others may require complete excision of all involved tissue [141]. Some of the more severe infections have a distinctive tissue plane involved by advancing inflammation and necrosis [141, 142]. These infections usually are not caused by opportunistic organisms per se but rather by the interaction between local tissue conditions and bacterial contamination [138, 141, 142]. Clinical clues that suggest the presence of these serious infections are prominent

Table 32-9. Deep, spreading soft-tissue infections

Characteristics	Crepitant cellulitis	Synergistic necrotizing cellulitis	Necrotizing fasciitis	Clostridial cellulitis	Clostridial myonecrosis
Predisposing conditions	Wounds, decubiti, peripheral vascular disease, diabetes	Diabetes, obesity, advanced age	Postoperative wounds, peri-anal infection, chronic cutaneous ulcers, IV drug use	Contaminated wound	Devitalized tissue, focal contamination
Onset	Gradual	Subacute, over several days	Variable, indolent to fulminant	Gradual, 4–5 days	Acute, 1–3 days
Pain/temperature	Mild	Severe	Minimal, sometimes hypesthesia	Mild	Severe, early
Systemic toxicity	Mild to moderate	Moderate to severe	Marked	Mild to moderate	Marked, early
Overlying skin	Minimal, discoloration brown to gray	Blue-gray, necrosis	Initially spared, then pale followed by gangrene	Minimal change, occasional blebs	Initially normal, then pale, bronze discoloration followed by necrosis
Exudate	Minimal, dark	Thin, reddish-brown	Rare, serious	Thin, dark	Serosanguinous
Odor	Foul	Foul	Foul	Rarely foul	"Mousy," slightly sweet
Gas formation	Abundant	Mild, up to 25%	Little	Abundant	Initially minimal, eventually moderate
Muscle involvement	No	Prominent feature, moderate spread	Rare, late	No	Prominent
Common pathogens	Anaerobes, Enterobacteriaceae	B. fragilis, streptococci, Enterobacteriaceae	Enterobacteriaceae, streptococci, Bacteroides, peptostreptococci	C. perfringens, C. septicum, C. novyi	C. perfringens, C. septicum, C. novyi

systemic toxicity, high fever, gas formation in soft tissues (crepitus), overlying skin necrosis, foul-smelling discharge, and bleb or bullae formation [138–142]. Skin necrosis is due to intravascular thrombosis of the perforating dermal blood vessels caused by the bacterial toxins and the host inflammatory response [142].

Several syndromes have been described on the basis of their clinical presentation and bacteriology.

Unfortunately the terminology may be confusing because of the existence of synonyms for the same clinical syndrome [138]. Likewise, while the various syndromes may have a distinctive picture in their pure state, many times the clinical presentation is confused, not always like the classic appearance (see Table 32-9). The presence of soft-tissue crepitus due to gas formation creates confusion, sometimes leading to the mislabeling of these pa-

Table 32-9. (continued)

Acute streptococcal hemolytic gangrene	Spontaneous streptococcal myositis	Anaerobic streptococcal myositis	Pyomyositis	Meleny's cellulitis
Minor trauma, IV drug use	None	Minor closed trauma	Tropics, malnutrition	Abdominal or thoracic surgery
1–4 days	Usually abrupt	Gradual, 1–4 days	Gradual	Gradual
Moderate to severe	Severe, early	Late	Moderate, early	Severe, early
Marked	Marked	Late	Fever, late	Fever, late
Erythema, followed by mottling and hemorrhagic blebs	Scattered or localized erythema	Early erythema and edema	Minimal early changes, later erythema	Shallow ulcer with erythematous red-purple margin
No	Minimal seropurulent	Seropurulent	Localized pus	Gray-yellow
Little	None	Sour to foul	No	No
Minimal to none	Minimal to none	Minimal to none	No	No
Sometimes	Characteristic	Characteristic	Characteristic	No
S. pyogenes, sometimes with S. aureus, S. epidermitidis	S. pyogenes	Peptostreptococci	S. aureus	Peptostreptococci, S. aureus, Enterobacteriaceae, Entamoeba histolytica

tients as gas gangrene [143–145]. Furthermore, gas formation cannot always be appreciated as crepitance on physical examination. Identification of air in the soft tissues may provide the first clue.

Rather than try to precisely classify patients into a defined syndrome, it is perhaps more important for the physician to take a unified approach, recognizing the life-threatening potential of these infections, instituting resuscitative therapy, instituting maximal, immediate broad-spectrum empiric antibiotic treatment, obtaining soft tissue x-rays for gas, and mobilizing appropriate surgical care [146, 147].

Empiric antibiotic therapy must be active against aerobic gram-positive and enteric gram-negative organisms as well as anaerobes. Imipenem is active against all classes of organisms listed above. An alternative regimen is clindamycin or metronidazole to cover aerobic gram-positive cocci and a third-generation cephalosporin for coverage of enteric gram negative bacilli as well as additional coverage against *S. aureus* and Streptococcal species. Clindamycin or metronidazole can be combined with an aminoglycoside. Aminoglycosides will initially sterilize the bloodstream, but are not active in situations with a low redox potential and acid pH. Furthermore renal toxicity is an important problem in this seriously ill population, especially in diabetics who may already have compromised renal function. The patient with a type I hypersensitivity to penicillin can be given metronidazole and aztreonam or clindamycin and an aminoglycoside (Table 32-10).

A Gram's stain that demonstrates organisms may guide initial therapy. If "boxcar" *Clostridia* species are seen, high-dose penicillin or imipenem is effective. Sheets of gram-positive cocci suggest *Streptococcus* species, for which penicillin, with or without clindamycin, is appropriate.

Crepitant (Gas-Forming) Infections

CREPITANT CELLULITIS

Crepitant cellulitis (also known as non-clostridial anaerobic cellulitis, anaerobic cellulitis, anaerobic aerogenic infections and gas abscess) is a gas-forming soft-tissue infection that results from the synergistic interaction of anaerobes (peptostreptococci

Table 32-10. Empiric antibiotic therapy for deep, spreading infections

Agent	Dosage
Imipenem	500–1000 mg q6h IV
Clindamycin + cefotaxime	900 mg q8h IV 2 g q6–8h IV
Metronidazole + cefotaxime	15 mg/kg loading dose, then 7.5 mg/kg q6h 2 g q6–8h IV
Penicillin Type I Hypersensitivity	
Vancomycin + metronidazole	1 g q12h IV 15 mg/kg loading dose, then 7.5 mg/kg q6h
Clindamycin + aztreonam	900 mg q8h IV 2 g q8h IV
Clindamycin + gentamicin	900 mg q8h IV 2 mg/kg IV loading dose, subsequent doses adjust for renal function

and *Bacteroides*) and *Enterobacteriaceae* infecting the subcutaneous tissues [138, 148], although occasional cases have only coliforms isolated [149]. Predisposing conditions of tissue damage (wounds, decubiti), ischemia (peripheral arterial disease), or defective host defenses (diabetes) are usually present [138, 148, 150].

This syndrome typically has a gradual onset, is associated with mild pain and tenderness, possesses only mild to moderate systemic toxicity, has minimal discoloration of overlying skin (brown to ashen gray), often a putrid odor to the discharge, and abundant gas formation with palpable crepitance [138, 148]. This infection goes by many other names, but more important, because of the abundant crepitance, it may be confused with clostridial myonecrosis (gas gangrene); soft-tissue crepitance is *not* diagnostic of gas gangrene [143–147].

Initial antibiotic treatment should be chosen to be effective against the likely pathogens: anaerobes and coliforms (see Table 32-10). Correction of fluid, electrolyte, and metabolic derangements may be necessary. Surgical therapy should include wide incision and careful examination of the fascia and muscle. In crepitant cellulitis the underlying muscle is not involved. The infected area should be opened widely, necrotic tissue débrided, and all pus drained [138, 141]. In diabetics with extremity involvement partial amputation may sometimes be required [148, 150].

SYNERGISTIC NECROTIZING CELLULITIS

Synergistic necrotizing cellulitis (also known as nonclostridial gas gangrene, synergistic nonclostridial anaerobic myonecrosis, perineal phlegmon, Fournier's gangrene or syndrome, necrotizing cutaneous myositis, and gram-negative anaerobic cutaneous gangrene) is a serious soft-tissue infection first described in 1972 [151]. This is a mixed infection resulting from bacterial synergism between *Enterobacteriaceae*, gram-positive cocci (usually aerobic or anaerobic streptococci), and anaerobes (especially *Bacteroides fragilis*) [138, 151–154]. In the cases reported to date diabetes is the predominant predisposing factor, followed by to obesity and advanced age [151–154].

This infection has a subacute onset over several days. The involved area is exquisitely tender, with large discrete areas of blue-gray necrotic skin separated by normal areas [151]. The discoloration is due to necrosis of the underlying fascia and muscle (see Color Plate 17). In synergistic necrotizing cellulitis primary muscle involvement is a characteristic feature, with the extremities or perineal area most commonly infected [138, 151]. A thin, reddish-brown, foul-smelling discharge (termed "dishwater" pus) is typical. Mild crepitance can be detected in about 25% of cases. Significant systemic toxicity and leukocytosis is the rule. Bacteremia has been detected in about 50% of cases and may be polymicrobial. Mortality is high, up to 75%, usually because of the wide-spread involvement and poor host condition.

Fournier's gangrene or syndrome is a necrotizing infection of the male genitals spreading along the fascial planes of the groin: Buck's (perineum), dartos (genitalia), Colle's (perineum), or Scarpa's (abdominal wall) fascia [155]. The precise classification of Fournier's gangrene is disputed; most authors consider it a variant of necrotizing fasciitis [156], while others classify it with synergistic necrotizing cellulitis [138]. The spreading infection of Fournier's gangrene interrupts the blood supply to the scrotum, producing extensive gangrene of the overlying skin. In Fournier's gangrene the process usually is precipitated by trauma or is spread from a urinary tract or perianal infection [155–157].

After cultures of blood and discharge from the wound, if present, have been obtained, broad-spectrum antibiotic therapy directed against the presumptive pathogens should be initiated in the emergency department (see Table 32-10) [146, 147, 151–154]. After significant fluid, electrolyte, and metabolic derangements have been corrected, the patient should be taken to the operating room for surgical incision, followed by blunt dissection to drain the pus and prudent débridement of clearly necrotic tissue [138, 151].

NECROTIZING FASCIITIS

Necrotizing fasciitis is a relatively rare infection that is usually due to the synergism between multiple organisms, both aerobic and anaerobic bacteria [158–163]. In a minority of cases of necrotizing fasciitis, only streptococci are found; the clinical syndrome is slightly different, is often classified separately, and is termed *acute streptococcal hemolytic gangrene* (see below). Case reports also document

the rare occurrence of necrotizing fasciitis due to *H. influenzae* [164].

Necrotizing fasciitis is distinctive for its necrosis of the superficial fascia and subcutaneous tissue, with extensive undermining of the skin [158–163]. The muscle is rarely involved and only late if at all. The majority of cases have one of the following as an inciting factor: (1) postoperative abdominal wounds, often with intra-abdominal sepsis, (2) acute perirectal infections, (3) chronic cutaneous ulcers, (4) IV drug abuse, or (5) orocervical infections [158–163, 165–169]. A delay in diagnosis or therapy is common, presumably because the relatively spared skin masks extensive subcutaneous involvement until systemic symptoms or signs call attention to the problem [138].

On diagnosis, patients usually are very ill, with marked systemic toxicity [158–163]. Because of the necrosis of the subcutaneous tissue along with its sensory nerves, there may be minimal local pain or sometimes even hypesthesia. The overlying skin initially is spared, but with thrombosis of the subcutaneous vessels, mottling, discoloration, and edema, sometimes with serosanguinous blebs, eventually occur [146, 147, 158]. Due to extensive undermining it is not possible to determine the extent of subcutaneous tissue necrosis by the external appearance. A putrid odor is common, but a purulent discharge is rare. Soft-tissue crepitance may be felt in up to 20% of cases, while gas formation is visible by plain radiograph in up to 80% [170]. The use of CT scanning may be helpful to determine the full extent of fascial spread [171]. Multiple complications have been observed: fluid loss, hemolysis, hypocalcemia, and shock. Despite medical treatment, overall mortality is about 30%–40% [142]. In patients with abdominal or perineal involvement, diabetes, atherosclerosis, or a delayed diagnosis, mortality can be as high as 80% [138, 142, 158–163].

Patients with necrotizing fasciitis require aggressive fluid resuscitation, prompt broad-spectrum antibiotics (see Table 32-10), red-cell transfusions when appropriate, and urgent surgery [172, 173]. Delay in operative treatment contributes to the high mortality seen in necrotizing fasciitis. In the operating room extensive longitudinal incisions are required to unroof all the undermined areas beyond the outermost extent of fascial involvement [141,

142]. A frozen-section biopsy may help the surgeon determine the extent of fascial involvement [163, 174]. The pathologic appearance of involved areas is fascial edema and necrosis with intravascular thrombosis and a dense dermal neutrophilic infiltrate, without significant changes in the epidermis. [163, 174]. Full débridement of involved skin is required, but perfused viable skin should be preserved [142]. Surgical wounds are left open with gauze that must be changed frequently during the next several days [141, 142].

One recent uncontrolled, nonrandomized study reported that the addition of hyperbaric oxygen (HBO) treatments reduced mortality and the number of repeated wound débridements required in patients with necrotizing fasciitis [175]. The role of HBO has yet to be determined in soft-tissue infections. HBO is expensive and time consuming with unproved efficacy.

CLOSTRIDIAL CELLULITIS

Clostridial cellulitis is a necrotizing infection of the subcutaneous tissues caused by one or more of the histotoxic strains of clostridia [138, 142, 143, 146, 147, 176–178]. Pathologically clostridial cellulitis differs from the more serious clostridial myonecrosis (gas gangrene) because it lacks muscle involvement [143, 176–178].

The incubation period for clostridial cellulitis is usually 4–5 days [178]. Skin changes are minimal, other than occasional bleb formation [138, 176]. Abundant gas formation in the soft tissues is typical. Any exudate is usually thin and dark red, usually without a significant foul odor. Gram's stains of the exudate will disclose the thick, gram-positive rods of the *Clostridium* bacillus. The infection can spread at a variable rate, but systemic toxicity is only mild to moderate [138, 146, 176].

Initial antibiotic treatment should include high doses of penicillin G, 10 million–20 million U/day for adults. Operative intervention requires extensive incision and drainage extending beyond the areas of involvement, similar to necrotizing fasciitis [141, 142].

CLOSTRIDIAL MYONECROSIS (GAS GANGRENE)

Clostridial myonecrosis is a serious infection due to one or more of the histotoxic strains of clostridia, with *Clostridium perfringens* being the most com-

mon isolate [179–180]. The three strains of clostridia that produce both cellular toxins and proteolytic enzymes (*C. perfringens*, *Clostridium septicum*, and *Clostridium novyi*) are found in the vast majority of cases.

Clostridial myonecrosis most commonly results from ischemic injury to skeletal muscle that becomes contaminated with clostridial spores, usually from the GI tract (Table 32-11) [180]. Rare cases have been reported without prior injury. Such spontaneous or occult cases are often associated with focal colonic lesions or cancer [181, 182]. The hypothesis is that colonic pathology allows for clostridia resident in the fecal stream to gain access to the circulation and localize in ischemic or damaged areas of skeletal muscle.

These histotoxic strains of clostridia produce at least 17 identified toxins, of which three contribute to the ability of this infection to spread rapidly and cause such systemic toxicity [180]. Alpha-toxin is a phospholipase C (lecithinase) that disrupts cell membranes, damaging red cells, platelets, and capillaries. Mu-toxin is a hyaluronidase that causes edema formation. Theta- (and alpha-) toxin experimentally produces profound depression of cardiac output, followed by hypotension, bradycardia, and eventually death [183].

When an inciting injury can be identified, the incubation period for gas gangrene is short, usually about 3 days [179, 180]. The onset typically is acute, with the initial symptoms being muscle heaviness and swelling, followed by severe pain [180]. Early systemic toxicity and changes in the sensorium are classic, with tachycardia out of proportion to the low-grade fever. Gas gangrene is predominately an infection of muscle, so the overlying skin may appear only pale early in the course, later displaying a bronze discoloration [180]. Ini-

Table 32-11. Classification of clostridial myonecrosis

Postinjury clostridial myonecrosis
   Trauma
   Surgery
Spontaneous clostridial myonecrosis
   Visceral cellulitis (e.g., uterus, gallbladder)
   Visceral cellulitis with spread to adjacent skeletal
     muscle
   Metastatic spread to skeletal muscle (occult
     myonecrosis)

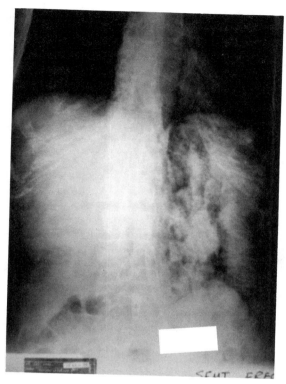

Fig. 32-3. Clostridial myonecrosis. Note feathery gas pattern evident radiographically over the chest and abdomen

tially crepitance is minimal, and gas formation is more reliably detected by radiographs (Fig. 32-3). Because gas is produced in the muscles, the pattern is longitudinal or feathery as gas dissects between the muscle fibers, as opposed to a bubble pattern seen when gas accumulates in the subcutaneous tissues [177]. Gas gangrene does not produce a significant leukocytic response, so any discharge is serosanguinous and relatively devoid of white cells. Absorption of alpha-toxin into the systemic circulation may produce intravascular hemolysis and thrombocytopenia. Bacteremia is uncommon, seen in less than 15% of cases.

An important fact about gas gangrene is that visual examination of the muscle is mandatory for diagnosis and must be done in the operating room [138, 141, 142, 180]. Fluid resuscitation needs to be prompt and aggressive. Red-cell transfusions may be required when hemolysis significantly diminishes oxygen-carrying capacity.

Current treatment for clostridial myonecrosis utilizes the combined modalities of antibiotics and surgical débridement [184]. The value of HBO has not yet been proved. Antibiotics need to be instituted as soon as possible. While antibiotics are not definitive therapy alone, they are important adjuncts in the treatment of gas gangrene. Experimental studies with animal models of gas gangrene have shown that antibiotics consistently augment survival [184, 185]. Penicillin G in high doses (20 million U/day in adults) is the standard agent [180]. However, because the diagnosis is not substantiated until the patient reaches the operating room, initial treatment with broad-spectrum agents or combinations is appropriate. Chloramphenicol, clindamycin, cephalothin, and metronidazole have all been used as single agents, and the combination of cefoxitin and gentamicin is also effective [179, 180, 184, 185]. The author recommends the regimens listed in Table 32-10. The key to antibiotic therapy is prompt administration at high doses.

Surgical débridement of all involved tissue is the second cornerstone of therapy, but the timing of surgery is less clear [179, 180, 184]. Some centers use HBO treatment prior to surgery, particularly if such treatment can be initiated within 1 hour of presentation [180, 184]. Initially in gas gangrene the muscle is edematous and pale but still bleeds when cut. With progression the muscle becomes beefy-red and noncontractile and does not bleed when cut. At surgery all involved muscle should be resected [142, 180]. Gas gangrene involving the distal extremities is treated most effectively by amputation [142, 180].

HBO treatment is the third part of the therapeutic triad for gas gangrene, but its utility has not been demonstrated. The generally accepted benefits of HBO include the following: (1) limitation in tissue necrosis; (2) better demarcation of viable from nonviable tissue at the time of surgery; and (3) reduction in mortality from systemic toxicity [179, 180, 184, 186, 187]. Because clostridia are strict anaerobes, it would be expected that their growth would be inhibited by the presence of oxygen, and this is indeed true. In vitro alpha-toxin production is suppressed at PO_2 around 80 torr, while PO_2 levels of 90 torr are bacteriocidal to bacillary forms of C. *perfringens*. While the PO_2 of arterial blood is usually at least 80 torr, or if not is easily increased by the institution of supplemental oxygen, the PO_2 in normal muscles is only 30–40 torr and even lower in those that are ischemic or infected by gas gangrene. To increase the P_{O_2} in these involved muscles requires the use of hyperbaric conditions [180, 186, 187]. Typical HBO regimens for gas gangrene use 2.4–3.0 absolute atmospheres (ATA) for 90–120 minutes [186, 187]. Usually two or three treatments are given during the first 24 hours, with subsequent treatments administered until there is clinical evidence of no further spread and systemic toxicity resolves.

Tetanus prophylaxis needs to be remembered [180]. The use of polyvalent gas gangrene antitoxin was controversial, and it is no longer commercially available [138].

There are about 1000 cases of gas gangrene in the United States each year [180]. Without treatment mortality approaches 100% within 48 hours. With treatment the overall mortality rate is 20%–30%, varying significantly according to the presentation, clinical circumstances, and area of involvement [184]. The majority of patients who present with an acute, fulminant course that develops over 24 hours will die. For patients who develop gas gangrene in an injured extremity, the mortality rate is about 20%. Patients who develop abdominal wall infection after surgery have a mortality rate of about 50%. Patients who present with metastatic skeletal muscle involvement have a reported mortality rate of 70% [181, 182].

Noncrepitant Infections

ACUTE STREPTOCOCCAL HEMOLYTIC GANGRENE

Acute streptococcal hemolytic gangrene (also known as streptococcal necrotizing fasciitis and gangrenous or necrotizing erysipelas) is probably a variant of necrotizing fasciitis in that it too spreads along the avascular plane of the superficial fascia. Rather than being a mixed infection, however, only beta-hemolytic streptococci, alone or in combination with staphylococci, are isolated [138, 142, 188–190]. Predisposing factors are reported to be minor trauma, attempted injection of illicit drugs, and the immediate postpartum period for neonates and women [188–190].

The initial lesion is cellulitic: hot, red, edematous, and painful [138, 188–190]. Within 1–4 days areas develop a dusky color (ischemic mot-

tling) and form hemorrhagic blebs (see Color Plate 18) [188,191]. Marked fever, systemic toxicity, and soft-tissue swelling are present. The swelling may be to the extent that mimics a compartment syndrome [192]. There is little odor and no detectable crepitance. Complications of septic shock, coagulopathy, and multiple organ failure may be seen. Muscle involvement, with myonecrosis and compartment syndrome, is possible. This syndrome may be as fulminant as gas gangrene, with a mortality of up to 50%, particularly in older patients [188, 189].

While isolation of beta-hemolytic streptococci is a consistent feature of this syndrome, animal experiments have found that synergism between these bacteria and alpha-lysine–producing strains of S. aureus is necessary to replicate the clinical appearance [193].

While high-dose penicillin G is effective for acute streptococcal hemolytic gangrene, broader antibiotic coverage should be initiated on the presumption of a mixed infection (see Table 32-10); it is not possible to predict accurately the pathogens from clinical appearance [146, 147]. The surgical treatment requires longitudinal incisions down to the superficial fascia with excision of necrotic areas. Decompressive fasciotomy is sometimes needed [188].

SPONTANEOUS STREPTOCOCCAL MYOSITIS

Spontaneous streptococcal myositis (also called spontaneous streptococcal gangrenous myositis, fulminant streptococcal myositis, and spontaneous gangrenous myositis) is a rare infection of skeletal muscle caused by S. pyogenes [194–198]. The varied clinical course has been categorized by Svane as: (1) malignant (or fulminant) with a rapid course, severe symptoms, and usually a fatal outcome; (2) acute, with a slower but progressive course, often with bacteremia and multiple areas of involvement; (3) subacute with gradual course; or (4) benign, essentially a localized muscle abscess [194].

This infection appears to develop without an inciting injury to skeletal muscle. The onset is usually abrupt, and in the malignant forms progression is rapid [196–198]. The involved muscle is painful and swollen. Because the lower extremities are more frequently involved, the patient may be misdiagnosed as having deep venous thrombosis

[197, 198]. The overlying skin has minimal changes, sometimes developing a bronze color followed by mottling later in the course. There is little gas formation within the muscle.

Treatment needs to be aggressive, with fluid resuscitation, antibiotics, and early surgical débridement of nonviable tissue [197]. Definitive therapy is maximal doses of penicillin and clindamycin. Empiric therapy regimens are listed in Table 32-10.

ANAEROBIC STREPTOCOCCAL MYOSITIS

Anaerobic streptococcal myositis (also called nonclostridial myositis, anaerobic streptococcal myonecrosis, nonclostridial gas gangrene, crepitant myositis) is an infection of skeletal muscle caused by anaerobic streptococci (peptostreptococci) that clinically partially resembles clostridial myonecrosis [199]. This infection usually follows closed trauma to the skeletal muscle. After an incubation period of 1–4 days the insidious development of local edema, cutaneous erythema, and a foul-smelling seropurulent exudate is noted. Pain or systemic toxicity is not prominent early. While gas formation within the soft tissues does occur, clinically it is not a prominent feature.

Broad-spectrum antibiotic coverage is appropriate initially (see Table 32-10), but can be adjusted to high-dose penicillin G (10–20 million U/day in adults) with the Gram's stain and culture results obtained from surgery [195, 199]. Surgical treatment starts with visual inspection of the muscle, which may be still contractile and viable. Incision and drainage of the involved fascia and muscle with removal of dark, nonviable, or necrotic muscle is required. Overall mortality depends on the clinical presentation; fulminant cases usually die despite antibiotics and surgery.

PYOMYOSITIS

Pyomyositis (also called tropical myositis) is an acute bacterial infection of the large skeletal muscles, 80%–90% of the time due to S. aureus [200–204]. This infection is endemic in tropical and subtropical areas, sometimes accounting for up to 4% of hospital admissions in these regions [195, 200, 202]. The first reported case of pyomyositis diagnosed in the United States was in 1971. The typical case seen in the United States is in a native of the tropics who has recently immigrated to North America [201–203], although occasional cases do occur without a tropical connection [205, 206].

Normally skeletal muscle is very resistant to bacterial infection, but presumably there is some inciting factor common to the tropics that renders these tissues susceptible to infection. The hypothesis that predisposing factors render the muscle susceptible to infection from a transient staphylococcal bacteremia is attractive but unproved [195, 202]. Factors common to the tropics that have been considered as predisposing conditions include local trauma, malnutrition, and parasitic infection.

These patients present with systemic manifestations of fever and malaise along with local manifestations of muscle infection [200–205]. Initially involved muscles are firm or indurated, followed by marked swelling, tenderness, and fluctuance as the area suppurates over the next 1–3 weeks. The large skeletal muscles are most commonly affected: quadriceps, gluteal, and truncal muscles [200–205]. Involvement of various muscle groups may mimic conditions such as acute abdomen or septic arthritis [208, 209]. Multiple sites of involvement are noted in up to 40% of cases [200]. Suppuration may not be initially apparent, because it takes time to develop [200–205]. Leukocytosis is seen in over 80% of cases, but bacteremia is detected in 5%–30% [200, 205].

The diagnosis is usually confirmed by detecting suppuration within the muscle, either by needle aspiration, ultrasound, or CT scanning [200–205, 208, 210]. The full extent of inflammation can be assessed by gallium scintigraphy or indium WBC scan [203, 205, 211]. Similar to other closed-space infections, incision and drainage of the pus are required. An appropriate antibiotic directed against S. aureus (beta-lactamase–resistant penicillin or cephalosporin) is indicated. Because this is a localized, albeit deep, infection with little tendency to spread, after appropriate treatment mortality is extremely low, less than 1%–2% [200].

Ulcerative Infection (Meleney's Cellulitis)

Meleney's cellulitis (also known as progressive bacterial synergistic cellulitis, bacterial synergistic gangrene, and postoperative progressive gangrene) is a slowly spreading, necrotizing infection of the skin and superficial subcutaneous tissues [138, 141, 142]. Classically microaerophilic or anaerobic streptococci (peptostreptococci) are isolated from the advancing edge, and S. *aureus* and/or *Enterobacteriaceae* organisms are found in the center of the lesion [138, 212]. It has been presumed that synergism between these bacteria is responsible for the slowly spreading ulcerative lesion. Recently Davson et al. argued that cutaneous amebiasis (*Entamoeba histolytica*) might be the heretofore unrecognized cause of Meleney's cellulitis [213].

Almost always this infection begins in an operative wound site, either thoracic or abdominal, often where retention sutures have been used [138, 141, 142, 212, 213]. The incubation period after surgery can vary from a few days to a few weeks. The initial symptoms are pain and tenderness, followed by induration and surrounding erythema [138, 213]. The lesion evolves into a shaggy ulcer with purple margins. The ulcer continues to spread unless treated. The infection involves primarily skin and superficial subcutaneous tissue; it rarely extends to fascia or muscle. There is little systemic toxicity or fever.

Routine diagnostic stains, cultures, and histopathologic studies will not detect cutaneous amebiasis [213]. If this diagnosis is to be accurately excluded, a search for the trophozoites has to be performed by wet-mount microscopy of the purulent exudate or periodic acid-Shiff stain of a biopsy from the ulcer edge [213].

Previous therapeutic recommendations included wide and complete excision of the involved area [142, 213]. Recent cases report cure with less radical surgery, using only simple débridement, removal of infected sutures, and antibiotics [212]. If cutaneous amebiasis is found, emetine is dramatically effective.

References

1. Bisno AL. Cutaneous infections: microbiologic and epidemiologic considerations. Am J Med 76:172, 1984.
2. Feingold DS, Hirschmann JV, Leyden JJ. Bacterial infections of the skin. J Am Acad Dermatol 20:469, 1989.
3. Finch R. Skin and soft-tissue infections. Lancet 1:164, 1988.
4. Kahn G. Bacterial infections of the skin of children. Pediatr Ann 11:199, 1982.
5. Schachner L et al. A therapeutic update of superficial skin infections. Pediatr Clin North Am 30:397, 1983.
6. Tunnessen WW. Cutaneous infections. Pediatr Clin North Am 30:515, 1983.
7. Tunnessen WW. Practical aspects of bacterial skin infections in children. Pediatr Dermatol 2:255, 1985.
8. Coskey RJ, Coskey LA. Diagnosis and treatment of impetigo. J Am Acad Dermatol 17:62, 1987.
9. Schachner L, Gonzalez A. Diagnosis and treatment of impetigo. J Am Acad Dermatol 20:132, 1989.
10. Dagan R, Bar-David Y. Comparison of amoxicillin and clavulanic acid (augmentin) for treatment of nonbullous impetigo. AJDC 143:916, 1989.
11. Demidovich CW et al. Impetigo. Current etiology and comparison of penicillin, erythromycin, and cephalexin therapies. AJDC 144:1313, 1990.
12. Dillon HC. Treatment of staphylococcal skin infections: a comparison of cephalexin and dicloxacillin. J Am Acad Dermatol 8:177, 1983.
13. Disney FA, Pichichero ME. Treatment of staphylococcal aureus infections in children in office practice. AJDC 137:361, 1983.
14. Rogers M et al. A three-year study of impetigo in Sydney. Med J Austr 147:63, 1987.
15. Baltimore RS. Treatment of impetigo: a review. Pediatr Infect Dis 4:597, 1985.
16. Fritsch WC. Therapy of impetigo and furunculosis. JAMA 214:1862, 1970.
17. Britton JW, Fajardo JE, Krafte-Jacobs B. Comparison of mupirocin and erythromycin in the treatment of impetigo. J Pediatr 117:827, 1990.
18. Buchvald J. An evaluation of topical mupirocin in moderately severe primary and secondary skin infections. J Internat Med Res 16:66, 1988.
19. Goldfarb J et al. Randomized clinical trial of topical mupirocin versus oral erythromycin for impetigo. Antimicrob Agents Chemother 32:1780, 1988.
20. Gratton D. Topical mupirocin versus oral erythromycin in the treatment of primary and secondary skin infections. Internat J Dermatol 26:472, 1987.
21. McLinn S. Topical mupirocin vs. systemic erythromycin treatment for pyoderma. Pediatr Infect Dis J 7:785, 1988.
22. Mertz PM et al. Topical mupirocin treatment is equal to oral erythromycin therapy. Arch Dermatol 125:1069, 1989.
23. Infectious Diseases and Immunization Committee. Mupirocin in the treatment of impetigo. Can Med Assoc J 142:543, 1990.

24. Linder CW. Treatment of impetigo and ecthyma. *J Fam Pract* 7:697, 1978.

25. Maddox JS, Ware JC, Dillon HC. The natural history of streptococcal skin infection: prevention with topical antibiotics. *J Am Acad Dermatol* 13:207, 1985.

26. Hewitt WD, Farrar WE. Bacteremia and ecthyma caused by *Streptococcus pyogenes* in a patient with acquired immunodeficiency syndrome. *Am J Med Sci* 295:52, 1988.

27. Turnbull D, Parry MF. Ecthyma-like skin lesions caused by *Staphylococcus aureus* [letter]. *Arch Intern Med* 141:689, 1981.

28. Kelly C, Taplin D, Allen AM. Streptococcal ecthyma. Treatment with benzathine penicillin G. *Arch Dermatol* 103:306, 1971.

29. Straus SE et al. NIH conference. Herpes simplex virus infection: biology, treatment, and prevention. *Ann Intern Med* 103:404, 1985.

30. Fiumara NJ. Herpes simplex. *Clin Dermatol* 7:23, 1989.

31. Corey L et al. Genital herpes simplex virus infections: clinical manifestations, course, and complications. *Ann Intern Med* 98:958, 1983.

32. Corey L, Holmes KK. Genital herpes simplex infections: current concepts on diagnosis, therapy, and prevention. *Ann Intern Med* 98:973, 1983.

33. Corey L, Spear PG. Infections with herpes simplex virus. *N Engl J Med* 314:686, 749, 1986.

34. Lafferty WE et al. Recurrences after oral and genital herpes simplex virus infection. Influence of site of infection and viral type. *N Engl J Med* 316:1444, 1987.

35. Bryson YJ et al. Treatment of first episodes of genital herpes simplex virus infection with oral acyclovir: randomized double-blind controlled trial in normal subjects. *N Engl J Med* 308:916, 1983.

36. Mertz GJ et al. Double-blind placebo-controlled trial of oral acyclovir in first episode genital herpes simplex virus infection. *JAMA* 252:1147, 1984.

37. Goldberg LH et al. Oral acyclovir for episodic treatment of recurrent genital herpes. Efficacy and safety. *J Am Acad Dermatol* 15:256, 1986.

38. Mindel A et al. Prophylactic oral acyclovir treatment in recurrent genital herpes. *Lancet* 2:57, 1984.

39. Luby JP et al. A collaborative study of patient-initiated treatment of recurrent genital herpes with topical acyclovir or placebo. *J Infect Dis* 150:1, 1984.

40. Straus SE et al. NIH conference. Varicella-zoster virus infections. Biology, natural history, treatment, and prevention. *Ann Intern Med* 108:221, 1988.

41. Strommen GL et al. Human infection with herpes zoster: etiology, pathophysiology, diagnosis, clinical course, and treatment. *Pharmacotherapy* 8:52, 1988.

42. Sadick NS et al. Comparison of detection of varicella-zoster virus by the Tzanck test, direct immunofluoroescence with a monoclonal antibody, and virus isolation. *J Am Acad Dermatol* 17:64, 1987.

43. Katz JA et al. Herpes zoster management. *Anesth Prog* 36:35, 1989.

44. Portenoy RK, Duma C, Foley KM. Acute herpetic and postherpetic neuralgia: clinical review and current management. *Ann Neurol* 20:651, 1986.

45. McKendrik MW et al. Oral acyclovir in acute herpes zoster. *Br Med J* 293:1529, 1986.

46. Shepp DH, Dandilker PS, Meyers JD. Treatment of varicella-zoster virus infection in severely immunocompromised patients: a randomized comparison of acyclovir and vidarabine. *N Engl J Med* 314:208, 1986.

47. Esmann V et al. Prenisolone does not prevent postherpetic neuralgia. *Lancet* 2:126, 1987.

48. Robertson DR, George CF. Treatment of post-herpetic neuralgia in the elderly. *Br Med Bull* 46:113, 1990.

49. Rowbotham MC, Fields HL. Topical lidocaine reduces pain in post-herpetic neuralgia. *Pain* 38:297, 1989.

50. Fleisher G, Ludwig S. Cellulitis: a prospective study. *Ann Emerg Med* 9:246, 1980.

51. Fleisher G et al. Cellulitis: initial management. *Ann Emerg Med* 10:356, 1981.

52. Fleisher G, Heeger P, Topf P. *Haemophilus influenzae* cellulitis. *Am J Emerg Med* 3:274, 1983.

53. Carter S, Feldman WE. Etiology and treatment of facial cellulitis in pediatric patients. *Pediatr Infect Dis* 2:222, 1983.

54. Baddour LM, Bisno AL. Non-group A beta-hemolytic streptococcal cellulitis. Association with venous and lymphatic compromise. *Am J Med* 79:155, 1985.

55. Paranka MS et al. Cellulitis at vein-donor sites [letter]. *Ann Intern Med* 101:881, 1984.

56. Pathak A, Hwu HH. Group B streptococcal cellulitis. *South Med J* 78:67, 1985.

57. Baddour LM, Bisno AL. Recurrent cellulitis after saphenous venectomy for coronary bypass surgery. *Ann Intern Med* 97:493, 1982.

58. Ginsberg MB. Cellulitis: analysis of 101 cases and review of the literature. *South Med J* 74:530, 1981.

59. Ho PWL, Pien FD, Hamburg D. Value of cultures in patients with acute cellulitis. *South Med J* 72:1402, 1979.

60. Szilagyi A, Mendelson J, Portnoy J. Cellulitis of the

skin: clinical observations of 50 cases. *Can Fam Physician* 28:1399, 1982.

61. Hook EW et al. Microbiologic evaluation of cutaneous cellulitis in adults. *Arch Intern Med* 146:295, 1986.

62. Uman SJ, Kunin CM. Needle aspiration in the diagnosis of soft tissue infections. *Arch Intern Med* 135:959, 1975.

63. Goldgeier MH. The microbial evaluation of acute cellulitis. *Cutis* 31:649, 1983.

64. Liles DK, Dall, LH. Needle aspiration for diagnosis of cellulitis. *Cutis* 36:63, 1985.

65. Lee PC, Turnidge J, McDonald PJ. Fine-needle aspiration biopsy in diagnosis of soft tissue infections. *J Clin Microbiol* 22:80, 1985.

66. Epperly TD. The value of needle aspiration in the management of cellulitis. *J Fam Pract* 23:337, 1986.

67. Howe PM, Fajardo JE, Orcutt MA. Etiologic diagnosis of cellulitis: comparison of aspirates obtained from the leading edge and the point of maximal inflammation. *Pediatr Infect Dis* 6:685, 1987.

68. Newell PM, Norden CW. Value of needle aspiration in bacteriologic diagnosis of cellulitis in adults. *J Clin Microbiol* 26:401, 1988.

69. Lutomski DM et al. Microbiology of adult cellulitis. *J Fam Pract* 26:45, 1988.

70. Sachs MK. The optimum use of needle aspiration in the bacteriologic diagnosis of cellulitis in adults. *Arch Intern Med* 150:1907, 1990.

71. Bernard P et al. Early detection of streptococcal group antigens in skin sampled by latex particle agglutination. *Arch Dermatol* 123:468, 1987.

72. Bernard P et al. Streptococcal cause of erysipelas and cellulitis in adults. A microbiologic study using a direct immunofluorescence technique. *Arch Dermatol* 125:779, 1989.

73. Haynes JH, Martin JC, Kurzweg FT. Erysipelas. *Am Fam Physician* 27:123, 1983.

74. Shama S, Calandra GB. Atypical erysipelas caused by group G streptococci in a patient with cured Hodgkin's disease. *Arch Dermatol* 118:934, 1982.

75. Dowsett EG et al. Outbreak of idiopathic erysipelas in a psychiatric hospital. *Br Med J* 1:500, 1975.

76. Shimoni Z et al. Changing patterns of erysipelas. *Israel J Med Sci* 20:242, 1984.

77. Barnett JH et al. Erysipeloid. *J Am Acad Dermatol* 9:116, 1983.

78. Reboli AC, Farrar WE. Erysipelothrix rhusiopathiae: an occupational pathogen. *Clin Microbiol Rev* 2:354, 1989.

79. Gorby GL, Peacock JE. Erysipelothrix rhusiopathiae endocarditis: microbiologic, epidemiologic, and clinical features of an occupational disease. *Rev Infect Dis* 10:317, 1988.

80. Howard RJ, Lieb S. Soft-tissue infections caused by halophilic marine vibrios. *Arch Surg* 123:245, 1988.

81. Auerbach PS. Natural microbiologic hazards of the aquatic environment. *Clin Dermatol* 5:52, 1987.

82. Zielinski CJ, Bora FW. Vibrio hand infections: a case report and review of the literature. *J Hand Surg* [AM] 9:754, 1984.

83. Morris JG, Black RE. Cholera and other vibrioses in the United States. *N Engl J Med* 312:343, 1985.

84. Jordan JH, Flynn T. Vibrio sepsis in a cirrhotic patient. *South Med J* 82:799, 1989.

85. Young DF, Barr RJ. Aeromonas hydrophilia infection of the skin. *Arch Dermatol* 117:244, 1981.

86. Freij BJ. Aermonas: biology of the organism and diseases in children. *Pediatr Infect Dis* 3:164, 1984.

87. Weber DJ et al. *Pasteurella multocida* infections, report of 34 cases and review of the literature. *Medicine* 63:133, 1984.

88. Callaham M. Wild and domestic animal bites. In PS Auerbach, EC Geehr (eds.), *Management of Wilderness and Environmental Emergencies* (2nd ed.). New York: McMillan, 1988.

89. Callaham M. Controversies in antibiotic choices for bite wounds. *Ann Emerg Med* 17:1321, 1988.

90. DeVillez RL, Lewis CW. Candidiasis seminar. *Cutis* 19:69, 1977.

91. Montes LF, Wilborn WH. Fungus-host relationship in candidiasis. A brief review. *Arch Dermatol* 121:119, 1985.

92. Sobel JD. Individualizing treatment of vaginal candidiasis. *J Am Acad Deramtol* 23:572, 1990.

93. Epstein JB. Antifungal therapy in oropharyngeal mycotic infections. *Oral Surg Oral Med Oral Pathol* 69:32, 1990.

94. Back O, Faergemann J, Hornqvist R. Pityrosporum folliculitis: a common disease of the young and middle-aged. *J Am Acad Dermatol* 12:56, 1985.

95. McCausland WJ, Cox PJ. Pseudomonas infection traced to motel whirlpool. *J Environ Health* 37:455, 1975.

96. Zacherle BJ, Silver DS. Hot tub folliculitis: a clinical syndrome. *West J Med* 137:191, 1982.

97. Silverman AR, Nieland ML. Hot tub dermatitis: a familial outbreak of pseudomonas folliculitis. *J Am Acad Dermatol* 8:153, 1983.

98. Huminer D et al. Home shower-bath pseudomonas folliculitis. *Israel J Med Sci* 25:44, 1989.

99. Kosatsky T, Kleeman J. Superficial and systemic illness related to a hot tub. *Am J Med* 79:10, 1985.

100. Pinkus H. Furuncle. *J Cutan Pathol* 6:517, 1979.

101. Dahl MV. Strategies for the management of recurrent furunculosis. *South Med J* 80:352, 1987.

102. Hedstrom SA. Treatment and prevention of recur-

rent staphylococcal furunculosis: clinical and bacteriologic follow-up. *Scand J Infect Dis* 17:55, 1985.

103. Recurrent staphylococcal furunculosis [editorial]. *Lancet* 2:81, 1985.

104. Zimakoff J et al. Recurrent staphylococcal furunculosis in families. *Scand J Infect Dis* 20:403, 1988.

105. Shah AM, Supe AN, Samsi AB. Carbuncle—a conservative approach. *J Postgrad Med* 33:55, 1987.

106. Simms MH et al. Treatment of acute abscesses in the casualty department. *Br Med J* 284:1827, 1982.

107. Llera JL, Levy RC, Staneck JL. Cutaneous abscesses: natural history and management in an outpatient facility. *J Emerg Med* 1:489, 1984.

108. Halvorsan GD, Halvorsan JE, Iserson KV. Abscess incision and drainage in the emergency department. *J Emerg Med* 3:227, 295, 1985.

109. Fine BC, Sheckman PR, Bartlett JC. Incision and drainage of soft-tissue abscesses and bacteremia. *Ann Intern Med* 103:645, 1985.

110. Stewart MPM, Laing MR, Krukowski ZH. Treatment of acute abscesses by incision, curettage and primary suture without antibiotics: a controlled trial. *Br J Surg* 72:66, 1985.

111. Llera JL, Levy RC. Treatment of cutaneous abscess: a double-blind clinical study. *Ann Emerg Med* 14:15, 1985.

112. Meislin HW et al. Cutaneous abscesses. Anaerobic and aerobic bacteriology and outpatient management. *Ann Intern Med* 87:145, 1977.

113. Brook I, Finegold SM. Aerobic and anaerobic bacteriology of cutaneous abscesses in children. *Pediatrics* 67:891, 1981.

114. Meislin HW. Pathogen identification of abscesses and cellulitis. *Ann Emerg Med* 15:329, 1986.

115. Carithers HA. Cat-scratch disease. An overview based on a study of 1200 patients. *AJDC* 139:1124, 1985.

116. Margileth AM, Wear DJ, English CK. Systemic cat scratch disease: report of 23 patients with prolonged or recurrent severe bacterial infection. *J Infect Dis* 155:390, 1987.

117. Carithers HA, Margileth AM. Cat-scratch disease. Acute encephalopathy and other neurologic manifestations. *AJDC* 145:98, 1991.

118. English CK et al. Cat-scratch disease. Isolation and culture of the bacterial agent. *JAMA* 259:1347, 1988.

119. Bogue CW et al. Antibiotic therapy for cat-scratch disease? *JAMA* 262:813, 1989.

120. Belknap BS. Sporotrichosis. *Dermatol Clin* 7:193, 1989.

121. Restrepo A et al. Itraconazole therapy in lymphatic and cutaneous sporotrichosis. *Arch Dermatol* 122:413, 1986.

122. Hay RJ. Chronic dermatophyte infections: clinical and mycological features. *Br J Dermatol* 106:1, 1982.

123. Ginsburg CM. Superficial fungal and mycobacterial infections of the skin. *Pediatr Infect Dis* 4:519, 1985.

124. Griffith ML, Flowers FP, Araujo OE. Superficial mycoses. Therapeutic agents and clinical applications. *Postgrad Med* 79:151, 1986.

125. Naftifine for fungal skin infections. *Med Lett Drugs Ther* 21:98, 1988.

126. Greer DL, Jolly HW. Treatment of tinea cruris with topical terbinafine. *J Am Acad Dermatol* 23:800, 1990.

127. Greer DL. Topical treatment for moccasin-type tinea pedis. *J Am Acad Dermatol* 16:554, 1987.

128. Pariser DM. Tinea vesicolor. A practical guide for primary care physicians. *Postgrad Med* 87:61, 1990.

129. Delescluse J. Itraconazole in tinea vesicolor: a review. *J Am Acad Dermatol* 23:551, 1990.

130. Hodson SB et al. Interdigital erythrasma. Part I: a review of the literature. *J Am Podiatric Med Assoc* 78:551, 1988.

131. Allen S et al. The Auckland skin clinic tinea pedis and erythrasma study. *NZ Med J* 103:391, 1990.

132. Highet AS. Viral warts. *Semin Dermatol* 7:53, 1988.

133. Cobb MW. Human papillomavirus infection. *J Am Acad Dermatol* 22:547, 1990.

134. Rees RB. The treatment of warts. *Clin Dermatol* 3:179, 1985.

135. Campbell BJ. The treatment of warts. *Prim Care* 13:465, 1986.

136. Taylor MB. Successful treatment of warts. Choosing the best method for each situation. *Postgrad Med* 84:126, 1988.

137. Wright TC, Richart RM. Role of human papillomavirus in the pathogenesis of genital tract warts and cancer. *Gyencol Oncol* 37:151, 1990.

138. Feingold DS. Gangrenous and crepitant cellulitis. *J Am Acad Dermatol* 6:289, 1982.

139. Furste W, Lobe TE, Botros NN. Gangrenous soft tissue infections. *Infect Surg* 4:837, 1985.

140. Davison AJ, Rotstein OD. The diagnosis and management of common soft-tissue infections. *Can J Surg* 31:333, 1988.

141. Baxter CR. Surgical management of soft tissue infections. *Surg Clin North Am* 52:1483, 1972.

142. Ahrenholz DH. Necrotizing soft-tissue infections. *Surg Clin North Am* 68:199, 1988.

143. Hedstrom SA. Differential diagnosis and treatment of gas-producing infections. *Acta Chir Scand* 141:582, 1975.

144. Vo NM, Watson S, Bryant LR. Infections of the

lower extremities due to gas-forming and non-gasforming organisms. *South Med J* 79:1493, 1986.

145. Chu DZ et al. Necrotizing gas-forming infections in cancer patients. *South Med J* 82:860, 1989.

146. Dellinger EP. Severe necrotizing soft-tissue infections: multiple disease entities requiring a common approach. *JAMA* 246:1717, 1981.

147. Freischlag JA, Ajalat G, Busuttil RW. Treatment of necrotizing soft tissue infections. The need for a new approach. *Am J Surg* 149:751, 1985.

148. Bessman AN, Wagner W. Nonclostridial gas gangrene. Report of 48 cases and review of the literature. *JAMA* 233:958, 1975.

149. Michowitz M et al. Crepitant cellulitis due to *Enterobacter aerogenes*. *Isr J Med Sci* 21:546, 1985.

150. Greenberg PM, Greenberg HH. Crepitant cellulitis. Polymicrobic infection of the diabetic lower extremity. *J Am Podiatr Med Assoc* 79:197, 1989.

151. Stone HH, Martin JD. Synergistic necrotizing cellulitis. *Ann Surg* 175:702, 1972.

152. Pizzo LJ. Synergistic necrotizing cellulitis of the head and neck. *Am J Otolaryngol* 3:452, 1982.

153. Archer CB et al. Progressive bacterial synergistic gangrene in patient with diabetes. *J R Soc Med* 77(suppl. 4):1, 1984.

154. VandeStadt J et al. Synergistic necrotizing cellulitis after pneumonectomy. *Intensive Care Med* 11:158, 1985.

155. Clayton MD et al. Causes, presentation and survival of fifty-seven patients with necrotizing fasciitis of the male genitalia. *Surg Gynecol Obstet* 170:49, 1990.

156. Hirn M, Niinikoski J. Management of perianal necrotizing fasciitis (Fournier's gangrene). *Ann Chir Gynaecol* 78:277, 1989.

157. DiFalco G et al. Fournier's gangrene following a perianal abscess. *Dis Colon Rectum* 29:582, 1986.

158. Brenner BE, Vitullo M, Simon RR. Necrotizing fasciitis. *Ann Emerg Med* 11:384, 1982.

159. Pessa ME, Howard RJ. Necrotizing fasciitis. *Surg Gynecol Obstet* 161:357, 1985.

160. Gozal D et al. Necrotizing fasciitis. *Arch Surg* 121:233, 1986.

161. Wilkerson R, Paull W, Coville FV. Necrotizing fasciitis. Review of the literature and case report. *Clin Orthop Relat Res* 216:187, 1987.

162. Ovesen OC, Arreskov AJ. Necrotizing fasciitis. A report of 3 cases. *Acta Orthop Scand* 59:191, 1988.

163. Umbert IJ et al. Necrotizing fasciitis: a clinical, microbiologic, and histopathologic study of 14 patients. *J Am Acad Dermatol* 20:774, 1989.

164. Collette CJ, Southerland D, Corrall CJ. Necrotizing fasciitis associated with *Haemophilus influenzae* type B. *AJDC* 141:1146, 1987.

165. Jacobson JM, Hirschman SZ. Necrotizing fasciitis complicating intravenous drug abuse. *Arch Intern Med* 142:634, 1982.

166. Svensson LG, Brookstone AJ, Wellsted M. Necrotizing fasciitis in contused areas. *J Trauma* 25:260, 1985.

167. Nallathambi MN et al. Craniocervical necrotizing fasciitis: critical factors in management. *Can J Surg* 30:61, 1987.

168. Farrell LD et al. Postoperative necrotizing fasciitis in children. *Pediatrics* 82:874, 1988.

169. Valko PC, Barrett SM, Campbell JP. Odontogenic cervical necrotizing fasciitis. *Ann Emerg Med* 19:568, 1990.

170. Fisher JR et al. Necrotizing fasciitis. Importance of roentgenographic studies for soft-tissue gas. *JAMA* 241:803, 1979.

171. Rogers JM et al. Usefulness of computerized tomography in evaluating necrotizing fasciitis. *South Med J* 77:782, 1984.

172. Majeski JA, Alexander JW. Early diagnosis, nutritional support, and immediate extensive débridement improve survival in necrotizing fasciitis. *Am J Surg* 145:784, 1983.

173. Sudarsky LA et al. Improved results from a standardized approach in treating patients with necrotizing fasciitis. *Ann Surg* 206:661, 1987.

174. Stamenkovic I, Lew PD. Early recognition of potentially fatal necrotizing fasciitis: the use of frozensection biopsy. *N Engl J Med* 310:1689, 1984.

175. Riseman JA et al. Hyperbaric oxygen therapy for necrotizing fasciitis reduces mortality and the need for débridements. *Surgery* 108:847, 1990.

176. Buggiani FP, Bredemeyer G. Clostridial myositis vs. clostridial cellulitis. *J Am Podiatry Assoc* 65:568, 1975.

177. Lindsey D. Clostridial cellulitis with gas. *Pediatr Infect Dis J* 9:679, 1990.

178. Moustoukas NM, Nichols RL, Voros D. Clostridial sepsis: unusual clinical presentations. *South Med J* 78:440, 1985.

179. Hart GB, Lamb RC, Strauss MB. Gas gangrene: I. A collective review. *J Trauma* 23:991, 1983.

180. Cline KA, Turnbull TL. Clostridial myonecrosis. *Ann Emerg Med* 14:459, 1985.

181. Nordkild P, Crone P. Spontaneous clostridial myonecrosis. A collective review and report of a case. *Ann Chir Gynaecol* 75:274, 1986.

182. Stevens DL et al. Spontaneous, nontraumatic gangrene due to *Clostridium septicum*. *Rev Infect Dis* 12:286, 1990.

183. Stevens DL et al. Lethal effects and cardiovascular effects of purified alpha- and theta-toxins from *Clostridium perfringens*. *J Infect Dis* 157:272, 1988.

184. Pierce EC. Gas gangrene: a critique of therapy. *Surg Rounds* 7:17, 1984.
185. Stevens DL et al. Comparison of clindamycin, tetracycline, metronidazole, and penicillin for efficacy in prevention of experimental gas gangrene due to *Clostridium perfringens*. *J Infect Dis* 155:220, 1987.
186. Gibson A, Davis FM. Hyperbaric oxygen in the management of *Clostridium perfringens* infections. *NZ Med J* 99:617, 1986.
187. Hirn M, Niinikoski J. Hyperbaric oxygen in the treatment of clostridial gas gangrene. *Ann Chir Gynaecol* 77:37, 1988.
188. Aitken DR, Mackett MC, Smith LL. The changing pattern of hemolytic streptococcal gangrene. *Arch Surg* 117:561, 1982.
189. Barker FG, Leppard BJ, Seal DV. Streptococcal necrotizing fasciitis: comparison between histological and clinical features. *J Clin Pathol* 40:335, 1987.
190. Riefler J et al. Necrotizing fasciitis in adults due to group B streptococcus. Report of a case and review of the literature. *Arch Intern Med* 148:727, 1988.
191. Gentry RH, Fitzpatrick JE. A peculiar purple bruise. Necrotizing fasciitis due to group-A beta-hemolytic streptococci. *Arch Dermatol* 126:816, 1990.
192. Bohn WW, Coleman CR. Streptococcal gangrene mimicking a compartment syndrome. A case report. *J Bone Joint Surg* 67:1125, 1985.
193. Seal DV, Kingston D. Streptococcal necrotizing fasciitis: development of an animal model to study its pathogenesis. *Br J Exp Pathol* 69:813, 1988.
194. Svane S. Peracute spontaneous streptococcal myositis. *Acta Chir Scand* 137:155, 1971.
195. Kallen PS et al. Infectious myositis and related syndromes. *Sem Arthritis Rheum* 11:421, 1982.
196. Yoder EL, Mendez J, Khatib R. Spontaneous gangrenous myositis induced by *Streptococcus pyogenes*: case report and review of the literature. *Rev Infect Dis* 9:382, 1987.
197. Doebbeling BN, Wenzel RP. Spontaneous streptococcal gangrenous myositis: survival with early débridement. *South Med J* 82:900, 1989.
198. Schattner A et al. Fulminant streptococcal myositis. *Ann Emerg Med* 18:320, 1989.
199. Anderson CB, Marr JJ, Jaffee BM. Anaerobic streptococcal infections simulating gas gangrene. *Arch Surg* 104:186, 1972.
200. Chiedozi LC. Pyomyositis: review of 205 cases in 112 patients. *Am J Surg* 137:255, 1979.
201. Schlech WF, Moulton P, Kaiser AB. Pyomyositis: tropical disease in a temperate climate. *Am J Med* 71:900, 1981.
202. Kallen P et al. Tropical pyomyositis. *Arthritis Rheum* 25:107, 1982.
203. Gibson RK, Rosenthal SJ, Lukert BP. Pyomyositis. Increasing recognition in temperate climates. *Am J Med* 77:768, 1984.
204. Duvie SO. Bacterial myositis and pyomyositis. *J R Coll Surg Edinb* 29:237, 1984.
205. Brown JD, Wheeler B. Pyomyositis. Report of 18 cases in Hawaii. *Arch Intern Med* 144:1749, 1984.
206. Muscat I, Anthony PP, Cruickshank JG. Nontropical pyomyositis. *J Clin Pathol* 39:1116, 1986.
207. Sarubbi FA, Gafford GD, Bishop DR. Gram-negative bacterial pyomyositis: unique case and review. *Rev Infect Dis* 11:789, 1989.
208. Kennedy CA, Mathisen G, Goetz MB. Tropical pyomyositis of the abdominal wall musculature mimicking acute abdomen. *West J Med* 152:296, 1990.
209. Andrew JG, Czyz WM. Pyomyositis presenting as septic arthritis. A report of 2 cases. *Acta Orthop Scand* 59:587, 1988.
210. Weinberg WG, Dembert ML. Tropical pyomyositis: delineation by gray scale ultrasound. *Am J Trop Med Hyg* 33:930, 1984.
211. Schiff RG, Silver L. Tropical pyomyositis. Demonstration of extent and distribution of disease by gallium scintigraphy. *Clin Nucl Med* 15:542, 1990.
212. Mbonu OO, Nwako FA. Synergistic bacterial gangrene and allied lesions: a unified etiological theory. *Int Surg* 68:122, 1984.
213. Davson J, Jones DM, Turner L. Diagnosis of Meleney's synergistic gangrene. *Br J Surg* 75:267, 1988.

33

Osteoarticular Infections

RONALD W. QUENZER

Individuals with acute or chronic infections of bones and joints often present to the emergency department. The emergency department physician must be alert to recognize the varied presentations in patients at risk for acute or chronic osteoarticular infections, informed of the appropriate diagnostic studies for the emergency department setting, knowledgeable of the initial medical and surgical options of management, and prudent in referral, consultation, and hospitalization decisions. This chapter discusses these and other issues of bone and joint infections. Diabetic foot infections are discussed in Chap. 11.

Infectious Arthritis

Septic arthritis is defined as the invasion of the synovial membrane by microorganisms, usually with extension into the joint space. Although the infection usually is not life threatening, delayed or improper treatment will leave the patient with a destroyed cartilage and permanent damage to the joint. Septic arthritis should be considered in any patient presenting to the emergency department with joint pain and must be distinguished from nonseptic arthritis. Patients with underlying joint disease from trauma, degeneration, rheumatoid ar-

thritis, surgery, or prosthesis are particularly prone to joint infection. Occasionally, septic arthritis is more than just an isolated infectious process; it may represent the presenting manifestation of a systemic disease or primary infection at another site, as in infective endocarditis, urinary tract infection, pneumonia, and disseminated gonococcal infection. The primary source for the bacteria is often unidentifiable in hematogenous septic arthritis. Symptoms and signs of a systemic infection may not be apparent.

The focus of this section is on the diagnosis and management considerations of septic arthritis in the emergency department setting.

Pathogenesis and Pathophysiology

The seriousness and the course of the infection depends on the virulence of the microorganism, underlying host factors, and the interval between the onset of disease and the time of diagnosis and treatment.

Septic arthritis may occur by (1) direct inoculation of the microorganism(s) into the joint, (2) contiguous spread from infected adjacent periarticular structures, or most commonly (3) from a distant site via the bloodstream.

The normal intact synovial membrane resists infectious agents by the phagocytic activity of synovial cells [1]. Penetration of the synovium by trauma, surgical incision, or needle puncture violates the normal protective barrier, putting the joint in jeopardy of infection. Rheumatologic diseases (e.g., rheumatoid arthritis, systemic lupus erythematosus) alter the local and systemic host defense mechanisms, permitting increased risk of septic arthritis. Decreased chemotaxis and phagocytosis of polymorphonuclear cells and decreased bactericidal activity of synovial fluid are relevant factors in patients with rheumatoid arthritis [2–5].

In infants and adults there is a vascular anastomosis between the metaphysis and the epiphysis and a common blood supply of the epiphysis and the synovium, allowing contiguous spread from infected bone (osteomyelitis) into the joint. In children and adults the anastomosis between the metaphysis and the epiphysis is not present, and the epiphyseal growth cartilage provides an effective barrier to vascular spread of infection. There are a few joints where the metaphysis lies within the joint—shoulder (proximeral humerus), hip (proximeral femur), elbow (proximal radius), and ankle (distal-lateral tibia). Spread of infection from metaphyseal-epiphyseal focus into the joint space may result in coexistant osteomyelitis and septic arthritis.

Joint cartilage is not destroyed by bacteria alone. The interaction of the infectious agent and the joint-space tissue induces a complex series of reactions, resulting in effusion and inflammation that may cause cartilage destruction [6, 7]. The reactions may occur rapidly with *Staphylococcus aureus* and other pyogenic bacteria. Untreated bacterial infection may lead to a permanently deformed and dysfunctional joint. The cartilage width decreases, pannus formation is seen, and erosions occur at the lateral margins of the cartilage. These changes deform and weaken the joint. Infection of the hip joint with a large effusion may result in vascular compromise and aseptic necrosis of the femoral head [8]. Early drainage and antibiotic therapy will diminish damage.

Etiology

The etiology of septic arthritis is primarily dependent on the patient's age and underlying host factors. *S. aureus*, group A streptococcus, *Streptococcus pneumoniae*, *Neisseria gonorrhoeae*, *Haemophilus influenzae*, and gram-negative bacilli are the organisms responsible for the majority of cases of bacterial arthritis (Table 33-1). *S. aureus* is responsible for more than 50% of nongonococcal-infected joints and is usually of hematogenous origin except when associated with a prosthetic joint infection [9, 10]. Streptococcal infections occur in all age groups and represent 15%–20% of cases [11]. *H. influenzae* is more frequent in young children than in adults. Enteric gram-negative bacilli occur predominantly in neonates, the elderly with underlying urinary tract infections, and IV drug users. The incidence of gram-negative arthritis is increasing from approximately 10% in the period 1947–1967 to 22%–26% currently [12, 13]. In sexually active individuals *N. gonorrhoeae* may cause an arthritis-dermatitis syndrome (e.g., disseminated gonococcal infection), consisting of fever, chills, pustular skin lesions, and polyarthralgia-polyarthritis usu-

Table 33-1. Etiology of bacterial arthritis percentages

Organism	<2 Years	2–15 Years	16–60 Years	>60 Years
Staphylococcus aureus	18	48	40	53
Streptococcus pneumoniae	12	05	04	05
Streptococci (other)	13	17	20	15
Haemophilus influenzae	48	05	04	05
Neisseria gonorrhoeae	—	15	75	—
Gram-negative bacilli	16	10	23	15

Sources: Composite of data from LeFrock JL, Kannangara DW. Bacterial arthritis. In EH Kass, R Platt (eds.), Current Therapy in Infectious Diseases. Philadelphia: Decker, 1983. Pp. 262–64; Goldenberg DL, Reed JI. Bacterial arthritis. *N Engl J Med* 312:764, 1985; McGurie NM, Kauffman CA. Septic arthritis in the elderly. *J Am Geriatr Soc* 33:170, 1985; Sharp JT et al. Infectious arthritis *Arch Intern Med* 139:1125, 1979.

ally accompanied by tenosynovitis [14]. Occasionally patients may present as any other pathogenic bacteria with monoarticular arthritis without skin lesions. Females, especially during menstruation or pregnancy, are particularly prone to disseminated gonococcal infection (DGI). Polymicrobial septic arthritis occurs in 5%–10% of patients and is associated with either penetrating trauma or extension of an intra-abdominal source [15]. Anaerobic organisms also are rare except in hip joint infections in association with enteric bacilli from an intra-abdominal source, traumatic injuries causing open wounds and fractures of the extremity, and arthroplasty [16].

Several nonpyogenic organisms also may cause infectious arthritis (Table 33-2). *Borrelia burgdorferi*, the agent of Lyme disease, causes chronic migratory polyarthritis of immunologic event. Rarely this organism can be isolated from the joint [17].

A number of viruses are causative agents for arthritis. Characteristically oligo- or polyarthritis develops concomitantly with the viral syndrome or, as is the case with hepatitis B virus (HBV) infection, manifests in the preicteric phase. Rubella, HBV, mumps, lymphocytic choriomeningitis, and human parvovirus (HPV) infections should be considered in all cases of polyarticular joint infection [18, 19]. Immigrants and travelers may have been exposed to arthropod-borne viruses of the togavirus family and develop a severe arthritis, usually of the large joints. The etiology of reactive arthritis is discussed later in this section.

Table 33-2. Nonpyogenic causes of infectious arthritis

Borrelia burgdorferi (Lyme disease)
Viruses
  Hepatitis B virus
  Rubella
  Lymphocytic choriomeningitis
  Human parvovirus
  Togaviruses
Mycobacteria
Fungi
  Sporothrix schenckii
  Histoplasma capsulatum
  Coccioioides immitis
  Blastomyces species
  Candida species
Nocardia species
Actinomycetes species

Mycobacteria produce a chronic monoarticular arthritis as a manifestation of extrapulmonary tuberculosis or as local joint infection by nontuberculous mycobacteria (*Mycobacterium kansasii*, *Mycobacterium avium-intracellulare*, *Mycobacterium marinum*, *Mycobacterium gordonae*, *Mycobacterium fortuitum*, *Mycobacterium chelonei*) [20]. Infection of the sacroiliac joint is extremely common, but any joint may be involved [21].

Sporothrix schenckii and several other fungi (*Histoplasma*, *Coccidioides*, *Blastomyces*, and *Candida* species) are also responsible for chronic infectious arthritis and cannot be differentiated from mycobacteria on clinical grounds alone [22]. Microbiologic and histologic confirmation are required. *Nocardia* and actinomycete are saprophytic organisms that also may cause infectious arthritis.

Clinical Features

The classic triad of fever, decreased range of motion, and joint pain provides the initial clue to the emergency department physician of infectious arthritis in most patients. The fever is usually low grade and present in 40%–90% of patients [23, 24]. Nearly all patients will have decreased active and passive range of motion of the involved extremity joint, and approximately 75% will complain of pain at the infected joint. The patient will usually recognize a gradual onset of these symptoms from a few days to 1–2 weeks. The patient should be questioned as to recent injury to the joint, prior surgery of the joint, underlying rheumatologic diseases, previous needle aspirations of the joint or corticosteroid injections into the joint, use of IV illicit drugs, recent diarrhea syndrome, and history of sexually transmitted diseases or exposure.

Signs characteristic of local infection (e.g., erythema, swelling, tenderness, and warmth) and limitation of joint motion should be sought. Joint effusions are present in 90% of patients [25]. Tenderness is also invariably present, but erythema and warmth may be imperceptible [26]. The pain and the physical findings usually are obvious and relate directly to the infected joint. However, the clinical features of infection of the spine, sacroiliac, or hip joints may be very atypical and poorly localized to the infected joint. Atypical presentations also are common in neonates, IV drug users, immunocompromised patients, and those with rheumatoid arthritis. Tenosynovitis, if present, suggests infection with gonococci, mycobacteria, or fungi. An infected tendon sheath is characterized by pain and tenderness to palpation along the path of the tendon. The pain is most accurately precipitated by stretching the respective muscle and tendon. Careful palpation of the tendon will also sometimes disclose thickening and erythema.

Nongonococcal pyogenic arthritis is monoarticular in 90% of cases [27]. In over half of the cases the knee is infected, followed by the hip, ankle, and elbow [28, 29]. Polyarticular infectious arthritis suggests infection due to gonococci, B. burgdorferi (e.g., Lyme disease), viruses (e.g., rubella or parvovirus), or organisms associated with "reactive" infectious arthritis. Polyarticular nongonococcal infection occurs in only about 10% of children and adults with septic arthritis [30–32]. The clinical features and the etiologic agents vary with certain predisposing factors, particularly age, the joint infected, and selected host situations.

Host-Pathogen Predispositions

Several predisposing factors increase the risk of septic arthritis (Table 33-3). Recognizing these factors will be helpful in the diagnosis and determining the probable causative microorganism.

AGE

Septic arthritis in the neonate and the infant is an acute, bacteremic event frequently involving multiple joints—hip, knee, and shoulder. Group B streptococcus, S. aureus, and coliform bacteria are the most common pathogens in neonates [33]. H. influenzae type B, followed by S. aureus, is the most common pathogen in infants and young children of preschool age [34]. Neonates and infants will usually be afebrile and present with pseudoparesis of the involved extremity and cry on passive or active movement of the joint. If the hip joint is infected, the infant may lie in a "frog-leg" position, with the thigh flexed, abducted, and externally rotated. The hip joint may be dislocated.

Septic arthritis in school-aged children is due to S. aureus, Streptococcus species, and Neisseria meningitidis. H. influenzae becomes less likely [35]. The knee, hip, ankle, and elbow are the most commonly involved joints in this age group.

Table 33-3. Host-pathogen associations in septic arthritis

Host	Pathogens
Neonates	Group B streptococci S. aureus Gram-negative coliforms
Infants	H. influenzae S. aureus Streptococcus sp
Children (>4 yr)	S. aureus Streptococcus sp N. meningitidis
Adolescents	N. gonorrhoeae S. aureus Streptococcus sp
Adults	N. gonorrhoeae S. aureus Streptococcus sp Gram-negative bacilli
Menstruating females	N. gonorrhoeae
Intravenous drug users	S. aureus P. aeruginosa Serratia sp Candida sp
Joint trauma/surgery	S. aureus Streptococcus sp Gram-negative bacilli Anaerobes
Dog/cat bite	P. multocida
Human bite	E. corrodans Streptococcus sp Anaerobes
Intra-articular aspiration/injection	S. aureus Gram-negative bacilli
Prosthetic joint	S. aureus Coagulase-negative staphylococcus Gram-negative bacilli
Sickle cell anemia	Salmonella sp S. pneumoniae
Diabetes mellitus	S. aureus Gram-negative bacilli
Myelogenous leukemia	Aeromonas hydrophila
Immunosuppressive Rx	Gram-negative bacilli
Cancer	Gram-negative bacilli
Rheumatoid arthritis	S. aureus

In sexually active adolescents and adults *N. gonorrhoeae* is the most frequent pathogen, representing nearly 75% of all cases. *S. aureus*, *Streptococcus* species, and gram-negative bacteria account for the remainder [36, 37].

Aged adults are more likely to be infected with *S. aureus*, *Streptococcus* species, *H. influenzae*, and gram-negative bacilli, the organisms of infancy.

GENDER

Patients with DGI may have infection of one or multiple joints. DGI is more common in women than in men and more often occurs around the time of menstruation [38]. A history of risk for sexually transmitted diseases should be sought. The patient is febrile and appears acutely ill. The gonococcal arthritis syndrome may have two stages. In the early stage of the gonococcal dermatitis-arthritis syndrome, polyarthralgia or polyarthritis with tenosynovitis is seen, but detectable synovial effusion usually is absent. A few pustular gonococcal skin lesions usually are evident on the extremities. Cultures for *N. gonorrhoeae* should be obtained from the cervix, rectum, throat, skin lesion, and blood. The joint fluid is usually sterile. The later stage is represented by a monoarthritis or oligoarthritis with negative blood and mucous membrane cultures for *N. gonorrhoeae* but positive synovial fluid cultures.

IV DRUG USE

Infectious complications of IV drug users are well known and were discussed in Chap. 18. Infectious arthritis and osteomyelitis frequently involve joints other than those of the extremities—sternoclavicular, sacroiliac, vertebral—due to hematogenous spread. The organisms also are less usual with a higher incidence of gram-negative organisms, especially *Pseudomonas aeruginosa* and *Serratia* species, as well as *S. aureus* and *Candida* species [39–41]. IV drug users also have a higher incidence of methicillin-resistant *S. aureus* infections in some communities than most other patient groups [42]. Septic arthritis in an IV drug user in particular may be a local manifestation of a more systemic disease, such as infective endocarditis.

JOINT TRAUMA OR SURGERY

Any joint that has been penetrated by animal or human bite will be infected and needs to be managed accordingly (see Chap. 13). Septic arthritis due to procedural contamination following joint aspiration or intra-articular corticosteroid injection may occur. The infection may be difficult to appreciate initially in patients with rheumatoid arthritis or other types of inflammatory joint disease. Asymmetry of inflammation, high fever, and joint fluid analysis are clues to an infected joint.

PROSTHETIC-JOINT INFECTIONS

An infected prosthetic joint should be strongly considered in any patient presenting to the emergency department with a history of fever with or without typical signs of joint inflammation. The incidence of postprosthetic septic arthritis is 2%–10% [43–46]. Approximately half of the infections are recognized within 1 month of surgery (e.g., early infection) and undoubtedly are the result of incidental contamination of the joint space at the time of surgery or from bacteremic spread from a distant site of infection (e.g., concurrent sepsis), such as a urinary tract infection. The delayed infections are due to hematogenous seeding.

The most common organisms are *S. aureus*, coagulase-negative staphylococcus, gram-negative bacilli, and anaerobes. Fungal prosthetic arthritis also occurs in this setting, with *Candida albicans* as the most common organism [47]. Normal postoperative changes of joint effusion, periarticular swelling, and limitation of joint movement may mask an early infectious process, but persistence of fever with joint tenderness and pain increases suspicion for infection. Diagnosis also may be delayed by reluctance to violate a prosthetic joint with needle aspiration to obtain fluid for microbiologic analysis. Patients presenting with a delayed infection generally will complain of pain at the prosthesis. Other clinical features include a synovial effusion, an elevated erythrocyte sedimentation rate, and a plain-film x-ray indicating loosening of the prosthesis. The indium 111-labeled WBC scan is most sensitive and specific in this situation at 86% and 100%, respectively [48]. The definitive diagnosis requires examination of the stains and cultures obtained by arthrocentesis or at surgery.

OTHER HOST-PATHOGEN RELATIONSHIPS

Establishing the diagnosis of septic arthritis in sickle cell anemia patients can be difficult. Bone and joint pains are a major symptom of the disease. However, these patients have a predilection for infection, including septic arthritis, by *S. pneumoniae* and *Salmonella* species [49, 50]. Several other host-pathogen relationships are not common, but to aid the clinician in early diagnosis and treatment, they are listed in Table 33-3.

Specific Joint Infections

SACROILIAC JOINTS

Bacterial sacroiliitis is relatively rare. A total of 166 cases were identified and reported in the world's literature between 1878 and 1990 [51]. Children, IV drug users, and pregnant women are particularly predisposed to pyogenic sacroiliitis [52–54]. Infection of the sacroiliac joint is almost always bacteremic in origin and unilateral in presentation. The patient will complain of pain in the low back, buttock, hip, upper thigh, or lower abdomen. Physical examination will elicit tenderness on palpation over the infected sacroiliac joint. The physician may be first impressed by the tenderness and pain in the abdomen, hip, or thigh and fail to carefully palpate the sacroiliac joints and therefore not correctly identify the site. In females the misdiagnosis of pelvic infection is likely. As the pain radiates into the buttock and hip, the patient may indeed protect the hip and the exam may suggest limited range of motion. Gentle manipulation of the hip and thigh will usually differentiate pyogenic sacroiliitis from a septic hip [55]. The Gaenslen maneuver (i.e., hyperextension of the hip and lower extremity with the patient lying on the side or prone) will generally produce pain in cases of pyogenic sacroiliitis. Patients with herniated nucleus of an intervertebral disc, vertebral osteomyelitis, or diskitis may also have a positive sign. Direct pressure applied to the sacroiliac joint while the patient is in the prone position will usually localize the infection.

HIP JOINTS

Patients with infected hip joints may not precisely localize the pain at the hip joint and often will complain of pain in the buttock, groin, anterior lateral thigh, or knee. Infants and adults with infected hip joints are unwilling to bear any weight on the leg. The Fabere maneuver will elicit pain at the hip site. Swelling and erythema are much less evident than in infection of most other joints. Depending on the pathogenesis of the infection, the organisms vary from *Enterobacteriaceae* and anaerobes if the infection extends from an intra-abdominal focus, staphylococcus coagulase negative if associated with a prosthetic hip joint, or *S. aureus* if hematogenous in a child or IV drug user.

SEPTIC BURSITIS

The two bursae most commonly involved are the olecranon and the prepatellar, although any bursae may become infected. Minor trauma to overlying skin is usually the precipitating event, although many patients cannot recall any injury. The patient will complain of swelling and local pain at the joint. Rarely will there be fever or other systemic symptoms. Examination will reveal swelling, cellulitis, and tenderness around the bursae. A differentiating finding from septic arthritis is that range of motion of the joint will not be compromised with septic bursitis. The bursae should be aspirated and the fluid gram-stained and cultured.

Acute septic bursitis nearly always is due to *S. aureus*; chronic infectious bursitis is seen with indolent organisms such as mycobacteria, *Nocardia* species, actinomycetes, and fungi [56–58]. These patients do not require hospitalization if parenteral antibiotics can be delivered in the outpatient setting, such as a home therapy program. Oral therapy initially is successful in some cases, but failure is more frequent than with parenteral treatment and is therefore discouraged. There is no need for injection of an antibiotic into the bursae space. Since most of the acute infections are secondary to *S. aureus*, cefazolin 2 g q8h IV or other comparable agent should be initiated in the emergency department. If the Gram's stain reveals gram-negative bacilli, then a third-generation cephalosporin (e.g., ceftriaxone 1–2 g q24h IV) should be used. The bursae should be completely aspirated of fluid, such as would be done with an infected joint space. Occasionally repeat aspirations are required. For persistent, relapsing, or chronic cases, incision and drainage or bursectomy is required. Antibiotics should be given intravenously initially for about 1 week, then oral therapy (e.g., dicloxacillin 2–4 g/day), if the physician elects, should be continued for 2 weeks.

Chronic Joint Infections

Whereas infection with pyogenic bacteria generally is an acute process, infections with mycobacteria,

Table 33-4. Musculoskeletal involvement with mycobacterial infections

Organism	Osteomyelitis	Synovitis	Tenosynovitis	Disseminated disease
Mycobacterium tuberculosis	Usually	Occasionally	Rarely	Occasionally
Mycobacterium kansasii	Rarely	Usually	Usually	Occasionally
Mycobacterium marinum	Occasionally	Occasionally	Usually	Never
Mycobacterium avium-intracellulare	Occasionally	Usually	Rarely	Usually
Mycobacterium fortuitum-chelonei	Usually	Rarely	Rarely	Never

fungi, and certain saprophytic bacteria typically present as chronic monoarticular arthritis. Patients will seek medical attention because of local pain, stiffness, and swelling of the joint but are seldom febrile or have significant constitutional symptoms unless the joint infection is part of a systemic infection.

Immunocompromised individuals are at higher risk for atypical pathogens. Patients with systemic lupus erythematosus, renal transplant and hemodialysis patients, and those with HIV disease may have an indolent course of infection from low-virulence organisms, so the emergency department physician must have a high index of suspicion in these situations.

MYCOBACTERIAL INFECTION

Mycobacterium tuberculosis, as well as the atypical mycobacteria, may cause septic arthritis (Table 33-4). The sites most often involved are the spine, hip, and knee [56]. One- to two-thirds of patients will have evidence of pulmonary disease [57]. Tenosynovitis may be associated with joint infections by mycobacteria and serves as a useful clue to the diagnosis. In many instances the diagnosis is delayed for months to years after the onset of symptoms. The diagnosis can be suspected in patients with chronic monoarthritis, a positive purified pro-

tein derivative (PPD) skin test, and radiographic changes showing soft-tissue swelling, subcondral cysts, and cortical and cartilage destruction. Immunocompromised and aged patients may not be skin-test positive. The diagnosis requires synovial fluid analysis for acid-fast bacilli and culture, which are positive in 20% and 80%, respectively. Synovial tissue samples by arthroscopy can increase the yield of the culture results to over 90% [58].

FUNGAL INFECTION

Septic arthritis caused by fungi is uncommon. All of the true pathogenic fungi associated with deep or systemic mycoses, as well as many opportunistic fungi, may cause osteoarticular infections. *Blastomyces dermatitidis*, *Candida* species, *Coccidioides immitis*, *Histoplasma capsulatum*, and *S. schenckii* are the most common fungal pathogens for arthritis. Detail to certain epidemiologic and host factors can identify individuals who may have a predilection for a fungal infection. A history of geographic exposures and preexisting joint surgery or trauma and identification of the underlying disease(s) and immune status of the patient may suggest that a certain fungal infection is probable. Selected clinical and epidemiologic features of joint infections with these organisms are listed in Table 33-5.

Blastomycosis is caused by the fungus *B. der-*

Table 33-5. Features of fungal arthritis

	Healthy patient	Immunocompromised patient	Joint surgery	Geographic location	Monoarticular	Polyarticular
Blastomyces	Yes	No	No	Yes	Yes	No
Candida	No	Yes	Yes	No	Yes	No
Coccidioides	Yes	Yes	No	Yes	Yes	Yes
Histoplasma	Yes	Yes	No	Yes	Yes	Yes
Sporothrix	No	Yes	No	No	Yes	Yes

matitidis. This fungus is found worldwide, but in the United States it is found especially along the Ohio and Mississippi Rivers and in the southeastern and south-central states. Pulmonary infection is the most common manifestation of blastomycosis. Approximately one-third of patients who have chronic blastomycosis will develop bone or joint infections. The long bones, spine, and ribs are most commonly involved. When arthritis is present, it occurs by extension from a contiguous infected bone. Radiographically the lesions are well circumscribed, lytic with or without periosteal reaction.

Candidal articular infection occurs with certain predisposing factors: prosthetic joint surgery, intra-articular corticosteroids, penetrating joint trauma, immunocompromised status, IV drug use, and candidemia [59–62]. Unique to most fungal joint infections, candidal infection may cause more rapid destruction of the joint. Larger joints are more commonly infected.

Osteoarticular infections by *C. immitis* may occur in perfectly healthy individuals during hematogenous dissemination of the fungi as well as in immunosuppressed patients. Most infections occur in semi-arid and arid regions of the southwestern United States. Coccidioidal arthritis is unique because a hypersensitivity arthritis occurs in patients with "valley fever." Migratory polyarthritis or polyarthralgia is usual [63]. The leading clinical clues are concomitant erythema multiforme or erythema nodosum and residence in or recent travel to the endemic area. The illness and arthritis will resolve on their own in 2–4 weeks without therapeutic intervention. Septic coccidioidal arthritis is uncommon, but it may result from disseminated disease or extension from a contiguous osteomyelitis and present as a chronic low-grade arthritis. The knee is involved in 70% of the cases.

H. capsulatum is found throughout the United States but primarily in the central region along the beds of the Ohio and Mississippi Rivers. Arthritis is rare in spite of near universal infection with serologic conversion of people living in the endemic areas. The onset is insidious and chronic without unique features.

Articular sporotrichosis, caused by *S. schenckii*, is uncommon. It may occur by direct inoculation into the joint, as a secondary infection to the lymphocutaneous form of disease (see Chap. 16), or as a result of hematogenous seeding from pulmonary infection [64, 65]. When extracutaneous disease does occur, the patient usually will have some underlying disease, such as alcoholism or myeloproliferative disorder, or be receiving immunosuppressive therapy [66, 67]. Polyarthritis occurs in half of the patients.

Diagnostic and therapeutic considerations are similar for all fungi. Definitive diagnosis of fungal septic arthritis requires identifying the organism in the synovial fluid or tissue. A synovial tissue biopsy for stains and cultures usually is required since the fluid is more often sterile except in candidal arthritis. An infectious disease specialist and an orthopedic surgeon must formulate a plan with the microbiology laboratory to ensure an accurate diagnosis.

LYME DISEASE

Lyme disease, caused by the tick-borne spirochete *B. burgdorferi*, also must be considered in patients presenting with chronic infectious arthritis. Migratory joint pains and myalgias may be seen as early as stage 2 (i.e., 3–21 weeks after the tick bite). But true arthritis of Lyme disease is not seen until stage 3, 6 weeks–2 years after the initial illness [68]. The knee joint and other large joints most often will be involved in a monarticular or oligoarticular fashion, but symmetric arthritis of the smaller joints resembling rheumatoid arthritis has been seen occasionally. Initially the arthritis lasts an average of 1 week with recurrences for years. Although the organism *B. burgdorferi* has been cultured from the joint fluid, it is rare. The diagnosis is based on serology and clinical findings (see Chap. 12). Patients with Lyme arthritis may have false-negative serology if they were treated early in stage 1 with antibiotics [69].

BRUCELLOSIS

Brucellosis is an uncommon disease in the United States today, with most cases reported in developing countries and in immigrants or travelers from such areas (see Chap. 19). Osteoarticular infection occurs in 10%–30% of patients with brucellosis, with the spine as the most common site. It may present as an acute arthritis or more commonly as a chronic systemic illness manifested as fever of unknown origin, generalized lymphadenopathy, hepatosplenomegaly, and monarticular or oligoarticular infection. Radiographic findings include

Table 33-6. Synovial fluid characteristics in infectious and noninfectious arthritis

Clinical condition	Color	Mucin clot	WBC at 1000 × mag.	Predominant cells	Stained smear
Normal	Straw–colored	Tight	<1	Mononuclear	Negative
Pyogenic bacteria	Yellow–turbid	Friable	10–100	Polymorphonuclear	Positive or negative
Inflammatory arthritis	Yellow	Friable	1–50	Polymorphonuclear	Negative
Nonseptic arthritis	Clear–yellow	Tight	<10	Mononuclear	Negative

subcortical osteopenia and reactive sclerosis. Articular infection is diagnosed from positive blood culture of *Brucella* species in acute infections, as well as a positive culture of the synovial fluid or tissue in chronic arthritis. Serologic testing for brucella agglutinin is helpful.

Laboratory Studies

Definitive diagnosis requires microbiologic confirmation. Each patient should have a peripheral cell count, and all joints suspected of infection should be aspirated for Gram's stain, culture, cell count with differential, and glucose and crystal analysis (Table 33-6). Two sets of blood cultures also should be obtained. All cultures should be set up for anaerobic and aerobic incubation. Synovial fluid should be sent to the laboratory in the sealed syringe. Blood culture bottles may be inoculated with fluid at the bedside in an effort to increase the yield. Peripheral leukocytosis will be present in 40%–60%, and blood cultures will be positive in 10%–40% of cases of acute bacterial arthritis [70]. The gross appearance of the synovial fluid will be helpful to the diagnosis. Normal synovial fluid is straw-colored in contrast to turbid infected fluid. Infected fluid leukocyte count ranges from 5,000–500,000/μl, with about 90% polymorphonuclear leukocytes in pyogenic bacterial infections and monocytes in mycobacterial and fungal infections. The synovial fluid glucose-to-blood glucose ratio will be lowered to less than the normal percentage of 90% but is nonspecific. The Gram's stain of the joint fluid will be positive in 50%–60% of the tests [71]. The culture positive rate of synovial fluid glucose is 60%. In cases of chronic joint infections, samples should also be sent for fungi and mycobacteria and the laboratory personnel informed of sus-

picion for slow-growing atypical organisms. Sexually active female patients should have rectal, pharyngeal, and cervical gonococcal cultures obtained unless the initial synovial fluid Gram's stain declares a nongonococcal organism.

Radiographic Findings

Plain film x-rays are most useful as a baseline for subsequent reference and in infants with infected hip in which hip displacement can be definitively determined. In most cases the x-ray reveals soft-tissue swelling. Widening or narrowing of the joint space from effusion or chronic cartilage destruction, respectively, will be seen occasionally. Further imaging studies are seldom necessary for septic arthritis except in cases of hip or sacroiliac joint infection. Technetium bone scans are highly sensitive but lack specificity so that, for example, a fracture of the femoral neck would show uptake not dissimilar from an infectious process. A normal bone scan is strong evidence against septic arthritis [72, 73]. Indium scans have increased specificity for infectious problems. MRI and CT scans have comparable sensitivity and remarkably improved anatomical resolution to technetium and indium or gallium scans and, in this author's opinion, either is preferential for hip joint infections [74].

Differential Diagnosis and Evaluation in the Emergency Department

Septic arthritis must be differentiated from other disorders with similar clinical and laboratory features. Many patients present to emergency physicians with arthralgia or arthritis with or without fever. Polyarthralgia may represent infected joints, noninfected inflamed joints, a periarticular pro-

Table 33-7. Differential diagnostic features of infectious arthritis and polyarthralgia

Disease	Acute	Chronic	Mono	Olio-Poly	Rash	Tenosynovitis	Tendonitis
Arthritis							
Nongonococcal bacterial (infants)	+ᵃ		+				
Gonococcal	+		+	+ +	+	+	
Viral	+		+		+/−ᵇ		
Reactive	+			+			+
Mycobacterial		+	+			+	
Fungal (coccidiodomycosis)	+	+	+	+	+		
Brucella		+	+	+ +			
Lyme disease		+	+	+ +			
Nocardia			+	+			
Actinomycetes							
Traumatic	+		+				
Collagen disorder	+	+ +		+ +	+/−		
Vasculitis	+	+ +		+	+/−		
Drug-induced		+		+	+/−		
Arthralgia							
Influenza	+			+			
Adenovirus	+			+	+/−		
Viral hemorrhagic fever	+			+	+		
Rocky Mountain spotted fever	+			+	+		
Erlichiosis	+			+			
Acute febrile illness	+			+			

ᵃ + = definitely
ᵇ +/− = possibly

cess, or a nonspecific rheumatologic symptom of an acute febrile illness. All causes of polyarthritis may initially manifest as polyarthralgia without noticeable increase in synovial effusion or other signs of infectious arthritis. In addition polyarthralgia is a frequent clinical feature of all rheumatologic disorders and several systemic infectious diseases. The presence or absence of a rash, tenosynovitis, insertional tendinitis, acute or chronic presentation, and mono- or polyarthritis is essential to establishing the diagnosis in the emergency department (Table 33-7).

All disorders that may cause joint inflammation should be considered in the differential diagnosis of each patient (Table 33-8). Perhaps differentiating traumatic effusions from septic arthritis is the most frequent dilemma for ED physicians. In most cases trauma to the joint will cause swelling within 24 hours, whereas it usually takes more than 24 hours from the time of injury for septic effusions to develop. Also the septic joint usually has a more restricted range of motion. Another common problem for emergency department physicians is in the patient presenting with an abrasion or cellulitis over a swollen joint, the patella, or ankle areas in particular. Is the joint infected? In most cases of severe soft-tissue infection around a joint, a small sterile sympathetic effusion develops. An uninfected joint will still maintain a good degree of mobility with less pain than in an infected joint. As a rule, a needle aspirate should not transgress an area of cellulitis, to avoid inoculating bacteria into the joint. After careful examination, if suspicion is still high for septic arthritis, the procedure can be done, followed by immediate institution of systemic antibiotics.

Table 33-8. Causes of joint inflammation

Infectious arthritis

Reactive arthritis: Reiter's disease, acute rheumatic fever, postmeningococcal arthritis, postintestinal bypass arthritis, postnongonococcal urethritis arthritis, enterocolitis syndrome, colitic arthritis of IBD

Primary rheumatologic disorders: rheumatoid arthritis, juvenile rheumatoid arthritis, collagen vascular diseases, gout, pseudogout, others

Whipple's disease

Acne conglobata

Hydradenitis suppurativa

Vasculitis

Drug-induced: Procainamide

Trauma

Reactive Arthritis

Reactive arthritis is a term applied to a sterile synovitis occurring in association with and usually following an infectious process at another body site. There are many arthritogenic organisms and syndromes that result in a reactive arthritis. Most cases are associated with sexually acquired (e.g., chlamydia) or enteric infections (e.g., enterocolitis syndrome) [75, 76]. The organisms most consistently associated with sterile arthritis are listed in Table 33-9. A few organisms, such as *H. influenzae*,

Table 33-9. Organisms associated with non-septic arthritis

Reactive Arthritis
Chlamydia trachomatis
Yersinia pseudotuberculosis
Yersinia enterocolitica
Salmonella species
Shigella flexneri
Campylobacter jejuni

Other Arthrides
Parasites (*Strongyloides, Taenia, Endolimax, Giardia, Schistosoma, Ascaris, Trichuris*)
Haemophilus influenzae (meningitis) *
Neisseria meningitidis (meningitis) *
Streptococcus pyogenes *
Mycoplasma species
Viruses (HBV, rubella)

* These organisms may cause septic or nonseptic arthritis.

N. meningitidis, and *Streptococcus pyogenes*, are known to cause either a septic or a reactive arthritis. The pathogenesis is a postinfectious immunologic reaction with a sterile synovitis. The emergency department physician should be familiar with these entities to differentiate from septic arthritis. Since 1972 it has been clear that the majority of patients with reactive arthritis share human leukocyte antigen (HLA) B27 [77]. The physician should search for a recent history of an acute diarrheal illness, viral exanthem, jaundice, urethral discharge, or dysuria, as well as evidence of a systemic disease such as rheumatic fever or infective endocarditis. Common clinical features are asymmetric distribution, predilection for large joints, oligoarthritis, and enthesopathy (e.g., insertional tendonitis) [78].

Therapeutic Approach

All patients with presumptive or proved septic arthritis should be hospitalized. Therapy consists of systemic antibiotics, closed or open drainage of the septic joint, and rehabilitation. Antibiotic treatment is initiated as soon as the appropriate samples have been obtained for the laboratory, and the joint fluid Gram's stain has been examined. It is appropriate to initiate antimicrobials in the emergency department once all sites have been cultured. Delay in therapy often results in incomplete recovery. Unless the Gram's stain of the synovial fluid or the clinical findings are sufficient for identification of the etiologic agent, presumptive (i.e., empiric) therapy for the most probable pathogen(s) will be required pending final culture information. Appropriate presumptive therapy should cover staphylococci, streptococci, and gram-negative bacilli (Table 33-10). Systemic therapy achieves adequate concentration in the joint space to obtain cure; therefore, intra-articular antibiotic administration is not indicated [79].

Oral therapy with quinolone agents shows promise for selected cases, particularly gram-negative infections. The ratio of the concentration of quinolones in synovial fluid to that of plasma varies from 0.9–1.2, which is substantially better than beta-lactam agents, aminoglycosides, or vancomycin. Oral ciprofloxacin, ofloxacin, and other quinolones have been used in experimental arthritis and clini-

Table 33-10. Therapy of infectious arthritis

Therapy	Antibiotic
Presumptive (No Bacteria Seen)	
Neonates	Nafcillin plus gentamicin
Infants	Cefotaxime
Children	Cefotaxime
Adolescents	Cefotaxime (or ceftriaxone)
Adults	Ceftriaxone 2 g q24h IV or cefotaxime 2 g q8h IV
Prosthetic joint	Vancomycin 1 g q12h IV plus ceftaxidime 1–2 g q8h IV
Penetrating injury	Ceftriaxone 2 g q24h IV or cefotaxime 1–2 g q8h IV + metronidazole 500 mg q8h IV (or PO)
S. aureus	Nafcillin 2 g q6h IV or cefazolin 2 g q8h IV
MRSA or MRSE	Vancomycin 1 g q12h IV
S. pneumoniae	Penicillin G 2,500,000 U q6h IV
S. pyogenes	Penicillin G 2,500,000 U q4–6h IV
Enterococcus species	Ampicillin 2 g q6h IV + gentamicin 3mg/kg/day IV
Enterobacteriaceae	Aztreonam 1–2 g q8h IV or third-generation cephalosporin or ciprofloxacin 400 mg q12h IV
Pseudomonas species	Tobramycin or gentamicin 5 mg/kg/day IV plus piperacillin 4 g q6h IV or ceftazidime 2 g q8h IV
Salmonella species	Ceftriaxone 2 g q24h IV or ciprofloxacin 400 mg q12h IV
N. gonorrhoeae	Ceftriaxone 1 g q24h IV
H. influenzae, amp-S	Ampicillin 2 g q6h IV
H. influenzae, amp-R	Cefotaxime 1 g q8h IV or other third-generation cephalosporin
B. burgdorferi	Ceftriaxone 2 g q24h IV or penicillin 20,000,000–24,000,000 U/day IV or doxycycline 100 mg bid PO or amoxicillin 500 mg tid PO

cal trials with comparable success to parenteral therapy [80–85]. Now that ciprofloxacin is available in parenteral form, other useful therapeutic strategies are available to the clinician. Quinolones may indeed become agents of choice for musculoskeletal infections.

Because of the numerous effective agents and the continuous introduction of newer antibiotics it is unrealistic to be dogmatic about the best choice of antibiotics for infected joints. More important, it is essential to select an agent that has an antibacterial spectrum appropriate for the presumed or determined microorganism(s). All beta-lactams and fluoroquinolones achieve adequate concentration in joint spaces. Aminoglycosides have been included in more traditional regimens, but with newer beta-lactams and quinolones clinicians now have other choices. The aminoglycosides' activity is diminished in an environment of low redox potential and increased acidity, as is found in infected joints. Possibly single-dose therapy with aminoglycosides

or local infusion via implantable pumps will overcome these disadvantages.

Delayed-onset prosthetic-joint infections are extremely difficult to cure without removing the device. Many strains of staphylococci produce slime-enhancing adhesion to the hardware and protect the organism from antibiotics. However, in early postprosthetic arthritis success may come with immediate arthrotomy with thorough débridement and irrigation, local antibiotic impregnated beads, and prolonged systemic antibiotics without removal of the device. Encouraging results were reported by administering local amikacin into acutely infected prosthetic joints (30 knees and 13 hips) via an implantable pump [86]. In this study pathogenic organisms included staphylococci, enterococci, and gram-negative bacilli. During therapy synovial fluid assays for amikacin levels were as high as 1100 µg/ml with nontoxic serum levels at all times. Without removing the prosthesis, 33 of 43 patients remained infection free at 9–60 months.

The standard length of treatment should be 1 week for DGI; 2 weeks for *Haemophilus* or streptococcal infections; 3 weeks or longer for gramnegative infections; and at least 4 weeks for *S. aureus* arthritis. Patients with associated osteomyelitis or prosthetic-joint involvement require longer therapy.

Management of chronic mycobacterial or fungal arthritis requires the combined efforts of an infectious disease specialist to select and guide the use of appropriate anti-infectives and an orthopedic surgeon to explore the joint, débride, and consider the need for synovectomy. The preferred agents for osteoarticular mycobacterial infections are the same as for pulmonary infections. Treatment regimens may be complex, with associated significant

adverse effects from the medication. The combination of INH, rifampin, and pyrazinamide or ethambutol is used initially. Streptomycin or amikacin or one or more of the second-line drugs may be required for certain atypical mycobacteria or resistant *M. tuberculosis* (Table 33-11).

. Amphotericin B is the mainstay of treatment for most fungal infections. Resistance has been noted in strains of *Candida*, *Coccidioides*, *Phycomycetes*, and *Pseudoallescheria*. The usual total dose for osteoarticular infections is 1.5–3.0 g. Refractory fungal arthritis can be treated with intra-articular infusions of 5–15 mg per dose. Ketoconazole serves as the alternative agent for most fungal infections. Failure is common at usual doses, even though the penetration into synovial fluid is excellent at con-

Table 33-11. Approach to presumptive treatment of mycobacterial infection of bones and joints

Organism	Drug combinations	Surgery
M. tuberculosis	1. INH + RIF + PZA for first 2 months, then 2. 2 drugs (INH + RIF) for 9–18 months 3. Add EMB if INH resistance suspected	1. Tissue for diagnosis 2. Drainage of very large abscesses 3. Decompression of spinal cord compression 4. Stabilization if unstable spinal lesion
M. avium-intracellulare	Variable resistance 1. INH + RIF + EMB 24–36 months + STR first 2–3 months	1. Surgical resection of localized disease necessary
M. kansasii	Variable resistance* 1. RIF + INH + EMB or STR for 12–18 months	1. Tissue for diagnosis 2. Excision of local disease
M. marinum	INH resistant 1. RIF + EMB 2. Cycloserine, amikacin, doxycycline, or kanamycin	1. Tissue for diagnosis 2. Débridement + drainage may be curative
M. gordonae	INH resistant 1. EMB + RIF	1. Tissue for diagnosis 2. Débridement 3. Remove prosthesis
M. fortuitum-chelonae	Usually resistant to most drugs 1. Amikacin + RIF or doxycycline or cefoxitin for 4–6 weeks	1. Excision of localized disease may be curative 2. Need wide incision + drainage
AFB organism but negative culture	1. INH + RIF + EMB	1. Tissue for diagnosis

Key: INH = isoniazid; RIF = rifampin; EMB = ethambutol; STR = streptomycin; ETN = ethionamide; CSR = cycloserine; KAN = kanamycin; CAP = capreomycin; VIO = viomycin; PZA = pyrazinamide.
* Resistant to conventional antituberculous drugs, requiring in vitro sensitivity testing of alternative antimicrobial agents.

centrations equal to plasma [87]. Failure may be due to the low bone concentration of only 20% of plasma. Although a saturated solution of potassium iodide is the treatment for lymphocutaneous sporotrichosis, amphotericin B is required for articular and other extracutaneous infections. The indications for fluconazole (and itraconazole) in osteoarticular infections have not been determined.

Treatment of Lyme arthritis should not be initiated casually, since many patients fail to respond and others have recurrent arthritis requiring repeated courses of therapy. Ceftriaxone or penicillin G for 14–21 days is currently the drug of choice for stage 3 disease. Doxycycline or amoxicillin over 4 weeks is an oral alternative. The response to therapy is slow or incomplete, with many patients receiving additional symptomatic relief with nonsteroidal anti-inflammatory agents. Acute brucellosis frequently resolves without treatment, at which time the patient may experience arthralgias and transient oligoarthritis. Chronic brucellosis requires prolonged therapy for 1–3 months. The preferred agents are doxycycline with rifampin. The main alternative treatment is doxycycline plus streptomycin.

Infected joints require repeat aspirations, arthroscopic débridement, or open surgical drainage. Each approach has its advocate [88–90].

Many patients, particularly those with gonococcal arthritis, will do very well with repeated joint aspirations. Therefore, the physician may decide to use arthroscopy to lyse adhesions and irrigate only those infected joints that are not responding after 2–3 days of therapy. Open surgical drainage is usual for infants with hip joint infections to reduce intracapsular pressure, thus avoiding ischemic destruction of the epiphyseal growth plate.

Prognosis

Prognosis is favorable for those patients with no underlying host compromise, penetrating injury, or infected prosthetic joint. Patients at extremes of age often have a more prolonged course than others, and those with infections from less sensitive microorganisms may require higher dosages and longer courses of therapy. A failure to initiate treatment within 7 days of onset seems to delay recovery and increase complications [91]. Persistence of joint

pain or limitation of movement is seen in about 27% of infants and children and up to half the adults with nongonococcal joint infection [92, 93]. All others can be expected to do well with early antimicrobial therapy and drainage.

Osteomyelitis

Osteomyelitis is defined as an infection of the bone marrow, trabeculae, and cortex. The causative agents of osteomyelitis can be bacteria, fungi, parasites, and rarely viruses. These organisms can cause acute or chronic bone infections. Medical therapy is key to the treatment of acute osteomyelitis; surgical therapy takes precedence for more chronic bone infections. As an aid to the clinician to determine the microbial etiology and the best therapeutic approach, it is useful to classify bone infections as acute or chronic, as well as community or hospital acquired infections, as is done with most other infectious diseases.

Acute osteomyelitis cases generally present with abrupt illness over a few days associated with systemic symptoms and generally with the infection present no longer than 2–4 weeks. Chronic osteomyelitis represents the remaining cases where the infection is indolent, slowly progressive with clinical features present for 4 or more weeks, and with minimal or no systemic symptoms or signs. Except in the cases of acute hematogenous and posttraumatic or postsurgical osteomyelitis, there can be only speculation as to the actual onset of the infection. Nonetheless, the emergency department is a common entry point for medical care for many of these patients, either because of an acute illness—with fever or pain, open fracture of an extremity, or an open wound—or lack of access to a primary-care physician.

Most acute community acquired cases of osteomyelitis occur in children by hematogenous seeding. These children may present to the emergency department with fever of unknown origin or with localized pain to the bone. Certain immunocompromised individuals (e.g., drug addicts, hemodialysis patients, patients with sickle cell anemia or AIDS) are predisposed to acute hematogenous bone infections.

More chronic community acquired cases are usually the result of trauma, such as in puncture wounds or open fractures, or associated with diabetic ulcerations and foot infections.

The incidence of acute and chronic bone infections that are hospital acquired is increasing due to joint replacement surgery and open reduction and internal fixation (ORIF) procedures for fractures. The incidence of joint replacement infection is now approximately 200 per 100,000 operated patients [94]. Long-term indwelling lines for parenteral nutrition, chemotherapy, or antimicrobials and Foley catheters also serve as a source from which organisms can spread to the bones. An ongoing centralized surveillance study in Denmark reported that 19% of cases of hematogenous osteomyelitis and 60% of contiguous osteomyelitis cases were hospital acquired in the 1984–1988 period [95].

Pathogenesis and Pathophysiology

Osteomyelitis may occur by hematogenous seeding, direct inoculation through an open wound, or contiguous spread from adjacent infected tissue. The pathogenesis of acute osteomyelitis is nearly always by bloodstream or direct inoculation, as may occur with an open bone fracture. In contrast, the pathogenesis of chronic infections usually is from spread of the organisms from contiguous structures, as is the case with osteomyelitis in diabetic feet.

Hematogenous osteomyelitis in infants and children usually localizes in the marrow of the metaphyseal portion of tubular long bones. In adults involvement of the spine and the pelvis is more common. Infection then spreads from the marrow into the epiphysis of infants or through the haversian and Volkmann canals to the subperiosteal region of the bone in children and adults [96]. Subperiosteal accumulation of pus lifts the periosteum and disrupts the periosteal blood supply, resulting in ischemia and localized bone death. The dead bone segment, a sequestrum, usually is microscopic, but it may be large enough to see on imaging studies or recognized at surgery. The sequestrum may harbor organisms for long periods of time, setting the stage for persistent or relapsing chronic osteomyelitis. The osteogenic layer of the periosteum forms new bone, the involucrum, surrounding the dead bone. The involucrum contains many small pores, or cloacae, through which microorganisms and inflammatory debris pass into the surrounding soft tissue and through sinus tracts that lead to the skin surface. The formation of sequestra, involucra, and sinus tracts characterizes the process as the chronic stage of osteomyelitis.

The pathogenesis of chronic contiguous osteomyelitis first involves the periosteum by spread from surrounding infected soft tissue. With time the infection extends through the periosteum to cortical and cancellous bone. The process usually is indolent and slow to provide clinical evidence of infection. Bacterial adhesion to bone and colonization of substrata, which initiates a localized immune response, eventually establishes the clinical features of chronic osteomyelitis [97]. The feet, hands, mandible, and skull are most often involved.

In the case of osseous infections microorganisms adhere to a substratum. Substrata may be organic (e.g., living or dead bone, allografts, or soft tissues) or nonorganic biomaterials (e.g., metals, synthetic polymers, or ceramics) [98]. Once in contact with a particular substratum many bacteria secrete proteinaceous adhesions and exopolysaccharide polymers (e.g., glycocalyx and "slime"), which help the organisms to adhere. Bacteria together with this glycocalyx form the biofilm. The biofilm offers the bacteria some form of resistance from antibiotics and immune response components. Within the biofilm is the microzone, the environment that promotes optimum growth of bacteria [99].

It should now be evident why osteoarticular infections that have reached the chronic stage or that are associated with nonorganic biomaterials are considered surgical infections requiring both surgical débridement, removal of the infected substratum, and appropriate antimicrobial administration. An understanding of these pathophysiologic processes will rationalize the management and improve the prognosis.

Acute Osteomyelitis

Acute osteomyelitis refers to infection presenting within 2–4 weeks of onset of initial symptoms. It is predominantly a disease of children aged 3–15 years, with European hospital incidence rates of 10–200 per 100,000 children at risk per year [100]. Male dominance of infection is noted in childhood with a relative risk of about 2.0 [101, 102]. The long bones of the extremities are the main sites in children, comprising two-thirds of the 440 infected bones in Nelson's series [103]. The most common sites are the metaphyses of the femur, tibia, and humerus [104, 105]. Pelvic osteomyelitis represents less than 10% of cases in children. In some instances of acute hematogenous osteomyelitis, the host defense mechanisms can contain the infection to a well-circumscribed area in a particular bone, usually the metaphysis of a long bone. This abscess represents a subacute manifestation of osteomyelitis and is called a Brodie's abscess.

Acute hematogenous osteomyelitis is less common in adults. However, the trend reported in Denmark is that of an increase in the number of adults over 50 years with acute hematogenous osteomyelitis since 1968 [106]. IV drug users experience acute hematogenous osteomyelitis but usually of the axial skeleton, particularly the vertebral, pelvic, and sternoclavicular areas [107, 108].

Nonhematogenous acute osteomyelitis is uncommon, but it may occur in patients with recently implanted bony hardware. Acute bone infection at the site of the donor or recipient bone graft may develop as a complication 7–10 days after surgery. Traumatic osteomyelitis associated with an open fracture or an ORIF procedure may present as an acute or chronic infection.

Chronic Osteomyelitis

Chronic osteomyelitis is the most difficult and frustrating disease the orthopedic surgeon and the infectious disease specialist are called on to treat. Before antibiotics chronic infection developed in 39%–50% of all cases of acute hematogenous osteomyelitis [109]. In modern times the cure rate in acute hematogenous osteomyelitis is over 90% [110, 111].

The vast majority of chronic cases in the antibiotic era result from contiguous soft-tissue infections, puncture wounds, open fractures, and osteoarticular prosthetic surgery. Diabetes mellitus and peripheral vascular disease are common predisposing factors for chronic contiguous osteomyelitis.

Relapses or recurrent infections plague chronic osteomyelitis. The incidence of recurrent infections should correlate with the appropriateness of the medical and surgical therapies, as well as selected host factors and the length of the follow-up period. Diabetics with vascular disease and orthopedic patients with bone fractures requiring ORIF have high relapse rates. Relapse rates increase with the duration of follow-up. Nearly a third of relapses in patients with acute hematogenous infections occurred more than 6 months after the initial infection [112]. Relapse rates in chronic infections are difficult to determine, since there is no agreement on what constitutes "cure." Relapse may occur years following clinical cure. However, in the author's experience as well as others, one disease-free year is strongly supportive of cure in about 85% of cases. It is better to think of the clinical status of infection in response to therapy for chronic osteomyelitis as active or inactive. Radiographic and histologic determinations for acute, chronic, suppressing, or relapsing status of bone infection are inaccurate. Only repeated microbiologic sampling of the site will give more valid information, but it cannot be justified in the majority of patients with evidence of clinical cure following therapy. Therefore, there is the possibility for relapse.

Tuberculous Osteomyelitis

Since 1985 the number of new cases of tuberculosis has increased each year. In 1990 there was a 9% increase from the previous year, in which 23,495 cases were reported. High rates of new infections occur in patients with AIDS and IV drug use, as well as in crowded populations of prisoners, homeless persons, and nursing home residents. Immigrants and minorities have an increased incidence. Skeletal osteomyelitis, established at the time of the initial infection through hematogenous dissemination, occurs in 1% of patients with tuberculosis. It is usual to have arthritis, as well as osteomyelitis. The spine (e.g., in Pott's disease), hip, and knee are most often involved [113]. Multiple bones and joints may be infected in severe disseminated disease. The gibbus formation of the spine is caused by the marked kyphosis, which results from the chronic indolent destruction of the intervertebral space and anterior portion of the adjacent vertebral bodies. Pus from the vertebral body characteristically ruptures anteriorly and may spread proximally and distally along the vertebrae and tissue planes. Granulomatous lesions with acid-fast bacilli and mycobacteria in culture obtained by surgical biopsy will confirm the diagnosis.

Vertebral Osteomyelitis

The axial skeleton is the area of predilection for acute hematogenous osteomyelitis in the adult. The main factor favoring bacteremic vertebral infection is the presence of rich cellular bone marrow with generous blood supply [114]. By way of peripheral and periosteal nutrient arteries of the spine and Batson's venous plexus, microorganisms gain access to these bones. Complications of spine or disk surgery, trauma, and contiguous spread of a paraspinal infection are also responsible for some cases of vertebral osteomyelitis. Once established extension of the infection across the disk space, along the longitudinal spinal ligaments, or through interconnecting spinal vessels occurs with time. It should be noted that the intervertebral disk is avascular in the skeletally mature adult, and accordingly the disk space is not primarily involved except in disk-space infections as a consequence of discogenic surgery. In infants the cartilaginous end plates of the intervertebral disk contain small blood vessels; distant infection may seed the disk space. The mean age of disk-space infection in children is 7 years, with the usual range of 1–16 years [115, 116].

Except in patients who have undergone surgical procedures of the spine, vertebral osteomyelitis occurs by bloodstream seeding from a distant infected focus. Hence, patients at greater risk are IV drug users, patients with infective endocarditis, and those with chronic or complicated genitourinary tract infections. The incidence is highest in IV drug abusers and the aged with a mean age of 60–70 years [117, 118].

Biomaterial-Centered Infections

Osteomyelitis can occur as a complication when nonorganic biomaterials (e.g., metals, synthetic polymers) or bone wax are used in the treatment of fractures or reconstructive surgery. An infectious process should be considered in any individual with foreign or prosthetic material presenting with fever, bone pain, or swelling. Many bacteria, especially staphylococci, through the secretion of slime (i.e., biofilm) adhere to polymers, polyethylene, poly-propylene, methylmethacrylate, and metallic surfaces regularly used in orthopedic surgery [119].

Etiology

The etiology of osteomyelitis varies considerably by age, site, host, and epidemiologic settings (Table 33-12). In children with acute hematogenous os-

Table 33-12. Osteomyelitis: etiologic agents

Situations	Organisms
Infants	Group B streptococcus
	S. aureus
	E. coli
Children	S. aureus
	S. pyogenes
Adults	S. aureus
	Gram-negative bacilli
Acute hematogenous	S. aureus
Vertebral	S. aureus
	Mycobacteria
	Fungi
IV drug users	S. aureus
	P. aeruginosa
	S. marcescens
	Candida species
Chronic	(Polymicrobial)
	S. aureus
	Streptococci
	Coagulase-negative staphylococci
	Gram-negative bacilli
	Anaerobes
	Mycobacteria
	Fungi
	Brucella species
Biomaterial	S. aureus
	Coagulase-negative staphylococci
	Corynebacterium species
	Gram-negative bacilli
Open fracture	S. aureus
	Gram-negative bacilli
Sickle cell disease	Salmonella species
Hemodialysis	S. aureus
Penetrating foot injury	P. aeruginosa
	S. aureus (polymicrobial)

teomyelitis the etiologic organism can be isolated in about 75% of the cases by obtaining blood [120]. S. aureus causes approximately half of these infections, with Streptococcus species the next most common pathogens. As in other infectious diseases of infants under 2 years of age, H. influenzae type B is common but is more likely to cause septic arthritis than osteomyelitis.

In the adult, pyogenic bacteria, brucella, mycobacteria, and fungi are responsible for the vast majority of acute hematogenous and vertebral osteomyelitis. S. aureus is responsible for more than half [121]. Gram-negative bacteria are responsible for nearly a third of cases, with Escherichia coli predominating, because the source is often the genitourinary tract with hematogenous seeding of the spine. The etiologic organism in the IV drug user is more difficult to predict. Pseudomonas aeruginosa, Serratia species, Enterobacter species, and C. albicans are as common as S. aureus [122].

In chronic contiguous osteomyelitis more than one pathogen is usually isolated, in contrast to monomicrobial etiology of acute hematogenous infections. S. aureus is most common, present in approximately 60% of cases, but coagulase-negative staphylococci, Streptococcus species, gram-negative bacilli, and anaerobes are often cultured as well [123]. Although rare Brucella species, Mycobacterium species, and certain fungi, especially C. immitis and B. dermatitidis should be considered in individuals from endemic areas and developing countries.

Postsurgical disk space infections usually are caused by S. aureus, coagulase-negative staphylococci, or occasionally P. aeruginosa [124, 125].

S. aureus and coagulase-negative staphylococci have a predilection for nonorganic biomaterials, because most strains secrete slime or glycocalyx and are a major part of human skin and mucous membrane microbiologic flora with easy access to these implanted foreign devices at the time of surgery. Corynebacterium species and gram-negative bacilli also have been associated with these infections.

Clinical Features

The clinical features of acute hematogenous infection are fever, increased heart rate, local pain, and tenderness at the site of infection. Muscle spasm may be present as a protective mechanism to prevent movement of the limb. In the infant, the aged, and patients with impaired immune status, any or all of these features may be absent or modified. These patients are always more difficult to evaluate clinically. In the neonate, infant, and child pseudoparalysis of the affected limb is a very sensitive sign of bone or joint infection [126]. To help localize the pain in a child, the physician should ask the youngster "to point to the place where it hurts." The physician should explore for recent dental work, IV drug use in the adolescent and adult, and procedural or surgical manipulations that could result in significant bacteremia.

The triad of fever, back pain, and local tenderness suggests vertebral osteomyelitis [127, 128]. Back pain is present in 85%–90% of cases but initially is poorly localized [129, 130]. The pain is usually of a chronic, persistent nature and with time becomes more localized. Local tenderness and fever occur in approximately 65% and 45%, respectively [131]. The emergency department physician must recognize the more atypical manifestations of vertebral infections, such as fever of unknown origin, arm, leg, or hip pain associated with nerve root compression, referred abdominal pain, and characteristic findings of cord compression [132]. In the infant refusal to walk or stand may be the key sign of disk-space infection. An older child may complain of back pain, hip and leg pain, or abdominal or meningeal irritation [133]. A chest x-ray should be obtained in each patient with suspected tuberculous vertebral osteomyelitis. Two-thirds of patients will demonstrate active pulmonary disease [134].

Pain of osteomyelitis is seldom a complaint in the diabetic with an insensate foot or the patient with spinal cord or other neuropathic disorders. Purulent discharge from an ulcer or sinus tract on the patient's sock or bedsheet is usually the first clue noticed by the patient or the care provider.

The examination in the emergency department will reveal fever in the majority of children and approximately half of adults with acute hematogenous osteomyelitis. Fever is uncommon in patients with chronic contiguous infections. The examination generally will show point tenderness at the infected site, but appreciable swelling, warmth, or erythema may not be evident due to the insulation and thickness of overlying soft tissues and skin. A subcutaneous abscess overlying bone is strongly suggestive of an underlying bone infection. Exposed bone visible to the eye is suspicious. In adults with acute hematogenous osteomyelitis involving the spine or the pelvis, the localizing clinical features usually are concealed. Clues to infection are rigidity of the spine to flexion or extension in about 15%–20% of patients, vertebral tenderness to a percussion hammer, a history of predisposing factors, and absence of any other source for the acute febrile illness. An abnormal erythrocyte sedimentation rate (ESR) and leukocyte count, although nonspecific, support an infection process but do not help determine if the infection is localized to the skin and soft tissue, deeper tissues, joint, or bone. A normal ESR does not rule out osteomyelitis. The large majority of patients with chronic localized osteomyelitis will have a normal leukocyte count.

Diagnosis by Imaging

Imaging techniques for diagnosis of acute and chronic osteomyelitis have undergone major changes in the past decade. Much is published on this subject, but controversy and confusion remain in regard to the best imaging study to diagnose osteomyelitis due in part to the scarcity of critical analysis and comparative studies. Plain films, gallium scans (Ga-67), 111-Indium scans (In-111), technetium bone scans (Tc-99m), CT scans, and MRI are available. Plain x-rays are insensitive for acute infections and lack specificity at fracture sites or in diabetics with Charcot's arthropathy. Vascular flow-dependent studies (e.g., Tc-99m bone scan, Ga-67 scan, and In-111 scan) have decreased sensitivity for bone infections in areas of severe peripheral vascular disease or bony sequestrations associated with chronic infection. Although the sensitivity is high, the specificity of Tc-99m bone scan for osteomyelitis is poor. CT scans offer relatively high sensitivity for osteomyelitis, but they have some difficulty in defining the extent of soft-tissue infection without IV contrast. MRI holds promise, but it may have limitations in sensitivity and specificity.

It is not the purpose of this section to review this controversy but rather to develop a reasonable radiographic approach for the emergency department

physician based on current understanding of the information available. In-depth reviews of imaging techniques in osteoarticular infections are available in several references [135–137].

PLAIN FILMS
The earliest radiographic sign by plain x-ray of osteomyelitis is blurring of the fascial planes of the involved site or soft-tissue swelling, which is usually present 3 days following the onset of symptoms. The first bone change, a periosteal reaction, does not appear for at least 10 days and may take up to 8 weeks. Over time the typical osteolytic changes develop. Plain-film tomograms increase the sensitivity of detecting bone lesions.

TECHNETIUM BONE SCANS
Technetium bone scans are reasonably sensitive but often lack specificity to permit a diagnosis of osteomyelitis with overlying cellulitis. Increased radionuclide uptake may be seen as early as 24–48 hours after the onset of infection. If osteoblastic activity is delayed or vascular flow to the infected site is severely compromised, then a false-negative finding will result [138, 139].

GALLIUM SCANS
The gallium scan is a modality with little utility in infectious diseases, replaced in favor by In-111, CT, and MRI scanning. Gallium-67 citrate binds to serum proteins and leukocytes and localizes to areas of inflammation [140]. The gallium scan is dependent on sufficient inflammatory activity and vascular flow to the infected site. Small sequestered infections, as is the usual case with osteomyelitis, and infections in poorly vascularized limbs may go undetected. The specificity is adversely affected by its increased uptake in areas of increased bone turnover, such as seen in neuropathic changes, tumor, fracture, or infection [141].

INDIUM-WBC SCANS
Indium-111–labeled leukocyte scans have essentially replaced gallium scanning in infectious diseases. The fact that patients' leukocytes are labeled with indium-111 improves the specificity for infections. Used alone the sensitivity is not optimal, ranging from 37%–100% in reported series. Localization of the isotope to bone or soft tissue is often

difficult to determine. However, when used in combination with the three-phase Tc-99m bone scan, the specificity significantly improves to 90% or greater [142, 143]. False-positive results have been observed in neuropathic diabetic feet, active rheumatoid arthritis, recent noninfected bone and joint surgery, recent fractures, and patients given antibiotics within the preceding month.

CT SCANS

The sensitivity of the CT scan may approach 90% in some series [144, 145]. The definition of cortical bone and early marrow changes by exudate makes CT scanning particularly useful [146]. It has better resolution of soft-tissue abnormalities when IV contrast is used.

MRI

The sensitivity of MRI has made it a useful modality to evaluate patients for suspected osteomyelitis [147]. MRI allows different imaging variables to detect an increase in water content in the bone marrow at the site of the infection and inflammatory reaction [148]. A decrease in the normal high marrow signal on T1 weighted images and the increase in the signal on T2 weighted images are compatible with osteomyelitis. This abnormal signal, however, is not specific for only an infectious process. Neoplastic bone lesions may disturb bone marrow and be easily detected with the MRI. However, characteristic radiographic features of infection versus tumor can usually distinguish these two entities [149, 150]. Several studies suggest MRI is at least as sensitive and as specific as scintigraphic studies [151–154].

The spatial resolution of MRI and CT scans for precise localization of the infection and demonstration of contiguous infection exceeds other imaging techniques. In general soft-tissue image of MRI is better than that of a CT scan. This information may be invaluable to the surgeon for accurate localization. The best technique may vary by location, type, and duration of infection (Table 33-13). The MRI alone and the Tc-99m and In-111 scans in combination seem to have comparable sensitivity and specificity for osteomyelitis. None of these imaging techniques has specific applicability in determining when the infection has been eradicated and therapy can be discontinued. Following treatment

Table 33-13. Diagnostic imaging for osteomyelitis

Stage or type of osteomyelitis	Imaging technique[*]
Acute hematogenous to limb	BS or MRI
Vertebral	MRI or CT
Chronic contiguous	MRI or BS + IN
Chronic (relapse)	MRI + IN
Hardware associated	IN
Post-traumatic fracture	MRI + IN

[*] Plain-film x-ray indicated in each; BS (Tc-99m), MRI (magnetic resonance imaging), CT (computed tomograms), IN (indium-111).

the MRI and bone scans stay positive for several months despite evidence of clinical cure. The In-111 scan will revert to normal with clinical cure, as well as with microbiologic suppression. Relapses may occur despite a negative scan at this stage. However, a positive posttreatment In-111 scan strongly suggests persistence of infection; therefore, this scan is useful in cases of osteomyelitis in which relapse is frequent (e.g., hardware-associated infections).

Histopathology

In acute osteomyelitis the tissue consists predominantly of polymorphonuclear leukocytes. In the chronic stage microscopy will reveal a mixture of lymphocytes, plasma cells, and histocytes. Fibroblastic activity and reactive new bone also are seen. Microorganisms are seldom seen on stain because of the relatively small number of organisms present in osteomyelitis. Granulomas suggest brucellosis, mycobacteriosis, or fungal infection.

Differential Diagnosis

The differential diagnosis includes all noninfectious diseases and disorders that commonly present with musculoskeletal pain. Benign diskitis of children and Scheuermann's disease (e.g., vertebral epiphysitis) of adolescents are of unknown etiology, but they may mimic acute hematogenous vertebral osteomyelitis in these age groups. Back pain in adults may represent neoplastic processes, trauma, disk herniation, musculoskeletal strain, herpes-zoster neuralgia, osteoporosis, or metabolic bone diseases. Taken collectively these conditions are more common than the infectious etiologies. The differential diagnosis of the diabetic foot is discussed in Chap. 11.

Workup in the Emergency Department

The definitive diagnosis of osteomyelitis is not always possible in the emergency department, but if the suspicion is present certain tests should be ordered or scheduled (Table 33-14). The most useful tests are blood cultures, the ESR, and imaging studies. A tuberculin skin test or serologic studies for coccidioidomycosis, blastomycosis, histoplasmosis, and brucellosis are indicated in selected patients. All patients with suspected acute hematogenous osteomyelitis should have blood cultures. Patients presenting with a subacute or chronic course infrequently have bacteremia. However, if fever or a history of fever is noted, blood cultures should be obtained. Only 20%–25% of patients will have positive blood cultures. The ESR may be significantly abnormal (more than twice the normal rate) in 80% of patients [155]. An elevated WBC count supports an active inflammatory process but is too insensitive and nonspecific to use alone for the diagnosis of acute or chronic osteomyelitis.

All patients should have a plain-film x-ray of the suspected site of infection, even though in acute cases the plain film may not reveal any bony abnor-mality. A plain tomogram will increase the sensitivity of findings. In IV drug users the cervical spine has a propensity to be infected, and the thoracic spine is most often involved in patients with tuberculous spondylitis. The decision to proceed with other imaging studies in the emergency department should be determined by the urgency of the problem and the advice of consultants. A CT scan or MRI has real value in delineating adjacent soft-tissue abscesses that would require urgent surgical attention. Granulomatous infections as seen with mycobacteria, *Brucella* species, and fungi are likely to be complicated by paravertebral extension and abscess formation.

The definitive diagnosis requires a closed needle or open surgical bone biopsy for microbiologic and histologic stains and cultures. The open approach allows direct visualization and larger sampling. Routine culturing of exudate from sinus tracts should be discouraged. The correlation of these more superficial cultures with bone biopsy culture results is poor. The exception is in the finding of *S. aureus* alone, for which there is an approximate 90% correlation [156]. Sinus-tract culture results, however, may be useful in identifying the pathogens responsible for an active cellulitis, if present.

Therapy

Medical and surgical therapies are determined by host factors, location and extent of the infectious process, and the etiologic organism(s). Surgical débridement of dead tissue and foreign material and biopsy of infected bone are essential to the therapeutic process. Initial antimicrobial selection is directed by Gram's stain, age, and clinical and epidemiologic factors. In patients presenting with acute hematogenous infection or with systemic signs of infection or sepsis, antimicrobials should be initiated in the emergency department after blood culture specimens have been obtained. Otherwise, antibiotics should be postponed following the bone biopsy. Patients with associated cellulitis or other concomitant infection may require earlier therapy. Standard and newer antimicrobial therapies for acute and chronic bacterial osteomyelitis are provided in Table 33-15. Newer antimicrobials, particularly the oral fluoroquinolones, provide some attractive options.

Table 33-14. Osteomyelitis workup in the emergency department

General
Erythrocyte sedimentation rate
Blood culture
Cell count
Chemistry panel (renal and hepatic functions)
Plain-film x-ray

Selected (Epidemiologic or Clinical Features)
PPD
Serology (brucella, fungi)
Chest x-ray (suspected TB or vertebral infection)
Other imaging studies (MRI, CT scan)

Table 33-15. Antibiotic regimens for bacterial osteomyelitis

Organism	Drug of choice	Adult dosage	Alternatives[*]
S. aureus	Nafcillin + rifampin	8–12 g/day 600 mg/d	Vancomycin, Cefazolin; clindamycin
S. aureus (MRSA)	Vancomycin + rifampin	2 g/day 600 mg/day	
S. epidermidis	Vancomycin ± rifampin	2 g/day 600 mg/day	Tetracycline PO; TMP-SMX PO, Cefazolin
Streptococci	Penicillin	12 million–24 million U/day	Cefazolin
Group D enterococci	Ampicillin + gentamicin	8 g/day 1–3 mg/kg/day	Vancomycin, ciprofloxacin, imipenem
H. influenzae	Ampicillin	8 g/day	Ciprofloxacin, ceftriaxone, cefotaxime, ampicillin-SB
Salmonella species	Ciprofloxacin	800 mg/day IV (1–2 g/day PO)	Ceftriaxone, cefotaxime
Gram-negative bacilli	Ceftriaxone	2 g/day	Gentamicin, cefotaxime, aztreonam, ciprofloxacin, ticarcillin-CA
P. aeruginosa	Gentamicin + piperacillin	3–6 mg/kg/day 18 g/day	Tobramycin, amikacin, ceftazidime, aztreonam, mezlocillin, ciprofloxacin
Anaerobes (PCNase +)	Metronidazole	1.5 g/day	Clindamycin, ampicillin-SB, ticarcillin-CA
Mixed aerobic and anaerobic	Ciprofloxacin + ticarcillin/CA	800 mg/day IV 1–2 g/day PO 12.4 g/day	Combinations: metronidazole, ampicillin-SB, clindamycin, cefotaxime, ceftriaxone

[*] Other third-generation cephalosporins may be used interchangeably with those listed; ciprofloxacin IV or PO (may substitute ofloxacin).

All patients with acute osteomyelitis or sepsis require parenteral therapy initially. After clinical stabilization, therapy with an appropriate oral agent may be utilized in selected cases. The total course of treatment in acute hematogenous infections is 4 weeks [157]. A relapse rate of 19% of infants and children treated for fewer than 21 days was noted [158]. The length of therapy for chronic osteomyelitis has been less clearly defined. Standard regimens recommend parenteral antibiotics for 4–8 weeks, followed in some cases by oral therapy for an additional 1–3 months. If the infected bone is largely resected, then a shorter course is adequate.

Oral antibiotic therapy from the outset or following a 2-to-3-week course of parenteral treatment is becoming popular with chronic osteomyelitis as well, because of the need to treat many of these patients for 6 weeks to several months, treatment that can be more easily and economically accomplished with oral agents at home [159]. The cost savings of an 8-week course of an oral agent as an alternative to injectable antimicrobial therapy for osteomyelitis is several thousand dollars [160]. Combination drug therapy and additional procedural and material cost of IV lines add substantially to this. Fluoroquinolones show much promise in the treatment of bacterial osteomyelitis because of their broad antimicrobial activity, low minimum bactericidal concentrations, and high degree of penetration into bone tissue [161–165]. Several clinical studies have shown excellent efficacy with oral fluoroquinolones [166–171]. Emerging resistance of some strains of *S. aureus* and *P. aeruginosa* has been seen with prolonged quinolone therapy and may be a caveat for these organisms [172].

Parenteral antibiotics with prolonged half-lives have attractive pharmacokinetic properties for outpatient treatment of osteomyelitis. Ceftriaxone in a single daily IV dose provides good serum and bone levels 12 and 24 hours after a 2-g dose [173]. Teicoplanin, a new glycopeptide antibiotic in the same class as vancomycin and yet to be approved in the United States, has favorable pharmacokinetics to permit single daily dosing [174].

Carefully selected oral therapies should be as successful as parenteral therapies except possibly in patients with diabetes mellitus or severe peripheral vascular diseases. In those cases all therapies to date have been disappointing, with a 1-year follow-up success rate of 66% or less [175].

The chemotherapy of skeletal tuberculosis is like pulmonary tuberculosis. The preferred drugs for initial therapy are isoniazid, rifampin, pyrazinamide, ethambutol HCl, and streptomycin sulfate (see Table 33-11). Second-line drugs may be required for patients intolerant of primary drug therapy, resistant organisms, and treatment failures.

Fungal or brucella bone infections are treated like joint infections.

Antibiotic Prophylaxis in Open Fractures

Osteomyelitis, as well as wound infections, frequently complicates open bone fractures [176]. Infection is the primary cause of nonunion in this situation [177]. The risk of infection directly correlates with the severity of the associated soft-tissue injury. Open fractures are graded (grades I–III) based on the degree of soft-tissue damage (Table 33-16). The reported risks of wound infection range from 0%–9% for grade I fractures, 1%–12% for grade II fractures, and 9%–55% for grade III fractures [178, 179]. Furthermore, severe grade IIIB fractures with associated vascular or extensive soft-tissue damage interfering with soft-tissue coverage of the fracture site have an infection rate 3–10

Table 33-16. Gustilo's grading system for open fractures

Grade I	Skin wound <1 cm; soft-tissue damage absent or minimal
Grade II	Large wounds; soft-tissue damage present
Grade IIIA	Open segmental fractures; soft-tissue damage extensive
Grade IIIB	Neurologic or vascular repair required

times higher than the less severe grade IIIA fractures [180, 181]. Such high infection rates should prompt the physician to consider the appropriateness of wound cultures, early wound débridement, and postcontamination, preinfection antibiotic administration in the emergency department.

Routine cultures of fracture wounds in animal studies and in a few clinical studies of humans show poor correlation in the initial culture results and subsequent cultures of established infections. Further studies are needed to better answer this issue, but it does seem irrelevant at this time to obtain preinfection open-fracture wound cultures in the emergency department. *S. aureus* is the most common pathogen to be involved in open-fracture infections. Streptococci and gram-negative rods are also seen in the more heavily contaminated and severe wounds. In soil-contaminant injuries, *Clostridium perfringens* and *Clostridium tetani* should be considered. The correlation of elapsed time from injury to débridement with the infection risk is still uncertain. Two studies have failed to show a significant reduction in the rate of infection with early (e.g., less than 3 hours) versus late initial débridement [182, 183]. Other studies describe a decisive period during which the wound infection rate can be diminished [184, 185]. In the presence of foreign material in an experimental model, a 6-hour lapse between bacterial inoculation and initiation of antibiotics led to failure to prevent infection [186]. Early postinjury preinfection antibiotic administration for all open fractures is recommended based on a review of controlled trials [187, 188]. Studies support the use of an agent (e.g., cefazolin) active against *S. aureus* and nonenterococcal streptococci species. More broad-spectrum regimens have not shown superiority [189–191]. Gram-negative bacilli are frequently recovered from grade III fractures, which has prompted many orthopedic surgeons to add an aminoglycoside or other agent to the cefazolin in those situations.

The duration of antibiotic treatment for non-established infections is uncertain, but studies comparing 6 hours to 5 days or longer have failed to show a correlation with the risk of infection. Rather than the need for prolonged therapy, the achievement of a high antibiotic level in the tissue early in the course of bacterial contamination may be most important in preventing an infection. A high dose (e.g., cefazolin 2 g IV) and a short duration of 24–48 hours administration are reasonable for grade I and II injuries and cefazolin plus gentamicin 3–5 mg/kg/day for grade III. If infection becomes apparent, specific therapy for the infecting organism(s) then should be instituted. For more information on antibiotic prophylaxis in orthopedic trauma and surgery the reader is referred to two excellent reviews, one by Norden, the other by Dellinger [192, 193].

Prognosis

Before the use of antibiotics acute hematogenous osteomyelitis had a mortality rate of approximately 20% and a 50% rate of complications [194–196]. The cure rate now exceeds 90%. Chronic osteomyelitis is well known for its high rate of recurrence. It is uncertain if delay in early treatment is an important factor in failure. Other factors probably correlate better with efficacy. Susceptible organism(s), adequate antimicrobial tissue (e.g., bone) levels, prolonged course of therapy, thorough surgical débridement, and absence of significant systemic or local immune or vascular host problems probably have a positive influence on outcome. The importance of such factors is currently under investigation and debate. A rare complication of chronic osteomyelitis is the development after 20–40 years of squamous cell carcinoma in a chronic draining sinus tract. This occurs in 1% of those patients with chronic disease. The nephrotic syndrome by membranoproliferative glomerulonephritis has been reported in association with chronic osteomyelitis [197]. Finally amyloidosis is now rarely seen as a complication.

References

1. Bhawan J. Ultrastructure of synovial membrane in pyogenic arthritis. Arch Pathol 96:155, 1973.
2. Karten I. Septic arthritis complicating rheumatoid arthritis. Ann Intern Med 70:1147, 1969.
3. Mowat AG, Baum J. Chemotaxis of polymorphonuclear leukocytes from patients with rheumatoid arthritis. J Clin Invest 50:2541, 1971.
4. Pruzanski W et al. Bacterial activity of sera and synovial fluid in rheumatoid arthritis and in osteoarthritis. Arthritis Rheum 17:207, 1974.
5. Mitchel WS et al. Septic arthritis in patients with rheumatoid disease: a still underdiagnosed complication. J Rheumatol 3:124, 1976.
6. Alderson M et al. Acute haematogenous osteomyelitis and septic arthritis-single disease. J Bone Joint Surg 68B:268, 1986.
7. Tesar JT, Dietz F. Mechanisms of inflammation infectious arthritis. Clin Rheum Dis 4:51, 1978.
8. Wilson NIL, DiPaola M. Acute septic arthritis in infancy and childhood. J Bone Joint Surg 68B:584, 1986.
9. Cooper C, Cawley MID. Bacterial arthritis in an English health district: a 10 year review. Ann Rheum Dis 45:458, 1986.
10. Goldenberg DL, Reed JI. Bacterial arthritis. N Engl J Med 312:764, 1985.
11. Kelly PJ, Martin WJ, Coventry MB. Bacterial (suppurative) arthritis in the adult. J Bone Joint Surg 52A:1595, 1970.
12. Goldenberg DL, Cohen AS. Acute infectious arthritis. Am J Med 60:369, 1976.
13. Goldenberg DL, Reed JI. Bacterial arthritis. N Engl J Med 312:764, 1985.
14. O'Brien JP, Goldenberg DL, Rice PA. Disseminated gonococcal infection: a prospective analysis of 49 patients and a review of pathophysiology and immune mechanisms. Medicine 62:395, 1983.
15. Newman ED, Davis DE, Harrington TM. Septic arthritis due to gram negative bacilli: older patients with good outcome. J Rheum 15:659, 1988.
16. Fitzgerald RH et al. Anaerobic septic arthritis. Clin Orthop 164:141, 1982.
17. Schmidli J et al. Cultivation of Borrelia burgdorferi from joint fluid three months after treatment of facial palsy due to Lyme borreliosis. J Infect Dis 158:905, 1988.
18. Smith JW, Sanford JP. Viral arthritis. Ann Intern Med 67:651, 1967.
19. Reid DM et al. Human parvovirus-associated arthritis: a clinical and laboratory description. Lancet 1:422, 1985.

20. Sutker WL, Lankford LL, Tompsett R. Granulomatous synovitis: the role of atypical mycobacteria. *Rev Infect Dis* 1:729, 1979.

21. Pouchot J et al. Tuberculosis of the sacroiliac joint: clinical features, outcome, and evaluation of closed needle biopsy in 11 consecutive cases. *Am J Med* 84:622, 1988.

22. Bayer AS, Scott VJ, and Guze LB. Fungal arthritis. III. Sporotrichal arthritis. *Semin Arthritis Rheum* 9:66, 1979.

23. Sharp JT et al. Infectious arthritis. *Arch Intern Med* 139:1125, 1979.

24. Goldenberg DL, Cohen AS. Acute infectious arthritis: a review of patients with non-gonococcal joint infections (with emphasis on therapy and prognosis). *Am J Med* 60:369, 1976.

25. Smith JW. Infectious arthritis. In GL Mandell, RG Douglas Jr, JE Bennett (eds.), *Principles and Practice of Infectious Diseases* (3rd ed.). New York: Churchill-Livingstone, 1990. P. 913.

26. Rosenthal J, Bole GG, Robinson WD. Acute non-gonococcal infectious arthritis. *Arthritis Rheum* 23:889, 1980.

27. Smith JW. Infectious arthritis. In GL Mandell, RG Douglas Jr, JE Bennett (eds.), *Principles and Practice of Infectious Diseases* (3rd ed.). New York: Churchill-Livingstone, 1990. P. 912.

28. Ho G, Su EY. Therapy for septic arthritis. *JAMA* 247:797, 1982.

29. Sharp JT et al. Infectious arthritis. *Arch Intern Med* 139:1125, 1979.

30. Sharp JT et al. Infectious arthritis. *Arch Intern Med* 139:1125, 1979.

31. Kelly PJ. Bacterial arthritis in the adult. *Orthop Clin North Am* 6:973, 1975.

32. Rosenthal J et al. Acute non-gonococcal infectious arthritis. Evaluation of risk factors, therapy and outcome. *Arthritis Rheum* 23:889, 1980.

33. McCracken GH. Septic arthritis in a neonate. *Hosp Pract* 14:158, 1979.

34. Hallow M, Chung SM, Plotkin SA. *Haemophilus influenzae* septic arthritis in infants and children. *Clin Pediatr* 14:1146, 1975.

35. Nelson JD. The bacterial etiology and antibiotic management of septic arthritis in infants and children. *Pediatrics* 50:437, 1972.

36. Rosenthal J et al. Acute nongonococcal infectious arthritis. Evaluation of risk factors, therapy and outcome. *Arthritis Rheum* 23:889, 1980.

37. Goldenberg DL, Cohen AS. Acute infectious arthritis. A review of patients with non-gonococcal joint infections (with emphasis on therapy and prognosis). *Am J Med* 60:369, 1976.

38. Goldenberg DL, Reed JI. Bacterial arthritis. *N Engl J Med* 312:764, 1985.

39. Bayer AS et al. Gram-negative bacillary septic arthritis: clinical, radiologic, therapeutic, and prognostic features. *Semin Arthritis Rheum* 7:123, 1977.

40. Goldin RH et al. Sternoarticular septic arthritis in heroin users. *N Engl J Med* 289:616, 1973.

41. Ross G, Baraff LJ, Quismorio FP. Serratia arthritis in heroin users. *J Bone Joint Surg* 57A:1158, 1975.

42. Ann-Fonte GZ, Rozboril MB, Thompson GR. Changes in nongonococcal septic arthritis: drug abuse and methicillin-resistant *Staphylococcus aureus*. *Arthritis Rheum* 28:210, 1985.

43. Andrews H, Arden G, Hart G. Deep infection after total hip replacement. *J Bone Joint Surg* 63B:53, 1981.

44. Fitzgerald RH. Problems associated with the infected total hip arthroplasty. *Clin Rheum Dis* 12:537, 1986.

45. Fitzgerald R, Jones D. Hip implant infection: treatment with resection arthroplasty and late total hip arthroplasty. *Am J Med* 78:225, 1985.

46. Surin V, Sundholm K, Backman L. Infection after total hip replacement. *J Bone Joint Surg* 65B:412, 1983.

47. Lambertus M, Thordarson D, Goetz MB. Fungal prosthetic arthritis: presentation of two cases and review of the literature. *Rev Infect Dis* 10:1038, 1988.

48. Fitzgerald RH Jr. The infected total hip arthroplasty: current concepts of treatment. *Hip* :347, 1984.

49. Ebong WW. The treatment of severely ill patients with sickle cell anemia and associated septic arthritis. *Clin Orthop* 149:145, 1980.

50. Syrogiannopoulos GA, McCracken GH, Nelson JD. Osteoarticular infections in children with sickle cell disease. *Pediatrics* 78:1090, 1986.

51. Vyskocil JJ et al. Pyogenic infection of the sacroiliac joint: case reports and review of the literature. *Medicine* 70:188, 1991.

52. Gordon G, Kabins SA. Pyogenic sacroiliitis. *Am J Med* 69:50, 1980.

53. Iczkovitz JM et al. Pyogenic sacroiliitis. *J Rheum* 8:157, 1981.

54. Schaad VB et al. Pyogenic arthritis of the sacroiliac joint in pediatric patients. *Pediatrics* 66:375, 1975.

55. Gordon G, Kabins SA. Pyogenic sacroiliitis. *Am J Med* 69:50, 1980.

56. Berney S, Goldstein M, Bishko F. Clinical and diagnostic features of tuberculous arthritis. *Am J Med* 53:36, 1972.

57. Alvarez S, McCabe WR. Extrapulmonary tuber-

culosis revisited: a review of experience at Boston city and other hospitals. *Medicine* 63:25, 1984.

58. Mahowald ML, Messner RP. Chronic infective arthritis. In D Schlossberg (ed.), *Orthopedic Infection: Clinical Topics in Infectious Disease*. New York: Springer-Verlag, 1988. Pp. 77–82.

59. Bayer AS, Guze LB. Fungal arthritis I. Candida arthritis: diagnostic and prognostic implications and therapeutic considerations. *Semin Arthritis Rheum* 8:142, 1978.

60. Katzenstein D. Isolated candida arthritis: report of a case and definition of a distinct clinical syndrome. *Arthritis Rheum* 28:1421, 1985.

61. Goodman JS et al. Fungal infection of prosthetic joints: report of two cases. *J Rheumatol* 10:494, 1983.

62. Dupont B, Drouhet E. Cutaneous, ocular, and osteoarticular candidiasis in heroin addicts: new clinical and therapeutic aspects in 38 patients. *J Infect Dis* 152:577, 1985.

63. Bayer AS, Guze LB. Fungal arthritis II. Coccidioidal synovitis. *Semin Arthritis Rheum* 8:200, 1979.

64. Bayer AS, Guze LB. Fungal arthritis III. Sporotrichal arthritis. *Semin Arthritis Rheum* 9:66, 1979.

65. Brook CJ, Ravikrishnan KP, Weg JG. Primary pulmonary and articular sporotrichosis. *Am Rev Respir Dis* 116:141, 1977.

66. Yao J, Penn RG, Ray S. Articular sporotrichosis. *Clin Orthop Rel Res* 204:207, 1986.

67. Gullberg RM et al. Sporotrichosis. Recurrent cutaneous, articular and CNS infection in a renal transplant patient. *Rev Infect Dis* 9:369, 1987.

68. Steere AC, Schoen RT, Taylor E. The clinical evolution of Lyme arthritis. *Ann Intern Med* 107:725, 1987.

69. Dattwyler RJ et al. Seronegative Lyme disease. Dissociation of specific T- and B-lymphocyte response to *Borrelia burgdorferi*. *N Engl J Med* 319:1441, 1988.

70. Sharp JT et al. Infectious arthritis. *Arch Intern Med* 139:1125, 1979.

71. Ward JR, Atcheson SG. Infectious arthritis. *Med Clin North Am* 61:313, 1977.

72. Namey TC, Halla JT. Radiographic and nucleographic techniques in the diagnosis of septic arthritis and osteomyelitis. *Clin Rheum Dis* 4:95, 1978.

73. Lisbona R, Rosenthal L. Observations on the sequential use of 99m Tc-phosphate complex and 67-Ga imaging in osteomyelitis, cellulitis and septic arthritis. *Radiology* 123:123, 1977.

74. Beltran J. Septic arthritis and tenosynovitis. In J Beltran, (ed.). *MRI: Musculoskeletal System*. Philadelphia: Lippincott, 1990. Pp. 10–11.

75. Ran RG, Ramsey KH, Hough AJ. Antibody-mediated modulation of arthritis induced by chlamydia. *Am J Pathol* 132:373, 1988.

76. Spra TJ, Kabins SA. Yersinia enterocolitica septicemia. *Arch Intern Med* 136:1305, 1976.

77. Brewerton DA et al. Ankylosing spondylitis and HL-A27. *Lancet* 1:904, 1973.

78. Aho K et al. Reactive arthritis. *Clin Rheum Dis* 11:25, 1985.

79. Parker RH, Schmid FR. Antibacterial activity of synovial fluid during treatment of septic arthritis. *Arthritis Rheum* 14:96, 1971.

80. Greenberg RN et al. Treatment of bone, joint, and soft-tissue infections with oral ciprofloxacin. *Antimicrob Agents Chemother* 31:151, 1987.

81. Black J et al. Oral antimicrobial therapy for adults with osteomyelitis or septic arthritis. *J Infect Dis* 155:968, 1987.

82. Waldvogel FA. Use of quinolones for the treatment of osteomyelitis and septic arthritis. *Rev Infect Dis* 11(suppl. 5):S1259, 1989.

83. Bayer AS, Norman D, Anderson D. Efficacy of ciprofloxacin in experimental arthritis caused by *Escherichia coli*—in vitro-in vivo correlations. *J Infect Dis* 152:811, 1985.

84. Peyramond D et al. Treatment of bacterial osteoarthritis with ofloxacin. *Rev Infect Dis* 10(suppl. 1):S187, 1988.

85. Bayer AS, Norman DC, Blumquist IK. Comparative efficacy of ciprofloxacin and ceftriaxone in experimental arthritis by *Escherichia coli*. *Rev Infect Dis* 10(suppl. 1):S184, 1988.

86. Perry CR. Administration of local antibiotics via an implantable pump in the treatment of orthopaedic infections. Abstract in Management of Non-unions and Orthopaedic Infections. At St. Louis, August 3–4, 1990.

87. Horsburgh CR, Cannady PB, Kirkpatrick CH. Treatment of fungal infections in the bones and joints with ketoconazole. *J Infect Dis* 147:1064, 1983.

88. Ivey M, Clark R. Arthroscopic débridement of the knee for septic arthritis. *Clin Orthop* 199:201, 1985.

89. Broy SB, Schmid FR. A comparison of medical drainage (needle aspiration) and surgical drainage (arthrotomy or arthroscopy) in the initial treatment of infected joints. *Clin Rheum Dis* 12:501, 1986.

90. Bynum DK et al. Pyogenic arthritis: emphasis on the need for surgical drainage of the infected joint. *South Med J* 75:1232, 1975.

91. Ward JR, Atcheson SG. Infectious arthritis. *Med Clin North Am* 61:313, 1977.

92. Howard JG, Highgenboten CL, Nelson JD. Residual effects of septic arthritis in infancy and childhood. *JAMA* 236:932, 1976.

93. Sharp JT et al. Infectious arthritis. *Arch Intern Med* 139:1125, 1979.

94. Lidwell OM. Air, antibiotics, and sepsis in replacement joints. *J Hosp Infect* 11(suppl. C):18, 1988.

95. Espersen F et al. Changing pattern of bone and joint infections due to *Staphylococcus aureus*: study of cases of bacteremia in Denmark, 1959–1988. *Rev Infect Dis* 13:347, 1991.

96. Kahn DS, Pritzker KPH. The pathophysiology of bone infection. *Clin Orthop* 96:12, 1973.

97. Gristina AG, Barth E, Webb LX. Microbes, metals, and other nonbiological substrata in man: substratum and substrate factors in infection. In RB Gustilo (ed.), *Orthopaedic Infection: Diagnosis and Treatment*. Philadelphia: Saunders, 1989. P. 26.

98. Gristina AG. Biomaterial-centered infection: microbial adhesion versus tissue integration. *Science* 237:1588, 1987.

99. Gristina AG, Barth E, Webb LX. Microbial adhesion and the pathogenesis of biomaterial-centered infections. In RB Gustilo (ed.), *Orthopaedic Infection: Diagnosis and Treatment*. Philadelphia: Saunders, 1989. P. 1.

100. Gillespie WJ, Nade S. Epidemiology. In WJ Gillespie, S Nade (eds.), *Musculoskeletal Infections*. New York: Blackwell, 1987. P. 33.

101. Vaughan PA, Newman NM, Rosman MA. Acute hematogenous osteomyelitis in children. *J Pediatr Orthop* 7:652, 1987.

102. LaMont RL et al. Acute hematogenous osteomyelitis in children. *J Pediatr Orthop* 7:579, 1987.

103. Nelson JD. Acute osteomyelitis in children. *Infect Dis Clin North Am* 4:513, 1990.

104. La Mont RL et al. Acute hematogenous osteomyelitis in children. *J Pediatr Orthop* 7:579, 1987.

105. Nade S. Acute haematogenous osteomyelitis in infancy and childhood. *J Bone Joint Surg* 65B:109, 1983.

106. Espersen F et al. Changing pattern of bone and joint infections due to *Staphylococcus aureus*: study of cases of bacteremia in Denmark, 1959–1988. *Rev Infect Dis* 13:347, 1991.

107. Chandrasekar PH, Narula AP. Bone and joint infections in intravenous drug abusers. *Rev Infect Dis* 8:904, 1986.

108. Sapico FL, Montgomerie JZ. Vertebral osteomyelitis in intravenous drug abusers: report of three cases and review of the literature. *Rev Infect Dis* 2:196, 1980.

109. Crossan ET. Haematogenous osteomyelitis. Collective review of the literature from 1932–1937. *Int Abst Surg* 66:176, 1938.

110. Syrogiannopoulos GA, Nelson JD. Duration of antimicrobial therapy for acute suppurative osteoarticular infections. *Lancet* 1:37, 1988.

111. Gillespie WJ, Mayo KM. The management of acute haematogenous osteomyelitis in the antibiotic era: a study of the outcome. *J Bone Joint Surg* 63B:126, 1981.

112. Gillespie WJ, Mayo KM. The management of acute haematogenous osteomyelitis in the antibiotic era: a study of outcome. *J Bone Joint Surg* 63B:126, 1981.

113. Davidson P, Horowitz I. Skeletal tuberculosis. *Am J Med* 48:77, 1970.

114. Wiley AM, Trueta J. The vascular anatomy of the spine and its relationship to pyogenic vertebral osteomyelitis. *J Bone Joint Surg* 41B:796, 1959.

115. Spiegel PG et al. Intervertebral disc-space inflammation in children. *J Bone Joint Surg* 54A:284, 1972.

116. Wenger DR, Bobechko WP, Gilday DZ. The spectrum of intervertebral disc space infection in children. *J Bone Joint Surg* 60A:100, 1978.

117. Waldvogel FA, Vasey H. Osteomyelitis: the past decade. *N Engl J Med* 303:360, 1980.

118. Sapico FL, Montgomerie JZ. Pyogenic vertebral osteomyelitis: report of nine cases and review of the literature. *Rev Infect Dis* 1:754, 1979.

119. Gristina AG. Biomaterial-centered infection: microbial adhesion versus tissue integration. *Science* 237:1588, 1987.

120. Nelson JD. Acute osteomyelitis in children. *Infect Dis Clin North Am* 4:513, 1990.

121. Sapico FL, Montgomerie JZ. Pyogenic vertebral osteomyelitis: report of nine cases and review of the literature. *Rev Infect Dis* 1:754, 1979.

122. Sapico FL, Montgomerie JZ. Vertebral osteomyelitis in intravenous drug abusers: report of three cases and review of the literature. *Rev Infect Dis* 2:196, 1980.

123. Gentry LO. Approach to the patient with chronic osteomyelitis. *Curr Clin Top Infect Dis* 8:62, 1987.

124. Thibodeau AA. Closed space infection following removal of lumbar intervertebral disc. *Clin Neurosurg* 14:337, 1966.

125. Fernand R, Lee CK. Postlaminectomy disc space infection. *Clin Orthop* (209):215, 1986.

126. Weissberg ED, Smith AL, Smith DH. Clinical features of neonatal osteomyelitis. *Pediatrics* 53:505, 1974.

127. Ross PM, Fleming JL. Vertebral body osteomyelitis: spectrum and natural history. *Clin Orthop* 118:190, 1976.

128. Musher DM et al. Vertebral osteomyelitis still a diagnostic pitfall. *Arch Intern Med* 136:105, 1976.

129. Waldvogel FA, Medoff G, Swartz MN. Osteomyelitis: a review of clinical features, therapeutic considerations and unusual aspects. *N Engl J Med* 282:198, 260, 316, 1970.

130. Abbey DM, Hosea SW. Diagnosis of vertebral osteomyelitis in a community hospital by using computed tomography. *Arch Intern Med* 149:2029, 1989.

131. Abbey DM, Hosea SW. Diagnosis of vertebral osteomyelitis in a community hospital by using computed tomography. *Arch Intern Med* 149:2029, 1989.

132. Stone DB, Bonfiglio M. Pyogenic vertebral osteomyelitis: a diagnostic pitfall for the internist. *Arch Intern Med* 112:491, 1963.

133. Rocco HD, Eyring EJ. Intervertebral disc infection in children. *AJDC* 123:448, 1972.

134. Silao JV et al. Profile of Pott's disease in PGH. *Acta Med Phil* 15A:4, 1980.

135. Murphy WA et al. Musculoskeletal system. In JKT Lee, SS Sagel, RJ Stanley (eds.), *Computed Body Tomography with MRI Correlation* (2nd ed.). New York: Raven, 1989.

136. Alazraki N. Radionuclide techniques. In D Resnick, G Niwayama (eds.), *Diagnosis of Bone and Joint Disorders* (2nd ed.). Philadelphia: Saunders, 1988.

137. Beltran J. *MRI Musculoskeletal System.* Philadelphia: Lippincott, 1990.

138. Teates CD, Williamson BRS. Hot and cold bone lesions in acute osteomyelitis. *AJR* 129:517, 1977.

139. Bonakdarpour A, Gains VD. The radiology of osteomyelitis. *Orthop Clin North Am* 14:21, 1983.

140. Hoffer P. Gallium mechanisms. *J Nucl Med* 21:282, 1980.

141. Glynn TP. Marked gallium accumulation in neuropathic arthopathy. *J Nucl Med* 22:1016, 1981.

142. Schauwecker DS et al. Combined bone scintigraphy and indium-111 leukocyte scans in neuropathic foot disease. *J Nucl Med* 29:1651, 1988.

143. Giamarellou H et al. Evaluation of Tc-MDP, Ga-Citrate and In-Chloride imaging in patients with confirmed chronic osteomyelitis. Interscience Congress on Antimicrobial Agents and Chemotherapy (ICAAC), Chicago, IL, 1991. Abstract in press.

144. Abbey DM, Hosea SW. Diagnosis of vertebral osteomyelitis in a community hospital by using computed tomography. *Arch Intern Med* 149:2029, 1989.

145. Kattapuram SV, Rosenthal DI. CT infections of the spine. *Curr Clin Topics Infect Dis* 7:311, 1986.

146. Wing VS et al. Chronic osteomyelitis examined by CT. *Radiology* 154:171, 1985.

147. Totty WG. Radiographic evaluation of osteomyelitis using magnetic resonance imaging. *Ortho Rev* 18:587, 1989.

148. Jacobson HG. Musculoskeletal applications of magnetic resonance imaging. *JAMA* 262:2420, 1989.

149. Porter BA. Low field, STIR advance MRI in clinical oncology. *Diagn Imag* 11:222, 1988.

150. Modic MT et al. Vertebral osteomyelitis: assessment using MR. *Radiology* 157:157, 1985.

151. Unger E et al. Diagnosis of osteomyelitis by MR imaging. *AJR* 150:605, 1988.

152. Beltran J et al. Experimental infections of the musculoskeletal system: evaluation with MR imaging and TC-99m MDP and Ga-67 scintigraphy. *Radiology* 167:167, 1988.

153. Meyers SP, Wiener SN. Diagnosis of hematogenous pyogenic vertebral osteomyelitis by magnetic resonance imaging. *Arch Intern Med* 151:683, 1991.

154. Quenzer R et al. Comparison of low-field MR imaging, bone scanning, and indium-labeled white blood cell scanning in diagnosis of osteomyelitis. Interscience Congress on Antimicrobial Agents and Chemotherapy (ICAAC), Chicago, IL, 1991. Abstract in press.

155. Abbey DM, Hosea SW. Diagnosis of vertebral osteomyelitis in a community hospital by using computed tomography. *Arch Intern Med* 149:2029, 1989.

156. Mackowiack PA, Jones SR, Smith JW. Diagnostic value of sinus-tract cultures in chronic osteomyelitis. *JAMA* 239:2772, 1978.

157. Waldvogel FA, Medoff G, Swartz MN. Osteomyelitis: a review of clinical features, therapeutic considerations, and unusual aspect. *N Engl J Med* 282:198, 260, 316, 1970.

158. Dich V, Nelson J, Haltalin K. Osteomyelitis in infants and children. *AJDC* 129:1273, 1975.

159. Gentry LO. Outpatient management of osteomyelitis in a DRG era. In GA Pankey (ed.), *Outpatient Antimicrobial Therapy.* Clifton, NJ: Oxford Health Care, 1989. P. 81.

160. Powers T, Bingham DH. Clinical and economic effect of ciprofloxacin as an alternative to injectable antimicrobial therapy. *Am J Hosp Pharm* 47:1781, 1990.

161. Parry MF, Panzer KB, Yukna ME. Quinolone resistance: susceptibility data from a 300-bed community hospital. *Am J Med* 87(5A):12S, 1989.

162. Wolfson JS, Hooper DC. The fluoroquinolones: structures, mechanisms of action and resistance, and spectra of activity in vitro. *Antimicrob Agents Chemother* 28:581, 1985.

163. Wise R, Donovan IA. Tissue penetration and metabolism of ciprofloxacin. *Am J Med* 82:103, 1987.

164. Schmidt HGK et al. Penetration of fleroxacin into bone and synovial fluid after administration of a single oral dose. *Rev Infect Dis* 11(S5):S1268, 1989.

165. Gerding DN, Hitt JA. Tissue penetration of the new quinolones in humans. *Rev Infect Dis* 11 (S5):S1046, 1989.

166. Etesse H, Dellamonica P, Lucht F. Treatment of bacterial osteomyelitis with ofloxacin. *Rev Infect Dis* 11(S5):S1269, 1989.

167. Gentry LO, Rodriguez GG. Oral ciprofloxacin compared with parenteral antibiotics in the treatment of osteomyelitis. *Antmicrob Agents Chemother* 34:40, 1990.

168. Waldvogel FA. Use of quinolones for the treatment of osteomyelitis and septic arthritis. *Rev Infect Dis* 11(S5):S1259, 1989.

169. Snydman DR et al. Randomized comparative trial of ciprofloxacin for treatment of patients with osteomyelitis. *Rev Infect Dis* 11(S5):S1271, 1989.

170. Gentry LO, Rodriguez-Gomez G. Ofloxacin versus parenteral therapy for chronic osteomyelitis. *Antimicrob Agents Chemother* 35:538, 1991.

171. Wispelwey B, Scheld WM. Ciprofloxacin in the treatment of *Staphylococcus aureus* osteomyelitis. A review. *Diag Microbiol Infect Dis* 13:169, 1990.

172. Parry MF, Panzer KB, Yukna ME. Quinolone resistance. *Am J Med* 87(S5A):12S, 1989.

173. Patel IH, Kaplan SA. Pharmacokinetic profile of ceftriaxone in man. *Am J Med* 77(S4C):17, 1984.

174. LeFrock JL et al. Teicoplanin in the treatment of acute bone and joint infections. In *Proceedings of the 17th International Congress of Chemotherapy*. Berlin, 1991. In press.

175. Peterson LR et al. Therapy of lower extremity infections with ciprofloxacin in patients with diabetes mellitus, peripheral vascular disease, or both. *Am J Med* 86:801, 1989.

176. Roth AI, Fry DE, Polk HJ Jr. Infectious morbidity in extremity fractures. *J Trauma* 28:757, 1986.

177. Dellinger EP et al. Risk of infection after open fracture of the arm or leg. *Arch Surg* 123:1320, 1988.

178. Dellinger EP. Antibiotic prophylaxis in trauma: penetrating abdominal injuries and open fractures. *Rev Infect Dis* 13(S10):S847, 1991.

179. Clansey BJ, Hansen ST. Open fractures of the tibia: a review of 102 cases. *J Bone Joint Surg* 60A:118, 1978.

180. Dellinger EP. Antibiotic prophylaxis in trauma: penetrating abdominal injuries and open fractures. *Rev Infect Dis* 13(S10):S847, 1991.

181. Gustilo RB, Mendoza RM, Williams DN. Problems in the management of type III (severe) open fractures: a new classification of type III open fractures. *J Trauma* 24:742, 1984.

182. Patzakis MJ, Wilkins J. Factors influencing infection rate in open fracture wounds. *Clin Orthop* 243:36, 1989.

183. Dellinger EP, Miller SD, Wertz MJ et al. Risk of infection after open fracture of the arm or leg. *Arch Surg* 123:1320, 1988.

184. Miles AA. Nonspecific defense reactions in bacterial infections. *Ann NY Acad Sci* 66:356, 1956.

185. Waldvogel FA et al. Perioperative antibiotic prophylaxis of wound and foreign body infections: microbial factors affecting efficacy. *Rev Infect Dis* 13(S10):S782, 1991.

186. Waldvogel FA et al. Perioperative antibiotic prophylaxis of wound and foreign body infections: microbial factors affecting efficacy. *Rev Infect Dis* 13(S10):S782, 1991.

187. Dellinger EP. Antibiotic prophylaxis in trauma: penetrating abdominal injuries and open fractures. *Rev Infect Dis* 13(S10):S847, 1991.

188. Tscherne H, Oestern HJ, Sturm J. Osteosynthesis of major fractures in polytrauma. *World J Surg* 7:80, 1983.

189. Dellinger EP et al. Duration of preventive antibiotic administration for open extremity fractures. *Arch Surg* 123:333, 1988.

190. Braun R, Enzler MA, Rittman WW. A double-blind clinical trial of prophylactic cloxacillin in open fractures. *J Orthop Trauma* 1:12, 1987.

191. Benson DR et al. Treatment of open fractures: a prospective study. *J Trauma* 23:25, 1983.

192. Norden CW. Antibiotic prophylaxis in orthopedic surgery. *Rev Infect Dis* 13(S10):S842, 1991.

193. Dellinger EP. Antibiotic prophylaxis in trauma: penetrating abdominal injuries and open fractures. *Rev Infect Dis* 13(S10):S847, 1991.

194. Espersen F et al. Changing pattern of bone and joint infections due to *Staphylococcus aureus*: study of cases of bacteremia in Denmark, 1959–1988. *Rev Infect Dis* 13:347, 1991.

195. Dickson FD. The clinical diagnosis, prognosis and treatment of acute hematogenous osteomyelitis. *JAMA* 127:212, 1945.

196. Trueta J, Morgan JD. Late results in the treatment of one hundred cases of acute haematogenous osteomyelitis. *Br J Surg* 41:449, 1954.

197. Boonshaft B, Maher J, Schreiner G. Nephrotic syndrome associated with osteomyelitis without secondary amyloidosis. *Arch Intern Med* 125:322, 1970.

THE HEAD AND NECK

34

Ear and Sinus Infections

FRED S. HERZON

Acute infectious diseases of the ear and the sinuses are frequently seen in an emergency department or urgent care center. The majority of patients with these complaints have uncomplicated infectious problems that will resolve with relatively straightforward treatment. It must be noted that all patients with an earache and a draining ear do not have acute infectious otitis media nor do those who have headache and a runny nose necessarily have a bacterial infection in their sinuses. This chapter uses classic acute infectious otitis media and sinusitis as the basic clinical disease process to which others are compared and contrasted. This will provide the foundation from which the more complicated aspects of the infectious diseases of these organ systems may be recognized and treated. Table 34-1 is a summary of the entities discussed in this chapter.

Ear Infections

Infectious Otologic Clinical Syndromes

EAR PAIN

Pain secondary to primary infections of the auricle, external canal, and middle ear is usually so severe that it frequently will be the chief complaint mo-tivating a patient to seek medical care in an emergency setting. Examination of the ear usually will reveal the infectious problem causing the pain. These primary infections are discussed later in this chapter.

Lesions of the tonsil, the base of tongue, the epiglotis, and the temporal mandibular joint commonly present as otalgia (Fig. 34-1). Infections in these areas rarely have ear pain as their sole presenting symptom but may have it as an associated complaint, which can lead to some confusion in the diagnosis. Adult epiglottitis with its normal oral pharyngeal examination is a prime example.

HEARING LOSS AND VERTIGO

Conductive hearing loss is a common complaint and finding in infectious otologic pathology presenting to an emergency department. Infections of the ear affect hearing through swelling and transudation of either the external canal or the middle ear space. It can be diagnosed using at least a 256-Hz, preferably a 512-Hz, fork to perform a Weber's test (placing the vibrating fork in the middle of the forehead). The patient will hear the fork best on the side of the conductive hearing loss. The Rinne test (comparing bone to air by placing the vibrating fork on the mastoid and then presenting the tines ap-

Table 34-1. Acute infections with ear pain or sinusitis

Infection	Signs and symptoms	Antibiotic	Dosage	Comment
Cellulitis/ perichondritis	Erythema, swelling, exposed cartilage	Dicloxacillin, erythromycin, cefaclor	PO for 10 days 250–500 mg q8h PO for 10 days	External drainage or pus, follow-up 24–48 hrs., IV antibiotics if no improvement
Acute otitis externa (bacterial)	Moisture-associated, erythema external canal, possible swelling and pus, pain on pinna traction	Broad-spectrum ototopical otic drops (cortisporin otic suspension)	2 gtts tid for 5–7 days	Use wick if canal is swollen shut
Fungal otitis externa	Less painful than bacterial otitis externa	Clotrimazole or n-cresyl acetate		Hyphae seen in canal
Malignant otitis externa	Immunocompromised, 3/5 signs (see text)	Ticarcillin or piperacillin + tobramycin, tobramycin + ceftazidime in penicillin allergy, ototopical drops	IV for 6–8 weeks	Admit
Myringitis granulosa	Sensation of hearing loss, occasional drainage, granular TM bumps, suppuration	None	NA	NA
Acute infectious otitis media	TM red, dull, bulging, non-mobile, perforation possible, fever	Amoxicillin	40 mg/kg/day ÷ tid PO for 10 days	14 day follow-up
		Erythromycin-sulfa, TMP-SMX	50/150 mg/kg qid, 8/40 mg/kg/day ÷ bid	
		First-generation cephalosporin (cefaclor), amoxicillin-clavulanate	40 mg/kg/day ÷ tid or 250 mg q8h	
Persistent middle ear effusion	Fussy child, TM red or brown, TM not bulging, afebrile	NA	NA	Chronic process requires scheduled ENT follow-up
Chronic infectious otitis media				
Without cholesteatoma	Chronic symptoms, no systemic response	Ototopical drops	Topical	ENT referral, evaluate for CNS complications
Chronic infectious otitis media	Chronic symptoms, TM thick-	Ototopical drops	Topical	ENT referral, evaluate for CNS com-

Table 34-1. (*continued*)

Infection	Signs and symptoms	Antibiotic	Dosage	Comment
With choles-teatoma	ened, perforated, ossicles calcified or necrotic, drainage (recurrent), cholesteatoma possible, confirmed by CT			plications
Mastoiditis	Antecendent otitis media, erythema, swelling or post-auricular abscess, + CAT scan	Cefuroxime + metronidazole	IV	Hospitalization ENT consult
Sinusitis	Nasal congestion, facial pain, headache, tenderness over sinus, fever	Amoxicillin Erythomycin-sulfa, TMP-SMX cefaclor	40 mg/kg/day ÷ tid PO for 10 days or 250 mg q8h 50/150 mg/kg ÷ qid, 8/40 mg/kg/day ÷ bid 40 mg/kg/day ÷ tid or 250 mg q8h	Topical decongestion; consider admission if patient toxic or with frontal or sphenoid sinusitis
Chronic infectious sinusitis	Complaints chronic, nasal congestion, facial pain, afebrile	None needed acutely	NA	CT scan, allergy evaluation, ENT referral

proximately 2 cm away from the external canal) will demonstrate that bone stimulation is perceived better than air conduction.

Although uncommon, nerve hearing loss may result either from a primary infection (mumps, measles, varicella-zoster, syphilis) of the cochlear-vestibular apparatus or secondary to bacterial or viral CNS infection, such as meningitis. The patient may present with hearing loss alone, hearing loss with vestibular symptoms, or any combination of these two associated with other CNS manifestations of infection. If the hearing loss is unilateral, the Weber test will lateralize away from the affected ear toward the "good" cochlea. The Rinne test will show air conduction greater than bone conduction.

If the vestibular system is involved, the patient may present with disabling vertigo, nausea, and vomiting as the primary complaints.

THE RED TYMPANIC MEMBRANE
Infectious entities causing abnormalities of the tympanic membrane are listed in Table 34-2.

Acute Infectious Pathology. The normal tympanic membrane is so thin that the middle ear space can be seen directly through it. Infections of the mucosa of the middle ear cause immediate erythema and edema of the drum. Early infections may cause only hyperemia of the tympanic membrane with little loss of landmarks. If the infection is allowed to progress, the tissues of the drum will

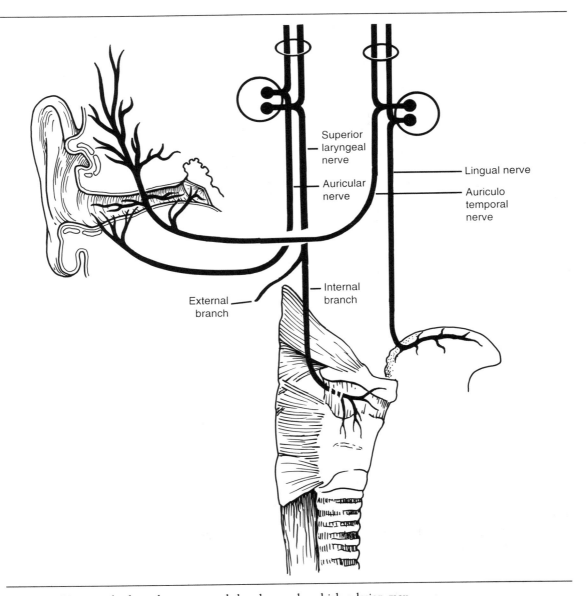

Fig. 34-1. Nerve paths from the tongue and the pharynx by which a lesion may cause ear pain. (Adapted with permission from MacComb WS, Fletcher GH. *Cancer of the Head and Neck,* 1967. P. 223)

weep fluid directly into the external canal without any evidence of a perforation.

Acute Noninfectious Pathology. Closed head trauma or acute pressure changes, which do not result in a ruptured ear drum, may result in erythematous changes in the tympanic membrane (TM). Barotrauma from eustachian-tube dysfunc-tion secondary to altitude change may result in a painful ear with a red drum. The patient usually will not have any associated systemic infectious signs, such as fever or an elevated white blood cell count.

The "No Landmark" Ear Drum. Commonly emergency department physicians will see a patient with a possible infectious problem related to the ear

Table 34-2. Infectious differential diagnosis of the abnormal tympanic membrane

Finding	Myringitis granulosa	Bullous myringitis	Acute infectious otitis media	Persistent middle ear effusion	Chronic infectious otitis media Without cholesteatoma	With cholesteatoma
Fever	No	No	Yes	No	No	No
Time course	Acute	Acute	Acute	Chronic	Chronic	Chronic
Tympanic membrane	Red, granular bumps	Vesicles	Red, bulging, wet	Red	Thickening	Pus
Perforation	No	No	Maybe	No	Yes	Yes
Drainage	No	No	No	No	Maybe	Yes
Hearing loss	No	No	Yes*	No	Yes	Yes
Etiology	Unclear	Mycoplasma	Bacterial, S. Pneumoniae, M. Catarrhalis	Bacterial, viral	Aerobic, anaerobic bacteria	Aerobic, anaerobic bacteria
Treatment	None	None	See Table 34-1	ENT follow-up	Otologic drops, ENT follow-up	Otologic drops, ENT follow-up

* Rarely measured.

and not be able to recognize landmarks on the tympanic membrane. This is usually either an acute infectious otitis media, in which the drum is so swollen without a perforation that no landmarks can be recognized, or a total TM perforation, in which the edges of the drum are not easily seen and one is looking at medial wall of the middle ear, which is made up primarily of the bulging basilar turn of the cochlea. In chronic infectious otitis media (which is discussed later) there will be no systemic signs of infection.

THE DRAINING EAR

The patient who presents to the emergency department with an infectious otologic problem frequently will have drainage and pain as the presenting complaints (Table 34-3). These symptoms may represent acute external otitis, necrotizing external otitis media, acute infectious otitis media, chronic infectious otitis media with or without a cholesteatoma, or even mastoiditis.

The first differential sign that should be noted is fever. This sign will often separate chronic infectious otitis media from external otitis, acute otitis

media, and mastoiditis, since the patient with the chronic process rarely has systemic toxicity. The presence of a large perforation will confirm the diagnosis of chronic infectious otitis media. Pain on auricular motion may be present in both otitis externa and mastoiditis but does not occur in acute infectious otitis media. A significant portion of otitis externa patients will not have fever or systemic toxicity, so they can be differentiated, leaving only the febrile external otitis and mastoiditis patients. Granulation tissue in the canal in a diabetic patient may point to malignant external otitis. Those patients with a postauricular abscess plus mastoiditis can then be identified. The external otitis patient will have a swollen external canal but an intact drum. The mastoiditis patient without a postauricular abscess will usually have a tympanic perforation or at least swelling of the posterior canal wall.

The Auricle

Cellulitis and perichondritis should be considered together, because their presentations are similar

Table 34-3. The draining ear

Finding	Chronic otitis media	Acute otitis media	Mastoiditis	External otitis	Malignant external otitis
Fever	−	+	+	±	±
Malaise	−	+	+	±	+
Immune problem	±	±	±	±	+
Auricular tenderness	−	−	±	+	+
Postauricular abscess	−	−	+	−	−
Swollen external canal	−	−	±	+	+
Perforation	+	+	+	−	−

and they are frequently difficult to differentiate. Historically cellulitis may have a more rapid onset and there may be no antecedent trauma, as is frequent in perichondritis. Pain, tenderness, and fever are common to both. Erythema, swelling, and tenderness of the auricle is seen in each (Fig. 34-2). Evidence of injury with exposed cartilage points to perichondritis. Practically, though, initial treatment consists of 10 days of oral antibiotics covering both *Staphylococcus* and *Streptococcus* organisms. Any drainage or possible fluctuant areas should be cultured if noted. *Pseudomonas* species may be seen in perichondritis but should not be treated without culture identification [1]. If there is no history or evidence of cartilaginous trauma, decrease in swelling, tenderness, and erythema should be evident in 24–48 hours. If that is not the case, otolaryngology consultation and possible hospitalization for IV antibiotic therapy should be considered.

The External Canal

GENERAL CONSIDERATIONS
The external canal is a bony and cartilaginous tube that is covered by a relatively thin layer of skin. Any swelling secondary to inflammation will fill the external canal, partially or completely obliterating any opening. Because there is little loose tissue, the swelling causes significant tension and therefore pain. Often the swelling is so severe that the tympanic membrane cannot be visualized, which raises the question of whether there is an associated middle ear infection. It is rare for acute or chronic infectious otitis media with perforation and drain-

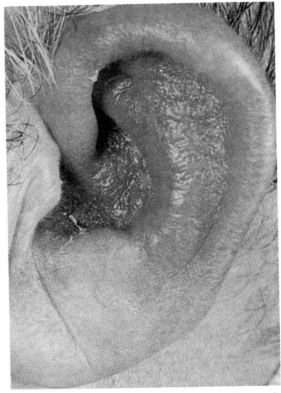

Fig. 34-2. Perichondritis of the auricle. Swelling and erythema of the upper two-thirds of the auricle as seen in perichondritis. (Reprinted with permission from Hawke M, Jahn AF. *Diseases of the Ear: Clinical and Pathologic Aspects.* Philadelphia: Lea & Febiger, 1987. Fig. 1.69)

age to have an associated external otitis; therefore, systemic treatment for an acute middle ear infection usually is unnecessary. Ototopical antibiotic drops usually are adequate for treatment of infections of the ear canal. These include polymyxin, a neomycin-and-hydrocortisone combination (Cortisporin otic), and dilute acetic acid or boric acid solutions.

OTITIS EXTERNA

Bacterial Infection. Bacterial infection of the external canal skin appears to have a significant correlation with moisture (swimming or humidity) and increased temperature. Incidence statistics show a clear increase during the summer months and in swimmers [1]. Pain, fullness, itching, and hearing loss are frequent complaints, depending on the degree of swelling of the external canal skin. Physical findings can range from mild erythema of the skin to marked swelling with pus, completely closing the external canal (Fig. 34-3). The pinna usually is normal and, most important, causes significant pain when gently pulled. Treatment is local, consisting of any of the broad-spectrum otitic drops (2 drops tid for 5 days). Suspensions are less irritating than solutions. Topical medication will not work if the canal is swollen shut. Under those circumstances a wick soaked with topical medication must be placed. Either a handmade cotton or manufactured wick (Otowick) can be used. Placement can be extremely painful to the patient, but the use of injectable local anesthesia is more painful than the wick placement itself.

Fungal Infection. Although much less common then bacterial otitis externa, fungal external otitis may present similarly. Most often the external canal skin is not completely swollen shut and usually is not as painful. Unaided visual examination often will reveal white or colored hyphae in the canal. Clotrimazole (lotrimin) or M-cresyl acetate should be prescribed. This is a local infection that rarely needs systemic antifungal agents for elimination.

Malignant External Otitis (Necrotizing Otitis Externa). This unusual life-threatening disease may present similarly to uncomplicated bacterial

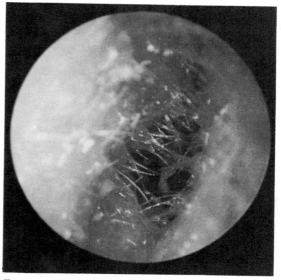

Fig. 34-3. Acute external otitis. Marked swelling and erythema of the skin of the external canal, which may be so marked that the tympanic membrane cannot be visualized. Also note clear, watery discharge. (Reprinted with permission from Hawke M, Jahn AF. *Diseases of the Ear: Clinical and Pathologic Aspects.* Philadelphia: Lea & Febiger, 1987. Fig. 2.51)

external otitits; the patient has pain, ear fullness, and drainage. The population, however, will usually have some sort of immunocompromised status, such as diabetes (80%) [2], and at least three of the five signs and symptoms of necrotizing otitis externa: (1) persistent external otitis, (2) granulation tissue in the external auditory canal, (3) CT scan confirmation of osteomyelitis of the external auditory canal, mastoid air cells, or skull base, (4) cranial nerve involvement, and (5) isolation of *Pseudomonas aeruginosa* from a culture of ear drainage [3]. Although it is not likely that culture results showing *Pseudomonas* species would be available to the emergency department physician, the history and the physical signs in this specific patient population should create a high index of suspicion for a diagnosis of malignant external otitis. This is a life-threatening infection that requires hospitalization, IV antipseudomonal antibiotic therapy for 6–8 weeks, and occasional surgical débridement of the temporal bone. Even newer broad-spectrum oral antibiotics are not appropriate for treating this very ill population.

The Tympanic Membrane

MYRINGITIS GRANULOSA

This presumed infectious disease of the tympanic membrane presents with ear pain, a sensation of hearing loss, and occasional drainage. Examination reveals multiple small, red, granular bumps on the tympanic membrane with surrounding or overlying suppuration. No perforation will be noted, the hearing will be normal, and the tympanic membrane will move normally on pneumatic examination. The etiology of this condition is not clear. Its clinical importance lies in confusing it for acute or chronic infectious otitis media. Any of the ototopical drops are adequate treatment for this problem.

BULLOUS MYRINGITIS

This acute process, which often is due to *Mycoplasma* bacteria, presents with the rapid onset of ear pain. There may be no associated systemic symptoms, or the patient may have symptoms of upper respiratory infection (URI). Clear vesicles are seen on the drum. Incising the vesicles with a needle usually will resolve the symptoms but requires an operating microscope. Systemic antibiotic therapy is not indicated for isolated myringitis, but ototopical antibiotics may prevent otitis externa [4].

The Middle Ear Cavity

ACUTE INFECTIOUS OTITIS MEDIA

In a recent epidemiologic study 90% of all children will have at least one episode of acute infectious otitis media by age 7, and 75% of this population will have had at least three or more episodes [5]. Otitis media becomes less common after 10 years of age. The cornerstone of this disease is a bacterial insult resulting in an acute inflammatory response. Pathologically this response is represented by such histologic findings as polymorphonuclear white cell accumulation, vascular dilation, and transudation of fluid.

The diagnosis in the adult is relatively straightforward. The patient will complain of ear pain, fever, and possibly hearing loss, ear popping or fullness, tinnitus, or vertigo. Symptoms of an URI

also may be present. The clinical symptoms in older children may be similar, but symptomatology is more subtle in infants and young children. Although rubbing or pulling of the ears may be present, this is not a reliable sign. Other symptoms are nonspecific, including irritability, crying, sleep problems, change in feeding, vomiting, and diarrhea. An antecedent URI is common. Fever may not be present and when present is generally low grade [6]. The presence of otitis media does not rule out more serious illness such as bacteria, pneumonia, or meningitis, especially in the presence of a very high fever (> 40°C). The physical examination in adults and older children generally is easier because the ear canal is wider than it is in young children. If cerumen obscures the tympanic membrane, it must be removed with a swab or a curette or by irrigation. Depending on what point in the infection the patient is examined, the physician may see a reddish, dull, nonmoving drum or a bulging, wet, red tympanic membrane, which on occasion will have ruptured, resulting in pus draining from the ear (Fig. 34-4). Mild vascular injection may occur in the child who has been crying. The infant's tympanic membrane normally may be dull without a light reflex.

Currently the most common organisms that cause acute infectious otitis media in children and adults are *Streptococcus pneumoniae* (30%–50%) and *H. influenzae* (20%–35%) [7]. Both group A streptococci and *Moraxella catarrhalis* also have been identified in this disease, but their incidence has not been as well established [8]. The aminopenicillins are still effective therapeutic modalities in this disease (amoxicillin 40–50 mg/kg/day divided tid). Ten days of therapy is usually adequate. Symptomatic improvement should be seen within 72 hours. If there is no improvement in 3 days, therapeutic failure at 10 days, penicillin allergy, or a high local incidence of ampicillin-resistant organisms, antibiotics that resist beta-lactamase, such as trimethoprim-sufamethoxazole, erythromycin and sulfamethoxazole, amoxicillin and clavulanate, or cefaclor would be appropriate [9]. There is no single drug of choice in this disease since social, epidemiologic, and economic factors must all be considered in the treatment decision.

Recurrent infections often are caused by the same organisms sensitive to the initial antibiotic. Nasal

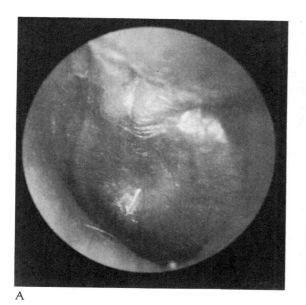
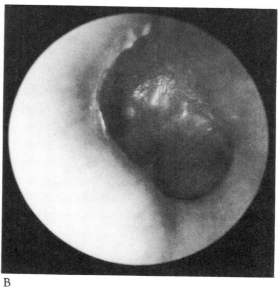

A   B

Fig. 34-4. Acute infectious otitis media. A. Early acute infectious otitis media showing mild erythema and minimal bulging of the tympanic membrane. B. Full-blown
acute infectious otitis media with classic bulging, wet, red tympanic membrane. Note
the white purulent fluid that can be seen accumulating behind the drum in the lower
portion of the middle ear. (Reprinted with permission from Hawke M, Jahn AF. *Diseases of the Ear: Clinical and Pathologic Aspects.* Philadelphia: Lea & Febiger, 1987.
Fig. 3.37)

decongestants may help nasal stuffiness, but they
have no effect on the outcome of the ear infection.
Myringotomy is rarely indicated in acute infectious
otitis media except in cases of an immunocompromised host, when accurate bacterial identification is mandatory. A child under 2 weeks of age
with otitis media must undergo a septic workup and
be admitted for observation. Extreme caution must
be used in a child less than 8 weeks of age to rule out
systemic illness. Cultures in these infants may yield
Escherichia coli, Klebsiella species, P. *aeruginosa*, and
other gram-negative bacteria [10]. All patients require follow-up in 10–14 days. The natural history
for the patient treated for otitis media is given in
Fig. 34-5.

THE DRAINING TYMPANOSTOMY TUBE
One of the most common medical procedures performed in the United States is placement of tympanostomy tubes. Up to 21% of children will have
at least one episode of otorrhea while tubes are in
place [11]. The child with a draining ear in the

presence of a tympanostomy tube may have pain or
discomfort but will rarely have fever or other systemic signs. No definitive studies have been accomplished defining the best treatment for this condition, except for Balkany's study showing that
ototopical drops decreased the incidence of otorrhea in the immediate postoperative period [12].
After that time a child seen in an urgent context
probably should be treated with oral antibiotics
similar to those used to treat acute otitis media.

PERSISTENT MIDDLE EAR EFFUSION
Often a child will present pulling on its ear, being
fussy, or crying who on physical examination will
have a red or brownish-appearing tympanic membrane. The drum will not be wet or bulging but may
be retracted. A conductive hearing loss will be
present. The child will be afebrile, and if obtained
the white blood cell count will be normal.

Although commonly diagnosed and treated as if
it were acute infectious otitis media except for pain
medication, persistent middle ear effusion does not

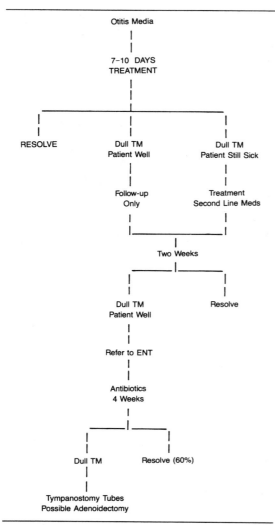

```
                    Otitis Media
                         |
                         |
                    7-10 DAYS
                    TREATMENT
                         |
                         |
        |_____|_____|
        |                |                |
        |                |                |
     RESOLVE          Dull TM          Dull TM
                    Patient Well     Patient Still Sick
                         |                |
                         |                |
                     Follow-up        Treatment
                       Only        Second Line Meds
                         |                |
                         |_____|
                                 |
                             Two Weeks
                      _____|_____
                     |                       |
                     |                       |
                  Dull TM                 Resolve
                Patient Well
                     |
                     |
               Refer to ENT
                     |
                 Antibiotics
                  4 Weeks
                     |
              _____|_____
             |              |
             |              |
          Dull TM      Resolve (60%)
             |
             |
      Tympanostomy Tubes
      Possible Adenoidectomy
```

Fig. 34-5. Common clinical course of an otherwise healthy child presenting with an initial episode of acute infectious otitis media.

require an emergency therapeutic intervention. A bacterial process has been implicated in about 50% of these situations [13]. Initiation in an emergency situation of any antimicrobial treatment for what is, in effect, a chronic process will not improve outcome. Elective otolaryngology follow-up is required for long-term management, which may include antibiotic therapy.

CHRONIC INFECTIOUS OTITIS MEDIA WITHOUT CHOLESTEATOMA

The word *chronic* can be related to either time or pathology. Many physicians use chronic as if it refers solely to time. This usage, however, does not give a complete picture of chronic infectious otitis media. Histologically the chronic inflammatory response includes fibrosis, necrosis, hyalinization, calcification, and hypertrophy, to name a few. On examination of an ear in which there is a chronic inflammatory response, the clinician may see evidence of all these processes. Clinically there would be a perforation and thickening of the middle ear mucosa (Fig. 34-6). Calcified and necrotic ossicles also may be evident. Drainage from either a long-standing bacterial infection or an acute exacerbation of the chronic process may be evident. Although the patient may have pain, it is unlikely that there will be any systemic response, such as fever or an elevated white blood cell count. What the examiner is looking at is, in effect, a walled-off abscess

Fig. 34-6. Chronic infectious otitis media. The surface of the drum and deep meatus is coated with a thick, brown, mucopurulent discharge. Through a posterosuperior perforation the head of the stapes is visible. The long process of the incus has undergone resorption and hence is not seen. (Reprinted with permission from Hawke M, Jahn AF. *Diseases of the Ear: Clinical and Pathologic Aspects.* Philadelphia: Lea & Febiger, 1987. Fig. 3.119)

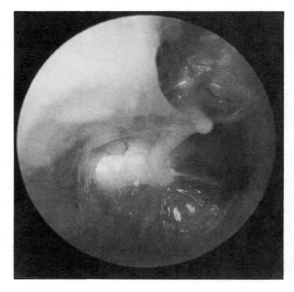

cavity. The bacteriology is that of a chronic infection, including both aerobic and anaerobic organisms such as *Pseudomonas* species, *S. aureus*, and *Bacteroides* species [14]. Both children and adults may present to the emergency department with a painful perforated draining ear, simulating an acute infectious otitis media. Questioning will most commonly elicit previous episodes of drainage over months or even years. The physical findings will be as just described, and the patient rarely will have any evidence of systemic toxicity. The acute drainage is merely an exacerbation of a chronic process. Emergency treatment requires little other than ototopical antibiotic drops, pain medication, and elective otologic referral. Systemic antibiotics are not indicated except occasionally in conjunction with definitive surgical therapy. These patients should be referred to an otolaryngologist.

CHRONIC INFECTIOUS OTITIS MEDIA WITH CHOLESTEATOMA

A cholesteatoma is an epithelial cyst that has grown into the middle ear or mastoid (Fig. 34-7). Its danger lies in it acting as a growing, frequently

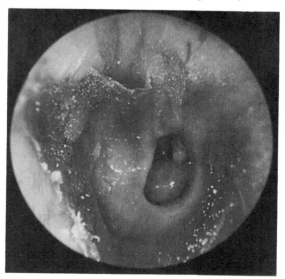

Fig. 34-7. Cholesteatoma. The white cyst visible behind the intact tympanic membrane is part of a cholesteatoma that extends around the ossicles. (Reprinted with permission from Hawke M, Jahn AF. *Diseases of the Ear: Clinical and Pathologic Aspects.* Philadelphia: Lea & Febiger, 1987. Fig. 3.163)

infected benign "tumor" in a closed space adjacent to many vital structures, such as the meninges, the eighth cranial nerve, the cochlea, and the semicircular canals. Diagnosis is difficult in the emergency department environment, since the patient usually will present with a painful ear full of pus. Microscopic otologic examination frequently is required to make the clinical diagnosis. Radiological evaluation, usually a CT scan, is used for confirmation rather than as a primary diagnostic tool. A defect in the drum containing epithelial debris supports the diagnosis of cholesteatoma. Emergency treatment is similar to that of chronic infectious otitis media without cholesteatoma. If a diagnosis of cholesteatoma is made in an emergent situation, the emergent physician should have a greater index of suspicion for the more serious complications of chronic infectious otitis media and look for the signs and symptoms described in the following sections. If the patient's only complaints and findings are a painful draining ear with some hearing loss, then elective otolaryngology referral is indicated.

Mastoiditis

MUCOSAL

The middle ear space is directly connected to the mastoid through a space in which lie the heads of the incus and the malleus. This passage leads directly to the antrum within the mastoid and from there connects to the remaining mastoid air cells (Fig. 34-8). All these contiguous chambers are mucosally lined. Any acute infection of the middle ear space commonly will involve the mucosa of part or all of the mastoid, thus giving rise to the term *mastoiditis*. This is *not* the bony-mastoid infection that has such serious consequences. Such an infection may be confused with bony osteitic mastoiditis if an x-ray is obtained that shows some fluid in the mastoid air cells and is returned to the emergency department with a radiologic diagnosis of "mastoiditis" (Fig. 34-9). Unless there is objective evidence of bony osteitic mastoiditis, such as a postauricular abscess (the auricle will be pushed forward by a fluctuant mass overlying the mastoid, as in Fig. 34-10), or radiologic evidence of breakdown of mastoid bony septa (coalescent mastoiditis), the clinician most likely is dealing with a straightforward acute otitis media with some mastoid mucosal ex-

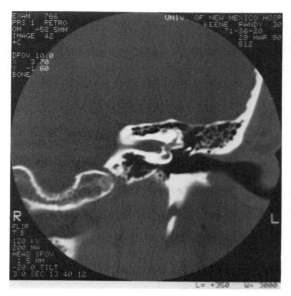

Fig. 34-8. Connection between the middle ear and the mastoid. Coronal CT scan of the temporal bone. Arrow shows the normal communication between the middle ear space and the mastoid

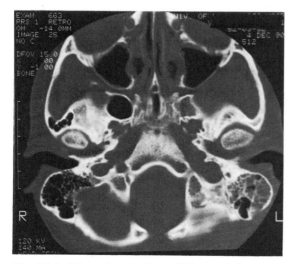

Fig. 34-9. Mucosal mastoiditis. CT scan of the mastoid air cells showing fluid secondary to acute infectious otitis media but no evidence of bony septal destruction

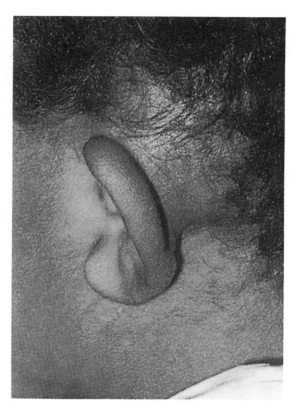

Fig. 34-10. Postauricular subperiosteal abscess secondary to mastoiditis. (Reprinted with permission from Hawke M, Jahn AF. *Diseases of the Ear: Clinical and Pathologic Aspects.* Philadelphia: Lea & Febiger, 1987. Fig. 3.52)

tension. Treatment is outpatient oral antibiotic therapy, as previously described.

OSTEITIS

For reasons not well known a small percentage of children and occasionally adults will develop a true osteitis secondary to an acute infectious otitis media. Before the antibiotic era 10% of children with acute infectious otitis media went on to develop bony mastoiditis. Today large urban medical centers rarely see more than 5–10 cases per year. Clinically these cases are characterized by a history of recently acquired or even treated acute otitis media. The illness persists, and the patient may become increasingly toxic. Physical findings will include a red and bulging tympanic membrane or posterior canal wall, and the drum may have perforated with pus present. There often will be postauricular erythema, swelling or a frank abscess (see Fig. 34-10). Radiologic evaluation (CT scan) should confirm that there is bony septal breakdown within the mastoid. The bacteriology of mastoiditis includes the standard organisms found in acute infectious otitis media plus additional aerobic species, including S. aureus and Proteus mirabilis, and various anaerobic organisms, such as Bacteroides, Clostridium, and Fusobacterium species [15]. This disease requires antibiotic treatment in the hospital and both pediatric and otologic consultation. Prior to culture results antibiotic treatment should include cefuroxime plus metronidazole. Once identification of the offending agent(s) has been made, therapy should be continued for 4–6 weeks, as in any bone infection.

Cochlear-Vestibular Infections

VIRAL INFECTIONS

Patients with acquired mumps, measles, and varicella-zoster may develop an acute neurosensory hearing loss during their illness, causing them to seek urgent medical evaluation. In measles and mumps the infection may affect both the cochlea and the vestibular systems, although hearing loss is more common. The hearing loss in mumps is unilateral in 80% of cases [16]. Varicella-zoster (herpes zoster oticus) produces painful auricular vesicles, followed shortly by a facial nerve paralysis. Auditory and vestibular symptoms are much less common in this infection. There is no effective treatment for any of these infections. Therapy with antivertiginous medications, such as meclazine or scopolamine dermal patches (Transderm-Scop), may provide symptomatic relief.

BACTERIAL INFECTION

Primary cochlear-vestibular bacterial infections do not occur. Secondary involvement of the inner ear is seen in meningitis and rarely may be associated with an acute or chronic infectious otitis media.

SYPHILIS

Congenital syphilis may cause neurosensory hearing loss early (0–3 years) or cause it to develop in the second or third decade [17]. Clinically the hearing loss develops gradually and should be an uncom-

monly seen chief complaint in an emergency department. On the other hand patients with acquired syphilis may develop nerve hearing loss during the second stage of the disease [17]. This loss is. sudden, may be bilateral, and usually has no associated vestibular symptoms. Diagnosis is made by identifying the high-risk patient and performing the appropriate clinical and serologic evaluation for secondary syphilis. This is one of the few neurosensory hearing losses that may respond to medical treatment, including antisyphilitic antibiotics and systemic steroids.

Infectious CNS Complications of Otologic Infection

MENINGITIS

Meningitis is the most common CNS complication of both acute and chronic infectious otitis media [18]. (For symptoms and diagnosis of meningitis see Chap. 7 and Chap. 31.) Otologic findings may be anything from an acute infectious otitis media to a cholesteatoma. Because any patient with an ear infection may present with fever and headache, the emergency physician must not overlook the possibility of CNS involvement (see Chap. 8 and Chap. 31).

BRAIN ABSCESS

Brain abscess is the second most common intracranial infectious problem secondary to suppurative ear disease. Up to 25% of all brain abscesses arise secondary to otologic infection [18]. As in meningitis the practitioner must have a relatively high index of suspicion for intracranial pathology in the patient presenting with headache and a draining ear. Most commonly brain abscess is associated with chronic infectious otitis media with or without cholesteatoma. Radiologic evaluation confirms the diagnosis (see Chap. 7 and Chap. 31).

SIGMOID SINUS THROMBOSIS

Sigmoid sinus thrombosis is an extremely uncommon disease. Like brain abscess it is associated with a chronic infectious otological problem. It also may present with CNS-associated symptoms such as headache, fever, nausea, and vomiting. There may be septic embolic phenomena manifesting by fever spikes, which may be helpful in suspecting the diagnosis. Cranial nerve involvement (IX, X, XI) and papilledema often are late clinical signs. A CT scan or an MRI is indicated if this diagnosis is suspected.

Sinusitis

Uncomplicated Acute Infectious Sinusitis

CLINICAL PRESENTATION AND EVALUATION

Most adults will present with some history of nasal congestion from either a URI or a worsening of an acute allergic problem. Other patients will have nasal polyps, nasal packing, an infected tooth root abutting the maxillary sinus, or barotrauma as a predisposing condition. Symptoms begin with facial pain, headache, rhinorrhea, and then fever. The pain may be stabbing or achy and a feeling of fullness noted. Bending, coughing, or straining may increase the pain. The location of the pain will be variable depending on the sinus or sinuses involved but often has some anatomic relationship to the infected cavity. Sinusitis occurs in order of frequency in the maxillary, ethmoid, frontal, and sphenoid sinuses. The pain of ethmoid or sphenoid sinusitis is vague.

Physical examination will reveal mucopurulent nasal drainage, but drainage may be prevented by completely blocked ostia. Tenderness may be elicited over an infected maxillary or frontal sinus. Facial and orbital swelling or skin erythema may occur but are not routine in the average case. Careful rhinoscopy with suction and magnification may reveal pus coming from the middle meatus, supporting the diagnosis of purulent sinusitis. This kind of nasal examination, however, rarely is available in an emergency department situation.

The history with mucopurulent nasal drainage, fever, facial pain, and tenderness provides the database on which a presumptive diagnosis of sinus infection can be made. The remaining evaluation question is whether a radiologic examination is necessary. In an otherwise healthy adult presenting with a typical history and physical examination, sinus radiographs usually will add little to the diagnosis while adding significantly to the cost of the medical encounter. Diagnostic radiology becomes more relevant in the minority of these "typical" patients if, after a reasonable therapeutic intervention, they do not have resolution of their disease. X-rays in acute sinusitis will demonstrate an air-fluid level or complete opacification of the involved sinus. In chronic sinusitis mucosal thickening or complete opacification will be found.

Children present less typical patterns than adults. Their "cold" is usually somewhat more severe than normal, with higher temperatures that do not resolve in the usual 5–7 days. They may not complain of pain but will usually have some facial swelling or erythema. Continued URI symptoms in a child beyond 10 days should alert the clinician to the possibility of a paranasal sinus infection. An x-ray demonstrating complete sinus opacification or an air-fluid level is useful in making the diagnosis [19].

NASAL CONGESTION AND FACIAL PAIN

Nasal congestion from any cause can precipitate midfacial pain and even tenderness that is often diagnosed as acute bacterial sinusitis, resulting in systemic antibiotic therapy. There is a group of patients who present this way but who have few systemic signs of toxicity, such as fever or an elevated white blood cell count. They usually have only obstruction of the osteomeatal complex with some air resorbtion and pressure in the maxillary sinus. Left untreated they may go on to an acute bacterial infection. At this stage all the patient may need is decongestion of the nasal mucous membranes and opening of the osteomeatal complex to allow air to flow into the maxillary sinus and restore pressure equalization. Oral and, more important, topical nasal decongestion should be used initially. Long-acting topical nasal spray should be used 3 times per day. The medication should be given in each nostril, then 3–5 minutes later applied again, aiming each time for the inner canthus of the eye. Within 24–48 hours this procedure will often open up the obstruction to the osteomeatal complex and eliminate the symptoms and may prevent the development of an acute bacterial sinusitis. The nasal spray usually can be discontinued in 3–5 days [20].

PATHOPHYSIOLOGY AND MICROBIOLOGY

Acute infectious sinusitis in an otherwise healthy patient is most commonly caused by obstruction of the osteomeatal complex (Fig. 34-11), which refers

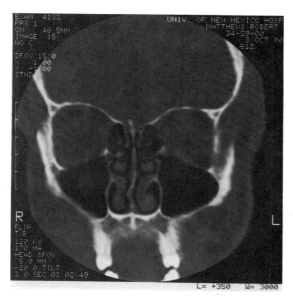

Fig. 34-11. CT scan of osteomeatal complex

to an area in the anterior portion of the middle meatus into which the maxillary, frontal, and anterior ethmoidal sinuses drain. This area is normally quite narrow, so any inflammation can easily cause obstruction of the ostea of these sinuses and result in acute infectious sinusitis. Either an acute viral rhinitis or a noninfectious inflammatory event such as allergic rhinitis can precipitate the infection. Up to 0.5% of patients with viral URIs may develop a sinusitis [21]. Since adults may develop two to three and children six to eight colds per year, sinusitis is a common diagnosis in an emergency outpatient setting [22]. In adults *H. influenzae* and *S. pneumoniae* are the most common organisms associated with this infection (65%). *Neisseria* species, *Streptococcus pyogenes*, alpha-hemolytic streptococcus, *Streptococcus viridans*, *Pseudomonas* species, *S. aureus*, *Enterobacteriaceae*, and viruses such as rhinovirus and influenza A also have been isolated [23, 24]. Children have a similar pattern of offending organisms except for the finding that *M. catarrhalis* has been noted in up to 19% of antral isolates [25, 26].

MAXILLARY ANTRUM

The maxillary antrum, which lies lateral to the nasal cavity and under the eye, may be the most commonly infected of the paranasal sinuses. It has been the most studied, since it is the most accessible. It is the only sinus that does not have a dural surface adjacent to it; therefore, its infections are rarely life threatening. Ten to 15% of maxillary sinusitis cases are of dental origin [27]. The maxillary antrum sinus is present from birth but is not clinically significant until the child is 1–2 years old [28]. When this sinus is infected, the patient will experience facial or upper maxillary dental pain. The sinus will be tender to palpation. Diagnostic aspiration can be performed with an 18-gauge trocar passed through the medial wall of the nose. It is a relatively easy procedure for an otolaryngologist to perform, even in an emergency department setting.

THE ETHMOIDAL SINUS

The ethmoidal sinus, or labyrinth (since it is not a single cavity but is made up of 3–15 separate cells), lies between the orbit and the nasal cavity. Its roof is the floor of the anterior cranial fossa, and its anterior and posterior margins are marked by the frontal and sphenoid sinuses, respectively. Because the roof of the sinus (fova ethmoidalis) is quite thick and the medial wall (lamina papyracea) so thin, most complications of ethmoidal infection manifest within the orbit. The ethmoids cannot be palpated from the face, so tenderness is not an associated physical finding in this disease. Pain is orbital or retrorbital and will be vague in nature. Periorbital erythema and swelling frequently may be seen. This sinus complex is present from birth and though less commonly infected then the maxillary, it is usually the origin of orbital complications of sinusitis in both children and adults [29].

THE FRONTAL SINUS

The frontal sinus, which develops late in childhood or early adolescence and is often absent in many patients, lies above the orbit and forms a portion of the anterior wall of the anterior cranial fossa. When the sinus is infected, the pain is frontal and tenderness can be elicited easily. Palpation should be accomplished just below the brow and above the medial canthus, because the wall of the sinus is thinnest at that point. The entire posterior wall of the sinus, which can be several square centimeters, is dural lined, putting anterior cranial fossa structures at risk for directed extension infectious complications.

THE SPHENOIDAL SINUS

The sphenoidal sinus, which is rarely solely infected, lies at the posterior superior border of the nasal cavity and has medial dural borders with the middle cranial fossa. Pain is rarely localizing and may be occipital when it does occur. Palpation is impossible. Radiologic evaluation is necessary for any accurate diagnosis of sphenoidal sinusitis. It, along with the frontal and the ethmoidal sinuses, does not easily lend itself to diagnostic aspiration.

TREATMENT

The antibiotic used should cover the most common organisms associated with maxillary sinusitis. Amoxicillin, ampicillin, trimethoprim-sulfamethoxazole, and cefaclor have all been shown to be approximately 80% effective in eliminating bacteria from an infected maxillary antrum [22]. The role of oral and topical decongestants in this disease is not clear. Symptomatic relief from the nasal congestion may be obtained from these agents. If obstruction of the osteomeatal complex is a primary etiologic factor in acute bacterial sinusitis, then relieving that obstruction should be a therapeutic aim. Topical decongestants can provide the most immediate effect on that obstruction. However, no controlled prospective study has proved that such therapy either negatively or positively affects the outcome of this disease. Until those data are forthcoming, topical and oral decongestants should be part of the medical therapy, so increased patient comfort may be achieved. Initiation and management of an uncomplicated maxillary or ethmoid sinusitis is appropriate in the urgent care setting. Acute frontal sinusitis, though less common, has been reported to have intracranial complications in up to 17% of cases in children and adolescents [30]. Adults also have a significant risk of intracranial problems [31]. Outpatient treatment as previously described and follow-up of a reliable patient who has no severe toxicity, swelling, or erythema over the frontal sinuses are possible. However, any patient who deviates from this clinical picture probably should be referred to otolaryngology for admission and IV antibiotic therapy.

Complicated Acute Infectious Sinusitis

THE IMMUNOCOMPROMISED PATIENT

Microbiological findings in this form of sinusitis do not follow typical patterns. Streptococcus, S. aureus, Staphylococcus epidermitidis, and assorted gram-negative bacilli have been found to be associated with sinusitis in diabetics [32]. No good data are available for AIDS patients. In these situations accurate cultures are necessary. Cultures must be obtained from antral puncture, because it has been shown in both children and adults that there is no correlation between nasal cultures and sinus aspirations [33, 34]. Close follow-up is mandatory, and hospitalization or parenteral antibiotic therapy should be considered.

NOSOCOMIAL SINUSITIS

Devices or packing placed intranasally during hospitalization may lead to sinusitis secondary to nosocomial bacteria such as P. aeruginosa, E. coli, K. pneumoniae, and Bacteroides melaninogenicus [35]. Should a patient who has been recently discharged from the hospital present with an acute sinusitis with a history of such nasal manipulations, then sinus aspiration is indicated to accurately define the microbiology for proper antibiotic therapy.

ORBITAL COMPLICATIONS OF SINUSITIS

The orbital septum is a connective tissue structure that extends from the orbital periosteum to the tarsal plates. It provides a protective barrier that helps prevent many of the lid and conjunctival inflammatory diseases from extending posteriorly to involve the orbit. The periosteum of the orbit provides a similar barrier for the rest of the intraorbital contents. That periosteum overlies the lamina papyracea of the ethmoids. In addition to the laminae parycea being extremely thin, there are natural dehiscences in it that allow direct infectious access to the orbit [36]. Orbital complications of sinusitis occur most frequently in children, and up to 75% of these infections appear to develop from an ethmoiditis [37]. Any patient with a suspected orbital complication of an acute infectious sinusitis should have a CT scan performed to define the extent of the disease. Orbital infection has been divided into various stages by Chandler [38] (Fig. 34-12). Although separated into various stages, orbital in-

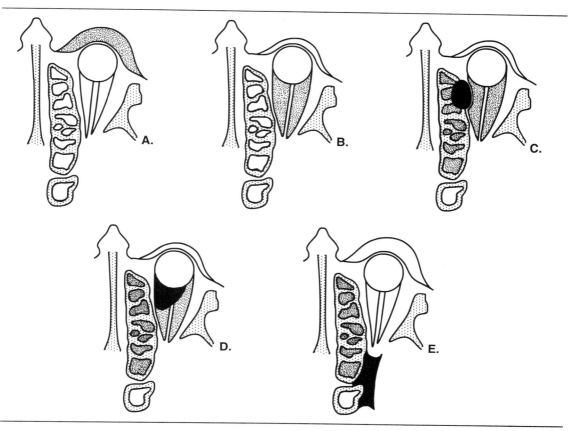

Fig. 34-12. Staging of orbital cellulitis and its complications. A. Periorbital cellulitis; B. Orbital cellulitis; C. Subperiosteal abscess; D. Orbital abscess; E. Cavernous sinus thrombosis. (Adapted with permission from Chandler J. Orbital cellulitis and its complications. In G Gates (ed.), *Current Therapy in Otolaryngology—Head and Neck Surgery* (4th ed.). Toronto: Decker, 1990. P. 267)

flammation is a continuum through which the infection moves. The following stagings provide diagnostic guidelines only and are not absolute.

Stage A: Periorbital Cellulitis. In this early stage of orbital infection the lids are primarily involved. The patient has erythema and edema of the skin. There is no visual or impaired ocular movement. Chemosis is lacking. If there is radiologic confirmation that the disease is limited to the preseptal area of the orbit, the offending sinus (most likely the ethmoid) is identified. If the patient or the family is considered reliable, outpatient medical treatment can be initiated. The organisms noted here are the same as for uncomplicated si-

nusitis. Daily follow-up is warranted until there is clear-cut disease resolution.

Stage B: Orbital Cellulitis. The infection is now within the orbit. There is diffuse infection of the orbital contents. Ocular motion and vision may be affected. Chemosis and exophthalmos may be present. The patient is febrile and appears sick. Hospitalization and administration of parenteral antibiotics are indicated at this point and in the following stages.

Stage C: Subperiosteal Abscess. An abscess has formed, usually under the periosteum overlying the lamina papyracea. The findings are similar to orbital cellulitis, except that the proptosis may be more extreme. A CT scan will usually confirm the diagnosis. In addition to medical therapy surgical intervention is indicated.

Stage D: Orbital Abscess. In this stage the abscess has formed in the orbital contents. In addition to the previously described signs the physician may see more severe ophthalmoplegia and vision impairment. If radiologic evaluation confirms the presence of an abscess, surgical intervention becomes necessary.

Stage E: Cavernous Sinus Thrombosis. Progression of the infection via thrombotic venous channels into the cavernous sinus heralds a life-threatening situation. Cranial nerve defects of the third, fourth, fifth, and sixth nerves may occur. Papilledema will be present, along with depression of the patient's mental status. Appropriate high-dose antibiotics and surgical intervention for sinus or abscess drainage are indicated. Any of the advanced orbital infections can progress to this stage if not treated, so prompt evaluation and diagnosis of any patient presenting to an emergency department with signs of sinusitis and orbital inflammation are of utmost importance.

FRONTAL BONE OSTEOMYELITIS

Quite rare today frontal bone osteomyelitis (Pott's puffy tumor) is occasionally seen presenting in an emergency department. An aggressive or untreated frontal sinusitis may involve the overlying bone. The skin over the sinus becomes swollen and erythematous. There may be abscess formation under the periosteum of the frontal bone. Bilateral periorbital inflammation is often present. CT evaluation is necessary for delineation of the extent of the disease. Hospitalization for medical and surgical therapy is indicated.

CNS COMPLICATIONS OF SINUSITIS

The walls of both the frontal and the sphenoidal sinus are dural lined, leading to the potential for the CNS spread of infection from these sinuses. Meningitis and subdural empyema are potential sequelae of sinus infection. The patient with frontal or sphenoidal sinusitis must undergo a careful neurologic evaluation for CNS infection. Close follow-up of patients with frontal and sphenoidal sinusitis is mandatory.

Chronic Infectious Sinusitis

Persons with chronic infectious sinusitis may not be seen in the urgent care setting per se, because their symptomatology is rarely acute. The patient complains of long-standing nasal congestion and/or obstruction. Headache or facial pain also may be present over several months or even years. Physical examination would reveal an afebrile patient in no severe distress. Nasal polyps, mucosal congestion, or septal deviation may be present. Workup in a routine ambulatory setting would include a CT scan of the sinuses plus allergic evaluation if warranted by the history. The bacteriology of chronic infectious sinusitis includes beta-hemolytic streptococci, S. aureus, and H. influenzae plus several strains of anaerobic organisms, such as Bacteroides and Fusobacterium species [39]. Treatment is directed at correcting the long-underlying problem by allergic management, correction of the deviated septum, surgically opening up an obstructed osteomeatal complex, and appropriate antibiotics.

References

1. Senturia BH, Marcus MD, Lecente FE. *Diseases of the External Ear.* New York: Grune & Stratton, 1980.
2. Kraus DH, Kinney SE. Necrotizing external otitis. In Gates (ed.), *Current Therapy in Otolaryngology-Head and Neck Surgery* (4th ed.). Toronto: Decker, 1990.
3. Kraus DH, Rehm SJ, Kinney SE. The evolving treatment of necrotizing otitis externa. *Laryngoscope* 98: 934, 1988.
4. Glasscock ME, Shambaugh GE, Johnson GD. Surgery of the ear. Philadelphia: Saunders, 1990.
5. Klein JO, Teele DV, Rosner B. Epidemiology of acute otitis media in Boston children from birth to seven years of age. In DJ Lim et al. (eds.), *Recent Advances in Otitis Media.* Toronto: Decker, 1988.
6. Howie VM, Schwartz RH. Acute otitis media one year in a general pediatric practice. *AJDC* 137:155, 1983.
7. Pelton SI, Klein JO. The draining ear: otitis media and externa. *Infect Dis Clin North Am* Vol 2(1):117, 1988.

8. Van Hare GF et al. Acute otitis media caused by *Branhamella catarrhalis:* biology and therapy. *Rev Infect Dis* 9:16, 1987.

9. Nelson JD. Changing trends in microbiology of acute otitis media. *Pediatr Infect Dis* 5:749, 1986.

10. Klein JO. Microbiology of otitis media. *Ann Otol Rhinol Laryngol* 65–77(Suppls.):98, 1980.

11. Healy G, Teele D. The microbiology of chronic middle ear effusions in children. *Laryngoscope* 87:1472, 1977.

12. Balkany TJ, Barkin RM, Suzuki BH. A prospective study of infection following tympanostomy and tube insertion. *Am J Otology* 4:288, 1983.

13. Mandel EM et al. Efficacy of amoxicillin in effusion. *N Engl J Med* 316:8, 1987.

14. Jonssson L et al. Aerobic and anaerobic bacteria in chronic supparative otitis media. A quantitative study. *Acta Otolaryngol* 102:410, 1986.

15. Maharaj D et al. Bacteriology in acute mastoiditis. *Arch Otolaryngol Head Neck Surg* 113:514, 1987.

16. Davis EL. Infections of the labyrinth. In CW Cummings et al. (eds.), *Otolaryngology—Head and Neck Surgery.* St. Louis: Mosby, 1986.

17. Saltiel P, Melmed CA, Portnoy D. Sensorineural deafness in early acquired syphilis. *Can J Neurol Sci* 10:114, 1983.

18. Kaplan RJ. Neurological complications of infections of the head and neck. *Otolaryngol Clin North Am* 9(3):729, 1976.

19. Wald ER. Acute sinusitis in children. *Pediatr Infect Dis* 2(1):61, 1983.

20. Herzon FH. Unpublished data, 1990.

21. Dingle JH, Badger GF, Jordan WS. Patterns of illness. In *Illness in the Home.* Cleveland: Western Reserve University, 1964. P. 347.

22. Gwaltney JM, Sydnor A, Sande MA. Etiology and antimicrobial treatment of acute sinusitis. *Ann of Otol* Suppl 25.

23. Evans FO et al. Sinusitis of the maxillary antrum. *N Engl J Med* 293:735, 1975.

24. Hamory BH et al. Etiology and antimicrobial therapy of acute maxillary sinusitis. *J Infect Dis* 139:197, 1979.

25. Bluestone CD. Sinusitis in children. In Gates (ed.), *Current Therapy in Otolaryngology—Head and Neck Surgery* (4th ed.). Toronto: Decker, 1990.

26. Wald ER et al. Acute maxillary sinusitis in children. *N Engl J Med* 304:749, 1981.

27. Dayal VS, Jones J, Noyek A. Management of odontogenic maxillary sinus disease. *Otolaryngol Clin North Am* 9(1):213, 1976.

28. Healy GB. Acute sinusitis in children. *N Engl J Med* 304:779, 1981.

29. Kogutt MS, Swischuk LE. Diagnosis of sinusitis in infants and children. *Pediatrics* 52:121, 1973.

30. Johnson DL et al. Treatment of intracranial abscesses associated with sinusitis in children and adolescents. *J Pediatr* 113(1):15, 1988.

31. Remmler D, Boles R. Intracranial complications of frontal sinusitis. *Laryngoscope* 90:1814, 1980.

32. Jackson RM, Rice DH. Acute bacterial sinusitis and diabetes mellitus. *Otolaryng Head and Neck Surgery* 97:469, 1987.

33. Wald ER et al. Acute maxillary sinusitis in children. *N Engl J Med* 304:749, 1981.

34. Ritter, FN. The paranasal sinuses: anatomy and surgical technique. St. Louis: Mosby, 1973.

35. Humphrey MA, Simpson GT, Gringlinger GA. Clinical characteristics of nosocomial sinusitis. *Ann Otol Rhinol Laryngol* 96:687, 1987.

36. Shahin J et al. Orbital complications of acute sinusitis. *J Otol* 16:23, 1987.

37. Chandler, Broffman. Orbital cellulitis and its complications. In Gates, GA (ed.), *Current Therapy in Otolaryngology—Head and Neck Surgery* (4th ed.). Toronto: Decker, 1990. P. 265.

38. Brook I. Pathogenic features of bacteroides. In ENT Infections, Infections in Medicine. Nov 1987. Pp. 413–21.

39. Brook, I. Bacteriologic features of chronic sinusitis in children. *JAMA* 246:967, 1981.

35

Ophthalmic Infections

THOMAS A. DEUTSCH

The majority of emergency eye problems require the experience and training of an ophthalmologist for optimal management. This is not true, however, for infectious ophthalmic emergencies. While the array of topical ophthalmic medications is somewhat confusing, some simple principles combined with an understanding of the microbiology and the pharmacology of ocular disease can turn any excellent physician into an ophthalmic infectious disease specialist.

Infectious Ophthalmic Emergencies

When faced with an infection in or around the eye, the emergency department physician must first determine which tissues are involved. From that information the disease process can be categorized and a differential diagnosis easily constructed.

Five tissue spaces must be differentiated in the evaluation of the patient with an infection in or around the eye. The spaces and the terms that refer to their respective inflammation are: (1) the skin and subcutaneous area (cellulitis), (2) the eyelids (blepharitis), (3) the conjunctiva (conjunctivitis), (4) the cornea (keratitis), and (5) the intraocular space (endophthalmitis). There are discrete differential diagnoses for each of these sites of potential

infection, and the microbiology of each of the infections is somewhat different. This chapter discusses each of these infections in turn.

Ophthalmologists are often surprised at how timid other physicians are when they attempt to examine the eye and the orbit of an emergency patient. Indeed, mere inspection is sufficient to determine the site of infection in almost all cases. Despite the great array of technological gadgets available to the ophthalmologist, most infectious diseases of the eye are diagnosed by using a hand-light.

The examiner should first decide which tissue or tissues are involved (Table 35-1). When cellulitis is present, the skin is erythematous, somewhat indurated, and warm. Blepharitis is characterized by inflammation of the eyelids and eyelid margins. There is sometimes an associated conjunctivitis, but this is usually much more prominent on the palpebral (eyelid) conjunctiva than the bulbar conjunctiva. When conjunctivitis is present, there is redness of the bulbar conjunctiva as well as the palpebral conjunctiva. In most cases this is a uniform redness, which is not any greater in one quadrant or area than any other. Keratitis is detected as cloudiness of the cornea, which may include a white dot obscuring the iris or the pupil. The eye is usually infected, but the redness may be confined

Table 35-1. Site-specific terminology in ocular infections

Site	Infection
Skin	Cellulitis
Eyelid	Blepharitis
Conjunctiva	Conjunctivitis
Cornea	Keratitis
Intraocular	Endophthalmitis

to an area close to the corneal lesion. Endophthalmitis is an overwhelming inflammatory condition associated with diffuse redness of the eye, haziness of the ocular media, including the anterior chamber and vitreous, and obscuration of retinal details.

Every patient who presents to the emergency room with an ocular problem should have documentation of the vital signs of the eye. These include a determination of visual acuity while wearing current-prescription glasses; examination of the pupil, including determination of the presence or absence of afferent pupillary defect (Marcus-Gunn pupil); and an attempt to visualize the optic nerve and macula using a direct ophthalmoscope.

With this information in hand, combined with a determination of the site of infection, an emergency physician is ready to tackle construction of a differential diagnosis, workup, and management.

Cellulitis

Cellulitis of the periocular tissues is similar to that seen anywhere else in the body. The major difference is the proximity to the eye, which is susceptible to injury from a contiguous mass (such as an abscess), and the presence of unvalved veins that lead to the intracranial sinuses. These anatomical considerations provide the potential for visual damage and even death from cellulitis [1].

Anatomical Classification

As a rule of thumb, the worst-looking cases of cellulitis are the most benign. The reason for this is

found in an understanding of the anatomy of the periocular spaces [1].

A fibrous septum extends from the bony rims of the orbit deep into both the upper and lower eyelids. Consequently any infectious process anterior to the septum will usually remain outside the orbit. Cellulitis of this type is referred to as *periorbital*, although the term *preseptal* is more descriptive and is preferred. When the site of infection is posterior to the orbital septum, the disease process is referred to as *orbital* or *postseptal*. Because of the poor drainage from the orbit there is a chance of the development of an orbital abscess, which can cause irreversible damage to the eye. The mechanism of action of this damage is primarily by compression of the blood supply or nerve supply to the globe. In addition infection in the subperiosteal space of the orbit can lead to compression of the optic nerve posteriorly with subsequent blindness.

Since the orbit is connected to the cavernous sinus via the superior orbital fissure, infection in this area can spread into the cavernous sinus and result in thrombosis, which can be fatal. It should be clear, therefore, that orbital cellulitis is a dangerous and life-threatening disease process and should be treated promptly and appropriately.

Presentation

Preseptal cellulitis is a progressive swelling and induration of the periorbital area. Often there has been some seemingly minor trauma that broke the skin in this area. Other times there is associated acute sinus disease noted up to 7 days prior to the onset of the cellulitis. Some children will appear toxic, but most patients will be well except for the area around the eye. In extreme cases, the lids will be so swollen that the eye will be shut, simulating decreased visual acuity.

In orbital cellulitis the skin around the eye is generally quiet. There may be some swelling of the eyelids, but this is usually only an illusion secondary to protrusion (proptosis) of the globe. The eye may be displaced in any direction, which can result in diplopia. The eye is sometimes red, although this is certainly not a constant finding. Compression of the optic nerve or vascular supply to the eye may result in abnormal pupil findings or decreased vision. These patients are sometimes quite ill, although many patients appear well other than their ocular findings.

Differential Diagnosis

While preseptal cellulitis may be an associated finding in some noninfectious processes, such as local neoplasms, in most cases it is an infectious, and usually bacterial process.

Orbital cellulitis presents primarily as a space-occupying lesion and may be mimicked by orbital tumors, thyroid disease, and pseudotumor of the orbit. The last of these is a nonneoplastic inflammatory syndrome that involves swelling of orbital tissues.

Diagnosis

Preseptal cellulitis is a clinical diagnosis and should be made by inspection. Since preseptal cellulitis rarely is associated with a concurrent orbital process, no imaging studies of the orbit are necessary. However, because preseptal cellulitis is often the result of acute sinus disease, it is worthwhile to do plain sinus films to rule out a treatable underlying disease.

As is obvious from this discussion, orbital cellulitis must be differentiated from other tumorfactions of the orbit. Therefore, orbital CT scanning using high-resolution, thin cuts should be done early. The scan should include the sinuses to determine whether sinus inflammation is present. The goal of the imaging study is to rule out other causes of orbital inflammation and to detect an orbital abscess, if present.

In preseptal cellulitis it is unwise to attempt aspiration of subcutaneous material for culture. The reason for this is that the orbital septum may be inadvertently perforated, leading to introduction of infected material into the orbit and a change from an otherwise benign extraorbital process to a complicated and dangerous intraorbital infection.

Likewise, it is unwise to aspirate material from the orbit, since the danger of ocular perforation is high when the tissue planes are distorted by inflammation or abscess. Also there is the risk of dragging infected material into the subcutaneous tissues of the face.

Complications

Preseptal cellulitis is essentially a cosmetic problem. Treated easily it is rarely associated with complications.

Orbital cellulitis can result in both visual and systemic complications. Both reversible and permanent blindness are well reported. Extreme morbidity from cavernous sinus thrombosis is rare, but it should be feared in every case of orbital cellulitis [2]. Development of a subdural empyema, bacterial meningitis, or even death are known sequelae of this disease.

Treatment and Disposition

Preseptal cellulitis should be treated with hot compresses and antibiotics. It is unnecessary to admit these patients unless they are either sick or unreliable. As a rule of thumb patients who appear capable of taking their medications and following up appropriately are treated as outpatients (Table 35-2).

The microbiology of both preseptal and orbital cellulitis is essentially the microbiology of acute sinus disease. Therefore, the most common organisms are staphylococci, streptococci, and *Haemophilus influenzae* [3, 4]. For outpatients being treated with oral antibiotics, a combination of amoxicillin and clavulanic acid covers virtually all the usual organisms.

In general orbital cellulitis requires admission to the hospital and IV antibiotics. Again it is prefer-

Table 35-2. Disposition of patients with cellulitis

Preseptal	Orbital
Oral antibiotics	Admission
Hot compresses	IV antibiotics
Paranasal sinus x-ray	
Admission only if patient is unreliable or septic	CT scan of orbit and paranasal sinuses
Reevaluation in 24–28 hours	Reevaluation in 12–24 hours
	Surgery if patient fails to improve or abscess forms

able to use a drug that covers the most predominant organisms. Currently the combination of ampicillin and sulbactam is efficacious against the most common organisms encountered in this disease process.

Both preseptal and orbital cellulitis should resolve rapidly with appropriate antibiotic treatment. Patients with preseptal cellulitis should be examined in 24–48 hours, and patients with orbital cellulitis in 12–18 hours for evidence of improvement. When preseptal cellulitis does not appear to improve, the physician should suspect that either the antibiotic is not appropriate or the diagnosis is incorrect. When orbital cellulitis fails to improve, the same thoughts should be entertained but in addition the presence of an orbital abscess should be sought. When an orbital abscess is present and fails to respond to therapy in 12–24 hours, surgical drainage of the abscess and any infected contiguous sinuses must be strongly considered.

Eyelid Infections (Blepharitis)

Eyelid infections are common problems that bring patients to the emergency department. The complaints range from discomfort and annoyance to unsightly cosmetic deformity. Indeed some cases of preseptal cellulitis begin as an eyelid infection.

Definitions

Inflammation of the eyelid is referred to as *blepharitis*. Blepharitis can be infectious or noninfectious. When an immunologic reaction is the cause of blepharitis, the antigen involved is often a component of the nonpathogenic *Staphylococcus* species that live as normal flora on the eyelid margin [5].

Chalazia are sterile inflammatory granulomas of the meibomian glands. These glands are located in the fibrous tarsus of the lid, each lid containing approximately 30 glands. A chalazion develops when there is poor drainage from a gland, and sebaceous material backs up into the gland itself. This incites a granulomatous reaction to the material, resulting in inflammation and swelling of the immediate area. The redness and swelling may be seen on the skin side, the conjunctival side, or

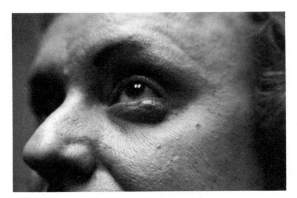

Fig. 35-1. Hordeolum ("stye")

both. Over time the inflammation abates, and the chalazion becomes hard and nodular.

A hordeolum is an acute inflammatory lesion of the external glands of the eyelid margin (Fig. 35-1). It is what generally is referred to as a "stye." Hordeola are often caused by gram-positive organisms, particularly staphylococci.

Treatment and Disposition

Eyelid infections are usually self-limited and are often the result of a reaction to nonpathogenic bacteria that live on the eyelid margins. For this reason lid hygiene is often the treatment of choice. Lid hygiene consists of hot compresses, using a washcloth soaked in running warm water, for approximately 5 minutes, 3 times a day. The soaking is followed by vigorous scrubbing of the eyelid margins for about ten seconds.

An antibiotic such as erythromycin ophthalmic ointment can be rubbed into the eyelid margin after soaking at bedtime to reduce the bacterial load in the eyelid margins. In addition some patients respond well to tetracycline 250 mg qid PO. The action of tetracycline is probably to change the composition of oils in the tear film in addition to its antiinfective role.

Nonophthalmologists should never use steroid-containing preparations, although it is tempting to do so in light of the inflammatory nature of eyelid infections. Any patient who fails to respond to lid hygiene should be referred to an ophthalmologist for further evaluation.

Conjunctivitis

Conjunctivitis refers to any inflammatory condition of the conjunctiva. Because the conjunctiva forms a continuous lining of both the inner eyelid and the external portion of the globe, conjunctivitis is usually associated with diffuse redness of the eye and inner lid.

Etiology

Inflammation of the conjunctiva (conjunctivitis) can be the result of infection by virus, bacteria, or chlamydia, or it can be an allergic reaction. Certain differentiating characteristics of these inflammations make it easy for an examiner with a handlight to come to a reasonable diagnosis (Fig. 35-2). For instance, the presence or absence of a preauricular node, the consistency of any discharge, and the duration of symptoms are clues for the examiner.

Viral conjunctivitis is accompanied by copious serous discharge and occasional photophobia. There is virtually always a tender preauricular node present on the affected side (see Chap. 10).

Bacterial conjunctivitis is associated with mucus and pus in the discharge, usually so heavy that the eyelids are stuck together in the morning and must be soaked to get them apart. No preauricular node is usually present. If the organism is gonococcus, the discharge is often so heavy that when it is wiped away it reaccumulates in 1–2 minutes.

Fig. 35-2. Bacterial conjunctivitis later proved to be secondary to gonococcus. The eye is diffusely inflamed, including both the palpebral and the bulbar conjunctiva

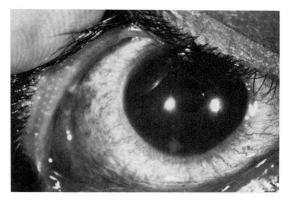

Chlamydial conjunctivitis presents with a several-week history of a bright, almost glowing redness of the conjunctiva. There is scant serous discharge and often the presence of a preauricular node. The history of several weeks of redness differentiates it from viral conjunctivitis, which is usually acute and fulminant and abates in 7–10 days.

Allergic conjunctivitis is associated with serous discharge, itching, and no pus. A preauricular node is not present.

Differentiation of the various forms of conjunctivitis can be made by scraping the conjunctiva and examining epithelial cells under the microscope after staining with Giemsa or other similar stain. Bacterial, viral, and chlamydial cultures also are useful. It is insufficient merely to culture the exudate or discharge, because this is reactive fluid and does not necessarily contain the infected organisms. The detection of eosinophils in the scraped material is diagnostic of allergic conjunctivitis.

Differential Diagnosis

The major differential diagnoses of conjunctivitis are conditions that cause redness of the eye without external inflammation.

Iritis is inflammation of the intraocular structures and usually appears as circumlimbal injection. There is pain, photophobia, and sometimes reduced vision. There should be no discharge and no preauricular node.

Acute angle-closure glaucoma is characterized by increased intraocular pressure with circumlimbal or diffuse redness of the bulbar conjunctiva. The palpebral conjunctiva should not be affected. There may be pain, nausea, and decreased vision. Palpation of the globe through the eyelid, when compared to the other eye, may allow the examiner to detect the greatly elevated intraocular pressure. There should, of course, be no discharge or preauricular node present.

Treatment

There is no antiinfective treatment of viral conjunctivitis. Patients should be instructed to use cold compresses, which seem to decrease the discomfort and swelling associated with the infection. In some cases antihistamine-containing eye drops can be prescribed, but this is best left to an ophthalmologist. The nonophthalmologist should never prescribe topical steroids.

Bacterial conjunctivitis should be treated with topical antibiotic drops or ointment. For most community acquired infections, erythromycin ophthalmic ointment or sulfacetamide 10% ophthalmic solution is more than sufficient treatment. Ophthalmologists tend to avoid preparations that contain neomycin, since over one-fourth of the population is sensitive to this antibiotic. Further redness of the eye may result for days following initiation of therapy, giving the impression that the infection is not responding to the antibiotic.

Chlamydial conjunctivitis should be treated with tetracycline 500 mg qid PO. Since chlamydia is a sexually transmitted infection, the patient's contacts also must be treated.

Keratitis

Inflammation of the cornea is referred to as *keratitis*. As in other parts of the body, disruption of the epithelium with underlying inflammation of the substantia propia is referred to as an *ulcer*. In the case of keratitis the stroma of the cornea is substantia propia. Therefore, a corneal ulcer is defined as a corneal epithelial defect with stromal inflammation.

Etiology

Corneal ulcers can be bacterial or viral or the result of a toxic reaction. The treatment in each case is quite different; therefore, it is essential that the proper diagnosis be made.

Bacterial keratitis presents as redness and pain. The examiner can detect a white lesion in the cornea. In some cases there is sufficient pus in the anterior chamber to result in a white fluid level, or hypopyon. Visual acuity is often reduced to 20/200 or worse. Both gram-negative and gram-positive organisms can be involved. *Staphylococcus* and *Streptococcus* species are the common gram-positive organisms. When there is a history of contact lens wear, particularly extended-wear soft contact

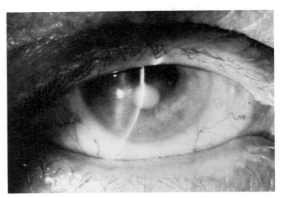

Fig. 35-3. Pseudomonas corneal ulcer in a patient wearing extended-wear soft contact lenses

lenses, gram-negative bacteria such as *Pseudomonas* species may cause a serious threat to vision (Fig. 35-3).

The most common viral etiology of a corneal ulcer is herpes simplex type I. In many cases the infection is localized to the epithelium in a dendritic form, although there is some underlying inflammation to qualify the lesion as an ulcer (Fig. 35-4). When the infection spreads into the corneal stroma, a serious situation ensues with the potential for recurrences, scarring, and sometimes permanent loss of vision. In many cases patients so infected require corneal transplantation. Patients who have purely epithelial infections almost invariably will develop stromal herpetic lesions if the cornea is treated with topical steroids. For that reason alone nonophthalmologists should never prescribe topical steroids under any circumstances.

Many conditions lead to toxic corneal ulcers.

Fig. 35-4. Keratitis caused by herpes simplex virus

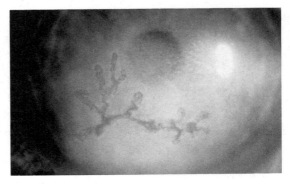

These include blepharitis, soft contact lens wear, and the chronic tuberculous infestation of the eyelids known as phlyctenulosis.

Diagnosis

Corneal ulcers are diagnosed by inspection that reveals redness of the bulbar conjunctiva, particularly in a circumlimbal or local orientation, with haziness of the cornea. A white corneal lesion may be noted. The patient should be referred to an ophthalmologist, who will scrape the cornea and make a culture of the epithelial cells.

Treatment and Disposition

Treatment should be instituted using intensive topical antibiotics if a bacterium is suspected or an antiviral agent such as trifluridine (Viroptic ophthalmic solution, 10%) if herpes simplex is suspected. These patients often require hospitalization to ensure that the drops are given on a timely basis. It has been shown that frequent, hourly or even half-hourly, topical antibiotic treatment of bacterial keratitis is more effective than subconjunctival or systemic administration of the antibiotics [6].

Endophthalmitis

Endophthalmitis is an overwhelming and catastrophic intraocular inflammatory process. When it is bacterial in origin, the condition can progress rapidly to blindness over the course of several hours.

Although endophthalmitis is defined as any intraocular inflammation, in its usual usage, the term refers to an overwhelming bacterial infection.

Common Clinical Situations

Bacterial endophthalmitis often occurs as a devastating complication of intraocular surgery. Although such surgery ordinarily is routine, increasing inflammation, pain, or reduced visual acuity are all warning signs that should be heeded in the early postoperative period. Unfortunately none of these is a constant finding, so every patient with even minor complaints within the first week or two after intraocular surgery should be examined and the

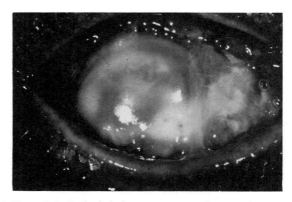

Fig. 35-5. Endophthalmitis in an eye 5 years after glaucoma surgery. This eye was completely quiet 24 hours prior to presentation

results compared to the most recent examination [7]. In addition any patient who has ever had glaucoma surgery is permanently at risk for the development of endophthalmitis because of the designed fistulization, which allows the external world into close proximity with the intraocular space [8] (Fig. 35-5).

The physical examination will reveal a red-hot eye, a pus-fluid level in the anterior chamber called a hypopyon, and an extremely limited view of the lens and fundus.

Unusual Endophthalmitis

Rarely endophthalmitis may be endogenous, the result of sepsis or an occult infection by bacteria, fungi, or viruses. Patients with overwhelming intraocular inflammation who have not had recent intraocular surgery should be suspected of having endogenous endophthalmitis, and an occult source of infection must be sought (Fig. 35-6).

Disposition

After the patient has been referred to an ophthalmologist, a culture of the intraocular contents should be taken. This procedure can be done in the clinic or the operating room, depending on the nature of the infection and other clinical circumstances. Treatment consists of a combination of intraocular antibiotics, systemic antibiotics, and in

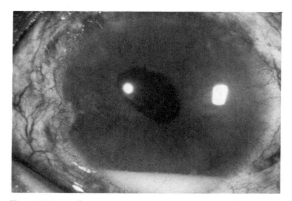

Fig. 35-6. A hypopyon in a patient with endogenous endophthalmitis secondary to overwhelming viral retinitis. This patient with AIDS was subsequently found to have CMV retinitis in the fellow eye

some cases removal of the vitreous itself (vitrectomy). Because of the urgency required in the management of endophthalmitis, an ophthalmologist should be consulted immediately when this diagnosis is suspected.

References

1. Jones DB, Steinkuller PG. Microbial preseptal and orbital cellulitis. In W Tasman, EA Jaeger (eds.), *Duane's Clinical Ophthalmology* (Vol. 4). Philadelphia: Lippincott, 1989. Chap. 25.
2. Harbour RC, Trobe JD, Ballinger WE. Septic cavernous sinus thrombosis associated with gingivitis and peripharyngeal abscess. *Arch Ophthalmol* 102:94–97, 1984.
3. Gellady AM, Shulman ST, Ayoub EM. Periorbital and orbital cellulitis in children. *Pediatrics* 61: 272–77, 1978.
4. Weiss A et al. Bacterial periorbital and orbital cellulitis in childhood. *Ophthalmology* 90:195–203, 1983.
5. Ostler HB. Blepharitis. In W Tasman, EA Jaeger (eds.), *Duane's Clinical Ophthalmology* (Vol. 4). Philadelphia: Lippincott, 1989. Chap. 22.
6. Baum J, Barza M. Topical vs. subconjunctival treatment of bacterial corneal ulcers. *Ophthalmology* 90:162–68, 1983.
7. Deutsch TA, Goldberg MF. Painless endophthalmitis. *Ophthalmic Surg* 15:837–40, 1984.
8. Lobue TD, Deutsch TA, Stein RM. *Moraxella nonliquefaciens* endophthalmitis after trabeculectomy. *Am J Ophthalmol* 99:343–45, 1985.

36

Mouth and Salivary Gland Infections

FRED S. HERZON

The oral cavity contains the dental apparatus and provides the terminal drainage point for the salivary glands. It is home to one of the most complex microbiologic habitats in the body. Over 200 bacterial species reside in the mouth [1]. There may be up to 10^{11} organisms per gram of collected material in some locations in the mouth [2]. Multiple excellent defense mechanisms prevent infections in the mouth and adjoining structures. These mechanisms include the epithelial barrier, the salivary flow, and the complex bacterial interaction of the resident organisms [3]. Additional protection comes from specific host defenses that include both humoral and cellular immunity [4]. Many of the oral, dental, and salivary gland infections that are commonly seen by physicians can be directly attributed to the breakdown of these protective barriers. Radiotherapy decreases vascular supply to oral tissue and permanently limits salivary flow. Poor dental hygiene can lead to perapical abscess, which in turn can invade the fascial spaces of the neck. Inadequate nutrition and hydration are prime etiologic factors in suppurative sialadenitis.

The Clinical Evaluation

History

As is true for any chief complaint, a good history must be obtained of any problem involving the mouth, the salivary glands, or the neck. Pain is probably the most common presenting symptom of infection, whether it originates on a mucosal surface, a dental structure, the neck, or a salivary gland. A history of trauma, factors that elicit pain, previous dental care, and previous antibiotic use is essential.

Examination

THE MOUTH

Proper evaluation of the mouth requires a good light, tongue blades, and gloves for palpation. The light can be a bright flashlight, a head mirror, or a head lamp. All mucosal surfaces and dental structures should be examined carefully and palpated if necessary. Palpation can reveal a loose tooth, tenderness, or fluctuance. Tooth percussion may elicit pain in infected teeth. Oral carcinoma may present with a relatively short history, have some ulceration with secondary infection, and manifest as a painful lesion. Short-term antibiotic treatment may relieve some of the symptoms but will not eliminate the lesion. Close follow-up of intraoral lesions is necessary to ensure that a malignancy will not be missed. Oral mucosal lesions can be caused by a variety of infectious agents and present from plaque-like lesions to ulcerative or vesicular lesions that are red to white in color. Table 36-1 provides a differential diagnosis of oral lesions by appearance.

THE NECK

Swelling of the neck or salivary glands is the most common sign of inflammation of these structures.

Table 36-1. Differential diagnosis by appearance of common oral mucosal lesions

Clinical description	Differential diagnosis	Presenting symptoms	Distinguishing features	Diagnostic tests
White lesions	Pseudomembranous candidiasis	Burning	Plaques wipe off easily	Culture, smear
	Hyperplastic candidiasis	—	Adherent plaques	Biopsy
	Trauma—physical, chemical, electrical	Pain	History, sloughing	—
	Bacterial—staphylococcal, streptococcal, diphtheria, Trepomema pallidum	Pain	Erythema, sloughing	Culture
	Benign keratosis	No pain	Homogeneous	Biopsy
	Dysplasia, squamous cell carcinoma	Mild or no pain	Irregular white patch	Biopsy
Red-white lesions	Candidiasis	Burning	Erythema, plaques	Culture, smear
	Mucositis	Burning, pain	Chemotherapy or irradiation	Culture, smear
	Bacterial—staphylococcal, streptococcal, others	Pain	Erythema, sloughing	Culture, smear
	Dysplasia, carcinoma	Minimal or no pain	Irregular red-white	Biopsy
Red lesions	Atrophic candidiasis	Burning	Depapillation of tongue, erythema	Culture, smear
	Mucositis	Burning	Chemotherapy or irradiation	Culture, smear
	Bacterial	Burning, pain	Erythema	Culture, smear
	Viral (CMV)	Burning	Mucosal erythema	Viral study
	Pemphigoid	Burning	Gingiva epithelial sloughing	Biopsy
	Lichen planus	Burning	Buccal mucosa, tongue	Biopsy
	Erythema multiforme	Burning	History, skin lesions	—
	Dysplasia, carcinoma	Minimal pain	Erythema	Biopsy

Vesicular lesions	HSV, primary	Pain, malaise	Lymphadenopathy, fever, gingival lesions	History, viral studies
	HSV, recurrent	Pain	Lip, gingiva	History
	Coxsackie	Pain	Oropharynx	History, viral studies
	VZV (chicken-pox)	Variable	Skin, oral mucosa	History, viral studies
	VZV (recurrent)	Pain	Neurologic pattern	History, viral studies
	Rubella	Systemic	Buccal mucosa	History
Ulcerative lesions	Viral	Pain	Round, 1–2 mm ulcers in clusters	Culture, viral studies
	Aphthous	Pain	Nonkeratinized mucosa, family history, regular borders	Biopsy
	Trauma	Pain	History, irregular borders	—
	Fungal—*candida*, *aspergillus*, others	Variable	Indurated ulcer	Culture, biopsy
	Malignancy	No or minimal pain	Indurated ulcer	History, biopsy
Pigmented lesions	Melanoma, vascular	No symptoms	Location, color	History, biopsy
Masses and Tumors	Malignancy	Variable	Size, texture, base, location	History, biopsy

Source: Reprinted with permission from Otolaryngologic Clinics of North America in A. Chow (ed.) Infectious Syndromes of the Head and Neck, Vol. 2(1). Philadelphia: Saunders. Table 1, pp. 188–89.

Fluctuance is an easily identifiable sign that confirms an abscess. Absence of fluctuation in an inflammatory neck mass does not rule out this process. Either needle aspiration or radiologic evaluation may be required for diagnosis.

THE SALIVARY GLANDS

Swelling and tenderness of the parotid and submandibular glands are the common manifestations of infection in these structures. Careful intraoral inspection may reveal pus coming from the major salivary duct openings opposite the second maxillary molar or in the anterior floor of the mouth. Obstruction of the ducts by a stone may prevent pus or saliva from flowing out of the ducts. This sign is difficult to observe with unaided vision.

The Mouth

Oral manifestations of infectious disease that does not arise from the teeth are heterogeneous. Viruses, particularly childhood enanthems, are frequent causes of oral lesions. Other viruses, such as as coxsackieviruses and herpes simplex virus, are also common. Oral lesions may be found in debilitated and immunosuppressed patients (candidiasis, gangrenous stomatitis). Sexually transmitted diseases are also considerations. Table 36-2 summarizes major infectious oral lesions by entity.

Noninfectious oral lesions also must be considered. Erythema multiforme may present with stomatitis, conjunctivitis, and rash. Stevens-Johnson syndrome is a severe form of erythema multiforme

Table 36-2. Nonodontogenic mouth lesions

Disease	Symptoms or history	Description	Antibiotics	Comments
Herpangina	Sore throat, odontophagia; in children refusal to eat	Vesicles on soft palate, tonsils, and uvula, up to 12 lesions	None	Symptomatic treatment
Hand-foot-mouth disease	Children: T = 38°–39°C, mouth pain, refusal to eat	Vesicles on buccal mucosa and tongue; peripheral rash	None	Symptomatic treatment
Herpes simplex virus infection	Generalized prodrome	Vesicles, extensive involvement of oral mucosa	None	Symptomatic treatment
Candidiasis	Infants, debilitated, immunosuppressed	Patchy white, plaques, erythema underlying plaques	Nystatin or clotrimazole troche	KOH stain of scraping
Gonorrhea	Recent antibiotic tx, exposure to STD, fever, malaise	Pharyngitis with exudate	Ceftriaxone (see Chap. 30)	
Syphilis	Exposure to STD		Penicillin (see Chap. 30)	
Primary	Extragenital lesion rare	Chancre on lip, tongue, tonsil		
Secondary		Mucous patch, pharyngitis		Highly infectious
Recurrent aphthous stomatitis	Oral burning, extreme pain 10–20 years	Ulcers 2–5 mm, buccal and labial mucosa, yellow-gray with red margins	None	Anesthetic topical paste

that involves mucous membranes extensively. Vesicles, bullae, and crusted or bleeding lesions may be noted about the mouth. This syndrome may be confused with severe herpetic gingivostomatitis, but lesions of Stevens-Johnson syndrome are more extensive. This is a medical emergency, and the patient should be hospitalized for observation.

Oral burns and other traumatic injuries must be considered, and an appropriate history elicited. Burns can be caused by hot foods, caustic substances, or electrical injury (e.g., a child biting an electric cord). Angular cheilosis, painful fissures at the mouth corners, can result from iron deficiency anemia, candidiasis, or local allergic reactions. Systemic lupus erythematosus can lead to oral ulcers and petechiae. Mucositis is suspected in the patient undergoing chemotherapy or irridation. Malignancy must be considered in lesions slow to resolve (see Table 36-1).

Coxsackievirus Infections

HERPANGINA

The majority of cases of herpangina are caused by coxsackie A viruses. The disease is often seasonal, seen frequently from June to October, with most cases being seen in children and adolescents. It appears less commonly in adults [5]. The presentation is similar to any viral pharyngitis, with fever, malaise, and sore throat. Physical examination will show small vesicles anywhere on the mucosal surface of the mouth but most commonly on the structures of the faucial arch (tonsillar pillars and soft palate). These vesicles rupture within a day or two, leaving shallow ulcers. The disease is self-limited, requiring only supportive care. The lesions are painful, so herpangina should be suspected in young children who will not eat.

HAND-FOOT-MOUTH DISEASE

Coxsackie A viruses are also responsible for hand-foot-mouth disease. In addition to the oral lesions there are vesicles or papules on the hands and the feet. Seventy-five percent of the cases will occur in children below the age of 4 years. The syndrome lasts 3–7 days [6].

ACUTE LYMPHONODULAR PHARYNGITIS

Acute lymphonodular pharyngitis is much less common then the other coxsackievirus infections.

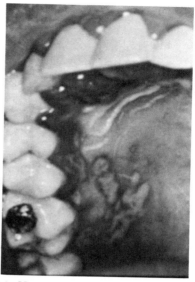

Fig. 36-1. Herpes simplex vesicles on the hard palate. (Reprinted with permission from Bengel W. *Differential Diagnosis of Diseases of the Oral Mucosa.* Lombard, IL: Quintessence, 1989. Fig. 6–10a)

The initial picture is similar to herpangina as seen in children, with complaints of sore throat, fever, anorexia, and perhaps some lymphadenitis. The lesions consist of raised whitish-yellow nodules located on the posterior pharyngeal wall. There are no oral lesions present. Symptoms last 1–2 weeks [7].

Herpes Simplex

Primary herpetic gingivostomatitis is most often caused by herpes simplex virus type 1 (HSV-1) [8]. The disease may be seen in all age groups, and the patient will present with a history of generalized prodromal symptoms of fever, headache, malaise, and possibly nausea, followed by development of oral lesions. Vesicles may be noted throughout the oral mucosa (Fig. 36-1), which, like those in cocksackievirus infections, will rupture and leave ulcers. They may coalesce into larger lesions. The gingivitis is more pronounced in the herpetic infection and may be helpful in the differential diagnosis [5]. In the healthy patient supportive care is the only treatment.

Candidiasis

Thrush is a superficial infection of the mucosa of the oral cavity that results in patchy whitish plaques consisting of desquamated epithelial and leukocytic cells. The mucosa surrounding the plaques may be erythematous, and the plaques are easily dislodged. Since candida is a normal inhabitant of the mouth, the infection is opportunistic. It is seen in all types of debilitated patients and may be secondary to antibiotic treatment for any manner of conditions. Several other infectious diseases appear clinically similar to oral candidiasis, so diagnosis depends on obtaining a history of prior antibiotic use or noting the characteristic oral lesions in a debilitated patient. Oral candidiasis is also seen in young children and may be associated with a candidal diaper rash. Breast-fed infants of mothers on antibiotics or with fungal infection in the nipples also may have thrush. Definitive diagnosis requires microscopic examination of the lesions and identification of the yeast. Oral topical nystatin or clotrimazole troches plus elimination of the predisposing factors will usually reverse acute oral candidiasis.

Sexually Transmitted Diseases

GONORRHEA

Gonococcal oropharyngitis is not physically distinguishable from any other acute bacterial oropharyngitis. The patient will present with sore throat, fever, and malaise. Oral examination will show erythema of the oropharynx and tonsils, with occasional mucopurulent exudate. Diagnosis depends on a good history to identify high-risk patients (e.g., homosexuals). Specific instructions to the laboratory requesting culture media (Thayer-Martin) to identify *Neisseria gonorrhoeae* are necessary to obtain accurate microbiological identification. Treatment is a single dose of ceftriaxone 250 mg IM.

SYPHILIS

Primary Syphilis. In primary syphilis chancre is rarely seen anywhere in the oral cavity. Extragenital oropharyngeal syphilitic chancres were not uncommon many years ago, being seen most commonly on the lip but also on the tongue and the tonsil [9].

Secondary Syphilis. Mucous patches may be seen anywhere in the oral cavity in secondary syphilis. These patches are considered the most highly infectious lesions of this disease [5]. The examiner also may see what appears to a prolonged pharyngitis, with the patient complaining of sore throat over a few weeks and physical examination showing only erythema of the oropharynx and tonsillitis. The appearance of secondary oral syphilis is not distinctive and, as in gonorrhea, requires a high index of suspicion to initiate the appropriate serologic testing to make the proper diagnosis.

Tertiary Syphilis. Gummatous lesions of the palate and the tongue are almost never seen.

AIDS

There are no unique oral manifestations of AIDS. Patients with this disease will complain of oral masses and difficult, painful swallowing. They will present with oral candidiasis, hairy leukoplakia, herpes simplex, Kaposi's sarcoma, intraoral ulcers, and benign follicular lymphoid hyperplasia (see Chap. 17) [10]. These problems rarely are the chief complaint of a patient with AIDS, so the systemic diagnosis usually will have been made. Oral candidiasis may be a marker for esophageal candidiasis [11]. If the diagnosis is AIDS appropriate referral is indicated.

Recurrent Aphthous Stomatitis

Recurrent aphthous stomatitis is a relatively common disease that is characterized by recurrent ulcers of the oral mucosa in patients who are otherwise well. Although commonly thought to be of viral etiology, it appears that this pathology is related to some form of an altered immune response rather than an overt infection [12, 13]. The disease often may start during adolescence with the individual noting some burning prior to the appearance of small, shallow, painful ulcers most commonly seen on the buccal and labial mucosa. The pharynx and the tonsils are not involved. The lesions are yellow-gray with raised red margins. Lymphadenopathy occurs only after secondary bacterial infection. There may be several lesions, which in most cases will resolve over several days. The patients are often uncomfortable, experiencing pain that may seem out of proportion to the observable lesions. Oral ulcers are also a feature of Behçet's disease, other features of which include genital ulcers and iritis. Treatment of aphthous ulcers is local, consisting of strict oral hygiene and medications containing steroids in a paste vehicle such as as Orabase. In more severe cases tetracycline mouthwashes (250 mg in 5 ml water qid) have been found to be helpful in decreasing the symptomatology and duration of the illness [14].

Symptomatic Relief of Oral Infections

Specific therapeutic intervention is the ideal way to deal with mucosal infections of the mouth. In addition the following symptomatic measures should be considered for the immediate relief of the patient's symptoms:

1. *Diet.* A bland soft diet without a high salt or acid content is useful. Consultation with a dietitian is useful.
2. *Mouth wash.* Simple saline or bicarbonate solutions are helpful in removing thickened secretions or necrotic debris from mucosal ulcers. Hydrogen peroxide in addition to mechanical cleansing of the mouth may be useful in helping periodontal infections in which anaerobic organisms may be involved [15].
3. *Topical anesthetics.* Any of the topical anesthetic agents, such as viscous lidocaine or benzocaine, can provide short-term improvement of symptoms. This is especially useful if the patient's oral discomfort is interfering with fluid and caloric intake.
4. *Coating agents.* Preparations such as milk of magnesia, kaolin-pectin, and amphogel can be used as a palliative oral swish when mucosal ulcerations are present [7]. A paste of kaolin-pectin, viscous xylocaine, and diphenhydramine elixir may be prepared.

Infections of Dental and Cervical Spaces

Odontogenic infections of the mouth are summarized in Table 36-3.

Dental Caries and Plaque

Dental caries and plaque, with their attendant microbiological components, are the most common "infectious disease" that affects the mouth. Over 90% of the population of the United States have had dental caries at some time in their lives, and there are close to 500 million untreated cavities in any given year [16, 17]. Although caries may be considered less then life threatening, they are re-

Table 36-3. Odontogenic mouth infections

Disease	Symptoms or history	Description	Treatment	Comments
Pulpitis/periapical abscess	Tooth pain	Localized gingival swelling, tooth percussion tenderness	Penicillin or erythromycin	Dental referral, abscess drainage
Simple gingivitis	Bleeding or pain on tooth brushing or eating	Diffuse gingival inflammation	Dental hygiene	
Acute necrotizing ulcerative gingivitis	Gum pain and bleeding, taste alteration, fever, malaise, lymphadenopathy	Shallow ulcers, gray membrane, fetid odor	Metronidazole or clindamycin or penicillin	Dental referral
Odontogenic cellulitis	History of dental infections, cheek pain and swelling	Buccal induration, tenderness, erythema	Penicillin or erythromycin	Dental referral, admission for extensive involvement

sponsible for a considerable amount of oral morbidity, which if severe enough can force a patient to seek help in an urgent care or emergency department facility. The primary complaint the patient will have is pain. Without proper radiologic and dental equipment, unavailable in most emergency departments, the diagnosis becomes one of exclusion. The emergency physician must rule out progression of the carious process to pulpitis or periapical abscess. If plaque and caries are left untreated, they become the basis for the more severe and often life-threatening fascial-space infections not uncommonly seen in emergency departments. The emergency physician must educate the patient to the need for dental follow-up and provide appropriate referral.

Pulpitis and Periapical Abscess

The pulp of the tooth is the central soft-tissue core containing connective tissue, blood vessels, and nerves, which enter through the apical foramen at the base of the tooth. This area can become infected when caries penetrate the center of the tooth, or when periodontitis allows egress of bacteria to the pulp via the perapical foramen. Once pulpitis occurs, the infection can spread out of the apical foramen and form a periapical abscess (Fig. 36-2). The patient will complain of pain. The pain may be excruciating as pressure builds within the unyielding enamel and bone, or it may be aching if drainage is occurring. Examination may show gingival swelling and erythema adjacent to the affected tooth, and occasionally pus will be coming from the tooth socket (Fig. 36-3). Percussion of the tooth may elicit tenderness. Compression of the gum over the root tip may also elicit pain. A panorex x-ray may show the periapical bone erosion typical of this process.

Treatment consists of antibiotics such as penicillin or erythromycin for the penicillin-allergic patient and referral for dental evaluation within 24 hours. Tooth extraction or a root canal may be necessary. If an abscess can be identified on the gingiva, dental consultation (if available) may be obtained to drain the abscess, but care must be taken if an abscess exists, to avoid dissemination of infection. Analgesia can be obtained with a regional dental block.

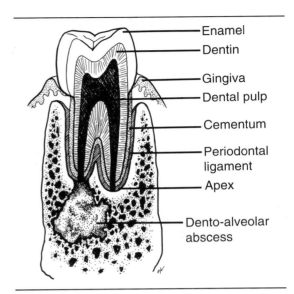

Enamel
Dentin
Gingiva
Dental pulp
Cementum
Periodontal ligament
Apex
Dento-alveolar abscess

Fig. 36-2. Anatomy of a tooth with periapical abscess

Periodontal Infection

SIMPLE GINGIVITIS

Simple gingivitis is an almost universally common disorder [18, 19] that manifests itself as either an acute or a chronic bacterial inflammation of the gingival tissue surrounding the teeth. Pain or bleeding on tooth brushing or eating may be noted. Over a long period of time it can result in periapical bone lose and ultimately loss of teeth. There is rarely acute symptomatology associated with this condition. This process is not usually seen as a primary diagnosis in an emergency department. Treatment is improved dental hygiene.

ACUTE NECROTIZING
ULCERATIVE GINGIVITIS

Acute necrotizing ulcerative gingivitis (ANUG), also referred to as Vincent's infection, trench mouth, and pseudomembranous angina, is an oral infection that appears rapidly over 24–48 hours. Its etiology is not absolutely clear, but there appears to be some relationship to stress [20]. It is seen in all age groups and may be associated with any debilitating illness. The onset of pain is acute and may interfere with eating. Taste alterations are noted, and bleeding is common. There is a fetid odor

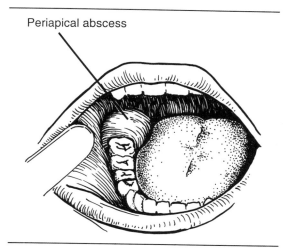

Periapical abscess

Fig. 36-3. Clinical appearance of periapical abscess

accompanying the infection. The patient has systemic symptoms, including fever, malaise, and regional lymphadenopathy. The lesions seen are shallow ulcers, usually covered by a gray membrane, on the gingival and oral surfaces. Multiple organisms are responsible for ANUG, including streptococci, oral treponemes, *Bacteroides melaninogenicus*, and *Fusobacterium* species [21]. Treatment includes local débridement, aggressive oral hygiene, and oral metronidazole, clindamycin, or penicillin. Decisions about hospitalization depend on the patient's circumstances rather than on the oral pathology.

Gangrenous stomatitis (Noma) no longer occurs in the United States, but it does occur in debilitated, malnourished children elsewhere. Although similar to ANUG it is more focal and destroys tissues deeper than the gingiva. The initial painful red spot or vesicle leads to a necrotic ulcer. Extension leads to cellulitis of the lips and cheeks. Admission and high-dose IV penicillin are required.

Cellulitis

The first manifestation of dental infection in the soft tissue of the face and neck is cellulitis close to the offending tooth. The microbiologic process (mixed aerobic and anaerobic), be it any of the previously discussed conditions, has moved from a localized dental infection to the tissues outside the oral cavity. The patient will present to the emergency department with the complaint of pain and swelling in the cheek or skin close to the mandible. The swelling may be intraoral or extraoral. The history should include questions about toothache, trauma, and difficulty with swallowing or talking. Physical examination will confirm the swelling, induration, and tenderness. There may be erythema of the skin, fever, and rarely mild trismus. The differential diagnosis includes nonodontogenic causes of lateral facial swelling. Trauma and trauma-related infections must be considered. In the young child purplish swelling may indicate *Haemophilus influenzae* cellulitis. Parotitis and insect bite also must be considered. Management includes penicillin, pain medication, and dental referral. Definitive treatment involves tooth extraction or a root canal. If the patient is already on penicillin, then a change to include broader-spectrum antistaphylococcal and antianaerobic antibiotics would be appropriate. Attention to the treatment of this disease is important, because the infection may be the precursor of more severe cervical fascial infections. If infection has spread beyond the buccal pouch, otolaryngologic, dental, or maxillofacial consultation is indicated. IV antibiotics or surgical drainage may be necessary.

Infections of the Cervical Fascial Spaces

Most infections of the deep cervical fascial spaces are secondary to sublingual IV drug abuse, odontogenic infections, and oropharyngeal infections. The most common symptoms seen are pain, fever, swelling, dysphagia, and odynophagia [22]. Table 36-4 summarizes these infections. Evaluation of the airway is the most important immediate initial assessment and should be made on any patient presenting with a serious head and neck space infection. Virtually any fascial-space infection or abscess discussed here can be complicated by airway obstruction. The security of the airway outweighs any choice of antibiotic or identification of the offending organism. Even if there is no airway compromise when the patient arrives in the emergency department, it can develop while the patient awaits evaluation by an emergency physician or is being seen by a specialty consultant. If there is any question about airway integrity on initial evaluation,

Table 36-4. Cervical fascial space infections

Infection	Symptoms or history	Location	Antibiotic	Comments
Submandibular abscess	Antecedent dental infection	Mass below and adjacent to jaw	Metronidazole or ampicillin-sulbactam or cefoxitin or cefotetan	Admission, surgical drainage
Ludwig's angina	Antecedent dental infection	Cellulitis of entire submandibular space, floor of mouth elevated and tongue pushed up	Metronidazole or ampicillin-sulbactam or cefoxitin or cefotetan	Admission, surgical drainage
Masticator infection	Antecedent dental infection	Swelling external to posterior mandible	Metronidazole or ampicillin-sulbactam or cefoxitin or cefotetan	Admission, surgical drainage
Pharyngomaxillary (lateral pharyngeal)	Antecedent phanyngitis	Swelling behind posterior pillar of tonsil	Penicillin or metronidazole or clindamycin	Admission, surgical drainage
Peritonsillar infection	Antecedent phanyngitis	Swelling superior to tonsil, uvular deviation	Penicillin or erythromycin or cefazolin	Needle aspiration in emergency department
Anterior visceral space	Esophageal perforation, attempts to place IV in internal jugular vein	Swelling midline and perimidline of neck	Ampicillin-sulbactam or penicillin + metronidazole or cefoxitin or cefotetan	Admission, incision and drainage, may replace with surgical drainage
Retropharyngeal prevertebral	Antecedent pharyngitis, pharyngeal perforation	Erythema, swelling of posterior pharyngeal wall	Ampicillin-sulbactam or penicillin + metronidazole or cefoxitin or cefotetan	Secure airway first, lateral neck x-ray or CT scan, admission, incision and drainage, may replace with surgical drainage

the airway should be secured by whatever appropriate means are available, be it endotracheal intubation or by surgical means. Tertiary-care centers should not allow transportation of these patients to their facility unless airway protection is assured.

Head and neck abscesses are caused by a wide variety of aerobic and anaeorbic organisms including streptococci, *staphylococcus aureus*, and *Peptostreptoccus* and *Bacteroides* species [19]. In children *S. aureus* and *Bacteroides* organisms are the pathogens most commonly identified [23]. Treatment of most of these infections requires hospitalization, IV antibiotics (penicillin and metronidazole or clindamycin, ampicillin-clavulonic acid, ampicillin-sulbactam, or chloramphenicol, if there is penicillin allergy) and surgical drainage. An understanding of the anatomy of the fascial spaces that may become infected is important in evaluating a patient presenting to the emergency department with this disease. Levitt's anatomic division of the neck based on the hyoid bone provides an excellent way of approaching these compartments [24].

SPACES ABOVE THE HYOID

The Submandibular Space. The submandibular space is divided by the mylohyoid into the sublingual (above) and submaxillary (below) spaces (Fig. 36-4 and Fig. 36-5). Because the submandibular space is adjacent to the mandible, it is most commonly infected secondary to dental infection.

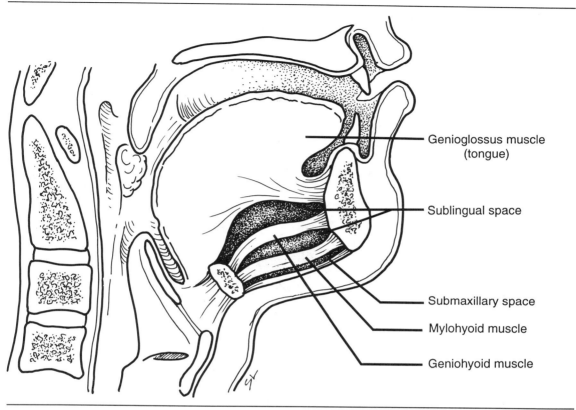

Fig. 36-4. Sagittal section through floor of mouth. Note submaxillary and sublingual spaces. (Adapted with permission from Paonessa DF, Goldstein JC. Anatomy and physiology of head and neck infections, infectious diseases of the head and neck. *Otolaryngol Clin North Am* 6(3):572, 1976.)

The space below the hyoid (submaxillary) is most commonly affected, representing approximately 25% of all neck infections seen in one study [19]. The inflammation usually begins from one of the teeth, progresses to a cellulitis, and finally develops into a full-blown abscess. Physically the swelling is obvious just below and adjacent to the jaw. Fluctuation may be difficult to define initially because of the tenseness of the skin. A needle aspiration usually will confirm the diagnosis. This procedure can be performed by emergency department personnel, but if the result is positive needle aspiration should not be used to empty the abscess cavity, since that could interfere with radiologic delineation of the disease. Hospitalization is indicated in all but the earliest of these infections. If the abscess is small and the patient is not toxic, then the abscess can be treated on an outpatient basis with needle aspiration and oral antibiotics [25]. This therapy should not be attempted by anyone without significant experience in the treatment of fascial-space infections of the head and neck.

Ludwig's angina is an infection that when advanced involves the complete submandibular space affecting the area bilaterally above and below the mylohyoid (see Fig. 36-4 and Fig. 36-5). There is a cellulitis throughout the tissues with little or no frank pus encountered [26]. Clinically there will be diffuse swelling of the entire submandibular space. The swelling will be woody without any apparent fluctuation. The mouth will be open with the tongue pushed up to the arch of the hard palate secondary to marked elevation of the floor of the mouth. The patient will have mild to severe respira-

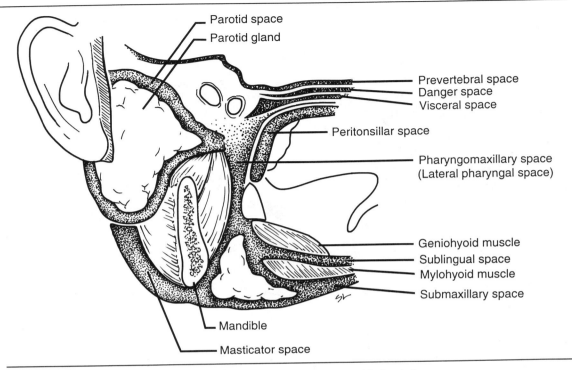

Fig. 36-5. Oblique section of the angle of the mandible. Note submandibular (sublingual and submaxillary) masticator and pharyngomaxillary spaces. (Adapted with permission from Paonessa DF, Goldstein JC. Anatomy and physiology of head and neck infections, infectious diseases of the head and neck. *Otolaryngol Clin North Am* 6(3):570, 1976)

tory distress, have trouble handling secretions, and appear toxic and have a fever. Treatment includes hospitalization, securing an airway (usually a tracheotomy), IV antibiotics, incision, and drainage. On a rare occasion this disease may be seen in a very early stage, in which the floor of the mouth is only mildly edematous, the tongue is not significantly raised, and there is no respiratory distress. Hospitalization for medical management and careful airway observation may suffice in that situation.

The Masticator Space. As indicated by its name, the masticator space involves all the muscles of mastication, including the masseter, the external and internal pterygoids, and the insertion of the temporalis on the mandible. The ramus and the posterior portion of the body of the mandible form the medial wall for this space (see Fig. 36-5). Dental infections are the antecedent cause for infec-

tion of the masticator space. Swelling is usually external, adjacent to the posterior body and the ramus of the mandible. Occasionally the infection may point intraorally if the medial portion of the space is involved. Trismus is prominent but airway obstruction uncommon, unless the patient does not seek treatment for several days. For most cases hospitalization and surgical drainage are indicated. A small subset of the patients who have an early lateral abscess may be treated as an outpatient basis with needle aspiration, oral antibiotics, pain medication, and close follow-up [24]. Referral to a head and neck specialist for this type of treatment is appropriate.

The Pharyngomaxillary Space (lateral pharyngeal). The pharyngomaxillary space may be visualized as an upside-down cone with its base sitting on the base of the skull and the rest of the cone narrowing to an apex at the hyoid bone. It is also known as the lateral pharyngeal or peripharyngeal space. Its medial wall borders the carotid sheath posteriorly and the tonsil and pharygeal wall anteriorly (see Fig. 36-5 and Fig. 21-2). The patient will present with a complaint of sore throat and difficulty swallowing. The key to diagnosis is severe trismus and evidence of swelling behind the posterior pillar of the tonsil, pushing the tonsillar fossa anteriorly and medially. This abscess may be easily confused with a peritonsillar abscess, both of which are discussed in detail in Chap. 21.

The Peritonsillar Space.

The peritonsillar space lies between the capsule of the tonsil, the superior constrictor muscle, and the anterior and posterior tonsillar pillars. Its infection is by far the most common abscess of the fascial spaces seen in the head and neck, accounting for approximately 70% of those seen [27]. This condition is also the easiest to treat in the emergency department setting. The abscess most often is preceded by a suppurative pharyngotonsillitis. Clinically patients will present to the emergency department complaining of severe sore throat. They will have fever, trismus, and a "hot potato" voice. Examination will reveal trismus and swelling of the superior peritonsillar tissue. The uvula will be moved toward the side opposite the infection. This condition is discussed in detail in Chap. 21.

SPACES BELOW THE HYOID

The Anterior Visceral Space. This fascial compartment surrounds the central visceral structures of the neck, including the larynx, trachea, and thyroid gland, and lies against the anterior wall of the esophagus (see Fig. 36-5 and Fig. 21-5). It extends from the top of the thyroid cartilage of the larynx down to the arch of the aorta. This space may become infected from an esophageal perforation or from attempts to utilize the internal jugular vein for IV drug use. Clinically there will be diffuse erythema, induration, and tenderness in the midline and perimidline of the neck. Dysphagia may be present because the larynx is mobile during deglutition. An abscess of this space is extremely dangerous because of it direct communication with the superior mediastinum. Hospitalization, IV antibiotics, and appropriate drainage are required.

SPACES TRAVERSING THE ENTIRE NECK

The Carotid Sheath. The carotid sheath by itself rarely becomes solely infected except in IV drug users. It can, however, provide a pathway for infection from various other fascial spaces to spread throughout the neck (see Chap. 21).

The Retropharyngeal-Prevertebral Space. Anatomically the retropharyngeal space, the prevertebral space, and the "danger" space between the deglutory tract and the vertebral column can be identified (see Fig. 21-2 and Fig. 21-5). These fascial spaces can be traced to the mediastinum and ultimately to the tip of the coccyx. If an infection develops initially in one of these spaces, the patient will complain of dysphagia and odontophagia. When seen in children (which is extremely rare today), the child will not extend the head or swallow saliva. Examination will show swelling and erythema of the posterior orpharyngeal wall. This condition is more completely discussed in Chap. 21.

The Superficial Cervical Space. There is a potential fascial space running from the mandible to the clavicle below the platysma. Isolated abscesses in this space are relatively rare and arise from suppurative breakdown of an infected lymph node or from neck trauma. Involvement more commonly is associated with other contiguous deep-space infections. Because of the superficial nature of this anatomic area, smaller abscesses occurring there lend themselves to outpatient medical and surgical treatment.

Salivary Glands

Infections of the salivary glands are summarized in Table 36-5.

Acute Infectious Sialadenitis

BACTERIAL INFECTIONS

The parotid and the submandibular (submaxillary) major salivary glands are the likely sites of suppurative sialadenitis. In adults the debilitated or postoperative state is the setting in which this disease is seen. Up to one-third of the cases of purulent

Table 36-5. Salivary gland infections

Infection	Symptoms or history	Location and signs	Antibiotic	Comments
Acute infectious sialadenitis	Debilitated, post-operative, children with history of viral parotitis	Pain, tenderness, erythema, fever	Dicloxacillin or cephazolin	Admission
		Parotid gland: swelling anterior and inferior to ear; submandibular gland: swelling inferior to body of mandible		
Mumps	Malaise, fever	Pus from salivary gland, bilateral gonadal or CNS involvement	None	
Sialolithiasis	Symptoms with eating	Usually submandibular involved, may be pus from salivary duct, fewer systemic symptoms than acute sialadenitis	None	Stone visualized on x-ray, sialogogues
Recurrent parotitis in children	Onset <6 years	Periodic unilateral or bilateral swelling	Penicillin	No stone

sialadenitis are associated with a postoperative condition [28]. Patients presenting to an emergency department are more likely to have dehydration or debilitation as their predisposing factors. Children with viral parotitis may also develop a secondary suppurative infection. In one study of 36 patients with septic parotitis all the patients were over 77 years of age. Penicillin-resistant *S. aureus* was the most common organism recovered, followed by an occasional *Streptococcus viridans* [29]. Clinical diagnosis is not difficult, because the patient will present with swelling in the confines of the specific gland involved, usually the parotid. There will be pain, tenderness, erythema, and possible fever. Pus coming from the intraoral opening of the gland duct will confirm the diagnosis. If no purulence is seen, then gentle pressure exerted on the skin overlying the swollen gland, moving from posterior to anterior, may produce a positive result. Mortality from this disease has been reported, so aggressive therapy

is indicated [28], usually hospitalization for treatment of the debilitation and for IV antibiotics effective against penicillin-resistant *S. aureus*. Rarely an abscess developing from a suppurative parotitis will require drainage.

VIRAL INFECTIONS
Mumps (paramyxovirus) was once the most common viral infection seen in the United States, with almost all cases seen in children or adolescents. Since the development of a vaccine in 1967 the number of cases has been reduced by up to 90% [5]. The disease is characterized by the sudden onset of bilateral parotid swelling associated with generalized malaise and fever. There may be associated gonadal and CNS involvement. Mumps used to be the most common cause of unilateral neurosensory deafness in children. Various other viruses, such as coxsackievirus A, parainfluenza, and echovirus, and lymphocytic choriomeningitis also have been

implicated in viral parotitis. Treatment is supportive.

SIALOLITHIASIS

Although not strictly an infectious disease, stones in the salivary glands quite frequently are complicated by secondary bacterial infection. Eighty to 90% of stones occur in the submandibular gland [30, 31]. Presentation includes acute swelling of the gland associated with severe pain. There may be a history of fluctuating swelling associated with eating. Systemic signs are variable, depending on whether secondary bacterial infection has occurred. An enlarged tender gland will be noted on examination. Intraoral examination of the duct orifice for pus will yield variable results depending on the completeness of the obstruction. Careful examination of the floor of the mouth by inspection or palpation may reveal a stone in the Wharton's duct. Approximately 80% of these stones are radiopaque. A periapical or occlusal x-ray will pick up most submandibular stones, and oblique views of the mandible are useful for the parotid gland. Sinlography is a somewhat complicated procedure that, in the author's experience, is not particularly valuable in making this diagnosis. Medical therapy includes antibiotics (antistaphylococcal) and sialogogues (hard candy) when no large stone is noted to stimulate salivation to wash the gland free of small minor stones. If a stone is large enough to be felt within the Wharton's duct, then referral for intraoral outpatient removal is indicated. Parenchymal stones may require surgical removal of the submaxillary or parotid glands.

Chronic Infectious Sialadenitis

There is an intimate relationship between sialolithiasis and chronic infectious sialadenitis. As previously noted, obstruction in the major salivary glands can lead to secondary bacterial infection. Often the secondary infection may resolve with antibiotic therapy, and the acute symptoms of swelling, pain, and tenderness may be relieved. If, however, the obstruction is not eliminated, then the process likely will be repeated in the future. This condition will evolve into a chronic bacterial process that eventually will be resistant to medical therapy and require the removal of the gland or stone for complete resolution.

Recurrent Parotitis in Children

This uncommon pediatric disease, which usually starts in children under the age of 6 years, presents with periodic recurrent unilateral or bilateral parotid swelling. Pathophysiologically there is diffuse sialectasis through the affected gland. The exact etiology of this condition is unknown and is probably a noninfectious inflammatory response. There is often secondary infection during the acute exacerbations, which should be treated with antibiotics. The initial diagnosis cannot be differentiated from any other acute parotitis. It is only over time that the recurrent nature of the disease becomes apparent. Stones are not seen in this disease, and in most cases the process ceases in the third decade of life. If the child is seen in an emergency department and the infection is the initial episode, treatment should include antibiotics (penicillin) and pain medication.

References

1. Mackowiak PA. The normal microbial flora. *N Engl J Med* 307:83, 1982.
2. Busch DF. Anaerobes in infections of the head and neck and ear, nose and throat. *Rev Infect Dis* 6 (Suppl. 1):S115, 1984.
3. Epstein JB, Truelove EL, Izutzu KT. Oral candidiasis: pathogenesis and host defense. *Rev Infect Dis* 6:96, 1984.
4. Epstein JB. The painful mouth—mucositis, gingivitis, and stomatitis. *Infect Dis Clin North Am* 2:183, 1988.
5. Lynch MA, Brightman VJ, Greenberg MS. *Burket's Oral Medicine*. Philadelphia: Lippincott, 1984. P. 169.
6. Adler JL et al. Epidemiologic investigation of hand-foot-and-mouth disease. *AJDC* 120:309–20, 1970.
7. Steigman AJ, Lipton MM, Braspennick H. Acute lymphonodular pharyngitis: a newly described condition due to coxsackie A virus. *J Pediatr* 61:331, 1962.
8. Nahmiias AJ, Roizman B. Infection with herpes simplex viruses 1 and 2. Part I. *N Engl J Med* 289:667–74, 1973.
9. Kampmeier RH. *Essentials of Syphilology.* Philadelphia: Lippincott, 1943.
10. Lucente FE, Meeteles LZ, Pincus RL. Bronchoesophageal manifestations of acquired immunodefi-

ciency syndrome. *Ann Otol Rhinol Laryngol* 97:530, 1988.

11. Tavitan A, Raufman JP, Rosenthal LE. Oral candidiasis as a marker for esophageal candidiasis in the acquired immunodeficiency syndrome. *Ann Intern Med* 104:54, 1986.

12. Dolby AE. Recurrent aphthous ulceration–effect of sera and peripheral blood lymphocytes upon oral epthelial tissue culture cells. *Immunology* 17:709, 1969.

13. Donatsky O, Dabelsteen E. An immunofluorescence study on the humoral immunity to strep 2A in recurrent aphthous stomatitis. *Acta Pathol Microbiol Scand* 82:107, 1974.

14. Guggenheimer J, Brightman, VJ. Ship II: effect of chlortetracycline mouthrinses on the healing of recurrent aphthous ulcers–a double blind controlled trial. *J Oral Ther Pharmacol* 4:406, 1968.

15. Daeffler R. Oral hygiene measures for patients with cancer (III). *Cancer Nurs* 4:29, 1981.

16. Kerr DA, Ash MM Jr. *Oral Pathology* (4th ed.). Philadelphia: Lea & Febiger, 1978. Pp. 183–203.

17. Schachtele CF. Dental caries. In GS Schuster (ed.), *Oral Microbiology and Infectious Disease*. Baltimore: Williams & Wilkins, 1983.

18. Courant PR. Periodontal disease. In WA Nolte (ed.), *Oral Microbiology*. St. Louis: Mosby, 1982.

19. Glickmen I. Periodontal disease. *N Engl J Med* 284:1071, 1971.

20. Farber PA, Miller AS. In D Scholossber, D (ed.), *Infections of the Head and Neck*. New York: Springer-Verlag, 1986.

21. Loesche WJ et al. The bacteriology of acute necrotizing ulcerative gingivitis. *J Periodontol* 53:223, 1982.

22. Tom MB, Rice DH. Presentation and management of neck abscess: a retrospective analysis. *Laryngoscope* 98:877, 1988.

23. Brook I. Microbiology of abscesses of the head and neck in children. *Ann Otol Rhinol Laryngol* 96:429, 1987.

24. Levitt GW. Cervical fascia and deep neck infections. *Otolaryngol Clin North Am* 9:703, 1976.

25. Herzon FH. Needle aspiration of nonperitonsillar abscesses. *Arch Otolaryngol Head Neck Surg* 114:1312, 1988.

26. Tschiassny K. Ludwig's angina: a surgical approach based on anatomical and pathological criteria. *Ann Otol* 56:937, 1947.

27. Herzon FH. Unpublished data.

28. Travis LW, Hecht DW. Acute and chronic inflammatory diseases of the salivary glands: diagnosis and management. *Otolaryngol Clin North Am* 110:329, 1970.

29. Speirs CF, Mason DK. Acute septic parotitis: incidence, etiology and management. *Scott Med J* 17:62, 1972.

30. Bahn SL, Tabachnick TT. Sialolithiasis of minor salivary glands. *Oral Surg* 32:371, 1971.

31. Jensen JL et al. Minor salivary gland calcui. A clinicopathologic study of forty-seven new cases. *Oral Surg* 47:44, 1979.

Index

DATE DUE

JAN - 6 1997			